OTHER PMIC TITLES OF INTEREST

PRACTICE MANAGEMENT

365 Ways to Manage the Business Called Private Practice
Achieving Profitability with a Medical Office System
Capitation: Tools, Trends, Traps & Techniques
Computerizing Your Medical Office
Critical Concepts in Medical Practice Management
Doctor Business
Encyclopedia of Practice and Financial Management
Getting Paid for What You Do
Health Information Management
The Managed Care Handbook
Managing Costs in the Physician's Office Laboratory
Managing Medical Office Personnel
Marketing Strategies for Physicians
McGraw-Hill Pocket Guide to Managed Care
Medical Marketing Handbook
Medical Office Policy Manual
Medical Practice Forms
Medical Practice Handbook
Medical Practice Pre-employment Tests Book
Medical Staff Privileges
Negotitating Managed Care Contracts
The New Practice Handbook
On-Line Systems: How to Access and Use Databases
Patient Satisfaction
Patients Build Your Practice
A Physician's Guide to Clinical Research Opportunities
Physician's Office Laboratory
Professional and Practice Development
Promoting Your Medical Practice
Starting in Medical Practice
Spanish/English Handbook for the Medical Professional
Surviving a Competitive Health Care Market

MEDICAL REFERENCE AND CLINICAL

Drugs of Abuse
Hematology: A Guide to the Diagnosis and Treatment of Blood Disorders
Medical Care of the Adolescent Athlete
Medical Procedures for Referral
Neurology: Problems in Primary Care
Patient Care Emergency Handbook
Patient Care Flowchart Manual
Patient Care Procedures for Your Practice
Questions and Answers on AIDS
Sexually Transmitted Diseases

AVAILABLE BY CALLING 1-800-MED-SHOP
OR BY VISITING HTTP://PMICONLINE.COM

OTHER PMIC TITLES OF INTEREST

CODING AND REIMBURSEMENT

Codelink® Guides to CPT and ICD-9-CM Code Linkages
Coder's Handbook
Collections Made Easy!
CPT Plus!
CPT & HCPCS Coding Made Easy!
E/M Coding Made Easy!
HCPCS Coders Choice®, Color Coded, Thumb Indexed
Health Insurance Carrier Directory
ICD-9-CM, Coders Choice®, Color Coded, Indexed
ICD-9-CM Coding For Physicians' Offices
ICD-9-CM Coding Made Easy!
Medicare Compliance Manual
Medicare Rules & Regulations
Medical Fees
Reimbursement Manual for the Medical Office
Working with Insurance and Managed Care Plans

FINANCIAL MANAGEMENT

Accounts Receivable Management for the Medical Practice
Business Ventures for Physicians
Financial Planning Workbook for Physicians
Financial Valuation of Your Practice
Pension Plan Strategies
Physician Financial Planning in a Changing Environment
Securing Your Assets
Selling or Buying a Medical Practice

RISK MANAGEMENT

Behavioral Types and the Art of Patient Management
Law, Liability and Ethics for Medical Office Personnel
Malpractice Depositions
Malpractice: Managing Your Defense
Medical Malpractice: A Physician's Guide
Testifying in Court

DICTIONARIES AND OTHER REFERENCE

Health and Medicine on the Interet
Medical Acronyms, Eponyms and Abbreviations
Medical Phrase Index
Medical Word Building
Medico-Legal Glossary
Spanish/English Handbook for Medical Professionals

**AVAILABLE BY CALLING 1-800-MED-SHOP
OR BY VISITING HTTP://PMICONLINE.COM**

ICD·9·CM

International Classification of Diseases
9th Revision

Clinical Modification
Sixth Edition

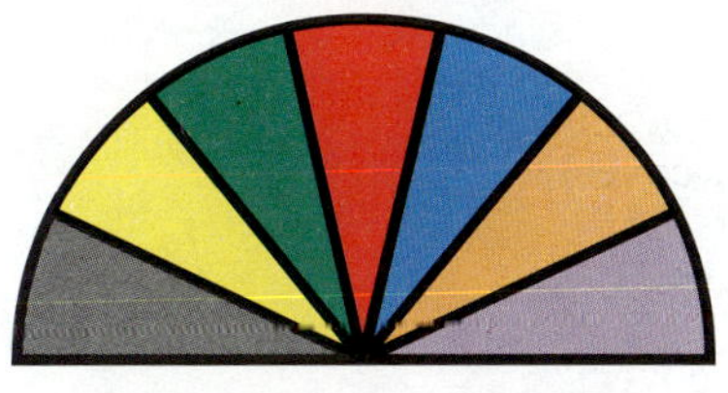

Color Coded

2003

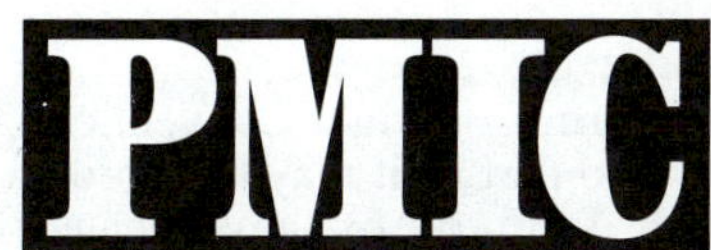

Volumes 1 & 2

ISBN 1-57066-258-4 (Soft cover)
ISBN 1-57066-262-2 (Hard cover)

Volumes 1, 2, & 3

ISBN 1-57066-259-2 (Soft cover)
ISBN 1-57066-261-4 (Timesaver Binder)

Non-indexed versions

ISBN 1-57066-257-6 (Volumes 1 & 2)
ISBN 1-57066-260-6 (Volumes 1, 2, & 3)

Practice Management Information Corporation [PMIC]
4727 Wilshire Boulevard, Suite 300
Los Angeles, California 90010
1-800-MED-SHOP
http://pmiconline.com/

Printed in China

Preface

Health care professionals have long used coding systems to describe procedures, services, and supplies. However, most described the reason for the procedure, service or supply with a diagnostic statement. Of those health care professionals who do code the diagnosis, either due to a requirement for a computer billing system and/or electronic claims filing, many do not code completely or accurately. With the passage of the Medicare Catastrophic Coverage Act of 1988, diagnostic coding using *ICD-9-CM* became mandatory for Medicare claims. In the area of health care reimbursement rules and regulations, the typical progression is that changes required for Medicare are followed shortly by similar changes for Medicaid and private insurance carriers.

To some professionals, the requirement to use diagnostic coding may have seemed like a burden or simply another excuse for Medicare intermediaries to delay or deny payment. However, it is important to understand that the proper use of coding systems for both procedures and diagnoses gives the professional absolute control over his or her billing and reimbursement. Accurate diagnosis coding is not easy. It requires a good working knowledge of medical terminology and a fundamental understanding of *ICD-9-CM*. In addition, the coder must know the rules and regulations required to comply with Medicare requirements for coding.

This edition of the *International Classification of Diseases, 9th Revision, Clinical Modification (ICD-9-CM)* is published by Practice Management Information Corporation in recognition of its responsibility to promulgate this classification throughout the United States for morbidity coding and billing purposes. The *International Classification of Diseases, 9th Revision*, originally published by the World Health Organization (WHO) is the foundation of the *ICD-9-CM* and continues to be the classification employed in cause-of-death coding in the United States.

The *ICD-9-CM* is recommended for use in all clinical settings, but is required for reporting diagnoses and diseases to all U.S. Public Health Service and Health Care Financing Administration programs. This version faithfully follows and contains the same information found in the U.S. Public Health Service and Health Care Financing Administration version of the *ICD-9-CM*.

All official authorized addenda effective October 1, 2002 have been included in this edition. A new revision will be available approximately September 15th of each year. Revised editions may be purchased from:

Practice Management Information Corporation
4727 Wilshire Boulevard, Suite 300
Los Angeles, California 90010
1-800-MED-SHOP

Or by contacting our web site at http://pmiconline.com/

Disclaimer

This publication is identical in content to U.S. Department of Health and Human Services Publication No. (PHS) 91-1260 with the exception that this publication includes special symbols to indicate additions and revisions from the previous edition and special symbols to facilitate identification of diagnostic codes that require 4th or 5th digit specificity, the use of color coding to alert the user to special coding considerations, and thumb indexing to make locating codes easier. This publication is revised annually so that we may present the most current information possible. Though all of the information is carefully researched and checked for accuracy and completeness, the publisher accepts no responsibility with regard to errors, omissions, misuse or misinterpretation.

Table of Contents

Table of Contents

Table of Contents

Table of Contents

(1) These listings appear only in the three volume edition

Introduction to ICD-9-CM

ICD-9-CM is an acronym for *International Classification of Diseases, 9th Revision, Clinical Modification*, published under different names since 1900. *ICD-9-CM* is a statistical classification system that arranges diseases and injuries into groups according to established criteria. Most *ICD-9-CM* codes are numeric and consist of three, four or five numbers and a description. The codes are revised approximately every 10 years by the World Health Organization and annual updates are published by the Centers for Medicare and Medicaid Services (CMS).

HISTORICAL PERSPECTIVE

The *International Classification of Diseases, 9th Revision, Clinical Modification (ICD-9-CM)* is based on the official version of the *World Health Organization's (WHO) 9th Revision, International Classification of Diseases (ICD-9)*. *ICD-9* is designed for the classification of morbidity and mortality information for statistical purposes, and for the indexing of medical records by disease and operations, and for data storage and retrieval. *ICD-9-CM* replaced the Eighth Revision International Classification of Diseases, Adapted for Use in the United States commonly referred to as *ICDA*.

The concept of extending the International Classification of Diseases for use in hospital indexing was originally developed in response to a need for a more efficient basis for storage and retrieval of diagnostic data. In 1950, the U.S. Public Health Service and the Veterans Administration began independent tests of the International Classification of Diseases for hospital indexing purposes. In the following year, the Columbia Presbyterian Medical Center in New York City adopted the International Classification of Diseases, 6th Revision for use in its medical record department. A few years later, the Commission on Professional and Hospital Activities adopted the International Classification of Diseases for use in hospitals participating in the Professional Activity Study (PAS).

In view of the growing interest in the use of the International Classification of Diseases for hospital indexing, a study was undertaken in 1956 by the American Medical Association and the American Medical Record Association of the relative efficiencies of coding systems for diagnostic indexing. Following this study, the major uses of the International Classification of Diseases for hospital indexing purposes consolidated their experiences and an adaptation was published in December 1959. A revision containing the first "Classification of Operations and Treatments" was published in 1962.

In 1968, following a study by the American Hospital Association, the United States Public Health Service published the Eighth Revision International Classification of Diseases, Adapted for Use in the United States. This publication became commonly known as ICDA, and served as the basis for coding diagnostic data for official morbidity and mortality statistics in the United States.

ICD-9-CM Background

In February 1977, a committee was convened by the National Center for Health Statistics to provide advice and counsel for the development of clinical modification of the ICD-9. The organizations represented on the committee included:

>American Association of Health Data Systems
>American Hospital Association
>American Medical Record Association
>Association for Health Records
>Council on Clinical Classifications, sponsored by:
>
>>American Academy of Pediatrics
>>American College of Obstetricians and Gynecologists
>>American College of Physicians
>>American College of Surgeons
>>American Psychiatric Association
>
>Commission on Professional and Hospital Activities
>Health Care Financing Administration
>WHO Center for Classification of Diseases

The resulting *ICD-9-CM* is a clinical modification of the *World Health Organization's International Classification of Diseases, 9th Revision (ICD-9)*. The term "clinical" is used to emphasize the modifications intent; namely, to serve as a useful tool in the area of classification of morbidity data for indexing of medical records, medical care review, ambulatory and other medical care programs, as well as for basic health statistics.

In use since January 1979, *ICD-9-CM* provides a diagnostic coding system that is more precise than those needed only for statistical groupings and trend analysis. Official addenda (updates) to *ICD-9-CM* are issued in October each year by the Health Care Financing Administration.

Use of ICD-9-CM Codes for Professional Billing

Until passage of the Medicare Catastrophic Coverage Act of 1988, health care professionals were not required to report *ICD-9-CM* codes when billing government or private insurance carriers for reimbursement. The exception to this requirement was for those health care professionals who filed insurance claims electronically and those who used "code driven" computer billing services or computer systems.

Most health care professionals simply included the text or description of the injury, illness, sign or symptom that was the reason for the encounter. Insurance carriers who used *ICD-9-CM* coding had to code the diagnostic statements prior to input into their computer systems for reimbursement processing.

A specific requirement of the Medicare Catastrophic Coverage Act of 1988 required health care professionals to include *ICD-9-CM* codes on their Medicare claim forms effective April 1, 1989. A two-month grace period, to June 1, 1989, was allowed at the request of the American Medical Association, to allow health care professionals additional time to develop the knowledge and systems necessary to implement the requirement.

TERMINOLOGY

There are terms used throughout this publication that are important for a proper understanding of *ICD-9-CM*. The following terms are defined specifically as they are used for *ICD-9-CM* with the knowledge that some terms may have other definitions and meanings.

acute	refers to the condition that is the primary reason for the current encounter.
addenda	official updates to *ICD-9-CM* published continuously since 1986, that become effective on October 1st of each year.
adverse	any response to a drug that is noxious and unintended and occurs with proper dosage.
aftercare	an encounter for something planned in advance, for example, cast removal.
AHFS	American Hospital Formulary Service.
alphabetic	the portion of *ICD-9-CM* that lists definitions and codes in alphabetic order. Also called Volume 2.
category	refers to diagnoses codes listed within a specific three-digit category, for example category 250, Diabetes Mellitus.
cause	that which brings about any condition or produces any effect.
chronic	continuing over a long period of time or recurring frequently.
CMS	Centers for Medicare and Medicaid Services (formerly HCFA), the government agency that administers the Medicare and Medicaid programs.
CMS1500	formerly HCFA1500, the uniform health insurance claim form used for billing services to Medicare and other insurance carriers
coding	the process of transferring written or verbal descriptions of diseases, injuries and procedures into numerical designations.
combination	a code that combines a diagnosis with an associated secondary process or complication.
complication	the occurrence of two or more diseases in the same patient at the same time.
concurrent	when a patient is being treated by more than one provider for different care conditions at the same time.
conventions	refers to the use of certain abbreviations, punctuation, symbols, type faces, and other instructions that must be clearly understood in order to use *ICD-9-CM*.
CPT	Current Procedural Terminology. Listing of codes and descriptions for procedures, services and supplies published by the American Medical Association. Used to bill insurance carriers.
diagnosis	a written description of the reason(s) for the procedure, service, supply or encounter.
down coding	the process where insurance carriers reduce the value of a procedure, and the resulting reimbursement, due to either 1) a mismatch of CPT code and description or 2) ICD-9-CM code does not justify the procedure or level of service.

E codes	specific ICD-9-CM codes used to identify the cause of injury, poisoning and other adverse effects.
eponyms	medical procedures or conditions named after a person or a place.
etiology	the cause(s) or origin of a disease.
HCFA	see CMS.
HCFA1500	see CMS1500.
hierarchy	a system that ranks items one above another.
ICD-9-CM	International Classification of Diseases, 9th Revision, Clinical Modification.
ICD-10	International Classification of Diseases, 10th Revision
late effect	a residual effect (condition produced) after the acute phase of an illness or injury has ended.
main term	refers to listings in the Alphabetic Index appearing BOLDFACE type.
manifestation	characteristic signs or symptoms of an illness.
multiple	refers to the need to use more than one ICD-9-CM code to fully identify coding a condition.
primary code	the ICD-9-CM code that defines the main reason for the current encounter.
residual	the long-term condition(s) resulting from a previous acute illness or injury.
rule out	refers to a method used to indicate that a condition is probable, suspected, or questionable but unconfirmed. ICD-9-CM has no provisions for the use of this term.
secondary	code(s) listed after the primary code that further indicate the cause(s) codefor the current encounter or define the need for higher levels of care.
sections	refers to portions of the Tabular List that are organized in groups of three-digit code numbers. For example, Malignant Neoplasm of Lip, Oral Cavity and Pharynx (140-149).
sequencing	the process of listing ICD-9-CM codes in the proper order.
specificity	refers to the requirement to code to the highest number of digits possible, 3, 4 or 5, when choosing an ICD-9-CM code.
sub term	refers to listings appearing in the Alphabetic Index under MAIN TERMS and always indented two spaces to the right.
subcategories	refers to groupings of four-digit codes listed under three-digit categories.
tabular list	the portion of ICD-9-CM that lists codes and definitions in numeric order. Also referred to as Volume 1.
V codes	specific ICD-9-CM codes used to identify encounters for reasons other than illness or injury, for example, immunization.
Volume 1	see TABULAR LIST
Volume 2	see ALPHABETIC INDEX
Volume 3	procedure codes used only for hospital coding. Volume 3 contains both a numeric listing and alphabetic index.

FORMAT OF ICD-9-CM

The *International Classification of Diseases, 9th Revision, Clinical Modification* was originally published as a three volume set (2nd edition). Newer versions of ICD-9-CM are available as either a two-volume set (Volume 1 and Volume 2) or as a three-volume set (Volumes 1, 2 and 3), depending on the publisher. It is also now available on CD-ROM from the U.S. Government.

The Third Edition of ICD-9-CM includes all official addenda from October 1986 through October 1988. The Fourth Edition of ICD-9-CM includes all official addenda from October 1986 through October 1994. This edition of ICD-9-CM includes all official addenda from October 1986 through October 2002.

The Tabular List (Volume 1)

The Tabular List (Volume 1) is a <u>numeric</u> listing of diagnosis codes and descriptions consisting of 17 chapters that classify diseases and injuries, two sections containing supplementary codes (V codes and E codes) and six appendices.

Classification of Diseases and Injuries

The Classification of Diseases and Injuries includes the following 17 chapters:

Chapter 1   Infectious and Parasitic Diseases (001-139)

Chapter 2   Neoplasms (140-239)

Chapter 3   Endocrine, Nutritional and Metabolic Diseases, and Immunity Disorders (240-279)

Chapter 4   Diseases of the Blood and Blood-Forming Organs (280-289)

Chapter 5   Mental Disorders (290-319)

Chapter 6   Diseases of the Nervous System and Sense Organs

Chapter 7   Diseases of the Circulatory System (390-459)

Chapter 8   Diseases of the Respiratory System (460-519)

Chapter 9   Diseases of the Digestive System (520-579)

Chapter 10   Diseases of the Genitourinary System (580-629)

Chapter 11   Complications of Pregnancy, Childbirth, and the Puerperium (630-676)

Chapter 12   Diseases of the Skin and Subcutaneous Tissue (680-709)

Chapter 13   Diseases of the Musculoskeletal System and Connective Tissue (710-739)

Chapter 14   Congenital Anomalies (740-759)

Chapter 15   Certain Conditions Originating in the Perinatal Period (760-779)

Chapter 16   Symptoms, Signs and Ill-defined Conditions (780-799)

Chapter 17   Injury and Poisoning (800-999)

Each chapter of the Tabular List (Volume 1) is structured into four components; namely:

Sections: groups of three-digit code numbers

Categories: three-digit code numbers

Subcategories: four-digit code numbers

Fifth-Digit Subclassifications: five-digit code numbers

Supplementary Classifications

There are two supplementary classifications included in the Tabular List (Volume 1). These are:

V Codes   Supplementary Classification of Factors Influencing Health Status and Contact with Health Services (V01-V83)

E Codes   Supplementary Classification of External Causes of Injury and Poisoning (E800-E999)

Appendices

The Tabular List (Volume 1) includes six appendices. These are:

Appendix 1   Morphology of Neoplasms

Appendix 2   Glossary of Mental Disorders

Appendix 3   Classification of Drugs by American Hospital Formulary Service List Number and their ICD-9-CM Equivalents

Appendix 4   Classification of Industrial Accidents According to Agency

Appendix 5   List of Three-Digit Categories

Appendix 6   Supplementary Classification of External Causes of Injury and Poisoning (E codes)

Specifications for the Tabular List

1. Three-digit rubrics and their contents are unchanged from *ICD-9*.

2. The sequence of three-digit rubrics is unchanged from *ICD-9*.

3. Three-digit rubrics are not added to the main body of the classification.

4.   Unsubdivided three-digit rubrics are subdivided where necessary to:

    a) Add clinical detail

    b) Isolate terms for clinical accuracy

5.   The modification in *ICD-9-CM* is accomplished by the addition of a fifth digit to existing *ICD-9* rubrics, except as noted under #7 below.

6.   Four-digit rubrics are added to subdivided three-digit codes only when there is no other means of achieving desired detail. These codes, unique to *ICD-9-CM* (28 three-digit categories) are marked with the symbol in the Tabular List.

7.   The optional dual classification in *ICD-9* is modified.

    a) Duplicate rubrics are deleted:

        1) Four-digit manifestation categories duplicating etiology entries.

        2) Manifestation inclusion terms duplicating etiology entries.

    b) Manifestations of diseases are identified, to the extent possible, by creating five digit codes in the etiology rubrics.

    c) When the manifestation of a disease cannot be included in the etiology rubrics, provision for its identification is made by retaining the *ICD-9* rubrics used for classifying manifestations of disease.

8.   The format of *ICD-9-CM* is revised from that used in *ICD-9*.

    a) American spelling of medical terms is used.

    b) Inclusion terms are indented beneath the titles of codes.

    c) Codes not to be used for primary tabulation of disease are printed in italics with the notation, "code also underlying disease."

The Alphabetical Index (Volume 2)

The Alphabetic Index (Volume 2) of ICD-9-CM consists of an alphabetic list of terms and codes, two supplementary Sections following the alphabetic listing, plus two special tables found within the alphabetic listing. The Alphabetic Index (Volume 2) is structured as follows:

MAIN TERMS: appear in **BOLDFACE** type

SUBTERMS: are always indented two spaces to the right under main terms

CARRY-OVER   are always indented more than two spaces from the level of the
LINES: preceding line

Supplementary Sections

The supplementary sections following the Alphabetic Index are:

TABLE OF DRUGS AND CHEMICALS

> This table contains a classification of drugs and other chemical substances to identify poisoning states and external causes of adverse effects.

INDEX TO EXTERNAL CAUSES OF INJURIES & POISONINGS (E-CODES)

> This section contains the index to the codes that classify environmental events, circumstances, and other conditions as the cause of injury and other adverse effects.

Special Tables

The two special tables, located within the Alphabetic Index, and found under the main terms as underlined below, are:

HYPERTENSION TABLE

NEOPLASM TABLE

Specifications for the Alphabetic Index

1. Format of the Alphabetic Index follows the format of the *ICD-9*.

2. Main terms in the Alphabetic Index are printed in bold face type.

3. When two codes are required to indicate etiology and manifestation, the optional manifestation code appears in brackets, e.g., diabetic cataract 250.5 *[366.41]*.

Procedures: Tabular List and Alphabetic Index (Volume 3)

Volume 3 consists of two sections, a tabular list of codes and an alphabetic index. These codes define procedures instead of diagnoses. Frequently used incorrectly by health care professionals, codes from Volume 3 are intended only for use by hospitals. The Fourth Edition of ICD-9-CM printed by the U.S. Government Printing Office did not include Volume 3. The Fifth Edition of ICD-9-CM issued by the U.S. Government included Volume 3 on a CD-ROM.

The ICD-9-CM Procedure Classification is a modification of WHO's "Fascicle V, Surgical Procedures," and is published as Volume 3 of ICD-9-CM. It contains both a Tabular List and an Alphabetic Index. Greater detail has been added to the ICD-9-CM Procedure Classification necessitating expansion of the codes from three to four digits. Approximately 90% of the rubrics refer to surgical procedures with the remaining 10% accounting for other investigative and therapeutic procedures.

Tabular List of Procedures

The Tabular List includes 16 chapters containing codes and descriptions for surgical procedures and miscellaneous diagnostic and therapeutic procedures.

Alphabetic Index to Procedures

The Alphabetic Index provides an alphabetic index to the Tabular List of Volume 3

Specifications for the Procedure Classification

1. The *ICD-9-CM* Procedure Classification is published in its own volume containing both a Tabular List and an Alphabetic Index.

2. The classification is a modification of Fascicle V "Surgical Procedures" of the *ICD-9* Classification of Procedures in Medicine, working from the draft dated Geneva, 30 September-6 October 1975, and labeled WHO/ICD-9/Rev. Conf. 75.4.

3. All three-digit rubrics in the range 01-86 are maintained as they appear in Fascicle V, whenever feasible.

4. Nonsurgical procedures are segregated from the surgical procedures and confined to the rubrics 87-99, whenever feasible.

5. Selected detail contained in the remaining fascicles of the *ICD-9 Classification of Procedures in Medicine* is accommodated where possible.

6. The structure of the classification is based on anatomy rather than surgical specialty.

7. The *ICD-9-CM* Procedure Classification is numeric only, i.e., no alphabetic characters are used.

8. The classification is based on a two-digit structure with two decimal digits where necessary.

9. Compatibility with the *ICD-9 Classification of Procedures in Medicine* was not maintained when a different axis was deemed more clinically appropriate.

CONVENTIONS USED IN THE TABULAR LIST

The ICD-9-CM Tabular List (Volume 1) makes use of certain abbreviations, punctuation, symbols, and other conventions that must be clearly understood. The purpose of these conventions is to first, provide special coding instructions, and second, to conserve space.

Abbreviations

NOS   Not Otherwise Specified. Equivalent to Unspecified. This abbreviation refers to a lack of sufficient detail in the statement of diagnosis to be able to assign it to a more specific sub division within the classification.

NEC   Not Elsewhere Classified. Used with ill-defined terms to alert the coder that a specified form of the condition is classified differently. The category number for the term including NEC is to be used only when the coder lacks the information necessary to code the term to a more specific category.

Punctuation

( )   PARENTHESIS are used to enclose supplementary words that may be present or absent in a statement of disease without effecting the code assignment.

[ ]   SQUARE BRACKETS are used to enclose synonyms, alternate wordings or explanatory phrases.

:   COLONS are used after an incomplete phrase or term that requires one or more of the modifiers indented under it to make it assignable to a given category. EXCEPTION to this rule pertains to the abbreviation NOS.

{ }   BRACES are used to connect a series of terms to a common stem. Each term on the left of the brace is incomplete and must be completed by a term to the right of the brace.

Symbols

•   A filled BLACK CIRCLE preceding a code indicates that the code is new to this revision of *ICD-9-CM*. A symbol key appears on all left-hand pages of the Tabular List, Volume 1.

▲   A filled BLACK TRIANGLE preceding a code indicates that there is a revision to the text or notes of an existing code. A symbol key appears on all left-hand pages of the Tabular List, Volume 1.

④ ⑤   A circle containing the number 4 or the number 5 preceding a code indicates that a fourth or fifth digit is required for coding to the highest level of specificity. Valid digits are in [brackets] under each code. Definitions of valid fifth digits are found under the major category.

Other conventions

Type Face:

BOLD: Bold type face is used for all codes and titles in the Tabular List.

Italics: Italicized type face is used for all exclusion notes and to identify those rubrics that are not to be used for primary tabulations of disease.

Format: *ICD-9-CM* uses an indented format for ease in reference.

Instructional Notations

Instructional terms define what is, or what is not, included in a given subdivision. This is accomplished by using both inclusion and exclusion terms.

INCLUDES: Indicates separate terms, such as, modifying adjectives, sites and conditions, entered under a subdivision, such as a category, to further define or give examples of, the content of the category.

Excludes: Exclusion terms are enclosed in a box and are printed in italics to draw attention to their presence. The importance of this instructional term is its use as a guideline to direct the coder to the proper code assignment. In other words, all terms following the word EXCLUDES: are to be coded elsewhere as indicated in each instance.

NOTES These are used to define terms and give coding instructions. Often used to list the fifth-digit subclassifications for certain categories.

SEE Acts as a cross reference and, is an explicit direction to look elsewhere. This instructional term must always be followed. (Cross references provide the user with other possible modifiers for a term, or, its synonyms.)

SEE CATEGORY A variation of the instructional term SEE. This refers the coder to a specific category. You must *always* follow this instructional term.

SEE ALSO A direction given to look elsewhere if the main term or subterm(s) are not sufficient to code the information you have.

CODE FIRST This instructional note is used for those codes not intended to be used as a principal diagnosis, or not to be sequenced before the underlying disease. The note requires that the underlying disease (etiology) be coded first with the code the note is applied to being coded second. This note appears only in the tabular list (Vol. 1).

USE ADDITIONAL CODE This instruction is placed in the Tabular List in those categories where the coder may wish to add further information, by using an additional code, to give a more complete picture of the diagnosis or procedure.

Related terms

AND Whenever this term appears in a title, it should be interpreted as "and/or."

WITH When this term is used in a title it indicates a requirement that both parts of the title must be present in the diagnostic statement.

COLOR CODING

All PMIC versions of *ICD-9-CM* include color-coding to alert the user to special coding situations or conditions that require additional attention. The use of color-coding is found in the Tabular List of Volume 1 and the Tabular List of Volume 3. The color is applied as solid rectangular bars over the codes only so that the descriptions remain clear and legible. The color codes and definitions are printed at the bottom of all right-sided pages of Volume 1 and Volume 3.

Volume 1

Three digit codes. Coding to fourth or fifth digit specificity is required.

Unspecified code. Descriptions include the term "unspecified". Use only if a more specific diagnosis is not known or available.

Nonspecific code. Descriptions include the term "nonspecific, unspecified, other specified or other". A report *may* be required by insurance carriers.

Manifestation codes. Used only to code the manifestation of an underlying disease. Code the underlying disease first.

Medicare secondary payer (MSP) alert. Diagnoses that may trigger a post-payment review by Medicare. Medicare is usually the secondary payer for these diagnoses.

Volume 3[*]

Noncovered operating room procedure. An operating room procedure that is not covered by Medicare.

Non-operating room procedure. A procedure that is not performed in the operating room that affects DRG assignment.

Bilateral procedure.

Valid operating room procedure. Prompts a change in DRG assignment.

Nonspecific operating room procedure. Choose a more precise code if possible.

*These colors appear only in the three-volume edition

MEDICARE REQUIREMENTS FOR ICD-9-CM CODING

The Medicare Catastrophic Coverage Act of 1988 (PL 100-330) requires that health care professionals submit an appropriate diagnosis code, using the *International Classification of Diseases, 9th Revision, Clinical Modification (ICD-9-CM)* for each procedure, service, or supply billed under Medicare Part B.

To comply with the regulations, health care professionals must convert the reason(s) for the procedures, services or supplies, performed or issued, from written diagnostic statements that may include specific diagnoses, signs, symptoms and/or complaints, into ICD-9-CM diagnosis codes. The Health Care Financing Administration (now the Centers for Medicare and Medicaid Services) originally set the implementation date for this requirement as April 1, 1989, however, it was subsequently delayed until June 1, 1989, at the request of the American Medical Association, to give health care providers additional time to prepare for the change.

HCFA Guidelines for Using ICD-9-CM Codes

The Center for Medicare and Medicaid Services (CMS, formerly HCFA) has prepared guidelines for using ICD-9-CM codes and instructions on how to report them on claim forms. In addition, CMS has directed your medicare intermediary to provide you with a written copy of these instructions. The basic guidelines are summarized below, however, it is very important that you obtain a copy of the guidelines from your Medicare intermediary as implementation of CMS requirements varies from one intermediary to another.

1. Indicate on the claim form or itemized statement the appropriate code(s) from the ICD-9-CM code range 001.0 through V83.02 to identify diagnoses, symptoms, conditions, problems, complaints or other reason(s) for the procedure, service or supply provided.

    A. In choosing codes to describe the reason for the encounter, the health care professional will frequently be using codes within the range from 001.0 through 999.9, the section of ICD-9-CM for the classification of diseases and injuries (e.g. infectious and parasitic diseases; neoplasms; signs, symptoms and ill-defined conditions). Codes that describe symptoms as opposed to diagnoses are acceptable if this is the highest level of certainty documented by the physician.

    B. ICD-9-CM also provides codes to deal with visits for circumstances other than a disease or injury, such as an encounter for a laboratory test only. These codes are found in the V-code section and range from V01.0 through V83.02.

2. The ICD-9-CM code for the diagnosis, condition, problem, or other reason for the encounter documented in the medical record as the main reason for the procedure, service or supply provided should be listed first. Additional ICD-9-CM codes that describe any current coexisting conditions are then listed. Do not include codes for conditions that were previously treated and no longer exist.

3.   ICD-9-CM codes should be used at their highest level of specificity.

    A.   Assign three digit codes only if there are no four digit codes within the coding category.

    B.   Assign four digit codes only if there is no fifth digit subclassification for that category.

    C.   Assign the fifth digit subclassification code for those categories where it exists.

Claims submitted with three or four digit codes where four and five digit codes are available may be returned to you by the Medicare intermediary for proper coding. It is recognized that a very specific diagnosis may not be known at the time of the initial encounter. However, that is not an acceptable reason to submit a three digit code when four or five digits are available.

For example, if the patient has chronic bronchitis, ICD-9-CM code 491, and the physician has not yet documented whether the bronchitis is simple, mucopurulent, or obstructive, the code for unspecified chronic bronchitis, ICD-9-CM code 491.9, should be listed.

4.   Diagnoses documented as "probable," "suspected," "questionable," or "rule out" should not be coded as if the diagnosis is confirmed. The condition(s) should be coded to the highest degree of certainty for the encounter, such as describing symptoms, signs, abnormal test results, or other reasons for the encounter.

5.   Chronic disease(s) treated on an ongoing basis may be coded and reported as many times as the patient receives treatment and care for the condition(s).

6.   When patients receive ancillary diagnostic services only during an encounter, the appropriate "V code" for the service should be listed first, and the diagnosis or problem for which the diagnostic procedures are being performed should be listed second.

    A.   V codes will be used frequently by radiologists who perform radiological examinations on referrals. For example, ICD-9-CM code V72.5, Radiological examination, not elsewhere classified, describes the reason for the encounter and should be listed first on the claim form or statement. If the reason for the referral is known, a second ICD-9-CM code that describes the signs or symptoms for which the examination was ordered should be listed.

    B.   Failure to list a second ICD-9-CM code in addition to the V code may result in claim delays or denials. The ICD-9-CM code V72.5, Radiological examination, not elsewhere classified, includes referrals for routine chest x-rays that are not covered by the Medicare program. Medicare intermediaries may establish screening programs to verify that the referrals were not for routine chest x-rays. By supplying a second ICD-9-CM code to describe the reason for the referral, these claims can be clearly identified by the Medicare intermediary as referrals to evaluate symptoms, signs or diagnoses. The mission of a second ICD-9-CM code may lead to requests for additional information from Medicare intermediaries prior to processing the claim.

7. For patients receiving only ancillary therapeutic services during an encounter, list the appropriate V code first, followed by the ICD-9-CM code for the diagnosis or problem for which the services are being performed. For example, a patient with multiple sclerosis presenting for rehabilitation services would be coded using either V57.1 Other physical therapy, or V57.89 Other care involving use of rehabilitation procedures, followed by code 340 Multiple sclerosis.

8. For surgical procedures, use the ICD-9-CM code for the diagnosis for which the surgery was performed. If the postoperative diagnosis is known to be different at the time the claim is filed, use the ICD-9-CM code for the post-operative diagnosis.

9. Code all documented conditions that coexist at the time of the visit that require or affect patient care, treatment or management. Do not code conditions that were previously treated and no longer exist.

Completing the CMS1500 Claim Form

Health care professionals using the Uniform Health Insurance Claim Form, CMS1500, to file claims for services provided to Medicare beneficiaries must list a minimum of one ICD-9-CM code and may list up to four total ICD-9-CM codes on the claim form.

The ICD-9-CM code for the diagnosis, condition, problem or other reason for the encounter is listed first, followed by up to three additional codes that describe any coexisting conditions. At times, there may be several conditions that equally resulted in the encounter. In these cases, the health care professional is free to select the one that will be listed first.

The ICD-9-CM codes are listed in Box 23 of the "old" CMS1500 (10/84) claim form and Box 21 of the "new" CMS1500 (12/90) claim form (see example). In addition, in Box 24 D of both versions of the form, you must indicate by a number from 1 to 4, or combination of numbers, which diagnoses from Box 23 support the procedure, service or supply listed in Box 24 C.

Due to space limitations on the claim form you may use only up to four ICD-9-CM codes for diagnoses, conditions, or signs and symptoms. Frequently the patient may have more than four conditions present at the time of the encounter, however, you must choose only four codes to be listed on the claim form.

If you strongly believe that additional diagnostic information is needed by the Medicare intermediary for proper claim processing you may attach additional supporting documentation to your manual claim. Keep in mind that in most cases the additional documentation will be ignored by the claims examiners, and, in other cases will result in reimbursement delay while someone reviews your documentation.

Medicare Penalties for Non-compliance

The Medicare Catastrophic Coverage Act of 1988 mandates submission of an appropriate ICD-9-CM diagnosis code or codes for each procedure, service, or supply furnished by the health care professional to Medicare Part B beneficiaries. The Act further specifies that compliance is mandatory and that penalties may be assessed for noncompliance.

The penalties for noncompliance differ depending upon whether or not the health care professional has agreed to accept assignment or not.

1. For health care professionals who accept assignment on a Medicare claim and who fail to include ICD-9-CM codes as required will have their claim(s) returned for proper coding and may be subject to post-payment review by the Medicare intermediary, as well as payment denials.

2. For health care professionals who do not accept assignment, the penalties are more severe.

    A. If the original claim form does not include ICD-9-CM codes as required, and the health care professional refuses to provide the codes promptly on request to the Medicare intermediary, the professional may be subject to a civil monetary penalty in an amount not to exceed $2,000, per claim.

    B. If the health care professional continuously fails to provide ICD-9-CM codes as requested, the professional may be subject to the sanction process described in section 1842 (j) (2) (A), that mandates that the professional may be barred from participation in the Medicare program for a period not to exceed five years.

CODING AND BILLING ISSUES

Diagnosis Codes Must Support Procedure Codes

Each service or procedure performed for a patient should be represented by a diagnosis that would substantiate those particular services or procedures as necessary in the investigation or treatment of their condition based on currently accepted standards of practice by the medical profession.

Place (Location) of Service

The actual setting that the services are rendered in for particular diagnoses plays an important part in reimbursement. Many people became accustomed to using Emergency Rooms for any type of illness or injury. By utilizing highly specialized places of service for conditions that were not true emergencies, third party payer were being billed with CPT codes indicating emergency services were rendered. Since the cost of services rendered on an emergency basis is considerably more expensive than those services in an non-emergency situation, third party payers began watching for those claims with diagnoses that did not indicate that a true emergency existed. Payment then was based on what the cost would have been had the patient been treated in the proper setting.

Level of Service Provided

The patient's condition and the treatment of that condition must be billed according to the criteria, as published by the AMA, for each level of service (i.e., minimal, brief, limited, intermediate, extended, comprehensive). Many practices bill the office visit level that they know will pay better rather than to consider the criteria that must be met to use a particular level of service. Again, the patient's diagnosis enters into this concept as well as it is often the diagnosis that indicates the complexity of the level of service to be used.

Frequency of Services

Many times claims are submitted for a patient with the same diagnosis and the same procedure(s) time after time. When the diagnosis indicates a chronic condition and the claims do not indicate any change in the patient's treatment or, give any indication that the patient's condition has been altered (i.e., exacerbated, other symptomology) the third party payer may deny payment based on the frequency of services for the reported condition.

Down Coding

Down coding is the process of reducing a code from one of a higher value to one of a lower value that results in lowered reimbursement. In the area of procedure coding, this process results in the loss of millions of dollars annually by health care professionals and their patients.

With procedure coding, down coding claims is easily resolved by either providing a procedure description that matches that of Current Procedural Terminology (CPT) exactly, or, even better, by eliminating all procedure descriptions from your claim forms, that forces the insurance carrier to allow full value for your procedure, service, or supply. With diagnosis coding, the issue is not mismatch of description to code, as the description is not required, but that the ICD-9-CM code(s) provide justification for the procedure, service or supply or the level of service provided.

A key point to remember is that if there are any current coexisting conditions that may complicate the treatment for the primary condition, it is very important to include the ICD-9-CM codes for the coexisting conditions that will help to justify the level of service provided.

Concurrent Care

Reimbursement problems often arise when a patient is being treated by different professionals, within the same billing entity (medical group or clinic), for different problems at the same time. This is known as concurrent care. For example, a patient may be hospitalized by a clinic's general surgeon for an operation and may also be seen while hospitalized by the group's cardiologist for an unrelated cardiac condition.

If you submit claims for daily hospital visits by both of the above professionals without explanation, most insurance carriers would reject one daily visit as an apparent "duplication" of service. Prior to publication of the 1992 edition of CPT, the key to obtaining proper reimbursement for concurrent care was first, to use the procedure modifier - 75, Concurrent Care, Services Rendered by More than One Physician, and second, to submit a different *ICD-9-CM* code for the services provided by each physician, that support and justify the need for those services.

Note that modifier -75 was deleted in the 1992 edition of CPT, therefore, when using the new CPT Evaluation and Management codes to bill Medicare, the *ICD-9-CM* code becomes the key factor for proper reimbursement of concurrent care.

ICD-10

Since 1948, the World Health Organization has revised the *International Classification of Diseases* approximately every 10 years, with a modified version appearing in the United States about one to three years following the WHO publication. Based on the regular schedule, *ICD-10* should have been released in 1987. However, due to difficulties in coordinating the international committees, the first volume of *ICD-10*, the Tabular List, was not published until June of 1992.

Implementation of ICD-10 in the United States

Prior to being implemented in the United States, *ICD-10* must be converted to "American" English and pass through a variety of private and government committees, agencies, associations and organizations. As of this printing, the official position of the Centers for Medicare and Medicaid Services (CMS) is that *ICD-10* will not be mandated for Medicare claims for several years.

WHERE TO GET ANSWERS TO QUESTIONS ABOUT ICD-9-CM

Questions regarding the use and interpretation of the *International Classification of Diseases, 9th Revision, Clinical Modification* should be directed in writing to any of the organizations listed below.

Coding Advice/Central Office on ICD-9-CM
American Hospital Association
One North Franklin
Chicago, Illinois 60606

World Health Organization Collaborating Center
for Classification of Diseases in North America
National Center for Health Statistics
Department of Health and Human Services
6525 Belcrest Road
Hyattsville, Maryland 20782

Morbidity Classification Branch
National Center for Health Statistics
Department of Health and Human Services
6525 Belcrest Road, Room 1100
Hyattsville, Maryland 20782

Centers for Medicare and Medicaid Services (CMS)
Division of Prospective Payment System
Mail Stop C4-07-07
7500 Security Blvd.
Baltimore, MD   21244-1850

Comments, questions or suggestions regarding the PMIC version of *ICD-9-CM* should be directed in writing to:

Managing Editor
Practice Management Information Corporation
4727 Wilshire Boulevard, Suite 300
Los Angeles, California 90010
http://pmiconline.com

ICD-9-CM CODING FUNDAMENTALS

Learning and following the basic steps of coding will increase your chances of better and faster reimbursement from third party payers, as well as establish meaningful profiles for future reimbursement rates. To become a proficient coder, two basic principles always must be considered.

First, it is imperative that you use both the Alphabetic Index (Volume 2) and the Tabular List (Volume 1) when locating and assigning codes. Coding only from the Alphabetic Index will cause you to miss any additional information provided only in the Tabular List, such as exclusions, instructions to use additional codes or the need for a fifth-digit.

Second, the level of specificity is important in all coding situations. A three-digit code that has subdivisions indicates you must use the appropriate subdivision code. Also, any time a fifth-digit subclassification is provided, you must use the fifth-digit code.

NINE STEPS FOR ACCURATE ICD-9-CM CODING

1.	Locate the main term within the diagnostic statement.

2.	Locate that main term in the Alphabetic Index (Volume 2). Keep in mind that the primary arrangement for main terms is by condition in the Alphabetic Index (Volume 2); main terms can be referred to in outmoded, ill-defined and lay terms as well as proper medical terms; main terms can be expressed in broad or specific terms, as nouns, adjectives or eponyms and can be with or without modifiers. Certain conditions may be listed under more than one main term.

3.	Remember to refer to all notes under the main term. Be guided by the instructions in any notes appearing in a box immediately after the main term.

4.	Examine any modifiers appearing in parentheses next to the main term. See if any of these modifiers apply to any of the qualifying terms used in the diagnostic statement.

5.	Take note of the subterms indented beneath the main term. Subterms differ from main terms in that they provide greater specificity, becoming more specific the further they are indented to the right of the main term in 2-space increments; also, they provide the anatomical sites affected by the disease or injury.

6.	Be sure to follow any cross reference instructions. These instructional terms ("see" or "see also") must be followed to locate the correct code.

7.	Confirm the code selection in the Tabular List (Volume 1). make certain you have selected the appropriate classification in accordance with the diagnosis.

8.	Follow instructional terms in the Tabular List (Volume 1). Watch for exclusion terms, notes and fifth-digit instructions that apply to the code number you are verifying. It is necessary to search not only the selected code number for instructions but also the category, section and chapter in which the code number is collapsible. Many times the instructional information is located one or more pages preceding the actual page you find the code number on.

9.	Finally, assign the code number you have determined to be correct.

ITALICIZED ENTRIES

During the process of designating a code to identify a principal diagnosis it is important to remember that italicized entries or codes in slanted brackets cannot be used. In these instances, it is required that the etiology code be sequenced first and the manifestation code be listed second even if the physician recorded them in the opposite order.

OTHER AND UNSPECIFIED CODES

Subcategories for diagnoses listed as "Other" and "Unspecified" are referred to as residual subcategories. Remember, the subdivisions are arranged in a hierarchy starting with the more specific and ending with the least specific. In the Tabular List (Volume 1), in most instances, the four-digit subcategory ".8" has been reserved for "Other" specified conditions not classifiable elsewhere and the four-digit subcategory ".9" has been reserved for "Unspecified" conditions. Following is an example demonstrating this principle.

005 Other food poisoning (bacterial)

Excludes: salmonella infections (003.0-003.9)
toxic effect of:
food contaminants (989.7)
noxious foodstuffs (988-0-988.9)

005.0   Staphylococcal food poisoning
Staphylococcal toxemia specified as due to food

005.1   Botulism
Food poisoning due to Clostridium botulinum

005.2   Food poisoning due to Clostridium perfringens [C. welchii]
Enteritis necroticans

005.3   Food poisoning due to other Clostridia

005.4   Food poisoning due to Vibrio parahaemolyticus

005.8   Other bacterial food poisoning

Excludes: salmonella food poisoning (003.0-003.9)

005.81   Food poisoning due to Vibrio vulnificus

005.89   Other bacterial food poisoning
Food poisoning due to Bacillus cereus

005.9   Food poisoning, unspecified

As you look at Category 005, note that codes 005.0-005.4 indicate that the food poisoning is related to specific types of organisms. Therefore, subcategories 005.0-005.4 are regarded as more specific than subcategory 005.9. Fifth-digit subclassification 005.89 *Other bacterial food poisoning* would include other specific types of <u>bacterial</u> food poisoning not classified elsewhere, as well as <u>bacterial</u> food poisoning NOS. Whereas subcategory 005.9 *Food poisoning unspecified* would be used for a diagnostic statement of "Food poisoning NOS" where the causative organism is not mentioned.

The hierarchy from more specific to less specific is not consistently maintained at the fifth-digit level. The level of specificity at the fifth-digit level is usually (not always) indicated by the use of 0 and 9. The digit 9 identifies the entry for "Other specified" while the digit 0 identifies the "Unspecified" entry. Below is an example.

279   Disorders involving the immune mechanism

    279.0   Deficiency of humoral immunity

        279.00   Hypogammaglobulinemia, unspecified
                          Agammaglobulinemia NOS

        279.01   Selective IgA immunodeficiency

        279.02   Selective IgM immunodeficiency

        279.03   Other selective immunoglobulin deficiencies
                          Selective deficiency of IgG

        279.04   Congenital hypogammaglobulinemia
                          Agammaglobulinemia:
                              Bruton's type
                              X-linked

        279.05   Immunodeficiency with increased IgM
                          Immunodeficiency with hyper-IgM:
                              autosomal recessive
                              X-linked

        279.06   Common variable immunodeficiency
                          Dysgammaglobulinemia (acquired)
                              (congenital) (primary)
                          Hypogammaglobulinemia:
                              acquired primary
                              congenital non-sex-linked
                              sporadic

        279.09   Other
                          Transient hypogammaglobulinemia of infancy

Notice that the fifth-digit 0 identifies "Unspecified" and the fifth-digit 9 identifies "Other specified."

ACUTE AND CHRONIC CODING

Whenever a particular condition is described as both acute and chronic, code according to the subentries in the Alphabetic Index (Volume 2) for the stated condition. The following directions should be considered.

1.   If there are separate subentries listed for acute, subacute and chronic, then use both codes, sequencing the code for the acute condition first.

2.   If there are no subentries to identify acute, subacute or chronic, ignore these adjectives when selecting the code for the particular condition.

3.   If a certain condition is described as a subacute condition and the index does not provide a subentry designating subacute, then code the condition as if it were acute.

CODING SUSPECTED CONDITIONS

Whenever the diagnosis is stated as "questionable," "probable," "likely," or "rule out," it is advisable to code documented symptoms or complaints by the patient. The reason for this is that you do not want an insurance carrier to include a disease code in the patient's history if in fact the "suspected" condition is never proven.

Keep in mind that there are no "rule out" codes per se in the ICD-9-CM coding system. If your diagnostic statement is "Rule out Breast Carcinoma" and you use code 174.9 *Malignant neoplasm of female breast, unspecified*, the code definition does not state "rule out." Therefore, the insurance carrier processes the code 174.9 as is, which results in the patient having an insurance history of breast cancer.

To avoid what could become a problem for you and your patient (including the potential of litigation), you should use codes for signs and symptoms in these cases. For example, use code 611.72 *Lump or mass in breast*, or 611.71 *Mastodynia (breast pain)* if these symptoms exist and this is the highest degree of certainty you can code to.

If the patient is asymptomatic but there is a family history of breast cancer then you should consider using a V-code, such as V16.3 *Family history of malignant neoplasm, breast* as your diagnosis code. There are also V-codes to indicate screening for a particular illness or disease. In the above example, code V76.1 *Special screening for malignant neoplasm, breast* could also have been used.

It is important to note that when you use a screening code from the V-code section you should also code signs or symptoms. The reason for doing so is because most health insurance carriers do not provide coverage for routine screening procedures or preventive medicine.

COMBINATION CODES

A combination code is used to fully identify an instance where two diagnoses or a diagnosis with an associated secondary process (manifestation) or complication is included in the description of a single code number. These combination codes are identified by referring to the subterms in the Alphabetic Index (Volume 2) and the inclusion and exclusion terms in the Tabular List (Volume 1).

Examples of commonly used combination codes include 034.0 *Streptococcal sore throat* and 404 *Hypertensive heart and renal disease*. Code 034.0 exists because the throat is often infected with Streptococcus and code 404 must be used whenever a patient has both heart and renal disease instead of assigning codes from categories 402 and 403.

Two main terms may be joined together by combination terms listed in the Alphabetic Index (Volume 2) as subterms such as:

associated with   *in*
complicated (by)   *secondary to*
due to   *with*
during   *without*
following

The listing for the above terms advises the coder to use one or two codes depending on the condition.

MULTIPLE CODING

The concept of multiple coding is encouraged when the use of more than one code number will fully identify a given condition. Thus, use of multiple codes allows all the components of a complex diagnosis to be identified. However, the statement of diagnosis must mention the presence of all the elements for each code number used.

When is multiple coding mandatory? Only if the instructional term "Code Also" appears in italics under an italicized subdivision in the Tabular List (Volume 1). In this instance, you should interpret mandatory as....requires the use of both codes, and that these codes must be sequenced with the code for the etiology being listed first and the code identifying the manifestation listed second. You will recognize mandatory multiple coding situations by instructional terms used in the Tabular List (Volume 1). Terms to watch for are: "Code also....," "Use additional code...," and "Note:..."

If you turn to Category 330 in the Tabular List (Volume 1), you will notice the instructional term cited: "Use additional code if desired, to identify associated mental retardation." The phrase "...identify associated mental retardation..." should be interpreted as "...identify associated mental retardation, if stated to be present in the diagnostic statement." With this understood, these diagnostic statements would be coded as below.

Coding Examples

Cerebral degeneration in childhood with mental retardation

    330.9   Unspecified cerebral degeneration in childhood

    319   Unspecified mental retardation

Cerebral degeneration in childhood

    330.9   Unspecified cerebral degeneration in childhood

In the Alphabetic Index (Volume 2), if two codes are listed, the first should be sequenced first with the code in italicized brackets listed second to indicate the additional code. However, the fact that two codes appear after a subterm in the Alphabetic Index does not automatically indicate mandatory multiple coding. It is necessary to verify both code numbers in the Tabular List. If, in the Tabular List, the code number is also in italics as in the Alphabetical Index and, the instructional term "Code also" appears in italics, then both criteria have been met for mandatory multiple coding.

Coding Example

Diabetic neuropathy

> **250.60** Diabetes with neurological manifestations
>
> **[357.2]** Polyneuropathy in diabetes
>
> In the Alphabetic Index (Volume 2) under "Diabetes," you will find "Neuropathy" listed followed by the codes 250.6 and [357.2] in brackets.

It should also be noted at this point, that even though mandatory multiple coding is always indicated by the presence of the instructional term "Code first" in italics beneath the italicized code number and title for the manifestation, this does not always hold true under the code number for the etiology. Multiple coding is not to be used in those instances when a combination code accurately identifies all of the elements within the diagnostic statement.

CODING LATE EFFECTS

You use late effects coding when coding diagnostic statements that identify a residual effect (condition produced) after the acute phase of an illness or injury has ended. The proper coding sequence is to list the code number identifying the residual (the current condition) first, with the code number identifying the cause (original illness/injury no longer present in its acute phase but which was the cause of the long term residual condition) listed second.

Coding Example

Hemiplegia due to previous cerebral vascular accident

> **342.90** Hemiplegia, unspecified, affecting unspecified side
>
> **438.20** Late effects of cerebrovascular disease, Hemiplegia affecting unspecified side
>
> The <u>residual</u> for this statement is "Hemiplegia" as it is the long term condition that resulted from a previous acute illness. The <u>cause</u> for this statement is "Cerebral vascular accident" as it is the original illness no longer in its acute phase but which did cause the long term residual condition now present.

How do you recognize when to use late effects coding and when not to? Often, the diagnostic statement will contain key words to help identify a late effects situation. Key words used in defining late effects include:

> *late*
> *due to an old injury*
> *due to a previous illness/injury*
> *due to an illness/injury occurring one year or more ago*

In cases where these key words (phrases) are not included within the diagnostic statement, an effect is considered to be late if sufficient time has elapsed between the occurrence of the acute illness/injury and the development of the residual effect.

Coding Example

Excessive scar tissue due to third degree burn, right leg

709.2   Scar conditions and fibrosis of skin

906.7   Late effect of burn of other extremities

The previous diagnostic statement does not indicate the time element with any modifying terms as "old" or "previous." The fact that enough time has elapsed for the development of scar tissue indicates that the acute phase of the injury has subsided and the scarring should be coded as a late effect.

If a diagnostic statement only specifies the cause of the late effect and does not indicate the residual, then use the code number for the cause.

Coding Example

Residuals of tuberculosis

137   Late effects of tuberculosis

The above statement does not identify the actual residuals, so you would use the code for the cause.

To find the code for such a statement in the Alphabetic Index (Volume 2), refer to the main term "LATE" and the subterm "EFFECTS OF." The only codes available for causes of late effects are:

137   Late effects of tuberculosis

138   Late effects of acute poliomyelitis

139   Late effects of other infectious and parasitic diseases

268.1   Rickets, late effects

326   Late effects of intracranial abscess or pyogenic infection

438   Late effects of cerebrovascular disease

677   Late effects of complication of pregnancy, childbirth and the puerperium

905   Late effects of musculoskeletal and connective tissue injuries

906   Late effects of injuries to skin and subcutaneous tissues

907   Late effects of injuries to the nervous system

908   Late effects of other and unspecified injuries

909   Late effects of other and unspecified external causes

E999   Late effect of injury due to war operations and terrorism

Be sure to distinguish between a late effect and a historical statement in a diagnosis. Whenever the statement uses the terms "effects of old...," "sequela of...," or "residuals of...," then code as late effects. If the diagnosis is expressed in terms as "history of...," these are coded to personal history of the illness or injury and are coded to the V-Codes (V-10 to V-15).

CODING INJURIES

Injuries comprise a major section of ICD-9-CM. Categories 800-959 include fractures, dislocations, sprains and various other types of injuries. Injuries are classified first according to the general type of injury and within each type there is a further breakdown by anatomical site.

In cases where a patient has multiple injuries, the most severe injury is the principal diagnosis. Where multiple sites of injury are specified in the diagnosis, you should interpret the term "with" as indicating involvement of both sites, and interpret the term "and" as indicating involvement of either or both sites. You will also note that fifth-digits are commonly used when coding injuries to provide information regarding level of consciousness, specific anatomical sites and severity of injuries.

Some general rules to apply when coding fractures follow. Fractures can either be "open" or "closed." An "open" fracture is when the skin has been broken and there is communication with the bone and the outside of the body. Whereas, with a "closed" fracture the bone does not have contact with the outside of the body.

Note the following descriptions as set forth in the ICD-9-CM at the four-digit subdivision level to help distinguish between an "open" and "closed" fracture.

Closed Fractures

comminuted	*simple*
linear	*greenstick*
fissured	*depressed*
spiral	*fractured NOS*
impacted	slipped epiphysis
elevated	

Open Fractures

compound	*with foreign body*
missile	*infected*
puncture	

Anytime that it is not indicated whether a fracture is open or closed, code it as if it were closed. Fracture-dislocations are classified as fractures. Pathological fractures are classified to the condition causing the fracture (i.e. osteoporosis) with the use of an additional code to identify the *Pathological fracture* (733.1).

When coding burns, code only the most severe degree of burns when the burns are of the same site but of different degrees. In cases of burns where it is noted that there is an infection, assign the code for the burn and also the code for the infection (958.3 *Posttraumatic wound infection NEC*).

The percentage of the body surface involved with burns is specified by using Category 948. This code may be used as a solo code when the site of the burn is unspecified. There is also a fifth-digit subclassification included in Category 948 to identify the percentage of the total body surface involved with third degree burns. Use Category 949 only when neither the site nor the percentage of the body surface involved is specified in the diagnosis.

POISONING AND ADVERSE EFFECTS OF DRUGS

There are two different sets of code numbers to use to differentiate between poisoning and adverse reactions to the correct substances properly administered. First, you must make the distinction between poisoning and adverse reaction. Poisoning by drugs includes:

Poisoning

Accidental

1.   Given in error during diagnostic or therapeutic procedures.

2.   Given in error by one person to another (for example, mother to child).

3.   Taken in error by self.

Purposeful

1.   Suicide attempt.

2.   Homicide attempt.

Adverse Reaction in Spite of Proper Administration of Correct Substance

1.   In therapeutic of diagnostic procedure.

2.   Taken by self or given to another as prescribed.

3.   Accumulative effect (intoxication due to....).

4.   Interaction of prescribed drugs.

5.   Synergistic reaction (enhancing the effect of another drug).

6.   Allergic reaction.

7.   Hypersensitivity.

To code poisoning by drugs, use the Alphabetic Index (Volume 2) which contains the Table of Drugs and Chemicals. This table includes one column to identify the poisoning code (960-989) and four columns of External Cause Codes to classify whether the poisoning was an accident, suicide, assault or undetermined.

The column labeled "Therapeutic Use" is not used for poisonings but in coding adverse reactions to correct substances properly administered. The External Cause Codes are optional but may be used if a facility's coding policy requires their use.

Note that in the Alphabetic Index (Volume 2) that the subterm entry "Drug" under the main term of "Poisoning" refers the coder to the Table of Drugs and Chemicals for the code assignment. Because the Table of Drugs and Chemicals is so extensive, it is acceptable to code directly from the Table without verifying the code obtained in Volume 1.

What if the drug which caused the poisoning is not listed in the Table of Drugs and Chemicals?

1.   Refer to Appendix C in Volume 1 (American Hospital Formulary Service) and locate the name of the drug.

2.   Note the AHFS category number listed.

3.   Turn to the Table of Drugs and Chemicals in the Alphabetic Index (Volume 2) of ICD-9-CM.

4.   Locate the term "Drug."

5.   Refer to the subterm "AHFS List."

6.   Look through the list until you find the AHFS Category Number determined in step 2 above. The AHFS Category Numbers are listed in numeric order.

7.   Assign the code.

How Do You Identify Poisoning by Drugs?

The statement of diagnosis will usually have descriptive terms that would indicate poisoning. Look for terms such as:

Intoxication	*Toxic effect*
Overdose	*Wrong drug given/taken in error*
Poisoning	*Wrong dosage given/taken in error*

Adverse effects of a medicine taken in combination with alcohol or from taking a prescribed drug in combination with a drug the patient took on his/her own initiative (for example antihistamines) are coded as poisonings. If you wish to code a manifestation of the poisoning as well, this code is always listed second, after listing the code identifying the poison first.

Adverse Effects of Drugs

The World Health Organization (WHO) defines adverse drug reaction as any response to a drug "which is noxious and unintended and which occurs at doses used in man for prophylaxis, diagnosis or therapy." Notice that this definition does not include the terms "overdose" or "poisoning."

Why does ICD-9-CM differentiate between poisoning and adverse drug reaction? Tabulation of statistical data indicates how often a drug reaction occurred because of the drug itself versus how often the drug was either not given or taken properly.

Two codes are required when coding adverse drug reactions to the correct substance properly administered. One code is used to identify the manifestation or the nature of the adverse reaction such as urticaria, vertigo, gastritis, etc. This code is assigned from Categories 001-799 in Volume 1.

Refer to the main term identifying the manifestation in the Alphabetic Index (Volume 2). But remember that the Table of Drugs and Chemicals is not used to locate the code for the manifestation, and the code used to identify the manifestation does not identify the drug responsible for the adverse reaction.

A second code is required to identify the drug causing the adverse reaction. In ICD-9-CM, the only codes provided to identify the drug causing an adverse reaction to a substance properly administered are E930 through E949. Anytime a code is selected from the E930-E949 range, it can never be sequenced first or stand as a solo code.

Locating the Proper E Code

How do you locate the proper E code to identify the drug which was responsible for causing an adverse reaction to a correct substance properly administered? Turn to the Table of Drugs and Chemicals in the Alphabetic Index (Volume 2). Earlier we noted that the column labeled "Therapeutic Use" was not used for coding instances involving poisoning. However, for adverse drug reactions to a correct substance properly administered, the "Therapeutic Use" column is used to find the proper code within the range E930 through E949 to identify the drug.

Drug Interactions Between Two or More Drugs

Drug interactions between two or more prescribed drugs are classified as adverse drug reactions to a correct substance properly administered. This holds true regardless of whether the drugs were prescribed by the same physician or different physicians.

Two types of drug interactions should be noted:

1. Synergistic interaction. One drug enhances the action of another drug so that the combined effect is greater than the sum of the effects of each used alone.

2. Antagonistic interaction. One drug represses the action of another drug.

To properly code drug interactions, first code the manifestation. Then code each drug involved in the interaction using the E codes from the column labeled "Therapeutic Use" from the Table of Drugs and Chemicals.

Coding Example

Gastritis due to interaction between Motrin and Procainamide

> **535.50** Unspecified gastritis and gastroduodenitis
> *List the manifestation first*

> **E935.8** Other specified analgesics and antipyretics

> **E942.0** Cardiac rhythm regulators

Coding Example

When a diagnostic statement does not state specifically the manifestation or nature of the adverse reaction, you should use the code provided to identify an adverse drug reaction of unspecified nature, 995.2 *Unspecified adverse effect of drug, medicinal and biological substance*. For example:

Allergic reaction to Motrin, proper dose

995.2   Unspecified adverse effect of drug medicinal and biological substance

E935.8 Other specified analgesics and antipyretics

Note in the above example that the code indicating the manifestation, although unspecified as to the nature, is listed first followed by the E code to identify the drug. When the drug causing an adverse effect is unknown or unspecified, use code E947.9 *Unspecified drug or medicinal substance*.

It is very important to remember that codes in the range 960 through 979 are never used in combination with codes in the range E930 through E949 because codes in the range 960-979 identify poisonings and codes in the range E930-E949 identify the external cause of adverse reactions to the correct substance properly administered.

CODING COMPLICATIONS OF MEDICAL AND SURGICAL CARE

A complication is when you have the occurrence of two or more diseases in the same patient. Recent studies have revealed serious deficiencies in properly coding complications for insurance claims processing. Often the complication is never mentioned. Complications are responsible for many of the procedures that are ordered for patients, therefore the complication should be coded and submitted on your insurance claims.

Postoperative complications that affect a specific anatomical site or body system are classified to the appropriate chapter 1 through 16 of the Tabular Index (Volume 1). Postoperative complications affecting more than one anatomical site or body system are classified in the chapter on injury and poisoning (Chapter 17, Categories 996-999). If the Alphabetic Index (Volume 2) does not provide a specific main term and subterm to identify a postoperative complication, classify the complication to categories 996-999.

Coding Example

Postcholecystectomy syndrome

576.0   Postcholecystectomy syndrome

The Alphabetic Index (Volume 2) specifically classifies the postoperative condition to one of the categories from 001 through 799. See main term "Complication," subterms "surgical procedure" and "postcholecystectomy syndrome."

Coding Examples

Postoperative wound infection

> **998.5**   Postoperative infection

The Alphabetic Index (Volume 2) has a main term "Infection" and subterms "wound, postoperative" for this condition. Note that this code appears in Chapter 17 within categories 996-999.

Postoperative atelectasis

> **997.3**   Respiratory complications

Refer to the main term "Atelectasis" in the Alphabetic Index (Volume 2). Note there is no subterm for postoperative beneath this main term. Therefore, you must presume this complication is classified to one of the categories in the range 969-999. You may also code 518.0 *Pulmonary collapse*, to identify the nature of the respiratory complication for statistical purposes; however, the code for the complication must be listed first.

COMPLICATIONS FROM MECHANICAL DEVICES

Subcategories in the range 996.0 through 996.5 are used to identify mechanical complications of devices. Mechanical complications are the result of a malfunction on the part of the internal prosthetic implant or device. What indicates a mechanical complication? Breakdown or obstruction, displacement, leakage, perforation or protrusion of the devices are all forms of mechanical complications.

Coding Examples

Displacement of cardiac pacemaker electrode

> **996.01**   Mechanical complication of cardiac device, implant, and graft due to cardiac pacemaker (electrode)

Protrusion of nail into acetabulum

> **996.4**   Mechanical complication of internal orthopedic device, implant, and graft

Other complications of devices, such as infection or hemorrhage, are due to an abnormal reaction of the body to an otherwise properly functioning device. All complications involving infection are coded to category 996.7 Other complications of internal prosthetic device, implant and graft.

Coding Examples

Infected arteriovenous shunt

> **996.6**   Infection and inflammatory reaction due to internal prosthetic device, implant, and graft

Anterior chamber hemorrhage due to displaced prosthetic lens

    996.7   Other complications of internal (biologic) (synthetic) prosthetic device, implant, and graft

CARDIAC COMPLICATIONS

In the case of cardiac complications, ICD-9-CM defines the "immediate postoperative period" as "the period between surgery and the time of discharge from the hospital." This definition is the basis of whether to code cardiac complications under subcategory 997.1 *Cardiac complications affecting specified body systems, not elsewhere classified,* or under subcategory 429.4 *Functional disturbances following cardiac surgery.*

Use 997.1 for a cardiac complication that occurs anytime between surgery and hospital discharge from any type of procedure performed. Use subcategory 429.4 to code long-term cardiac complications resulting from cardiac surgery.

It is important to distinguish between complications and aftercare. Aftercare is usually an encounter for something planned in advance (example, removal of Kirshner wire). Aftercare is classified using codes in the range of V51-V58. An encounter for a complication occurs from unforeseen circumstances, such as wound infection, resulting in complication of the patient's condition.

SPECIAL CODING SITUATIONS

As you become an experienced coder you will encounter situations where the standard rules do not seem to apply, or which require a special understanding in order to code properly. These situations include coding of circulatory diseases, diabetes, mental disorders, infectious diseases, manifestations, neoplasms, and pregnancy and childbirth. The following sections address these specific special coding situations.

CODING CIRCULATORY DISEASES

Because of the variety of terms and phrases used by physicians to identify diseases of the circulatory system, you will often experience difficulty in coding. To accurately code disorders of the circulatory system, it is imperative that the coder carefully read all inclusion, exclusion and "use additional code" notations contained in the Tabular List (Volume 1).

Fifth digit subclassifications are also frequently used to code combination disorders or to provide further specificity in this section. Even those in specialties other than cardiology will frequently find themselves coding circulatory system diagnoses due to the prevalence of circulatory disorders in this country.

Chapter 7 of the Tabular List (Volume 1), titled Diseases of the Circulatory System, contains the following major sections:

    Acute Rheumatic Fever (390-392)

    Chronic Rheumatic Heart Disease (393-398)

Hypertensive Disease (401-405)

Ischemic Heart Disease (410-414)

Diseases of Pulmonary Circulation (415-417)

Other Forms of Heart Disease (420-429)

Cerebrovascular Disease (430-438)

Diseases of Arteries, Arterioles, and Capillaries (440-448)

Diseases of Veins, Lymphatics, and Ohter Diseases of the Circulatory System (451-459)

Diseases of Mitral and Aortic Valves

Certain diseases of the mitral valve of unspecified etiology are presumed to be of rheumatic origin and others are not. None of the disorders of the aortic valve of unspecified etiology are presumed to be of rheumatic origin. When you have disorders involving both the mitral and aortic valves of unspecified etiology, then they are presumed to be of rheumatic origin.

Coding Examples

Mitral valve insufficiency

> **424.0**   Mitral valve disorders
>
> Refer to the main term "Insufficiency" in the Alphabetic Index (Volume 2). Note the subterm "mitral (valve)."

Mitral valve stenosis

> **394.0**   Mitral stenosis
>
> Refer to the main term "Stenosis" and the sub-term "mitral (valve)" in the Alphabetic Index (Volume 2).

Aortic valve insufficiency

> **424.1**   Aortic valve disorders

Aortic valve stenosis

> **424.1**   Aortic valve disorders
>
> Look up the main term "Stenosis" and the subterm "aortic" in the Alphabetic Index (Volume 2). Remember that aortic valve disorders of unspecified etiology are not considered rheumatic in nature or origin.

Insufficiency of mitral and aortic valves

396.3 Mitral valve insufficiency and aortic valve insufficiency

Under the main term "Insufficiency" in the Alphabetic Index (Volume 2) you will find the subterm "aortic." Further review will locate "with," "mitral valve disease," "insufficiency, incompetence or regurgitation" which directs you to code 396.3

Ischemic Heart Disease

In ischemic heart disease, the manifestations are due to a lack of blood flow to the heart rather than to the anatomical lesion of the coronary arteries. The most common cause of coronary heart disease is coronary atherosclerosis. However, ischemic heart disease can be due to non-coronary disease, such as aortic valvular stenosis, as well. There are many synonyms used to indicate ischemic heart disease such as: coronary artery heart disease, ASHD, and coronary ischemia. Categories in the range 410-414, Ischemic Heart Disease, includes that with mention of hypertension. Use an additional code to identify the presence of hypertension.

Coding Examples

Angina pectoris

413.9 Other and unspecified angina pectoris

As no mention of hypertension is made in the diagnostic statement, a single code is all that is required.

Angina pectoris with essential hypertension

413.9 Other and unspecified angina pectoris

401.9 Essential hypertension, unspecified

In this example, the mention of hypertension in the diagnostic statement requires the use of a second code.

Myocardial Infarction

A myocardial infarction is classified as acute if it is either specified as "acute" in the diagnostic statement or with a stated duration of eight weeks or less. When a myocardial infarction is specified as "chronic" or with symptoms after eight weeks from the date of the onset, it should be coded to subcategory 414.8 *Other specified forms of chronic ischemic heart disease.* If a myocardial infarction is specified as old or healed or has been diagnosed by special investigation (EKG) but is currently not presenting any symptoms, code using category 412 *Old myocardial infarction.*

Coding Examples

Myocardial infarction three weeks ago

410.92 Acute myocardial infarction, unspecified site

Chronic myocardial infarction with angina

414.8   Other specified forms of chronic ischemic heart disease

413.9   Other and unspecified angina pectoris

Myocardial infarction diagnoses by EKG, symptomatic

412   Old myocardial infarction

Arteriosclerotic Cardiovascular Disease (ASCVD)

Arteriosclerotic cardiovascular disease (ASCVD) is classified to subcategory 429.2 *Cardiovascular disease, unspecified.* You should use an additional code to identify the presence of arteriosclerosis when coding ASCVD. For example, the diagnostic statement "generalized arteriosclerotic cardiovascular disease" should be coded using 429.2 followed by 440.9 *Generalized and unspecified atherosclerosis.*

"Other forms of heart disease", categories 420-429, are used for multiple coding purposes to fully identify a stated diagnosis. The exception to this rule is if the Alphabetic Index (Volume 2) or Tabular List (Volume 1) specifically instructs you otherwise.

Coding Examples

Arteriosclerotic heart disease with acute pulmonary edema

428.1   Left heart failure

414.0   Coronary atherosclerosis

Note that the code for ASHD (414.0) is listed second as a possible underlying cause of the acute situation.

Arteriosclerotic heart disease with congestive heart failure

428.0   Congestive heart failure, unspecified

414.0   Coronary atherosclerosis

Cerebrovascular Disease

When coding cerebrovascular disease (codes 430-438), you should code the component parts of the diagnostic statement identifying the cerebrovascular disease, unless specifically instructed to do otherwise in the Alphabetic Index (Volume 2) or Tabular List (Volume 1).

Coding Examples

Cerebrovascular arteriosclerosis with subarachnoid hemorrhage

430   Subarachnoid hemorrhage

437.0   Cerebral atherosclerosis

Cerebrovascular accident secondary to thrombosis

> **434.00** Cerebral thrombosis, without mention of cerebral infarction

> In this example, you use only one code because of the instructions in the Alphabetic Index (Volume 2). When you look up the main term "Accident" with subterm "cerebrovascular," you are instructed to "(*see also* Disease, cerebrovascular, acute) 436". When you locate the main term "Disease" and subterms "cerebrovascular," "acute" and "thrombotic," you are further instructed to "*see* Thrombosis, brain". This is where you finally locate the single code for this diagnosis, 434.0. When you look up the code in the Tabular List (Volume 1), you are instructed to add a fifth digit "0" if it is without mention of cerebral infarction, and "1" if it is with cerebral infarction.

Whenever there are conditions resulting from the acute cerebrovascular disease, code them if they are stated to be residual(s). If the resulting condition is stated to be transient, do not code them.

Coding Examples

Cerebrovascular accident with residual aphasia

> **436**   Acute, but ill-defined, cerebrovascular disease

> **784.3**   Aphasia

Cerebrovascular accident with transient hemiparesis

> **436**   Acute, but ill-defined, cerebrovascular disease

Hypertensive Disease

As demonstrated earlier with ischemic heart disease, conditions that are classified to cerebrovascular disease (codes 430-438) include that with mention of hypertension, but you must identify the hypertension with another code (401-405) and list it second.

Hypertensive disease is classified to the categories 401-405. The Table of Hypertension is located in the Alphabetic Index (Volume 2) under the main term "Hypertension." This Table contains subterms to identify types of hypertension and complications as well as three columns labeled "malignant," "benign," and "unspecified."

Hypertension is frequently the cause of various forms of heart and vascular disease. However, the mention of hypertension with some heart conditions should not be interpreted as a combination resulting in hypertensive heart disease. The combination is only to be made if there is a cause-and-effect relationship between hypertension and a heart condition classified to subcategories 425.8, 428.0-428.9, 429.0-429.3 and 429.8-429.9.

First you need to be able to make a distinction between conditions specified as "due to" or "with" hypertension. Keep in mind that the phrase "due to hypertension" and the word "hypertensive" are considered synonymous.

Coding Examples

Hypertensive heart disease

> **402.90** Hypertensive heart disease, unspecified, without heart failure

Heart disease due to hypertension

> **402.90** Hypertensive heart disease, unspecified, without heart failure

Each of the above diagnostic statements indicate clearly a cause-and-effect relationship between hypertension and the condition by specifying that the condition is "due to." Therefore, both statements are coded using 402.90.

If the phrase "with hypertension" is stated or, the diagnostic statement mentions the conditions separately, then you code the conditions separately.

Coding Example

Myocarditis with hypertension

> **429.0** Myocarditis, unspecified

> **401.9** Essential hypertension, unspecified

As a cause-and-effect relationship is not indicated in the diagnostic statement, the conditions are coded separately.

High Blood Pressure Versus Elevated Blood Pressure

With the ICD-9-CM coding system there is a differentiation made between high blood pressure (hypertension) and elevated blood pressure without a diagnosis of hypertension. If the diagnostic statement indicates elevated blood pressure without the diagnosis of hypertension, it is coded to subcategory 796.2 *Elevated blood pressure reading without diagnosis of hypertension*. If the diagnostic statement indicates high blood pressure or hypertension, it is coded to category 401 *Essential hypertension*.

DIABETES MELLITUS CODING (250)

In 1980, the American Diabetic Association reclassified the types of diabetes mellitus to signify whether or not the patient is dependent on insulin for survival of life. In 1994, additional classifications were added. Note the revisions (bracketed portions) of the statements below for the fifth-digit subclassification.

0   type II [non-insulin dependent type] [NIDDM type] [adult-onset type] or unspecified type, not stated as uncontrolled

    Fifth digit 0 is for use with type II, adult onset diabetic patients, even if the patient requires insulin

1   type I [insulin dependent type] [IDDM] [juvenile type], not stated as uncontrolled

2   type II [non-insulin dependent type] [NIDDM] [adult-onset type] or unspecified type, uncontrolled

         Fifth digit 2 is for use with type II, adult onset diabetic patients, even if the patient requires insulin

3   type I [insulin dependent type][IDDM][juvenile type], uncontrolled

Do not assume a patient has insulin-dependent diabetes simply because the patient is receiving insulin, as some non-dependent diabetics may require temporary use when they encounter stressful situations such as surgery or physical or mental illness.

Anytime diabetes is described as "brittle" or "uncontrolled" you should interpret it as diabetes mellitus complicated and assign code 250.9 with the appropriate fifth-digit, 0, 1, 2 or 3. However, if there is also a specific complication present, then assign the code identifying that specific complication, for example, Diabetes mellitus, brittle, with ketoacidosis would be 250.13.

CODING MENTAL DISORDERS

You should be aware of the existence of the glossary of mental disorders in Appendix B of the Tabular List (Volume 1). This glossary is not used for coding purposes but rather as a guide to provide a common frame of reference for statistical comparisons. It is simply an alphabetized listing of mental disorders with definitions.

The coder should choose code assignments based on the terminology used by the physician or psychiatrist and not by the coder's impression of the content of the categories and subcategories. The chapter on mental disorders has many fifth digit subclassifications to watch for when selecting your code.

INFECTIOUS AND PARASITIC DISEASES

There are two categories for identifying the organism causing diseases classified elsewhere. These codes may be used as either additional codes, or as solo codes depending on the diagnostic statement.

      041   Bacterial infection in conditions classified elsewhere and of unspecified site

      079   Viral and chlamydial infection in conditions classified elsewhere and of unspecified site

Coding Examples

Acute UTI due to Escherchia coli

      599.0   Urinary tract infection, site not specified

      041.4   Escherchia coli

Staphylococcus infection

      041.11   Staphylococcus aureus

Bacterial infection

> **041.9**   Bacterial infection, unspecified

The basic coding principles regarding combination codes (one code accurately identifies the components of the condition) applies throughout the chapter on Infectious and Parasitic Diseases.

In the Alphabetic Index (Volume 2), a subterm that identifies an infectious organism takes precedence in code assignment over a subterm at the same indentation level that identifies a site or other descriptive term.

Coding Example

Chronic syphilitic cystitis

> **095.8**   Other specified forms of late symptomatic syphilis

Using the Alphabetic Index (Volume 2) to look up the main term "Cystitis (bacillary)," you will note the subterms "chronic 595.2" and "syphilitic 095.8" at the same indentation level under the main term. Therefore, code 095.8 is assigned to this diagnostic statement, as the organism has precedence over other descriptive terms or anatomical sites.

MANIFESTATIONS

Manifestations are characteristic signs or symptoms of an illness. Signs and symptoms that point rather definitely to a given diagnosis are assigned to the appropriate chapter of ICD-9-CM. For example, hematuria is assigned to the Genitourinary System chapter. However, Chapter 16 *Symptoms, Signs and Ill-Defined Conditions* (780-799), includes ill-defined conditions and symptoms that may suggest two or more diseases or may point to two or more systems of the body, and are used in cases lacking the necessary study to make a final diagnosis.

Conditions allocated to Chapter 16 include:

1.   Cases for which no more specific diagnosis can be made even after all facts bearing on the case have been investigated; for example code 784.0 *Headache.*

2.   Signs or symptoms existing at the time of initial encounter that proved to be transient and whose cause could not be determined; for example code 780.2 *Syncope and collapse.*

3.   Provisional diagnoses in a patient who failed to return for further investigation or care; for example code 782.4 *Jaundice, unspecified, not of newborn.*

4.   Cases referred elsewhere for investigation or treatment before the diagnosis was made; for example code 782.5 *Cyanosis.*

5.   Cases in which a more precise diagnosis was not available for any other reason; for example code 780.4 *Dizziness and giddiness.*

6.   Certain symptoms which represent important problems in medical care and which it might be desired to classify in addition to a known cause; for example, code 780.01 *Coma.*

In the last case, if the cause of a symptom or sign is stated in the diagnosis, assign the code identifying the cause. An additional code may be assigned to further identify this symptom or sign if there is a need to further identify the symptom or sign. In such cases, the code identifying the cause will ordinarily be listed as the principal diagnosis.

CODING OF NEOPLASMS

The coding of neoplasms requires a good understanding of medical terminology. All neoplasms are classified in the Tabular List (Volume 1) in Chapter 2 *Neoplasms* 140-239 which contains the following broad groups:

140-195	Malignant neoplasms, stated or presumed to be primary, of specified sites, except of lymphatic and hematopoietic tissue
196-198	Malignant neoplasms, stated or presumed to be secondary, of specified sites
199	Malignant neoplasms, without specification of site
200-208	Malignant neoplasms, stated or presumed to be primary of lymphatic and hematopoietic tissue
210-229	Benign neoplasms
230-234	Carcinoma in situ
235-238	Neoplasms of uncertain behavior
239	Neoplasms of unspecified nature

Table of Neoplasms

The Table of Neoplasms appears in the Alphabetic Index (Volume 2) under the main term "Neoplasms." This table gives the code numbers for neoplasms of anatomical site. For each anatomical site there are six possible code numbers according to whether the neoplasm in questions is either:

    Malignant:
      Primary
      Secondary
      Ca in situ
    Benign
    Of uncertain behavior
    Of unspecified nature

Definitions of Site and Behaviors of Neoplasms

Primary	Identifies the stated or presumed site of origin.
Secondary	Identifies site(s) to which the primary site has spread (direct extension) or metastasized by lymphatic spread, invading local blood vessels, or by implantation as tumor cells shed into body cavities.

In-situ — Tumor cells that are undergoing malignant changes but are still confined to the point of origin without invasion of surrounding normal tissue (non-infiltrating, non-invasive or pre-invasive carcinoma).

Benign — Tumor does not invade adjacent structures or spread to distant sites but may displace or exert pressure on adjacent structures.

Of Uncertain Behavior — The pathologist is not able to determine whether the tumor is benign or malignant because some features of each are present.

Of Unspecified Nature — Neither the behavior nor the histological type of tumors are specified in the diagnostic statement. This type of diagnosis may be encountered when the patient has been treated elsewhere and comes in terminally ill without accompanying information, is referred elsewhere for work-up, or no work-up is performed because of advanced age or poor condition of the patient.

Steps to Coding Neoplasms

1. ICD-9-CM disregards classification of neoplasms by histological type (according to tissue origin) with the exception of lymphatic and hematopoietic neoplasms, malignant melanoma of skin, lipoma, and a few common tumors of bone, uterus, ovary, etc. All other tumors are classified by system, organ or site. The existence of these exceptions makes it necessary to first consult the Alphabetic Index (Volume 2) to determine whether a specific code has been assigned to a specified histological type. For example, *Malignant melanoma of skin of scalp* is coded 172.4 although the code specified in the "Malignant: Primary Column" of the Neoplasm Table for skin of scalp is 173.4.

2. The General Alphabetical Index (Volume 2) also provides guidance to the appropriate column for neoplasms which are not assigned a specific code by histological type. For example, if you look up *Lipomyoma, specified site* in the Alphabetic Index (Volume 2), you will find "*see* Neoplasm, connective tissue, benign."

   The guidance in the Alphabetic Index (Volume 2) can be over-ridden if a descriptor is present. For example, *Malignant adenoma of colon* is coded as 153.9 and not as 211.3 because the adjective "malignant" overrides the entry "adenoma — *see also* Neoplasm, benign."

3. The Neoplasm Table may be consulted directly if a specific neoplasm diagnosis indicates which column of the table is appropriate but does not delineate a specific type of tumor.

4. Sites marked with an asterisk (*), such as buttock NEC* or calf*, should be classified to malignant neoplasm of skin of these sites if the variety of neoplasm is a squamous cell carcinoma or an epidermoid carcinoma and to benign neoplasm of skin of these sites if the variety of neoplasm is a papilloma (of any type).

5. Primary malignant neoplasms are classified to the site of origin of the neoplasm. In some cases, it may not be possible to identify the site of origin, such as malignant neoplasms originating from contiguous sites.

    Neoplasms with overlapping site boundaries are classified to the fourth-digit subcategory .8 "other." For example, code 151.8 *Malignant neoplasm of contiguous or overlapping sites of stomach* whose point of origin cannot be determined.

6. Neoplasms which demonstrate functional activity require an additional code to identify the functional activity.

    Coding Example

    Cushing's syndrome due to malignant pheochromocytoma

    > **194.0**   Malignant neoplasm of adrenal gland

    > **255.0**   Disorders of adrenal glands; Cushing's syndrome

    Code sequencing depends on the circumstances of the encounter.

7. Two categories in the malignant neoplasm section represent departures from the usual principles of classification in that the fourth-digit subdivisions in each case are not mutually exclusive. These categories are 150 *Malignant neoplasm of esophagus* and 201 *Hodgkin's disease*. The dual axis is provided to account for differing terminology, for there is no uniform international agreement on the use of these terms.

    Coding Example

    Malignant neoplasm of the esophagus

    > **150.0**   Cervical esophagus

    > **150.1**   Thoracic esophagus

    > **150.2**   Abdominal esophagus

    or using alternate coding

    > **150.3**   Upper third of esophagus

    > **150.4**   Middle third of esophagus

    > **150.5**   Lower third of esophagus

8. When the treatment is directed at the primary site of the malignancy, designate the primary site as the principal diagnosis, except when the encounter or hospital admission is solely for *Radiotherapy* (V58.0) or, for *Chemotherapy* (V58.1).

9. When surgical intervention for removal of a primary site or secondary site malignancy is followed by adjunct chemotherapy or radiotherapy, code the malignancy using codes in the 140-198 series, or, where appropriate, in the

200-203 series as long as chemotherapy or radiotherapy is being actively administered. If the admission is for chemotherapy or radiotherapy, the malignancy code is listed second.

10.   When the primary malignancy has been previously excised or eradicated from its site and there is no adjunct treatment directed to that site, and there is no evidence of any remaining malignancy at the primary site, use the appropriate code from the V10 series to indicate the site of the primary malignancy. Any mention of extension, invasion or metastasis to a nearby structure or organ, or to a distant site, is coded as a secondary malignant neoplasm to that site and may be the principal diagnosis in the absence of the primary site.

11.   If the patient has no secondary malignancy and if the reason for admission or for the visit is follow-up of the malignancy, two codes are used and sequenced.

Coding Example

Follow-up of breast cancer treated with chemotherapy. No evidence of recurrence.

> **V67.2**   Follow-up examination following chemotherapy
>
> **V10.3**   Personal history of carcinoma of breast

12.   Malignancies of hematopoietic and lymphatic tissue are always coded to the 200.0-208.9 series unless specified as "in remission." If they are in remission, they are coded as V10.60-V10.79.

13.   If the primary malignant neoplasm previously excised or eradicated has recurred, code it as primary malignancy of the stated site unless the Alphabetic Index (Volume 2) directs you to do otherwise.

Coding Examples

Recurrence of prostate carcinoma

> **185**   Malignant neoplasm of prostate

Recurrence of breast carcinoma in mastectomy site

> **198.2**   Secondary malignant neoplasm of other specified sites, skin of breast

Make sure to code any mention of secondary site(s).

14.   Terminology referring to metastatic cancer is often ambiguous, so when there is doubt as to the meaning intended, the following rules should be used:

A. Cancer described as metastatic "from" a site should be interpreted as primary of that site.

B. Cancer described as metastatic "to" a site should be interpreted as secondary of that site.

Coding Examples

Carcinoma in axillary lymph nodes and lungs metastatic from breast

      174.9   Malignant neoplasm of female breast, unspecified

      196.3   Secondary and unspecified malignant neoplasm of lymph nodes of axilla and upper limb

      197.0   Secondary malignant neoplasm of lung

Adenocarcinoma of colon with extension to peritoneum

      153.9   Malignant neoplasm of colon, unspecified

      197.6   Secondary malignant neoplasm of retroperitoneum and peritoneum

15.   Diagnostic statements when only one site is identified as metastatic:

A. Code to the category for "primary of unspecified site" for the morphological type concerned UNLESS the code thus obtained is either 199.0 or 199.1.

B. If the code obtained in the above step is 199.0 or 199.1, then code the site qualified as "metastatic" as for a primary malignant neoplasm of the stated site EXCEPT for the sites listed below, which should always be coded as secondary neoplasm of the state site:

Bone	Mediastinum
Brain	Meninges
Diaphragm	Peritoneum
Heart	Pleura
Liver	Retroperitoneum
Lymph nodes	Spinal cord

Sites classifiable to 195

C. Also assign the appropriate code for primary or secondary malignant neoplasm of specified or unspecified site, depending on the diagnostic statement you are coding.

Coding Examples

Metastatic renal cell carcinoma of lung

      189.0   Malignant neoplasm of kidney, except pelvis

      197.0   Secondary malignant neoplasm of lung

Metastatic carcinoma of lung

> **162.9**   Malignant neoplasm of bronchus and lung, unspecified
>
> **199.1**   Malignant neoplasm without specification of site, other

This code is assigned to identify "secondary neoplasm of unspecified site" per the instructions in step C above.

Metastatic carcinoma of brain

> **198.3**   Secondary malignant neoplasm of other specified sites, brain and spinal cord
>
> **199.1**   Malignant neoplasm without specification of site, other

In this case, the brain is one of the sites listed in Step B as an exception. So for this diagnostic statement, the code assignment is for secondary neoplasm of the brain and primary malignant neoplasm of unspecified site.

16. When two or more sites are stated in the diagnostic statement and all are qualified to be "metastatic," you should code as for "primary site unknown" and code the stated sites as secondary neoplasms of those sites.

Coding Example

Metastatic melanoma of lung and liver

> **172.9**   Malignant melanoma of skin, site unspecified
>
> **197.0**   Secondary malignant neoplasm of lung
>
> **197.7**   Secondary malignant neoplasm of liver, specified as secondary

17. When there is no site specified in the diagnostic statement, but the morphological type is qualified as "metastatic," code as for "primary site unknown." Then assign the code for secondary neoplasms of unspecified site.

Coding Example

Metastatic apocrine adenocarcinoma

> **173.9**   Other malignant neoplasms of skin, site unspecified
>
> **199.1**   Malignant neoplasm without specification of site, other

18. When two or more sites are stated in the diagnosis and only some are qualified as "metastatic" while others are not, code as for "primary site unknown." However, you should interpret the following sites as secondary neoplasms:

> *Bone*   *Meninges*
> *Brain*   *Peritoneum*
> *Diaphragm*   *Pleura*
> *Heart*   *Retroperitoneum*
> *Liver*   *Spinal Cord*

> *Sites classifiable to category 195*

Coding Example

Carcinoma of lung, metastatic, and brain

198.3   Secondary malignant neoplasm of brain and spinal cord

197.0   Secondary malignant neoplasm of lung

199.1   Malignant neoplasm without specification of site, other

Pregnancy, Childbirth, and the Puerperium

Chapter 11 of the Tabular List (Volume 1) uses fifth-digit subclassifications extensively. In general, the fifth digit is not given in the Alphabetic Index (Volume 2), so each code must be verified in the Tabular List (Volume 1).

The codes for Ectopic and Molar Pregnancy (630-633), do not require the fifth digit. Note also that for the codes 634-638, there is a "common" set of fourth-digit subcategory codes to include complications. Be aware of the use of section marks with categories 634-637 to indicate the need for a fifth digit. All other codes, 640-676 require the use of a fifth digit with the single exception of code 650 *Normal delivery*.

Coding Example

Pregnancy, 3 months gestation complicated by benign essential hypertension

642.03   Benign essential hypertension complicating pregnancy, childbirth, and the puerperium, antepartum condition or complication

Categories 647 and 648 are used for conditions that are usually classified elsewhere, but which have been classified here because they are complications of pregnancy. The interaction of certain conditions with the pregnant state complicates the pregnancy and/or aggravates the non-obstetrical condition (i.e., diabetes mellitus, drug dependence, thyroid dysfunction) and are the main reasons for the obstetrical care provided.

Coding Examples

Rubella in woman, 7 months gestation

647.53   Infectious and parasitic conditions in the mother classifiable elsewhere, but complicating pregnancy, childbirth or the puerperium, rubella, antepartum condition or complication

Pregnancy with diabetes mellitus

648.03   Other current conditions in the mother classifiable elsewhere, but complicating pregnancy, childbirth or the puerperium, diabetes mellitus, antepartum condition or complication

If greater detail is needed for the complication, use an additional code to identify the complication more completely.

Coding Example

Pregnancy with pernicious anemia

648.23   Other current conditions in the mother classifiable elsewhere, but complicating pregnancy, childbirth or the puerperium, anemia, antepartum condition or complication

281.0   Pernicious anemia

Using V Codes

V-codes are used to identify encounters with the health care setting for reasons other than an illness or injury, for example, immunization. V-codes are also used to identify encounters of persons who are injured or ill and whose injury or illness is influenced by some circumstance or problem classified to the V-codes, for example, a person with a functioning pacemaker who requires emergency gastrointestinal surgery. V-codes fall into one of three categories: problems, services or factual.

Problem
: These v-codes identify a circumstance or problem that could affect a patient's overall health status but is not itself a current illness or injury. In other words, you may note that a patient has a drug allergy to sulfonamides by using code V14.2 *Personal history of allergy to sulfonamides.* Although this allergy is not considered an illness or a problem in a healthy person, it may affect how the physician will actually care for the patient. You would only use a problem V-code when the problem has a potential effect on the patient's current diagnosis and the physician's treatment plan for management of the illness or injury.

Service
: These v-codes describe circumstances other than an illness or injury which prompt the patient's visit. This type of visit often occurs when the patient has a chronic disease but is not acutely ill. An example would be a patient with a known neoplasm that has sought care to receive chemotherapy. In this instance, you would assign V58.1 *Maintenance chemotherapy* as the primary code on your claim and list the code to identify the known neoplasm second.

Factual
: These v-codes are used to describe certain facts that do not fall into the "problem" or "service" categories. For example, coding the type of birth using code V30.1 *Single liveborn, born before admission to hospital.*

V-codes can be used as a solo code, a principal code or as a secondary code. It is important to use V-codes properly. If a complication is present, the complication should be coded to categories 001-799 instead of to a V-code.

Coding Example

Colostomy status with colostomy malfunction

> **569.60** Colostomy and enterostomy complications, unspecified

> Code V44.3 *Artificial opening status, colostomy* would not be used in this case because of the complication.

Key words found in diagnostic statements which may result in selection of a V code include:

Admission for	*Health or healthy*
Aftercare	*History (of)*
Attention to	*Maintenance*
Care (of)	*Maladjustment*
Carrier	*Observation*
Checking/checkup	*Problem (with)*
Contact	*Prophylactic*
Contraception	*Replacement (by)(of)*
Counseling	*Screening*
Dialysis	*Status*
Donor	*Supervision (of)*
Examination	*Test*
Fitting of	*Transplant*
Follow up	*Vaccination*

Using E Codes

E-codes permit the classification of environmental events, circumstances and conditions as the cause of injury, poisoning and other adverse effects. The use of E-codes together with the code identifying the injury or condition provides additional information of particular concern to industrial medicine, insurance carriers, national safety programs and public health agencies.

The E-codes may be assigned with any of the codes in the main classification 001-999 to identify the external cause of an injury or condition. E-codes are *never* used as solo codes or as principal diagnostic codes.

When using E-codes, search the Alphabetic Index (Volume 2) for the main term identifying the cause such as "accident," "fire," "shooting," "fall," or "collision." To find the E-code for an adverse reaction to surgical or medical treatment, use the main term "reaction."

Coding Example

Burns to right arm, occurred while burning trash

> **943.00** Burn of upper limb, except wrist and hand, unspecified degree

> **E897** Accident caused by controlled fire not in building or structure

E-codes are important for providing the details of an accident to an insurance carrier to enable them to issue faster and more accurate reimbursement. Most insurance carriers want to be sure they reimburse only for services covered under their policy and not for services covered under worker's compensation, automobile or homeowner's insurance. A clear understanding of the circumstances will eliminate questions from the insurance carrier which cause delays in reimbursements.

Coding Example

Fractured ribs due to fall from ladder at home

807.00 Fracture of ribs, closed, unspecified

E881.0 Fall from ladder

E849.0 Place of occurrence, home

Using the above E-codes to provide important information regarding the circumstances of the injury to the insurance carrier eliminates any doubt about the insurer's responsibility for coverage.

When using E-codes always list the E-codes as secondary or supplemental to the code(s) describing the injury.

Anatomical Illustrations

A fundamental knowledge and understanding of basic human anatomy and physiology is a prerequisite for accurate diagnosis coding. While a comprehensive treatment of anatomy and physiology is beyond the scope of this text, the large scale, full color anatomical illustrations on the following pages are designed to facilitate the diagnosis coding process for both beginning and experienced coders.

The illustrations provide an anatomical perspective of diagnosis coding by providing a side-by-side view of the major systems of the human body and a corresponding list of the most common diagnoses categories used to support medical, surgical and diagnostic services performed on the illustrated system.

The diagnostic categories listed on the left facing page of each anatomical illustration are three-digit categories and may not be used for coding. These categories are provided as "pointers" to the appropriate section of the ICD-9-CM Volume 1 where the complete listings, including 4th and 5th digits if appropriate, may be found.

PLATE 1. SKIN AND SUBCUTANEOUS TISSUE - MALE

Viral diseases accompanied by exanthem 050-057

Neoplasms

Malignant melanoma of skin	172
Other malignant neoplasm of skin	173
Malignant neoplasm of male breast	175
Kaposi's sarcoma	176
Benign neoplasm of skin	216
Carcinoma in situ of skin	232

Infections of skin and subcutaneous tissue

Carbuncle and furuncle	680
Cellulitis and abscess of finger and toe	681
Other cellulitis and abscess	682
Acute lymphadenitis	683
Impetigo	684
Pilonidal cyst	685
Other local infections of skin and subcutaneous tissue	686

Other inflammatory conditions of skin and subcutaneous tissue

Erythematosquamous dermatosis	690
Atopic dermatitis and related conditions	691
Contact dermatitis and other eczema	692
Dermatitis due to substances taken internally	693
Bullous dermatoses	694
Erythematous conditions	695
Psoriasis and similar disorders	696
Lichen	697
Pruritus and related conditions	698

Other diseases of skin and subcutaneous tissue

Corns and callosities	700
Other hypertrophic and atrophic conditions of skin	701
Diseases of nail	703
Diseases of hair and hair follicles	704
Disorders of sweat glands	705
Diseases of sebaceous glands	706
Chronic ulcer of skin	707
Urticaria	708
Other disorders of skin and subcutaneous tissue	709
Symptoms involving skin and other integumentary tissue	782

Symptoms, signs and ill-defined conditions 780-799

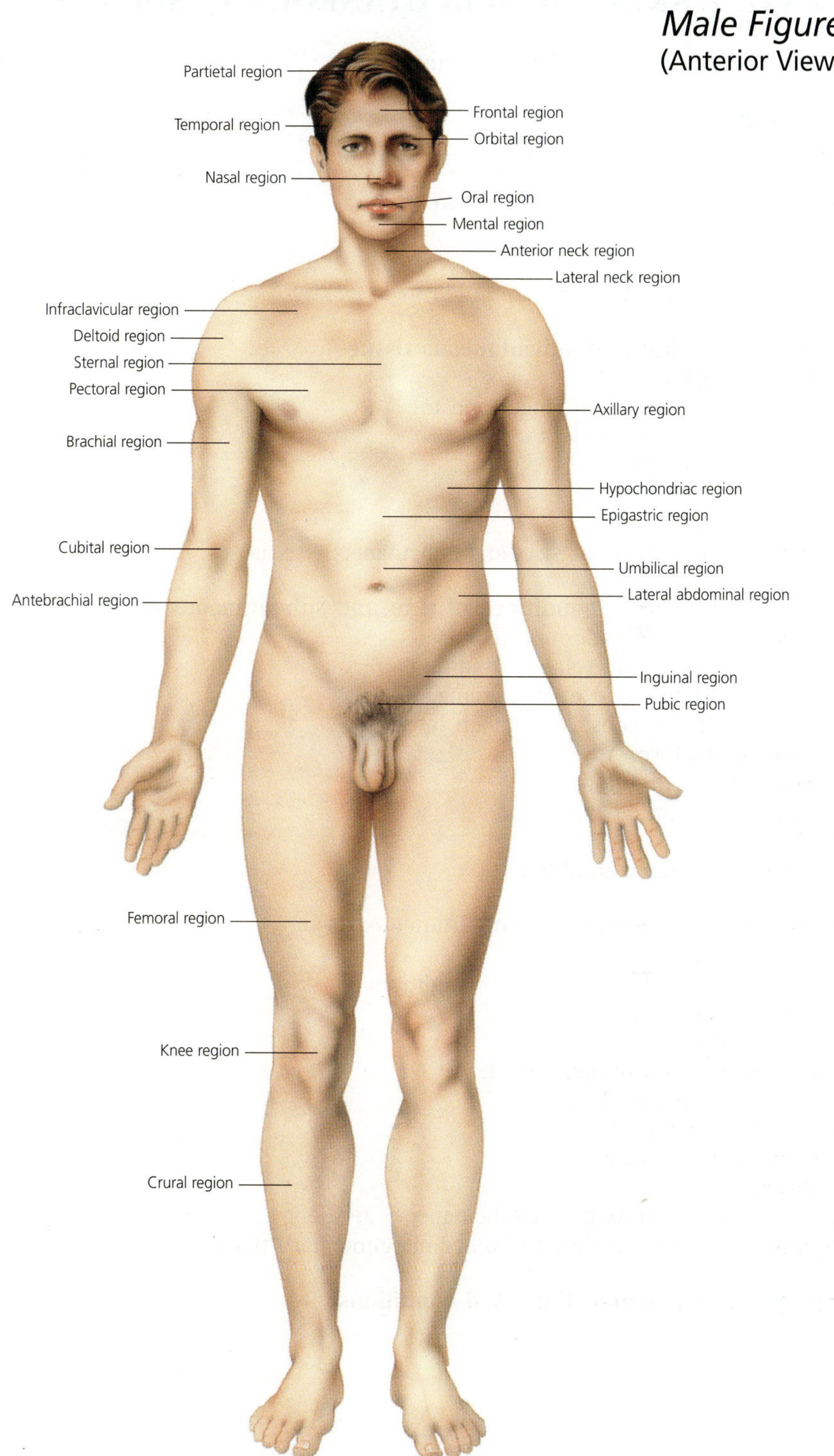
Male Figure
(Anterior View)
Partietal region
Temporal region
Nasal region
Frontal region
Orbital region
Oral region
Mental region
Anterior neck region
Lateral neck region
Infraclavicular region
Deltoid region
Sternal region
Pectoral region
Axillary region
Brachial region
Hypochondriac region
Epigastric region
Cubital region
Antebrachial region
Umbilical region
Lateral abdominal region
Inguinal region
Pubic region
Femoral region
Knee region
Crural region

PLATE 2. SKIN AND SUBCUTANEOUS TISSUE - FEMALE

Viral diseases accompanied by exanthem   050-057

Neoplasms
Malignant melanoma of skin   172
Other malignant neoplasm of skin   173
Malignant neoplasm of female breast   174
Kaposi's sarcoma   176
Benign neoplasm of skin   216
Carcinoma in situ of skin   232

Infections of skin and subcutaneous tissue
Carbuncle and furuncle   680
Cellulitis and abscess of finger and toe   681
Other cellulitis and abscess   682
Acute lymphadenitis   683
Impetigo   684
Pilonidal cyst   685
Other local infections of skin and subcutaneous tissue   686

Other inflammatory conditions of skin and subcutaneous tissue
Erythematosquamous dermatosis   690
Atopic dermatitis and related conditions   691
Contact dermatitis and other eczema   692
Dermatitis due to substances taken internally   693
Bullous dermatoses   694
Erythematous conditions   695
Psoriasis and similar disorders   696
Lichen   697
Pruritus and related conditions   698

Other diseases of skin and subcutaneous tissue
Corns and callosities   700
Other hypertrophic and atrophic conditions of skin   701
Other dermatoses   702
Diseases of nail   703
Diseases of hair and hair follicles   704
Disorders of sweat glands   705
Diseases of sebaceous glands   706
Chronic ulcer of skin   707
Urticaria   708
Other disorders of skin and subcutaneous tissue   709
Symptoms involving skin and other integumentary tissue   782

Symptoms, signs and ill-defined conditions   780-799

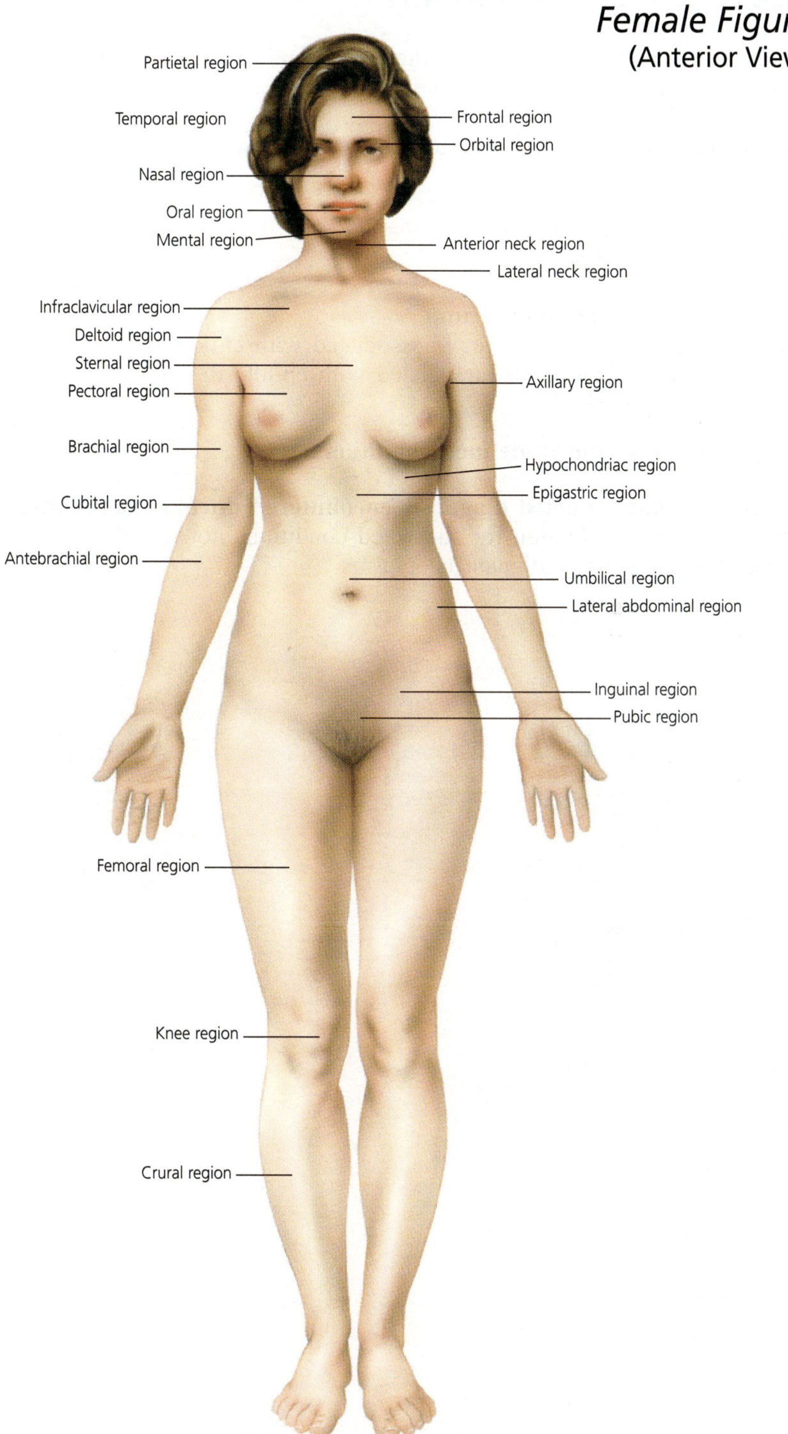

Female Figure
(Anterior View)
Partietal region
Temporal region
Frontal region
Orbital region
Nasal region
Oral region
Mental region
Anterior neck region
Lateral neck region
Infraclavicular region
Deltoid region
Sternal region
Pectoral region
Axillary region
Brachial region
Hypochondriac region
Epigastric region
Cubital region
Antebrachial region
Umbilical region
Lateral abdominal region
Inguinal region
Pubic region
Femoral region
Knee region
Crural region

PLATE 3. FEMALE BREAST

Female Breast

59

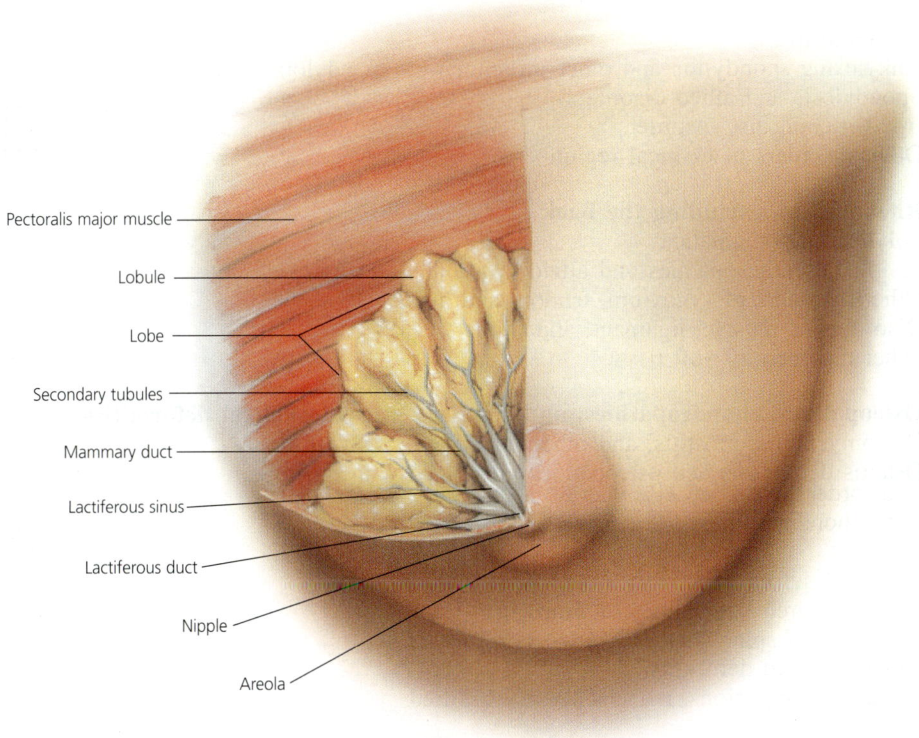

PLATE 4. MUSCULAR SYSTEM AND CONNECTIVE TISSUE - ANTERIOR VIEW

Arthropathies and related disorders

Diffuse diseases of connective tissue	710
Arthropathy associated with infections	711
Crystal arthropathies	712
Arthropathy associated with other disorders classified elsewhere	713
Rheumatoid arthritis and other inflammatory polyarthropathies	714
Osteoarthrosis and allied disorders	715
Internal derangement of knee	717
Other derangement of joint	718

Dorsopathies

Ankylosing spondylitis and other inflammatory spondylopathies	720
Spondylosis and allied disorders	721
Intervertebral disc disorders	722
Other disorders of cervical region	723

Rheumatism, excluding the back

Polymyalgia rheumatica	725
Peripheral enthesopathies and allied syndromes	726
Other disorders of synovium, tendon, and bursa	727
Disorders of muscle, ligament, and fascia	728
Other disorders of soft tissues	729

Osteopathies, chondropathies, and acquired musculoskeletal deformities

Osteomyelitis, periostitis, and other infections involving bone	730
Osteitis deformans and osteopathies associated with other disorders classified elsewhere	731
Osteochondropathies	732
Flat foot	734
Acquired deformities of toe	735
Other acquired deformities of limbs	736
Curvature of spine	737
Other acquired deformity	738
Nonallopathic lesions, not elsewhere classified	739

Symptoms, signs and ill-defined conditions 780-799

Muscular System
(Anterior View)

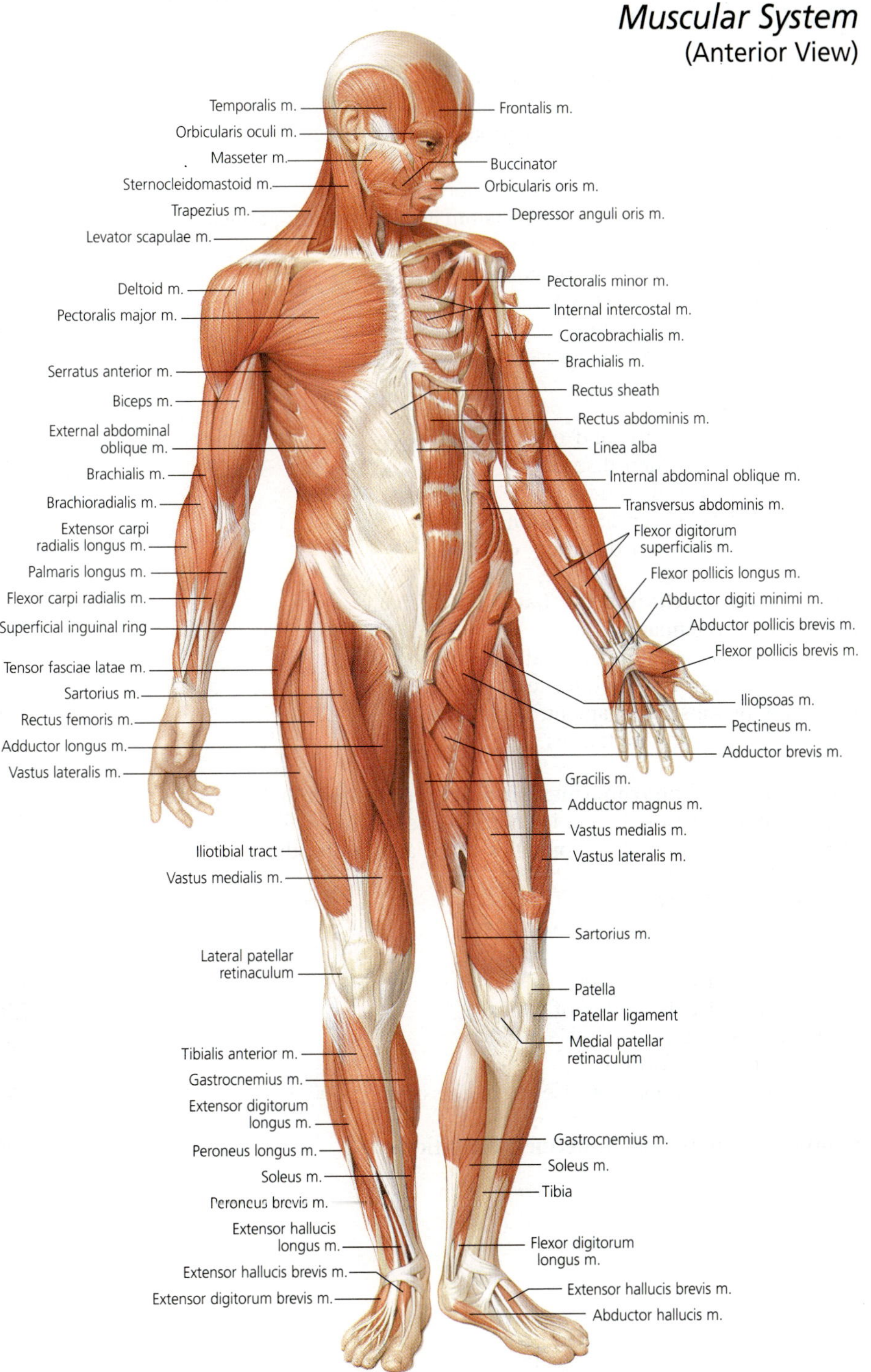

PLATE 5. MUSCULAR SYSTEM AND CONNECTIVE TISSUE - POSTERIOR VIEW

Arthropathies and related disorders	
Diffuse diseases of connective tissue	710
Arthropathy associated with infections	711
Crystal arthropathies	712
Arthropathy associated with other disorders classified elsewhere	713
Rheumatoid arthritis and other inflammatory polyarthropathies	714
Osteoarthrosis and allied disorders	715
Other and unspecified arthropathies	716
Internal derangement of knee	717
Other derangement of joint	718
Other and unspecified disorders of joint	719
Dorsopathies	
Ankylosing spondylitis and other inflammatory spondylopathies	720
Spondylosis and allied disorders	721
Intervertebral disc disorders	722
Other disorders of cervical region	723
Other and unspecified disorders of back	724
Rheumatism, excluding the back	
Polymyalgia rheumatica	725
Peripheral enthesopathies and allied syndromes	726
Other disorders of synovium, tendon, and bursa	727
Disorders of muscle, ligament, and fascia	728
Other disorders of soft tissues	729
Osteopathies, chondropathies, and acquired musculoskeletal deformities	
Osteomyelitis, periostitis, and other infections involving bone	730
Osteitis deformans and osteopathies associated with other disorders classified elsewhere	731
Osteochondropathies	732
Other disorders of bone and cartilage	733
Flat foot	734
Acquired deformities of toe	735
Other acquired deformities of limbs	736
Curvature of spine	737
Other acquired deformity	738
Nonallopathic lesions, not elsewhere classified	739
Symptoms, signs and ill-defined conditions	780-799

Muscular System
(Posterior View)

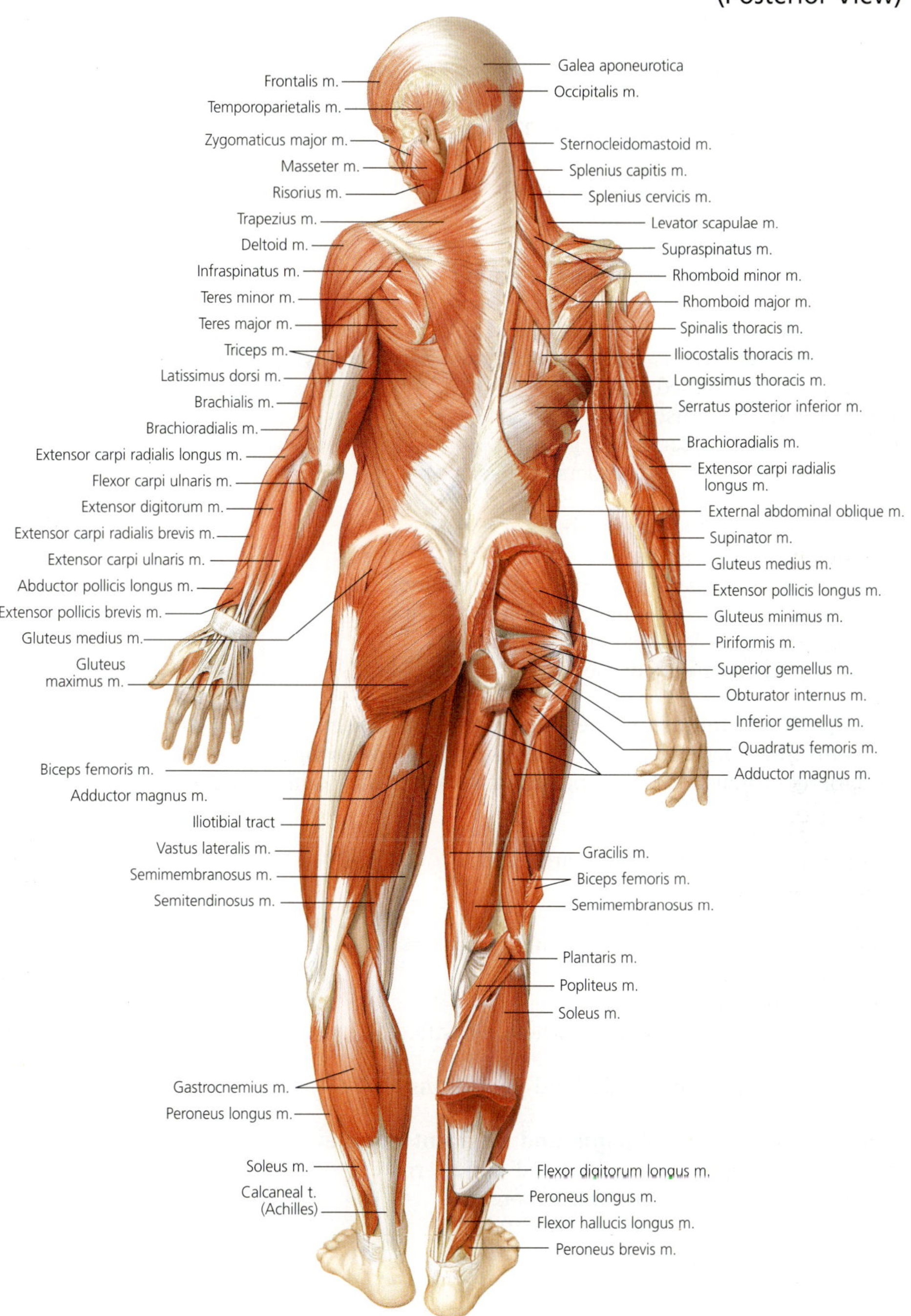

PLATE 6. MUSCULAR SYSTEM - SHOULDER AND ELBOW

Arthropathies and related disorders

Diffuse diseases of connective tissue	710
Arthropathy associated with infections	711
Crystal arthropathies	712
Arthropathy associated with other disorders classified elsewhere	713
Rheumatoid arthritis and other inflammatory polyarthropathies	714
Osteoarthrosis and allied disorders	715
Other and unspecified arthropathies	716
Internal derangement of knee	717
Other derangement of joint	718
Other and unspecified disorders of joint	719

Dorsopathies

Ankylosing spondylitis and other inflammatory spondylopathies	720
Spondylosis and allied disorders	721
Intervertebral disc disorders	722
Other disorders of cervical region	723
Other and unspecified disorders of back	724

Rheumatism, excluding the back

Polymyalgia rheumatica	725
Peripheral enthesopathies and allied syndromes	726
Other disorders of synovium, tendon, and bursa	727
Disorders of muscle, ligament, and fascia	728
Other disorders of soft tissues	729

Osteopathies, chondropathies, and acquired musculoskeletal deformities

Osteomyelitis, periostitis, and other infections involving bone	730
Osteitis deformans and osteopathies associated with other disorders classified elsewhere	731
Osteochondropathies	732
Other disorders of bone and cartilage	733
Flat foot	734
Acquired deformities of toe	735
Other acquired deformities of limbs	736
Curvature of spine	737
Other acquired deformity	738
Nonallopathic lesions, not elsewhere classified	739

Symptoms, signs and ill-defined conditions	780-799

Sprains and strains of joints and adjacent muscles

Sprains and strains of shoulder and upper arm	840
Sprains and strains of elbow and forearm	841
Other and ill-defined sprains and strains	848

Shoulder and Elbow
(Anterior View)

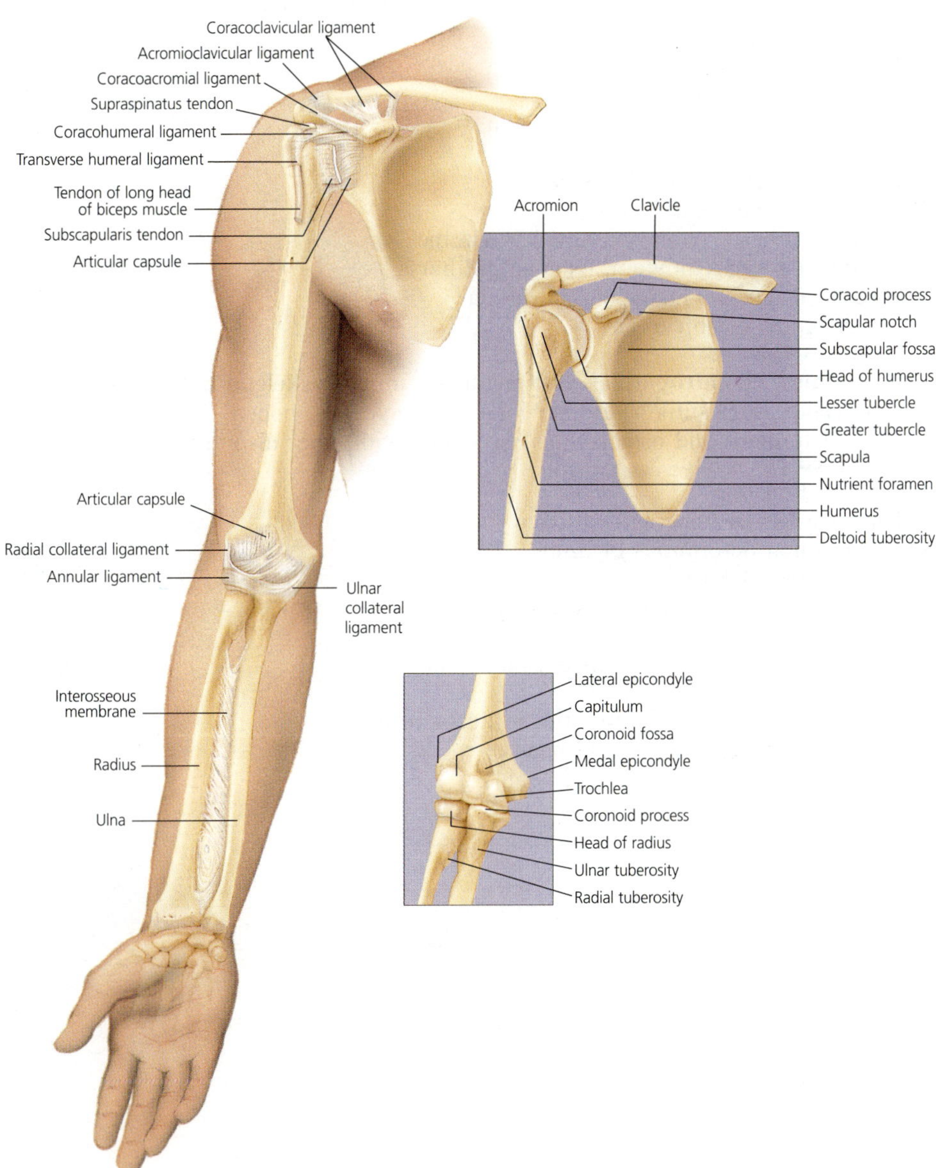

PLATE 7. MUSCULAR SYSTEM - HAND AND WRIST

Hand and Wrist

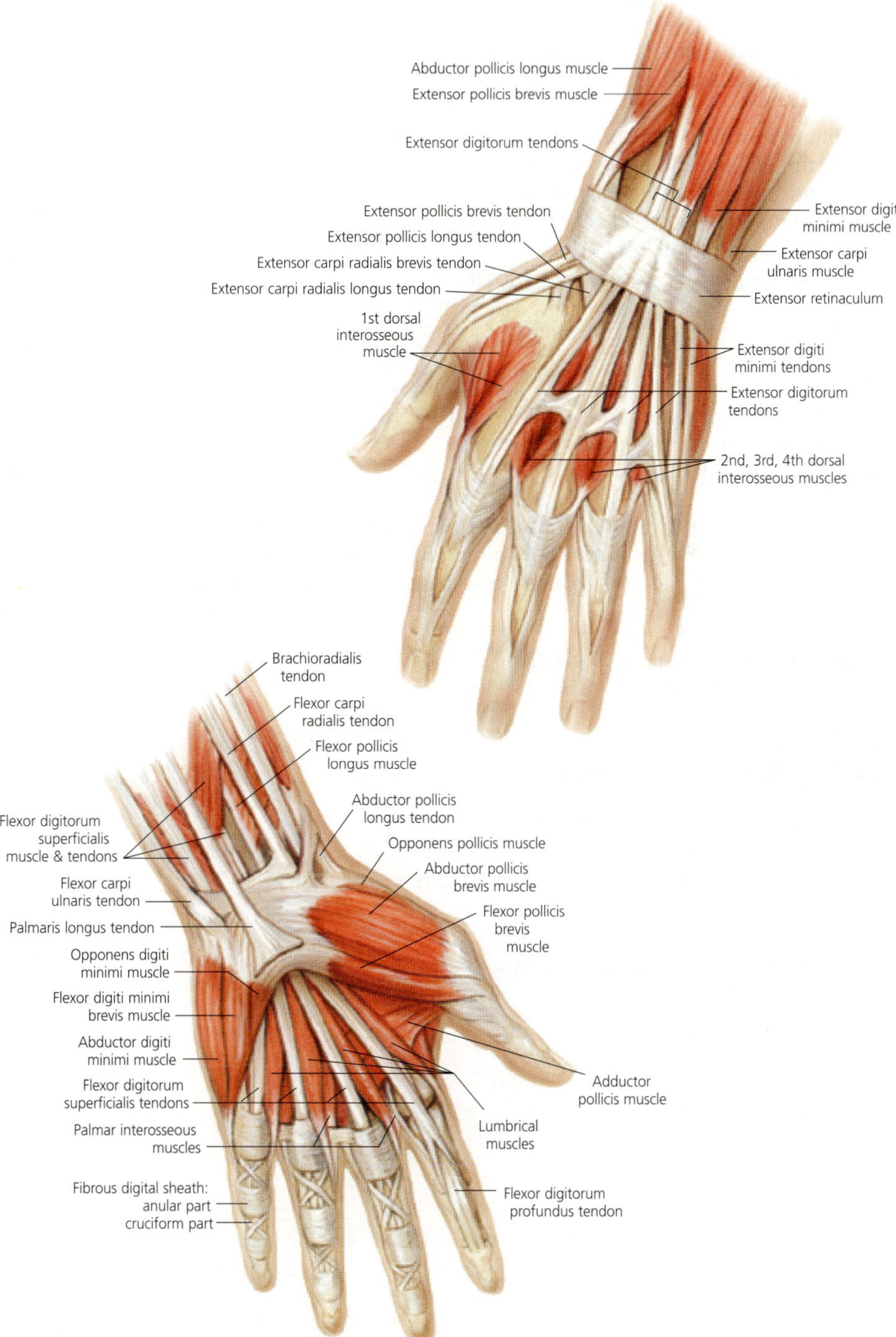

PLATE 8. MUSCULOSKELETAL SYSTEM - HIP AND KNEE

Hip and Knee
(Anterior View)

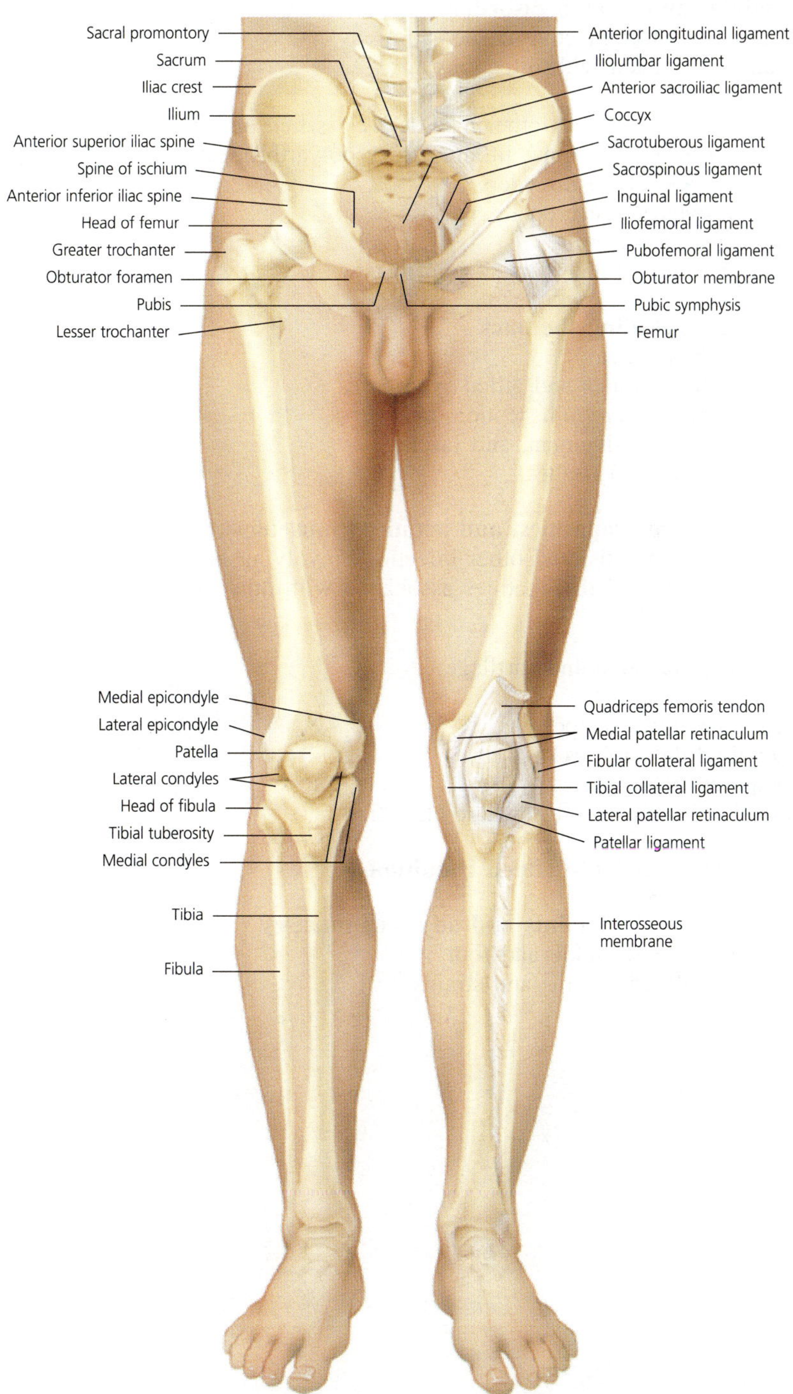

©Practice Management Information Corp., Los Angeles, CA

PLATE 9. MUSCULOSKELETAL SYSTEM - FOOT AND ANKLE

Foot and Ankle

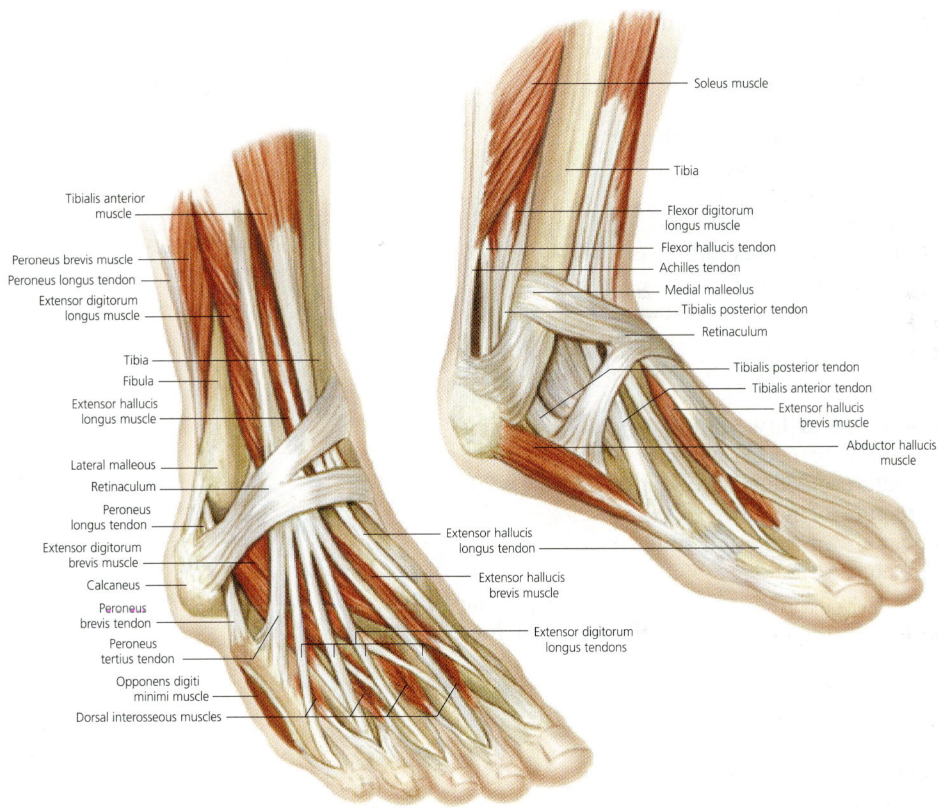

PLATE 10. SKELETAL SYSTEM - ANTERIOR VIEW

Symptoms, signs and ill-defined conditions 780-799

Fracture of skull

Fracture of vault of skull	800
Fracture of base of skull	801
Fracture of face bones	802
Multiple fractures involving skull or face with other bones	804

Fracture of neck and trunk

Fracture of vertebral column without mention of spinal cord injury	805
Fracture of vertebral column with spinal cord injury	806
Fracture of rib(s), sternum, larynx and trachea	807
Fracture of pelvis	808

Fracture of upper limb

Fracture of clavicle	810
Fracture of scapula	811
Fracture of humerus	812
Fracture of radius and ulna	813
Fracture of carpal bone(s)	814
Fracture of metacarpal bone(s)	815
Fracture of one or more phalanges of hand	816
Multiple fractures of hand bones	817

Fracture of lower limb

Fracture of neck of femur	820
Fracture of other and unspecified parts of femur	821
Fracture of patella	822
Fracture of tibia and fibula	823
Fracture of ankle	824
Fracture of one or more tarsal and metatarsal bones	825
Fracture of one or more phalanges of foot	826

Dislocation

Dislocation of jaw	830
Dislocation of shoulder	831
Dislocation of elbow	832
Dislocation of wrist	833
Dislocation of finger	834
Dislocation of hip	835
Dislocation of knee	836
Dislocation of ankle	837
Dislocation of foot	838

Skeletal System
(Anterior View)
Frontal bone
Parietal bone
Temporal bone
Orbit
Nasal conchae
Zygomatic bone
Maxilla
Nasal septum
Manubrium of sternum
Mandible
Coracoid process
Hyoid bone
Acromion
Clavicle
Greater tubercle
Coracoclavicular ligament
Head of humerus
Supraspinatus tendon
Scapula
Subscapularis tendon
Humerus
Body of sternum
True ribs (1–7)
Xiphoid process
False ribs (8–12)
Costal cartilages
Medial epicondyle
Anterior longitudinal ligament
Lateral epicondyle
Ulnar collateral ligament
Radius
Radial collateral ligament
Ulna
Annular ligament
Sacrum
Iliac crest
Anterior superior iliac spine
Anterior sacroiliac ligament
Head of femur
Interosseous membrane
Greater trochanter
Inguinal ligament
Coccyx
Iliofemoral ligament
Pubic symphysis
Metacarpals
Proximal phalanges
Middle phalanges
Femur
Distal phalanges
L3
1
2
3
4
5
6
7
8
9
10
11
12
Key to Carpal Bones
A Scaphoid
B Trapezium
C Trapezoid
D Capitate
E Lunate
F Pisiform
G Triquetral
H Hamate
Medial epicondyle
Quadriceps femoris tendon
Lateral epicondyle
Tibial collateral ligament
Patella
Fibular collateral ligament
Head of fibula
Patellar ligament
Tibial tuberosity
Tibia
Fibula
Interosseous membrane
Medial malleolus
Lateral malleolus
Key to Tarsal Bones
J Intermediate cuneiform
K Lateral cuneiform
L Cuboid
M Talus
N Navicular
O Calcaneus
P Medial cuneiform

PLATE 11. SKELETAL SYSTEM - POSTERIOR VIEW

Symptoms, signs and ill-defined conditions 780-799

Fracture of skull

Fracture of vault of skull	800
Fracture of base of skull	801
Fracture of face bones	802
Multiple fractures involving skull or face with other bones	804

Fracture of neck and trunk

Fracture of vertebral column without mention of spinal cord injury	805
Fracture of vertebral column with spinal cord injury	806
Fracture of rib(s), sternum, larynx and trachea	807
Fracture of pelvis	808

Fracture of upper limb

Fracture of clavicle	810
Fracture of scapula	811
Fracture of humerus	812
Fracture of radius and ulna	813
Fracture of carpal bone(s)	814
Fracture of metacarpal bone(s)	815
Fracture of one or more phalanges of hand	816
Multiple fractures of hand bones	817

Fracture of lower limb

Fracture of neck of femur	820
Fracture of other and unspecified parts of femur	821
Fracture of patella	822
Fracture of tibia and fibula	823
Fracture of ankle	824
Fracture of one or more tarsal and metatarsal bones	825
Fracture of one or more phalanges of foot	826

Dislocation

Dislocation of jaw	830
Dislocation of shoulder	831
Dislocation of elbow	832
Dislocation of wrist	833
Dislocation of finger	834
Dislocation of hip	835
Dislocation of knee	836
Dislocation of ankle	837
Dislocation of foot	838

Skeletal System
(Posterior View)

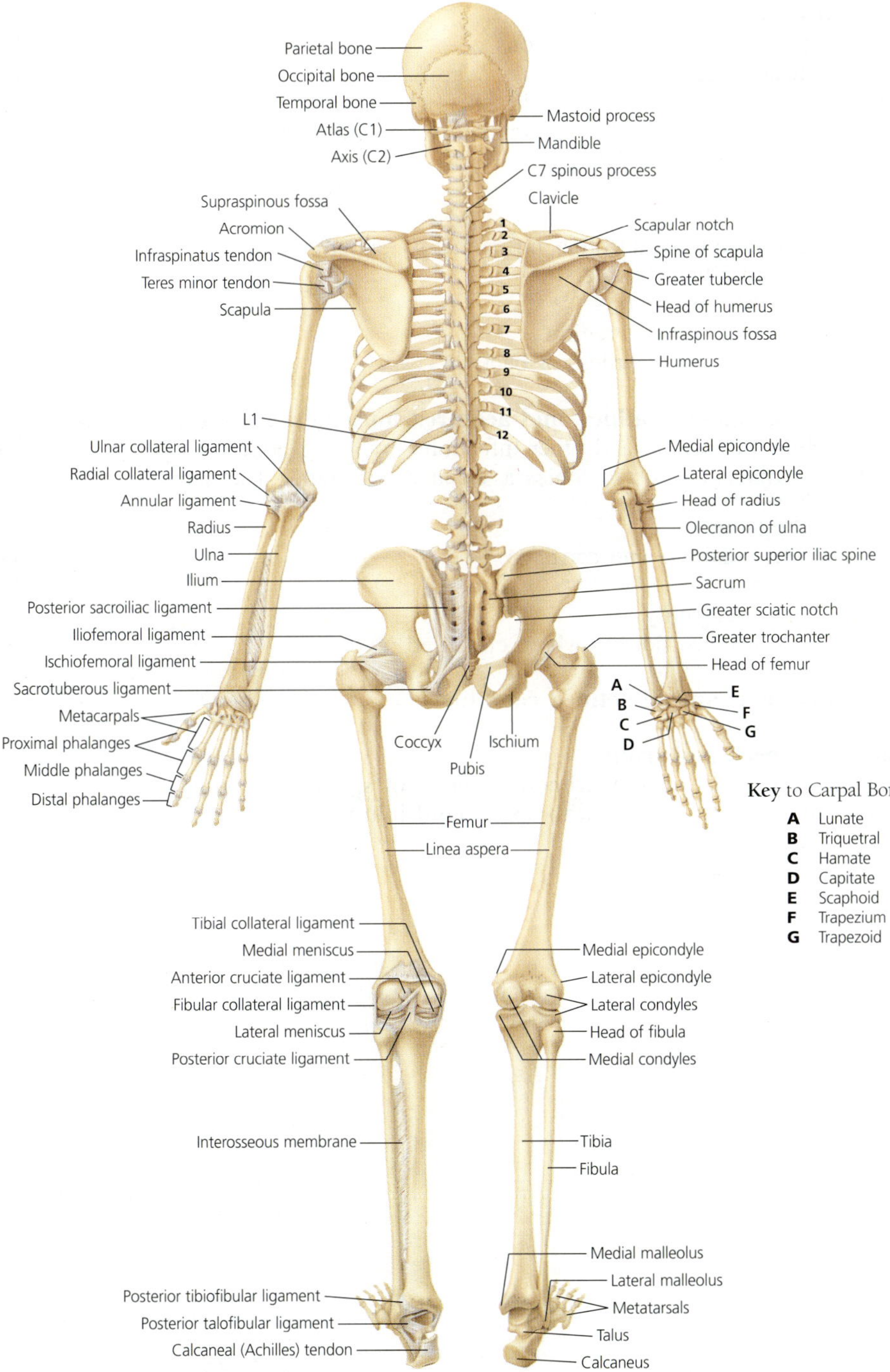

Key to Carpal Bones

A Lunate
B Triquetral
C Hamate
D Capitate
E Scaphoid
F Trapezium
G Trapezoid

PLATE 12. SKELETAL SYSTEM - VERTEBRAL COLUMN

Vertebral Column
(Lateral View)

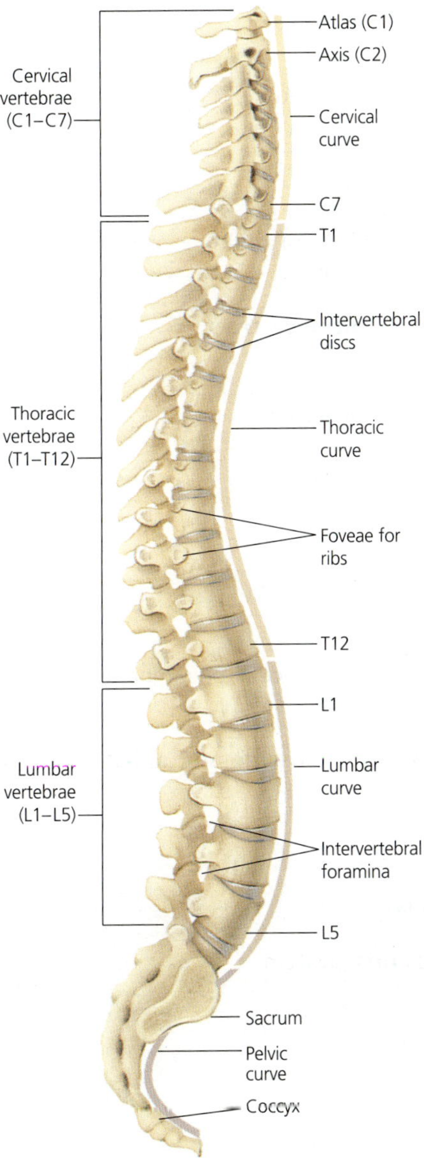

PLATE 13. RESPIRATORY SYSTEM

Respiratory System

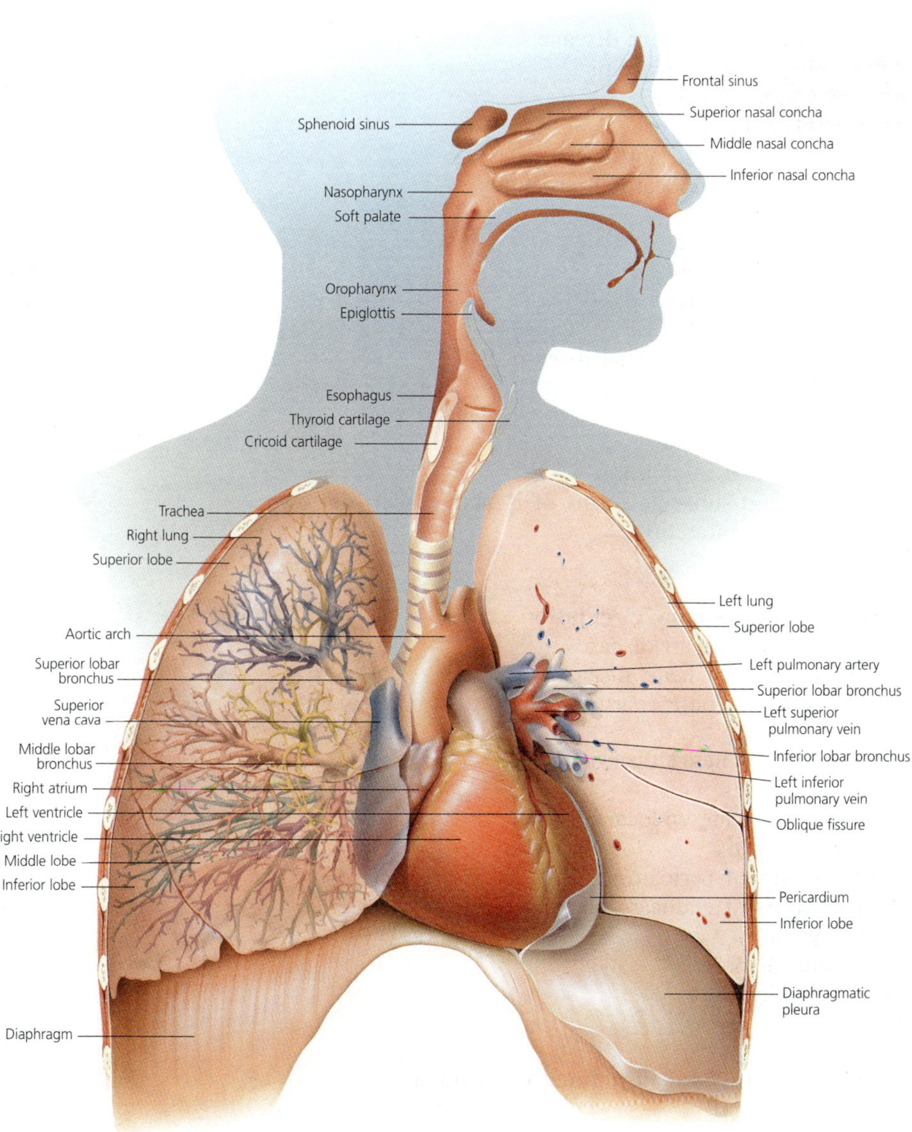

PLATE 14. HEART AND PERICARDIUM

Heart
(External View)

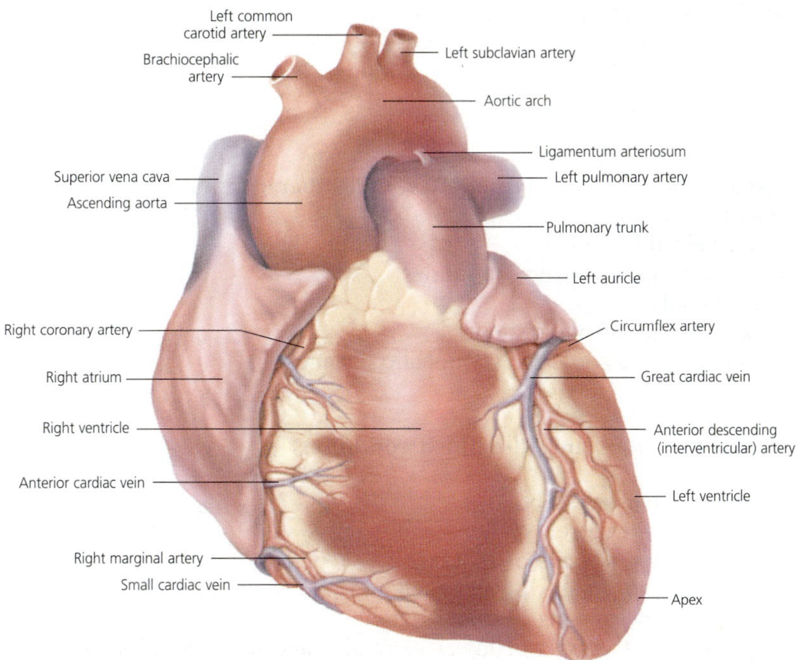

Heart
(Internal View)

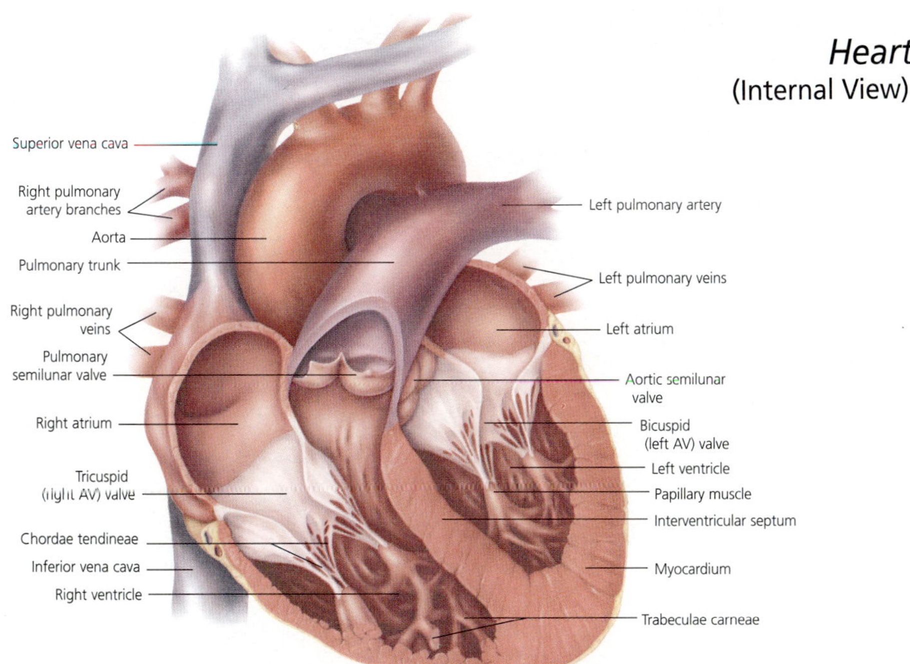

PLATE 15. CIRCULATORY SYSTEM

Vascular System

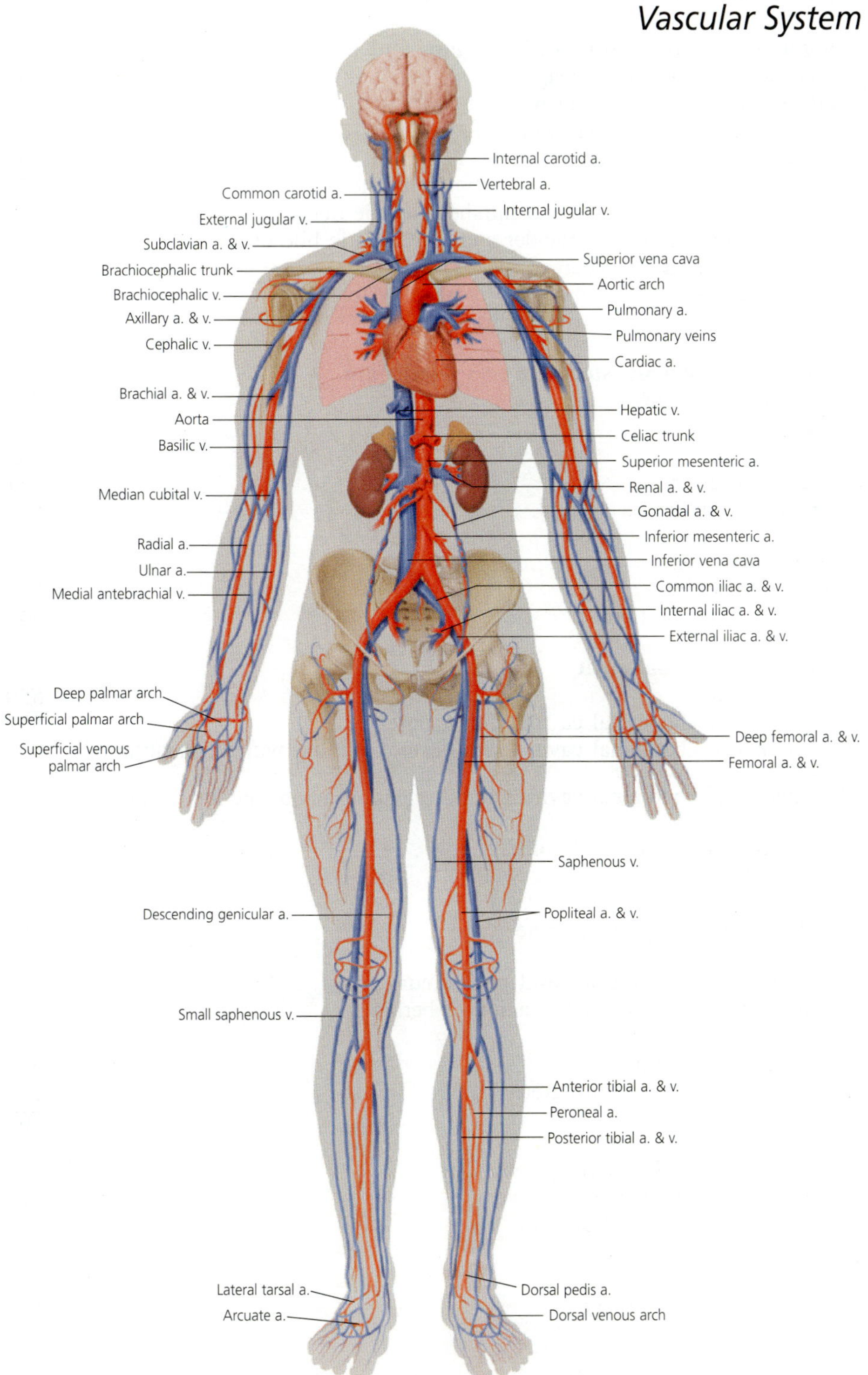

PLATE 16. DIGESTIVE SYSTEM

Digestive System

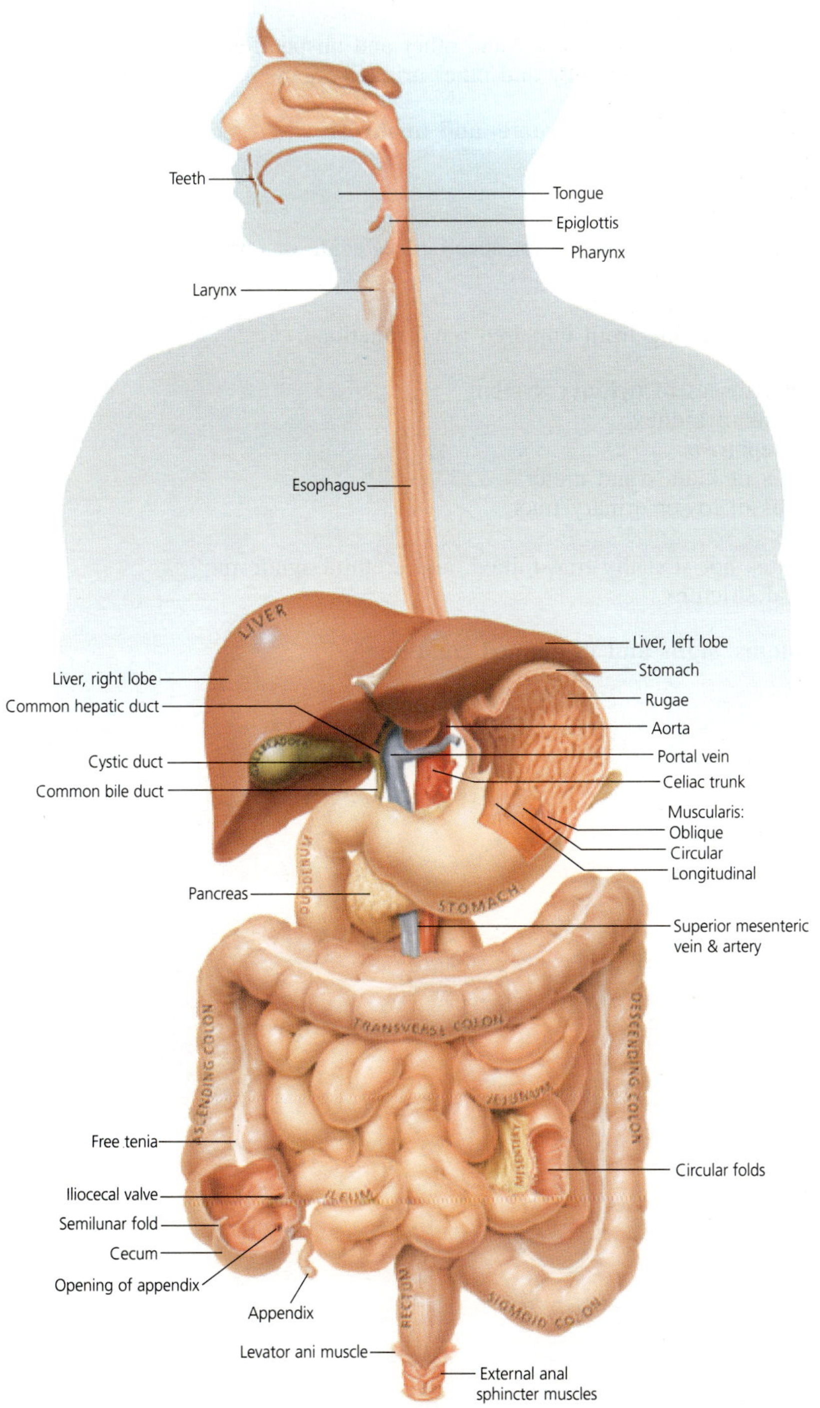

PLATE 17. GENITOURINARY SYSTEM

Neoplasms

Nephritis, nephrotic syndrome, and nephrosis

Other diseases of urinary system

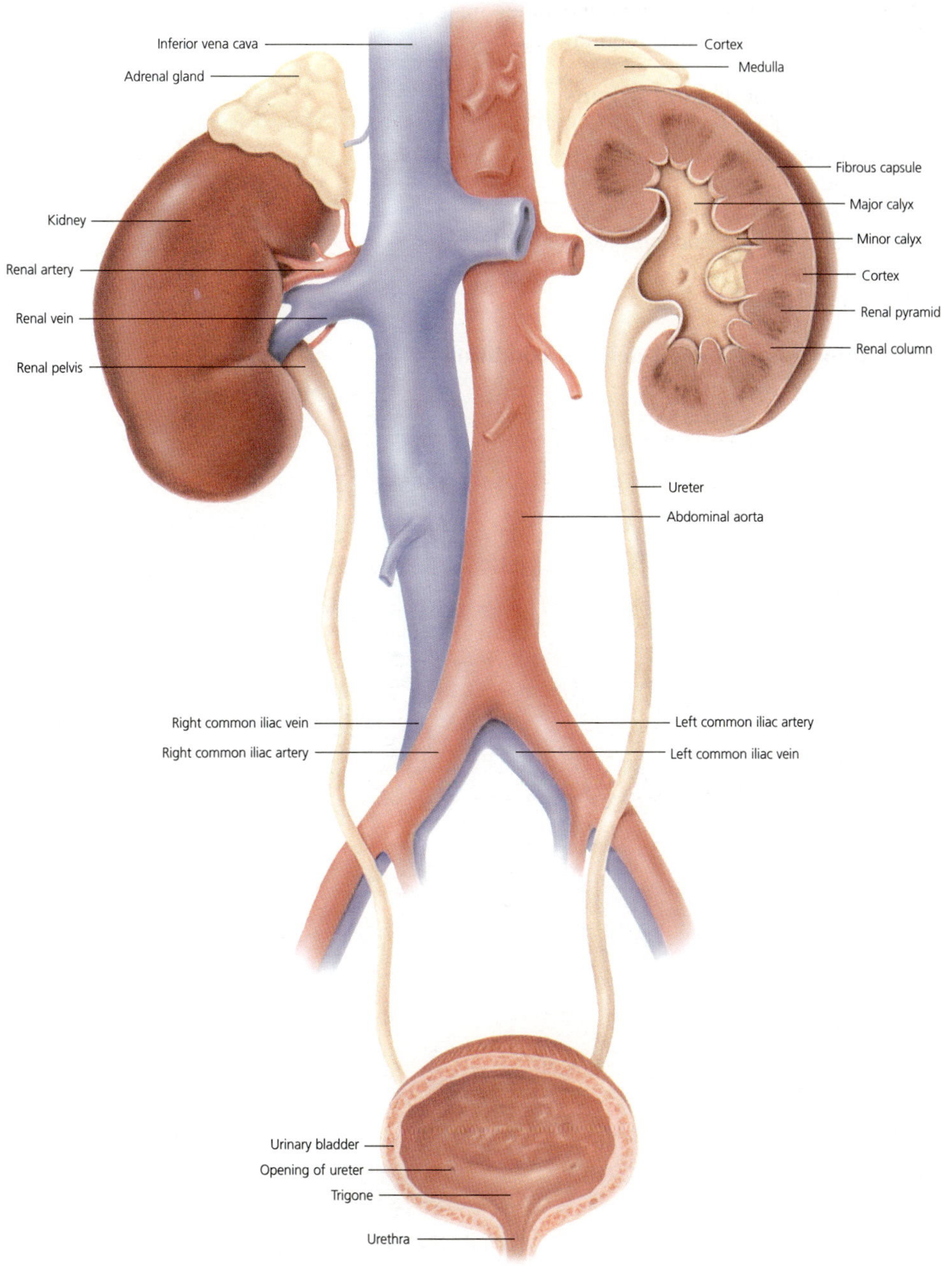

Urinary System

PLATE 18. MALE GENITAL ORGANS

Male Reproductive System

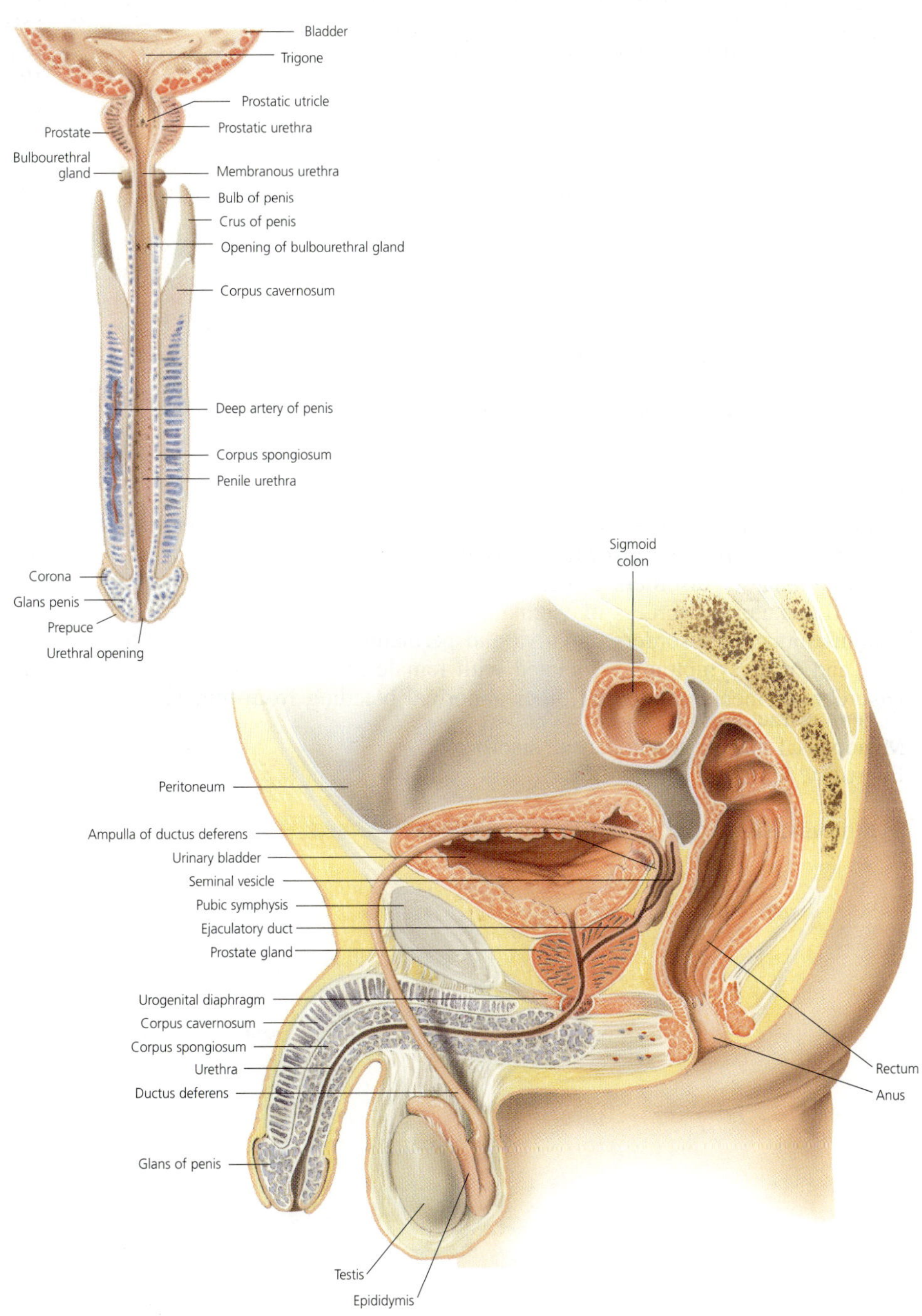

PLATE 19. FEMALE GENITAL ORGANS

Female Reproductive System

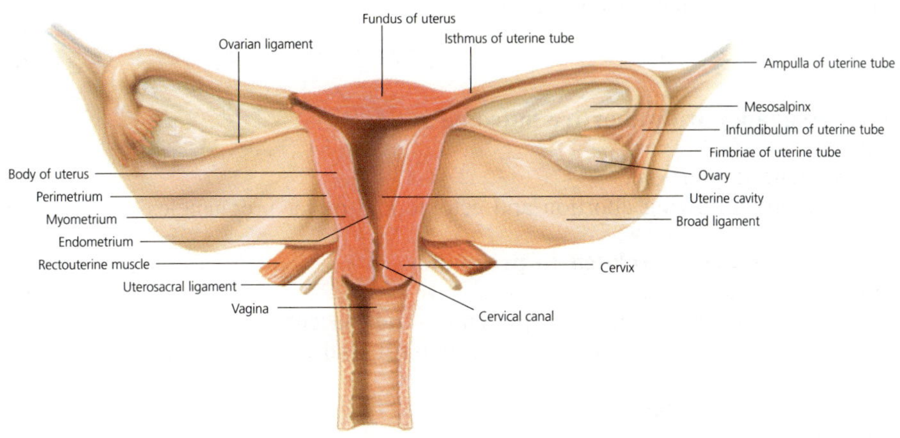

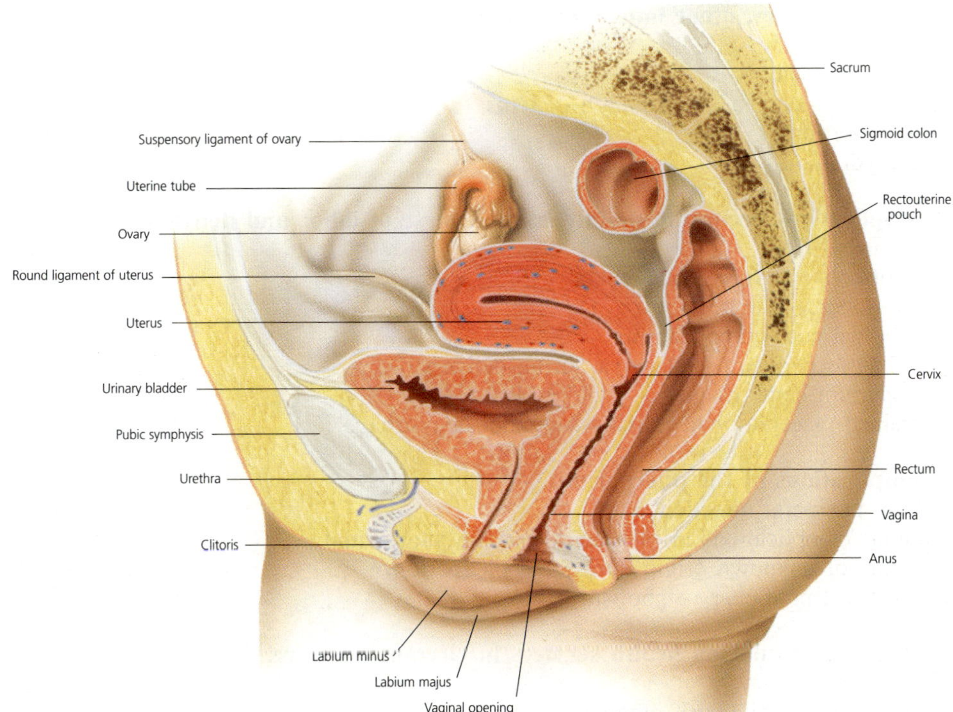

PLATE 20. PREGNANCY, CHILDBIRTH AND THE PUERPERIUM

Female Reproductive System: Pregnancy
(Lateral View)

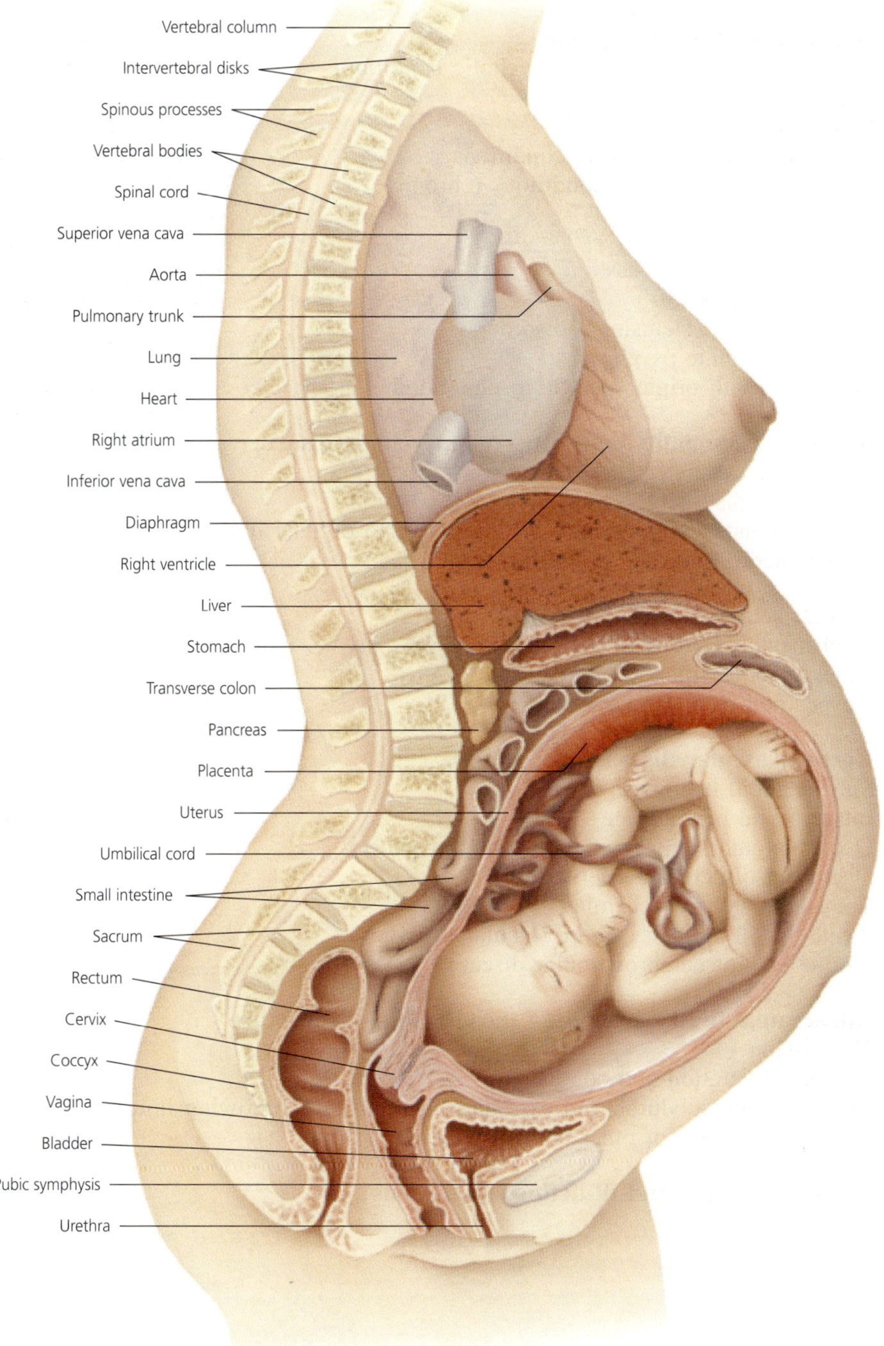

PLATE 21. NERVOUS SYSTEM - BRAIN

Brain
(Base View)

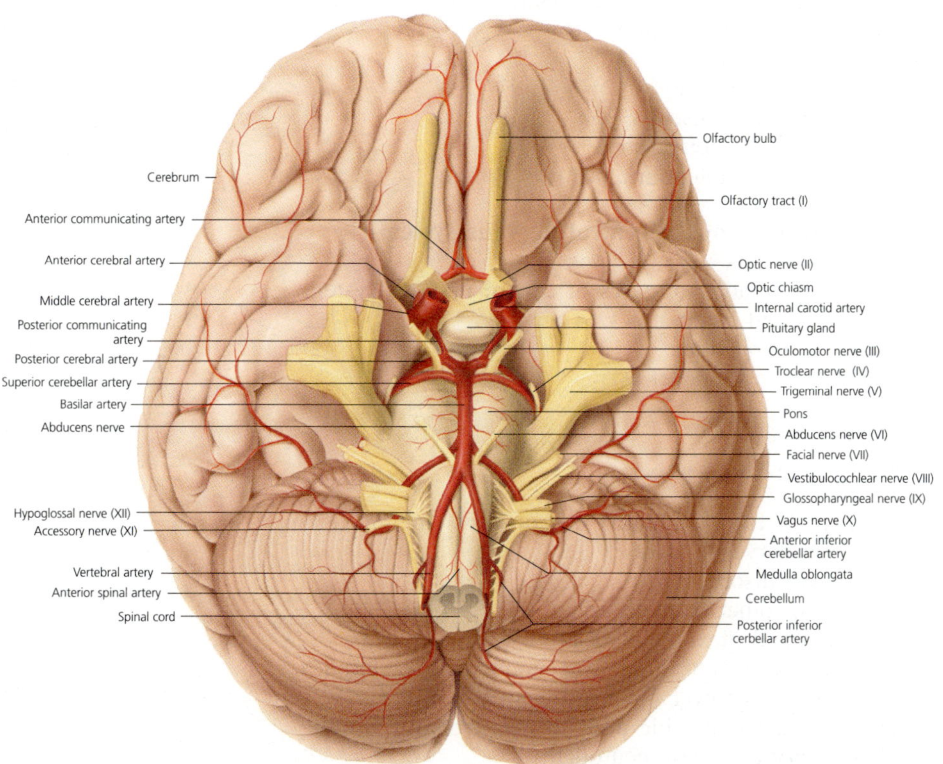

PLATE 22. NERVOUS SYSTEM

Nervous System

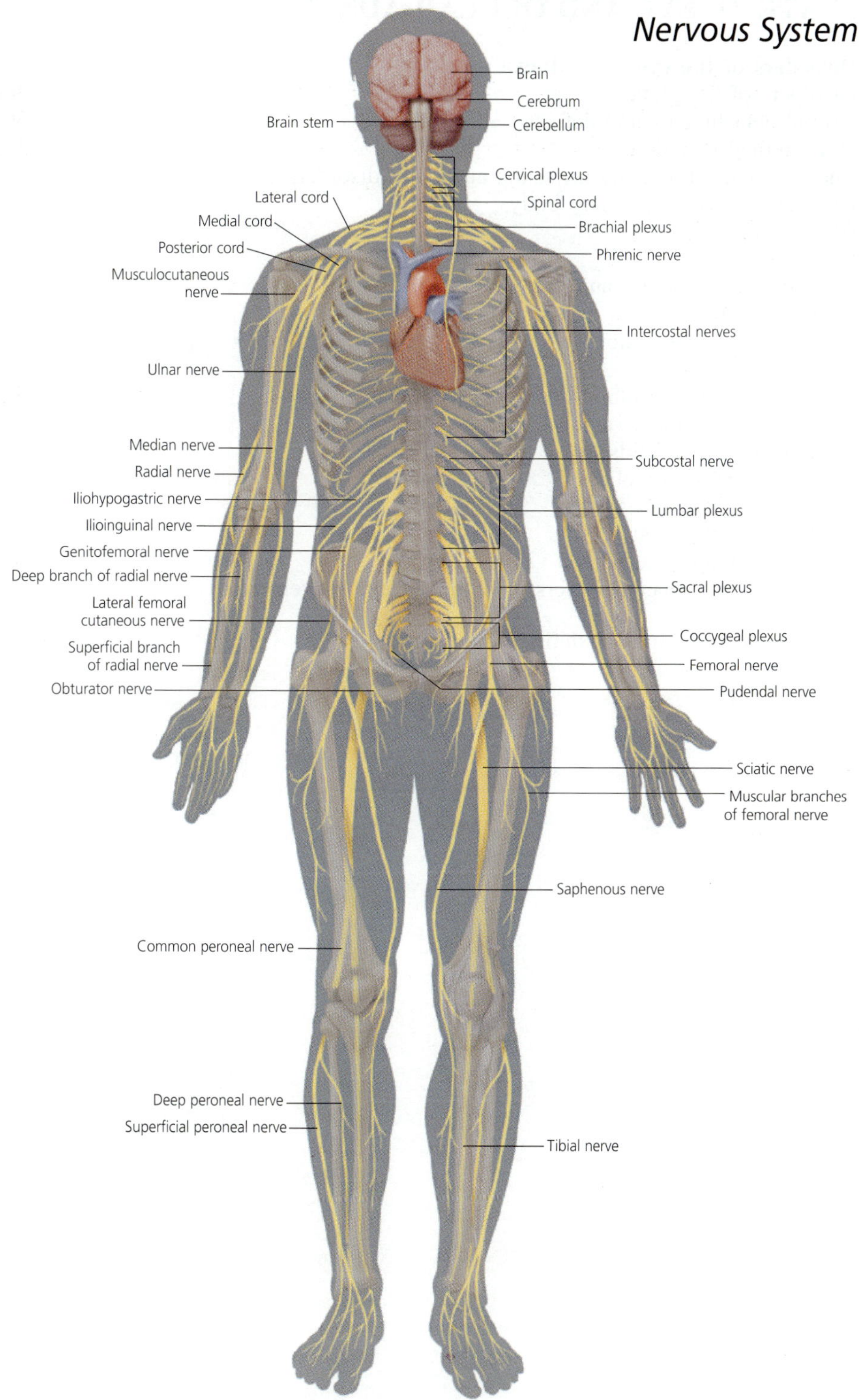

PLATE 23. EYE AND OCULAR ADNEXA

Right Eye
(Horizontal Section)

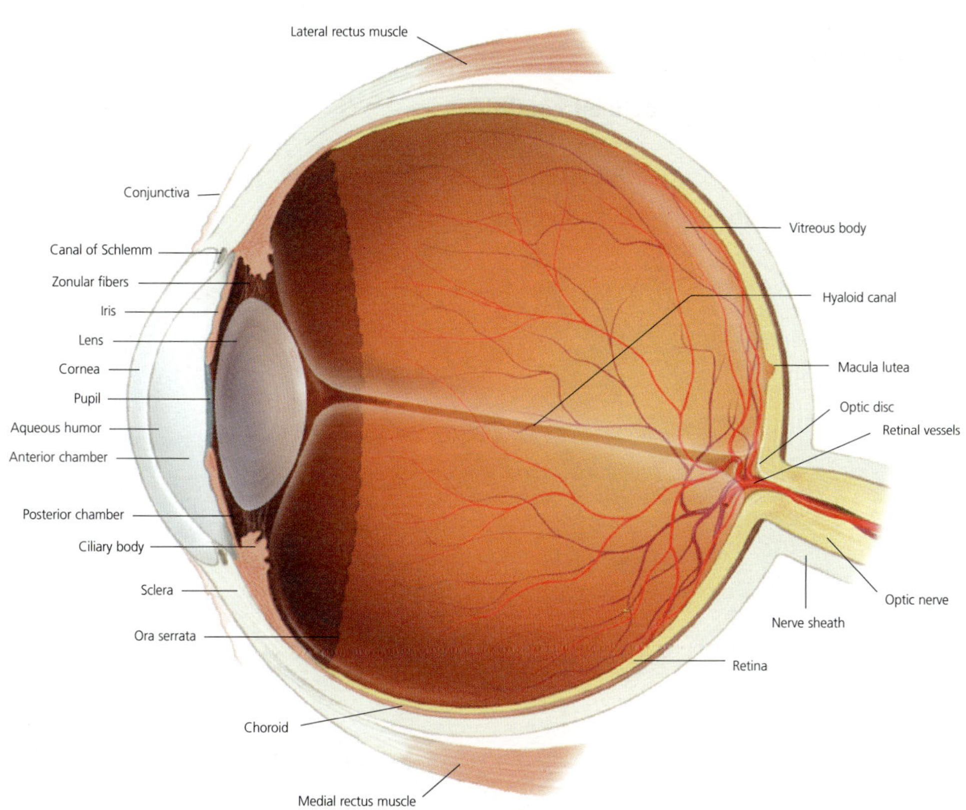

PLATE 24. AUDITORY SYSTEM

Diseases of the ear and mastoid process

The Ear

Temporalis bone
Temporalis muscle
Cartilage
Auricle
External auditory canal
Middle ear
Semicircular canals
Cochlea
Cochlear nerve
Eustachian tube
Cartilage
Nasopharynx
Ossicles:
Stapes
Incus
Malleus
Tympanic membrane

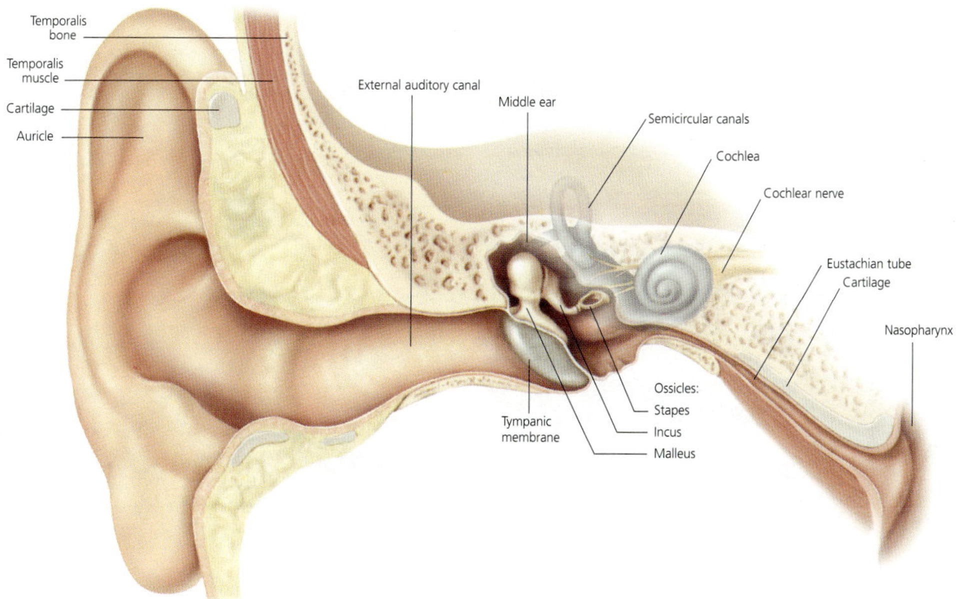

102

DISEASES: TABULAR LIST
VOLUME 1

1. INFECTIOUS AND PARASITIC DISEASES (001-139)

Note: Categories for "late effects" of infectious and parasitic diseases are to be found at 137-139.
Includes: diseases generally recognized as communicable or transmissible as well as a few diseases of unknown but possibly infectious origin

Excludes: *acute respiratory infections (460-466)*

carrier or suspected carrier of infectious organism (V02.0-V02.9)
certain localized infections
influenza (487.0-487.8)

INTESTINAL INFECTIOUS DISEASES (001-009)

Excludes: *helminthiases (120.0-129)*

001 Cholera

001.0 Due to Vibrio cholerae

001.1 Due to Vibrio cholerae el tor

001.9 Cholera, unspecified

002 Typhoid and paratyphoid fevers

002.0 Typhoid fever
Typhoid (fever) (infection) [any site]

002.1 Paratyphoid fever A

002.2 Paratyphoid fever B

002.3 Paratyphoid fever C

002.9 Paratyphoid fever, unspecified

003 Other salmonella infections
Includes: infection or food poisoning by Salmonella [any serotype]

003.0 Salmonella gastroenteritis
Salmonellosis

003.1 Salmonella septicemia

⑤ **003.2 Localized salmonella infections**

    003.20 Localized salmonella infection, unspecified

    003.21 Salmonella meningitis

    003.22 Salmonella pneumonia

    003.23 Salmonella arthritis

    003.24 Salmonella osteomyelitis

    003.29 Other

003.8 Other specified salmonella infections

003.9 Salmonella infection, unspecified

004 Shigellosis
Includes: bacillary dysentery

004.0 Shigella dysenteriae
Infection by group A Shigella (Schmitz) (Shiga)

004.1 Shigella flexneri
Infection by group B Shigella

004.2 Shigella boydii
Infection by group C Shigella

004.3 Shigella sonnei
Infection by group D Shigella

004.8 Other specified shigella infections

004.9 Shigellosis, unspecified

005 Other food poisoning (bacterial)

Excludes: *salmonella infections (003.0-003.9)*

toxic effect of:
food contaminants (989.7)
noxious foodstuffs (988.0-988.9)

005.0 Staphylococcal food poisoning
Staphylococcal toxemia specified as due to food

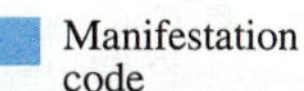

Add 4th or 5th digit	Nonspecific code	Unspecified code	Manifestation code

005.1 Botulism
Food poisoning due to Clostridium botulinum

005.2 Food poisoning due to Clostridium perfringens [C. welchii]
Enteritis necroticans

005.3 Food poisoning due to other Clostridia

005.4 Food poisoning due to Vibrio parahaemolyticus

⑤ **005.8 Other bacterial food poisoning**

$\boxed{\textit{Excludes:}}$ *salmonella food poisoning (003.0-003.9)*

 005.81 Food poisoning due to Vibrio vulnificus
 005.89 Other bacterial food poisoning
 Food poisoning due to Bacillus cereus

005.9 Food poisoning, unspecified

006 Amebiasis
Includes: infection due to Entamoeba histolytica

$\boxed{\textit{Excludes:}}$ *amebiasis due to organisms other than Entamoeba histolytica (007.8)*

006.0 Acute amebic dysentery without mention of abscess
Acute amebiasis

006.1 Chronic intestinal amebiasis without mention of abscess
Chronic:
 amebiasis
 amebic dysentery

006.2 Amebic nondysenteric colitis

006.3 Amebic liver abscess
Hepatic amebiasis

006.4 Amebic lung abscess
Amebic abscess of lung (and liver)

006.5 Amebic brain abscess
Amebic abscess of brain (and liver) (and lung)

006.6 Amebic skin ulceration
Cutaneous amebiasis

006.8 Amebic infection of other sites
Amebic: Ameboma
 appendicitis
 balanitis

$\boxed{\textit{Excludes:}}$ *specific infections by free-living amebae (136.2)*

006.9 Amebiasis, unspecified
Amebiasis NOS

007 Other protozoal intestinal diseases
Includes: protozoal:
 colitis
 diarrhea
 dysentery

007.0 Balantidiasis
Infection by Balantidium coli

007.1 Giardiasis
Infection by Giardia lamblia
Lambliasis

007.2 Coccidiosis
Infection by Isospora belli and Isospora hominis
Isosporiasis

007.3 Intestinal trichomoniasis

007.4 Cryptosporidiosis

007.5 Cyclosporiasis

007.8 Other specified protozoal intestinal diseases
Amebiasis due to organisms other than Entamoeba histolytica

007.9 Unspecified protozoal intestinal disease
Flagellate diarrhea   Protozoal dysentery NOS

● Code new   ▲ Revision of   ④ ⑤ Fourth or fifth
  to this edition   existing code   digit required

008 Intestinal infections due to other organisms
Includes: any condition classifiable to 009.0-009.3 with mention of the responsible organisms

Excludes: *food poisoning by these organisms (005.0-005.9)*

⑤ **008.0 Escherichia coli [E. coli]**

008.00 E. coli, unspecified
E. coli enteritis NOS

008.01 Enteropathogenic E. coli

008.02 Enterotoxigenic E. coli

008.03 Enteroinvasive E. coli

008.04 Enterohemorrhagic E. coli

008.09 Other intestinal E. coli infections

008.1 Arizona group of paracolon bacilli

008.2 Aerobacter aerogenes
Enterobacter aerogenes

008.3 Proteus (mirabilis) (morganii)

⑤ **008.4 Other specified bacteria**

008.41 Staphylococcus
Staphylococcal enterocolitis

008.42 Pseudomonas

008.43 Campylobacter

008.44 Yersinia enterocolitica

008.45 Clostridium difficile
Pseudomembranous colitis

008.46 Other anaerobes
Anaerobic enteritis NOS
Gram-negative anaerobes
Bacteroides (fragilis)

008.47 Other Gram-negative bacteria
Gram-negative enteritis NOS

Excludes: *Gram-negative anaerobes (008.46)*

008.49 Other

008.5 Bacterial enteritis, unspecified

⑤ **008.6 Enteritis due to specified virus**

008.61 Rotavirus

008.62 Adenovirus

008.63 Norwalk virus
Norwalk-like agent

008.64 Other small round viruses [SRV's]
Small round virus NOS

008.65 Calcivirus

008.66 Astrovirus

008.67 Enterovirus NEC
Coxsackie virus
Echovirus

Excludes: *poliovirus (045.0-045.9)*

008.69 Other viral enteritis
Torovirus

008.8 Other organism, not elsewhere classified
Viral:
enteritis NOS
gastroenteritis

Excludes: *influenza with involvement of gastrointestinal tract (487.8)*

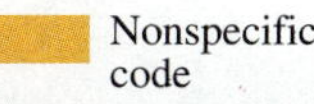

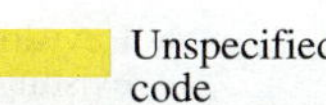

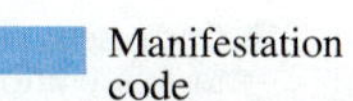

009 Ill-defined intestinal infections

> _Excludes:_ _diarrheal disease or intestinal infection due to specified organism (001.0-008.8)_
> _diarrhea following gastrointestinal surgery (564.4)_
> _intestinal malabsorption (579.0-579.9)_
> _ischemic enteritis (557.0-557.9)_
> _other noninfectious gastroenteritis and colitis (558.1-558.9)_
> _regional enteritis (555.0-555.9)_
> _ulcerative colitis (556)_

009.0 Infectious colitis, enteritis, and gastroenteritis

Colitis		Dysentery:
Enteritis	} septic	NOS
Gastroenteritis		catarrhal
		hemorrhagic

009.1 Colitis, enteritis, and gastroenteritis of presumed infectious origin

> _Excludes:_ _colitis NOS (558.9)_
> _enteritis NOS (558.9)_
> _gastroenteritis NOS (558.9)_

009.2 Infectious diarrhea

Diarrhea: Infectious diarrheal disease NOS
  dysenteric
  epidemic

009.3 Diarrhea of presumed infectious origin

> _Excludes:_ _diarrhea NOS (787.91)_

TUBERCULOSIS (010-018)

Includes: infection by Mycobacterium tuberculosis (human) (bovine)

> _Excludes:_ _congenital tuberculosis (771.2)_
> _late effects of tuberculosis (137.0-137.4)_

The following fifth-digit subclassification is for use with categories 010-018:

0 **unspecified**

1 **bacteriological or histological examination not done**

2 **bacteriological or histological examination unknown (at present)**

3 **tubercle bacilli found (in sputum) by microscopy**

4 **tubercle bacilli not found (in sputum) by microscopy, but found by bacterial culture**

5 **tubercle bacilli not found by bacteriological examination, but tuberculosis confirmed histologically**

6 **tubercle bacilli not found by bacteriological or histological examination but tuberculosis confirmed by other methods [inoculation of animals]**

⑤ **010 Primary tuberculous infection**

> _Excludes:_ _nonspecific reaction to tuberculin skin test without active tuberculosis (795.5)_
> _positive PPD (795.5)_
> _positive tuberculin skin test without active tuberculosis (795.5)_

⑤ **010.0 Primary tuberculous complex**

⑤ **010.1 Tuberculous pleurisy in primary progressive tuberculosis**

⑤ **010.8 Other primary progressive tuberculosis**

> _Excludes:_ _tuberculous erythema nodosum (017.1)_

⑤ **010.9 Primary tuberculous infection, unspecified**

⑤ **011 Pulmonary tuberculosis**

Use additional code, if desired, to identify any associated silicosis (502)

⑤ **011.0 Tuberculosis of lung, infiltrative**

⑤ **011.1 Tuberculosis of lung, nodular**

⑤ **011.2 Tuberculosis of lung with cavitation**

⑤ **011.3 Tuberculosis of bronchus**

> _Excludes:_ _isolated bronchial tuberculosis (012.2)_

⑤ **011.4 Tuberculous fibrosis of lung**

⑤ **011.5 Tuberculous bronchiectasis**

| ● Code new to this edition | ▲ Revision of existing code | ④ ⑤ Fourth or fifth digit required |

⑤ **011.6   Tuberculous pneumonia [any form]**

⑤ **011.7   Tuberculous pneumothorax**

⑤ **011.8   Other specified pulmonary tuberculosis**

⑤ **011.9   Pulmonary tuberculosis, unspecified**
Respiratory tuberculosis NOS
Tuberculosis of lung NOS

⑤ **012   Other respiratory tuberculosis**

> *Excludes:* respiratory tuberculosis, unspecified (011.9)

⑤ **012.0   Tuberculous pleurisy**
Tuberculosis of pleura   Tuberculous hydrothorax
Tuberculous empyema

> *Excludes:* pleurisy with effusion without mention of cause (511.9)
>
> tuberculous pleurisy in primary progressive tuberculosis (010.1)

⑤ **012.1   Tuberculosis of intrathoracic lymph nodes**
Tuberculosis of lymph nodes:
  hilar
  mediastinal
  tracheobronchial
Tuberculous tracheobronchial adenopathy

> *Excludes:* that specified as primary (010.0-010.9)

⑤ **012.2   Isolated tracheal or bronchial tuberculosis**

⑤ **012.3   Tuberculous laryngitis**
Tuberculosis of glottis

⑤ **012.8   Other specified respiratory tuberculosis**
Tuberculosis of: Tuberculosis of:
  mediastinum   nose (septum)
  nasopharynx   sinus [any nasal]

⑤ **013   Tuberculosis of meninges and central nervous system**

⑤ **013.0   Tuberculous meningitis**
Tuberculosis of meninges   Tuberculous:
  (cerebral) (spinal)   leptomeningitis
                                   meningoencephalitis

> *Excludes:* tuberculoma of meninges (013.1)

⑤ **013.1   Tuberculoma of meninges**

⑤ **013.2   Tuberculoma of brain**
Tuberculosis of brain (current disease)

⑤ **013.3   Tuberculous abscess of brain**

⑤ **013.4   Tuberculoma of spinal cord**

⑤ **013.5   Tuberculous abscess of spinal cord**

⑤ **013.6   Tuberculous encephalitis or myelitis**

⑤ **013.8   Other specified tuberculosis of central nervous system**

⑤ **013.9   Unspecified tuberculosis of central nervous system**
Tuberculosis of central nervous system NOS

⑤ **014   Tuberculosis of intestines, peritoneum, and mesenteric glands**

⑤ **014.0   Tuberculous peritonitis**
Tuberculous ascites

⑤ **014.8   Other**
Tuberculosis (of):   Tuberculous enteritis
  anus
  intestine (large) (small)
  mesenteric glands
  rectum
  retroperitoneal (lymph nodes)

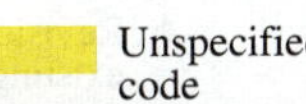

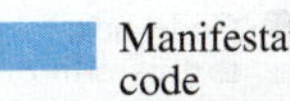

⑤ **015 Tuberculosis of bones and joints**
Use additional code, if desired, to identify manifestation, as:
  tuberculous:
    arthropathy (711.4)
    necrosis of bone (730.8)
    osteitis (730.8)
    osteomyelitis (730.8)
    synovitis (727.01)
    tenosynovitis (727.01)

⑤ **015.0 Vertebral column**
    Pott's disease
Use additional code, if desired, to identify manifestation, as:
    curvature of spine [Pott's] (737.4)
    kyphosis (737.4)
    spondylitis (720.81)

⑤ **015.1 Hip**

⑤ **015.2 Knee**

⑤ **015.5 Limb bones**
    Tuberculous dactylitis

⑤ **015.6 Mastoid**
    Tuberculous mastoiditis

⑤ **015.7 Other specified bone**

⑤ **015.8 Other specified joint**

⑤ **015.9 Tuberculosis of unspecified bones and joints**

⑤ **016 Tuberculosis of genitourinary system**

⑤ **016.0 Kidney**
    Renal tuberculosis
Use additional code, if desired, to identify manifestation, as:
    tuberculous:
      nephropathy (583.81)
      pyelitis (590.81)
      pyelonephritis (590.81)

⑤ **016.1 Bladder**

⑤ **016.2 Ureter**

⑤ **016.3 Other urinary organs**

⑤ **016.4 Epididymis**

⑤ **016.5 Other male genital organs**
Use additional code, if desired, to identify manifestation, as:
    tuberculosis of:
      prostate (601.4)
      seminal vesicle (608.81)
      testis (608.81)

⑤ **016.6 Tuberculous oophoritis and salpingitis**

⑤ **016.7 Other female genital organs**
    Tuberculous:
      cervicitis
      endometritis

⑤ **016.9 Genitourinary tuberculosis, unspecified**

⑤ **017 Tuberculosis of other organs**

⑤ **017.0 Skin and subcutaneous cellular tissue**

Lupus:	Tuberculosis:
exedens	colliquativa
vulgaris	cutis
Scrofuloderma	lichenoides
	papulonecrotica
	verrucosa cutis

Excludes:	*lupus erythematosus (695.4)*
	disseminated (710.0)
	lupus NOS (710.0)
	nonspecific reaction to tuberculin skin test without active tuberculosis (795.5)
	positive PPD (795.5)
	positive tuberculin skin test without active tuberculosis (795.5)

  ● Code new
    to this edition
  ▲ Revision of
    existing code
  ④ ⑤ Fourth or fifth
     digit required

⑤ **017.1 Erythema nodosum with hypersensitivity reaction in tuberculosis**

    Bazin's disease   Tuberculosis indurativa
    Erythema:
      induratum
      nodosum, tuberculous

    Excludes: *erythema nodosum NOS (695.2)*

⑤ **017.2 Peripheral lymph nodes**

    Scrofula   Tuberculous adenitis
    Scrofulous abscess

    Excludes: *tuberculosis of lymph nodes:*
          bronchial and mediastinal (012.1)
          mesenteric and retroperitoneal (014.8)
          tuberculous tracheobronchial adenopathy (012.1)

⑤ **017.3 Eye**

Use additional code, if desired, to identify manifestation, as:
    tuberculous:
      chorioretinitis, disseminated (363.13)
      episcleritis (379.09)
      interstitial keratitis (370.59)
      iridocyclitis, chronic (364.11)
      keratoconjunctivitis (phlyctenular) (370.31)

⑤ **017.4 Ear**

    Tuberculosis of ear
    Tuberculous otitis media

    Excludes: *tuberculous mastoiditis (015.6)*

⑤ **017.5 Thyroid gland**

⑤ **017.6 Adrenal glands**

    Addison's disease, tuberculous

⑤ **017.7 Spleen**

⑤ **017.8 Esophagus**

⑤ **017.9 Other specified organs**

Use additional code, if desired, to identify manifestation, as:
    tuberculosis of:
      endocardium [any valve] (424.91)
      myocardium (422.0)
      pericardium (420.0)

⑤ **018 Miliary tuberculosis**

    Includes: tuberculosis:
      disseminated
      generalized
      miliary, whether of a single specified site, multiple sites, or unspecified site
      polyserositis

⑤ **018.0 Acute miliary tuberculosis**

⑤ **018.8 Other specified miliary tuberculosis**

⑤ **018.9 Miliary tuberculosis, unspecified**

ZOONOTIC BACTERIAL DISEASES (020-027)

020 Plague

    Includes: infection by Yersinia [Pasteurella] pestis

020.0 Bubonic

020.1 Cellulocutaneous

020.2 Septicemic

020.3 Primary pneumonic

020.4 Secondary pneumonic

020.5 Pneumonic, unspecified

020.8 Other specified types of plague

    Abortive plague   Pestis minor
    Ambulatory plague

020.9 Plague, unspecified

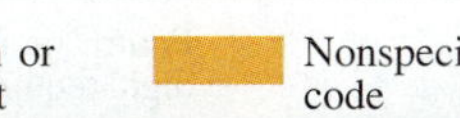

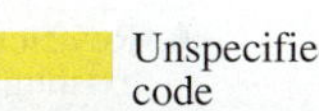

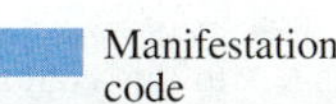

021 Tularemia
Includes: deerfly fever
infection by Francisella [Pasteurella] tularensis
rabbit fever

021.0 Ulceroglandular tularemia

021.1 Enteric tularemia
Tularemia:
cryptogenic
intestinal
typhoidal

021.2 Pulmonary tularemia
Bronchopneumonic tularemia

021.3 Oculoglandular tularemia

021.8 Other specified tularemia
Tularemia:
generalized or disseminated
glandular

021.9 Unspecified tularemia

022 Anthrax

022.0 Cutaneous anthrax
Malignant pustule

022.1 Pulmonary anthrax
Respiratory anthrax   Wool-sorters' disease

022.2 Gastrointestinal anthrax

022.3 Anthrax septicemia

022.8 Other specified manifestations of anthrax

022.9 Anthrax, unspecified

023 Brucellosis
Includes: fever:
Malta
Mediterranean
undulant

023.0 Brucella melitensis

023.1 Brucella abortus

023.2 Brucella suis

023.3 Brucella canis

023.8 Other brucellosis
Infection by more than one organism

023.9 Brucellosis, unspecified

024 Glanders
Infection by: Farcy
Actinobacillus mallei   Malleus
Malleomyces mallei
Pseudomonas mallei

025 Melioidosis
Infection by:
Malleomyces pseudomallei
Pseudomonas pseudomallei
Whitmore's bacillus
Pseudoglanders

026 Rat-bite fever

026.0 Spirillary fever
Rat-bite fever due to Spirillum minor [S. minus]
Sodoku

026.1 Streptobacillary fever
Epidemic arthritic erythema
Haverhill fever
Rat-bite fever due to Streptobacillus moniliformis

026.9 Unspecified rat-bite fever

027 Other zoonotic bacterial diseases

● Code new   ▲ Revision of   ④ ⑤ Fourth or fifth
to this edition   existing code   digit required

027.0 Listeriosis
> Infection
> Septicemia } by Listeria monocytogenes

Use additional code, if desired, to identify manifestation, as meningitis (320.7)

> Excludes: congenital listeriosis (771.2)

027.1 Erysipelothrix infection
> Erysipeloid (of Rosenbach)
> Infection
> Septicemia } by Erysipelothrix insidiosa [E. rhusiopathiae]

027.2 Pasteurellosis
> Pasteurella pseudotuberculosis infection
> Mesenteric adenitis
> Septic infection (cat bite) (dog bite) } by Pasteurella multocida [P. septica]

> Excludes: infection by:
> > Francisella [Pasteurella] tularensis (021.0-021.9)
> > Yersinia [Pasteurella] pestis (020.0-020.9)

027.8 Other specified zoonotic bacterial diseases

027.9 Unspecified zoonotic bacterial disease

OTHER BACTERIAL DISEASES (030-041)

> Excludes: bacterial venereal diseases (098.0-099.9)
> > bartonellosis (088.0)

030 Leprosy
> Includes: Hansen's disease
> infection by Mycobacterium leprae

030.0 Lepromatous [type L]
> Lepromatous leprosy (macular) (diffuse) (infiltrated) (nodular) (neuritic)

030.1 Tuberculoid [type T]
> Tuberculoid leprosy (macular) (maculoanesthetic) (major) (minor) (neuritic)

030.2 Indeterminate [group I]
> Indeterminate [uncharacteristic] leprosy (macular) (neuritic)

030.3 Borderline [group B]
> Borderline or dimorphous leprosy (infiltrated) (neuritic)

030.8 Other specified leprosy

030.9 Leprosy, unspecified

031 Diseases due to other mycobacteria

031.0 Pulmonary
> Infection by Mycobacterium:
> > avium
> > intracellulare [Battey bacillus]
> > kansasii
> Battey disease

031.1 Cutaneous
> Buruli ulcer
> Infection by Mycobacterium:
> > marinum [M. balnei]
> > ulcerans

031.2 Disseminated
> Disseminated mycobacterium avium-intracellulare complex (DMAC)
> Mycobacterium avium-intracellulare complex (MAC) bacteremia

031.8 Other specified mycobacterial diseases

031.9 Unspecified diseases due to mycobacteria
> Atypical mycobacterium infection NOS

032 Diphtheria
> Includes: infection by Corynebacterium diphtheriae

032.0 Faucial diphtheria
> Membranous angina, diphtheritic

032.1 Nasopharyngeal diphtheria

032.2 Anterior nasal diphtheria

032.3 Laryngeal diphtheria
> Laryngotracheitis, diphtheritic

Add 4th or 5th digit | Nonspecific code | Unspecified code | Manifestation code

⑤ **032.8 Other specified diphtheria**

    032.81 Conjunctival diphtheria
        Pseudomembranous diphtheritic conjunctivitis

    032.82 Diphtheritic myocarditis

    032.83 Diphtheritic peritonitis

    032.84 Diphtheritic cystitis

    032.85 Cutaneous diphtheria

    032.89 Other

032.9 Diphtheria, unspecified

033 Whooping cough
    Includes: pertussis

Use additional code, if desired, to identify any associated pneumonia (484.3)

033.0 Bordetella pertussis [B. pertussis]

033.1 Bordetella parapertussis [B. parapertussis]

033.8 Whooping cough due to other specified organism
    Bordetella bronchiseptica [B. bronchiseptica]

033.9 Whooping cough, unspecified organism

034 Streptococcal sore throat and scarlet fever

034.0 Streptococcal sore throat
    Septic: Streptococcal:
      angina   angina
        sore throat   laryngitis
                              pharyngitis
                              tonsillitis

034.1 Scarlet fever
    Scarlatina

    Excludes: *parascarlatina (057.8)*

035 Erysipelas

    Excludes: *postpartum or puerperal erysipelas (670)*

036 Meningococcal infection

036.0 Meningococcal meningitis
    Cerebrospinal fever   Meningitis:
      (meningococcal)   cerebrospinal
                                epidemic

036.1 Meningococcal encephalitis

036.2 Meningococcemia
    Meningococcal septicemia

036.3 Waterhouse-Friderichsen syndrome, meningococcal
    Meningococcal hemorrhagic adrenalitis
    Meningococcic adrenal syndrome
    Waterhouse-Friderichsen syndrome NOS

⑤ **036.4 Meningococcal carditis**

    036.40 Meningococcal carditis, unspecified

    036.41 Meningococcal pericarditis

    036.42 Meningococcal endocarditis

    036.43 Meningococcal myocarditis

⑤ **036.8 Other specified meningococcal infections**

    036.81 Meningococcal optic neuritis

    036.82 Meningococcal arthropathy

    036.89 Other

036.9 Meningococcal infection, unspecified
    Meningococcal infection NOS

● Code new   ▲ Revision of   ④ ⑤ Fourth or fifth
   to this edition   existing code   digit required

037 Tetanus

> *Excludes:* *tetanus:*
>
>> *complicating:*
>>> *abortion (634-638 with .0, 639.0)*
>>> *ectopic or molar pregnancy (639.0)*
>> *neonatorum (771.3)*
>> *puerperal (670)*

038 Septicemia

> *Excludes:* *bacteremia (790.7)*
>> *during labor (659.3)*
>> *following ectopic or molar pregnancy (639.0)*
>> *following infusion, injection, transfusion, or vaccination (999.3)*
>> *postpartum, puerperal (670)*
>> *septicemia (sepsis) of newborn (771.81)*
>> *that complicating abortion (634-638 with .0, 639.0)*

038.0 Streptococcal septicemia

⑤ **038.1 Staphylococcal septicemia**

> **038.10 Staphylococcal septicemia, unspecified**
>
> **038.11 Staphylococcus aureus septicemia**
>
> **038.19 Other staphylococcal septicemia**

038.2 Pneumococcal septicemia

038.3 Septicemia due to anaerobes
Septicemia due to bacteroides

> *Excludes:* *gas gangrene (040.0)*
>> *that due to anaerobic streptococci (038.0)*

⑤ **038.4 Septicemia due to other gram-negative organisms**

> **038.40 Gram-negative organism, unspecified**
> Gram-negative septicemia NOS
>
> **038.41 Hemophilus influenzae [H. influenzae]**
>
> **038.42 Escherichia coli [E. coli]**
>
> **038.43 Pseudomonas**
>
> **038.44 Serratia**
>
> **038.49 Other**

038.8 Other specified septicemias

> *Excludes:* *septicemia (due to):*
>> *anthrax (022.3)*
>> *gonococcal (098.89)*
>> *herpetic (054.5)*
>> *meningococcal (036.2)*
>> *septicemic plague (020.2)*

038.9 Unspecified septicemia
Septicemia NOS

> *Excludes:* *bacteremia NOS (790.7)*

039 Actinomycotic infections
Includes: actinomycotic mycetoma
infection by Actinomycetales, such as species of Actinomyces, Actinomadura,
Nocardia, Streptomyces
maduromycosis (actinomycotic)
schizomycetoma (actinomycotic)

039.0 Cutaneous
Erythrasma   Trichomycosis axillaris

039.1 Pulmonary
Thoracic actinomycosis

039.2 Abdominal

039.3 Cervicofacial

039.4 Madura foot

> *Excludes:* *madura foot due to mycotic infection (117.4)*

039.8 Of other specified sites

Add 4th or 5th digit	Nonspecific code	Unspecified code	Manifestation code

039.9 Of unspecified site
Actinomycosis NOS Nocardiosis NOS
Maduromycosis NOS

040 Other bacterial diseases

> *Excludes:* *bacteremia NOS (790.7)*
> *bacterial infection NOS (041.9)*

040.0 Gas gangrene
Gas bacillus infection Malignant edema
  or gangrene Myonecrosis, clostridial
Infection by Clostridium: Myositis, clostridial
  histolyticum
  oedematiens
  perfringens [welchii]
  septicum
  sordellii

040.1 Rhinoscleroma

040.2 Whipple's disease
Intestinal lipodystrophy

040.3 Necrobacillosis

⑤ **040.8 Other specified bacterial diseases**

040.81 Tropical pyomyositis

● **040.82 Toxic shock syndrome**
Use additional code to identify the organism

040.89 Other

041 Bacterial infection in conditions classified elsewhere and of unspecified site
Note: This category is provided to be used as an additional code where it is desired to identify the bacterial agent in diseases classified elsewhere. This category will also be used to classify bacterial infections of unspecified nature or site.

> *Excludes:* *bacteremia NOS (790.7)*
> *septicemia (038.0-038.9)*

⑤ **041.0 Streptococcus**

041.00 Streptococcus, unspecified

041.01 Group A

041.02 Group B

041.03 Group C

041.04 Group D [Enterococcus]

041.05 Group G

041.09 Other Streptococcus

⑤ **041.1 Staphylococcus**

041.10 Staphylococcus, unspecified

041.11 Staphylococcus aureus

041.19 Other Staphylococcus

041.2 Pneumococcus

041.3 Friedländer's bacillus
Infection by Klebsiella pneumoniae

041.4 Escherichia coli [E. coli]

041.5 Hemophilus influenzae [H. influenzae]

041.6 Proteus (mirabilis) (morganii)

041.7 Pseudomonas

⑤ **041.8 Other specified bacterial infections**

041.81 Mycoplasma
Eaton's agent
Pleuropneumonia-like organisms [PPLO]

041.82 Bacillus fragilis

041.83 Clostridium perfringens

● Code new ▲ Revision of ④ ⑤ Fourth or fifth
to this edition   existing code   digit required

041.84   **Other anaerobes**
Gram-negative anaerobes
Bacteroides (fragilis)

Excludes: Helicobacter pylori (041.86)

041.85   **Other Gram-negative organisms**
Aerobacter aerogenes
Gram-negative bacteria NOS
Mima polymorpha
Serratia

Excludes: Gram-negative anaerobes (041.84)

041.86   **Helicobacter pylori (H. pylori)**

041.89   **Other specified bacteria**

041.9   **Bacterial infection, unspecified**

HUMAN IMMUNODEFICIENCY VIRUS (HIV) INFECTION (042)

042   Human immunodeficiency virus [HIV] disease
Acquired immune deficiency syndrome
Acquired immunodeficiency syndrome
AIDS
AIDS-like syndrome
AIDS-related complex
ARC
HIV infection, symptomatic

Use additional code(s) to identify all manifestations of HIV

Use additional code, if desired, to identify HIV-2 infection (079.53)

Excludes: asymptomatic HIV infection status (V08)
exposre to HIV virus (V01.7)
nonspecific serologic evidence of HIV (795.71)

POLIOMYELITIS AND OTHER NON-ARTHROPOD-BORNE VIRAL DISEASES OF CENTRAL NERVOUS SYSTEM (045-049)

⑤ **045   Acute poliomyelitis**

Excludes: late effects of acute poliomyelitis (138)

The following fifth-digit subclassification is for use with category 045:

0   **poliovirus, unspecified type**

1   **poliovirus type I**

2   **poliovirus type II**

3   **poliovirus type III**

⑤ **045.0   Acute paralytic poliomyelitis specified as bulbar**
Infantile paralysis (acute)
Poliomyelitis (acute) (anterior) } specified as bulbar
Polioencephalitis (acute) (bulbar)
Polioencephalomyelitis (acute) (anterior) (bulbar)

⑤ **045.1   Acute poliomyelitis with other paralysis**
Paralysis:
  acute atrophic, spinal infantile, paralytic
Poliomyelitis (acute) }
  anterior } with paralysis except bulbar
  epidemic

⑤ **045.2   Acute nonparalytic poliomyelitis**
Poliomyelitis (acute) }
  anterior } specified as nonparalytic
  epidemic

⑤ **045.9   Acute poliomyelitis, unspecified**
Infantile paralysis
Poliomyelitis (acute) } unspecified whether paralytic or nonparalytic
  anterior
  epidemic

046   Slow virus infection of central nervous system

046.0   Kuru

046.1   Jakob-Creutzfeldt disease
Subacute spongiform encephalopathy

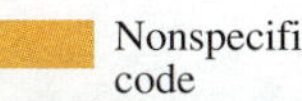

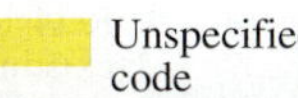

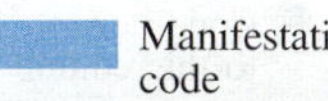

Manifestation
code

046.2 Subacute sclerosing panencephalitis
Dawson's inclusion body encephalitis
Van Bogaert's sclerosing leukoencephalitis

046.3 Progressive multifocal leukoencephalopathy
Multifocal leukoencephalopathy NOS

046.8 Other specified slow virus infection of central nervous system

046.9 Unspecified slow virus infection of central nervous system

047 Meningitis due to enterovirus
Includes: meningitis:
abacterial
aseptic
viral

Excludes: meningitis due to:
adenovirus (049.1)
arthropod-borne virus (060.0-066.9)
leptospira (100.81)
virus of:
herpes simplex (054.72)
herpes zoster (053.0)
lymphocytic choriomeningitis (049.0)
mumps (072.1)
poliomyelitis (045.0-045.9)
any other infection specifically classified elsewhere

047.0 Coxsackie virus

047.1 ECHO virus
Meningo-eruptive syndrome

047.8 Other specified viral meningitis

047.9 Unspecified viral meningitis
Viral meningitis NOS

048 Other enterovirus diseases of central nervous system
Boston exanthem

049 Other non-arthropod-borne viral diseases of central nervous system

Excludes: late effects of viral encephalitis (139.0)

049.0 Lymphocytic choriomeningitis
Lymphocytic:
meningitis (serous) (benign)
meningoencephalitis (serous) (benign)

049.1 Meningitis due to adenovirus

049.8 Other specified non-arthropod-borne viral diseases of central nervous system
Encephalitis: Encephalitis:
acute: lethargica
inclusion body   Rio Bravo
necrotizing   von Economo's disease
epidemic

049.9 Unspecified non-arthropod-borne viral diseases of central nervous system
Viral encephalitis NOS

VIRAL DISEASES ACCOMPANIED BY EXANTHEM (050-057)

Excludes: arthropod-borne viral diseases (060.0-066.9)
Boston exanthem (048)

050 Smallpox

050.0 Variola major
Hemorrhagic (pustular)   Malignant smallpox
smallpox   Purpura variolosa

050.1 Alastrim
Variola minor

050.2 Modified smallpox
Varioloid

050.9 Smallpox, unspecified

● Code new   ▲ Revision of   ④ ⑤ Fourth or fifth
to this edition   existing code   digit required

051 Cowpox and paravaccinia

051.0 Cowpox
Vaccinia not from vaccination

Excludes: vaccinia (generalized) (from vaccination) (999.0)

051.1 Pseudocowpox
Milkers' node

051.2 Contagious pustular dermatitis
Ecthyma contagiosum   Orf

051.9 Paravaccinia, unspecified

052 Chickenpox

052.0 Postvaricella encephalitis
Postchickenpox encephalitis

052.1 Varicella (hemorrhagic) pneumonitis

052.7 With other specified complications

052.8 With unspecified complication

052.9 Varicella without mention of complication
Chickenpox NOS
Varicella NOS

053 Herpes zoster
Includes: shingles
                  zona

053.0 With meningitis

⑤ **053.1 With other nervous system complications**

053.10   With unspecified nervous system complication

053.11   Geniculate herpes zoster
Herpetic geniculate ganglionitis

053.12   Postherpetic trigeminal neuralgia

053.13   Postherpetic polyneuropathy

053.19   Other

⑤ **053.2 With ophthalmic complications**

053.20   Herpes zoster dermatitis of eyelid
Herpes zoster ophthalmicus

053.21   Herpes zoster keratoconjunctivitis

053.22   Herpes zoster iridocyclitis

053.29   Other

⑤ **053.7 With other specified complications**

053.71   Otitis externa due to herpes zoster

053.79   Other

053.8 With unspecified complication

053.9 Herpes zoster without mention of complication
Herpes zoster NOS

054 Herpes simplex

Excludes: congenital herpes simplex (771.2)

054.0 Eczema herpeticum
Kaposi's varicelliform eruption

⑤ **054.1 Genital herpes**

054.10   Genital herpes, unspecified
Herpes progenitalis

054.11   Herpetic vulvovaginitis

054.12   Herpetic ulceration of vulva

054.13   Herpetic infection of penis

054.19   Other

054.2 Herpetic gingivostomatitis

054.3 Herpetic meningoencephalitis
Herpes encephalitis   Simian B disease

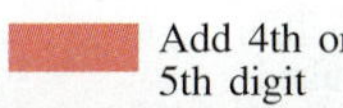
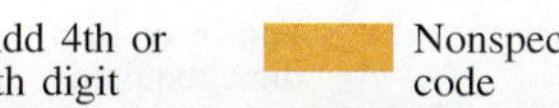
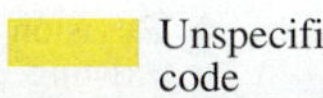
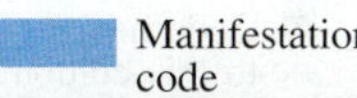

Add 4th or
5th digit   Nonspecific
                        code   Unspecified
                                            code   Manifestation
                                                              code

⑤ **054.4 With ophthalmic complications**

　　054.40 With unspecified ophthalmic complication

　　054.41 Herpes simplex dermatitis of eyelid

　　054.42 Dendritic keratitis

　　054.43 Herpes simplex disciform keratitis

　　054.44 Herpes simplex iridocyclitis

　　054.49 Other

054.5 Herpetic septicemia

054.6 Herpetic whitlow
　　Herpetic felon

⑤ **054.7 With other specified complications**

　　054.71 Visceral herpes simplex

　　054.72 Herpes simplex meningitis

　　054.73 Herpes simplex otitis externa

　　054.79 Other

054.8 With unspecified complication

054.9 Herpes simplex without mention of complication

055 Measles
　　Includes: morbilli
　　　　　　　rubeola

055.0 Postmeasles encephalitis

055.1 Postmeasles pneumonia

055.2 Postmeasles otitis media

⑤ **055.7 With other specified complications**

　　055.71 Measles keratoconjunctivitis
　　　　Measles keratitis

　　055.79 Other

055.8 With unspecified complication

055.9 Measles without mention of complication

056 Rubella
　　Includes: German measles

　　Excludes: congenital rubella (771.0)

⑤ **056.0 With neurological complications**

　　056.00 With unspecified neurological complication

　　056.01 Encephalomyelitis due to rubella
　　　　Encephalitis
　　　　Meningoencephalitis　　　} due to rubella

　　056.09 Other

⑤ **056.7 With other specified complications**

　　056.71 Arthritis due to rubella

　　056.79 Other

056.8 With unspecified complications

056.9 Rubella without mention of complication

057 Other viral exanthemata

057.0 Erythema infectiosum [fifth disease]

057.8 Other specified viral exanthemata
　　Dukes (-Filatow) disease　　Parascarlatina
　　Exanthema subitum　　　　　Pseudoscarlatina
　　　[sixth disease]　　　　　　Roseola infantum
　　Fourth disease

057.9 Viral exanthem, unspecified

● Code new
　to this edition　　　　　▲ Revision of
　　　　　　　　　　　　　existing code　　　　④ ⑤ Fourth or fifth
　　　　　　　　　　　　　　　　　　　　　　　digit required

ARTHROPOD-BORNE VIRAL DISEASES (060-066)

Use additional code, if desired, to identify any associated meningitis (321.2)

Excludes: *late effects of viral encephalitis (139.0)*

060 Yellow fever

060.0 Sylvatic
Yellow fever:
  jungle
  sylvan

060.1 Urban

060.9 Yellow fever, unspecified

061 Dengue
Breakbone fever

Excludes: *hemorrhagic fever caused by dengue virus (065.4)*

062 Mosquito-borne viral encephalitis

062.0 Japanese encephalitis
Japanese B encephalitis

062.1 Western equine encephalitis

062.2 Eastern equine encephalitis

Excludes: *Venezuelan equine encephalitis (066.2)*

062.3 St. Louis encephalitis

062.4 Australian encephalitis
Australian arboencephalitis
Australian X disease
Murray Valley encephalitis

062.5 California virus encephalitis
Encephalitis: Tahyna fever
  California
  La Crosse

062.8 Other specified mosquito-borne viral encephalitis
Encephalitis by Ilheus virus

Excludes: *West Nile virus (066.4)*

062.9 Mosquito-borne viral encephalitis, unspecified

063 Tick-borne viral encephalitis
Includes: diphasic meningoencephalitis

063.0 Russian spring-summer [taiga] encephalitis

063.1 Louping ill

063.2 Central European encephalitis

063.8 Other specified tick-borne viral encephalitis
Langat encephalitis   Powassan encephalitis

063.9 Tick-borne viral encephalitis, unspecified

064 Viral encephalitis transmitted by other and unspecified arthropods
Arthropod-borne viral encephalitis, vector unknown
Negishi virus encephalitis

Excludes: *viral encephalitis NOS (049.9)*

065 Arthropod-borne hemorrhagic fever

065.0 Crimean hemorrhagic fever [CHF Congo virus]
Central Asian hemorrhagic fever

065.1 Omsk hemorrhagic fever

065.2 Kyasanur Forest disease

065.3 Other tick-borne hemorrhagic fever

065.4 Mosquito-borne hemorrhagic fever
Chikungunya hemorrhagic fever
Dengue hemorrhagic fever

Excludes: *Chikungunya fever (066.3)*
  dengue (061)
  yellow fever (060.0-060.9)

Add 4th or 5th digit | Nonspecific code | Unspecified code | Manifestation code

065.8 **Other specified arthropod-borne hemorrhagic fever**
Mite-borne hemorrhagic fever

065.9 **Arthropod-borne hemorrhagic fever, unspecified**
Arbovirus hemorrhagic fever NOS

066 **Other arthropod-borne viral diseases**

066.0 **Phlebotomus fever**
Changuinola fever   Sandfly fever

066.1 **Tick-borne fever**
Nairobi sheep disease   Tick fever:
Tick fever: Kemerovo
  American mountain   Quaranfil
  Colorado

066.2 **Venezuelan equine fever**
Venezuelan equine encephalitis

066.3 **Other mosquito-borne fever**
Fever (viral):   Fever (viral):
  Bunyamwera   Oropouche
  Bwamba   Pixuna
  Chikungunya   Rift valley
  GuamaR Mayaro   Ross river
  Mucambo   Wesselsbron
  O'nyong-nyong   Zika

Excludes: dengue (061)
      yellow fever (060.0-060.9)

● **066.4** **West Nile fever**
West Nile encephalitis
West Nile encephalomyelitis
West Nile virus

066.8 **Other specified arthropod-borne viral diseases**
Chandipura fever   Piry fever

066.9 **Arthropod-borne viral disease, unspecified**
Arbovirus infection NOS

OTHER DISEASES DUE TO VIRUSES AND CHLAMYDIAE (070-079)

070 **Viral hepatitis**
Includes: viral hepatitis (acute) (chronic)

Excludes: cytomegalic inclusion virus hepatitis (078.5)

The following fifth-digit subclassification is for use with categories 070.2 and 070.3:

  0 **acute or unspecified, without mention of hepatitis delta**

  1 **acute or unspecified, with hepatitis delta**

  2 **chronic, without mention of hepatitis delta**

  3 **chronic, with hepatitis delta**

070.0 **Viral hepatitis A with hepatic coma**

070.1 **Viral hepatitis A without mention of hepatic coma**
Infectious hepatitis

⑤ **070.2** **Viral hepatitis B with hepatic coma**

⑤ **070.3** **Viral hepatitis B without mention of hepatic coma**
Serum hepatitis

⑤ **070.4** **Other specified viral hepatitis with hepatic coma**

  070.41 **Acute or unspecified hepatitis C with hepatic coma**

  070.42 **Hepatitis delta without mention of active hepatitis B disease with hepatic coma**
Hepatitis delta with hepatitis B carrier state

  070.43 **Hepatitis E with hepatic coma**

  070.44 **Chronic hepatitis C with hepatic coma**

  070.49 **Other specified viral hepatitis with hepatic coma**

⑤ **070.5** **Other specified viral hepatitis without mention of hepatic coma**

  070.51 **Acute or unspecified hepatitis C without mention of hepatic coma**

  070.52 **Hepatitis delta without mention of active hepatitis B disease or hepatic coma**

  070.53 **Hepatitis E without mention of hepatic coma**

● Code new   ▲ Revision of   ④ ⑤ Fourth or fifth
  to this edition   existing code   digit required

070.54   **Chronic hepatitis C without mention of hepatic coma**

070.59   **Other specified viral hepatitis without mention of hepatic coma**

070.6   **Unspecified viral hepatitis with hepatic coma**

070.9   **Unspecified viral hepatitis without mention of hepatic coma**
Viral hepatitis NOS

071   Rabies
Hydrophobia   Lyssa

072   Mumps

072.0   Mumps orchitis

072.1   Mumps meningitis

072.2   Mumps encephalitis
Mumps meningoencephalitis

072.3   Mumps pancreatitis

⑤ **072.7   Mumps with other specified complications**

072.71   **Mumps hepatitis**

072.72   **Mumps polyneuropathy**

072.79   **Other**

072.8   **Mumps with unspecified complication**

072.9   Mumps without mention of complication
Epidemic parotitis   Infectious parotitis

073   Ornithosis
Includes: parrot fever
psittacosis

073.0   With pneumonia
Lobular pneumonitis due to ornithosis

073.7   **With other specified complications**

073.8   **With unspecified complication**

073.9   **Ornithosis, unspecified**

074   Specific diseases due to Coxsackie virus

Excludes: *Coxsackie virus:*

infection NOS (079.2)
meningitis (047.0)

074.0   Herpangina
Vesicular pharyngitis

074.1   Epidemic pleurodynia
Bornholm disease   Epidemic:
Devil's grip   myalgia
myositis

⑤ **074.2   Coxsackie carditis**

074.20   **Coxsackie carditis, unspecified**

074.21   **Coxsackie pericarditis**

074.22   **Coxsackie endocarditis**

074.23   **Coxsackie myocarditis**
Aseptic myocarditis of newborn

074.3   Hand, foot, and mouth disease
Vesicular stomatitis and exanthem

074.8   **Other specified diseases due to Coxsackie virus**
Acute lymphonodular pharyngitis

075   Infectious mononucleosis
Glandular fever   Pfeiffer's disease
Monocytic angina

076   Trachoma

Excludes: *late effect of trachoma (139.1)*

076.0   Initial stage
Trachoma dubium

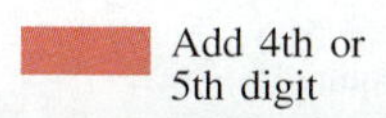

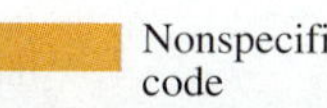

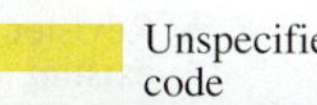

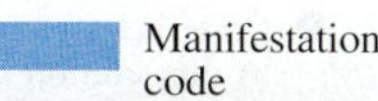

076.1 Active stage
    Granular conjunctivitis (trachomatous)
    Trachomatous:
      follicular conjunctivitis
      pannus

076.9 Trachoma, unspecified
    Trachoma NOS

077 Other diseases of conjunctiva due to viruses and Chlamydiae

    Excludes: *ophthalmic complications of viral diseases classified elsewhere*

077.0 Inclusion conjunctivitis
    Paratrachoma
    Swimming pool conjunctivitis

    Excludes: *inclusion blennorrhea (neonatal) (771.6)*

077.1 Epidemic keratoconjunctivitis
    Shipyard eye

077.2 Pharyngoconjunctival fever
    Viral pharyngoconjunctivitis

077.3 Other adenoviral conjunctivitis
    Acute adenoviral follicular conjunctivitis

077.4 Epidemic hemorrhagic conjunctivitis
    Apollo:
      conjunctivitis
      disease
    Conjunctivitis due to enterovirus type 70
    Hemorrhagic conjunctivitis (acute) (epidemic)

077.8 Other viral conjunctivitis
    Newcastle conjunctivitis

⑤ **077.9 Unspecified diseases of conjunctiva due to viruses and Chlamydiae**

    077.98 Due to Chlamydiae

    077.99 Due to viruses
      Viral conjunctivitis NOS

078 Other diseases due to viruses and Chlamydiae

    Excludes: *viral infection NOS (079.0-079.9)*
          viremia NOS (790.8)

078.0 Molluscum contagiosum

⑤ **078.1 Viral warts**
    Viral warts due to Human papillomavirus

    078.10 Viral warts, unspecified
      Condyloma NOS
      Verruca:
        NOS
        vulgaris
      Warts (infectious)

    078.11 Condyloma acuminatum

    078.19 Other specified viral warts
      Genital warts NOS
      Verruca:
        plana
        plantaris

078.2 Sweating fever
    Miliary fever   Sweating disease

078.3 Cat-scratch disease
    Benign lymphoreticulosis (of inoculation)
    Cat-scratch fever

078.4 Foot and mouth disease
    Aphthous fever
    Epizootic:
      aphthae
      stomatitis

    ● Code new to this edition   ▲ Revision of existing code   ④ ⑤ Fourth or fifth digit required

078.5 Cytomegaloviral disease
Cytomegalic inclusion disease
Salivary gland virus disease
Use additional code, if desired, to identify manifestation, as:
cytomegalic inclusion virus:
hepatitis (573.1)
pneumonia (484.1)

Excludes: *congenital cytomegalovirus infection (771.1)*

078.6 Hemorrhagic nephrosonephritis
Hemorrhagic fever: Hemorrhagic fever:
  epidemic   Russian
  Korean   with renal syndrome

078.7 Arenaviral hemorrhagic fever
Hemorrhagic fever: Hemorrhagic fever:
  Argentine   Junin virus
  Bolivian   Machupo virus

⑤ **078.8 Other specified diseases due to viruses and Chlamydiae**

Excludes: *epidemic diarrhea (009.2)*
lymphogranuloma venereum (099.1)

    078.81 Epidemic vertigo

    078.82 Epidemic vomiting syndrome
        Winter vomiting disease

    078.88 Other specified diseases due to Chlamydiae

    078.89 Other specified diseases due to viruses
        Epidemic cervical myalgia
        Marburg disease
        Tanapox

079 Viral and chlamydial infection in conditions classified elsewhere and of unspecified site
Note: This category is provided to be used as an additional code where it is desired to identify the viral agent in diseases classifiable elsewhere. This category will also be used to classify virus infection of unspecified nature or site.

079.0 Adenovirus

079.1 ECHO virus

079.2 Coxsackievirus

079.3 Rhinovirus

079.4 Human papillomavirus

⑤ **079.5 Retrovirus**

Excludes: *human immunodeficiency virus, type 1 [HIV-1] (042)*
human T-cell lymphotrophic virus, type III [HTLV-III] (042)
lymphadenopathy-associated virus [LAV] (042)

    079.50 Retrovirus, unspecified

    079.51 Human T-cell lymphotrophic virus, type I [HTLV-I]

    079.52 Human T-cell lymphotrophic virus, type II [HTLV-II]

    079.53 Human immunodeficiency virus, type 2 [HIV-2]

    079.59 Other specified retrovirus

079.6 Respiratory syncytial virus (RSV)

⑤ **079.8 Other specified viral and chlamydial infections**

    079.81 Hantavirus

    079.88 Other specified chlamydial infection

    079.89 Other specified viral infection

⑤ **079.9 Unspecified viral and chlamydial infections**

Excludes: *viremia NOS (790.8)*

    079.98 Unspecified chlamydial infection
        Chlamydial infection NOS

    079.99 Unspecified viral infection
        Viral infection NOS

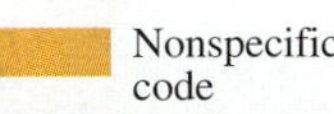

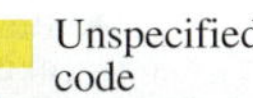

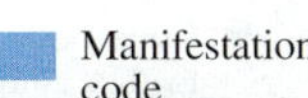

Manifestation
code

RICKETTSIOSES AND OTHER ARTHROPOD-BORNE DISEASES (080-088)

> **Excludes:** *arthropod-borne viral diseases (060.0-066.9)*

080 Louse-borne [epidemic] typhus
Typhus (fever):   Typhus (fever):
  classical   exanthematic NOS
  epidemic   louse-borne

081 Other typhus

  081.0 Murine [endemic] typhus
    Typhus (fever):
     endemic
     flea-borne

  081.1 Brill's disease
    Brill-Zinsser disease
    Recrudescent typhus (fever)

  081.2 Scrub typhus
    Japanese river fever   Mite-borne typhus
    Kedani fever   Tsutsugamushi

  081.9 Typhus, unspecified
    Typhus (fever) NOS

082 Tick-borne rickettsioses

  082.0 Spotted fevers
    Rocky mountain spotted fever
    São Paulo fever

  082.1 Boutonneuse fever
    African tick typhus   Marseilles fever
    India tick typhus   Mediterranean tick fever
    Kenya tick typhus

  082.2 North Asian tick fever
    Siberian tick typhus

  082.3 Queensland tick typhus

  ⑤ **082.4 Ehrlichiosis**
    082.40 Ehrlichiosis, unspecified
    082.41 Ehrlichiosis chafeensis (*E. chafeensis*)
    082.49 Other ehrlichiosis

  082.8 Other specified tick-borne rickettsioses
    Lone star fever

  082.9 Tick-borne rickettsiosis, unspecified
    Tick-borne typhus NOS

083 Other rickettsioses

  083.0 Q fever

  083.1 Trench fever
    Quintan fever   Wolhynian fever

  083.2 Rickettsialpox
    Vesicular rickettsiosis

  083.8 Other specified rickettsioses

  083.9 Rickettsiosis, unspecified

084 Malaria

Note: Subcategories 084.0-084.6 exclude the listed conditions with mention of pernicious complications (084.8-084.9).

> **Excludes:** *congenital malaria (771.2)*

  084.0 Falciparum malaria [malignant tertian]
    Malaria (fever):
     by Plasmodium falciparum
     subtertian

  084.1 Vivax malaria [benign tertian]
    Malaria (fever) by Plasmodium vivax

  084.2 Quartan malaria
    Malaria (fever) by Plasmodium malariae
    Malariae malaria

● Code new to this edition   ▲ Revision of existing code   ④ ⑤ Fourth or fifth digit required

084.3 Ovale malaria
Malaria (fever) by Plasmodium ovale

084.4 Other malaria
Monkey malaria

084.5 Mixed malaria
Malaria (fever) by more than one parasite

084.6 Malaria, unspecified
Malaria (fever) NOS

084.7 Induced malaria
Therapeutically induced malaria

> *Excludes:* *accidental infection from syringe, blood transfusion, etc. (084.0-084.6, above, according to parasite species)*
> *transmission from mother to child during delivery (771.2)*

084.8 Blackwater fever
Hemoglobinuric: Malarial hemoglobinuria
  fever (bilious)
  malaria

084.9 Other pernicious complications of malaria
Algid malaria
Cerebral malaria

Use additional code, if desired, to identify complication, as:
  malarial:
    hepatitis (573.2)
    nephrosis (581.81)

085 Leishmaniasis

085.0 Visceral [kala-azar]
Dumdum fever   Leishmaniasis:
Infection by Leishmania: dermal, post-kala-azar
  donovani   Mediterranean
  infantum   visceral (Indian)

085.1 Cutaneous, urban
Aleppo boil   Leishmaniasis, cutaneous:
Baghdad boil   dry form
Delhi boil   late
Infection by Leishmania   recurrent
  tropica (minor)   ulcerating
                                 Oriental sore

085.2 Cutaneous, Asian desert
Infection by Leishmania tropica major
Leishmaniasis, cutaneous:
  acute necrotizing
  rural
  wet form
  zoonotic form

085.3 Cutaneous, Ethiopian
Infection by Leishmania ethiopica
Leishmaniasis, cutaneous:
  diffuse
  lepromatous

085.4 Cutaneous, American
Chiclero ulcer
Infection by Leishmania mexicana
Leishmaniasis tegumentaria diffusa

085.5 Mucocutaneous (American)
Espundia
Infection by Leishmania braziliensis
Uta

085.9 Leishmaniasis, unspecified

086 Trypanosomiasis
Use additional code, if desired, to identify manifestations, as:
  trypanosomiasis:
    encephalitis (323.2)
    meningitis (321.3)

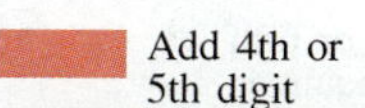

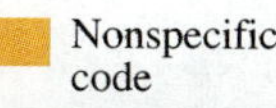

086.0 Chagas' disease with heart involvement
American trypanosomiasis
Infection by Trypanosoma cruzi   } with heart involvement
Any condition classifiable to 086.2

086.1 Chagas' disease with other organ involvement
American trypanosomiasis
Infection by Trypanosoma cruzi   } with involvement of organ other
Any condition classifiable to 086.2   than heart

086.2 Chagas' disease without mention of organ involvement
American trypanosomiasis
Infection by Trypanosoma cruzi

086.3 Gambian trypanosomiasis
Gambian sleeping sickness
Infection by Trypanosoma gambiense

086.4 Rhodesian trypanosomiasis
Infection by Trypanosoma rhodesiense
Rhodesian sleeping sickness

086.5 African trypanosomiasis, unspecified
Sleeping sickness NOS

086.9 Trypanosomiasis, unspecified

087 Relapsing fever
Includes: recurrent fever

087.0 Louse-borne

087.1 Tick-borne

087.9 Relapsing fever, unspecified

088 Other arthropod-borne diseases

088.0 Bartonellosis
Carrión's disease   Verruga peruana
Oroya fever

⑤ **088.8 Other specified arthropod-borne diseases**

088.81 Lyme Disease
Erythema chronicum migrans

088.82 Babesiosis
Babesiasis

088.89 Other

088.9 Arthropod-borne disease, unspecified

SYPHILIS AND OTHER VENEREAL DISEASES (090-099)

Excludes: *nonvenereal endemic syphilis (104.0)*
urogenital trichomoniasis (131.0)

090 Congenital syphilis

090.0 Early congenital syphilis, symptomatic
Congenital syphilitic: Syphilitic (congenital):
choroiditis   epiphysitis
coryza (chronic)   osteochondritis
hepatomegaly   pemphigus
mucous patches   Any congenital syphilitic condition specified as early
periostitis   or manifest less than two years after birth
splenomegaly

090.1 Early congenital syphilis, latent
Congenital syphilis without clinical manifestations, with positive serological reaction
and negative spinal fluid test, less than two years after birth

090.2 Early congenital syphilis, unspecified
Congenital syphilis NOS, less than two years after birth

090.3 Syphilitic interstitial keratitis
Syphilitic keratitis:
parenchymatous
punctata profunda

Excludes: *interstitial keratitis NOS (370.50)*

⑤ **090.4 Juvenile neurosyphilis**
Use additional code, if desired, to identify any associated mental disorder

---

    ● Code new   ▲ Revision of   ④ ⑤ Fourth or fifth
to this edition   existing code   digit required

090.40 **Juvenile neurosyphilis, unspecified**
Congenital neurosyphilis
Dementia paralytica juvenilis
Juvenile:
    general paresis
    tabes
    taboparesis

090.41 **Congenital syphilitic encephalitis**

090.42 **Congenital syphilitic meningitis**

090.49 **Other**

090.5 **Other late congenital syphilis, symptomatic**
Gumma due to congenital syphilis
Hutchinson's teeth
Syphilitic saddle nose
Any congenital syphilitic condition specified as late or manifest two years or more after
    birth

090.6 **Late congenital syphilis, latent**
Congenital syphilis without clinical manifestations, with positive serological reaction and
    negative spinal fluid test, two years or more after birth

090.7 **Late congenital syphilis, unspecified**
Congenital syphilis NOS, two years or more after birth

090.9 **Congenital syphilis, unspecified**

091 **Early syphilis, symptomatic**

> *Excludes:*   *early cardiovascular syphilis (093.0-093.9)*
>   *early neurosyphilis (094.0-094.9)*

091.0 **Genital syphilis (primary)**
Genital chancre

091.1 **Primary anal syphilis**

091.2 **Other primary syphilis**

Primary syphilis of:	Primary syphilis of:
breast	lip
fingers	tonsils

091.3 **Secondary syphilis of skin or mucous membranes**

Condyloma latum	Secondary syphilis of:
Secondary syphilis of:	skin
anus	tonsils
mouth	vulva
pharynx	

091.4 **Adenopathy due to secondary syphilis**
Syphilitic adenopathy (secondary)
Syphilitic lymphadenitis (secondary)

⑤ **091.5** **Uveitis due to secondary syphilis**

    091.50 **Syphilitic uveitis, unspecified**

    091.51 **Syphilitic chorioretinitis (secondary)**

    091.52 **Syphilitic iridocyclitis (secondary)**

⑤ **091.6** **Secondary syphilis of viscera and bone**

    091.61 **Secondary syphilitic periostitis**

    091.62 **Secondary syphilitic hepatitis**
        Secondary syphilis of liver

    091.69 **Other viscera**

091.7 **Secondary syphilis, relapse**
Secondary syphilis, relapse (treated) (untreated)

⑤ **091.8** **Other forms of secondary syphilis**

    091.81 **Acute syphilitic meningitis (secondary)**

    091.82 **Syphilitic alopecia**

    091.89 **Other**

091.9 **Unspecified secondary syphilis**

092 **Early syphilis, latent**
Includes: syphilis (acquired) without clinical manifestations, with positive serological reaction
        and negative spinal fluid test, less than two years after infection

Add 4th or 5th digit	Nonspecific code	Unspecified code	Manifestation code

092.0 Early syphilis, latent, serological relapse after treatment

092.9 Early syphilis, latent, unspecified

093 Cardiovascular syphilis

093.0 Aneurysm of aorta, specified as syphilitic
Dilatation of aorta, specified as syphilitic

093.1 Syphilitic aortitis

⑤ **093.2 Syphilitic endocarditis**

093.20 Valve, unspecified
Syphilitic ostial coronary disease

093.21 Mitral valve

093.22 Aortic valve
Syphilitic aortic incompetence or stenosis

093.23 Tricuspid valve

093.24 Pulmonary valve

⑤ **093.8 Other specified cardiovascular syphilis**

093.81 Syphilitic pericarditis

093.82 Syphilitic myocarditis

093.89 Other

093.9 Cardiovascular syphilis, unspecified

094 Neurosyphilis
Use additional code, if desired, to identify any associated mental disorder

094.0 Tabes dorsalis
Locomotor ataxia (progressive)
Posterior spinal sclerosis (syphilitic)
Tabetic neurosyphilis
Use additional code, if desired, to identify manifestation, as:
neurogenic arthropathy [Charcot's joint disease] (713.5)

094.1 General paresis
Dementia paralytica   Paretic neurosyphilis
General paralysis (of the   Taboparesis
insane) (progressive)

094.2 Syphilitic meningitis
Meningovascular syphilis

Excludes: acute syphilitic meningitis (secondary) (091.81)

094.3 Asymptomatic neurosyphilis

⑤ **094.8 Other specified neurosyphilis**

094.81 Syphilitic encephalitis

094.82 Syphilitic Parkinsonism

094.83 Syphilitic disseminated retinochoroiditis

094.84 Syphilitic optic atrophy

094.85 Syphilitic retrobulbar neuritis

094.86 Syphilitic acoustic neuritis

094.87 Syphilitic ruptured cerebral aneurysm

094.89 Other

094.9 Neurosyphilis, unspecified
Gumma (syphilitic)
Syphilis (early) (late) } of central nervous system NOS
Syphiloma

095 Other forms of late syphilis, with symptoms
Includes: gumma (syphilitic)
syphilis, late, tertiary, or unspecified stage

095.0 Syphilitic episcleritis

095.1 Syphilis of lung

095.2 Syphilitic peritonitis

095.3 Syphilis of liver

095.4 Syphilis of kidney

   ● Code new   ▲ Revision of   ④ ⑤ Fourth or fifth
to this edition   existing code   digit required

095.5 Syphilis of bone

095.6 Syphilis of muscle
Syphilitic myositis

095.7 Syphilis of synovium, tendon, and bursa
Syphilitic:
  bursitis
  synovitis

095.8 Other specified forms of late symptomatic syphilis

> Excludes: *cardiovascular syphilis (093.0-093.9)*
> *neurosyphilis (094.0-094.9)*

095.9 Late symptomatic syphilis, unspecified

096 Late syphilis, latent
Syphilis (acquired) without clinical manifestations, with positive serological reaction and negative spinal fluid test, two years or more after infection

097 Other and unspecified syphilis

097.0 Late syphilis, unspecified

097.1 Latent syphilis, unspecified
Positive serological reaction for syphilis

097.9 Syphilis, unspecified
Syphilis (acquired) NOS

> Excludes: *syphilis NOS causing death under two years of age (090.9)*

098 Gonococcal infections

098.0 Acute, of lower genitourinary tract
Gonococcal: Gonorrhea (acute):
  Bartholinitis (acute)   NOS
  urethritis (acute)   genitourinary (tract) NOS
  vulvovaginitis (acute)

⑤ **098.1 Acute, of upper genitourinary tract**

098.10 Gonococcal infection (acute) of upper genitourinary tract, site unspecified

098.11 Gonococcal cystitis (acute)
Gonorrhea (acute) of bladder

098.12 Gonococcal prostatitis (acute)

098.13 Gonococcal epididymo-orchitis (acute)
Gonococcal orchitis (acute)

098.14 Gonococcal seminal vesiculitis (acute)
Gonorrhea (acute) of seminal vesicle

098.15 Gonococcal cervicitis (acute)
Gonorrhea (acute) of cervix

098.16 Gonococcal endometritis (acute)
Gonorrhea (acute) of uterus

098.17 Gonococcal salpingitis, specified as acute

098.19 Other

098.2 Chronic, of lower genitourinary tract
Gonococcal:
  Bartholinitis
  urethritis
  vulvovaginitis
Gonorrhea: } specified as chronic or with
  NOS   duration of two months or more
  genitourinary (tract)
Any condition classifiable
  to 098.0

⑤ **098.3 Chronic, of upper genitourinary tract**
Includes: any condition classifiable to 098.1 stated as chronic or with a duration of two months or more

098.30 Chronic gonococcal infection of upper genitourinary tract, site unspecified

098.31 Gonococcal cystitis, chronic
Any condition classifiable to 098.11, specified as chronic
Gonorrhea of bladder, chronic

098.32 Gonococcal prostatitis, chronic
Any condition classifiable to 098.12, specified as chronic

098.33 Gonococcal epididymo-orchitis, chronic
Any condition classifiable to 098.13, specified as chronic
Chronic gonococcal orchitis

098.34 Gonococcal seminal vesiculitis, chronic
Any condition classifiable to 098.14, specified as chronic
Gonorrhea of seminal vesicle, chronic

098.35 Gonococcal cervicitis, chronic
Any condition classifiable to 098.15, specified as chronic
Gonorrhea of cervix, chronic

098.36 Gonococcal endometritis, chronic
Any condition classifiable to 098.16, specified as chronic

098.37 Gonococcal salpingitis (chronic)

098.39 Other

⑤ **098.4 Gonococcal infection of eye**

098.40 Gonococcal conjunctivitis (neonatorum)
Gonococcal ophthalmia (neonatorum)

098.41 Gonococcal iridocyclitis

098.42 Gonococcal endophthalmia

098.43 Gonococcal keratitis

098.49 Other

098.5 Gonococcal infection of joint

098.50 Gonococcal arthritis
Gonococcal infection of joint NOS

098.51 Gonococcal synovitis and tenosynovitis

098.52 Gonococcal bursitis

098.53 Gonococcal spondylitis

098.59 Other
Gonococcal rheumatism

098.6 Gonococcal infection of pharynx

098.7 Gonococcal infection of anus and rectum
Gonococcal proctitis

⑤ **098.8 Gonococcal infection of other specified sites**

098.81 Gonococcal keratosis (blennorrhagica)

098.82 Gonococcal meningitis

098.83 Gonococcal pericarditis

098.84 Gonococcal endocarditis

098.85 Other gonococcal heart disease

098.86 Gonococcal peritonitis

098.89 Other
Gonococcemia

099 Other venereal diseases

099.0 Chancroid

Bubo (inguinal):	Chancre:
chancroidal	Ducrey's
due to Hemophilus ducreyi	simple
	soft
	Ulcus molle (cutis) (skin)

099.1 Lymphogranuloma venereum

Climatic or tropical bubo	Esthiomene
(Durand-) Nicolas- Favre	Lymphogranuloma inguinale
disease	

099.2 Granuloma inguinale

Donovanosis	Granuloma venereum
Granuloma pudendi	Pudendal ulcer
(ulcerating)	

● Code new to this edition   ▲ Revision of existing code   ④ ⑤ Fourth or fifth digit required

099.3 Reiter's disease
Reiter's syndrome
Use additional code for associated:
arthropathy (711.1)
conjunctivitis (372.33)

⑤ **099.4 Other nongonococcal urethritis [NGU]**

`099.40` **Unspecified**
Nonspecific urethritis

`099.41` **Chlamydia trachomatis**

`099.49` **Other specified organism**

⑤ **099.5 Other venereal diseases due to Chlamydia trachomatis**

Excludes: *Chlamydia trachomatis infection of conjunctiva (076.0-076.9, 077.0, 077.9)*
Lymphogranuloma venereum (099.1)

`099.50` **Unspecified site**

`099.51` **Pharynx**

`099.52` **Anus and rectum**

`099.53` **Lower genitourinary sites**

Excludes: *urethra (099.41)*
Use additional code, if desired, to specify site of infection, such as:
bladder (595.4)
cervix (616.0)
vagina and vulva (616.11)

`099.54` **Other genitourinary sites**
Use additional code, if desired, to specify site of infection, such as:
pelvic inflammatory disease NOS (614.9)
testis and epididymis (604.91)

`099.55` **Unspecified genitourinary site**

`099.56` **Peritoneum**
Perihepatitis

`099.59` **Other specified site**

`099.8` **Other specified venereal diseases**

`099.9` **Venereal disease, unspecified**

OTHER SPIROCHETAL DISEASES (100-104)

`100` **Leptospirosis**

100.0 Leptospirosis icterohemorrhagica
Leptospiral or spirochetal jaundice (hemorrhagic)
Weil's disease

⑤ **100.8 Other specified leptospiral infections**

`100.81` **Leptospiral meningitis (aseptic)**

`100.89` **Other**

Fever:	Infection by Leptospira:
Fort Bragg	australis
pretibial	bataviae
swamp	pyrogenes

`100.9` **Leptospirosis, unspecified**

101 Vincent's angina

Acute necrotizing ulcerative:	Spirochetal stomatitis
gingivitis	Trench mouth
stomatitis	Vincent's:
Fusospirochetal pharyngitis	gingivitis
	infection [any site]

`102` **Yaws**
Includes: frambesia
pian

102.0 Initial lesions

Chancre of yaws	Initial frambesial ulcer
Frambesia, initial or primary	Mother yaw

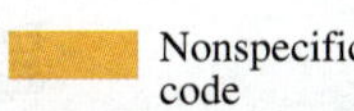

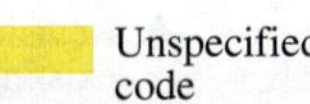

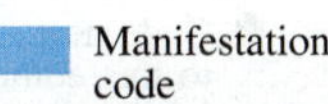

102.1 Multiple papillomata and wet crab yaws
Butter yaws   Planter or palmer papilloma of yaws
Frambesioma
Pianoma

102.2 Other early skin lesions
Early yaws (cutaneous) (macular) (papular) (maculopapular) (micropapular)
Frambeside of early yaws
Cutaneous yaws, less than five years after infection

102.3 Hyperkeratosis
Ghoul hand
Hyperkeratosis, palmer or plantar (early) (late) due to yaws
Worm-eaten soles

102.4 Gummata and ulcers
Nodular late yaws (ulcerated)
Gummatous frambeside

102.5 Gangosa
Rhinopharyngitis mutilans

102.6 Bone and joint lesions
Goundou
Gumma, bone   } of yaws (late)
Gummatous osteitis or periostitis

Hydrarthrosis
Osteitis   } of yaws (early) (late)
Periostitis (hypertrophic)

102.7 Other manifestations
Juxta-articular nodules of yaws
Mucosal yaws

102.8 Latent yaws
Yaws without clinical manifestations, with positive serology

102.9 Yaws, unspecified

103 Pinta

103.0 Primary lesions
Chancre (primary)
Papule (primary)   } of pinta [carate]
Pintid

103.1 Intermediate lesions
Erythematous plaques
Hyperchromic lesions   } of pinta [carate]
Hyperkeratosis

103.2 Late lesions
Cardiovascular lesions
Skin lesions:
  achromic
  cicatricial   } of pinta [carate]
  dyschromic
Vitiligo

103.3 Mixed lesions
Achromic and hyperchromic skin lesions of pinta [carate]

103.9 Pinta, unspecified

104 Other spirochetal infection

104.0 Nonvenereal endemic syphilis
Bejel   Njovera

104.8 Other specified spirochetal infections
Excludes: *relapsing fever (087.0-087.9)*
syphilis (090.0-097.9)

104.9 Spirochetal infection, unspecified

● Code new   ▲ Revision of   ④ ⑤ Fourth or fifth
  to this edition   existing code   digit required

MYCOSES (110-118)

Use additional code, if desired, to identify manifestation, as:
arthropathy (711.6)
meningitis (321.0-321.1)
otitis externa (380.15)

Excludes: *infection by Actinomycetales, such as species of Actinomyces, Actinomadura, Nocardia, Streptomyces (039.0-039.9)*

110 Dermatophytosis
Includes:

infection by species of Epidermophyton, Microsporum, and Trichophyton
tinea, any type except those in 111

110.0 Of scalp and beard
Kerion
Sycosis, mycotic
Trichophytic tinea [black dot tinea], scalp

110.1 Of nail
Dermatophytic onychia   Tinea unguium
Onychomycosis

110.2 Of hand
Tinea manuum

110.3 Of groin and perianal area
Dhobie itch   Tinea cruris
Eczema marginatum

110.4 Of foot
Athlete's foot   Tinea pedis

110.5 Of the body
Herpes circinatus
Tinea imbricata [Tokelau]

110.6 Deep seated dermatophytosis
Granuloma trichophyticum
Majocchi's granuloma

110.8 Of other specified sites

110.9 Of unspecified site
Favus NOS   Ringworm NOS
Microsporic tinea NOS

111 Dermatomycosis, other and unspecified

111.0 Pityriasis versicolor
Infection by Malassezia [Pityrosporum] furfur
Tinea flava
Tinea versicolor

111.1 Tinea nigra
Infection by   Microsporosis nigra
    Cladosporium species   Pityriasis nigra
Keratomycosis nigricans   Tinea palmaris nigra

111.2 Tinea blanca
Infection by Trichosporon (beigelii) cutaneum
White piedra

111.3 Black piedra
Infection by Piedraia hortai

111.8 Other specified dermatomycoses

111.9 Dermatomycosis, unspecified

112 Candidiasis
Includes: infection by Candida species
moniliasis

Excludes: *neonatal monilial infection (771.7)*

112.0 Of mouth
Thrush (oral)

112.1 Of vulva and vagina
Candidal vulvovaginitis   Monilial vulvovaginitis

112.2 Of other urogenital sites
Candidal balanitis

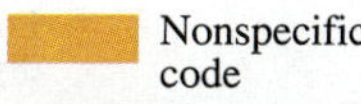

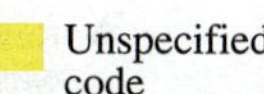

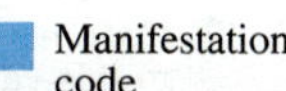

112.3 Of skin and nails
Candidal intertrigo
Candidal onychia
Candidal perionyxis [paronychia]

112.4 Of lung
Candidal pneumonia

112.5 Disseminated
Systemic candidiasis

⑤ **112.8 Of other specified sites**

    112.81 Candidal endocarditis

    112.82 Candidal otitis externa
      Otomycosis in moniliasis

    112.83 Candidal meningitis

    112.84 Candidal esophagitis

    112.85 Candidal enteritis

    112.89 Other

112.9 Of unspecified site

114 Coccidioidomycosis
Includes: infection by Coccidioides (immitis)
Posada-Wernicke disease

114.0 Primary coccidioidomycosis (pulmonary)
Acute pulmonary coccidioidomycosis
Coccidioidomycotic pneumonitis
Desert rheumatism
Pulmonary coccidioidomycosis
San Joaquin Valley fever

114.1 Primary extrapulmonary coccidioidomycosis
Chancriform syndrome
Primary cutaneous coccidioidomycosis

114.2 Coccidioidal meningitis

114.3 Other forms of progressive coccidioidomycosis
Coccidioidal granuloma
Disseminated coccidioidomycosis

114.4 Chronic pulmonary coccidioidomycosis

114.5 Pulmonary coccidioidomycosis, unspecified

114.9 Coccidioidomycosis, unspecified

⑤ **115 Histoplasmosis**
The following fifth-digit subclassification is for use with category 115:

    0 without mention of manifestation

    1 meningitis

    2 retinitis

    3 pericarditis

    4 endocarditis

    5 pneumonia

    9 other

⑤ **115.0 Infection by Histoplasma capsulatum**
American histoplasmosis
Darling's disease
Reticuloendothelial cytomycosis
Small form histoplasmosis

⑤ **115.1 Infection by Histoplasma duboisii**
African histoplasmosis
Large form histoplasmosis

⑤ **115.9 Histoplasmosis, unspecified**
Histoplasmosis NOS

116 Blastomycotic infection

● Code new
  to this edition

▲ Revision of
  existing code

④ ⑤ Fourth or fifth
    digit required

116.0 Blastomycosis
Blastomycotic dermatitis
Chicago disease
Cutaneous blastomycosis
Disseminated blastomycosis
Gilchrist's disease
Infection by Blastomyces [Ajellomyces] dermatitidis
North American blastomycosis
Primary pulmonary blastomycosis

116.1 Paracoccidioidomycosis
Brazilian blastomycosis
Infection by Paracoccidioides [Blastomyces] brasiliensis
Lutz-Splendore-Almeida disease
Mucocutaneous-lymphangitic paracoccidioidomycosis
Pulmonary paracoccidioidomycosis
South American blastomycosis
Visceral paracoccidioidomycosis

116.2 Lobomycosis
Infections by Loboa [Blastomyces] loboi
Keloidal blastomycosis
Lobo's disease

117 Other mycoses

117.0 Rhinosporidiosis
Infection by Rhinosporidium seeberi

117.1 Sporotrichosis
Cutaneous sporotrichosis
Disseminated sporotrichosis
Infection by Sporothrix [Sporotrichum] schenckii
Lymphocutaneous sporotrichosis
Pulmonary sporotrichosis
Sporotrichosis of the bones

117.2 Chromoblastomycosis
Chromomycosis
Infection by Cladosporidium carrionii, Fonsecaea compactum, Fonsecaea pedrosoi,
Phialophora verrucosa

117.3 Aspergillosis
Infection by Aspergillus species, mainly A. fumigatus, A. flavus group, A. terreus group

117.4 Mycotic mycetomas
Infection by various genera and species of Ascomycetes and Deuteromycetes, such as
Acremonium [Cephalosporium] falciforme, Neotestudina rosatii, Madurella grisea,
Madurella mycetomii, Pyrenochaeta romeroi, Zopfia [Leptosphaeria] senegalensis
Madura foot, mycotic
Maduromycosis, mycotic

Excludes: *actinomycotic mycetomas (039.0-039.9)*

117.5 Cryptococcosis

Busse-Buschke's disease	Pulmonary cryptococcosis
European cryptococcosis	Systemic cryptococcosis
Infection by Cryptococcus neoformans	Torula

117.6 Allescheriosis [Petriellidosis]
Infections by Allescheria [Petriellidium] boydii [Monosporium apiospermum]

Excludes: *mycotic mycetoma (117.4)*

117.7 Zygomycosis [Phycomycosis or Mucormycosis]
Infection by species of Absidia, Basidiobolus, Conidiobolus, Cunninghamella,
Entomophthora, Mucor, Rhizopus, Saksenaea

117.8 Infection by dematiacious fungi, [Phaehyphomycosis]
Infection by dematiacious fungi, such as Cladosporium trichoides [bantianum], Dreschlera
hawaiiensis, Phialophora gougerotii, Phialophora jeanselmi

117.9 Other and unspecified mycoses

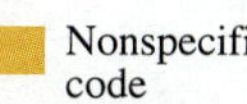
Add 4th or
5th digit

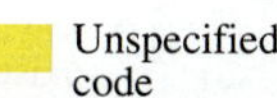
Nonspecific
code

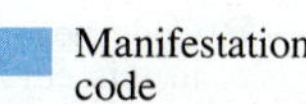
Unspecified
code

Manifestation
code

118 Opportunistic mycoses

Infection of skin, subcutaneous tissues, and/or organs by a wide variety of fungi generally considered to be pathogenic to compromised hosts only (e.g., infection by species of Alternaria, Dreschlera, Fusarium)

HELMINTHIASES (120-129)

120 Schistosomiasis [bilharziasis]

120.0 Schistosoma haematobium

Vesical schistosomiasis NOS

120.1 Schistosoma mansoni

Intestinal schistosomiasis NOS

120.2 Schistosoma japonicum

Asiatic schistosomiasis NOS
Katayama disease or fever

120.3 Cutaneous

Cercarial dermatitis

Schistosome dermatitis

Infection by cercariae

Swimmers' itch

of Schistosoma

120.8 Other specified schistosomiasis

Infection by Schistosoma:

Infection by Schistosoma spindale

bovis

Schistosomiasis chestermani

intercalatum
mattheii

120.9 Schistosomiasis, unspecified

Blood flukes NOS

Hemic distomiasis

121 Other trematode infections

121.0 Opisthorchiasis

Infection by:
cat liver fluke
Opisthorchis (felineus) (tenuicollis) (viverrini)

121.1 Clonorchiasis

Biliary cirrhosis due to clonorchiasis
Chinese liver fluke disease
Hepatic distomiasis due to Clonorchis sinensis
Oriental liver fluke disease

121.2 Paragonimiasis

Infection by Paragonimus

Pulmonary distomiasis

Lung fluke disease (oriental)

121.3 Fascioliasis

Infection by Fasciola:

Liver flukes NOS

gigantica

Sheep liver fluke infection

hepatica

121.4 Fasciolopsiasis

Infection by Fasciolopsis [buski]
Intestinal distomiasis

121.5 Metagonimiasis

Infection by Metagonimus yokogawai

121.6 Heterophyiasis

Infection by:
Heterophyes heterophyes
Stellantchasmus falcatus

121.8 Other specified trematode infections

Infection by:
Dicrocoelium dendriticum
Echinostoma ilocanum
Gastrodiscoides hominis

121.9 Trematode infection, unspecified

Distomiasis NOS

Fluke disease NOS

122 Echinococcosis

Includes: echinococciasis
hydatid disease
hydatidosis

122.0 Echinococcus granulosus infection of liver

122.1 Echinococcus granulosus infection of lung

● Code new
to this edition

▲ Revision of
existing code

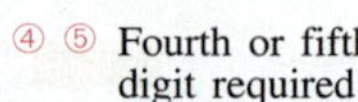
④ ⑤ Fourth or fifth
digit required

122.2 Echinococcus granulosus infection of thyroid

122.3 Echinococcus granulosus infection, other

122.4 Echinococcus granulosus infection, unspecified

122.5 Echinococcus multilocularis infection of liver

122.6 Echinococcus multilocularis infection, other

122.7 Echinococcus multilocularis infection, unspecified

122.8 Echinococcosis, unspecified, of liver

122.9 Echinococcosis, other and unspecified

123 Other cestode infection

123.0 Taenia solium infection, intestinal form
Pork tapeworm (adult) (infection)

123.1 Cysticercosis
Cysticerciasis
Infection by Cysticercus cellulosae [larval form of Taenia solium]

123.2 Taenia saginata infection
Beef tapeworm (infection)
Infection by Taeniarhynchus saginatus

123.3 Taeniasis, unspecified

123.4 Diphyllobothriasis, intestinal
Diphyllobothrium (adult) (latum) (pacificum) infection
Fish tapeworm (infection)

123.5 Sparganosis [larval diphyllobothriasis]
Infection by:
Diphyllobothrium larvae
Sparganum (mansoni) (proliferum)
Spirometra larvae

123.6 Hymenolepiasis
Dwarf tapeworm (infection)
Hymenolepis (diminuta) (nana) infection
Rat tapeworm (infection)

123.8 Other specified cestode infection
Diplogonoporus (grandis) ⎫
Dipylidium (caninum)   ⎬ infection
Dog tapeworm (infection) ⎭

123.9 Cestode infection, unspecified
Tapeworm (infection) NOS

124 Trichinosis
Trichinella spiralis infection   Trichinellosis
Trichiniasis

125 Filarial infection and dracontiasis

125.0 Bancroftian filariasis
Chyluria   ⎫
Elephantiasis   ⎪
Infection   ⎬ due to Wuchereria bancrofti
Lymphadenitis   ⎪
Lymphangitis   ⎭
Wuchereriasis

125.1 Malayan filariasis
Brugia filariasis ⎫
Chyluria   ⎪
Elephantiasis   ⎬ due to Brugia [Wuchereria] malayi
Infection   ⎪
Lymphadenitis   ⎪
Lymphangitis   ⎭

125.2 Loiasis
Eyeworm disease of Africa
Loa loa infection

125.3 Onchocerciasis
Onchocerca volvulus infection
Onchocercosis

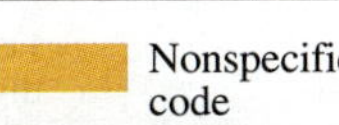

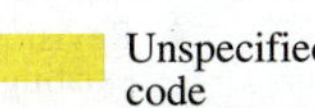

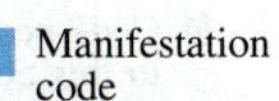

125.4 Dipetalonemiasis
Infection by:
    Acanthocheilonema perstans
    Dipetalonema perstans

125.5 Mansonella ozzardi infection
Filariasis ozzardi

125.6 Other specified filariasis
Dirofilaria infection
Infection by:
    Acanthocheilonema streptocerca
    Dipetalonema streptocerca

125.7 Dracontiasis
Guinea-worm infection
Infection by Dracunculus medinensis

125.9 Unspecified filariasis

126 Ancylostomiasis and necatoriasis
Includes: cutaneous larva migrans due to Ancylostoma
                hookworm (disease) (infection)
                uncinariasis

126.0 Ancylostoma duodenale

126.1 Necator americanus

126.2 Ancylostoma braziliense

126.3 Ancylostoma ceylanicum

126.8 Other specified Ancylostoma

126.9 Ancylostomiasis and necatoriasis, unspecified
Creeping eruption NOS
Cutaneous larva migrans NOS

127 Other intestinal helminthiases

127.0 Ascariasis
Ascaridiasis
Infection by Ascaris lumbricoides
Roundworm infection

127.1 Anisakiasis
Infection by Anisakis larva

127.2 Strongyloidiasis
Infection by Strongyloides stercoralis

> *Excludes:* *trichostrongyliasis (127.6)*

127.3 Trichuriasis
Infection by Trichuris trichiuria
Trichocephaliasis
Whipworm (disease) (infection)

127.4 Enterobiasis
Infection by Enterobius vermicularis
Oxyuriasis
Oxyuris vermicularis infection
Pinworn (disease) (infection)
Threadworm infection

127.5 Capillariasis
Infection by Capillaria philippinensis

> *Excludes:* *infection by Capillaria hepatica (128.8)*

127.6 Trichostrongyliasis
Infection by Trichostrongylus species

127.7 Other specified intestinal helminthiasis
Infection by:
    Oesophagostomum apiostomum and related species
    Ternidens diminutus
    other specified intestinal helminth
Physalopteriasis

127.8 Mixed intestinal helminthiasis
Infection by intestinal helminths classified to more than one of the categories
    120.0-127.7
Mixed helminthiasis NOS

● Code new
   to this edition   ▲ Revision of
                                existing code   ④ ⑤ Fourth or fifth
                                                              digit required

127.9 Intestinal helminthiasis, unspecified

128 Other and unspecified helminthiases

128.0 Toxocariasis
Larva migrans visceralis
Toxocara (canis) (cati) infection
Visceral larva migrans syndrome

128.1 Gnathostomiasis
Infection by Gnathostoma spinigerum and related species

128.8 Other specified helminthiasis
Infection by:
Angiostrongylus cantonensis
Capillaria hepatica
other specified helminth

128.9 Helminth infection, unspecified
Helminthiasis NOS   Worms NOS

129 Intestinal parasitism, unspecified

OTHER INFECTIOUS AND PARASITIC DISEASES (130-136)

130 Toxoplasmosis
Includes: infection by toxoplasma gondii
toxoplasmosis (acquired)

Excludes: *congenital toxoplasmosis (771.2)*

130.0 Meningoencephalitis due to toxoplasmosis
Encephalitis due to acquired toxoplasmosis

130.1 Conjunctivitis due to toxoplasmosis

130.2 Chorioretinitis due to toxoplasmosis
Focal retinochoroiditis due to acquired toxoplasmosis

130.3 Myocarditis due to toxoplasmosis

130.4 Pneumonitis due to toxoplasmosis

130.5 Hepatitis due to toxoplasmosis

130.7 Toxoplasmosis of other specified sites

130.8 Multisystemic disseminated toxoplasmosis
Toxoplasmosis of multiple sites

130.9 Toxoplasmosis, unspecified

131 Trichomoniasis
Includes: infection due to Trichomonas (vaginalis)

⑤ **131.0 Urogenital trichomoniasis**

131.00 Urogenital trichomoniasis, unspecified
Fluor (vaginalis)   ⎱ trichomonal or due to Trichomonas
Leukorrhea (vaginalis)   ⎰   (vaginalis)

131.01 Trichomonal vulvovaginitis
Vaginitis, trichomonal or due to Trichomonas (vaginalis)

131.02 Trichomonal urethritis

131.03 Trichomonal prostatitis

131.09 Other

131.8 Other specified sites

Excludes: *intestinal (007.3)*

131.9 Trichomoniasis, unspecified

132 Pediculosis and phthirus infestation

132.0 Pediculus capitis [head louse]

132.1 Pediculus corporis [body louse]

132.2 Phthirus pubis [pubic louse]
Pediculus pubis

132.3 Mixed infestation
Infestation classifiable to more than one of the categories 132.0-132.2

132.9 Pediculosis, unspecified

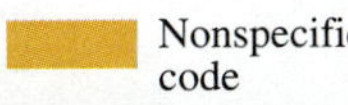

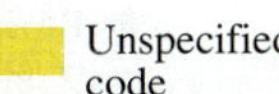

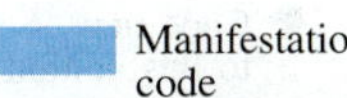

Manifestation
code

133 Acariasis

    133.0 Scabies
        Infestation by Sarcoptes   Norwegian scabies
          scabiei   Sarcoptic itch

    133.8 Other acariasis
        Chiggers
        Infestation by:
          Demodex folliculorum
          Trombicula

    133.9 Acariasis, unspecified
        Infestation by mites NOS

134 Other infestation

    134.0 Myiasis
        Infestation by: Infestation by:
          Dermatobia (hominis)   maggots
          fly larvae   Oestrus ovis
          Gasterophilus (intestinalis)

    134.1 Other arthropod infestation
        Infestation by: Jigger disease
          chigoe   Scarabiasis
          sand flea   Tungiasis
          Tunga penetrans

    134.2 Hirudiniasis
        Hirudiniasis (external) (internal)
        Leeches (aquatic) (land)

    134.8 Other specified infestations

    134.9 Infestation, unspecified
        Infestation (skin) NOS   Skin parasites NOS

135 Sarcoidosis
    Besnier-Boeck- Schaumann disease   Sarcoid (any site):
    Lupoid (miliary) of Boeck   NOS
    Lupus pernio (Besnier)   Boeck
    Lymphogranulomatosis, benign   Darier-Roussy
        (Schaumann's)   Uveoparotid fever

136 Other and unspecified infectious and parasitic diseases

    136.0 Ainhum
        Dactylolysis spontanea

    136.1 Behçet's syndrome

    136.2 Specific infections by free-living amebae
        Meningoencephalitis due to Naegleria

    136.3 Pneumocystosis
        Pneumonia due to Pneumocystis carinii

    136.4 Psorospermiasis

    136.5 Sarcosporidiosis
        Infection by Sarcocystis lindemanni

    136.8 Other specified infectious and parasitic diseases
        Candiru infestation

    136.9 Unspecified infectious and parasitic diseases
        Infectious disease NOS
        Parasitic disease NOS

LATE EFFECTS OF INFECTIOUS AND PARASITIC DISEASES (137-139)

137 Late effects of tuberculosis

    Note: This category is to be used to indicate conditions classifiable to 010-018 as the cause of late effects, which are themselves classified elsewhere. The "late effects" include those specified as such, as sequelae, or as due to old or inactive tuberculosis, without evidence of active disease.

    137.0 Late effects of respiratory or unspecified tuberculosis

    137.1 Late effects of central nervous system tuberculosis

    137.2 Late effects of genitourinary tuberculosis

    137.3 Late effects of tuberculosis of bones and joints

    137.4 Late effects of tuberculosis of other specified organs

● Code new to this edition   ▲ Revision of existing code   ④ ⑤ Fourth or fifth digit required

138 Late effects of acute poliomyelitis

> Note: This category is to be used to indicate conditions classifiable to 045 as the cause of late effects, which are themselves classified elsewhere. The "late effects" include conditions specified as such, or as sequelae, or as due to old or inactive poliomyelitis, without evidence of active disease.

139 Late effects of other infectious and parasitic diseases

> Note: This category is to be used to indicate conditions classifiable to categories 001-009, 020-041, 046-136 as the cause of late effects, which are themselves classified elsewhere. The "late effects" include conditions specified as such; they also include sequela of diseases classifiable to the above categories if there is evidence that the disease itself is no longer present.

139.0 Late effects of viral encephalitis
> Late effects of conditions classifiable to 049.8-049.9, 062-064

139.1 Late effects of trachoma
> Late effects of conditions classifiable to 076

139.8 Late effects of other and unspecified infectious and parasitic diseases

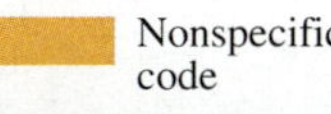

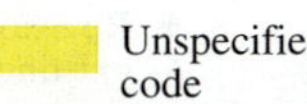

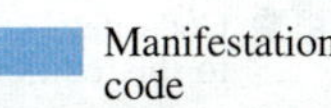

● Code new
to this edition

▲ Revision of
existing code

④ ⑤ Fourth or fifth
digit required

2. NEOPLASMS (140-239)

Notes:

1. Content
This chapter contains the following broad groups:

140-195 **Malignant neoplasms, stated or presumed to be primary, of specified sites, except of lymphatic and hematopoietic tissue**

196-198 **Malignant neoplasms, stated or presumed to be secondary, of specified sites**

199 **Malignant neoplasms, without specification of site**

200-208 **Malignant neoplasms, stated or presumed to be primary, of lymphatic and hematopoietic tissue**

210-229 **Benign neoplasms**

230-234 **Carcinoma in situ**

235-238 **Neoplasms of uncertain behavior [see Note, page 92]**

239 **Neoplasms of unspecified nature**

2. Functional activity
All neoplasms are classified in this chapter, whether or not functionally active. An additional code from Chapter 3 may be used, if desired, to identify such functional activity associated with any neoplasm, e.g.:

catecholamine-producing malignant pheochromocytoma of adrenal:
code 194.0, additional code 255.6
basophil adenoma of pituitary with Cushing's syndrome:
code 227.3, additional code 255.0

3. Morphology [Histology]
For those wishing to identify the histological type of neoplasms, a comprehensive coded nomenclature, which comprises the morphology rubrics of the ICD-Oncology, is given on pages 529-542.

4. Malignant neoplasms overlapping site boundaries
Categories 140-195 are for the classification of primary malignant neoplasms according to their point of origin. A malignant neoplasm that overlaps two or more subcategories within a three-digit rubric and whose point of origin cannot be determined should be classified to the subcategory .8 "Other." For example, "carcinoma involving tip and ventral surface of tongue" should be assigned to 141.8. On the other hand, "carcinoma of tip of tongue, extending to involve the ventral surface" should be coded to 141.2, as the point of origin, the tip, is known. Three subcategories (149.8, 159.8, 165.8) have been provided for malignant neoplasms that overlap the boundaries of three-digit rubrics within certain systems. Overlapping malignant neoplasms that cannot be classified as indicated above should be assigned to the appropriate subdivision of category 195 (Malignant neoplasm of other and ill-defined sites).

MALIGNANT NEOPLASM OF LIP, ORAL CAVITY, AND PHARYNX (140-149)

> Excludes: *carcinoma in situ (230.0)*

140 **Malignant neoplasm of lip**

> Excludes: *skin of lip (173.0)*

140.0 Upper lip, vermilion border
Upper lip:
NOS
external
lipstick area

140.1 Lower lip, vermilion border
Lower lip:
NOS
external
lipstick area

140.3 Upper lip, inner aspect

Upper lip:	Upper lip:
buccal aspect	mucosa
frenulum	oral aspect

140.4 Lower lip, inner aspect

Lower lip:	Lower lip:
buccal aspect	mucosa
frenulum	oral aspect

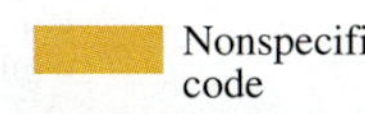

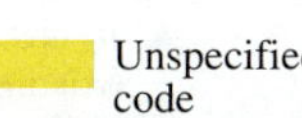

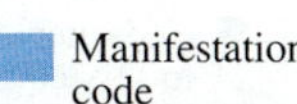

140.5 Lip, unspecified, inner aspect
>Lip, not specified whether upper or lower:
>>buccal aspect
>>frenulum
>>mucosa
>>oral aspect

140.6 Commissure of lip
>Labial commissure

140.8 Other sites of lip
>Malignant neoplasm of contiguous or overlapping sites of lip whose point of origin cannot be determined

140.9 Lip, unspecified, vermilion border
>Lip, not specified as upper or lower:
>>NOS
>>external
>>lipstick area

141 Malignant neoplasm of tongue

141.0 Base of tongue
>Dorsal surface of base of tongue
>Fixed part of tongue NOS

141.1 Dorsal surface of tongue
>Anterior two-thirds of tongue, dorsal surface
>Dorsal tongue NOS
>Midline of tongue

>*Excludes:* dorsal surface of base of tongue (141.0)

141.2 Tip and lateral border of tongue

141.3 Ventral surface of tongue
>Anterior two-thirds of tongue, ventral surface
>Frenulum linguae

141.4 Anterior two-thirds of tongue, part unspecified
>Mobile part of tongue NOS

141.5 Junctional zone
>Border of tongue at junction of fixed and mobile parts at insertion of anterior tonsillar pillar

141.6 Lingual tonsil

141.8 Other sites of tongue
>Malignant neoplasm of contiguous or overlapping sites of tongue whose point of origin cannot be determined

141.9 Tongue, unspecified
>Tongue NOS

142 Malignant neoplasm of major salivary glands
>Includes: salivary ducts

>*Excludes:* malignant neoplasm of minor salivary glands:
>>NOS (145.9)
>>buccal mucosa (145.0)
>>soft palate (145.3)
>>tongue (141.0-141.9)
>>tonsil, palatine (146.0)

142.0 Parotid gland

142.1 Submandibular gland
>Submaxillary gland

142.2 Sublingual gland

142.8 Other major salivary glands
>Malignant neoplasm of contiguous or overlapping sites of salivary glands and ducts whose point of origin cannot be determined

142.9 Salivary gland, unspecified
>Salivary gland (major) NOS

● Code new
to this edition

▲ Revision of
existing code

④ ⑤ Fourth or fifth
digit required

143 **Malignant neoplasm of gum**
Includes: alveolar (ridge) mucosa
gingiva (alveolar) (marginal)
interdental papillae

Excludes: malignant odontogenic neoplasms (170.0-170.1)

143.0 **Upper gum**

143.1 **Lower gum**

143.8 **Other sites of gum**
Malignant neoplasm of contiguous or overlapping sites of gum whose point of origin cannot be determined

143.9 **Gum, unspecified**

144 **Malignant neoplasm of floor of mouth**

144.0 **Anterior portion**
Anterior to the premolar-canine junction

144.1 **Lateral portion**

144.8 **Other sites of floor of mouth**
Malignant neoplasm of contiguous or overlapping sites of floor of mouth whose point of origin cannot be determined

144.9 **Floor of mouth, part unspecified**

145 **Malignant neoplasm of other and unspecified parts of mouth**

Excludes: mucosa of lips (140.0-140.9)

145.0 **Cheek mucosa**
Buccal mucosa   Cheek, inner aspect

145.1 **Vestibule of mouth**
Buccal sulcus (upper) (lower)
Labial sulcus (upper) (lower)

145.2 **Hard palate**

145.3 **Soft palate**

Excludes: nasopharyngeal [posterior] [superior] surface of soft palate (147.3)

145.4 **Uvula**

145.5 **Palate, unspecified**
Junction of hard and soft palate
Roof of mouth

145.6 **Retromolar area**

145.8 **Other specified parts of mouth**
Malignant neoplasm of contiguous or overlapping sites of mouth whose point of origin cannot be determined

145.9 **Mouth, unspecified**
Buccal cavity NOS
Minor salivary gland, unspecified site
Oral cavity NOS

146 **Malignant neoplasm of oropharynx**

146.0 **Tonsil**
Tonsil:
NOS
faucial
palatine

Excludes: lingual tonsil (141.6)
pharyngeal tonsil (147.1)

146.1 **Tonsillar fossa**

146.2 **Tonsillar pillars (anterior) (posterior)**
Faucial pillar   Palatoglossal arch
Glossopalatine fold   Palatopharyngeal arch

146.3 **Vallecula**
Anterior and medial surface of the pharyngoepiglottic fold

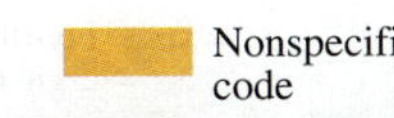

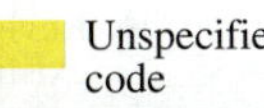

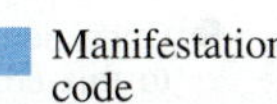

146.4 Anterior aspect of epiglottis
Epiglottis, free border [margin] Glossoepiglottic fold(s)

Excludes: *epiglottis:*
NOS (161.1)
suprahyoid portion (161.1)

146.5 Junctional region
Junction of the free margin of the epiglottis, the aryepiglottic fold, and the pharyngoepiglottic fold

146.6 Lateral wall of oropharynx

146.7 Posterior wall of oropharynx

146.8 Other specified sites of oropharynx
Branchial cleft
Malignant neoplasm of contiguous or overlapping sites of oropharynx whose point of origin cannot be determined

146.9 Oropharynx, unspecified

147 Malignant neoplasm of nasopharynx

147.0 Superior wall
Roof of nasopharynx

147.1 Posterior wall
Adenoid   Pharyngeal tonsil

147.2 Lateral wall
Fossa of Rosenmüller   Pharyngeal recess
Opening of auditory tube

147.3 Anterior wall
Floor of nasopharynx
Nasopharyngeal [posterior] [superior] surface of soft palate
Posterior margin of nasal septum and choanae

147.8 Other specified sites of nasopharynx
Malignant neoplasm of contiguous or overlapping sites of nasopharynx whose point of origin cannot be determined

147.9 Nasopharynx, unspecified
Nasopharyngeal wall NOS

148 Malignant neoplasm of hypopharynx

148.0 Postcricoid region

148.1 Pyriform sinus
Pyriform fossa

148.2 Aryepiglottic fold, hypopharyngeal aspect
Aryepiglottic fold or interarytenoid fold:
NOS
marginal zone

Excludes: *aryepiglottic fold or interarytenoid fold, laryngeal aspect (161.1)*

148.3 Posterior hypopharyngeal wall

148.8 Other specified sites of hypopharynx
Malignant neoplasm of contiguous or overlapping sites of hypopharynx whose point of origin cannot be determined

148.9 Hypopharynx, unspecified
Hypopharyngeal wall NOS   Hypopharynx NOS

149 Malignant neoplasm of other and ill-defined sites within the lip, oral cavity, and pharynx

149.0 Pharynx, unspecified

149.1 Waldeyer's ring

149.8 Other
Malignant neoplasms of lip, oral cavity, and pharynx whose point of origin cannot be assigned to any one of the categories 140-148

Excludes: *"book leaf" neoplasm [ventral surface of tongue and floor of mouth] (145.8)*

149.9 Ill-defined

● Code new to this edition   ▲ Revision of existing code   ④ ⑤ Fourth or fifth digit required

MALIGNANT NEOPLASM OF DIGESTIVE ORGANS AND PERITONEUM (150-159)

Excludes: carcinoma in situ (230.1-230.9)

150 Malignant neoplasm of esophagus

150.0 Cervical esophagus

150.1 Thoracic esophagus

150.2 Abdominal esophagus

Excludes: adenocarcinoma (151.0)
cardio-esophageal junction (151.0)

150.3 Upper third of esophagus
Proximal third of esophagus

150.4 Middle third of esophagus

150.5 Lower third of esophagus
Distal third of esophagus

Excludes: adenocarcinoma (151.0)
cardio-esophageal junction (151.0)

150.8 Other specified part
Malignant neoplasm of contiguous or overlapping sites of esophagus whose point of origin cannot be determined

150.9 Esophagus, unspecified

151 Malignant neoplasm of stomach

151.0 Cardia
Cardiac orifice Cardio-esophageal junction

Excludes: squamous cell carcinoma (150.2, 150.5)

151.1 Pylorus
Prepylorus Pyloric canal

151.2 Pyloric antrum
Antrum of stomach NOS

151.3 Fundus of stomach

151.4 Body of stomach

151.5 Lesser curvature, unspecified
Lesser curvature, not classifiable to 151.1-151.4

151.6 Greater curvature, unspecified
Greater curvature, not classifiable to 151.0-151.4

151.8 Other specified sites of stomach
Anterior wall, not classifiable to 151.0-151.4
Posterior wall, not classifiable to 151.0-151.4
Malignant neoplasm of contiguous or overlapping sites of stomach whose point of origin cannot be determined

151.9 Stomach, unspecified
Carcinoma ventriculi Gastric cancer

152 Malignant neoplasm of small intestine, including duodenum

152.0 Duodenum

152.1 Jejunum

152.2 Ileum

Excludes: ileocecal valve (153.4)

152.3 Meckel's diverticulum

152.8 Other specified sites of small intestine
Duodenojejunal junction
Malignant neoplasm of contiguous or overlapping sites of small intestine whose point of origin cannot be determined

152.9 Small intestine, unspecified

153 Malignant neoplasm of colon

153.0 Hepatic flexure

153.1 Transverse colon

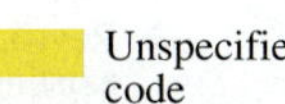
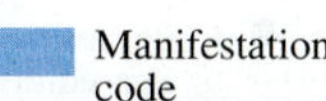

153.2 Descending colon
Left colon

153.3 Sigmoid colon
Sigmoid (flexure)

Excludes: rectosigmoid junction (154.0)

153.4 Cecum
Ileocecal valve

153.5 Appendix

153.6 Ascending colon
Right colon

153.7 Splenic flexure

153.8 Other specified sites of large intestine
Malignant neoplasm of contiguous or overlapping sites of colon whose point of origin
cannot be determined

Excludes: ileocecal valve (153.4)
rectosigmoid junction (154.0)

153.9 Colon, unspecified
Large intestine NOS

154 Malignant neoplasm of rectum, rectosigmoid junction, and anus

154.0 Rectosigmoid junction
Colon with rectum   Rectosigmoid (colon)

154.1 Rectum
Rectal ampulla

154.2 Anal canal
Anal sphincter

Excludes: skin of anus (172.5, 173.5)

154.3 Anus, unspecified

Excludes: anus:
margin (172.5, 173.5)
skin (172.5, 173.5)
perianal skin (172.5, 173.5)

154.8 Other
Anorectum
Cloacogenic zone
Malignant neoplasm of contiguous or overlapping sites of rectum, rectosigmoid
junction, and anus whose point of origin cannot be determined

155 Malignant neoplasm of liver and intrahepatic bile ducts

155.0 Liver, primary
Carcinoma:
liver, specified as primary
hepatocellular
liver cell
Hepatoblastoma

155.1 Intrahepatic bile ducts
Canaliculi biliferi   Intrahepatic:
Interlobular: biliary passages
bile ducts   canaliculi
biliary canals   gall duct

Excludes: hepatic duct (156.1)

155.2 Liver, not specified as primary or secondary

156 Malignant neoplasm of gallbladder and extrahepatic bile ducts

156.0 Gallbladder

156.1 Extrahepatic bile ducts
Biliary duct or passage NOS   Cystic duct
Common bile duct   Hepatic duct
Sphincter of Oddi

156.2 Ampulla of Vater

● Code new   ▲ Revision of   ④ ⑤ Fourth or fifth
to this edition   existing code   digit required

156.8 Other specified sites of gallbladder and extrahepatic bile ducts
Malignant neoplasm of contiguous or overlapping sites of gallbladder and extrahepatic bile ducts whose point of origin cannot be determined

156.9 Biliary tract, part unspecified
Malignant neoplasm involving both intrahepatic and extrahepatic bile ducts

157 Malignant neoplasm of pancreas

157.0 Head of pancreas

157.1 Body of pancreas

157.2 Tail of pancreas

157.3 Pancreatic duct
Duct of:
Santorini
Wirsung

157.4 Islets of Langerhans
Islets of Langerhans, any part of pancreas
Use additional code, if desired, to identify any functional activity

157.8 Other specified sites of pancreas
Ectopic pancreatic tissue
Malignant neoplasm of contiguous or overlapping sites of pancreas whose point of origin cannot be determined

157.9 Pancreas, part unspecified

158 Malignant neoplasm of retroperitoneum and peritoneum

158.0 Retroperitoneum
Periadrenal tissue
Perinephric tissue
Perirenal tissue
Retrocecal tissue

158.8 Specified parts of peritoneum
Cul-de-sac (of Douglas)
Mesentery
Mesocolon
Omentum
Malignant neoplasm of contiguous or overlapping sites of retroperitoneum and peritoneum whose point of origin cannot be determined
Peritoneum:
parietal
pelvic
Rectouterine pouch

158.9 Peritoneum, unspecified

159 Malignant neoplasm of other and ill-defined sites within the digestive organs and peritoneum

159.0 Intestinal tract, part unspecified
Intestine NOS

159.1 Spleen, not elsewhere classified
Angiosarcoma
Fibrosarcoma
} of spleen

Excludes: *Hodgkin's disease (201.0-201.9)*
lymphosarcoma (200.1)
reticulosarcoma (200.0)

159.8 Other sites of digestive system and intra-abdominal organs
Malignant neoplasm of digestive organs and peritoneum whose point of origin cannot be assigned to any one of the categories 150-158

Excludes: *anus and rectum (154.8)*
cardio-esophageal junction (151.0)
colon and rectum ORANGE (154.0)

159.9 Ill-defined
Alimentary canal or tract NOS
Gastrointestinal tract NOS

Excludes: *abdominal NOS (195.2)*
intra-abdominal NOS (195.2)

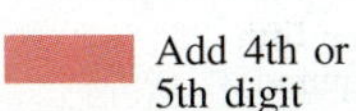

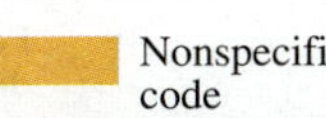

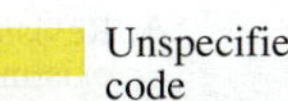

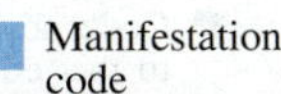

MALIGNANT NEOPLASM OF RESPIRATORY AND INTRATHORACIC ORGANS (160-165)

> *Excludes:* carcinoma in situ (231.0-231.9)

160 Malignant neoplasm of nasal cavities, middle ear, and accessory sinuses

160.0 Nasal cavities

Cartilage of nose	Septum of nose
Conchae, nasal	Vestibule of nose
Internal nose	

> *Excludes:* nasal bone (170.0)
> nose NOS (195.0)
> olfactory bulb (192.0)
> posterior margin of septum and choanae (147.3)
> skin of nose (172.3, 173.3)
> turbinates (170.0)

160.1 Auditory tube, middle ear, and mastoid air cells

Antrum tympanicum	Tympanic cavity
Eustachian tube	

> *Excludes:* auditory canal (external) (172.2, 173.2)
> bone of ear (meatus) (170.0)
> cartilage of ear (171.0)
> ear (external) (skin) (172.2, 173.2)

160.2 Maxillary sinus
Antrum (Highmore) (maxillary)

160.3 Ethmoidal sinus

160.4 Frontal sinus

160.5 Sphenoidal sinus

160.8 Other
Malignant neoplasm of contiguous or overlapping sites of nasal cavities, middle ear, and accessory sinuses whose point of origin cannot be determined

160.9 Accessory sinus, unspecified

161 Malignant neoplasm of larynx

161.0 Glottis

Intrinsic larynx	True vocal cord
Laryngeal commissure	Vocal cord NOS
(anterior) (posterior)	

161.1 Supraglottis
Aryepiglottic fold or interarytenoid fold, laryngeal aspect
Epiglottis (suprahyoid portion) NOS
Extrinsic larynx
False vocal cords
Posterior (laryngeal) surface of epiglottis
Ventricular bands

> *Excludes:* anterior aspect of epiglottis (146.4)
> aryepiglottic fold or interarytenoid fold:
>   NOS (148.2)
>   hypopharyngeal aspect (148.2)
>   marginal zone (148.2)

161.2 Subglottis

161.3 Laryngeal cartilages

Cartilage:	Cartilage:
arytenoid	cuneiform
cricoid	thyroid

161.8 Other specified sites of larynx
Malignant neoplasm of contiguous or overlapping sites of larynx whose point of origin cannot be determined

161.9 Larynx, unspecified

162 Malignant neoplasm of trachea, bronchus, and lung

162.0 Trachea

Cartilage	} of trachea
Mucosa	

● Code new
 to this edition   ▲ Revision of
 existing code   ④ ⑤ Fourth or fifth
 digit required

162.2 Main bronchus
      Carina   Hilus of lung

162.3 Upper lobe, bronchus or lung

162.4 Middle lobe, bronchus or lung

162.5 Lower lobe, bronchus or lung

162.8 Other parts of bronchus or lung
      Malignant neoplasm of contiguous or overlapping sites of bronchus or lung whose point of origin cannot be determined

162.9 Bronchus and lung, unspecified

163 Malignant neoplasm of pleura

163.0 Parietal pleura

163.1 Visceral pleura

163.8 Other specified sites of pleura
      Malignant neoplasm of contiguous or overlapping sites of pleura whose point of origin cannot be determined

163.9 Pleura, unspecified

164 Malignant neoplasm of thymus, heart, and mediastinum

164.0 Thymus

164.1 Heart
      Endocardium   Myocardium
      Epicardium   Pericardium

      Excludes: *great vessels (171.4)*

164.2 Anterior mediastinum

164.3 Posterior mediastinum

164.8 Other
      Malignant neoplasm of contiguous or overlapping sites of thymus, heart, and mediastinum whose point of origin cannot be determined

164.9 Mediastinum, part unspecified

165 Malignant neoplasm of other and ill-defined sites within the respiratory system and intrathoracic organs

165.0 Upper respiratory trace, part unspecified

165.8 Other
      Malignant neoplasm of respiratory and intrathoracic organs whose point of origin cannot be assigned to any one of the categories 160-164

165.9 Ill-defined sites within the respiratory system
      Respiratory tract NOS

      Excludes: *intrathoracic NOS (195.1)*
                thoracic NOS (195.1)

MALIGNANT NEOPLASM OF BONE, CONNECTIVE TISSUE, SKIN, AND BREAST (170-176)

      Excludes: *carcinoma in situ:*
                breast (233.0)
                skin (232.0-232.9)

170 Malignant neoplasm of bone and articular cartilage
      Includes: cartilage (articular) (joint)
                periosteum

      Excludes: *bone marrow NOS (202.9)*
                cartilage:
                  ear (171.0)
                  eyelid (171.0)
                  larynx (161.3)
                  nose (160.0)
                synovia (171.0-171.9)

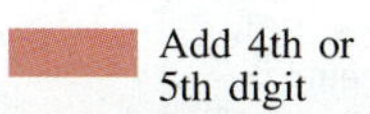

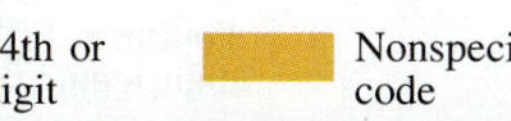

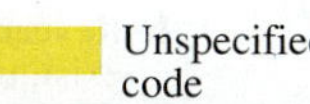

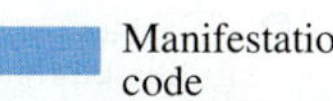

170.0 Bones of skull and face, except mandible

Bone:	Bone:
ethmoid	sphenoid
frontal	temporal
malar	zygomatic
nasal	Maxilla (superior)
occipital	Turbinate
orbital	Upper jaw bone
parietal	Vomer

> *Excludes:* *carcinoma, any type except intraosseous or odontogenic:*
> *maxilla, maxillary (sinus) (160.2)*
> *upper jaw bone (143.0)*
> *jaw bone (lower) (170.1)*

170.1 Mandible

Inferior maxilla	Lower jaw bone
Jaw bone NOS	

> *Excludes:* *carcinoma, any type except intraosseous or odontogenic:*
> *jaw bone NOS (143.9)*
> *lower (143.1)*
> *upper jaw bone (170.0)*

170.2 Vertebral column, excluding sacrum and coccyx

Spinal column	Vertebra
Spine	

> *Excludes:* *sacrum and coccyx (170.6)*

170.3 Ribs, sternum, and clavicle

Costal cartilage	Xiphoid process
Costovertebral joint	

170.4 Scapula and long bones of upper limb

Acromion	Radius
Bones NOS of upper limb	Ulna
Humerus	

170.5 Short bones of upper limb

Carpal	Scaphoid (of hand)
Cuneiform, wrist	Semilunar or lunate
Metacarpal	Trapezium
Navicular, of hand	Trapezoid
Phalanges of hand	Unciform
Pisiform	

170.6 Pelvic bones, sacrum, and coccyx

Coccygeal vertebra	Pubic bone
Ilium	Sacral vertebra
Ischium	

170.7 Long bones of lower limb

Bones NOS of lower limb	Fibula
Femur	Tibia

170.8 Short bones of lower limb

Astragalus [talus]	Navicular (of ankle)
Calcaneus	Patella
Cuboid	Phalanges of foot
Cuneiform, ankle	Tarsal
Metatarsal	

170.9 Bone and articular cartilage, site unspecified

● Code new
to this edition

▲ Revision of
existing code

④ ⑤ Fourth or fifth
digit required

171 Malignant neoplasm of connective and other soft tissue
    Includes: blood vessel
                bursa
                fascia
                fat
                ligament, except uterine
                muscle
                peripheral, sympathetic, and parasympathetic nerves and ganglia
                synovia
                tendon (sheath)

       Excludes: *cartilage (of):*
                    articular (170.0-170.9)
                    larynx (161.3)
                    nose (160.0)
              connective tissue:
                breast (174.0-175.9)
                internal organs—code to malignant neoplasm of the site [e.g., leiomyosarcoma of
                    stomach, 151.9]
                heart (164.1)
                uterine ligament (183.4)

171.0 Head, face, and neck
    Cartilage of:
      ear
      eyelid

171.2 Upper limb, including shoulder

Arm	Forearm
Finger	Hand

171.3 Lower limb, including hip

Foot	Thigh
Leg	Toe
Popliteal space	

171.4 Thorax

Axilla	Great vessels
Diaphragm	

       Excludes: *heart (164.1)*
                mediastinum (164.2-164.9)
                thymus (164.0)

171.5 Abdomen

Abdominal wall	Hypochondrium

       Excludes: *peritoneum (158.8)*
                retroperitoneum (158.0)

171.6 Pelvis

Buttock	Inguinal region
Groin	Perineum

       Excludes: *pelvic peritoneum (158.8)*
                retroperitoneum (158.0)
                uterine ligament, any (183.3-183.5)

171.7 Trunk, unspecified

Back NOS	Flank NOS

171.8 Other specified sites of connective and other soft tissue
    Malignant neoplasm of contiguous or overlapping sites of connective tissue whose point
      of origin cannot be determined

171.9 Connective and other soft tissue, site unspecified

172 Malignant melanoma of skin
    Includes: melanocarcinoma
                melanoma (skin) NOS

       Excludes: *skin of genital organs (184.0-184.9, 187.1-187.9)*
                sites other than skin—code to malignant neoplasm of the site

172.0 Lip

       Excludes: *vermilion border of lip (140.0-140.1, 140.9)*

172.1 Eyelid, including canthus

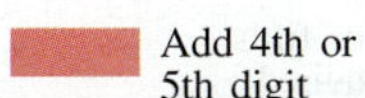
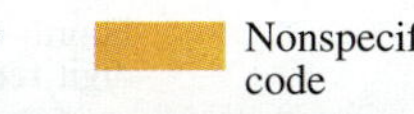

	Add 4th or 5th digit		Nonspecific code		Unspecified code		Manifestation code

172.2 **Ear and external auditory canal**
Auricle (ear)
Auricular canal, external
External [acoustic] meatus
Pinna

172.3 **Other and unspecified parts of face**
Cheek (external)   Forehead
Chin   Nose, external
Eyebrow   Temple

172.4 **Scalp and neck**

172.5 **Trunk, except scrotum**
Axilla   Perianal skin
Breast   Perineum
Buttock   Umbilicus
Groin

    Excludes: *anal canal (154.2)*
        anus NOS (154.3)
        scrotum (187.7)

172.6 **Upper limb, including shoulder**
Arm   Forearm
Finger   Hand

172.7 **Lower limb, including hip**
Ankle   Leg
Foot   Popliteal area
Heel   Thigh
Knee   Toe

172.8 **Other specified sites of skin**
Malignant melanoma of contiguous or overlapping sites of skin whose point of origin cannot be determined

172.9 **Melanoma of skin, site unspecified**

173 **Other malignant neoplasm of skin**
Includes: malignant neoplasm of:
sebaceous glands
sudoriferous, sudoriparous glands
sweat glands

    Excludes: *Kaposi's sarcoma (176.0-176.9)*
        malignant melanoma of skin (172.0-172.9)
        skin of genital organs (184.0-184.9, 187.1-187.9)

173.0 **Skin of lip**

    Excludes: *vermilion border of lip (140.0-140.1, 140.9)*

173.1 **Eyelid, including canthus**

    Excludes: *cartilage of eyelid (171.0)*

173.2 **Skin of ear and external auditory canal**
Auricle (ear)   External meatus
Auricular canal, external Pinna

    Excludes: *cartilage of ear (171.0)*

173.3 **Skin of other and unspecified parts of face**
Cheek, external   Forehead
Chin   Nose, external
Eyebrow   Temple

173.4 **Scalp and skin of neck**

● Code new   ▲ Revision of   ④ ⑤ Fourth or fifth
  to this edition   existing code   digit required

173.5 Skin of trunk, except scrotum

Axillary fold	Skin of:
Perianal skin	buttock
Skin of:	chest wall
abdominal wall	groin
anus	perineum
back	Umbilicus
breast	

> *Excludes:* *anal canal (154.2)*
> *anus NOS (154.3)*
> *skin of scrotum (187.7)*

173.6 Skin of upper limb, including shoulder

Arm	Forearm
Finger	Hand

173.7 Skin of lower limb, including hip

Ankle	Leg
Foot	Popliteal area
Heel	Thigh
Knee	Toe

173.8 Other specified sites of skin
Malignant neoplasm of contiguous or overlapping sites of skin whose point of origin cannot be determined

173.9 Skin, site unspecified

174 Malignant neoplasm of female breast
Includes:

breast (female)	Paget's disease of:
connective tissue	breast
soft parts	nipple

> *Excludes:* *skin of breast (172.5, 173.5)*

174.0 Nipple and areola

174.1 Central portion

174.2 Upper-inner quadrant

174.3 Lower-inner quadrant

174.4 Upper-outer quadrant

174.5 Lower-outer quadrant

174.6 Axillary tail

174.8 Other specified sites of female breast

Ectopic sites	Midline of breast
Inner breast	Outer breast
Lower breast	Upper breast

Malignant neoplasm of contiguous or overlapping sites of breast whose point of origin cannot be determined

174.9 Breast (female), unspecified

175 Malignant neoplasm of male breast

> *Excludes:* *skin of breast (172.5, 173.5)*

175.0 Nipple and areola

175.9 Other and unspecified sites of male breast
Ectopic breast tissue, male

176 Kaposi's sarcoma

176.0 Skin

176.1 Soft Tissue
Includes:

blood vessel	ligament
connective tissue	lymphatic(s) NEC
fascia	muscle

> *Excludes:* *lymph glands and nodes (176.5)*

176.2 Palate

176.3 Gastrointestinal sites

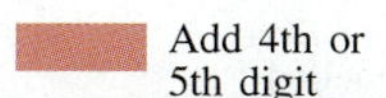

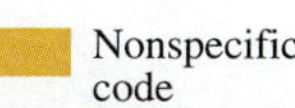

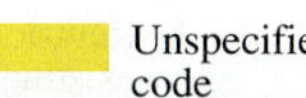

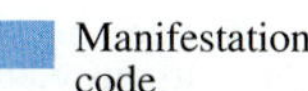

176.4 Lung

176.5 Lymph nodes

176.8 Other specified sites
Includes: oral cavity NEC

176.9 Unspecified
Viscera NOS

MALIGNANT NEOPLASM OF GENITOURINARY ORGANS (179-189)

Excludes: carcinoma in situ (233.1-233.9)

179 Malignant neoplasm of uterus, part unspecified

180 Malignant neoplasm of cervix uteri
Includes: invasive malignancy [carcinoma]

Excludes: carcinoma in situ (233.1)

180.0 Endocervix
Cervical canal NOS   Endocervical gland
Endocervical canal

180.1 Exocervix

180.8 Other specified sites of cervix
Cervical stump
Squamocolumnar junction of cervix
Malignant neoplasm of contiguous or overlapping sites of cervix uteri whose point of
origin cannot be determined

180.9 Cervix uteri, unspecified

181 Malignant neoplasm of placenta
Choriocarcinoma NOS   Chorioepithelioma NOS

Excludes: chorioadenoma (destruens) (236.1)
hydatidiform mole (630)
malignant (236.1)
invasive mole (236.1)
male choriocarcinoma NOS (186.0-186.9)

182 Malignant neoplasm of body of uterus

Excludes: carcinoma in situ (233.2)

182.0 Corpus uteri, except isthmus
Cornu   Fundus
Endometrium   Myometrium

182.1 Isthmus
Lower uterine segment

182.8 Other specified sites of body of uterus
Malignant neoplasm of contiguous or overlapping sites of body of uterus whose point
of origin cannot be determined

Excludes: uterus NOS (179)

183 Malignant neoplasm of ovary and other uterine adnexa

Excludes: Douglas' cul-de-sac (158.8)

183.0 Ovary
Use additional code, if desired, to identify any functional activity

183.2 Fallopian tube
Oviduct   Uterine tube

183.3 Broad ligament
Mesovarium   Parovarian region

183.4 Parametrium
Uterine ligament NOS   Uterosacral ligament

183.5 Round ligament

183.8 Other specified sites of uterine adnexa
Tubo-ovarian
Utero-ovarian
Malignant neoplasm of contiguous or overlapping sites of ovary and other uterine
adnexa whose point of origin cannot be determined

183.9 Uterine adnexa, unspecified

● Code new   ▲ Revision of   ④ ⑤ Fourth or fifth
to this edition   existing code   digit required

184 Malignant neoplasm of other and unspecified female genital organs

> Excludes: carcinoma in situ (233.3)

184.0 Vagina
Gartner's duct　　　　　　　　Vaginal vault

184.1 Labia majora
Greater vestibular [Bartholin's] gland

184.2 Labia minora

184.3 Clitoris

184.4 Vulva, unspecified
External female genitalia NOS
Pudendum

184.8 Other specified sites of female genital organs
Malignant neoplasm of contiguous or overlapping sites of female genital organs whose point of origin cannot be determined

184.9 Female genital organ, site unspecified
Female genitourinary tract NOS

185 Malignant neoplasm of prostate

> Excludes: seminal vesicles (187.8)

186 Malignant neoplasm of testis
Use additional code, if desired, to identify any functional activity

186.0 Undescended testis
Ectopic testis　　　　　　　　Retained testis

186.9 Other and unspecified testis
Testis:
 NOS
 descended
 scrotal

187 Malignant neoplasm of penis and other male genital organs

187.1 Prepuce
Foreskin

187.2 Glans penis

187.3 Body of penis
Corpus cavernosum

187.4 Penis, part unspecified
Skin of penis NOS

187.5 Epididymis

187.6 Spermatic cord
Vas deferens

187.7 Scrotum
Skin of scrotum

187.8 Other specified sites of male genital organs
Seminal vesicle
Tunica vaginalis
Malignant neoplasm of contiguous or overlapping sites of penis and other male genital organs whose point of origin cannot be determined

187.9 Male genital organ, site unspecified
Male genital organ or tract NOS

188 Malignant neoplasm of bladder

> Excludes: carcinoma in situ (233.7)

188.0 Trigone of urinary bladder

188.1 Dome of urinary bladder

188.2 Lateral wall of urinary bladder

188.3 Anterior wall of urinary bladder

188.4 Posterior wall of urinary bladder

188.5 Bladder neck
Internal urethral orifice

188.6 Ureteric orifice

188.7 Urachus

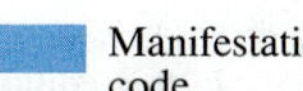

Add 4th or 5th digit	Nonspecific code	Unspecified code	Manifestation code

188.8 Other specified sites of bladder
Malignant neoplasm of contiguous or overlapping sites of bladder whose point of origin cannot be determined

188.9 Bladder, part unspecified
Bladder wall NOS

189 Malignant neoplasm of kidney and other and unspecified urinary organs

189.0 Kidney, except pelvis
Kidney NOS   Kidney parenchyma

189.1 Renal pelvis
Renal calyces   Ureteropelvic junction

189.2 Ureter

Excludes: ureteric orifice of bladder (188.6)

189.3 Urethra

Excludes: urethral orifice of bladder (188.5)

189.4 Paraurethral glands

189.8 Other specified sites of urinary organs
Malignant neoplasm of contiguous or overlapping sites of kidney and other urinary organs whose point of origin cannot be determined

189.9 Urinary organ, site unspecified
Urinary system NOS

MALIGNANT NEOPLASM OF OTHER AND UNSPECIFIED SITES (190-199)

Excludes: carcinoma in situ (234.0-234.9)

190 Malignant neoplasm of eye

Excludes: carcinoma in situ (234.0)
        eyelid (skin) (172.1, 173.1)
         cartilage (171.0)
        optic nerve (192.0)
        orbital bone (170.0)

190.0 Eyeball, except conjunctiva, cornea, retina, and choroid
Ciliary body   Sclera
Crystalline lens   Uveal tract
Iris

190.1 Orbit
Connective tissue of orbit
Extraocular muscle
Retrobulbar

Excludes: bone of orbit (170.0)

190.2 Lacrimal gland

190.3 Conjunctiva

190.4 Cornea

190.5 Retina

190.6 Choroid

190.7 Lacrimal duct
Lacrimal sac   Nasolacrimal duct

190.8 Other specified sites of eye
Malignant neoplasm of contiguous or overlapping sites of eye whose point of origin cannot be determined

190.9 Eye, part unspecified

191 Malignant neoplasm of brain

Excludes: cranial nerves (192.0)
        retrobulbar area (190.1)

191.0 Cerebrum, except lobes and ventricles
Basal ganglia   Globus pallidus
Cerebral cortex   Hypothalamus
Corpus striatum   Thalamus

191.1 Frontal lobe

● Code new
to this edition   ▲ Revision of
existing code   ④ ⑤ Fourth or fifth
digit required

191.2 Temporal lobe
    Hippocampus   Uncus

191.3 Parietal lobe

191.4 Occipital lobe

191.5 Ventricles
    Choroid plexus   Floor of ventricle

191.6 Cerebellum NOS
    Cerebellopontine angle

191.7 Brain stem
    Cerebral peduncle   Midbrain
    Medulla oblongata   Pons

191.8 Other parts of brain
    Corpus callosum
    Tapetum
    Malignant neoplasm of contiguous or overlapping sites of brain whose point of origin
        cannot be determined

191.9 Brain, unspecified
    Cranial fossa NOS

192 Malignant neoplasm of other and unspecified parts of nervous system

> *Excludes:* *peripheral, sympathetic, and parasympathetic nerves and ganglia (171.0-171.9)*

192.0 Cranial nerves
    Olfactory bulb

192.1 Cerebral meninges
    Dura (mater)   Meninges NOS
    Falx (cerebelli) (cerebri)   Tentorium

192.2 Spinal cord
    Cauda equina

192.3 Spinal meninges

192.8 Other specified sites of nervous system
    Malignant neoplasm of contiguous or overlapping sites of other parts of nervous system
        whose point of origin cannot be determined

192.9 Nervous system, part unspecified
    Nervous system (central) NOS

> *Excludes:* *meninges NOS (192.1)*

193 Malignant neoplasm of thyroid gland
    Sipple's syndrome   Thyroglossal duct
Use additional code, if desired, to identify any functional activity

194 Malignant neoplasm of other endocrine glands and related structures
Use additional code, if desired, to identify any functional activity

> *Excludes:* *islets of Langerhans (157.4)*
>   *ovary (183.0)*
>   *testis (186.0-186.9)*
>   *thymus (164.0)*

194.0 Adrenal gland
    Adrenal cortex   Suprarenal gland
    Adrenal medulla

194.1 Parathyroid gland

194.3 Pituitary gland and craniopharyngeal duct
    Craniobuccal pouch   Rathke's pouch
    Hypophysis   Sella turcica

194.4 Pineal gland

194.5 Carotid body

194.6 Aortic body and other paraganglia
    Coccygeal body   Para-aortic body
    Glomus jugulare

194.8 Other
    Pluriglandular involvement NOS
Note: If the sites of multiple involvements are known, they should be coded separately.

194.9 Endocrine gland, site unspecified

195 **Malignant neoplasm of other and ill-defined sites**
Includes: malignant neoplasms of contiguous sites, not elsewhere classified, whose point of origin cannot be determined

Excludes: malignant neoplasm:
lymphatic and hematopoietic tissue (200.0-208.9)
secondary sites (196.0-198.8)
unspecified site (199.0-199.1)

195.0 Head, face, and neck
Cheek NOS
Jaw NOS
Nose NOS
Supraclavicular region NOS

195.1 Thorax
Axilla
Chest (wall) NOS
Intrathoracic NOS

195.2 Abdomen
Intra-abdominal NOS

195.3 Pelvis
Groin
Inguinal region NOS
Presacral region
Sacrococcygeal region
Sites overlapping systems within pelvis, as:
rectovaginal (septum)
rectovesical (septum)

195.4 Upper limb

195.5 Lower limb

195.8 Other specified sites
Back NOS
Flank NOS
Trunk NOS

196 **Secondary and unspecified malignant neoplasm of lymph nodes**

Excludes: any malignant neoplasm of lymph nodes, specified as primary (200.0-202.9)
Hodgkin's disease (201.0-201.9)
lymphosarcoma (200.1)
reticulosarcoma (200.0)
other forms of lymphoma (202.0-202.9)

196.0 Lymph nodes of head, face, and neck
Cervical
Cervicofacial
Scalene
Supraclavicular

196.1 Intrathoracic lymph nodes
Bronchopulmonary
Intercostal
Mediastinal
Tracheobronchial

196.2 Intra-abdominal lymph nodes
Intestinal
Mesenteric
Retroperitoneal

196.3 Lymph nodes of axilla and upper limb
Brachial
Epitrochlear
Infraclavicular
Pectoral

196.5 Lymph nodes of inguinal region and lower limb
Femoral
Groin
Popliteal
Tibial

196.6 Intrapelvic lymph nodes
Hypogastric
Iliac
Obturator
Parametrial

196.8 Lymph nodes of multiple sites

196.9 Site unspecified
Lymph nodes NOS

197 **Secondary malignant neoplasm of respiratory and digestive systems**

Excludes: lymph node metastasis (196.0-196.9)

197.0 Lung
Bronchus

197.1 Mediastinum

197.2 Pleura

● Code new
to this edition

▲ Revision of
existing code

④ ⑤ Fourth or fifth
digit required

197.3 Other respiratory organs
  Trachea

197.4 Small intestine, including duodenum

197.5 Large intestine and rectum

197.6 Retroperitoneum and peritoneum

197.7 Liver, specified as secondary

197.8 Other digestive organs and spleen

198 Secondary malignant neoplasm of other specified sites

> *Excludes:* lymph node metastasis (196.0-196.9)

198.0 Kidney

198.1 Other urinary organs

198.2 Skin
  Skin of breast

198.3 Brain and spinal cord

198.4 Other parts of nervous system
  Meninges (cerebral) (spinal)

198.5 Bone and bone marrow

198.6 Ovary

198.7 Adrenal gland
  Suprarenal gland

⑤ **198.8 Other specified sites**

> **198.81 Breast**

> *Excludes:* skin of breast (198.2)

> **198.82 Genital organs**

> **198.89 Other**

> *Excludes:* retroperitoneal lymph nodes (196.2)

199 Malignant neoplasm without specification of site

199.0 Disseminated
  Carcinomatosis
  Generalized:
    cancer
    malignancy
  Multiple cancer } unspecified site (primary) (secondary)

199.1 Other
  Cancer
  Carcinoma
  Malignancy } unspecified site (primary) (secondary)

MALIGNANT NEOPLASM OF LYMPHATIC AND HEMATOPOIETIC TISSUE (200-208)

> *Excludes:* secondary neoplasm of:
>   bone marrow (198.5)
>   spleen (197.8)
>   secondary and unspecified neoplasm of lymph nodes (196.0-196.9)

The following fifth-digit subclassification is for use with categories 200-202:

0 unspecified site, extranodal and solid organ sites

1 lymph nodes of head, face, and neck

2 intrathoracic lymph nodes

3 intra-abdominal lymph nodes

4 lymph nodes of axilla and upper limb

5 lymph nodes of inguinal region and lower limb

6 intrapelvic lymph nodes

7 spleen

8 lymph nodes of multiple sites

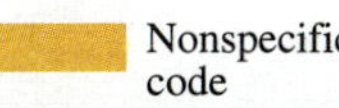

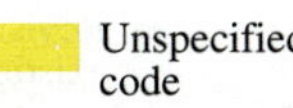

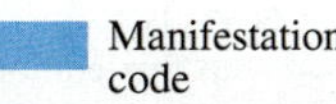

Manifestation
code

⑤ **200** **Lymphosarcoma and reticulosarcoma**

⑤ **200.0** **Reticulosarcoma**
    Lymphoma (malignant):
      histiocytic (diffuse):
        nodular
        pleomorphic cell type
      reticulum cell type
    Reticulum cell sarcoma:
      NOS
      pleomorphic cell type

⑤ **200.1** **Lymphosarcoma**
    Lymphoblastoma (diffuse)   Lymphosarcoma:
    Lymphoma (malignant):   NOS
      lymphoblastic (diffuse)   diffuse NOS
      lymphocytic (cell type)   lymphoblastic (diffuse)
        (diffuse)   lymphocytic (diffuse)
      lymphosarcoma type   prolymphocytic

    Excludes: *lymphosarcoma:*
        follicular or nodular (202.0)
        mixed cell type (200.8)
        lymphosarcoma cell leukemia (207.8)

⑤ **200.2** **Burkitt's tumor or lymphoma**
    Malignant lymphoma, Burkitt's type

⑤ **200.8** **Other named variants**
    Lymphoma (malignant):
      lymphoplasmacytoid type
      mixed lymphocytic-histiocytic (diffuse)
    Lymphosarcoma, mixed cell type (diffuse)
    Reticulolymphosarcoma (diffuse)

⑤ **201** **Hodgkin's disease**

⑤ **201.0** **Hodgkin's paragranuloma**

⑤ **201.1** **Hodgkin's granuloma**

⑤ **201.2** **Hodgkin's sarcoma**

⑤ **201.4** **Lymphocytic-histiocytic predominance**

⑤ **201.5** **Nodular sclerosis**
    Hodgkin's disease, nodular sclerosis:
      NOS
      cellular phase

⑤ **201.6** **Mixed cellularity**

⑤ **201.7** **Lymphocytic depletion**
    Hodgkin's disease, lymphocytic depletion:
      NOS
      diffuse fibrosis
      reticular type

⑤ **201.9** **Hodgkin's disease, unspecified**
    Hodgkin's: Malignant:
      disease NOS   lymphogranuloma
      lymphoma NOS   lymphogranulomatosis

⑤ **202** **Other malignant neoplasms of lymphoid and histiocytic tissue**

⑤ **202.0** **Nodular lymphoma**
    Brill-Symmers disease   Lymphosarcoma:
    Lymphoma: follicular (giant)
      follicular (giant)   nodular
      lymphocytic, nodular   Reticulosarcoma, follicular or nodular

⑤ **202.1** **Mycosis fungoides**

⑤ **202.2** **Sézary's disease**

⑤ **202.3** **Malignant histiocytosis**
    Histiocytic medullary reticulosis
    Malignant:
      reticuloendotheliosis
      reticulosis

⑤ **202.4** **Leukemic reticuloendotheliosis**
    Hairy-cell leukemia

● Code new to this edition   ▲ Revision of existing code   ④ ⑤ Fourth or fifth digit required

⑤ **202.5 Letterer-Siwe disease**
Acute:
differentiated progressive histiocytosis
histiocytosis X (progressive)
infantile reticuloendotheliosis
reticulosis of infancy

Excludes: *Hand-Schüller-Christian disease (277.8)*
histiocytosis (acute) (chronic) (277.8)
histiocytosis X (chronic) (277.8)

⑤ **202.6 Malignant mast cell tumors**
Malignant: Mast cell sarcoma
  mastocytoma   Systemic tissue mast cell disease
  mastocytosis

Excludes: *mast cell leukemia (207.8)*

⑤ **202.8 Other lymphomas**
Lymphoma (malignant):
NOS
diffuse

Excludes: *benign lymphoma (229.0)*

⑤ **202.9 Other and unspecified malignant neoplasms of lymphoid and histiocytic tissue**
Malignant neoplasm of bone marrow NOS

⑤ **203 Multiple myeloma and immunoproliferative neoplasms**
The following fifth-digit subclassification is for use with category 203

  0 **without mention of remission**

  1 **in remission**

⑤ **203.0 Multiple myeloma**
Kahler's disease   Myelomatosis

Excludes: *solitary myeloma (238.6)*

⑤ **203.1 Plasma cell leukemia**
Plasmacytic leukemia

⑤ **203.8 Other immunoproliferative neoplasms**

⑤ **204 Lymphoid leukemia**
Includes:
leukemia: leukemia:
  lymphatic   lymphocytic
  lymphoblastic   lymphogenous
The following fifth-digit subclassification is for use with category 204

  0 **without mention of remission**

  1 **in remission**

⑤ **204.0 Acute**

Excludes: *acute exacerbation of chronic lymphoid leukemia (204.1)*

⑤ **204.1 Chronic**

⑤ **204.2 Subacute**

⑤ **204.8 Other lymphoid leukemia**
Aleukemic leukemia:
lymphatic
lymphocytic
lymphoid

⑤ **204.9 Unspecified lymphoid leukemia**

⑤ **205 Myeloid leukemia**
Includes:
leukemia: leukemia:
  granulocytic   myelomonocytic
  myeloblastic   myelosclerotic
  myelocytic   myelosis
  Tmyelogenous
The following fifth-digit subclassification is for use with category 205

  0 **without mention of remission**

  1 **in remission**

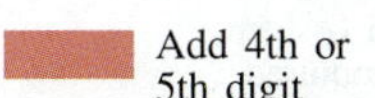

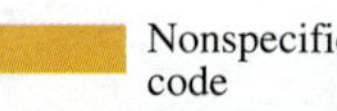

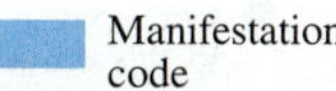

⑤ **205.0 Acute**
Acute promyelocytic leukemia

Excludes: acute exacerbation of chronic myeloid leukemia (205.1)

⑤ **205.1 Chronic**
Eosinophilic leukemia   Neutrophilic leukemia

⑤ **205.2 Subacute**

⑤ **205.3 Myeloid sarcoma**
Chloroma
Granulocytic sarcoma

⑤ **205.8 Other myeloid leukemia**
Aleukemic leukemia:
    granulocytic
    myelogenous
    myeloid
Aleukemic myelosis

⑤ **205.9 Unspecified myeloid leukemia**

⑤ **206 Monocytic leukemia**
Includes: leukemia:
         histiocytic
         monoblastic
         monocytoid

The following fifth-digit subclassification is for use with category 206

    0   without mention of remission

    1   in remission

⑤ **206.0 Acute**

Excludes: acute exacerbation of chronic monocytic leukemia (206.1)

⑤ **206.1 Chronic**

⑤ **206.2 Subacute**

⑤ **206.8 Other monocytic leukemia**
Aleukemic:
    monocytic leukemia
    monocytoid leukemia

⑤ **206.9 Unspecified monocytic leukemia**

⑤ **207 Other specified leukemia**

Excludes: leukemic reticuloendotheliosis (202.4)
         plasma cell leukemia (203.1)

The following fifth-digit subclassification is for use with category 207

    0   without mention of remission

    1   in remission

⑤ **207.0 Acute erythremia and erythroleukemia**
Acute erythremic myelosis   Erythremic myelosis
Di Guglielmo's disease

⑤ **207.1 Chronic erythremia**
Heilmeyer-Schöner disease

⑤ **207.2 Megakaryocytic leukemia**
Megakaryocytic myelosis   Thrombocytic leukemia

⑤ **207.8 Other specified leukemia**
Lymphosarcoma cell leukemia

⑤ **208 Leukemia of unspecified cell type**
The following fifth-digit subclassification is for use with category 208

    0   without mention of remission

    1   in remission

⑤ **208.0 Acute**
Acute leukemia NOS   Stem cell leukemia
Blast cell leukemia

Excludes: acute exacerbation of chronic unspecified leukemia (208.1)

⑤ **208.1 Chronic**
Chronic leukemia NOS

   ● Code new   ▲ Revision of   ④ ⑤ Fourth or fifth
     to this edition   existing code   digit required

⑤ **208.2** **Subacute**
Subacute leukemia NOS

⑤ **208.8** **Other leukemia of unspecified cell type**

⑤ **208.9** **Unspecified leukemia**
Leukemia NOS

BENIGN NEOPLASMS (210-229)

210 **Benign neoplasm of lip, oral cavity, and pharynx**

> *Excludes:* *cyst (of):*
> *jaw (526.0-526.2, 526.89)*
> *oral soft tissue (528.4)*
> *radicular (522.8)*

210.0 **Lip**
Frenulum labii
Lip (inner aspect) (mucosa) (vermilion border)

> *Excludes:* *labial commissure (210.4)*
> *skin of lip (216.0)*

210.1 **Tongue**
Lingual tonsil

210.2 **Major salivary glands**
Gland:
   parotid
   sublingual
   submandibular

> *Excludes:* *benign neoplasms of minor salivary glands:*
> *NOS (210.4)*
> *buccal mucosa (210.4)*
> *lips (210.0)*
> *palate (hard) (soft) (210.4)*
> *tongue (210.1)*
> *tonsil, palatine (210.5)*

210.3 **Floor of mouth**

210.4 **Other and unspecified parts of mouth**
Gingiva   Oral mucosa
Gum (upper) (lower)   Palate (hard) (soft)
Labial commissure   Uvula
Oral cavity NOS

> *Excludes:* *benign odontogenic neoplasms of bone (213.0-213.1)*
> *developmental odontogenic cysts (526.0)*
> *mucosa of lips (210.0)*
> *nasopharyngeal [posterior] [superior] surface of soft palate (210.7)*

210.5 **Tonsil**
Tonsil (faucial) (palatine)

> *Excludes:* *lingual tonsil (210.1)*
> *pharyngeal tonsil (210.7)*
> *tonsillar:*
> *fossa (210.6)*
> *pillars (210.6)*

210.6 **Other parts of oropharynx**
Branchial cleft or vestiges
Epiglottis, anterior aspect
Fauces NOS
Mesopharynx NOS
Tonsillar:
   fossa
   pillars
Vallecula

> *Excludes:* *epiglottis:*
> *NOS (212.1)*
> *suprahyoid portion (212.1)*

210.7 **Nasopharynx**
Adenoid tissue   Pharyngeal tonsil
Lymphadenoid tissue   Posterior nasal septum

210.8 Hypopharynx
    Arytenoid fold   Postcricoid region
    Laryngopharynx   Pyriform fossa

210.9 Pharynx, unspecified
    Throat NOS

211 Benign neoplasm of other parts of digestive system

211.0 Esophagus

211.1 Stomach
    Body   ⎫   Cardiac orifice
    Cardia   ⎬ stomach Pylorus
    Fundus ⎭

211.2 Duodenum, jejunum, and ileum
    Small intestine NOS

> *Excludes:* *ampulla of Vater (211.5)*
>   *ileocecal valve (211.3)*

211.3 Colon
    Appendix   Ileocecal valve
    Cecum   Large intestine NOS

> *Excludes:* *rectosigmoid junction (211.4)*

211.4 Rectum and anal canal
    Anal canal or sphincter   Rectosigmoid junction
    Anus NOS

> *Excludes:* *anus:*
>   *margin (216.5)*
>   *skin (216.5)*
>   *perianal skin (216.5)*

211.5 Liver and biliary passages
    Ampulla of Vater   Gallbladder
    Common bile duct   Hepatic duct
    Cystic duct   Sphincter of Oddi

211.6 Pancreas, except islets of Langerhans

211.7 Islets of Langerhans
    Islet cell tumor

Use additional code, if desired, to identify any functional activity

211.8 Retroperitoneum and peritoneum
    Mesentery   Omentum
    Mesocolon   Retroperitoneal tissue

211.9 Other and unspecified site
    Alimentary tract NOS   Intestinal tract NOS
    Digestive system NOS   Intestine NOS
    Gastrointestinal tract NOS Spleen, not elsewhere classified

212 Benign neoplasm of respiratory and intrathoracic organs

212.0 Nasal cavities, middle ear, and accessory sinuses
    Cartilage of nose   Sinus:
    Eustachian tube   ethmoidal
    Nares   frontal
    Septum of nose   maxillary
                       sphenoidal

> *Excludes:* *auditory canal (external) (216.2)*
>   *bone of:*
>   *ear (213.0)*
>   *nose [turbinates] (213.0)*
>   *cartilage of ear (215.0)*
>   *ear (external) (skin) (216.2)*
>   *nose NOS (229.8)*
>   *skin (216.3)*
>   *olfactory bulb (225.1)*
>   *polyp of:*
>   *accessory sinus (471.8)*
>   *ear (385.30-385.35)*
>   *nasal cavity (471.0)*
>   *posterior margin of septum and choanae (210.7)*

212.1 Larynx

Cartilage:	Epiglottis (suprahyoid portion) NOS
arytenoid	Glottis
cricoid	Vocal cords (false) (true)
cuneiform	
thyroid	

Excludes: *epiglottis, anterior aspect (210.6)*
polyp of vocal cord or larynx (478.4)

212.2 Trachea

212.3 Bronchus and lung
Carina   Hilus of lung

212.4 Pleura

212.5 Mediastinum

212.6 Thymus

212.7 Heart

Excludes: *great vessels (215.4)*

212.8 Other specified sites

212.9 Site unspecified
Respiratory organ NOS
Upper respiratory tract NOS

Excludes: *intrathoracic NOS (229.8)*
thoracic NOS (229.8)

213 Benign neoplasm of bone and articular cartilage
Includes: cartilage (articular) (joint)
periosteum

Excludes: *cartilage of:*
ear (215.0)
eyelid (215.0)
larynx (212.1)
nose (212.0)
exostosis NOS (726.91)
synovia (215.0-215.9)

213.0 Bones of skull and face

Excludes: *lower jaw bone (213.1)*

213.1 Lower jaw bone

213.2 Vertebral column, excluding sacrum and coccyx

213.3 Ribs, sternum, and clavicle

213.4 Scapula and long bones of upper limb

213.5 Short bones of upper limb

213.6 Pelvic bones, sacrum, and coccyx

213.7 Long bones of lower limb

213.8 Short bones of lower limb

213.9 Bone and articular cartilage, site unspecified

214 Lipoma
Includes: angiolipoma
fibrolipoma
hibernoma
lipoma (fetal) (infiltrating) (intramuscular)
myelolipoma
myxolipoma

214.0 Skin and subcutaneous tissue of face

214.1 Other skin and subcutaneous tissue

214.2 Intrathoracic organs

214.3 Intra-abdominal organs

214.4 Spermatic cord

214.8 Other specified sites

214.9 Lipoma, unspecified site

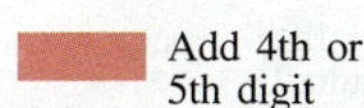

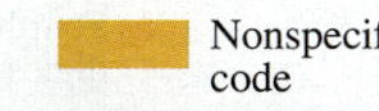

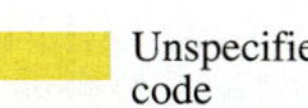

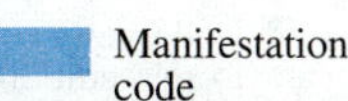

215 Other benign neoplasm of connective and other soft tissue

Includes:

blood vessel	peripheral, sympathetic, and parasympathetic nerves
bursa	and ganglia
fascia	synovia
ligament	tendon (sheath)
muscle	

Excludes: *cartilage:*
   articular (213.0-213.9)
   larynx (212.1)
   nose (212.0)
connective tissue of:
   breast (217)
   *internal organ, except lipoma and hemangioma — code to benign neoplasm of
      the site*
lipoma (214.0-214.9)

215.0 Head, face, and neck

215.2 Upper limb, including shoulder

215.3 Lower limb, including hip

215.4 Thorax

Excludes: *heart (212.7)*
   mediastinum (212.5)
   thymus (212.6)

215.5 Abdomen

Abdominal wall   Hypochondrium

215.6 Pelvis

Buttock   Inguinal region
Groin   Perineum

Excludes: *uterine:*
   leiomyoma (218.0-218.9)
   ligament, any (221.0)

215.7 Trunk, unspecified

Back NOS   Flank NOS

215.8 Other specified sites

215.9 Site unspecified

216 Benign neoplasm of skin

Includes:

blue nevus	pigmented nevus
dermatofibroma	syringoadenoma
hydrocystoma	syringoma

Excludes: *skin of genital organs (221.0-222.9)*

216.0 Skin of lip

Excludes: *vermilion border of lip (210.0)*

216.1 Eyelid, including canthus

Excludes: *cartilage of eyelid (215.0)*

216.2 Ear and external auditory canal

Auricle (ear)   External meatus
Auricular canal, external   Pinna

Excludes: *cartilage of ear (215.0)*

216.3 Skin of other and unspecified parts of face

Cheek, external   Nose, external
Eyebrow   Temple

216.4 Scalp and skin of neck

● Code new   ▲ Revision of   ④ ⑤ Fourth or fifth
   to this edition   existing code   digit required

216.5 Skin of trunk, except scrotum

Axillary fold
Perianal skin
Skin of:
    abdominal wall
    anus
    back
    breast
Skin of:
    buttock
    chest wall
    groin
    perineum
Umbilicus

> *Excludes:* *anal canal (211.4)*
> *anus NOS (211.4)*
> *skin of scrotum (222.4)*

216.6 Skin of upper limb, including shoulder

216.7 Skin of lower limb, including hip

216.8 Other specified sites of skin

216.9 Skin, site unspecified

217 Benign neoplasm of breast

Breast (male) (female)
    connective tissue
    glandular tissue
    soft parts

> *Excludes:* *adenofibrosis (610.2)*
> *benign cyst of breast (610.0)*
> *fibrocystic disease (610.1)*
> *skin of breast (216.5)*

218 Uterine leiomyoma

Includes: fibroid (bleeding) (uterine)
    uterine:
        fibromyoma
        myoma

218.0 Submucous leiomyoma of uterus

218.1 Intramural leiomyoma of uterus
Interstitial leiomyoma of uterus

218.2 Subserous leiomyoma of uterus
Subperitoneal leiomyoma of uterus

218.9 Leiomyoma of uterus, unspecified

219 Other benign neoplasm of uterus

219.0 Cervix uteri

219.1 Corpus uteri
Endometrium   Myometrium
Fundus

219.8 Other specified parts of uterus

219.9 Uterus, part unspecified

220 Benign neoplasm of ovary

Use additional code, if desired, to identify any functional activity (256.0-256.1)

> *Excludes:* *cyst:*
> *corpus albicans (620.2)*
> *corpus luteum (620.1)*
> *endometrial (617.1)*
> *follicular (atretic) (620.0)*
> *graafian follicle (620.0)*
> *ovarian NOS (620.2)*
> *retention (620.2)*

221 Benign neoplasm of other female genital organs

Includes: adenomatous polyp
    benign teratoma

> *Excludes:* *cyst:*
> *epoophoron (752.11)*
> *fimbrial (752.11)*
> *Gartner's duct (752.11)*
> *parovarian (752.11)*

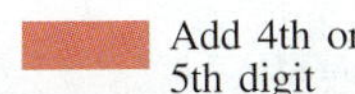

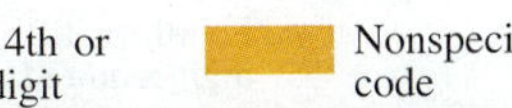

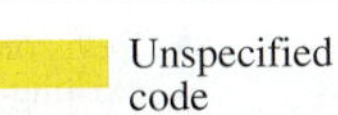

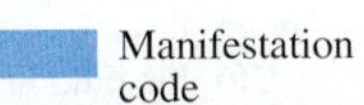

221.0 Fallopian tube and uterine ligaments
Oviduct
Parametrium
Uterine ligament (broad) (round) (uterosacral)
Uterine tube

221.1 Vagina

221.2 Vulva
Clitoris
External female genitalia NOS
Greater vestibular [Bartholin's] gland
Labia (majora) (minora)
Pudendum

Excludes: *Bartholin's (duct) (gland) cyst (616.2)*

221.8 Other specified sites of female genital organs

221.9 Female genital organ, site unspecified
Female genitourinary tract NOS

222 Benign neoplasm of male genital organs

222.0 Testis
Use additional code, if desired, to identify any functional activity

222.1 Penis
Corpus cavernosum
Glans penis
Prepuce

222.2 Prostate

Excludes: *adenomatous hyperplasia of prostate (600.2)*
prostatic:
adenoma (600.2)
enlargement (600.0)
hypertrophy (600.0)

222.3 Epididymis

222.4 Scrotum
Skin of scrotum

222.8 Other specified sites of male genital organs
Seminal vesicle
Spermatic cord

222.9 Male genital organ, site unspecified
Male genitourinary tract NOS

223 Benign neoplasm of kidney and other urinary organs

223.0 Kidney, except pelvis
Kidney NOS

Excludes: *renal:*
calyces (223.1)
pelvis (223.1)

223.1 Renal pelvis

223.2 Ureter

Excludes: *ureteric orifice of bladder (223.3)*

223.3 Bladder

⑤ **223.8 Other specified sites of urinary organs**

223.81 Urethra

Excludes: *urethral orifice of bladder (223.3)*

223.89 Other
Paraurethral glands

223.9 Urinary organ, site unspecified
Urinary system NOS

224 Benign neoplasm of eye

Excludes: *cartilage of eyelid (215.0)*
eyelid (skin) (216.1)
optic nerve (225.1)
orbital bone (213.0)

224.0 Eyeball, except conjunctiva, cornea, retina, and choroid
Ciliary body
Iris
Sclera
Uveal tract

● Code new to this edition   ▲ Revision of existing code   ④ ⑤ Fourth or fifth digit required

224.1 Orbit

Excludes: *bone of orbit (213.0)*

224.2 Lacrimal gland

224.3 Conjunctiva

224.4 Cornea

224.5 Retina

Excludes: *hemangioma of retina (228.03)*

224.6 Choroid

224.7 Lacrimal duct
Lacrimal sac   Nasolacrimal duct

224.8 Other specified parts of eye

224.9 Eye, part unspecified

225 Benign neoplasm of brain and other parts of nervous system

Excludes: *hemangioma (228.02)*
neurofibromatosis (237.7)
peripheral, sympathetic, and parasympathetic nerves and ganglia (215.0-215.9)
retrobulbar (224.1)

225.0 Brain

225.1 Cranial nerves

225.2 Cerebral meninges
Meninges NOS   Meningioma (cerebral)

225.3 Spinal cord
Cauda equina

225.4 Spinal meninges
Spinal meningioma

225.8 Other specified sites of nervous system

225.9 Nervous system, part unspecified
Nervous system (central) NOS

Excludes: *meninges NOS (225.2)*

226 Benign neoplasm of thyroid glands
Use additional code, if desired, to identify any functional activity

227 Benign neoplasm of other endocrine glands and related structures
Use additional code, if desired, to identify any functional activity

Excludes: *ovary (220)*
pancreas (211.6)
testis (222.0)

227.0 Adrenal gland
Suprarenal gland

227.1 Parathyroid gland

227.3 Pituitary gland and craniopharyngeal duct (pouch)
Craniobuccal pouch   Rathke's pouch
Hypophysis   Sella turcica

227.4 Pineal gland
Pineal body

227.5 Carotid body

227.6 Aortic body and other paraganglia
Coccygeal body   Para aortic body
Glomus jugulare

227.8 Other

227.9 Endocrine gland, site unspecified

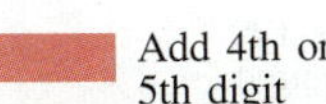

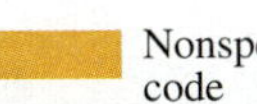

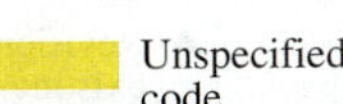

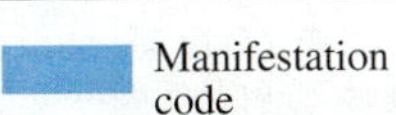

228 Hemangioma and lymphangioma, any site
Includes: angioma (benign) (cavernous) (congenital) NOS
cavernous nevus
glomus tumor
hemangioma (benign) (congenital)

Excludes: *benign neoplasm of spleen, except hemangioma and lymphangioma (211.9)*
glomus jugulare (227.6)
nevus:
NOS (216.0-216.9)
blue or pigmented (216.0-216.9)
vascular (757.32)

⑤ **228.0 Hemangioma, any site**

228.00 Of unspecified site

228.01 Of skin and subcutaneous tissue

228.02 Of intracranial structures

228.03 Of retina

228.04 Of intra-abdominal structures
Peritoneum   Retroperitoneal tissue

228.09 Of other sites
Systemic angiomatosis

228.1 Lymphangioma, any site
Congenital lymphangioma   Lymphatic nevus

229 Benign neoplasm of other and unspecified sites

229.0 Lymph nodes

Excludes: *lymphangioma (228.1)*

229.8 Other specified sites
Intrathoracic NOS   Thoracic NOS

229.9 Site unspecified

CARCINOMA IN SITU (230-234)

Includes: Bowen's disease
erythroplasia
Queyrat's erythroplasia

Excludes: *leukoplakia—see Alphabetic Index*

230 Carcinoma in situ of digestive organs

230.0 Lip, oral cavity, and pharynx
Gingiva   Oropharynx
Hypopharynx   Salivary gland or duct
Mouth [any part]   Tongue
Nasopharynx

Excludes: *aryepiglottic fold or interarytenoid fold, laryngeal aspect (231.0)*
epiglottis:
NOS (231.0)
suprahyoid portion (231.0)
skin of lip (232.0)

230.1 Esophagus

230.2 Stomach
Body
Cardia   } of stomach   Cardiac orifice
Fundus   Pylorus

230.3 Colon
Appendix   Ileocecal valve
Cecum   Large intestine NOS

Excludes: *rectosigmoid junction (230.4)*

230.4 Rectum
Rectosigmoid junction

230.5 Anal canal
Anal sphincter

● Code new   ▲ Revision of   ④ ⑤ Fourth or fifth
to this edition   existing code   digit required

230.6 Anus, unspecified

> *Excludes:* *anus:*
>> *margin (232.5)*
>> *skin (232.5)*
>> *perianal skin (232.5)*

230.7 Other and unspecified parts of intestine

Duodenum   Jejunum
Ileum   Small intestine NOS

> *Excludes:* *ampulla of Vater (230.8)*

230.8 Liver and biliary system

Ampulla of Vater   Gallbladder
Common bile duct   Hepatic duct
Cystic duct   Sphincter of Oddi

230.9 Other and unspecified digestive organs

Digestive organ NOS   Pancreas
Gastrointestinal tract NOS   Spleen

231 Carcinoma in situ of respiratory system

231.0 Larynx

Cartilage: Epiglottis:
  arytenoid   NOS
  cricoid   posterior surface
  cuneiform   suprahyoid portion
  thyroid   Vocal cords (false) (true)

> *Excludes:* *aryepiglottic fold or interarytenoid fold:*
>> *NOS (230.0)*
>> *hypopharyngeal aspect (230.0)*
>> *marginal zone (230.0)*

231.1 Trachea

231.2 Bronchus and lung

Carina   Hilus of lung

231.8 Other specified parts of respiratory system

Accessory sinuses   Nasal cavities
Middle ear   Pleura

> *Excludes:* *ear (external) (skin) (232.2)*
>> *nose NOS (234.8)*
>> *skin (232.3)*

231.9 Respiratory system, part unspecified

Respiratory organ NOS

232 Carcinoma in situ of skin

Includes: pigment cells

232.0 Skin of lip

> *Excludes:* *vermilion border of lip (230.0)*

232.1 Eyelid, including canthus

232.2 Ear and external auditory canal

232.3 Skin of other and unspecified parts of face

232.4 Scalp and skin of neck

232.5 Skin of trunk, except scrotum

Anus, margin   Skin of:
Axillary fold   breast
Perianal skin   buttock
Skin of: chest wall
  abdominal wall   groin
  anus   perineum
  back   Umbilicus

> *Excludes:* *anal canal (230.5)*
>> *anus NOS (230.6)*
>> *skin of genital organs (233.3, 233.5-233.6)*

232.6 Skin of upper limb, including shoulder

232.7 Skin of lower limb, including hip

232.8 Other specified sites of skin

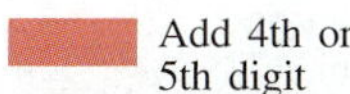

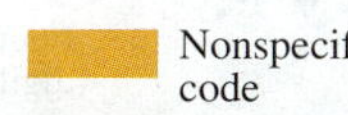

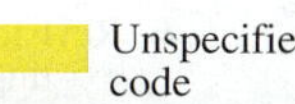

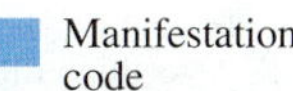

232.9 Skin, site unspecified

233 Carcinoma in situ of breast and genitourinary system

233.0 Breast

> Excludes: *Paget's disease (174.0-174.9)*
> *skin of breast (232.5)*

233.1 Cervix uteri

233.2 Other and unspecified parts of uterus

233.3 Other and unspecified female genital organs

233.4 Prostate

233.5 Penis

233.6 Other and unspecified male genital organs

233.7 Bladder

233.9 Other and unspecified urinary organs

234 Carcinoma in situ of other and unspecified sites

234.0 Eye

> Excludes: *cartilage of eyelid (234.8)*
> *eyelid (skin) (232.1)*
> *optic nerve (234.8)*
> *orbital bone (234.8)*

234.8 Other specified sites

Endocrine gland [any]

234.9 Site unspecified

Carcinoma in situ NOS

NEOPLASMS OF UNCERTAIN BEHAVIOR (235-238)

Note: Categories 235-238 classify by site certain histo-morphologically well-defined neoplasms, the subsequent behavior of which cannot be predicted from the present appearance.

235 Neoplasm of uncertain behavior of digestive and respiratory systems

235.0 Major salivary glands

Gland:
  parotid
  sublingual
  submandibular

> Excludes: *minor salivary glands (235.1)*

235.1 Lip, oral cavity, and pharynx

Gingiva	Nasopharynx
Hypopharynx	Oropharynx
Minor salivary glands	Tongue
Mouth	

> Excludes: *aryepiglottic fold or interarytenoid fold, laryngeal aspect (235.6)*
> *epiglottis:*
> *NOS (235.6)*
> *suprahyoid portion (235.6)*
> *skin of lip (238.2)*

235.2 Stomach, intestines, and rectum

235.3 Liver and biliary passages

Ampulla of Vater	Gallbladder
Bile ducts [any]	Liver

235.4 Retroperitoneum and peritoneum

235.5 Other and unspecified digestive organs

Anal:	Esophagus
canal	Pancreas
sphincter	Spleen
Anus NOS	

> Excludes: *anus:*
> *margin (238.2)*
> *skin (238.2)*
> *perianal skin (238.2)*

● Code new to this edition ▲ Revision of existing code ④ ⑤ Fourth or fifth digit required

235.6 Larynx

> *Excludes:* *aryepiglottic fold or interarytenoid fold:*
> *NOS (235.1)*
> *hypopharyngeal aspect (235.1)*
> *marginal zone (235.1)*

235.7 Trachea, bronchus, and lung

235.8 Pleura, thymus, and mediastinum

235.9 Other and unspecified respiratory organs

Accessory sinuses	Nasal cavities
Middle ear	Respiratory organ NOS

> *Excludes:* *ear (external) (skin) (238.2)*
> *nose (238.8)*
> *skin (238.2)*

236 Neoplasm of uncertain behavior of genitourinary organs

236.0 Uterus

236.1 Placenta
Chorioadenoma (destruens)
Invasive mole
Malignant hydatid(iform) mole

236.2 Ovary
Use additional code, if desired, to identify any functional activity

236.3 Other and unspecified female genital organs

236.4 Testis
Use additional code, if desired, to identify any functional activity

236.5 Prostate

236.6 Other and unspecified male genital organs

236.7 Bladder

236.9 Other and unspecified urinary organs

> **236.90 Urinary organ, unspecified**
>
> **236.91 Kidney and ureter**
>
> **236.99 Other**

237 Neoplasm of uncertain behavior of endocrine glands and nervous system

237.0 Pituitary gland and craniopharyngeal duct
Use additional code, if desired, to identify any functional activity

237.1 Pineal gland

237.2 Adrenal gland
Suprarenal gland
Use additional code, if desired, to identify any functional activity

237.3 Paraganglia

Aortic body	Coccygeal body
Carotid body	Glomus jugulare

237.4 Other and unspecified endocrine glands

Parathyroid gland	Thyroid gland

237.5 Brain and spinal cord

237.6 Meninges
Meninges:
NOS
cerebral
spinal

237.7 Neurofibromatosis
von Recklinghausen's disease

> **237.70 Neurofibromatosis, unspecified**
>
> **237.71 Neurofibromatosis, Type I [von   Recklinghausen's disease]**
>
> **237.72 Neurofibromatosis, Type II [acoustic neurofibromatosis]**

237.9 Other and unspecified parts of nervous system
Cranial nerves

> *Excludes:* *peripheral, sympathetic, and parasympathetic nerves and ganglia (238.1)*

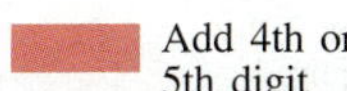

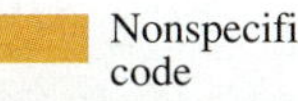

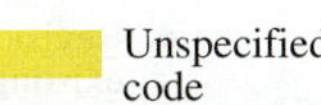

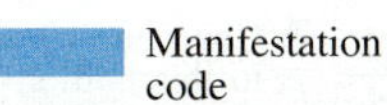

238 Neoplasm of uncertain behavior of other and unspecified sites and tissues

238.0 Bone and articular cartilage

> *Excludes:* *cartilage:*
> *ear (238.1)*
> *eyelid (238.1)*
> *larynx (235.6)*
> *nose (235.9)*
> *synovia (238.1)*

238.1 Connective and other soft tissue
Peripheral, sympathetic, and parasympathetic nerves and ganglia

> *Excludes:* *cartilage (of):*
> *articular (238.0)*
> *larynx (235.6)*
> *nose (235.9)*
> *connective tissue of breast (238.3)*

238.2 Skin

> *Excludes:* *anus NOS (235.5)*
> *skin of genital organs (236.3, 236.6)*
> *vermilion border of lip (235.1)*

238.3 Breast

> *Excludes:* *skin of breast (238.2)*

238.4 Polycythemia vera

238.5 Histiocytic and mast cells
Mast cell tumor NOS   Mastocytoma NOS

238.6 Plasma cells
Plasmacytoma NOS   Solitary myeloma

238.7 Other lymphatic and hematopoietic tissues
Disease:
 lymphoproliferative (chronic) NOS
 myeloproliferative (chronic) NOS
Idiopathic thrombocythemia
Megakaryocytic myelosclerosis
Myelodysplastic syndrome
Myelosclerosis with myeloid metaplasia
Panmyelosis (acute)

> *Excludes:* *myelofibrosis (289.8)*
> *myelosclerosis NOS (289.8)*
> *myelosis:*
> *NOS (205.9)*
> *megakaryocytic (207.2)*

238.8 Other specified sites
Eye   Heart

> *Excludes:* *eyelid (skin) (238.2)*
> *cartilage (238.1)*

238.9 Site unspecified

NEOPLASMS OF UNSPECIFIED NATURE (239)

239 Neoplasms of unspecified nature
Note: Category 239 classifies by site neoplasms of unspecified morphology and behavior. The term "mass," unless otherwise stated, is not to be regarded as a neoplastic growth.
Includes: "growth" NOS
neoplasm NOS
new growth NOS
tumor NOS

239.0 Digestive system

> *Excludes:* *anus:*
> *margin (239.2)*
> *skin (239.2)*
> *perianal skin (239.2)*

239.1 Respiratory system

  ● Code new   ▲ Revision of   ④ ⑤ Fourth or fifth
to this edition   existing code   digit required

239.2 **Bone, soft tissue, and skin**

Excludes: *anal canal (239.0)*
anus NOS (239.0)
bone marrow (202.9)
cartilage:
　larynx (239.1)
　nose (239.1)
connective tissue of breast (239.3)
skin of genital organs (239.5)
vermilion border of lip (239.0)

239.3 **Breast**

Excludes: *skin of breast (239.2)*

239.4 **Bladder**

239.5 **Other genitourinary organs**

239.6 **Brain**

Excludes: *cerebral meninges (239.7)*
cranial nerves (239.7)

239.7 **Endocrine glands and other parts of nervous system**

Excludes: *peripheral, sympathetic, and parasympathetic nerves and ganglia (239.2)*

239.8 **Other specified sites**

Excludes: *eyelids (skin) (239.2)*
　cartilage (239.2)
great vessels (239.2)
optic nerve (239.7)

239.9 **Site unspecified**

● Code new
to this edition

▲ Revision of
existing code

④ ⑤ Fourth or fifth
digit required

3. ENDOCRINE, NUTRITIONAL AND METABOLIC DISEASES, AND IMMUNITY DISORDERS (240-279)

> *Excludes:* *endocrine and metabolic disturbances specific to the fetus and newborn (775.0-775.9)*

Note: All neoplasms, whether functionally active or not, are classified in Chapter 2. Codes in Chapter 3 (i.e., 242.8, 246.0, 251-253, 255-259) may be used, if desired, to identify such functional activity associated with any neoplasm, or by ectopic endocrine tissue.

DISORDERS OF THYROID GLAND (240-246)

240 Simple and unspecified goiter

240.0 Goiter, specified as simple
Any condition classifiable to 240.9, specified as simple

240.9 Goiter, unspecified

Enlargement of thyroid	Goiter or struma:
Goiter or struma:	hyperplastic
NOS	nontoxic (diffuse)
diffuse colloid	parenchymatous
endemic	sporadic

> *Excludes:* *congenital (dyshormonogenic) goiter (246.1)*

241 Nontoxic nodular goiter

> *Excludes:* *adenoma of thyroid (226)*
> *cystadenoma of thyroid (226)*

241.0 Nontoxic uninodular goiter
Thyroid nodule
Uninodular goiter (nontoxic)

241.1 Nontoxic multinodular goiter
Multinodular goiter (nontoxic)

241.9 Unspecified nontoxic nodular goiter
Adenomatous goiter
Nodular goiter (nontoxic) NOS
Struma nodosa (simplex)

⑤ 242 Thyrotoxicosis with or without goiter

> *Excludes:* *neonatal thyrotoxicosis (775.3)*

The following fifth-digit subclassification is for use with category 242:

   0 without mention of thyrotoxic crisis or storm

   1 with mention of thyrotoxic crisis or storm

⑤ 242.0 Toxic diffuse goiter
Basedow's disease
Exophthalmic or toxic goiter NOS
Graves' disease
Primary thyroid hyperplasia

⑤ 242.1 Toxic uninodular goiter
Thyroid nodule
Uninodular goiter } toxic or with hyperthyroidism

⑤ 242.2 Toxic multinodular goiter
Secondary thyroid hyperplasia

⑤ 242.3 Toxic nodular goiter, unspecified
Adenomatous goiter
Nodular goiter } toxic or with hyperthyroidism
Struma nodosa
Any condition classifiable to 241.9 specified as toxic or with hyperthyroidism

⑤ 242.4 Thyrotoxicosis from ectopic thyroid nodule

⑤ 242.8 Thyrotoxicosis of other specified origin
Overproduction of thyroid-stimulating hormone [TSH]
Thyrotoxicosis:
  factitia
  from ingestion of excessive thyroid material
Use additional E code to identify cause, if drug-induced

⑤ 242.9 Thyrotoxicosis without mention of goiter or other cause
Hyperthyroidism NOS   Thyrotoxicosis NOS

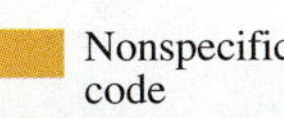

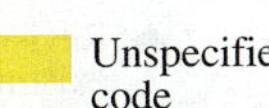

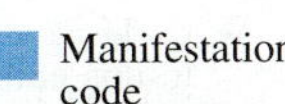

Manifestation
code

243 Congenital hypothyroidism
  Congenital thyroid insufficiency
  Cretinism (athyrotic) (endemic)

Use additional code to identify associated mental retardation

> *Excludes:* congenital (dyshormonogenic) goiter (246.1)

244 Acquired hypothyroidism
  Includes: athyroidism (acquired)
             hypothyroidism (acquired)
             myxedema (adult) (juvenile)
             thyroid (gland) insufficiency (acquired)

244.0 Postsurgical hypothyroidism

244.1 Other postablative hypothyroidism
  Hypothyroidism following therapy, such as irradiation

244.2 Iodine hypothyroidism
  Hypothyroidism resulting from administration or ingestion of iodide

Use additional E code to identify drug

244.3 Other iatrogenic hypothyroidism
  Hypothyroidism resulting from:
    P-aminosalicylic acid [PAS]
    Phenylbutazone
    Resorcinol
  Iatrogenic hypothyroidism NOS

Use additional E code to identify drug

244.8 Other specified acquired hypothyroidism
  Secondary hypothyroidism NEC

244.9 Unspecified hypothyroidism
  Hypothyroidism ⎫
  Myxedema   ⎬ primary or NOS

245 Thyroiditis

245.0 Acute thyroiditis
  Abscess of thyroid
  Thyroiditis:
    nonsuppurative, acute
    pyogenic
    suppurative

Use additional code to identify organism

245.1 Subacute thyroiditis
  Thyroiditis: Thyroiditis:
    de Quervain's   granulomatous
    giant cell   viral

245.2 Chronic lymphocytic thyroiditis
  Hashimoto's disease   Thyroiditis:
  Struma lymphomatosa   autoimmune
                                  lymphocytic (chronic)

245.3 Chronic fibrous thyroiditis
  Struma fibrosa
  Thyroiditis:
    invasive (fibrous)
    ligneous
    Riedel's

245.4 Iatrogenic thyroiditis
Use additional code to identify cause

245.8 Other and unspecified chronic thyroiditis
  Chronic thyroiditis:
    NOS
    nonspecific

245.9 Thyroiditis, unspecified
  Thyroiditis NOS

246 Other disorders of thyroid

246.0 Disorders of thyrocalcitonin secretion
  Hypersecretion of calcitonin or thyrocalcitonin

● Code new   ▲ Revision of   ④ ⑤ Fourth or fifth
  to this edition   existing code   digit required

246.1 Dyshormonogenic goiter
Congenital (dyshormonogenic) goiter
Goiter due to enzyme defect in synthesis of thyroid hormone
Goitrous cretinism (sporadic)

246.2 Cyst of thyroid

Excludes: cystadenoma of thyroid (226)

246.3 Hemorrhage and infarction of thyroid

246.8 Other specified disorders of thyroid
Abnormality of   Hyper-TBG-nemia
  thyroid-binding globulin   Hypo-TBG-nemia
Atrophy of thyroid

246.9 Unspecified disorder of thyroid

DISEASES OF OTHER ENDOCRINE GLANDS (250-259)

250 Diabetes mellitus

Excludes: gestational diabetes (648.8)
  hyperglycemia NOS (790.6)
  neonatal diabetes mellitus (775.1)
  nonclinical diabetes (790.2)

The following fifth-digit subclassification is for use with category 250:

0 type II [non-insulin dependent type] [NIDDM type] [adult-onset type] or unspecified type, not stated as uncontrolled

Fifth-digit 0 is for use with type II, adult-onset diabetic patients, even if the patient requires insulin

1 type I [insulin dependent type] [IDDM] [juvenile type], not stated as uncontrolled

2 type II [non-insulin dependent type] [NIDDM type] [adult-onset type] or unspecified type, uncontrolled

Fifth-digit 2 is for use with type II, adult-onset diabetic patients, even if the patient requires insulin

3 type I [insulin dependent type] [IDDM] [juvenile type], uncontrolled

250.0 Diabetes mellitus without mention of complication
Diabetes mellitus without mention of complication or manifestation classifiable to
  250.1-250.9
Diabetes (mellitus) NOS

250.1 Diabetes with ketoacidosis
Diabetic:
  acidosis
  ketosis   } without mention of coma

250.2 Diabetes with hyperosmolarity
Hyperosmolar (nonketotic) coma

250.3 Diabetes with other coma
Diabetic coma (with ketoacidosis)
Diabetic hypoglycemic coma
Insulin coma NOS

Excludes: diabetes with hyperosmolar coma (250.2)

250.4 Diabetes with renal manifestations
Use additional code to identify manifestation, as:
  diabetic:
    nephropathy NOS (583.81)
    nephrosis (581.81)
  intercapillary glomerulosclerosis (581.81)
  Kimmelstiel-Wilson syndrome (581.81)

250.5 Diabetes with ophthalmic manifestations
Use additional code to identify manifestation, as:
  diabetic:
    blindness (369.00-369.9)
    cataract (366.41)
    glaucoma (365.44)
    retinal edema (362.83)
    retinopathy (362.01-362.02)

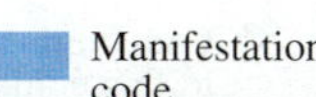

⑤ **250.6 Diabetes with neurological manifestations**

Use additional code to identify manifestation, as:
>>diabetic:
>>>amyotrophy (358.1)
>>>mononeuropathy (354.0-355.9)
>>>neurogenic arthropathy (713.5)
>>>peripheral autonomic neuropathy (337.1)
>>>polyneuropathy (357.2)

⑤ **250.7 Diabetes with peripheral circulatory disorders**

Use additional code to identify manifestation, as:
>>diabetic:
>>>gangrene (785.4)
>>>peripheral angiopathy (443.81)

⑤ **250.8 Diabetes with other specified manifestations**
>>Diabetic hypoglycemia
>>Hypoglycemic shock

Use additional code to identify manifestation, as:
>>any associated ulceration (707.10-707.9)
>>diabetic bone changes (731.8)

Use additional E code to identify cause, if drug-induced

⑤ **250.9 Diabetes with unspecified complication**

251 Other disorders of pancreatic internal secretion

251.0 Hypoglycemic coma
>>Iatrogenic hyperinsulinism   Non-diabetic insulin coma

Use additional E code to identify cause, if drug-induced

> *Excludes:* *hypoglycemic coma in diabetes mellitus (250.3)*

251.1 Other specified hypoglycemia

Use additional E code to identify cause, if drug-induced
>>Hyperinsulinism:
>>>NOS
>>>ectopic
>>>functional
>>Hyperplasia of pancreatic islet beta cells NOS

> *Excludes:* *hypoglycemia in diabetes mellitus (250.8)*
>>*hypoglycemia in infant of diabetic mother (775.0)*
>>*hypoglycemic coma (251.0)*
>>*neonatal hypoglycemia (775.6)*

251.2 Hypoglycemia, unspecified
>>Hypoglycemia:
>>>NOS
>>>reactive
>>>spontaneous

> *Excludes:* *hypoglycemia:*
>>*with coma (251.0)*
>>*in diabetes mellitus (250.8)*
>*leucine-induced (270.3)*

251.3 Postsurgical hypoinsulinemia
>>Hypoinsulinemia following complete or partial pancreatectomy
>>Postpancreatectomy hyperglycemia

251.4 Abnormality of secretion of glucagon
>>Hyperplasia of pancreatic islet alpha cells with glucagon excess

251.5 Abnormality of secretion of gastrin
>>Hyperplasia of pancreatic alpha cells with gastrin excess
>>Zollinger-Ellison syndrome

251.8 Other specified disorders of pancreatic internal secretion

251.9 Unspecified disorder of pancreatic internal secretion
>>Islet cell hyperplasia NOS

● Code new
to this edition   ▲ Revision of
existing code   ④ ⑤ Fourth or fifth
digit required

252 Disorders of parathyroid gland

252.0 Hyperparathyroidism
Hyperplasia of parathyroid
Osteitis fibrosa cystica generalisata
von Recklinghausen's disease of bone

Excludes: *ectopic hyperparathyroidism (259.3)*
secondary hyperparathyroidism (of renal origin) (588.8)

252.1 Hypoparathyroidism
Parathyroiditis (autoimmune)
Tetany:
  parathyroid
  parathyroprival

Excludes: *pseudohypoparathyroidism (275.4)*
pseudo-pseudohypoparathyroidism (275.4)
tetany NOS (781.7)
transitory neonatal hypoparathyroidism (775.4)

252.8 Other specified disorders of parathyroid gland
Cyst
Hemorrhage } of parathyroid gland

252.9 Unspecified disorder of parathyroid gland

253 Disorders of the pituitary gland and its hypothalamic control
Includes: the listed conditions whether the disorder is in the pituitary or the hypothalamus

Excludes: *Cushing's syndrome (255.0)*

253.0 Acromegaly and gigantism
Overproduction of growth hormone

253.1 Other and unspecified anterior pituitary hyperfunction
Forbes-Albright syndrome

Excludes: *overproduction of:*
  ACTH (255.3)
  thyroid-stimulating hormone [TSH] (242.8)

253.2 Panhypopituitarism
Cachexia, pituitary
Necrosis of pituitary
  (postpartum)
Pituitary insufficiency NOS

Sheehan's syndrome
Simmonds' disease

Excludes: *iatrogenic hypopituitarism (253.7)*

253.3 Pituitary dwarfism
Isolated deficiency of (human) growth hormone [HGH]
Lorain-Levi dwarfism

253.4 Other anterior pituitary disorders
Isolated or partial deficiency of an anterior pituitary hormone, other than growth hormone
Prolactin deficiency

253.5 Diabetes insipidus
Vasopressin deficiency

Excludes: *nephrogenic diabetes insipidus (588.1)*

253.6 Other disorders of neurohypophysis
Syndrome of inappropriate secretion of antidiuretic hormone [ADH]

Excludes: *ectopic antidiuretic hormone secretion (259.3)*

253.7 Iatrogenic pituitary disorders
Hypopituitarism:
  hormone-induced
  hypophysectomy-induced
  postablative
  radiotherapy-induced

Use additional E code to identify cause

253.8 Other disorders of the pituitary and other syndromes of diencephalohypophyseal origin
Abscess of pituitary
Adiposogenital dystrophy

Cyst of Rathke's pouch
Fröhlich's syndrome

Excludes: *craniopharyngioma (237.0)*

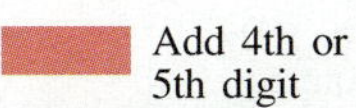

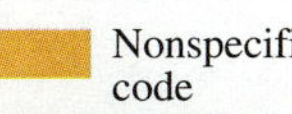

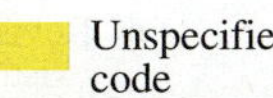

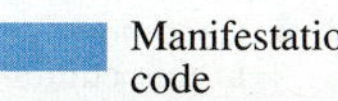

253.9 Unspecified
Dyspituitarism

254 Diseases of thymus gland

Excludes: *aplasia or dysplasia with immunodeficiency (279.2)*
hypoplasia with immunodeficiency (279.2)
myasthenia gravis (358.0)

254.0 Persistent hyperplasia of thymus
Hypertrophy of thymus

254.1 Abscess of thymus

254.8 Other specified diseases of thymus gland
Atrophy
Cyst } of thymus

Excludes *thymoma (212.6)*

254.9 Unspecified disease of thymus gland

255 Disorders of adrenal glands
Includes: the listed conditions whether the basic disorder is in the adrenals or is
pituitary-induced

255.0 Cushing's syndrome
Adrenal hyperplasia due to   Ectopic ACTH syndrome
excess ACTH   Iatrogenic syndrome of excess cortisol
Cushing's syndrome: Overproduction of cortisol
NOS
iatrogenic
idiopathic
pituitary-dependent

Use additional E code to identify cause, if drug-induced

Excludes: *congenital adrenal hyperplasia (255.2)*

255.1 Hyperaldosteronism
Aldosteronism (primary)   Bartter's syndrome
(secondary)   Conn's syndrome

255.2 Adrenogenital disorders
Adrenogenital syndromes, virilizing or feminizing, whether acquired or associated with
congenital adrenal hyperplasia consequent on inborn enzyme defects in hormone
synthesis
Achard-Thiers syndrome
Congenital adrenal hyperplasia
Female adrenal pseudohermaphroditism
Male:
macrogenitosomia praecox
sexual precocity with adrenal hyperplasia
Virilization (female) (suprarenal)

Excludes: *adrenal hyperplasia due to excess ACTH (255.0)*
isosexual virilization (256.4)

255.3 Other corticoadrenal overactivity
Acquired benign adrenal androgenic overactivity
Overproduction of ACTH

255.4 Corticoadrenal insufficiency
Addisonian crisis   Adrenal:
Addison's disease NOS   crisis
Adrenal: hemorrhage
atrophy (autoimmune)   infarction
calcification   insufficiency NOS

Excludes: *tuberculous Addison's disease (017.6)*

255.5 Other adrenal hypofunction
Adrenal medullary insufficiency

Excludes: *Waterhouse-Friderichsen syndrome (meningococcal) (036.3)*

255.6 Medulloadrenal hyperfunction
Catecholamine secretion by pheochromocytoma

255.8 Other specified disorders of adrenal glands
Abnormality of cortisol-binding globulin

255.9 Unspecified disorder of adrenal glands

● Code new   ▲ Revision of   ④ ⑤ Fourth or fifth
to this edition   existing code   digit required

256 Ovarian dysfunction

256.0 Hyperestrogenism

256.1 Other ovarian hyperfunction
Hypersecretion of ovarian androgens

256.2 Postablative ovarian failure
Ovarian failure:
  iatrogenic
  postirradiation
  postsurgical

Use additional code for states associated with artificial menopause (627.4)

Excludes:	asymptomatic age-related (natural) postmenopausal status (V49.81)
	acquired absence of ovary (V45.77)

⑤ **256.3 Other ovarian failure**
Use additional code for states associated with natural menopause (627.2)

Excludes:	asymptomatic age-related (natural) postmenopausal status (V49.81)

    256.31 Premature menopause

    256.39 Other ovarian failure
      Delayed menarche
      Ovarian hypofunction
      Primary ovarian failure NOS

256.4 Polycystic ovaries
Isosexual virilization   Stein-Leventhal syndrome

256.8 Other ovarian dysfunction

256.9 Unspecified ovarian dysfunction

257 Testicular dysfunction

257.0 Testicular hyperfunction
Hypersecretion of testicular hormones

257.1 Postablative testicular hypofunction
Testicular hypofunction:
  iatrogenic
  postirradiation
  postsurgical

257.2 Other testicular hypofunction
Defective biosynthesis of testicular androgen
Eunuchoidism:
  NOS
  hypogonadotropic
Failure:
  Leydig's cell, adult
  seminiferous tubule, adult
Testicular hypogonadism

Excludes:	azoospermia (606.0)

257.8 Other testicular dysfunction
Goldberg-Maxwell syndrome
Male pseudohermaphroditism with testicular feminization
Testicular feminization

257.9 Unspecified testicular dysfunction

258 Polyglandular dysfunction and related disorders

258.0 Polyglandular activity in multiple endocrine adenomatosis
Wermer's syndrome

258.1 Other combinations of endocrine dysfunction
Lloyd's syndrome   Schmidt's syndrome

258.8 Other specified polyglandular dysfunction

258.9 Polyglandular dysfunction, unspecified

259 Other endocrine disorders

259.0 Delay in sexual development and puberty, not elsewhere classified
Delayed puberty

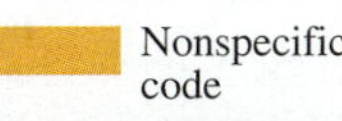
Add 4th or
5th digit

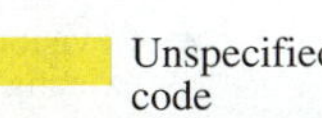
Nonspecific
code

Unspecified
code

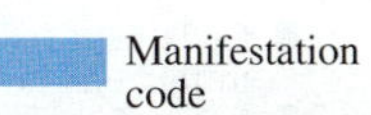
Manifestation
code

259.1 Precocious sexual development and puberty, not elsewhere classified
Sexual precocity:
NOS
constitutional
cryptogenic
idiopathic

259.2 Carcinoid syndrome
Hormone secretion by carcinoid tumors

259.3 Ectopic hormone secretion, not elsewhere classified
Ectopic:
antidiuretic hormone secretion [ADH]
hyperparathyroidism

Excludes: ectopic ACTH syndrome (255.0)

259.4 Dwarfism, not elsewhere classified
Dwarfism:
NOS
constitutional

Excludes: dwarfism:
achondroplastic (756.4)
intrauterine (759.7)
nutritional (263.2)
pituitary (253.3)
renal (588.0)
progeria (259.8)

259.8 Other specified endocrine disorders
Pineal gland dysfunction   Werner's syndrome
Progeria

259.9 Unspecified endocrine disorder
Disturbance: Infantilism NOS
endocrine NOS
hormone NOS

NUTRITIONAL DEFICIENCIES (260-269)

Excludes: deficiency anemias (280.0-281.9)

260 Kwashiorkor
Nutritional edema with dyspigmentation of skin and hair

261 Nutritional marasmus
Nutritional atrophy   Severe malnutrition NOS
Severe calorie deficiency

262 Other severe protein-calorie malnutrition
Nutritional edema without mention of dyspigmentation of skin and hair

263 Other and unspecified protein-calorie malnutrition

263.0 Malnutrition of moderate degree

263.1 Malnutrition of mild degree

263.2 Arrested development following protein-calorie malnutrition
Nutritional dwarfism
Physical retardation due to malnutrition

263.8 Other protein-calorie malnutrition

263.9 Unspecified protein-calorie malnutrition
Dystrophy due to malnutrition
Malnutrition (calorie) NOS

Excludes: nutritional deficiency NOS (269.9)

264 Vitamin A deficiency

264.0 With conjunctival xerosis

264.1 With conjunctival xerosis and Bitot's spot
Bitot's spot in the young child

264.2 With corneal xerosis

264.3 With corneal ulceration and xerosis

264.4 With keratomalacia

264.5 With night blindness

264.6 With xerophthalmic scars of cornea

● Code new
to this edition

▲ Revision of
existing code

④ ⑤ Fourth or fifth
digit required

264.7 Other ocular manifestations of vitamin A deficiency
Xerophthalmia due to vitamin A deficiency

264.8 Other manifestations of vitamin A deficiency
Follicular keratosis
Xeroderma } due to vitamin A deficiency

264.9 Unspecified vitamin A deficiency
Hypovitaminosis A NOS

265 Thiamine and niacin deficiency states

265.0 Beriberi

265.1 Other and unspecified manifestations of thiamine deficiency
Other vitamin B_1 deficiency states

265.2 Pellagra
Deficiency:
niacin (-tryptophan)
nicotinamide
nicotinic acid
vitamin PP
Pellagra (alcoholic)

266 Deficiency of B-complex components

266.0 Ariboflavinosis
Riboflavin [vitamin B_2] deficiency

266.1 Vitamin B_6 deficiency
Deficiency: Vitamin B_6 deficiency syndrome
pyridoxal
pyridoxamine
pyridoxine

Excludes: *vitamin B_6-responsive sideroblastic anemia (285.0)*

266.2 Other B-complex deficiencies
Deficiency:
cyanocobalamin
folic acid
vitamin B_{12}

Excludes: *combined system disease with anemia (281.0-281.1)*
deficiency anemias (281.0-281.9)
subacute degeneration of spinal cord with anemia (281.0-281.1)

266.9 Unspecified vitamin B deficiency

267 Ascorbic acid deficiency
Deficiency of vitamin C   Scurvy

Excludes: *scorbutic anemia (281.8)*

268 Vitamin D deficiency

Excludes: *vitamin D-resistant:*
osteomalacia (275.3)
rickets (275.3)

268.0 Rickets, active

Excludes: *celiac rickets (579.0)*
renal rickets (588.0)

268.1 Rickets, late effect
Any condition specified as due to rickets and stated to be a late effect or sequela of
rickets

Use additional code to identify the nature of late effect

268.2 Osteomalacia, unspecified

268.9 Unspecified vitamin D deficiency
Avitaminosis D

269 Other nutritional deficiencies

269.0 Deficiency of vitamin K

Excludes: *deficiency of coagulation factor due to vitamin K deficiency (286.7)*
vitamin K deficiency of newborn (776.0)

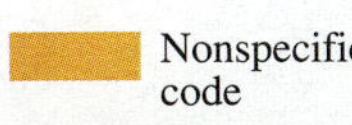

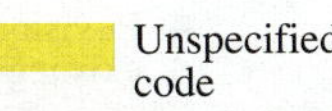

Unspecified
code

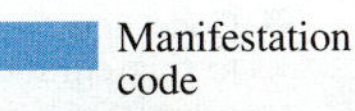

269.1 **Deficiency of other vitamins**
Deficiency:
vitamin E
vitamin P

269.2 **Unspecified vitamin deficiency**
Multiple vitamin deficiency NOS

269.3 **Mineral deficiency, not elsewhere classified**
Deficiency:
calcium, dietary
iodine

> *Excludes:* *deficiency:*
> *calcium NOS (275.4)*
> *potassium (276.8)*
> *sodium (276.1)*

269.8 **Other nutritional deficiency**

> *Excludes:* *adult failure to thrive (783.7)*
> *failure to thrive in childhood (783.41)*
> *feeding problems (783.3)*
> *newborn (779.3)*

269.9 **Unspecified nutritional deficiency**

OTHER METABOLIC AND IMMUNITY DISORDERS (270-279)

Use additional code to identify any associated mental retardation

270 **Disorders of amino-acid transport and metabolism**

> *Excludes:* *abnormal findings without manifest disease (790.0-796.9)*
> *disorders of purine and pyrimidine metabolism (277.1-277.2)*
> *gout (274.0-274.9)*

270.0 **Disturbances of amino-acid transport**
Cystinosis
Cystinuria
Fanconi (-de Toni) (-Debré) syndrome
Glycinuria (renal)
Hartnup disease

270.1 **Phenylketonuria [PKU]**
Hyperphenylalaninemia

270.2 **Other disturbances of aromatic amino-acid metabolism**

Albinism	Hypertyrosinemia
Alkaptonuria	Indicanuria
Alkaptonuric ochronosis	Kynureninase defects
Disturbances of metabolism	Oasthouse urine disease
of tyrosine and tryptophan	Ochronosis
Homogentisic acid defects	Tyrosinosis
Hydroxykynureninuria	Tyrosinuria
	Waardenburg syndrome

> *Excludes:* *vitamin B$_6$-deficiency syndrome (266.1)*

270.3 **Disturbances of branched-chain amino-acid metabolism**
Disturbances of metabolism of leucine, isoleucine, and valine
Hypervalinemia
Intermittent branched-chain ketonuria
Leucine-induced hypoglycemia
Leucinosis
Maple syrup urine disease

270.4 **Disturbances of sulphur-bearing amino-acid metabolism**
Cystathioninemia
Cystathioninuria
Disturbances of metabolism of methionine, homocystine, and cystathionine
Homocystinuria
Hypermethioninemia
Methioninemia

270.5 **Disturbances of histidine metabolism**

Carnosinemia	Hyperhistidinemia
Histidinemia	Imidazole aminoaciduria

● Code new to this edition   ▲ Revision of existing code   ④ ⑤ Fourth or fifth digit required

270.6 Disorders of urea cycle metabolism
Argininosuccinic aciduria
Citrullinemia
Disorders of metabolism of ornithine, citrulline, argininosuccinic acid, arginine, and
ammonia
Hyperammonemia
Hyperornithinemia

270.7 Other disturbances of straight-chain amino-acid metabolism
Glucoglycinuria
Glycinemia (with methyl-
malonic acidemia)
Hyperglycinemia
Hyperlysinemia
Pipecolic acidemia
Saccharopinuria
Other disturbances of metabolism of glycine, threonine,
serine, glutamine, and lysine

270.8 Other specified disorders of amino-acid metabolism
Alaninemia
Ethanolaminuria
Glycoprolinuria
Hydroxyprolinemia
Hyperprolinemia
Iminoacidopathy
Prolinemia
Prolinuria
Sarcosinemia

270.9 Unspecified disorder of amino-acid metabolism

271 Disorders of carbohydrate transport and metabolism

> *Excludes:* *abnormality of secretion of glucagon (251.4)*
> *diabetes mellitus (250.0-250.9)*
> *hypoglycemia NOS (251.2)*
> *mucopolysaccharidosis (277.5)*

271.0 Glycogenosis
Amylopectinosis
Glucose-6-phosphatase
deficiency
Glycogen storage disease
McArdle's disease
Pompe's disease
von Gierke's disease

271.1 Galactosemia
Galactose-1-phosphate uridyl transferase deficiency
Galactosuria

271.2 Hereditary fructose intolerance
Essential benign fructosuria
Fructosemia

271.3 Intestinal disaccharidase deficiencies and disaccharide malabsorption
Intolerance or malabsorption (congenital) (of):
glucose-galactose
lactose
sucrose-isomaltose

271.4 Renal glycosuria
Renal diabetes

271.8 Other specified disorders of carbohydrate transport and metabolism
Essential benign pentosuria
Fucosidosis
Glycolic aciduria
Hyperoxaluria (primary)
Mannosidosis
Oxalosis
Xylosuria
Xylulosuria

271.9 Unspecified disorder of carbohydrate transport and metabolism

272 Disorders of lipoid metabolism

> *Excludes:* *localized cerebral lipidoses (330.1)*

272.0 Pure hypercholesterolemia
Familial hypercholesterolemia
Fredrickson Type IIa hyperlipoproteinemia
Hyperbetalipoproteinemia
Hyperlipidemia, Group A
Low-density-lipoid-type [LDL] hyperlipoproteinemia

272.1 Pure hyperglyceridemia
Endogenous hyperglyceridemia
Frederickson Type IV hyperlipoproteinemia
Hyperlipidemia, Group B
Hyperprebetalipoproteinemia
Hypertriglyceridemia, essential
Very-low-density-lipoid-type [VLDL] hyperlipoproteinemia

Add 4th or 5th digit	Nonspecific code	Unspecified code	Manifestation code

272.2 Mixed hyperlipidemia
Broad- or floating-betalipoproteinemia
Fredrickson Type IIb or III hyperlipoproteinemia
Hypercholesterolemia with endogenous hyperglyceridemia
Hyperbetalipoproteinemia with prebetalipoproteinemia
Tubo-eruptive xanthoma
Xanthoma tuberosum

272.3 Hyperchylomicronemia
Bürger-Grütz syndrome   Hyperlipidemia, Group D
Fredrickson type I or V   Mixed hyperglyceridemia
    hyperlipoproteinemia

272.4 Other and unspecified hyperlipidemia
Alpha-lipoproteinemia   Hyperlipidemia NOS
Combined hyperlipidemia   Hyperlipoproteinemia NOS

272.5 Lipoprotein deficiencies
Abetalipoproteinemia
Bassen-Kornzweig syndrome
High-density lipoid deficiency
Hypoalphalipoproteinemia
Hypobetalipoproteinemia (familial)

272.6 Lipodystrophy
Barraquer-Simons disease
Progressive lipodystrophy
Use additional E code to identify cause, if iatrogenic

Excludes: intestinal lipodystrophy (040.2)

272.7 Lipidoses
Chemically-induced lipidosis   Disease:
Disease: triglyceride storage, Type I or II
  Anderson's   Wolman's or triglyceride storage, Type III
  Fabry's   Mucolipidosis II
  Gaucher's   Primary familial xanthomatosis
  I cell [mucolipidosis I]
  lipoid storage NOS
  Neimann-Pick
  pseudo-Hurler's or
    mucolipidosis III

Excludes: cerebral lipidoses (330.1)
          Tay-Sachs disease (330.1)

272.8 Other disorders of lipoid metabolism
Hoffa's disease or liposynovitis prepatellaris
Launois-Bensaude's lipomatosis
Lipoid dermatoarthritis

272.9 Unspecified disorder of lipoid metabolism

273 Disorders of plasma protein metabolism

Excludes: agammaglobulinemia and hypogammaglobulinemia (279.0 -279.2)
          coagulation defects (286.0-286.9)
          hereditary hemolytic anemias (282.0-282.9)

273.0 Polyclonal hypergammaglobulinemia
Hypergammaglobulinemic purpura:
  benign primary
  Waldenström's

273.1 Monoclonal paraproteinemia
Benign monoclonal hypergammaglobulinemia [BMH]
Monoclonal gammopathy:
  NOS
  associated with lymphoplasmacytic dyscrasias
  benign
Paraproteinemia:
  benign (familial)
  secondary to malignant or inflammatory disease

273.2 Other paraproteinemias
Cryoglobulinemic: Mixed cryoglobulinemia
  purpura
  vasculitis

     ● Code new   ▲ Revision of   ④ ⑤ Fourth or fifth
         to this edition   existing code   digit required

273.3 Macroglobulinemia
Macroglobulinemia (idiopathic) (primary)
Waldenström's macroglobulinemia

273.8 Other disorders of plasma protein metabolism
Abnormality of transport protein
Bisalbuminemia

273.9 Unspecified disorder of plasma protein metabolism

274 Gout

Excludes: lead gout (984.0-984.9)

274.0 Gouty arthropathy

⑤ **274.1 Gouty nephropathy**

   274.10 Gouty nephropathy, unspecified

   274.11 Uric acid nephrolithiasis

   274.19 Other

⑤ **274.8 Gout with other specified manifestations**

   274.81 Gouty tophi of ear

   274.82 Gouty tophi of other sites
   Gouty tophi of heart

   274.89 Other
   Use additional code to identify manifestations, as:
      gouty:
         iritis (364.11)
         neuritis (357.4)

274.9 Gout, unspecified

275 Disorders of mineral metabolism

Excludes: abnormal findings without manifest disease (790.0-796.9)

275.0 Disorders of iron metabolism
Bronzed diabetes   Pigmentary cirrhosis (of liver)
Hemochromatosis

Excludes: anemia:
         iron deficiency (280.0-280.9)
         sideroblastic (285.0)

275.1 Disorders of copper metabolism
Hepatolenticular degeneration
Wilson's disease

275.2 Disorders of magnesium metabolism
Hypermagnesemia   Hypomagnesemia

275.3 Disorders of phosphorus metabolism
Familial hypophosphatemia
Hypophosphatasia
Vitamin D-resistant:
   osteomalacia
   rickets

⑤ **275.4 Disorders of calcium metabolism**

Excludes: parathyroid disorders (252.0-252.9)
         vitamin D deficiency (268.0-268.9)

   275.40 Unspecified disorder of calcium metabolism

   275.41 Hypocalcemia

   275.42 Hypercalcemia

   275.49 Other disorders of calcium metabolism
   Nephrocalcinosis
   Pseudohypoparathyroidism
   Pseudopseudohypoparathyroidism

275.8 Other specified disorders of mineral metabolism

275.9 Unspecified disorder of mineral metabolism

276 Disorders of fluid, electrolyte, and acid-base balance

Excludes: diabetes insipidus (253.5)
         familial periodic paralysis (359.3)

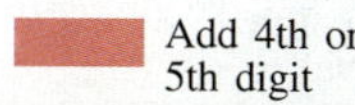

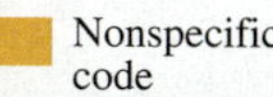

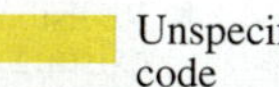

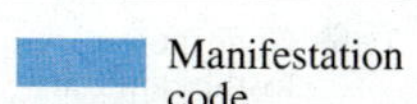

276.0 Hyperosmolality and/or hypernatremia
Sodium [Na] excess   Sodium [Na] overload

276.1 Hyposmolality and/or hyponatremia
Sodium [Na] deficiency

276.2 Acidosis
Acidosis:
NOS
lactic
metabolic
respiratory

Excludes: *diabetic acidosis (250.1)*

276.3 Alkalosis
Alkalosis:
NOS
metabolic
respiratory

276.4 Mixed acid-base balance disorder
Hypercapnia with mixed acid-base disorder

276.5 Volume depletion
Dehydration
Depletion of volume of plasma or extracellular fluid
Hypovolemia

Excludes: *hypovolemic shock:*
postoperative (998.0)
traumatic (958.4)

276.6 Fluid overload
Fluid retention

Excludes: *ascites (789.5)*
localized edema (782.3)

276.7 Hyperpotassemia
Hyperkalemia
Potassium [K]:
excess
intoxication
overload

276.8 Hypopotassemia
Hypokalemia   Potassium [K] deficiency

276.9 Electrolyte and fluid disorders not elsewhere classified
Electrolyte imbalance   Hypochloremia
Hyperchloremia

Excludes: *electrolyte imbalance:*
associated with hyperemesis gravidarum (643.1)
complicating labor and delivery (669.0)
following abortion and ectopic or molar pregnancy (634-638 with .4, 639.4)

277 Other and unspecified disorders of metabolism

⑤ **277.0 Cystic fibrosis**
Fibrocystic disease of the pancreas
Mucoviscidosis

277.00 Without mention of meconium ileus
Cystic fibrosis NOS

277.01 With meconium ileus
Meconium:
ileus (of newborn)
obstruction of intestine in mucoviscidosis

● **277.02 With pulmonary manifestations**
Cystic fibrosis with pulmonary exacerbation
Use additional code to identify any infectious organism present, such as:
pseudomonas (041.7)

● **277.03 With gastrointestinal manifestations**

Excludes: *with meconium ileus (277.01)*

● **277.09 With other manifestations**

● Code new   ▲ Revision of   ④ ⑤ Fourth or fifth
to this edition   existing code   digit required

277.1 Disorders of porphyrin metabolism
Hematoporphyria
Hematoporphyrinuria
Hereditary coproporphyria
Porphyria
Porphyrinuria
Protocoproporphyria
Protoporphyria
Pyrroloporphyria

277.2 Other disorders of purine and pyrimidine metabolism
Hypoxanthine-guanine-phosphoribosyltransferase deficiency [HG-PRT deficiency]
Lesch-Nyhan syndrome
Xanthinuria

Excludes: gout (274.0-274.9)
orotic aciduric anemia (281.4)

277.3 Amyloidosis
Amyloidosis:
  NOS
  inherited systemic
  nephropathic
  neuropathic (Portuguese) (Swiss)
  secondary
Benign paroxysmal peritonitis
Familial Mediterranean fever
Hereditary cardiac amyloidosis

277.4 Disorders of bilirubin excretion
Hyperbilirubinemia:
  congenital
  constitutional
Syndrome:
  Crigler-Najjar
  Dubin-Johnson
  Gilbert's
  Rotor's

Excludes: hyperbilirubinemias specific to the perinatal period (774.0-774.7)

277.5 Mucopolysaccharidosis
Gargoylism
Hunter's syndrome
Hurler's syndrome
Lipochondrodystrophy
Maroteaux-Lamy syndrome
Morquio-Brailsford disease
Osteochondrodystrophy
Sanfilippo's syndrome
Scheie's syndrome

277.6 Other deficiencies of circulating enzymes
Alpha 1-antitrypsin deficiency
Hereditary angioedema

277.7 Dysmetabolic syndrome X
Use additional code for associated manifestations, such as:
    cardiovascular disease (414.00-414.06)
    obesity (278.00-278.01)

277.8 Other specified disorders of metabolism
Hand-Schüller-Christian disease
Histiocytosis (acute) (chronic)
Histiocytosis X (chronic)

Excludes: histiocytosis:
    acute differentiated progressive (202.5)
    X, acute (progressive) (202.5)

277.9 Unspecified disorder of metabolism
Enzymopathy NOS

278 Obesity and other hyperalimentation

Excludes: hyperalimentation NOS (783.6)
    poisoning by vitamins NOS (963.5)
    polyphagia (783.6)

⑤ **278.0 Obesity**

Excludes: adiposogenital dystrophy (253.8)
    obesity of endocrine origin NOS (259.9)

278.00 Obesity, unspecified
Obesity NOS

278.01 Morbid obesity

278.1 Localized adiposity
Fat pad

278.2 Hypervitaminosis A

	Add 4th or 5th digit		Nonspecific code		Unspecified code		Manifestation code

278.3 Hypercarotinemia

278.4 Hypervitaminosis D

278.8 Other hyperalimentation

279 Disorders involving the immune mechanism

⑤ **279.0 Deficiency of humoral immunity**

279.00 Hypogammaglobulinemia, unspecified
Agammaglobulinemia NOS

279.01 Selective IgA immunodeficiency

279.02 Selective IgM immunodeficiency

279.03 Other selective immunoglobulin deficiencies
Selective deficiency of IgG

279.04 Congenital hypogammaglobulinemia
Agammaglobulinemia:
Bruton's type
X-linked

279.05 Immunodeficiency with increased IgM
Immunodeficiency with hyper-IgM:
autosomal recessive
X-linked

279.06 Common variable immunodeficiency
Dysgammaglobulinemia (acquired) (congenital) (primary)
Hypogammaglobulinemia:
acquired primary
congenital non-sex-linked
sporadic

279.09 Other
Transient hypogammaglobulinemia of infancy

⑤ **279.1 Deficiency of cell-mediated immunity**

279.10 Immunodeficiency with predominant T-cell defect, unspecified

279.11 DiGeorge's syndrome
Pharyngeal pouch syndrome
Thymic hypoplasia

279.12 Wiskott-Aldrich syndrome

279.13 Nezelof's syndrome
Cellular immunodeficiency with abnormal immunoglobulin deficiency

279.19 Other

Excludes: *ataxia-telangiectasia (334.8)*

279.2 Combined immunity deficiency
Agammaglobulinemia:
autosomal recessive
Swiss-type
x-linked recessive
Severe combined immunodeficiency [SCID]
Thymic:
alymphoplasia
aplasia or dysplasia with immunodeficiency

Excludes: *thymic hypoplasia (279.11)*

279.3 Unspecified immunity deficiency

279.4 Autoimmune disease, not elsewhere classified
Autoimmune disease NOS

Excludes: *transplant failure or rejection (996.80-996.89)*

279.8 Other specified disorders involving the immune mechanism
Single complement [C_1-C_9] deficiency or dysfunction

279.9 Unspecified disorder of immune mechanism

● Code new
to this edition

▲ Revision of
existing code

④ ⑤ Fourth or fifth
digit required

4. DISEASES OF THE BLOOD AND BLOOD-FORMING ORGANS (280-289)

Excludes: anemia complicating pregnancy or the puerperium (648.2)

280 Iron deficiency anemias

Includes: anemia:
asiderotic
hypochromic-microcytic
sideropenic

Excludes: familial microcytic anemia (282.4)

280.0 Secondary to blood loss (chronic)
Normocytic anemia due to blood loss

Excludes: acute posthemorrhagic anemia (285.1)

280.1 Secondary to inadequate dietary iron intake

280.8 Other specified iron deficiency anemias
Paterson-Kelly syndrome
Plummer-Vinson syndrome
Sideropenic dysphagia

280.9 Iron deficiency anemia, unspecified
Anemia:
achlorhydric
chlorotic
idiopathic hypochromic
iron [Fe] deficiency NOS

281 Other deficiency anemias

281.0 Pernicious anemia
Anemia: Congenital intrinsic factor [Castle's] deficiency
Addison's
Biermer's
congenital pernicious

Excludes: combined system disease without mention of anemia (266.2)
subacute degeneration of spinal cord without mention of anemia (266.2)

281.1 Other vitamin B_{12} deficiency anemia
Anemia:
vegan's
vitamin B_{12} deficiency (dietary)
due to selective vitamin B_{12} malabsorption with proteinuria
Syndrome:
Imerslund's
Imerslund-Gräsbeck

Excludes: combined system disease without mention of anemia (266.2)
subacute degeneration of spinal cord without mention of anemia (266.2)

281.2 Folate-deficiency anemia
Congenital folate malabsorption
Folate or folic acid deficiency anemia:
NOS
dietary
drug-induced
Goat's milk anemia
Nutritional megaloblastic anemia (of infancy)
Use additional E code, if desired, to identify drug

281.3 Other specified megaloblastic anemias not elsewhere classified
Combined B_{12} and folate-deficiency anemia
Refractory megaloblastic anemia

281.4 Protein-deficiency anemia
Amino-acid-deficiency anemia

281.8 Anemia associated with other specified nutritional deficiency
Scorbutic anemia

281.9 Unspecified deficiency anemia
Anemia: Anemia:
dimorphic   nutritional NOS
macrocytic   simple chronic
megaloblastic NOS

Add 4th or 5th digit • Nonspecific code • Unspecified code • Manifestation code

282 Hereditary hemolytic anemias

282.0 Hereditary spherocytosis
Acholuric (familial) jaundice
Congenital hemolytic anemia (spherocytic)
Congenital spherocytosis
Minkowski-Chauffard syndrome
Spherocytosis (familial)

> *Excludes:* *hemolytic anemia of newborn (773.0-773.5)*

282.1 Hereditary elliptocytosis
Elliptocytosis (congenital)
Ovalocytosis (congenital) (hereditary)

282.2 Anemias due to disorders of glutathione metabolism
Anemia:
6-phosphogluconic dehydrogenase deficiency
enzyme deficiency, drug-induced
erythrocytic glutathione deficiency
glucose-6-phosphate dehydrogenase [G-6-PD] deficiency
glutathione-reductase deficiency
hemolytic nonspherocytic (hereditary), type I
Disorder of pentose phosphate pathway
Favism

282.3 Other hemolytic anemias due to enzyme deficiency
Anemia:
hemolytic nonspherocytic (hereditary), type II
hexokinase deficiency
pyruvate kinase [PK] deficiency
triosephosphate isomerase deficiency

282.4 Thalassemias
Cooley's anemia
Hereditary leptocytosis
Mediterranean anemia (with other hemoglobinopathy)
Microdrepanocytosis
Sickle-cell thalassemia
Thalassemia (alpha) (beta) (intermedia) (major) (minima) (minor) (mixed) (trait) (with other hemoglobinopathy)
Thalassemia-Hb-S disease

> *Excludes:* *sickle-cell:*
> *anemia (282.60-282.69)*
> *trait (282.5)*

282.5 Sickle-cell trait
Hb-AS genotype
Hemoglobin S [Hb-S] trait
Heterozygous:
hemoglobin S
Hb-S

> *Excludes:* *that with other hemoglobinopathy (282.60-282.69)*
> *that with thalassemia (282.4)*

⑤ **282.6 Sickle-cell anemia**

> *Excludes:* *sickle-cell thalassemia (282.4)*
> *sickle-cell trait (282.5)*

282.60 Sickle-cell anemia, unspecified

282.61 Hb-S disease without mention of crisis

282.62 Hb-S disease with mention of crisis
Sickle-cell crisis NOS

282.63 Sickle-cell/Hb-C disease
Hb-S/Hb-C disease

282.69 Other
Disease:
Hb-S/Hb-D
Hb-S/Hb-E
Disease:
sickle-cell/Hb-D
sickle-cell/Hb-E

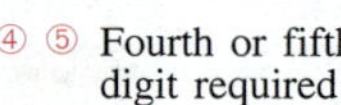

● Code new to this edition   ▲ Revision of existing code   ④ ⑤ Fourth or fifth digit required

282.7 Other hemoglobinopathies
Abnormal hemoglobin NOS
Congenital Heinz-body anemia
Disease:
  Hb-Bart's
  hemoglobin C [Hb-C]
  hemoglobin D [Hb-D]
  hemoglobin E [Hb-E]
  hemoglobin Zurich [Hb-Zurich]
Hemoglobinopathy NOS
Hereditary persistence of fetal hemoglobin [HPFH]
Unstable hemoglobin hemolytic disease

Excludes: *familial polycythemia (289.6)*
  hemoglobin M [Hb-M] disease (289.7)
  high-oxygen-affinity hemoglobin (289.0)

282.8 Other specified hereditary hemolytic anemias
Stomatocytosis

282.9 Hereditary hemolytic anemia, unspecified
Hereditary hemolytic anemia NOS

283 Acquired hemolytic anemias

283.0 Autoimmune hemolytic anemias
Autoimmune hemolytic anemias (cold type) (warm type)
Chronic cold hemagglutinin disease
Cold agglutinin disease or hemoglobinuria
Hemolytic anemia:
  cold type (secondary) (symptomatic)
  drug-induced
  warm type (secondary) (symptomatic)

Use additional E code, if desired, to identify cause, if drug-induced

Excludes: *Evans' syndrome (287.3)*
  hemolytic disease of newborn (773.0-773.5)

⑤ **283.1 Non-autoimmune hemolytic anemias**

283.10 Non-autoimmune hemolytic anemia, unspecified

283.11 Hemolytic-uremic syndrome

283.19 Other non-autoimmune hemolytic anemias
Hemolytic anemia:
  mechanical
  microangiopathic
  toxic
Use additional E code, if desired, to identify cause

283.2 Hemoglobinuria due to hemolysis from external causes
Acute intravascular hemolysis
Hemoglobinuria:
  from exertion
  march
  paroxysmal (cold) (nocturnal)
  due to other hemolysis
Marchiafava-Micheli syndrome

Use additional E code, if desired, to identify cause

283.9 Acquired hemolytic anemia, unspecified
Acquired hemolytic anemia NOS
Chronic idiopathic hemolytic anemia

284 Aplastic anemia

284.0 Constitutional aplastic anemia
Aplasia, (pure) red cell: Familial hypoplastic anemia
  congenital   Fanconi's anemia
  of infants   Pancytopenia with malformations
  primary
Blackfan-Diamond syndrome

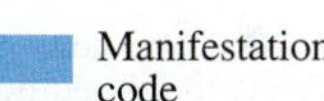

284.8 **Other specified aplastic anemias**

Aplastic anemia (due to):
chronic systemic disease
drugs
infection
radiation
toxic (paralytic)

Pancytopenia (acquired)
Red cell aplasia (acquired) (adult) (pure) (with thymoma)

Use additional E code, if desired, to identify cause

284.9 **Aplastic anemia, unspecified**

Anemia:
aplastic (idiopathic) NOS
aregenerative
hypoplastic NOS

Anemia:
nonregenerative
refractory
Medullary hypoplasia

285 **Other and unspecified anemias**

285.0 **Sideroblastic anemia**

Anemia:
hypochromic with iron loading
sideroachrestic
sideroblastic
acquired
congenital
hereditary
primary
refractory
secondary (drug-induced) (due to disease)
sex-linked hypochromic
vitamin B_6-responsive
Pyridoxine-responsive (hypochromic) anemia

Use additional E code, if desired, to identify cause, if drug induced

285.1 **Acute posthemorrhagic anemia**

Anemia due to acute blood loss

Excludes: *anemia due to chronic blood loss (280.0)*
blood loss anemia NOS (280.0)

⑤ **285.2** **Anemia in chronic illness**

285.21 **Anemia in end-stage renal disease**

285.22 **Anemia in neoplastic disease**

285.29 **Anemia of other chronic illness**

285.8 **Other specified anemias**

Anemia:
dyserythropoietic (congenital)
dyshematopoietic (congenital)
leukoerythroblastic
von Jaksch's
Infantile pseudoleukemia

285.9 **Anemia, unspecified**

Anemia:
NOS
essential
normocytic, not due to blood
loss

Anemia:
profound
progressive
secondary
Oligocythemia

Excludes: *anemia (due to):*
blood loss:
acute (285.1)
chronic or unspecified (280.0)
iron deficiency (280.0-280.9)

● Code new
to this edition

▲ Revision of
existing code

④ ⑤ Fourth or fifth
digit required

286 **Coagulation defects**

286.0 Congenital factor VIII disorder

Antihemophilic globulin
  [AHG]
  deficiency
Factor VIII (functional)
  deficiency
Hemophilia:
  NOS
  A
  classical
  familial
  hereditary
Subhemophilia

Excludes: factor VIII deficiency with vascular defect (286.4)

286.1 Congenital factor IX disorder

Christmas disease
Deficiency:
  factor IX (functional)
  plasma thromboplastin component [PTC]
Hemophilia B

286.2 Congenital factor XI deficiency

Hemophilia C
Plasma thromboplastin antecedent [PTA] deficiency
Rosenthal's disease

286.3 Congenital deficiency of other clotting factors

Congenital afibrinogenemia
Deficiency:
  AC globulin factor:
    I [fibrinogen]
    II [prothrombin]
    V [labile]
    VII [stable]
    X [Stuart-Prower]
    XII [Hageman]
    XIII [fibrin stabilizing]
Deficiency:
  Laki-Lorand factor
  proaccelerin
Disease:
  Owren's
  Stuart-Prower
Dysfibrinogenemia (congenital)
Dysprothrombinemia (constitutional)
Hypoproconvertinemia
Hypoprothrombinemia (hereditary)
Parahemophilia

286.4 von Willebrand's disease

Angiohemophilia (A) (B)
Constitutional thrombopathy
Factor VIII deficiency with vascular defect
Pseudohemophilia type B
Vascular hemophilia
von Willebrand's (-Jürgens') disease

Excludes: factor VIII deficiency:
  NOS (286.0)
   with functional defect (286.0)
  hereditary capillary fragility (287.8)

286.5 Hemorrhagic disorder due to circulating anticoagulants

Antithrombinemia
Antithromboplastinemia
Antithromboplastinogenemia
Hyperheparinemia
Increase in:
  anti-VIIIa
  anti-IXa
  anti-Xa
  anti-XIa
  antithrombin
Systemic lupus erythematosus [SLE] inhibitor

Use additional E code, if desired, to identify cause, if drug induced

286.6 Defibrination syndrome

Afibrinogenemia, acquired
Consumption coagulopathy
Diffuse or disseminated intravascular coagulation [DIC syndrome]
Fibrinolytic hemorrhage, acquired
Hemorrhagic fibrinogenolysis
Pathologic fibrinolysis
Purpura:
  fibrinolytic
  fulminans

Excludes: that complicating:
  abortion (634-638 with .1, 639.1)
  pregnancy or the puerperium (641.3, 666.3)
  disseminated intravascular coagulation in newborn (776.2)

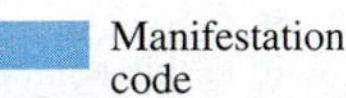

286.7 Acquired coagulation factor deficiency
Deficiency of coagulation factor due to:
  liver disease
  vitamin K deficiency
Hypoprothrombinemia, acquired

| *Excludes:* | *vitamin K deficiency of newborn (776.0)* |

Use additional E-code, if desired, to identify cause, if drug induced

286.9 Other and unspecified coagulation defects
Defective coagulation NOS
Deficiency, coagulation factor NOS
Delay, coagulation
Disorder:
  coagulation
  hemostasis

Excludes:	*abnormal coagulation profile (790.92)*
	hemorrhagic disease of newborn (776.0)
	that complicating:
	abortion (634-638 with .1, 639.1)
	pregnancy or the puerperium (641.3, 666.3)

287 Purpura and other hemorrhagic conditions

| *Excludes:* | *hemorrhagic thrombocythemia (238.7)* |
| | *purpura fulminans (286.6)* |

287.0 Allergic purpura
Peliosis rheumatica   Purpura:
Purpura: nonthrombocytopenic:
  anaphylactoid   hemorrhagic
  autoimmune   idiopathic
  Henoch's   rheumatica
                                                 Schönlein-Henoch
                                                 vascular
                                              Vasculitis, allergic

| *Excludes:* | *hemorrhagic purpura (287.3)* |
| | *purpura annularis telangiectodes (709.1)* |

287.1 Qualitative platelet defects
Thrombasthenia (hemorrhagic) (hereditary)
Thrombocytasthenia
Thrombocytopathy (dystrophic)
Thrombopathy (Bernard-Soulier)

| *Excludes:* | *von Willebrand's disease (286.4)* |

287.2 Other nonthrombocytopenic purpuras
Purpura:
  NOS
  senile
  simplex

287.3 Primary thrombocytopenia
Evans' syndrome   Thrombocytopenia:
Megakaryocytic hypoplasia   congenital
Purpura, thrombocytopenic   hereditary
  congenital   primary
  hereditary   Tidal platelet dysgenesis
  idiopathic

| *Excludes:* | *thrombotic thrombocytopenic purpura (446.6)* |
| | *transient thrombocytopenia of newborn (776.1)* |

287.4 Secondary thrombocytopenia
Posttransfusion purpura
Thrombocytopenia (due to):
  dilutional
  drugs
  extracorporeal circulation of blood
  massive blood transfusion
  platelet alloimmunization

Use additional E code, if desired, to identify cause

| *Excludes:* | *transient thrombocytopenia of newborn (776.1)* |

● Code new   ▲ Revision of   ④ ⑤ Fourth or fifth
  to this edition   existing code   digit required

287.5 Thrombocytopenia, unspecified

287.8 Other specified hemorrhagic conditions
Capillary fragility (hereditary)
Vascular pseudohemophilia

287.9 Unspecified hemorrhagic conditions
Hemorrhagic diathesis (familial)

288 Diseases of white blood cells

> *Excludes:* *leukemia (204.0-208.9)*

288.0 Agranulocytosis
Infantile genetic agranulo-
  cytosis
Kostmann's syndrome
Neutropenia:
  NOS
  cyclic

Neutropenia:
  drug-induced
  immune
  periodic
  toxic
Neutropenic splenomegaly

Use additional E code, if desired, to identify drug or other cause

> *Excludes:* *transitory neonatal neutropenia (776.7)*

288.1 Functional disorders of polymorphonuclear neutrophils
Chronic (childhood) granulomatous disease
Congenital dysphagocytosis
Job's syndrome
Lipochrome histiocytosis (familial)
Progressive septic granulomatosis

288.2 Genetic anomalies of leukocytes
Anomaly (granulation) (granulocyte) or syndrome:
  Alder's (-Reilly)
  Chédiak-Steinbrinck (-Higashi)
  Jordan's
  May-Hegglin
  Pelger-Huet
Hereditary:
  hypersegmentation
  hyposegmentation
  leukomelanopathy

288.3 Eosinophilia
Eosinophilia
  allergic
  hereditary
  idiopathic
  secondary
Eosinophilic leukocytosis

> *Excludes:* *Löffler's syndrome (518.3)*
> *pulmonary eosinophilia (518.3)*

288.8 Other specified disease of white blood cells
Leukemoid reaction
  lymphocytic
  monocytic
  myelocytic
Leukocytosis
Lymphocytopenia

Lymphocytosis (symptomatic)
Lymphopenia
Monocytosis (symptomatic)
Plasmacytosis

> *Excludes:* *immunity disorders (279.0-279.9)*

288.9 Unspecified disease of white blood cells

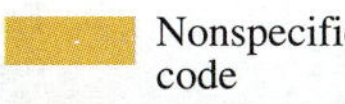
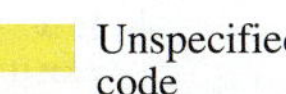

Add 4th or 5th digit   Nonspecific code   Unspecified code   Manifestation code

289 **Other diseases of blood and blood-forming organs**

289.0 **Polycythemia, secondary**

High-oxygen-affinity
hemoglobin
Polycythemia:
acquired
benign
due to:
fall in plasma volume
high altitude

Polycythemia:
emotional
erythropoietin
hypoxemic
nephrogenous
relative
spurious
stress

Excludes: *polycythemia:*
neonatal (776.4)
primary (238.4)
vera (238.4)

289.1 **Chronic lymphadenitis**

Chronic:
adenitis
lymphadenitis } any lymph node, except mesenteric

Excludes: *acute lymphadenitis (683)*
mesenteric (289.2)
enlarged glands NOS (785.6)

289.2 **Nonspecific mesenteric lymphadenitis**

Mesenteric lymphadenitis (acute) (chronic)

289.3 **Lymphadenitis, unspecified, except mesenteric**

289.4 **Hypersplenism**

"Big spleen" syndrome   Hypersplenia
Dyssplenism

Excludes: *primary splenic neutropenia (288.0)*

⑤ **289.5** **Other diseases of spleen**

289.50 **Disease of spleen, unspecified**

289.51 **Chronic congestive splenomegaly**

289.59 **Other**

Lien migrans
Perisplenitis
Splenic:
abscess
atrophy
cyst

Splenic:
fibrosis
infarction
rupture, nontraumatic
Splenitis
Wandering spleen

Excludes: *bilharzial splenic fibrosis (120.0-120.9)*
hepatolienal fibrosis (571.5)
splenomegaly NOS (789.2)

289.6 **Familial polycythemia**

Familial:
benign polycythemia
erythrocytosis

289.7 **Methemoglobinemia**

Congenital NADH [DPNH]-methemoglobin-reductase deficiency
Hemoglobin M [Hb-M] disease
Methemoglobinemia:
NOS
acquired (with sulfhemoglobinemia)
hereditary
toxic
Stokvis' disease
Sulfhemoglobinemia

Use additional E code, if desired, to identify cause

289.8 **Other specified diseases of blood and blood-forming organs**

Hypergammaglobulinemia   Pseudocholinesterase deficiency
Myelofibrosis

289.9 **Unspecified diseases of blood and blood-forming organs**

Blood dyscrasia NOS   Erythroid hyperplasia

● Code new
to this edition

▲ Revision of
existing code

④ ⑤ Fourth or fifth
digit required

5. MENTAL DISORDERS (290-319)

In the International Classification of Diseases, 9th Revision (*ICD-9*), the corresponding Chapter V, "Mental Disorders," includes a glossary which defines the contents of each category. The introduction to Chapter V in *ICD-9* indicates that the glossary is intended so that psychiatrists can make the diagnosis based on the descriptions provided rather than from the category titles. Lay coders are instructed to code whatever diagnosis the physician records.

Chapter 5, "Mental Disorders," in *ICD-9-CM* uses the standard classification format with inclusion and exclusion terms, omitting the glossary as part of the main text.

The mental disorders section of *ICD-9-CM* has been expanded to incorporate additional psychiatric disorders not listed in *ICD-9*. The glossary from *ICD-9* does not contain all these terms. It now appears in Appendix B, pages 543-564 which also contains descriptions and definitions for the terms added in *ICD-9-CM*. Some of these were provided by the American Psychiatric Association's Task Force on Nomenclature and Statistics who are preparing the *Diagnostic and Statistical Manual*, Third Edition (DSM-III), and others from *A Psychiatric Glossary*.

The American Psychiatric Association provided invaluable assistance in modifying Chapter 5 of *ICD-9-CM* to incorporate detail useful to American clinicians and gave permission to use material from the aforementioned sources.

1. **Manual of the *International Statistical Classification of Diseases, Injuries, and Causes of Death*, 9th Revision, World Health Organization, Geneva, Switzerland, 1975.**

2. **American Psychiatric Association, Task Force on Nomenclature and Statistics, Robert L. Spitzer, M.D., Chairman.**

3. ***A Psychiatric Glossary*, Fourth Edition, American Psychiatric Association, Washington, D.C., 1975.**

PSYCHOSES (290-299)

> | *Excludes:* | *mental retardation (317-319)* |

ORGANIC PSYCHOTIC CONDITIONS (290-294)

> Includes: psychotic organic brain syndrome

> | *Excludes:* | *nonpsychotic syndromes of organic etiology (310.0-310.9)* |

> *psychoses classifiable to 295-298 and without impairment of orientation, comprehension, calculation, learning capacity, and judgement, but associated with physical disease, injury, or condition affecting the brain [e.g., following childbirth] (295.0-298.8)*

290 Senile and presenile organic psychotic conditions
Code first the associated neurological condition

> | *Excludes:* | *dementia not classified as senile, presenile, or arteriosclerotic (294.10-294.11)* |

> *psychoses classifiable to 295-298 occurring in the senium without dementia or delirium (295.0-298.8)*
> *senility with mental changes of nonpsychotic severity (310.1)*
> *transient organic psychotic conditions (293.0-293.9)*

290.0 Senile dementia, uncomplicated
Senile dementia:
  NOS
  simple type

> | *Excludes:* | *mild memory disturbances, not amounting to dementia, associated with senile brain disease (310.1)* |

> *senile dementia with:*
>   *delirium or confusion (290.3)*
>   *delusional [paranoid] features (290.20)*
>   *depressive features (290.21)*

⑤ 290.1 Presenile dementia
Brain syndrome with presenile brain disease

> | *Excludes:* | *arteriosclerotic dementia (290.40-290.43)* |

> *dementia associated with other cerebral conditions (294.10-294.11)*

290.10 Presenile dementia, uncomplicated
Presenile dementia:
  NOS
  simple type

290.11 Presenile dementia with delirium
Presenile dementia with acute confusional state

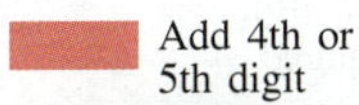

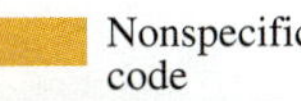

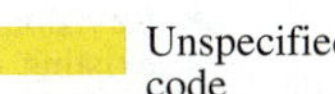

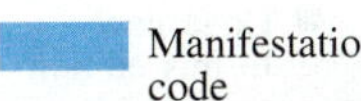

290.12 Presenile dementia with delusional features
Presenile dementia, paranoid type

290.13 Presenile dementia with depressive features
Presenile dementia, depressed type

⑤ **290.2 Senile dementia with delusional or depressive features**

| Excludes: | senile dementia:
NOS (290.0)
with delirium and/or confusion (290.3)

290.20 Senile dementia with delusional features
Senile dementia, paranoid type
Senile psychosis NOS

290.21 Senile dementia with depressive features

290.3 Senile dementia with delirium
Senile dementia with acute confusional state

| Excludes: | senile:

dementia NOS (290.0)
psychosis NOS (290.20)

⑤ **290.4 Arteriosclerotic dementia**
Multi-infarct dementia or psychosis

Use additional code to identify cerebral atherosclerosis (437.0)

| Excludes: | suspected cases with no clear evidence of arteriosclerosis (290.9)

290.40 Arteriosclerotic dementia, uncomplicated
Arteriosclerotic dementia:
NOS
simple type

290.41 Arteriosclerotic dementia with delirium
Arteriosclerotic dementia with acute confusional state

290.42 Arteriosclerotic dementia with delusional features
Arteriosclerotic dementia, paranoid type

290.43 Arteriosclerotic dementia with depressive features
Arteriosclerotic dementia, depressed type

290.8 Other specified senile psychotic conditions
Presbyophrenic psychosis

290.9 Unspecified senile psychotic condition

291 Alcoholic psychoses

| Excludes: | alcoholism without psychosis (303.0-303.9)

291.0 Alcohol withdrawal delirium
Alcoholic delirium   Delirium tremens

| Excludes: | alcohol withdrawal (291.81)

291.1 Alcohol amnestic syndrome
Alcoholic polyneuritic psychosis
Korsakoff's psychosis, alcoholic
Wernicke-Korsakoff syndrome (alcoholic)

291.2 Other alcoholic dementia
Alcoholic dementia NOS
Alcoholism associated with dementia NOS
Chronic alcoholic brain syndrome

291.3 Alcohol withdrawal hallucinosis
Alcoholic:
hallucinosis (acute)
psychosis with hallucinosis

| Excludes: | alcohol withdrawal with delirium (291.0)

schizophrenia (295.0-295.9) and paranoid states (297.0-297.9) taking the form of
chronic hallucinosis with clear consciousness in an alcoholic

     ● Code new   ▲ Revision of   ④ ⑤ Fourth or fifth
      to this edition   existing code   digit required

291.4 Idiosyncratic alcohol intoxication
Pathologic:
alcohol intoxication
drunkenness

Excludes: *acute alcohol intoxication (305.0)*
in alcoholism (303.0)
simple drunkenness (305.0)

291.5 Alcoholic jealousy
Alcoholic:
paranoia
psychosis, paranoid type

Excludes: *nonalcoholic paranoid states (297.0-297.9)*
schizophrenia, paranoid type (295.3)

⑤ **291.8 Other specified alcoholic psychosis**

291.81 Alcohol withdrawal
Alcohol:
withdrawal syndrome or symptoms
abstinence syndrome or symptoms

Excludes: *alcohol withdrawal:*
delirium (291.0)
hallucinosis (291.3)
delirium tremens (291.0)

291.89 Other

291.9 Unspecified alcoholic psychosis
Alcoholic:
mania NOS
psychosis NOS
Alcoholism (chronic) with psychosis

292 Drug psychoses
Includes: drug-induced mental disorders
organic brain syndrome associated with consumption of drugs

Use additional code for any associated drug dependence (304.0-304.9)

Use additional E code, if desired, to identify drug

292.0 Drug withdrawal syndrome
Drug:
abstinence syndrome or symptoms
withdrawal syndrome or symptoms

⑤ **292.1 Paranoid and/or hallucinatory states induced by drugs**

292.11 Drug-induced organic delusional syndrome
Paranoid state induced by drugs

292.12 Drug-induced hallucinosis
Hallucinatory state induced by drugs

Excludes: *states following LSD or other hallucinogens, lasting only a few days or less ["bad trips"] (305.3)*

292.2 Pathological drug intoxication
Drug reaction:
NOS
idiosyncratic } resulting in brief psychotic states
pathologic

Excludes: *expected brief psychotic reactions to hallucinogens ["bad trips"] (305.3)*
physiological side-effects of drugs (e.g., dystonias)

⑤ **292.8 Other specified drug-induced mental disorders**

292.81 Drug-induced delirium

292.82 Drug-induced dementia

292.83 Drug-induced amnestic syndrome

292.84 Drug-induced organic affective syndrome
Depressive state induced by drugs

292.89 Other
Drug-induced organic personality syndrome

292.9 Unspecified drug-induced mental disorder
Organic psychosis NOS due to or associated with drugs

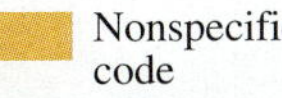
Add 4th or 5th digit   Nonspecific code

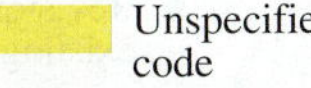
Unspecified code   Manifestation code

293 Transient organic psychotic conditions
Includes: transient organic mental disorders not associated with alcohol or drugs
Code first the associated physical or neurological condition

Excludes: *confusional state or delirium superimposed on senile dementia (290.3)*
dementia due to:
alcohol (291.0-291.9)
arteriosclerosis (290.40-290.43)
drugs (292.82)
senility (290.0)

293.0 Acute delirium
Acute:
confusional state
infective psychosis
organic reaction
posttraumatic organic
psychosis
psycho-organic syndrome

Acute psychosis associated with endocrine, metabolic,
or cerebrovascular disorder
Epileptic:
confusional state
twilight state

293.1 Subacute delirium
Subacute:
confusional state
infective psychosis
organic reaction
posttraumatic organic
psychosis

Subacute:
psycho-organic syndrome
psychosis associated with endocrine or metabolic
disorder

⑤ **293.8 Other specified transient organic mental disorders**

293.81 Organic delusional syndrome
Transient organic psychotic condition, paranoid type

293.82 Organic hallucinosis syndrome
Transient organic psychotic condition, hallucinatory type

293.83 Organic affective syndrome
Transient organic psychotic condition, depressive type

293.84 Organic anxiety syndrome

293.89 Other

293.9 Unspecified transient organic mental disorder
Organic psychosis:
infective NOS
posttraumatic NOS
transient NOS

Psycho-organic syndrome

294 Other organic psychotic conditions (chronic)
Includes: organic psychotic brain syndromes (chronic), not elsewhere classified

294.0 Amnestic syndrome
Korsakoff's psychosis or syndrome (nonalcoholic)

Excludes: *alcoholic:*
amnestic syndrome (291.1)
Korsakoff's psychosis (291.1)

⑤ **294.1 Dementia in conditions classified elsewhere**
Code first any underlying physical condition, as:
dementia in:
Alzheimer's disease (331.0)
cerebral lipidoses (330.1)
epilepsy (345.0-345.9)
general paresis [syphilis] (094.1)
hepatolenticular degeneration (275.1)
Huntington's chorea (333.4)
Jakob-Creutzfeldt disease (046.1)
multiple sclerosis (340)
Pick's disease of the brain (331.1)
polyarteritis nodosa (446.0)
syphilis (094.1)

Excludes: *dementia:*
arteriosclerotic (290.40-290.43)
presenile (290.10-290.13)
senile (290.0)
epileptic psychosis NOS (294.8)

● Code new
to this edition
▲ Revision of
existing code
④ ⑤ Fourth or fifth
digit required

294.10 ***Dementia in conditions classified elsewhere without behavioral disturbance***
Dementia in conditions classified elsewhere NOS

294.11 ***Dementia in conditions classified elsewhere with behavioral disturbance***
Aggressive behavior
Combative behavior
Violent behavior
Wandering off

294.8 **Other specified organic brain syndromes (chronic)**
Epileptic psychosis NOS
Mixed paranoid and affective organic psychotic states
Use additional code for associated epilepsy (345.0-345.9)

Excludes: *mild memory disturbances, not amounting to dementia (310.1)*

294.9 **Unspecified organic brain syndrome (chronic)**
Organic psychosis (chronic)

OTHER PSYCHOSES (295-299)

Use additional code to identify any associated physical disease, injury, or condition affecting the brain with psychoses classifiable to 295-298

295 **Schizophrenic disorders**
Includes: schizophrenia of the types described in 295.0-295.9 occurring in children

Excludes: *childhood type schizophrenia (299.9)*

infantile autism (299.0)

The following fifth-digit subclassification is for use with category 295:

0 **unspecified**

1 **subchronic**

2 **chronic**

3 **subchronic with acute exacerbation**

4 **chronic with acute exacerbation**

5 **in remission**

295.0 **Simple type**
Schizophrenia simplex

Excludes: *latent schizophrenia (295.5)*

295.1 **Disorganized type**
Hebephrenia
Hebephrenic type schizophrenia

295.2 **Catatonic type**

Catatonic (schizophrenia):
agitation
excitation
excited type
stupor
withdrawn type

Schizophrenic:
catalepsy
catatonia
flexibilitas cerea

295.3 **Paranoid type**
Paraphrenic schizophrenia

Excludes: *involutional paranoid state (297.2)*

paranoia (297.1)
paraphrenia (297.2)

295.4 **Acute schizophrenic episode**
Oneirophrenia
Schizophreniform:
attack
disorder
psychosis, confusional type

Excludes: *acute forms of schizophrenia of:*

catatonic type (295.2)
hebephrenic type (295.1)
paranoid type (295.3)
simple type (295.0)
undifferentiated type (295.8)

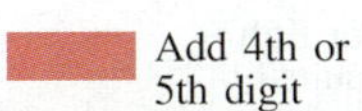 Add 4th or 5th digit

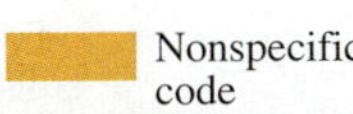 Nonspecific code

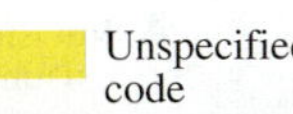 Unspecified code

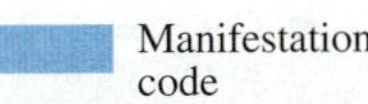 Manifestation code

⑤ **295.5 Latent schizophrenia**

Latent schizophrenic reaction   Schizophrenia:
Schizophrenia: prepsychotic
  borderline   prodromal
  incipient   pseudoneurotic
                                       pseudopsychopathic

Excludes: schizoid personality (301.20-301.22)

⑤ **295.6 Residual schizophrenia**

Chronic undifferentiated schizophrenia
Restzustand (schizophrenic)
Schizophrenic residual state

⑤ **295.7 Schizo-affective type**

Cyclic schizophrenia
Mixed schizophrenic and affective psychosis
Schizo-affective psychosis
Schizophreniform psychosis, affective type

⑤ **295.8 Other specified types of schizophrenia**

Acute (undifferentiated) schizophrenia
Atypical schizophrenia
Cenesthopathic schizophrenia

Excludes: infantile autism (299.0)

⑤ **295.9 Unspecified schizophrenia**

Schizophrenia: Schizophrenic reaction NOS
  NOS   Schizophreniform psychosis NOS
  mixed NOS
  undifferentiated NOS

296 Affective psychoses

Includes: episodic affective disorders

Excludes: neurotic depression (300.4)
           reactive depressive psychosis (298.0)
           reactive excitation (298.1)

The following fifth-digit subclassification is for use with categories 296.0-296.6:

0 unspecified

1 mild

2 moderate

3 severe, without mention of psychotic behavior

4 severe, specified as with psychotic behavior

5 in partial or unspecified remission

6 in full remission

⑤ **296.0 Manic disorder, single episode**

Hypomania (mild) NOS
Hypomanic psychosis
Mania (monopolar) NOS   } single episode or unspecified
Manic-depressive psychosis or reaction:
  hypomanic
  manic

Excludes: circular type, if there was a previous attack of depression (296.4)

⑤ **296.1 Manic disorder, recurrent episode**

Any condition classifiable to 296.0, stated to be recurrent

Excludes: circular type, if there was a previous attack of depression (296.4)

⑤ **296.2 Major depressive disorder, single episode**

Depressive psychosis
Endogenous depression
Involutional melancholia
Manic-depressive psychosis or reaction,   } single episode or unspecified
  depressed type
Monopolar depression
Psychotic depression

● Code new   ▲ Revision of   ④ ⑤ Fourth or fifth
  to this edition   existing code   digit required

> *Excludes:* *circular type, if previous attack was of manic type (296.5)*
> *depression NOS (311)*
> *reactive depression (neurotic) (300.4)*
> *psychotic (298.0)*

⑤ **296.3 Major depressive disorder, recurrent episode**
Any condition classifiable to 296.2, stated to be recurrent

> *Excludes:* *circular type, if previous attack was of manic type (296.5)*
> *depression NOS (311)*
> *reactive depression (neurotic) (300.4)*
> *psychotic (298.0)*

⑤ **296.4 Bipolar affective disorder, manic**
Bipolar disorder, now manic
Manic-depressive psychosis, circular type but currently manic

> *Excludes:* *brief compensatory or rebound mood swings (296.99)*

⑤ **296.5 Bipolar affective disorder, depressed**
Bipolar disorder, now depressed
Manic-depressive psychosis, circular type but currently depressed

> *Excludes:* *brief compensatory or rebound mood swings (296.99)*

⑤ **296.6 Bipolar affective disorder, mixed**
Manic-depressive psychosis, circular type, mixed

296.7 Bipolar affective disorder, unspecified
Atypical bipolar affective disorder NOS
Manic-depressive psychosis, circular type, current condition not specified as either manic or depressive

⑤ **296.8 Manic-depressive psychosis, other and unspecified**

296.80 Manic-depressive psychosis, unspecified
Manic-depressive:
reaction NOS
syndrome NOS

296.81 Atypical manic disorder

296.82 Atypical depressive disorder

296.89 Other
Manic-depressive psychosis, mixed type

⑤ **296.9 Other and unspecified affective psychoses**

> *Excludes:* *psychogenic affective psychoses (298.0-298.8)*

296.90 Unspecified affective psychosis
Affective psychosis NOS
Melancholia NOS

296.99 Other specified affective psychoses
Mood swings:
brief compensatory
rebound

297 Paranoid states (Delusional disorders)
Includes: paranoid disorders

> *Excludes:* *acute paranoid reaction (298.3)*
> *alcoholic jealousy or paranoid state (291.5)*
> *paranoid schizophrenia (295.3)*

297.0 Paranoid state, simple

297.1 Paranoia
Chronic paranoid psychosis
Sander's disease
Systematized delusions

> *Excludes:* *paranoid personality disorder (301.0)*

297.2 Paraphrenia
Involutional paranoid state
Late paraphrenia
Paraphrenia (involutional)

297.3 Shared paranoid disorder
Folie à deux
Induced psychosis or paranoid disorder

297.8 Other specified paranoid states
      Paranoia querulans
      Sensitiver Beziehungswahn

    Excludes: *acute paranoid reaction or state (298.3)*
             senile paranoid state (290.20)

297.9 Unspecified paranoid state
      Paranoid: Paranoid:
        disorder NOS   reaction NOS
        psychosis   state NOS

298 Other nonorganic psychoses
     Includes: psychotic conditions due to or provoked by:
            emotional stress
            environmental factors as major part of etiology

298.0 Depressive type psychosis
      Psychogenic depressive psychosis
      Psychotic reactive depression
      Reactive depressive psychosis

    Excludes: *manic-depressive psychosis, depressed type (296.2-296.3)*
             neurotic depression (300.4)
             reactive depression NOS (300.4)

298.1 Excitative type psychosis
      Acute hysterical psychosis   Reactive excitation
      Psychogenic excitation

    Excludes: *manic-depressive psychosis, manic type (296.0-296.1)*

298.2 Reactive confusion
      Psychogenic confusion
      Psychogenic twilight state

    Excludes: *acute confusional state (293.0)*

298.3 Acute paranoid reaction
      Acute psychogenic paranoid psychosis
      Bouffée délirante

    Excludes: *paranoid states (297.0-297.9)*

298.4 Psychogenic paranoid psychosis
      Protracted reactive paranoid psychosis

298.8 Other and unspecified reactive psychosis
      Brief reactive psychosis NOS
      Hysterical psychosis
      Psychogenic psychosis NOS
      Psychogenic stupor

    Excludes: *acute hysterical psychosis (298.1)*

298.9 Unspecified psychosis
      Atypical psychosis   Psychosis NOS

⑤ **299 Psychoses with origin specific to childhood**
     Includes: pervasive developmental disorders

    Excludes: *adult type psychoses occurring in childhood, as:*
             affective disorders (296.0-296.9)
             manic-depressive disorders (296.0-296.9)
             schizophrenia (295.0-295.9)

The following fifth-digit subclassification is for use with category 299:

    0   **current or active state**

    1   **residual state**

⑤ **299.0 Infantile autism**
      Childhood autism   Kanner's syndrome
      Infantile psychosis

    Excludes: *disintegrative psychosis (299.1)*
             Heller's syndrome (299.1)
             schizophrenic syndrome of childhood (299.9)

    ● Code new   ▲ Revision of   ④ ⑤ Fourth or fifth
       to this edition   existing code   digit required

⑤ **299.1 Disintegrative psychosis**
    Heller's syndrome
Use additional code to identify any associated neurological disorder

> | *Excludes:* | *infantile autism (299.0)* |
> | | *schizophrenic syndrome of childhood (299.9)* |

⑤ **299.8 Other specified early childhood psychoses**
    Atypical childhood psychosis
    Borderline psychosis of childhood

> | *Excludes:* | *simple stereotypies without psychotic disturbance (307.3)* |

⑤ **299.9 Unspecified**
    Child psychosis NOS
    Schizophrenia, childhood type NOS
    Schizophrenic syndrome of childhood NOS

> | *Excludes:* | *schizophrenia of adult type occurring in childhood (295.0-295.9)* |

NEUROTIC DISORDERS, PERSONALITY DISORDERS, AND OTHER NONPSYCHOTIC MENTAL DISORDERS (300-316)

300 Neurotic disorders

⑤ **300.0 Anxiety states**

> | *Excludes:* | *anxiety in:* |
> | | *acute stress reaction (308.0)* |
> | | *transient adjustment reaction (309.24)* |
> | | *neurasthenia (300.5)* |
> | | *psychophysiological disorders (306.0-306.9)* |
> | | *separation anxiety (309.21)* |

    300.00 Anxiety state, unspecified
        Anxiety:
          neurosis
          reaction
          state (neurotic)
        Atypical anxiety disorder

    300.01 Panic disorder
        Panic:
          attack
          state

    300.02 Generalized anxiety disorder

    300.09 Other

⑤ **300.1 Hysteria**

> | *Excludes:* | *adjustment reaction (309.0-309.9)* |
> | | *anorexia nervosa (307.1)* |
> | | *gross stress reaction (308.0-308.9)* |
> | | *hysterical personality (301.50-301.59)* |
> | | *psychophysiologic disorders (306.0-306.9)* |

    300.10 Hysteria, unspecified

    300.11 Conversion disorder
        Astasia-abasia, hysterical
        Conversion hysteria or reaction
        Hysterical:
          blindness
          deafness
          paralysis

    300.12 Psychogenic amnesia
        Hysterical amnesia

    300.13 Psychogenic fugue
        Hysterical fugue

    300.14 Multiple personality
        Dissociative identity disorder

    300.15 Dissociative disorder or reaction, unspecified

    300.16 Factitious illness with psychological symptoms
        Compensation neurosis
        Ganser's syndrome, hysterical

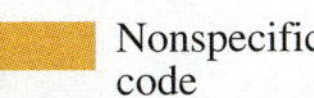 Add 4th or 5th digit   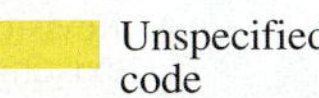 Nonspecific code   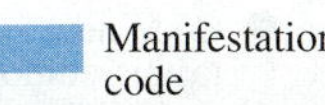 Unspecified code   Manifestation code

300.19 Other and unspecified factitious illness
Factitious illness (with physical symptoms) NOS

Excludes: *multiple operations or hospital addiction syndrome (301.51)*

⑤ **300.2 Phobic disorders**

Excludes: *anxiety state not associated with a specific situation or object (300.0-300.09)*
obsessional phobias (300.3)

300.20 Phobia, unspecified
Anxiety-hysteria NOS
Phobia NOS

300.21 Agoraphobia with panic attacks
Fear of:
open spaces
streets   } with panic attacks
travel

300.22 Agoraphobia without mention of panic attacks
Any condition classifiable to 300.21 without mention of panic attacks

300.23 Social phobia
Fear of:
eating in public
public speaking
washing in public

300.29 Other isolated or simple phobias
Acrophobia   Claustrophobia
Animal phobias   Fear of crowds

300.3 Obsessive-compulsive disorders
Anancastic neurosis   Obsessional phobia [any]
Compulsive neurosis

Excludes: *obsessive-compulsive symptoms occurring in:*
endogenous depression (296.2-296.3)
organic states (e.g., encephalitis)
schizophrenia (295.0-295.9)

300.4 Neurotic depression
Anxiety depression   Dysthymic disorder
Depression with anxiety   Neurotic depressive state
Depressive reaction   Reactive depression

Excludes: *adjustment reaction with depressive symptoms (309.0-309.1)*
depression NOS (311)
manic-depressive psychosis, depressed type (296.2-296.3)
reactive depressive psychosis (298.0)

300.5 Neurasthenia
Fatigue neurosis   Psychogenic:
Nervous debility   asthenia
                               general fatigue

Use additional code to identify any associated physical disorder

Excludes: *anxiety state (300.00-300.09)*
neurotic depression (300.4)
psychophysiological disorders (306.0-306.9)
specific nonpsychotic mental disorders following organic brain damage
(310.0-310.9)

300.6 Depersonalization syndrome
Depersonalization disorder
Derealization (neurotic)
Neurotic state with depersonalization episode

Excludes: *depersonalization associated with:*
anxiety (300.00-300.09)
depression (300.4)
manic-depressive disorder or psychosis (296.0-296.9)
schizophrenia (295.0-295.9)

● Code new   ▲ Revision of   ④ ⑤ Fourth or fifth
to this edition   existing code   digit required

300.7 Hypochondriasis
Body dysmorphic disorder

Excludes: *hypochondriasis in:*
hysteria (300.10-300.19)
manic-depressive psychosis, depressed type (296.2-296.3)
neurasthenia (300.5)
obsessional disorder (300.3)
schizophrenia (295.0-295.9)

⑤ **300.8 Other neurotic disorders**

300.81 Somatization disorder
Briquet's disorder
Severe somatoform disorder

300.82 Undifferentiated somatoform disorder
Atypical somatoform disorder
Somatoform disorder NOS

300.89 Other
Occupational neurosis, including writers' cramp
Psychasthenia
Psychasthenic neurosis

300.9 Unspecified neurotic disorder
Neurosis NOS   Psychoneurosis NOS

301 Personality disorders
Includes: character neurosis

Use additional code to identify any associated neurosis or psychosis, or physical condition

Excludes: *nonpsychotic personality disorder associated with organic brain syndromes*
(310.0-310.9)

301.0 Paranoid personality disorder
Fanatic personality
Paranoid personality (disorder)
Paranoid traits

Excludes: *acute paranoid reaction (298.3)*
alcoholic paranoia (291.5)
paranoid schizophrenia (295.3)
paranoid states (297.0-297.9)

⑤ **301.1 Affective personality disorder**

Excludes: *affective psychotic disorders (296.0-296.9)*
neurasthenia (300.5)
neurotic depression (300.4)

301.10 Affective personality disorder, unspecified

301.11 Chronic hypomanic personality disorder
Chronic hypomanic disorder
Hypomanic personality

301.12 Chronic depressive personality disorder
Chronic depressive disorder
Depressive character or personality

301.13 Cyclothymic disorder
Cycloid personality
Cyclothymia
Cyclothymic personality

⑤ **301.2 Schizoid personality disorder**

Excludes: *schizophrenia (295.0-295.9)*

301.20 Schizoid personality disorder, unspecified

301.21 Introverted personality

301.22 Schizotypal personality

301.3 Explosive personality disorder
Aggressive: Emotional instability (excessive)
personality   Pathological emotionality
reaction   Quarrelsomeness
Aggressiveness

Excludes: *dyssocial personality (301.7)*
hysterical neurosis (300.10-300.19)

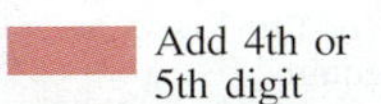

301.4 Compulsive personality disorder
Anancastic personality
Obsessional personality

Excludes:	*obsessive-compulsive disorder (300.3)*
	phobic state (300.20-300.29)

⑤ **301.5 Histrionic personality disorder**

Excludes:	*hysterical neurosis (300.10-300.19)*

301.50 Histrionic personality disorder, unspecified
Hysterical personality NOS

301.51 Chronic factitious illness with physical symptoms
Hospital addiction syndrome
Multiple operations syndrome
Munchausen syndrome

301.59 Other histrionic personality disorder
Personality:
emotionally unstable
labile
psychoinfantile

301.6 Dependent personality disorder
Asthenic personality   Passive personality
Inadequate personality

Excludes:	*neurasthenia (300.5)*
	passive-aggressive personality (301.84)

301.7 Antisocial personality disorder
Amoral personality
Asocial personality
Dyssocial personality
Personality disorder with predominantly sociopathic or asocial manifestation

Excludes:	*disturbance of conduct without specifiable personality disorder (312.0-312.9)*
	explosive personality (301.3)

⑤ **301.8 Other personality disorders**

301.81 Narcissistic personality

301.82 Avoidant personality

301.83 Borderline personality

301.84 Passive-aggressive personality

301.89 Other
Personality: Personality:
eccentric   masochistic
"haltlose" type   psychoneurotic
immature

Excludes:	*psychoinfantile personality (301.59)*

301.9 Unspecified personality disorder
Pathological personality   Psychopathic:
NOS   constitutional state
Personality disorder NOS   personality (disorder)

302 Sexual deviations and disorders

Excludes:	*sexual disorder manifest in:*
	organic brain syndrome (290.0-294.9, 310.0-310.9)
	psychosis (295.0-298.9)

302.0 Ego-dystonic homosexuality
Ego-dystonic lesbianism
Homosexual conflict disorder

Excludes:	*homosexual pedophilia (302.2)*

302.1 Zoophilia
Bestiality

302.2 Pedophilia

302.3 Transvestism

Excludes:	*trans-sexualism (302.5)*

302.4 Exhibitionism

● Code new   ▲ Revision of   ④ ⑤ Fourth or fifth
to this edition   existing code   digit required

⑤ **302.5 Trans-sexualism**

> *Excludes:* *transvestism (302.3)*

    302.50 **With unspecified sexual history**

    302.51 **With asexual history**

    302.52 **With homosexual history**

    302.53 **With heterosexual history**

302.6 Disorders of psychosexual identity
    Feminism in boys
    Gender identity disorder of childhood

> *Excludes:* *gender identity disorder in adult (302.85)*
> *homosexuality (302.0)*
> *trans-sexualism (302.50-302.53)*
> *transvestism (302.3)*

⑤ **302.7 Psychosexual dysfunction**

> *Excludes:* *impotence of organic origin (607.84)*
> *normal transient symptoms from ruptured hymen*
> *transient or occasional failures of erection due to fatigue, anxiety, alcohol, or drugs*

    302.70 **Psychosexual dysfunction, unspecified**

    302.71 **With inhibited sexual desire**

    302.72 **With inhibited sexual excitement**
        Frigidity   Impotence

    302.73 **With inhibited female orgasm**

    302.74 **With inhibited male orgasm**

    302.75 **With premature ejaculation**

    302.76 **With functional dyspareunia**
        Dyspareunia, psychogenic

    302.79 **With other specified psychosexual dysfunctions**

⑤ **302.8 Other specified psychosexual disorders**

    302.81 **Fetishism**

    302.82 **Voyeurism**

    302.83 **Sexual masochism**

    302.84 **Sexual sadism**

    302.85 **Gender identity disorder of adolescent or adult life**

    302.89 **Other**
        Nymphomania   Satyriasis

302.9 Unspecified psychosexual disorder
    Pathologic sexuality NOS   Sexual deviation NOS

⑤ **303 Alcohol dependence syndrome**
Use additional code to identify any associated condition, as:
    alcoholic psychoses (291.0-291.9)
    drug dependence (304.0-304.9)
    physical complications of alcohol, such as:
        cerebral degeneration (331.7)
        cirrhosis of liver (571.2)
        epilepsy (345.0-345.9)
        gastritis (535.3)
        hepatitis (571.1)
        liver damage NOS (571.3)

> *Excludes:* *drunkenness NOS (305.0)*

The following fifth-digit subclassification is for use with category 303:

    0 **unspecified**

    1 **continuous**

    2 **episodic**

    3 **in remission**

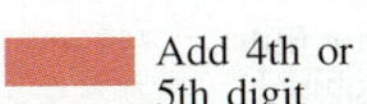

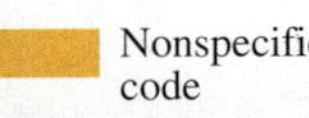

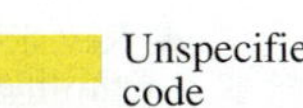

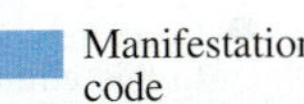

⑤ **303.0 Acute alcoholic intoxication**
Acute drunkenness in alcoholism

⑤ **303.9 Other and unspecified alcohol dependence**
Chronic alcoholism   Dipsomania

⑤ **304 Drug dependence**

> Excludes: *nondependent abuse of drugs (305.1-305.9)*

The following fifth-digit subclassification is for use with category 304:

0 **unspecified**

1 **continuous**

2 **episodic**

3 **in remission**

⑤ **304.0 Opioid type dependence**
Heroin   Opium alkaloids and their derivatives
Meperidine   Synthetics with morphine-like effects
Methadone
Morphine
Opium

⑤ **304.1 Barbiturate and similarly acting sedative or hypnotic dependence**
Barbiturates
Nonbarbiturate sedatives and tranquilizers with a similar effect:
chlordiazepoxide
diazepam
glutethimide
meprobamate
methaqualone

⑤ **304.2 Cocaine dependence**
Coca leaves and derivatives

⑤ **304.3 Cannabis dependence**
Hashish   Marihuana
Hemp

⑤ **304.4 Amphetamine and other psychostimulant dependence**
Methylphenidate   Phenmetrazine

⑤ **304.5 Hallucinogen dependence**
Dimethyltryptamine [DMT]
Lysergic acid diethylamide [LSD] and derivatives
Mescaline
Psilocybin

⑤ **304.6 Other specified drug dependence**
Absinthe addiction   Glue sniffing

> Excludes: *tobacco dependence (305.1)*

⑤ **304.7 Combinations of opioid type drug with any other**

⑤ **304.8 Combinations of drug dependence excluding opioid type drug**

⑤ **304.9 Unspecified drug dependence**
Drug addiction NOS   Drug dependence NOS

⑤ **305 Nondependent abuse of drugs**
Note: Includes cases where a person, for whom no other diagnosis is possible, has come under medical care because of the maladaptive effect of a drug on which he is not dependent and that he has taken on his own initiative to the detriment of his health or social functioning.

> Excludes: *alcohol dependence syndrome (303.0-303.9)*
> *drug dependence (304.0-304.9)*
> *drug withdrawal syndrome (292.0)*
> *poisoning by drugs or medicinal substances (960.0-979.9)*

The following fifth-digit subclassification is for use with codes 305.0, 305.2-305.9:

0 **unspecified**

1 **continuous**

2 **episodic**

3 **in remission**

● Code new to this edition   ▲ Revision of existing code   ④ ⑤ Fourth or fifth digit required

⑤ **305.0 Alcohol abuse**
 Drunkenness NOS
 Excessive drinking of alcohol NOS
 "Hangover" (alcohol)
 Inebriety NOS

 Excludes: acute alcohol intoxication in alcoholism (303.0)
     alcoholic psychoses (291.0-291.9)

305.1 Tobacco use disorder
 Tobacco dependence

 Excludes: history of tobacco use (V15.82)

⑤ **305.2 Cannabis abuse**

⑤ **305.3 Hallucinogen abuse**
 Acute intoxication from hallucinogens ["bad trips"]
 LSD reaction

⑤ **305.4 Barbiturate and similarly acting sedative or hypnotic abuse**

⑤ **305.5 Opioid abuse**

⑤ **305.6 Cocaine abuse**

⑤ **305.7 Amphetamine or related acting sympathomimetic abuse**

⑤ **305.8 Antidepressant type abuse**

⑤ **305.9 Other, mixed, or unspecified drug abuse**
 "Laxative habit"
 Misuse of drugs NOS
 Nonprescribed use of drugs or patent medicinals

306 Physiological malfunction arising from mental factors
 Includes: psychogenic:
     physical symptoms
     physiological manifestations } not involving tissue damage

 Excludes: hysteria (300.11-300.19)

    physical symptoms secondary to a psychiatric disorder classified elsewhere
    psychic factors associated with physical conditions involving tissue damage
     classified elsewhere (316)
    specific nonpsychotic mental disorders following organic brain damage (310.0-310.9)

306.0 Musculoskeletal
 Psychogenic paralysis   Psychogenic torticollis

 Excludes: Gilles de la Tourette's syndrome (307.23)

    paralysis as hysterical or conversion reaction (300.11)
    tics (307.20-307.22)

306.1 Respiratory
 Psychogenic:
  air hunger
  cough
  hiccough
 Psychogenic:
  hyperventilation
  yawning

 Excludes: psychogenic asthma (316 and 493.9)

306.2 Cardiovascular
 Cardiac neurosis
 Cardiovascular neurosis
 Neurocirculatory asthenia
 Psychogenic cardiovascular disorder

 Excludes: psychogenic paroxysmal tachycardia (316 and 427.2)

306.3 Skin
 Psychogenic pruritus

 Excludes: psychogenic:

    alopecia (316 and 704.00)
    dermatitis (316 and 692.9)
    eczema (316 and 691.8 or 692.9)
    urticaria (316 and 708.0-708.9)

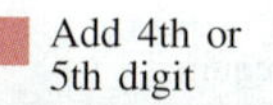

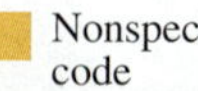

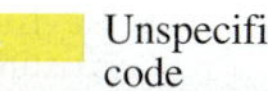

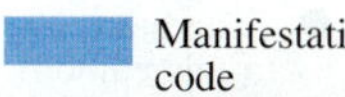

306.4 Gastrointestinal
Aerophagy
Cyclical vomiting, psychogenic

Diarrhea, psychogenic
Nervous gastritis
Psychogenic dyspepsia

Excludes: *cyclical vomiting NOS (536.2)*
globus hystericus (300.11)
mucous colitis (316 and 564.9)
psychogenic:
cardiospasm (316 and 530.0)
duodenal ulcer (316 and 532.0-532.9)
gastric ulcer (316 and 531.0-531.9)
peptic ulcer NOS (316 and 533.0-533.9)
vomiting NOS (307.54)

⑤ **306.5 Genitourinary**

Excludes: *enuresis, psychogenic (307.6)*
frigidity (302.72)
impotence (302.72)
psychogenic dyspareunia (302.76)

306.50 Psychogenic genitourinary malfunction, unspecified

306.51 Psychogenic vaginismus
Functional vaginismus

306.52 Psychogenic dysmenorrhea

306.53 Psychogenic dysuria

306.59 Other

306.6 Endocrine

306.7 Organs of special sense

Excludes: *hysterical blindness or deafness (300.11)*
psychophysical visual disturbances (368.16)

306.8 Other specified psychophysiological malfunction
Bruxism   Teeth grinding

306.9 Unspecified psychophysiological malfunction
Psychophysiologic disorder NOS
Psychosomatic disorder NOS

307 Special symptoms or syndromes, not elsewhere classified
Note: This category is intended for use if the psychopathology is manifested by a single specific symptom or group of symptoms which is not part of an organic illness or other mental disorder classifiable elsewhere.

Excludes: *those due to mental disorders classified elsewhere*
those of organic origin

307.0 Stammering and stuttering

Excludes: *dysphasia (784.5)*
lisping or lalling (307.9)
retarded development of speech (315.31-315.39)

307.1 Anorexia nervosa

Excludes: *eating disturbance NOS (307.50)*
feeding problem (783.3)
of nonorganic origin (307.59)
loss of appetite (783.0)
of nonorganic origin (307.59)

⑤ **307.2 Tics**

Excludes: *nail-biting or thumb-sucking (307.9)*
stereotypies occurring in isolation (307.3)
tics of organic origin (333.3)

307.20 Tic disorder, unspecified

307.21 Transient tic disorder of childhood

307.22 Chronic motor tic disorder

307.23 Gilles de la Tourette's disorder
Motor-verbal tic disorder

● Code new to this edition   ▲ Revision of existing code   ④ ⑤ Fourth or fifth digit required

307.3 Stereotyped repetitive movements

Body-rocking   Spasmus nutans
Head banging   Stereotypies NOS

Excludes: *tics (307.20-307.23)*
of organic origin (333.3)

⑤ **307.4 Specific disorders of sleep of nonorganic origin**

Excludes: *narcolepsy (347)*
those of unspecified cause (780.50-780.59)

307.40 Nonorganic sleep disorder, unspecified

307.41 Transient disorder of initiating or maintaining sleep

Hyposomnia
Insomnia   } associated with acute or intermittent emotional reactions
Sleeplessness   } or conflicts

307.42 Persistent disorder of initiating or maintaining sleep

Hyposomnia, insomnia, or sleeplessness associated with:
  anxiety
  conditioned arousal
  depression (major) (minor)
  psychosis

307.43 Transient disorder of initiating or maintaining wakefulness

Hypersomnia associated with acute or intermittent emotional reactions or
  conflicts

307.44 Persistent disorder of initiating or maintaining wakefulness

Hypersomnia associated with depression (major) (minor)

307.45 Phase-shift disruption of 24-hour sleep-wake cycle

Irregular sleep-wake rhythm, nonorganic origin
Jet lag syndrome
Rapid time-zone change
Shifting sleep-work schedule

307.46 Somnambulism or night terrors

307.47 Other dysfunctions of sleep stages or arousal from sleep

Nightmares: Sleep drunkenness
  NOS
  REM-sleep type

307.48 Repetitive intrusions of sleep

Repetitive intrusion of sleep with:
  atypical polysomnographic features
  environmental disturbances
  repeated REM-sleep interruptions

307.49 Other

"Short-sleeper"
Subjective insomnia complaint

⑤ **307.5 Other and unspecified disorders of eating**

Excludes: *anorexia:*
  nervosa (307.1)
  of unspecified cause (783.0)
overeating, of unspecified cause (783.6)
vomiting:
  NOS (787.0)
  cyclical (536.2)
    psychogenic (306.4)

307.50 Eating disorder, unspecified

307.51 Bulimia

Overeating of nonorganic origin

307.52 Pica

Perverted appetite of nonorganic origin

307.53 Psychogenic rumination

Regurgitation, of nonorganic origin, of food with reswallowing

Excludes: *obsessional rumination (300.3)*

307.54 Psychogenic vomiting

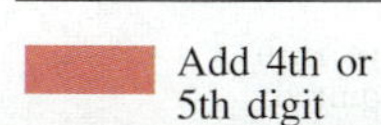

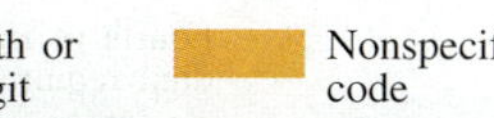

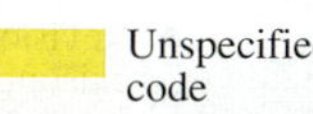

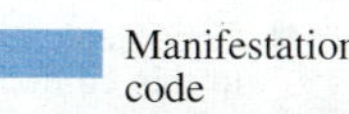

307.59 **Other**
Infantile feeding disturbances
Loss of appetite
} of nonorganic origin

307.6 **Enuresis**
Enuresis (primary) (secondary) of nonorganic origin

Excludes: *enuresis of unspecified cause (788.3)*

307.7 **Encopresis**
Encopresis (continuous) (discontinuous) of nonorganic origin

Excludes: *encopresis of unspecified cause (787.6)*

⑤ **307.8** **Psychalgia**

307.80 **Psychogenic pain, site unspecified**

307.81 **Tension headache**

Excludes: *headache:*
NOS (784.0)
migraine (346.0-346.9)

307.89 **Other**
Psychogenic backache

Excludes: *pains not specifically attributable to a psychological cause (in):*
back (724.5)
joint (719.4)
limb (729.5)
lumbago (724.2)
rheumatic (729.0)

307.9 **Other and unspecified special symptoms or syndromes, not elsewhere classified**
Hair plucking   Masturbation
Lalling   Nail-biting
Lisping   Thumb-sucking

308 **Acute reaction to stress**
Includes: catastrophic stress
combat fatigue
gross stress reaction (acute)
transient disorders in response to exceptional physical or mental stress which
usually subside within hours or days

Excludes: *adjustment reaction or disorder (309.0-309.9)*
chronic stress reaction (309.1-309.9)

308.0 **Predominant disturbance of emotions**
Anxiety
Emotional crisis   } as acute reaction to exceptional [gross] stress
Panic state

308.1 **Predominant disturbance of consciousness**
Fugues as acute reaction to exceptional [gross] stress

308.2 **Predominant psychomotor disturbance**
Agitation states   } as acute reaction to exceptional [gross] stress
Stupor

308.3 **Other acute reactions to stress**
Acute situational disturbance
Brief or acute posttraumatic stress disorder

Excludes: *prolonged posttraumatic emotional disturbance (309.81)*

308.4 **Mixed disorders as reaction to stress**

308.9 **Unspecified acute reaction to stress**

309 **Adjustment reaction**
Includes: adjustment disorders
reaction (adjustment) to chronic stress

Excludes: *acute reaction to major stress (308.0-308.9)*
neurotic disorders (300.0-300.9)

● Code new
to this edition

▲ Revision of
existing code

④ ⑤ Fourth or fifth
digit required

309.0 Brief depressive reaction
Adjustment disorder with depressed mood
Grief reaction

Excludes: *affective psychoses (296.0-296.9)*
neurotic depression (300.4)
prolonged depressive reaction (309.1)
psychogenic depressive psychosis (298.0)

309.1 Prolonged depressive reaction

Excludes: *affective psychoses (296.0-296.9)*
brief depressive reaction (309.0)
neurotic depression (300.4)
psychogenic depressive psychosis (298.0)

⑤ **309.2 With predominant disturbance of other emotions**

309.21 Separation anxiety disorder

309.22 Emancipation disorder of adolescence and early adult life

309.23 Specific academic or work inhibition

309.24 Adjustment reaction with anxious mood

309.28 Adjustment reaction with mixed emotional features
Adjustment reaction with anxiety and depression

309.29 Other
Culture shock

309.3 With predominant disturbance of conduct
Conduct disturbance ⎱
Destructiveness ⎰ as adjustment reaction

Excludes: *destructiveness in child (312.9)*
disturbance of conduct NOS (312.9)
dyssocial behavior without manifest psychiatric disorder (V71.01-V71.02)
personality disorder with predominantly sociopathic or asocial manifestations (301.7)

309.4 With mixed disturbance of emotions and conduct

⑤ **309.8 Other specified adjustment reactions**

309.81 Prolonged posttraumatic stress disorder
Chronic posttraumatic stress disorder
Concentration camp syndrome

Excludes: *posttraumatic brain syndrome:*
nonpsychotic (310.2)
psychotic (293.0-293.9)

309.82 Adjustment reaction with physical symptoms

309.83 Adjustment reaction with withdrawal
Elective mutism as adjustment reaction
Hospitalism (in children) NOS

309.89 Other

309.9 Unspecified adjustment reaction
Adaptation reaction NOS   Adjustment reaction NOS

310 Specific nonpsychotic mental disorders due to organic brain damage

Excludes: *neuroses, personality disorders, or other nonpsychotic conditions occurring in a*
form similar to that seen with functional disorders but in association with a
physical condition (300.0-300.9, 301.0-301.9)

310.0 Frontal lobe syndrome
Lobotomy syndrome
Postleucotomy syndrome [state]

Excludes: *postcontusion syndrome (310.2)*

310.1 Organic personality syndrome
Cognitive or personality change of other type, of nonpsychotic severity
Mild memory disturbance
Organic psychosyndrome of nonpsychotic severity
Presbyophrenia NOS
Senility with mental changes of nonpsychotic severity

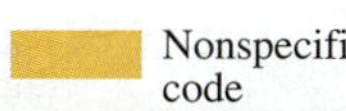

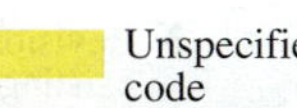

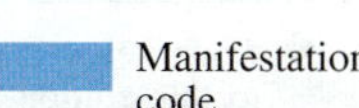

310.2 Postconcussion syndrome
Postcontusion syndrome or encephalopathy
Posttraumatic brain syndrome, nonpsychotic
Status postcommotio cerebri

Excludes: *frontal lobe syndrome (310.0)*
postencephalitic syndrome (310.8)
any organic psychotic conditions following head injury (293.0—294.0)

310.8 Other specified nonpsychotic mental disorders following organic brain damage
Postencephalitic syndrome
Other focal (partial) organic psychosyndromes

310.9 Unspecified nonpsychotic mental disorder following organic brain damage

311 Depressive disorder, not elsewhere classified
Depressive disorder NOS
Depressive state NOS   Depression NOS

Excludes: *acute reaction to major stress with depressive symptoms (308.0)*
affective personality disorder (301.10-301.13)
affective psychoses (296.0-296.9)
brief depressive reaction (309.0)
depressive states associated with stressful events (309.0-309.1)
disturbance of emotions specific to childhood and adolescence, with misery and
unhappiness (313.1)
mixed adjustment reaction with depressive symptoms (309.4)
neurotic depression (300.4)
prolonged depressive adjustment reaction (309.1)
psychogenic depressive psychosis (298.0)

312 Disturbance of conduct, not elsewhere classified

Excludes: *adjustment reaction with disturbance of conduct (309.3)*
drug dependence (304.0-304.9)
dyssocial behavior without manifest psychiatric disorder (V71.01-V71.02)
personality disorder with predominantly sociopathic or asocial manifestations
(301.7)
sexual deviations (302.0-302.9)

The following fifth-digit subclassification is for use with categories 312.0-312.2:

0 unspecified

1 mild

2 moderate

3 severe

⑤ **312.0 Undersocialized conduct disorder, aggressive type**
Aggressive outburst   Unsocialized aggressive disorder
Anger reaction

⑤ **312.1 Undersocialized conduct disorder, unaggressive type**
Childhood truancy,   Solitary stealing
unsocialized   Tantrums

⑤ **312.2 Socialized conduct disorder**
Childhood truancy, socialized
Group delinquency

Excludes: *gang activity without manifest psychiatric disorder (V71.01)*

⑤ **312.3 Disorders of impulse control, not elsewhere classified**

312.30 Impulse control disorder, unspecified

312.31 Pathological gambling

312.32 Kleptomania

312.33 Pyromania

312.34 Intermittent explosive disorder

312.35 Isolated explosive disorder

312.39 Other

312.4 Mixed disturbance of conduct and emotions
Neurotic delinquency

Excludes: *compulsive conduct disorder (312.3)*

⑤ **312.8 Other specified disturbances of conduct, not elsewhere classified**

   ● Code new   ▲ Revision of   ④ ⑤ Fourth or fifth
to this edition   existing code   digit required

312.81 **Conduct disorder, childhood onset type**

312.82 **Conduct disorder, adolescent onset type**

312.89 **Other conduct disorder**

312.9 **Unspecified disturbance of conduct**
Delinquency (juvenile)

313 **Disturbance of emotions specific to childhood and adolescence**

Excludes: *adjustment reaction (309.0-309.9)*
emotional disorder of neurotic type (300.0-300.9)
masturbation, nail-biting, thumb-sucking, and other isolated symptoms (307.0-307.9)

313.0 **Overanxious disorder**
Anxiety and fearfulness } of childhood and adolescence
Overanxious disorder

Excludes: *abnormal separation anxiety (309.21)*
anxiety states (300.00-300.09)
hospitalism in children (309.83)
phobic state (300.20-300.29)

313.1 **Misery and unhappiness disorder**

Excludes: *depressive neurosis (300.4)*

⑤ 313.2 **Sensitivity, shyness, and social withdrawal disorder**

Excludes: *infantile autism (299.0)*
schizoid personality (301.20-301.22)
schizophrenia (295.0-295.9)

313.21 **Shyness disorder of childhood**
Sensitivity reaction of childhood or adolescence

313.22 **Introverted disorder of childhood**
Social withdrawal } of childhood or adolescence
Withdrawal reaction

313.23 **Elective mutism**

Excludes: *elective mutism as adjustment reaction (309.83)*

313.3 **Relationship problems**
Sibling jealousy

Excludes: *relationship problems associated with aggression, destruction, or other forms of*
conduct disturbance (312.0-312.9)

⑤ 313.8 **Other or mixed emotional disturbances of childhood or adolescence**

313.81 **Oppositional disorder**

313.82 **Identity disorder**

313.83 **Academic underachievement disorder**

313.89 **Other**

313.9 **Unspecified emotional disturbance of childhood or adolescence**

314 **Hyperkinetic syndrome of childhood**

Excludes: *hyperkinesis as symptom of underlying disorder—code the underlying disorder*

⑤ 314.0 **Attention deficit disorder**
Adult
Child

314.00 **Without mention of hyperactivity**
Predominantly inattentive type

314.01 **With hyperactivity**
Combined type
Overactivity NOS
Predominantly hyperactive/impulsive type
Simple disturbance of attention with overactivity

314.1 **Hyperkinesis with developmental delay**
Developmental disorder of hyperkinesis
Use additional code to identify any associated neurological disorder

314.2 **Hyperkinetic conduct disorder**
Hyperkinetic conduct disorder without developmental delay

Excludes: *hyperkinesis with significant delays in specific skills (314.1)*

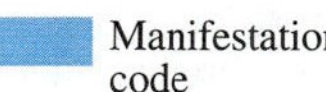

314.8 Other specified manifestations of hyperkinetic syndrome

314.9 Unspecified hyperkinetic syndrome
Hyperkinetic reaction of childhood or adolescence NOS
Hyperkinetic syndrome NOS

315 Specific delays in development

Excludes: that due to a neurological disorder (320.0-389.9)

⑤ **315.0 Specific reading disorder**

315.00 Reading disorder, unspecified

315.01 Alexia

315.02 Developmental dyslexia

315.09 Other
Specific spelling difficulty

315.1 Specific arithmetical disorder
Dyscalculia

315.2 Other specific learning difficulties

Excludes: specific arithmetical disorder (315.1)
specific reading disorder (315.00-315.09)

⑤ **315.3 Developmental speech or language disorder**

315.31 Developmental language disorder
Developmental aphasia
Expressive language disorder
Word deafness

Excludes: acquired aphasia (784.3)
elective mutism (309.83, 313.0, 313.23)

315.32 Receptive language disorder (mixed)
Receptive expressive language disorder

315.39 Other
Developmental articulation disorder
Dyslalia

Excludes: lisping and lalling (307.9)
stammering and stuttering (307.0)

315.4 Coordination disorder
Clumsiness syndrome
Dyspraxia syndrome
Specific motor development disorder

315.5 Mixed development disorder

315.8 Other specified delays in development

315.9 Unspecified delay in development
Developmental disorder NOS

316 Psychic factors associated with diseases classified elsewhere
Psychologic factors in physical conditions classified elsewhere
Use additional code to identify the associated physical condition, as:
psychogenic:
asthma (493.9)
dermatitis (692.9)
duodenal ulcer (532.0-532.9)
eczema (691.8, 692.9)
gastric ulcer (531.0-531.9)
mucous colitis (564.9)
paroxysmal tachycardia (427.2)
ulcerative colitis (556)
urticaria (708.0-708.9)
psychosocial dwarfism (259.4)

Excludes: physical symptoms and physiological malfunctions, not involving tissue damage, of
mental origin (306.0-306.9)

● Code new
to this edition   ▲ Revision of
existing code   ④ ⑤ Fourth or fifth
digit required

MENTAL RETARDATION (317-319)

Use additional code(s) to identify any associated psychiatric or physical condition(s)

317 Mild mental retardation   Mild mental subnormality
High-grade defect
IQ 50-70

318 Other specified mental retardation

318.0 Moderate mental retardation   Moderate mental subnormality
IQ 35-49

318.1 Severe mental retardation
IQ 20-34
Severe mental subnormality

318.2 Profound mental retardation   Profound mental subnormality
IQ under 20

319 Unspecified mental retardation   Mental subnormality NOS
Mental deficiency NOS

Add 4th or 5th digit   Nonspecific code   Unspecified code   Manifestation code

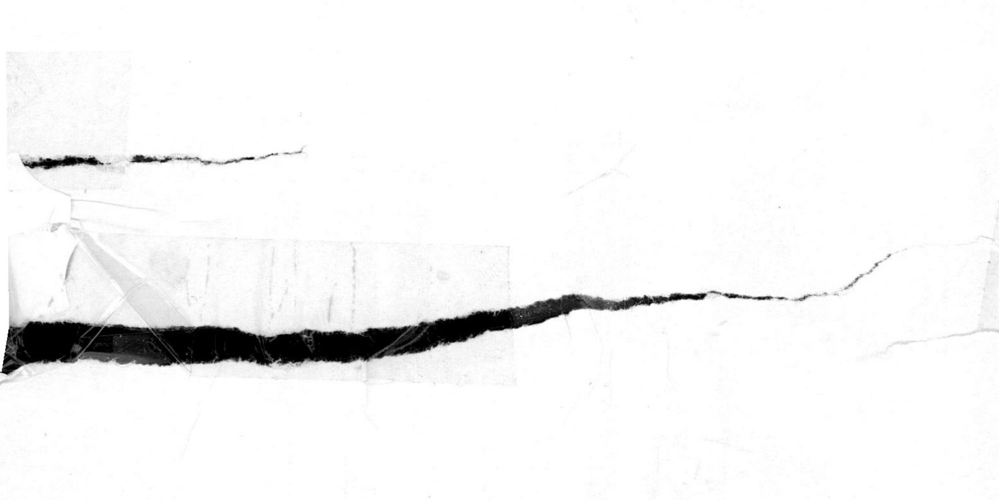

● Code new
to this edition

▲ Revision of
existing code

④ ⑤ Fourth or fifth
digit required

6. DISEASES OF THE NERVOUS SYSTEM AND SENSE ORGANS (320-389)

INFLAMMATORY DISEASES OF THE CENTRAL NERVOUS SYSTEM (320-326)

320 Bacterial meningitis

Includes:

arachnoiditis
leptomeningitis
meningitis
meningoencephalitis } bacterial
meningomyelitis
pachymeningitis

320.0 Hemophilus meningitis

Meningitis due to Hemophilus influenzae [H. influenzae]

320.1 Pneumococcal meningitis

320.2 Streptococcal meningitis

320.3 Staphylococcal meningitis

320.7 *Meningitis in other bacterial diseases classified elsewhere*

Code first underlying disease, as:
actinomycosis (039.8)
listeriosis (027.0)
typhoid fever (002.0)
whooping cough (033.0-033.9)

Excludes: *meningitis (in):*

epidemic (036.0)
gonococcal (098.82)
meningococcal (036.0)
salmonellosis (003.21)
syphilis:
  NOS (094.2)
  congenital (090.42)
  meningovascular (094.2)
  secondary (091.81)
tuberculous (013.0)

⑤ **320.8 Meningitis due to other specified bacteria**

320.81 Anaerobic meningitis

Bacteroides (fragilis)
Gram-negative anaerobes

320.82 Meningitis due to Gram-negative bacteria, not elsewhere classified

Aerobacter aerogenes
Escherichia coli [E. coli]
Friedlander bacillus
Klebsiella pneumoniae
Proteus morganii
Pseudomonas

Excludes: *Gram-negative anaerobes (320.81)*

320.89 Meningitis due to other specified bacteria

Bacillus pyocyaneus

320.9 Meningitis due to unspecified bacterium

Meningitis:
  bacterial NOS
  purulent NOS

Meningitis:
  pyogenic NOS
  suppurative NOS

321 Meningitis due to other organisms

Includes:

arachnoiditis due to organisms other than bacteria
leptomeningitis due to organisms other than bacteria
meningitis due to organisms other than bacteria
pachymeningitis due to organisms other than bacteria

321.0 *Cryptococcal meningitis*

Code first underlying disease (117.5)

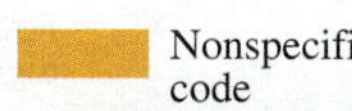

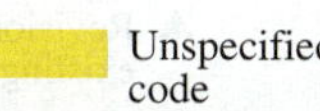

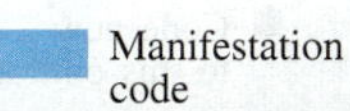

321.1 *Meningitis in other fungal diseases*
  Code first underlying disease (110.0-118)

  Excludes: *meningitis in:*
      candidiasis (112.83)
      coccidioidomycosis (114.2)
      histoplasmosis (115.01, 115.11, 115.91)

321.2 *Meningitis due to viruses not elsewhere classified*
  Code first underlying disease, as:
    meningitis due to arbovirus (060.0-066.9)

  Excludes: *meningitis (due to):*
      abacterial (047.0-047.9)
      adenovirus (049.1)
      aseptic NOS (047.9)
      Coxsackie (virus) (047.0)
      ECHO virus (047.1)
      enterovirus (047.0-047.9)
      herpes simplex virus (054.72)
      herpes zoster virus (053.0)
      lymphocytic choriomeningitis virus (049.0)
      mumps (072.1)
      viral NOS (047.9)
    meningo-eruptive syndrome (047.1)

321.3 *Meningitis due to trypanosomiasis*
  Code first underlying disease (086.0-086.9)

321.4 *Meningitis in sarcoidosis*
  Code first underlying disease (135)

321.8 *Meningitis due to other nonbacterial organisms classified elsewhere*
  Code first underlying disease

  Excludes: *leptospiral meningitis (100.81)*

322 **Meningitis of unspecified cause**
  Includes:

    arachnoiditis
    leptomeningitis   } with no organism specified as cause
    meningitis
    pachymeningitis

322.0 **Nonpyogenic meningitis**
  Meningitis with clear cerebrospinal fluid

322.1 **Eosinophilic meningitis**

322.2 **Chronic meningitis**

322.9 **Meningitis, unspecified**

323 **Encephalitis, myelitis, and encephalomyelitis**
  Includes: acute disseminated encephalomyelitis
    meningoencephalitis, except bacterial
    meningomyelitis, except bacterial
    myelitis (acute):
      ascending
      transverse

  Excludes: *bacterial:*
      meningoencephalitis (320.0-320.9)
      meningomyelitis (320.0-320.9)

● Code new   ▲ Revision of   ④ ⑤ Fourth or fifth
  to this edition   existing code   digit required

323.0 *Encephalitis in viral diseases classified elsewhere*
Code first underlying disease, as:
cat-scratch disease (078.3)
infectious mononucleosis (075)
ornithosis (073.7)

Excludes: *encephalitis (in):*

arthropod-borne viral (062.0-064)
herpes simplex (054.3)
mumps (072.2)
poliomyelitis (045.0-045.9)
rubella (056.01)
slow virus infections of central nervous system (046.0-046.9)
other viral diseases of central nervous system (049.8-049.9)
viral NOS (049.9)

323.1 *Encephalitis in rickettsial diseases classified elsewhere*
Code first underlying disease (080-083.9)

323.2 *Encephalitis in protozoal diseases classified elsewhere*
Code first underlying disease, as:
malaria (084.0-084.9)
trypanosomiasis (086.0-086.9)

323.4 *Other encephalitis due to infection classified elsewhere*
Code first underlying disease

Excludes: *encephalitis (in):*

meningococcal (036.1)
syphilis:
NOS (094.81)
congenital (090.41)
toxoplasmosis (130.0)
tuberculosis (013.6)
meningoencephalitis due to free-living ameba [Naegleria] (136.2)

323.5 Encephalitis following immunization procedures
Encephalitis
Encephalomyelitis } postimmunization or postvaccinal

Use additional E code, if desired, to identify vaccine

323.6 *Postinfectious encephalitis*
Code first underlying disease

Excludes: *encephalitis:*

postchickenpox (052.0)
postmeasles (055.0)

323.7 *Toxic encephalitis*
Code first underlying cause, as:
carbon tetrachloride (982.1)
hydroxyquinoline derivatives (961.3)
lead (984.0-984.9)
mercury (985.0)
thallium (985.8)

323.8 Other causes of encephalitis

323.9 Unspecified cause of encephalitis

324 Intracranial and intraspinal abscess

324.0 Intracranial abscess
Abscess (embolic):   Abscess (embolic) of brain [any part]:
cerebellar   epidural
cerebral   extradural
                    otogenic
                    subdural

Excludes: *tuberculous (013.3)*

324.1 Intraspinal abscess
Abscess (embolic) of spinal cord [any part]:
epidural
extradural
subdural

Excludes: *tuberculous (013.5)*

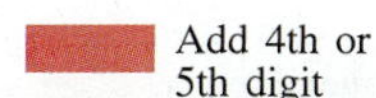

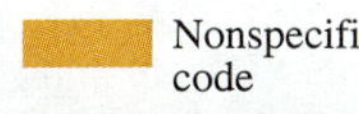

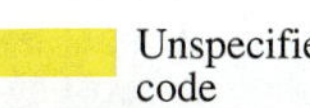

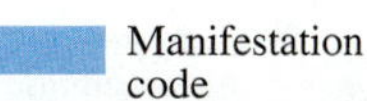

324.9 Of unspecified site
Extradural or subdural abscess NOS

325 Phlebitis and thrombophlebitis of intracranial venous sinuses
Embolism
Endophlebitis
Phlebitis, septic or suppurative
Thrombophlebitis
Thrombosis
} of cavernous, lateral, or other intracranial or
unspecified intracranial venous sinus

> *Excludes:* *that specified as:*
> *complicating pregnancy, childbirth, or the puerperium (671.5)*
> *of nonpyogenic origin (437.6)*

326 Late effects of intracranial abscess or pyogenic infection
Note: This category is to be used to indicate conditions whose primary classification is to 320-325 [excluding 320.7, 321.0-321.8, 323.0-323.4, 323.6-323.7] as the cause of late effects, themselves classifiable elsewhere. The "late effects" include conditions specified as such, or as sequelae, which may occur at any time after the resolution of the causal condition.

Use additional code, if desired, to identify condition, as:
hydrocephalus (331.4)
paralysis (342.0-342.9, 344.0-344.9)

HEREDITARY AND DEGENERATIVE DISEASES OF THE CENTRAL NERVOUS SYSTEM (330-337)

> *Excludes:* *hepatolenticular degeneration (275.1)*
> *multiple sclerosis (340)*
> *other demyelinating diseases of central nervous system (341.0-341.9)*

330 Cerebral degenerations usually manifest in childhood
Use additional code, if desired, to identify associated mental retardation

330.0 Leukodystrophy
Krabbe's disease
Leukodystrophy:
NOS
globoid cell
Leukodystrophy:
metachromatic
sudanophilic
Pelizaeus-Merzbacher disease
Sulfatide lipidosis

330.1 Cerebral lipidoses
Amaurotic (familial) idiocy
Disease:
Batten
Jansky-Bielschowsky
Disease:
Kufs'
Spielmeyer-Vogt
Tay-Sachs
Gangliosidosis

330.2 Cerebral degeneration in generalized lipidoses
Code first underlying disease, as:
Fabry's disease (272.7)
Gaucher's disease (272.7)
Neimann-Pick disease (272.7)
sphingolipidosis (272.7)

330.3 Cerebral degeneration of childhood in other diseases classified elsewhere
Code first underlying disease, as:
Hunter's disease (277.5)
mucopolysaccharidosis (277.5)

330.8 Other specified cerebral degenerations in childhood
Alpers' disease or gray-matter degeneration
Infantile necrotizing encephalomyelopathy
Leigh's disease
Subacute necrotizing encephalopathy or encephalomyelopathy

330.9 Unspecified cerebral degeneration in childhood

331 Other cerebral degenerations

331.0 Alzheimer's disease

331.1 Pick's disease

331.2 Senile degeneration of brain

> *Excludes:* *senility NOS (797)*

331.3 Communicating hydrocephalus

> *Excludes:* *congenital hydrocephalus (741.0, 742.3)*

● Code new
to this edition   ▲ Revision of
existing code   ④ ⑤ Fourth or fifth
digit required

331.4 Obstructive hydrocephalus
Acquired hydrocephalus NOS

Excludes: *congenital hydrocephalus (741.0, 742.3)*

331.7 *Cerebral degeneration in diseases classified elsewhere*
Code first underlying disease, as:
alcoholism (303.0-303.9)
beriberi (265.0)
cerebrovascular disease (430-438)
congenital hydrocephalus (741.0, 742.3)
neoplastic disease (140.0-239.9)
myxedema (244.0-244.9)
vitamin B_{12} deficiency (266.2)

Excludes: *cerebral degeneration in:*

Jakob-Creutzfeldt disease (046.1)
progressive multifocal leukoencephalopathy (046.3)
subacute spongiform encephalopathy (046.1)

⑤ **331.8 Other cerebral degeneration**

331.81 Reye's syndrome

331.89 Other
Cerebral ataxia

331.9 Cerebral degeneration, unspecified

332 Parkinson's disease

332.0 Paralysis agitans
Parkinsonism or Parkinson's disease:
NOS
idiopathic
primary

332.1 Secondary Parkinsonism
Parkinsonism due to drugs

Use additional E code, if desired, to identify drug, if drug-induced

Excludes: *Parkinsonism (in):*

Huntington's disease (333.4)
progressive supranuclear palsy (333.0)
Shy-Drager syndrome (333.0)
syphilitic (094.82)

333 Other extrapyramidal disease and abnormal movement disorders
Includes: other forms of extrapyramidal, basal ganglia, or striatopallidal disease

Excludes: *abnormal movements of head NOS (781.0)*

333.0 Other degenerative diseases of the basal ganglia
Atrophy or degeneration:
olivopontocerebellar [Déjérine-Thomas syndrome]
pigmentary pallidal [Hallervorden-Spatz disease]
striatonigral
Parkinsonian syndrome associated with:
idiopathic orthostatic hypotension
symptomatic orthostatic hypotension
Progressive supranuclear ophthalmoplegia
Shy-Drager syndrome

333.1 Essential and other specified forms of tremor
Benign essential tremor   Familial tremor

Use additional E code, if desired, to identify drug, if drug-induced

Excludes: *tremor NOS (781.0)*

333.2 Myoclonus
Familial essential myoclonus
Progressive myoclonic epilepsy
Unverricht-Lundborg disease

Use additional E code, if desired, to identify drug, if drug-induced

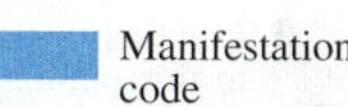

333.3 Tics of organic origin

> Excludes: *Gilles de la Tourette's syndrome (307.23)*
> *habit spasm (307.22)*
> *tic NOS (307.20)*

Use additional E code, if desired, to identify drug, if drug-induced

333.4 Huntington's chorea

333.5 Other choreas
    Hemiballism(us)
    Paroxysmal choreo-athetosis

> Excludes: *Sydenham's or rheumatic chorea (392.0-392.9)*

Use additional E code, if desired, to identify drug, if drug-induced

333.6 Idiopathic torsion dystonia
    Dystonia:
      deformans progressiva
      musculorum deformans
    (Schwalbe-) Ziehen-Oppenheim disease

333.7 Symptomatic torsion dystonia
    Athetoid cerebral palsy [Vogt's disease]
    Double athetosis (syndrome)

Use additional E code, if desired, to identify drug, if drug-induced

⑤ **333.8 Fragments of torsion dystonia**

Use additional E code, if desired, to identify drug, if drug-induced

    333.81 Blepharospasm

    333.82 Orofacial dyskinesia

    333.83 Spasmodic torticollis

> Excludes: *torticollis:*
> *NOS (723.5)*
> *hysterical (300.11)*
> *psychogenic (306.0)*

    333.84 Organic writers' cramp

> Excludes: *psychogenic (300.89)*

    333.89 Other

⑤ **333.9 Other and unspecified extrapyramidal diseases and abnormal movement disorders**

    333.90 Unspecified extrapyramidal disease and abnormal movement disorder

    333.91 Stiff-man syndrome

    333.92 Neuroleptic malignant syndrome
      Use additional E code to identify drug

    333.93 Benign shuddering attacks

    333.99 Other
      Restless legs

334 Spinocerebellar disease

> Excludes: *olivopontocerebellar degeneration (333.0)*
> *peroneal muscular atrophy (356.1)*

334.0 Friedreich's ataxia

334.1 Hereditary spastic paraplegia

334.2 Primary cerebellar degeneration
    Cerebellar ataxia:
      Marie's
      Sanger-Brown
    Dyssynergia cerebellaris myoclonica
    Primary cerebellar degeneration:
      NOS
      hereditary
      sporadic

334.3 Other cerebellar ataxia
    Cerebellar ataxia NOS

Use additional E code, if desired, to identify drug, if drug-induced

● Code new to this edition   ▲ Revision of existing code   ④ ⑤ Fourth or fifth digit required

334.4 Cerebellar ataxia in diseases classified elsewhere
Code first underlying disease, as:
    alcoholism (303.0-303.9)
    myxedema (244.0-244.9)
    neoplastic disease (140.0-239.9)

334.8 Other spinocerebellar diseases
    Ataxia-telangiectasia [Louis-Bar syndrome]
    Corticostriatal-spinal degeneration

334.9 Spinocerebellar disease, unspecified

335 Anterior horn cell disease

335.0 Werdnig-Hoffmann disease
    Infantile spinal muscular atrophy
    Progressive muscular atrophy of infancy

⑤ **335.1 Spinal muscular atrophy**

335.10 Spinal muscular atrophy, unspecified

335.11 Kugelberg-Welander disease
    Spinal muscular atrophy:
        familial
        juvenile

335.19 Other
    Adult spinal muscular atrophy

⑤ **335.2 Motor neuron disease**

335.20 Amyotrophic lateral sclerosis
    Motor neuron disease (bulbar) (mixed type)

335.21 Progressive muscular atrophy
    Duchenne-Aran muscular atrophy
    Progressive muscular atrophy (pure)

335.22 Progressive bulbar palsy

335.23 Pseudobulbar palsy

335.24 Primary lateral sclerosis

335.29 Other

335.8 Other anterior horn cell diseases

335.9 Anterior horn cell disease, unspecified

336 Other diseases of spinal cord

336.0 Syringomyelia and syringobulbia

336.1 Vascular myelopathies
    Acute infarction of spinal cord (embolic) (nonembolic)
    Arterial thrombosis of spinal cord
    Edema of spinal cord
    Hematomyelia
    Subacute necrotic myelopathy

336.2 Subacute combined degeneration of spinal cord in diseases classified elsewhere
Code first underlying disease, as:
    pernicious anemia (281.0)
    other vitamin B_{12} deficiency anemia (281.1)
    vitamin B_{12} deficiency (266.2)

336.3 Myelopathy in other diseases classified elsewhere
Code first underlying disease, as:
    myelopathy in neoplastic disease (140.0-239.9)

Excludes: myelopathy in:
        intervertebral disc disorder (722.70-722.73)
        spondylosis (721.1, 721.41-721.42, 721.91)

336.8 Other myelopathy
    Myelopathy:
        drug-induced
        radiation-induced

Use additional E code, if desired, to identify cause

336.9 Unspecified disease of spinal cord
    Cord compression NOS   Myelopathy NOS

Excludes: myelitis (323.0-323.9)
        spinal (canal) stenosis (723.0, 724.00-724.09)

Add 4th or 5th digit	Nonspecific code	Unspecified code	Manifestation code

235

337 Disorders of the autonomic nervous system
Includes: disorders of peripheral autonomic, sympathetic, parasympathetic, or vegetative system
Excludes: *familial dysautonomia [Riley-Day syndrome] (742.8)*

337.0 Idiopathic peripheral autonomic neuropathy
Carotid sinus syncope or syndrome
Cervical sympathetic dystrophy or paralysis

337.1 *Peripheral autonomic neuropathy in disorders classified elsewhere*
Code first underlying disease, as:
amyloidosis (277.3)
diabetes (250.6)

⑤ **337.2 Reflex sympathetic dystrophy**

337.20 Reflex sympathetic dystrophy, unspecified

337.21 Reflex sympathetic dystrophy of the upper limb

337.22 Reflex sympathetic dystrophy of the lower limb

337.29 Reflex sympathetic dystrophy of other specified site

337.3 Autonomic dysreflexia
Use additional code to identify the cause, such as:
decubitus ulcer (707.0)
fecal impaction (560.39)
urinary tract infection (599.0)

337.9 Unspecified disorder of autonomic nervous system

OTHER DISORDERS OF THE CENTRAL NERVOUS SYSTEM (340-349)

340 Multiple sclerosis
Disseminated or multiple sclerosis:
NOS
brain stem
cord
generalized

341 Other demyelinating diseases of central nervous system

341.0 Neuromyelitis optica

341.1 Schilder's disease
Baló's concentric sclerosis
Encephalitis periaxialis:
concentrica [Baló's]
diffusa [Schilder's]

341.8 Other demyelinating diseases of central nervous system
Central demyelination of corpus callosum
Central pontine myelinosis
Marchiafava (-Bignami) disease

341.9 Demyelinating disease of central nervous system, unspecified

⑤ **342 Hemiplegia and hemiparesis**
Excludes: *congenital (343.1)*
hemiplegia due to late effect of cerebrovascular accident (438.20-438.22)
infantile NOS (343.4)

Note: This category is to be used when hemiplegia (complete) (incomplete) is reported without further specification, or is stated to be old or long-standing but of unspecified cause. The category is also for use in multiple coding to identify these types of hemiplegia resulting from any cause.

The following fifth-digits are for use with codes 342.0-342.9

0 affecting unspecified site

1 affecting dominant site

2 affecting nondominant site

⑤ **342.0 Flaccid hemiplegia**

⑤ **342.1 Spastic hemiplegia**

⑤ **342.8 Other specified hemiplegia**

⑤ **342.9 Hemiplegia, unspecified**

● Code new
to this edition

▲ Revision of
existing code

④ ⑤ Fourth or fifth
digit required

343 Infantile cerebral palsy

Includes: cerebral:
  palsy NOS
  spastic infantile paralysis
congenital spastic paralysis (cerebral)
Little's disease
paralysis (spastic) due to birth injury:
  intracranial
  spinal

Excludes: *hereditary cerebral paralysis, such as:*
  hereditary spastic paraplegia (334.1)
  Vogt's disease (333.7)
  spastic paralysis specified as noncongenital or noninfantile (344.0-344.9)

343.0 Diplegic
Congenital diplegia   Congenital paraplegia

343.1 Hemiplegic
Congenital hemiplegia

Excludes: *infantile hemiplegia NOS (343.4)*

343.2 Quadriplegic
Tetraplegic

343.3 Monoplegic

343.4 Infantile hemiplegia
Infantile hemiplegia (postnatal) NOS

343.8 Other specified infantile cerebral palsy

343.9 Infantile cerebral palsy, unspecified
Cerebral palsy NOS

344 Other paralytic syndromes

Note: This category is to be used when the listed conditions are reported without further
specification or are stated to be old or long-standing but of unspecified cause. The category
is also for use in multiple coding to identify these conditions resulting from any cause.
Includes: paralysis (complete) (incomplete), except as classifiable to 342 and 343

Excludes: *congenital or infantile cerebral palsy (343.0-343.9)*
  hemiplegia (342.0-342.9)
  congenital or infantile (343.1, 343.4)

⑤ **344.0 Quadriplegia and quadriparesis**

  344.00 Quadriplegia, unspecified

  344.01 C1-C4, complete

  344.02 C1-C4, incomplete

  344.03 C5-C7, complete

  344.04 C5-C7, incomplete

  344.09 Other

344.1 Paraplegia
Paralysis of both lower limbs
Paraplegia (lower)

344.2 Diplegia of upper limbs
Diplegia (upper)
Paralysis of both upper limbs

⑤ **344.3 Monoplegia of lower limb**
Paralysis of lower limb

Excludes: *monoplegia of lower limb due to late effect of cerebrovascular accident*
  (438.40-438.42)

  344.30 affecting unspecified side

  344.31 affecting dominant side

  344.32 affecting nondominant side

⑤ **344.4 Monoplegia of upper limb**
Paralysis of upper limb

Excludes: *monoplegia of upper limb due to late effect of cerebrovascular accident*
  (438.30-438.32)

  344.40 affecting unspecified side

	Add 4th or 5th digit		Nonspecific code		Unspecified code		Manifestation code

344.41 affecting dominant side

344.42 affecting nondominant side

344.5 Unspecified monoplegia

⑤ **344.6 Cauda equina syndrome**

344.60 Without mention of neurogenic bladder

344.61 With neurogenic bladder
Acontractile bladder
Autonomic hyperreflexia of bladder
Cord bladder
Detrusor hyperreflexia

⑤ **344.8 Other specified paralytic syndromes**

344.81 Locked-in state

344.89 Other specified paralytic syndrome

344.9 Paralysis, unspecified

345 Epilepsy
The following fifth-digit subclassification is for use with categories 345.0, 345.1, 345.4-345.9:

0 without mention of intractable epilepsy

1 with intractable epilepsy

Excludes: *progressive myoclonic epilepsy (333.2)*

⑤ **345.0 Generalized nonconvulsive epilepsy**

Absences:	Pykno-epilepsy
atonic	Seizures:
typical	akinetic
Minor epilepsy	atonic
Petit mal	

⑤ **345.1 Generalized convulsive epilepsy**

Epileptic seizures:	Grand mal
clonic	Major epilepsy
myoclonic	
tonic	
tonic-clonic	

Excludes: *convulsions:*
NOS (780.3)
infantile (780.3)
newborn (779.0)
infantile spasms (345.6)

345.2 Petit mal status
Epileptic absence status

345.3 Grand mal status
Status epilepticus NOS

Excludes: *epilepsia partialis continua (345.7)*
status:
psychomotor (345.7)
temporal lobe (345.7)

⑤ **345.4 Partial epilepsy, with impairment of consciousness**
Epilepsy:
limbic system
partial:
secondarily generalized
with memory and ideational disturbances
psychomotor
psychosensory
temporal lobe
Epileptic automatism

⑤ **345.5 Partial epilepsy, without mention of impairment of consciousness**

Epilepsy:	Epilepsy:
Bravais-Jacksonian NOS	sensory-induced
focal (motor) NOS	somatomotor
Jacksonian NOS	somatosensory
motor partial	visceral
partial NOS	visual

● Code new
to this edition

▲ Revision of
existing code

④ ⑤ Fourth or fifth
digit required

⑤ **345.6 Infantile spasms**
Hypsarrhythmia Salaam attacks
Lightning spasms

Excludes: salaam tic (781.0)

⑤ **345.7 Epilepsia partialis continua**
Kojevnikov's epilepsy

⑤ **345.8 Other forms of epilepsy**
Epilepsy:
  cursive [running]
  gelastic

⑤ **345.9 Epilepsy, unspecified**
Epileptic convulsions, fits, or seizures NOS

Excludes: convulsive seizure or fit NOS (780.3)

⑤ **346 Migraine**

The following fifth-digit subclassification is for use with category 346:

0 without mention of intractable migraine

1 with intractable migraine, so stated

⑤ **346.0 Classical migraine**
Migraine preceded or accompanied by transient focal neurological phenomena
Migraine with aura

⑤ **346.1 Common migraine**
Atypical migraine Sick headache

⑤ **346.2 Variants of migraine**
Cluster headache Migraine:
Histamine cephalgia   lower half
Horton's neuralgia   retinal
Migraine: Neuralgia:
  abdominal   ciliary
  basilar   migrainous

⑤ **346.8 Other forms of migraine**
Migraine:
  hemiplegic
  ophthalmoplegic

⑤ **346.9 Migraine, unspecified**

347 Cataplexy and narcolepsy

348 Other conditions of brain

348.0 Cerebral cysts
Arachnoid cyst Porencephaly, acquired
Porencephalic cyst Pseudoporencephaly

Excludes: porencephaly (congenital) (742.4)

348.1 Anoxic brain damage

Excludes: that occurring in:
    abortion (634-638 with .7, 639.8)
    ectopic or molar pregnancy (639.8)
    labor or delivery (668.2, 669.4)
   that of newborn (767.0, 768.0-768.9, 772.1-772.2)

Use additional E code, if desired, to identify cause

348.2 Benign intracranial hypertension
Pseudotumor cerebri

Excludes: hypertensive encephalopathy (437.2)

348.3 Encephalopathy, unspecified

348.4 Compression of brain
Compression
Herniation } brain (stem)
Posterior fossa compression syndrome

348.5 Cerebral edema

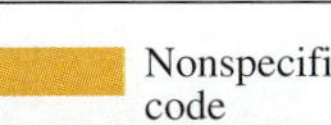

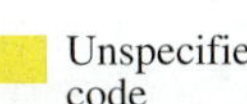

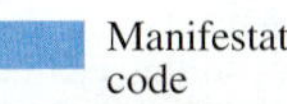

348.8 Other conditions of brain
Cerebral:
  calcification
  fungus

348.9 Unspecified condition of brain

349 Other and unspecified disorders of the nervous system

349.0 Reaction to spinal or lumbar puncture
Headache following lumbar puncture

349.1 Nervous system complications from surgically implanted device

Excludes: *immediate postoperative complications (997.00-997.09)*
mechanical complications of nervous system device (996.2)

349.2 Disorders of meninges, not elsewhere classified
Adhesions, meningeal (cerebral) (spinal)
Cyst, spinal meninges
Meningocele, acquired
Pseudomeningocele, acquired

⑤ **349.8 Other specified disorders of nervous system**

349.81 Cerebrospinal fluid rhinorrhea

Excludes: *cerebrospinal fluid otorrhea (388.61)*

349.82 Toxic encephalopathy
Use additional E code, if desired, to identify cause

349.89 Other

349.9 Unspecified disorders of nervous system
Disorder of nervous system (central) NOS

DISORDERS OF THE PERIPHERAL NERVOUS SYSTEM (350-359)

Excludes: *diseases of:*
acoustic [8th] nerve (388.5)
oculomotor [3rd, 4th, 6th] nerves (378.0-378.9)
optic [2nd] nerve (377.0-377.9)
peripheral autonomic nerves (337.0-337.9)
neuralgia
neuritis } *NOS or "rheumatic" (729.2)*
radiculitis
peripheral neuritis in pregnancy (646.4)

350 Trigeminal nerve disorders
Includes: disorders of 5th cranial nerve

350.1 Trigeminal neuralgia
Tic douloureux   Trigeminal neuralgia NOS
Trifacial neuralgia

Excludes: *postherpetic (053.12)*

350.2 Atypical face pain

350.8 Other specified trigeminal nerve disorders

350.9 Trigeminal nerve disorder, unspecified

351 Facial nerve disorders
Includes: disorders of 7th cranial nerve

Excludes: *that in newborn (767.5)*

351.0 Bell's palsy
Facial palsy

351.1 Geniculate ganglionitis
Geniculate ganglionitis NOS

Excludes: *herpetic (053.11)*

351.8 Other facial nerve disorders
Facial myokymia   Melkersson's syndrome

351.9 Facial nerve disorder, unspecified

352 Disorders of other cranial nerves

352.0 Disorders of olfactory [1st] nerve

352.1 Glossopharyngeal neuralgia

● Code new
to this edition

▲ Revision of
existing code

④ ⑤ Fourth or fifth
digit required

352.2 Other disorders of glossopharyngeal [9th] nerve

352.3 Disorders of pneumogastric [10th] nerve
Disorders of vagal nerve

Excludes: *paralysis of vocal cords or larynx (478.30-478.34)*

352.4 Disorders of accessory [11th] nerve

352.5 Disorders of hypoglossal [12th] nerve

352.6 Multiple cranial nerve palsies
Collet-Sicard syndrome   Polyneuritis cranialis

352.9 Unspecified disorder of cranial nerves

353 Nerve root and plexus disorders

Excludes: *conditions due to:*
intervertebral disc disorders (722.0-722.9)
spondylosis (720.0-721.9)
vertebrogenic disorders (723.0-724.9)

353.0 Brachial plexus lesions
Cervical rib syndrome   Thoracic outlet syndrome
Costoclavicular syndrome
Scalenus anticus syndrome

Excludes: *brachial neuritis or radiculitis NOS (723.4)*
that in newborn (767.6)

353.1 Lumbosacral plexus lesions

353.2 Cervical root lesions, not elsewhere classified

353.3 Thoracic root lesions, not elsewhere classified

353.4 Lumbosacral root lesions, not elsewhere classified

353.5 Neuralgic amyotrophy
Parsonage-Aldren-Turner syndrome

353.6 Phantom limb (syndrome)

353.8 Other nerve root and plexus disorders

353.9 Unspecified nerve root and plexus disorder

354 Mononeuritis of upper limb and mononeuritis multiplex

354.0 Carpal tunnel syndrome
Median nerve entrapment   Partial thenar atrophy

354.1 Other lesion of median nerve
Median nerve neuritis

354.2 Lesion of ulnar nerve
Cubital tunnel syndrome   Tardy ulnar nerve palsy

354.3 Lesion of radial nerve
Acute radial nerve palsy

354.4 Causalgia of upper limb

Excludes: *causalgia:*
NOS (355.9)
lower limb (355.71)

354.5 Mononeuritis multiplex
Combinations of single conditions classifiable to 354 or 355

354.8 Other mononeuritis of upper limb

354.9 Mononeuritis of upper limb, unspecified

355 Mononeuritis of lower limb and unspecified site

355.0 Lesion of sciatic nerve

Excludes: *sciatica NOS (724.3)*

355.1 Meralgia paresthetica
Lateral cutaneous femoral nerve of thigh compression or syndrome

355.2 Other lesion of femoral nerve

355.3 Lesion of lateral popliteal nerve
Lesion of common peroneal nerve

355.4 Lesion of medial popliteal nerve

355.5 Tarsal tunnel syndrome

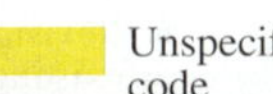

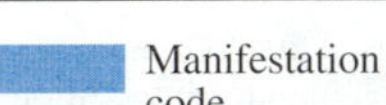

Manifestation
code

355.6 Lesion of plantar nerve
Morton's metatarsalgia, neuralgia, or neuroma

⑤ **355.7 Other mononeuritis of lower limb**

355.71 Causalgia of lower limb

| *Excludes:* | causalgia: |

NOS (355.9)
upper limb (354.4)

355.79 Other mononeuritis of lower limb

355.8 Mononeuritis of lower limb, unspecified

355.9 Mononeuritis of unspecified site
Causalgia NOS

| *Excludes:* | causalgia: |

lower limb (355.71)
upper limb (354.4)

356 Hereditary and idiopathic peripheral neuropathy

356.0 Hereditary peripheral neuropathy
Déjérine-Sottas disease

356.1 Peroneal muscular atrophy
Charcot-Marie-Tooth disease
Neuropathic muscular atrophy

356.2 Hereditary sensory neuropathy

356.3 Refsum's disease
Heredopathia atactica polyneuritiformis

356.4 Idiopathic progressive polyneuropathy

356.8 Other specified idiopathic peripheral neuropathy
Supranuclear paralysis

356.9 Unspecified

357 Inflammatory and toxic neuropathy

357.0 Acute infective polyneuritis
Guillain-Barré syndrome
Postinfectious polyneuritis

357.1 *Polyneuropathy in collagen vascular disease*
Code first underlying disease, as:
disseminated lupus erythematosus (710.0)
polyarteritis nodosa (446.0)
rheumatoid arthritis (714.0)

357.2 *Polyneuropathy in diabetes*
Code first underlying disease (250.6)

357.3 *Polyneuropathy in malignant disease*
Code first underlying disease (140.0-208.9)

357.4 *Polyneuropathy in other diseases classified elsewhere*
Code first underlying disease, as:
amyloidosis (277.3)
beriberi (265.0)
deficiency of B vitamins (266.0-266.9)
diphtheria (032.0-032.9)
hypoglycemia (251.2)
pellagra (265.2)
porphyria (277.1)
sarcoidosis (135)
uremia (585)

| *Excludes:* | polyneuropathy in: |

herpes zoster (053.13)
mumps (072.72)

357.5 Alcoholic polyneuropathy

357.6 Polyneuropathy due to drugs
Use additional E code, if desired, to identify drug

357.7 Polyneuropathy due to other toxic agents
Use additional E code, if desired, to identify toxic agent

● Code new
to this edition
▲ Revision of
existing code
④ ⑤ Fourth or fifth
digit required

⑤ **357.8 Other**

● **357.81   Chronic inflammatory demyelinating polyneuritis**

● **357.82   Critical illness polyneuropathy**
Acute motor neuropathy

● **357.89   Other inflammatory and toxic neuropathy**

357.9 Unspecified

358 Myoneural disorders

358.0 Myasthenia gravis

358.1 *Myasthenic syndromes in diseases classified elsewhere*
Amyotrophy
Eaton-Lambert syndrome } from stated cause classified elsewhere
Code first underlying disease, as:
botulism (005.1)
diabetes mellitus (250.6)
hypothyroidism (244.0-244.9)
malignant neoplasm (140.0-208.9)
pernicious anemia (281.0)
thyrotoxicosis (242.0-242.9)

358.2 Toxic myoneural disorders
Use additional E code, if desired, to identify toxic agent

358.8 Other specified myoneural disorders

358.9 Myoneural disorders, unspecified

359 Muscular dystrophies and other myopathies
Excludes: *idiopathic polymyositis (710.4)*

359.0 Congenital hereditary muscular dystrophy
Benign congenital myopathy
Central core disease
Centronuclear myopathy
Myotubular myopathy
Nemaline body disease

Excludes: *arthrogryposis multiplex congenita (754.89)*

359.1 Hereditary progressive muscular dystrophy

Muscular dystrophy:
NOS
distal
Duchenne
Erb's
fascioscapulohumeral

Muscular dystrophy:
Gower's
Landouzy-Déjérine
limb-girdle
ocular
oculopharyngeal

359.2 Myotonic disorders

Dystrophia myotonica
Eulenburg's disease
Myotonia congenita

Paramyotonia congenita
Steinert's disease
Thomsen's disease

359.3 Familial periodic paralysis
Hypokalemic familial periodic paralysis

359.4 Toxic myopathy
Use additional E code, if desired, to identify toxic agent

359.5 *Myopathy in endocrine diseases classified elsewhere*
Code first underlying disease, as:
Addison's disease (255.4)
Cushing's syndrome (255.0)
hypopituitarism (253.2)
myxedema (244.0 244.9)
thyrotoxicosis (242.0-242.9)

| Add 4th or 5th digit | Nonspecific code | Unspecified code | Manifestation code |

359.6 *Symptomatic inflammatory myopathy in diseases classified elsewhere*
    Code first underlying disease, as:
      amyloidosis (277.3)
      disseminated lupus erythematosus (710.0)
      malignant neoplasm (140.0-208.9)
      polyarteritis nodosa (446.0)
      rheumatoid arthritis (714.0)
      sarcoidosis (135)
      scleroderma (710.1)
      Sjögren's disease (710.2)

⑤ **359.8 Other myopathies**

  ● **359.81 Critical illness myopathy**
      Acute necrotizing myopathy
      Acute quadriplegic myopathy
      Intensive care (ICU) myopathy
      Myopathy of critical illness

  ● **359.89 Other myopathies**

359.9 Myopathy, unspecified

DISORDERS OF THE EYE AND ADNEXA (360-379)

360 **Disorders of the globe**
    Includes: disorders affecting multiple structures of eye

⑤ **360.0 Purulent endophthalmitis**

  360.00 Purulent endophthalmitis, unspecified

  360.01 Acute endophthalmitis

  360.02 Panophthalmitis

  360.03 Chronic endophthalmitis

  360.04 Vitreous abscess

⑤ **360.1 Other endophthalmitis**

  360.11 Sympathetic uveitis

  360.12 Panuveitis

  360.13 Parasitic endophthalmitis NOS

  360.14 Ophthalmia nodosa

  360.19 Other
      Phacoanaphylactic endophthalmitis

⑤ **360.2 Degenerative disorders of globe**

  360.20 Degenerative disorder of globe, unspecified

  360.21 Progressive high (degenerative) myopia
      Malignant myopia

  360.23 Siderosis

  360.24 Other metallosis
      Chalcosis

  360.29 Other

  Excludes: *xerophthalmia (264.7)*

⑤ **360.3 Hypotony of eye**

  360.30 Hypotony, unspecified

  360.31 Primary hypotony

  360.32 Ocular fistula causing hypotony

  360.33 Hypotony associated with other ocular disorders

  360.34 Flat anterior chamber

⑤ **360.4 Degenerated conditions of globe**

  360.40 Degenerated globe or eye, unspecified

  360.41 Blind hypotensive eye
      Atrophy of globe   Phthisis bulbi

  360.42 Blind hypertensive eye
      Absolute glaucoma

  360.43 Hemophthalmos, except current injury

  Excludes: *traumatic (871.0-871.9, 921.0-921.9)*

  ● Code new to this edition   ▲ Revision of existing code   ④ ⑤ Fourth or fifth digit required

360.44   **Leucocoria**

⑤ **360.5**   **Retained (old) intraocular foreign body, magnetic**

> *Excludes:* *current penetrating injury with magnetic foreign body (871.5)*
> *retained (old) foreign body of orbit (376.6)*

360.50   **Foreign body, magnetic, intraocular, unspecified**

360.51   **Foreign body, magnetic, in anterior chamber**

360.52   **Foreign body, magnetic, in iris or ciliary body**

360.53   **Foreign body, magnetic, in lens**

360.54   **Foreign body, magnetic, in vitreous**

360.55   **Foreign body, magnetic, in posterior wall**

360.59   **Foreign body, magnetic, in other or multiple sites**

⑤ **360.6**   **Retained (old) intraocular foreign body, nonmagnetic**
Retained (old) foreign body:
  NOS
  nonmagnetic

> *Excludes:* *current penetrating injury with (nonmagnetic) foreign body (871.6)*
> *retained (old) foreign body in orbit (376.6)*

360.60   **Foreign body, intraocular, unspecified**

360.61   **Foreign body in anterior chamber**

360.62   **Foreign body in iris or ciliary body**

360.63   **Foreign body in lens**

360.64   **Foreign body in vitreous**

360.65   **Foreign body in posterior wall**

360.69   **Foreign body in other or multiple sites**

⑤ **360.8**   **Other disorders of globe**

360.81   **Luxation of globe**

360.89   **Other**

360.9   **Unspecified disorder of globe**

361   **Retinal detachments and defects**

⑤ **361.0**   **Retinal detachment with retinal defect**
Rhegmatogenous retinal detachment

> *Excludes:* *detachment of retinal pigment epithelium (362.42-362.43)*
> *retinal detachment (serous) (without defect) (361.2)*

361.00   **Retinal detachment with retinal defect, unspecified**

361.01   **Recent detachment, partial, with single defect**

361.02   **Recent detachment, partial, with multiple defects**

361.03   **Recent detachment, partial, with giant tear**

361.04   **Recent detachment, partial, with retinal dialysis**
Dialysis (juvenile) of retina (with detachment)

361.05   **Recent detachment, total or subtotal**

361.06   **Old detachment, partial**
Delimited old retinal detachment

361.07   **Old detachment, total or subtotal**

⑤ **361.1**   **Retinoschisis and retinal cysts**

> *Excludes:* *juvenile retinoschisis (362.73)*
> *microcystoid degeneration of retina (362.62)*
> *parasitic cyst of retina (360.13)*

361.10   **Retinoschisis, unspecified**

361.11   **Flat retinoschisis**

361.12   **Bullous retinoschisis**

361.13   **Primary retinal cysts**

361.14   **Secondary retinal cysts**

361.19   **Other**
Pseudocyst of retina

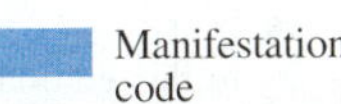

Add 4th or 5th digit	Nonspecific code	Unspecified code	Manifestation code

361.2 Serous retinal detachment
Retinal detachment without retinal defect

Excludes: *central serous retinopathy (362.41)*
retinal pigment epithelium detachment (362.42-362.43)

⑤ **361.3 Retinal defects without detachment**

Excludes: *chorioretinal scars after surgery for detachment (363.30-363.35)*
peripheral retinal degeneration without defect (362.60-362.66)

361.30 Retinal defect, unspecified
Retinal break(s) NOS

361.31 Round hole of retina without detachment

361.32 Horseshoe tear of retina without detachment
Operculum of retina without mention of detachment

361.33 Multiple defects of retina without detachment

⑤ **361.8 Other forms of retinal detachment**

361.81 Traction detachment of retina
Traction detachment with vitreoretinal organization

361.89 Other

361.9 Unspecified retinal detachment

362 Other retinal disorders

Excludes: *chorioretinal scars (363.30-363.35)*
chorioretinitis (363.0-363.2)

⑤ ***362.0 Diabetic retinopathy***
Code first diabetes (250.5)

362.01 Background diabetic retinopathy
Diabetic retinal microaneurysms
Diabetic retinopathy NOS

362.02 Proliferative diabetic retinopathy

⑤ **362.1 Other background retinopathy and retinal vascular changes**

362.10 Background retinopathy, unspecified

362.11 Hypertensive retinopathy

362.12 Exudative retinopathy
Coats' syndrome

362.13 Changes in vascular appearance
Vascular sheathing of retina
Use additional code for any associated atherosclerosis (440.8)

362.14 Retinal microaneurysms NOS

362.15 Retinal telangiectasia

362.16 Retinal neovascularization NOS
Neovascularization:
choroidal
subretinal

362.17 Other intraretinal microvascular abnormalities
Retinal varices

362.18 Retinal vasculitis
Eales' disease　　　　　Retinal:
Retinal:　　　　　　　　perivasculitis
arteritis　　　　　　　phlebitis
endarteritis

⑤ **362.2 Other proliferative retinopathy**

362.21 Retrolental fibroplasia

362.29 Other nondiabetic proliferative retinopathy

⑤ **362.3 Retinal vascular occlusion**

362.30 Retinal vascular occlusion, unspecified

362.31 Central retinal artery occlusion

362.32 Arterial branch occlusion

● Code new
to this edition　　　　　▲ Revision of
existing code　　　　　④ ⑤ Fourth or fifth
digit required

362.33 **Partial arterial occlusion**
Hollenhorst plaque   Retinal microembolism

362.34 **Transient arterial occlusion**
Amaurosis fugax

362.35 **Central retinal vein occlusion**

362.36 **Venous tributary (branch) occlusion**

362.37 **Venous engorgement**
Occlusion:
incipient
partial } of retinal vein

⑤ **362.4** **Separation of retinal layers**

Excludes: *retinal detachment (serous) (361.2)*
rhegmatogenous (361.00-361.07)

362.40 **Retinal layer separation, unspecified**

362.41 **Central serous retinopathy**

362.42 **Serous detachment of retinal pigment epithelium**
Exudative detachment of retinal pigment epithelium

362.43 **Hemorrhagic detachment of retinal pigment epithelium**

⑤ **362.5** **Degeneration of macula and posterior pole**

Excludes: *degeneration of optic disc (377.21-377.24)*
hereditary retinal degeneration [dystrophy] (362.70-362.77)

362.50 **Macular degeneration (senile), unspecified**

362.51 **Nonexudative senile macular degeneration**
Senile macular degeneration:
atrophic
dry

362.52 **Exudative senile macular degeneration**
Kuhnt-Junius degeneration
Senile macular degeneration:
disciform
wet

362.53 **Cystoid macular degeneration**
Cystoid macular edema

362.54 **Macular cyst, hole, or pseudohole**

362.55 **Toxic maculopathy**
Use additional E code, if desired, to identify drug, if drug induced

362.56 **Macular puckering**
Preretinal fibrosis

362.57 **Drusen (degenerative)**

⑤ **362.6** **Peripheral retinal degenerations**

Excludes: *hereditary retinal degeneration [dystrophy] (362.70-362.77)*
retinal degeneration with retinal defect (361.00-361.07)

362.60 **Peripheral retinal degeneration, unspecified**

362.61 **Paving stone degeneration**

362.62 **Microcystoid degeneration**
Blessig's cysts   Iwanoff's cysts

362.63 **Lattice degeneration**
Palisade degeneration of retina

362.64 **Senile reticular degeneration**

362.65 **Secondary pigmentary degeneration**
Pseudoretinitis pigmentosa

362.66 **Secondary vitreoretinal degenerations**

⑤ **362.7** **Hereditary retinal dystrophies**

362.70 **Hereditary retinal dystrophy, unspecified**

362.71 ***Retinal dystrophy in systemic or cerebroretinal lipidoses***
Code first underlying disease, as:
cerebroretinal lipidoses (330.1)
systemic lipidoses (272.7)

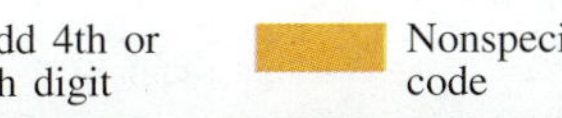

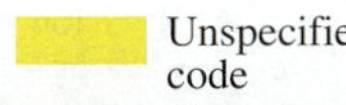

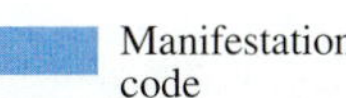

Manifestation
code

362.72 Retinal dystrophy in other systemic disorders and syndromes
Code first underlying disease, as:
    Bassen-Kornzweig syndrome (272.5)
    Refsum's disease (356.3)

362.73 Vitreoretinal dystrophies
Juvenile retinoschisis

362.74 Pigmentary retinal dystrophy
Retinal dystrophy, albipunctate
Retinitis pigmentosa

362.75 Other dystrophies primarily involving the sensory retina
Progressive cone (-rod) dystrophy
Stargardt's disease

362.76 Dystrophies primarily involving the retinal pigment epithelium
Fundus flavimaculatus
Vitelliform dystrophy

362.77 Dystrophies primarily involving Bruch's membrane
Dystrophy:
    hyaline
    pseudoinflammatory foveal
Hereditary drusen

⑤ **362.8 Other retinal disorders**

Excludes: chorioretinal inflammations (363.0-363.2)
    chorioretinal scars (363.30-363.35)

362.81 Retinal hemorrhage
Hemorrhage:
    preretinal
    retinal (deep) (superficial)
    subretinal

362.82 Retinal exudates and deposits

362.83 Retinal edema
Retinal:
    cotton wool spots
    edema (localized) (macular) (peripheral)

362.84 Retinal ischemia

362.85 Retinal nerve fiber bundle defects

362.89 Other retinal disorders

362.9 Unspecified retinal disorder

363 Chorioretinal inflammations, scars, and other disorders of choroid

⑤ **363.0 Focal chorioretinitis and focal retinochoroiditis**

Excludes: focal chorioretinitis or retinochoroiditis in:
    histoplasmosis (115.02, 115.12, 115.92)
    toxoplasmosis (130.2)
      congenital infection (771.2)

363.00 Focal chorioretinitis, unspecified
Focal:
    choroiditis or chorioretinitis NOS
    retinitis or retinochoroiditis NOS

363.01 Focal choroiditis and chorioretinitis, juxtapapillary

363.03 Focal choroiditis and chorioretinitis of other posterior pole

363.04 Focal choroiditis and chorioretinitis, peripheral

363.05 Focal retinitis and retinochoroiditis, juxtapapillary
Neuroretinitis

363.06 Focal retinitis and retinochoroiditis, macular or paramacular

363.07 Focal retinitis and retinochoroiditis of other posterior pole

363.08 Focal retinitis and retinochoroiditis, peripheral

⑤ **363.1 Disseminated chorioretinitis and disseminated retinochoroiditis**

Excludes: disseminated choroiditis or chorioretinitis in secondary syphilis (091.51)
    neurosyphilitic disseminated retinitis or retinochoroiditis (094.83)
    retinal (peri)vasculitis (362.18)

  ● Code new
    to this edition
  ▲ Revision of
    existing code
  ④ ⑤ Fourth or fifth
    digit required

363.10 **Disseminated chorioretinitis, unspecified**
Disseminated:
choroiditis or chorioretinitis NOS
retinitis or retinochoroiditis NOS

363.11 **Disseminated choroiditis and chorioretinitis, posterior pole**

363.12 **Disseminated choroiditis and chorioretinitis, peripheral**

363.13 *Disseminated choroiditis and chorioretinitis, generalized*
Code first any underlying disease, as:
tuberculosis (017.3)

363.14 **Disseminated retinitis and retinochoroiditis, metastatic**

363.15 **Disseminated retinitis and retinochoroiditis, pigment epitheliopathy**
Acute posterior multifocal placoid pigment epitheliopathy

⑤ **363.2** **Other and unspecified forms of chorioretinitis and retinochoroiditis**
Excludes: *panophthalmitis (360.02)*
sympathetic uveitis (360.11)
uveitis NOS (364.3)

363.20 **Chorioretinitis, unspecified**
Choroiditis NOS
Retinitis NOS
Uveitis, posterior NOS

363.21 **Pars planitis**
Posterior cyclitis

363.22 **Harada's disease**

⑤ **363.3** **Chorioretinal scars**
Scar (postinflammatory) (postsurgical) (posttraumatic):
choroid
retina

363.30 **Chorioretinal scar, unspecified**

363.31 **Solar retinopathy**

363.32 **Other macular scars**

363.33 **Other scars of posterior pole**

363.34 **Peripheral scars**

363.35 **Disseminated scars**

⑤ **363.4** **Choroidal degenerations**

363.40 **Choroidal degeneration, unspecified**
Choroidal sclerosis NOS

363.41 **Senile atrophy of choroid**

363.42 **Diffuse secondary atrophy of choroid**

363.43 **Angioid streaks of choroid**

⑤ **363.5** **Hereditary choroidal dystrophies**
Hereditary choroidal atrophy:
partial [choriocapillaris]
total [all vessels]

363.50 **Hereditary choroidal dystrophy or atrophy, unspecified**

363.51 **Circumpapillary dystrophy of choroid, partial**

363.52 **Circumpapillary dystrophy of choroid, total**
Helicoid dystrophy of choroid

363.53 **Central dystrophy of choroid, partial**
Dystrophy, choroidal:
central areolar
circinate

363.54 **Central choroidal atrophy, total**
Dystrophy, choroidal:
central gyrate
serpiginous

363.55 **Choroideremia**

363.56 **Other diffuse or generalized dystrophy, partial**
Diffuse choroidal sclerosis

363.57 **Other diffuse or generalized dystrophy, total**
Generalized gyrate atrophy, choroid

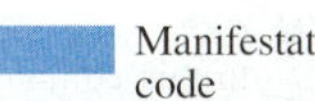

⑤ **363.6 Choroidal hemorrhage and rupture**

  363.61 Choroidal hemorrhage, unspecified

  363.62 Expulsive choroidal hemorrhage

  363.63 Choroidal rupture

⑤ **363.7 Choroidal detachment**

  363.70 Choroidal detachment, unspecified

  363.71 Serous choroidal detachment

  363.72 Hemorrhagic choroidal detachment

363.8 Other disorders of choroid

363.9 Unspecified disorder of choroid

364 Disorders of iris and ciliary body

⑤ **364.0 Acute and subacute iridocyclitis**
  Anterior uveitis
  Cyclitis ⎫ acute
  Iridocyclitis ⎬ subacute
  Iritis ⎭

  | Excludes: | gonococcal (098.41)
  herpes simplex (054.44)
  herpes zoster (053.22)

  364.00 Acute and subacute iridocyclitis, unspecified

  364.01 Primary iridocyclitis

  364.02 Recurrent iridocyclitis

  364.03 Secondary iridocyclitis, infectious

  364.04 Secondary iridocyclitis, noninfectious
    Aqueous:
      cells
      fibrin
      flare

  364.05 Hypopyon

⑤ **364.1 Chronic iridocyclitis**

  | Excludes: | posterior cyclitis (363.21)

  364.10 Chronic iridocyclitis, unspecified

  364.11 Chronic iridocyclitis in diseases classified elsewhere
    Code first underlying disease, as:
      sarcoidosis (135)
      tuberculosis (017.3)

  | Excludes: | syphilitic iridocyclitis (091.52)

⑤ **364.2 Certain types of iridocyclitis**

  | Excludes: | posterior cyclitis (363.21)
  sympathetic uveitis (360.11)

  364.21 Fuchs' heterochromic cyclitis

  364.22 Glaucomatocyclitic crises

  364.23 Lens-induced iridocyclitis

  364.24 Vogt-Koyanagi syndrome

364.3 Unspecified iridocyclitis
  Uveitis NOS

⑤ **364.4 Vascular disorders of iris and ciliary body**

  364.41 Hyphema
    Hemorrhage of iris or ciliary body

  364.42 Rubeosis iridis
    Neovascularization of iris or ciliary body

⑤ **364.5 Degenerations of iris and ciliary body**

  364.51 Essential or progressive iris atrophy

  364.52 Iridoschisis

● Code new
to this edition

▲ Revision of
existing code

④ ⑤ Fourth or fifth
digit required

364.53 **Pigmentary iris degeneration**
Acquired heterochromia
Pigment dispersion syndrome } of iris
Translucency

364.54 **Degeneration of pupillary margin**
Atrophy of sphincter } of iris
Ectropion of pigment epithelium

364.55 **Miotic cysts of pupillary margin**

364.56 **Degenerative changes of chamber angle**

364.57 **Degenerative changes of ciliary body**

364.59 **Other iris atrophy**
Iris atrophy (generalized) (sector shaped)

⑤ **364.6** **Cysts of iris, ciliary body, and anterior chamber**

Excludes: *miotic pupillary cyst (364.55)*
parasitic cyst (360.13)

364.60 **Idiopathic cysts**

364.61 **Implantation cysts**
Epithelial down-growth, anterior chamber
Implantation cysts (surgical) (traumatic)

364.62 **Exudative cysts of iris or anterior chamber**

364.63 **Primary cyst of pars plana**

364.64 **Exudative cyst of pars plana**

⑤ **364.7** **Adhesions and disruptions of iris and ciliary body**

Excludes: *flat anterior chamber (360.34)*

364.70 **Adhesions of iris, unspecified**
Synechiae (iris) NOS

364.71 **Posterior synechiae**

364.72 **Anterior synechiae**

364.73 **Goniosynechiae**
Peripheral anterior synechiae

364.74 **Pupillary membranes**
Iris bombé
Pupillary:
occlusion
seclusion

364.75 **Pupillary abnormalities**
Deformed pupil   Rupture of sphincter, pupil
Ectopic pupil

364.76 **Iridodialysis**

364.77 **Recession of chamber angle**

364.8 **Other disorders of iris and ciliary body**
Prolapse of iris NOS

Excludes: *prolapse of iris in recent wound (871.1)*

364.9 **Unspecified disorder of iris and ciliary body**

365 **Glaucoma**

Excludes: *blind hypertensive eye [absolute glaucoma] (360.42)*
congenital glaucoma (743.20-743.22)

⑤ **365.0** **Borderline glaucoma [glaucoma suspect]**

365.00 **Preglaucoma, unspecified**

365.01 **Open angle with borderline findings**
Open angle with:
borderline intraocular pressure
cupping of optic discs

365.02 **Anatomical narrow angle**

365.03 **Steroid responders**

365.04 **Ocular hypertension**

⑤ **365.1** **Open-angle glaucoma**

    365.10 **Open-angle glaucoma, unspecified**
        Wide-angle glaucoma NOS

    365.11 **Primary open angle glaucoma**
        Chronic simple glaucoma

    365.12 **Low tension glaucoma**

    365.13 **Pigmentary glaucoma**

    365.14 **Glaucoma of childhood**
        Infantile or juvenile glaucoma

    365.15 **Residual stage of open angle glaucoma**

⑤ **365.2** **Primary angle-closure glaucoma**

    365.20 **Primary angle-closure glaucoma, unspecified**

    365.21 **Intermittent angle-closure glaucoma**
        Angle-closure glaucoma:
          interval
          subacute

    365.22 **Acute angle-closure glaucoma**

    365.23 **Chronic angle-closure glaucoma**

    365.24 **Residual stage of angle-closure glaucoma**

⑤ **365.3** **Corticosteroid-induced glaucoma**

    365.31 **Glaucomatous stage**

    365.32 **Residual stage**

⑤ **365.4** **Glaucoma associated with congenital anomalies, dystrophies, and systemic syndromes**

    365.41 *Glaucoma associated with chamber angle anomalies*
        Code first associated disorder, as:
          Axenfeld's anomaly (743.44)
          Rieger's anomaly or syndrome (743.44)

    365.42 *Glaucoma associated with anomalies of iris*
        Code first associated disorder, as:
          aniridia (743.45)
          essential iris atrophy (364.51)

    365.43 *Glaucoma associated with other anterior segment anomalies*
        Code first associated disorder, as:
          microcornea (743.41)

    365.44 *Glaucoma associated with systemic syndromes*
        Code first associated disease, as:
          neurofibromatosis (237.7)
          Sturge-Weber (-Dimitri) syndrome (759.6)

⑤ **365.5** **Glaucoma associated with disorders of the lens**

    365.51 **Phacolytic glaucoma**
        Use additional code for associated hypermature cataract (366.18)

    365.52 **Pseudoexfoliation glaucoma**
        Use additional code for associated pseudoexfoliation of capsule (366.11)

    365.59 **Glaucoma associated with other lens disorders**
        Use additional code for associated disorder, as:
          dislocation of lens (379.33-379.34)
          spherophakia (743.36)

⑤ **365.6** **Glaucoma associated with other ocular disorders**

    365.60 **Glaucoma associated with unspecified ocular disorder**

    365.61 **Glaucoma associated with pupillary block**
        Use additional code for associated disorder, as:
          seclusion of pupil [iris bombé] (364.74)

    365.62 **Glaucoma associated with ocular inflammations**
        Use additional code for associated disorder, as:
          glaucomatocyclitic crises (364.22)
          iridocyclitis (364.0-364.3)

    365.63 **Glaucoma associated with vascular disorders**
        Use additional code for associated disorder, as:
          central retinal vein occlusion (362.35)
          hyphema (364.41)

● Code new to this edition   ▲ Revision of existing code   ④ ⑤ Fourth or fifth digit required

365.64 Glaucoma associated with tumors or cysts
Use additional code for associated disorder, as:
    benign neoplasm (224.0-224.9)
    epithelial down-growth (364.61)
    malignant neoplasm (190.0-190.9)

365.65 Glaucoma associated with ocular trauma
Use additional code for associated condition, as:
    contusion of globe (921.3)
    recession of chamber angle (364.77)

⑤ **365.8 Other specified forms of glaucoma**

    365.81 Hypersecretion glaucoma

    365.82 Glaucoma with increased episcleral venous pressure

    ● **365.83 Aqueous misdirection**
        Malignant glaucoma

    365.89 Other specified glaucoma

365.9 Unspecified glaucoma

366 Cataract

    Excludes: congenital cataract (743.30-743.34)

⑤ **366.0 Infantile, juvenile, and presenile cataract**

    366.00 Nonsenile cataract, unspecified

    366.01 Anterior subcapsular polar cataract

    366.02 Posterior subcapsular polar cataract

    366.03 Cortical, lamellar, or zonular cataract

    366.04 Nuclear cataract

    366.09 Other and combined forms of nonsenile cataract

⑤ **366.1 Senile cataract**

    366.10 Senile cataract, unspecified

    366.11 Pseudoexfoliation of lens capsule

    366.12 Incipient cataract
        Cataract: Water clefts
          coronary
          immature NOS
          punctate

    366.13 Anterior subcapsular polar senile cataract

    366.14 Posterior subcapsular polar senile cataract

    366.15 Cortical senile cataract

    366.16 Nuclear sclerosis
        Cataracta brunescens
        Nuclear cataract

    366.17 Total or mature cataract

    366.18 Hypermature cataract
        Morgagni cataract

    366.19 Other and combined forms of senile cataract

⑤ **366.2 Traumatic cataract**

    366.20 Traumatic cataract, unspecified

    366.21 Localized traumatic opacities
        Vossius' ring

    366.22 Total traumatic cataract

    366.23 Partially resolved traumatic cataract

⑤ **366.3 Cataract secondary to ocular disorders**

    366.30 Cataracts complicata, unspecified

    366.31 *Glaucomatous flecks (subcapsular)*
        Code first underlying glaucoma (365.0-365.9)

    366.32 *Cataract in inflammatory disorders*
        Code first underlying condition, as:
        chronic choroiditis (363.0-363.2)

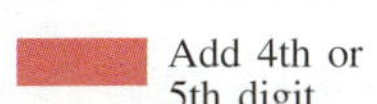

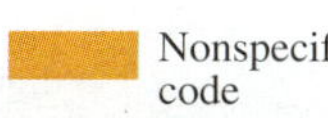

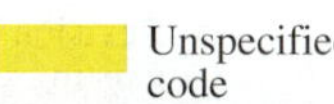

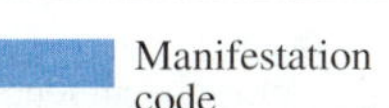

366.33 *Cataract with neovascularization*
  Code first underlying condition, as:
    chronic iridocyclitis (364.10)

366.34 *Cataract in degenerative disorders*
  Sunflower cataract
  Code first underlying condition, as:
    chalcosis (360.24)
    degenerative myopia (360.21)
    pigmentary retinal dystrophy (362.74)

⑤ **366.4 Cataract associated with other disorders**

366.41 *Diabetic cataract*
  Code first diabetes (250.5)

366.42 *Tetanic cataract*
  Code first underlying disease, as:
    calcinosis (275.4)
    hypoparathyroidism (252.1)

366.43 *Myotonic cataract*
  Code first underlying disorder (359.2)

366.44 *Cataract associated with other syndromes*
  Code first underlying condition, as:
    craniofacial dysostosis (756.0)
    galactosemia (271.1)

366.45 Toxic cataract
  Drug-induced cataract
  Use additional E code, if desired, to identify drug or other toxic substance

366.46 Cataract associated with radiation and other physical influences
  Use additional E code, if desired, to identify cause

⑤ **366.5 After-cataract**

366.50 After-cataract, unspecified
  Secondary cataract NOS

366.51 Soemmering's ring

366.52 Other after-cataract, not obscuring vision

366.53 After-cataract, obscuring vision

366.8 Other cataract
  Calcification of lens

366.9 Unspecified cataract

367 Disorders of refraction and accommodation

367.0 Hypermetropia
  Far-sightedness   Hyperopia

367.1 Myopia
  Near-sightedness

⑤ **367.2 Astigmatism**

367.20 Astigmatism, unspecified

367.21 Regular astigmatism

367.22 Irregular astigmatism

⑤ **367.3 Anisometropia and aniseikonia**

367.31 Anisometropia

367.32 Aniseikonia

367.4 Presbyopia

⑤ **367.5 Disorders of accommodation**

367.51 Paresis of accommodation
  Cycloplegia

367.52 Total or complete internal ophthalmoplegia

367.53 Spasm of accommodation

⑤ **367.8 Other disorders of refraction and accommodation**

367.81 Transient refractive change

367.89 Other
  Drug-induced disorders of refraction and accommodation
  Toxic disorders of refraction and accommodation

● Code new to this edition   ▲ Revision of existing code   ④ ⑤ Fourth or fifth digit required

367.9 Unspecified disorder of refraction and accommodation

368 Visual disturbances

> Excludes: electrophysiological disturbances (794.11-794.14)

⑤ **368.0** Amblyopia ex anopsia

368.00 Amblyopia, unspecified

368.01 Strabismic amblyopia
Suppression amblyopia

368.02 Deprivation amblyopia

368.03 Refractive amblyopia

⑤ **368.1** Subjective visual disturbances

368.10 Subjective visual disturbance, unspecified

368.11 Sudden visual loss

368.12 Transient visual loss
Concentric fading   Scintillating scotoma

368.13 Visual discomfort
Asthenopia   Photophobia
Eye strain

368.14 Visual distortions of shape and size
Macropsia   Micropsia
Metamorphopsia

368.15 Other visual distortions and entoptic phenomena
Photopsia   Visual halos
Refractive:
diplopia
polyopia

368.16 Psychophysical visual disturbances
Visual:
agnosia
disorientation syndrome
hallucinations

368.2 Diplopia
Double vision

⑤ **368.3** Other disorders of binocular vision

368.30 Binocular vision disorder, unspecified

368.31 Suppression of binocular vision

368.32 Simultaneous visual perception without fusion

368.33 Fusion with defective stereopsis

368.34 Abnormal retinal correspondence

⑤ **368.4** Visual field defects

368.40 Visual field defect, unspecified

368.41 Scotoma involving central area
Scotoma:
central
centrocecal
paracentral

368.42 Scotoma of blind spot area
Enlarged: Paracecal scotoma
angioscotoma
blind spot

368.43 Sector or arcuate defects
Scotoma:
arcuate
Bjerrum
Seidel

368.44 Other localized visual field defect
Scotoma: Visual field defect:
NOS   nasal step
ring   peripheral

368.45 Generalized contraction or constriction

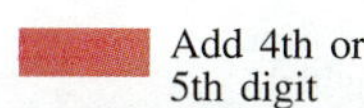

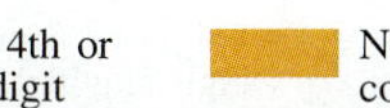

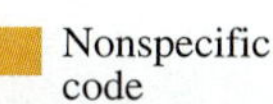

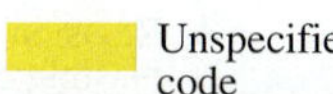

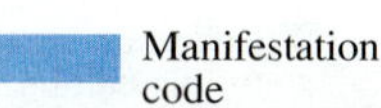

368.46 Homonymous bilateral field defects
Hemianopsia (altitudinal) (homonymous)
Quadrant anopia

368.47 Heteronymous bilateral field defects
Hemianopsia:
  binasal
  bitemporal

⑤ **368.5 Color vision deficiencies**
Color blindness

368.51 Protan defect
Protanomaly   Protanopia

368.52 Deutan defect
Deuteranomaly   Deuteranopia

368.53 Tritan defect
Tritanomaly   Tritanopia

368.54 Achromatopsia
Monochromatism (cone) (rod)

368.55 Acquired color vision deficiencies

368.59 Other color vision deficiencies

⑤ **368.6 Night blindness**
Nyctalopia

368.60 Night blindness, unspecified

368.61 Congenital night blindness
Hereditary night blindness
Oguchi's disease

368.62 Acquired night blindness

Excludes: *that due to vitamin A deficiency (264.5)*

368.63 Abnormal dark adaptation curve
Abnormal threshold   }
Delayed adaptation   } of cones or rods

368.69 Other night blindness

368.8 Other specified visual disturbances
Blurred vision NOS

368.9 Unspecified visual disturbance

369 Blindness and low vision
Note: Visual impairment refers to a functional limitation of the eye (e.g., limited visual acuity or visual field). It should be distinguished from visual disability, indicating a limitation of the abilities of the individual (e.g., limited reading skills, vocational skills), and from visual handicap, indicating a limitation of personal and socioeconomic independence (e.g., limited mobility, limited employability.)

The levels of impairment defined in the table on page 174 are based on the recommendations of the WHO Study Group on Prevention of Blindness (Geneva, November 6-10, 1972; WHO Technical Report Series 518), and of the International Council of Ophthalmology (1976).

Note that definitions of blindness vary in different settings.

For international reporting WHO defines blindness as profound impairment. This definition can be applied to blindness of one eye (369.1, 369.6) and to blindness of the individual (369.0).

For determination of benefits in the U.S.A., the definition of legal blindness as severe impairment is often used. This definition applies to blindness of the individual only.

Excludes: *correctable impaired vision due to refractive errors (367.0-367.9)*

⑤ **369.0 Profound impairment, both eyes**

369.00 Impairment level not further specified
Blindness:
  NOS according to WHO definition
  both eyes

369.01 Better eye: total impairment;
lesser eye: total impairment

● Code new   ▲ Revision of   ④ ⑤ Fourth or fifth
   to this edition   existing code   digit required

369.02   **Better eye: near-total impairment;**
     lesser eye: not further specified

369.03   **Better eye: near-total impairment;**
     lesser eye: total impairment

369.04   **Better eye: near-total impairment;**
     lesser eye: near-total impairment

369.05   **Better eye: profound impairment;**
     lesser eye: not further specified

369.06   **Better eye: profound impairment;**
     lesser eye: total impairment

369.07   **Better eye: profound impairment;**
     lesser eye: near-total impairment

369.08   **Better eye: profound impairment;**
     lesser eye: profound impairment

⑤ **369.1   Moderate or severe impairment, better eye, profound impairment lesser eye**

369.10   **Impairment level not further specified**
     Blindness, one eye, low vision other eye

369.11   **Better eye: severe impairment;**
     lesser eye: blind, not further specified

369.12   **Better eye: severe impairment;**
     lesser eye: total impairment

369.13   **Better eye: severe impairment;**
     lesser eye: near-total impairment

369.14   **Better eye: severe impairment;**
     lesser eye: profound impairment

369.15   **Better eye: moderate impairment;**
     lesser eye: blind, not further specified

369.16   **Better eye: moderate impairment;**
     lesser eye: total impairment

369.17   **Better eye: moderate impairment;**
     lesser eye: near-total impairment

369.18   **Better eye: moderate impairment;**
     lesser eye: profound impairment

⑤ **369.2   Moderate or severe impairment, both eyes**

369.20   **Impairment level not further specified**
     Low vision, both eyes NOS

369.21   **Better eye: severe impairment;**
     lesser eye: not further specified

369.22   **Better eye: severe impairment;**
     lesser eye: severe impairment

369.23   **Better eye: moderate impairment;**
     lesser eye: not further specified

369.24   **Better eye: moderate impairment;**
     lesser eye: severe impairment

369.25   **Better eye: moderate impairment;**
     lesser eye: moderate impairment

369.3   Unqualified visual loss, both eyes

> *Excludes:* *blindness NOS:*
>   *legal [U.S.A. definition] (369.4)*
>   *WHO definition (369.00)*

369.4   Legal blindness, as defined in U.S.A.
     Blindness NOS according to U.S.A. definition

> *Excludes:* *legal blindness with specification of impairment level (369.01-369.08,*
>   *369.11-369.14, 369.21-369.22)*

⑤ **369.6   Profound impairment, one eye**

369.60   **Impairment level not further specified**
     Blindness, one eye

369.61   **One eye: total impairment; other eye: not specified**

369.62   **One eye: total impairment; other eye: near-normal vision**

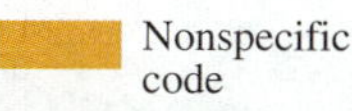

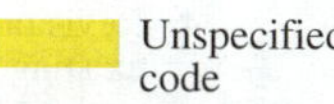

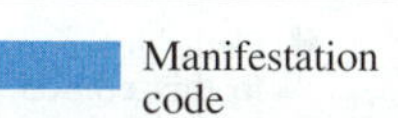

Manifestation
code

369.63 One eye: total impairment; other eye: normal vision

369.64 One eye: near-total impairment; other eye: not specified

369.65 One eye: near-total impairment; other eye: near-normal vision

369.66 One eye: near-total impairment; other eye: normal vision

369.67 One eye: profound impairment; other eye: not specified

369.68 One eye: profound impairment; other eye: near-normal vision

369.69 One eye: profound impairment; other eye: normal vision

⑤ **369.7 Moderate or severe impairment, one eye**

369.70 **Impairment level not further specified**
Low vision, one eye

369.71 One eye: severe impairment; other eye: not specified

369.72 One eye: severe impairment; other eye: near-normal vision

369.73 One eye: severe impairment; other eye: normal vision

369.74 One eye: moderate impairment; other eye: not specified

Classification		LEVELS OF VISUAL IMPAIRMENT					Additional Descriptors which may be encountered
"legal"	WHO	Visual Acuity and/or Visual Field Limitation (*whichever is worse*)					
	(NEAR-) NORMAL VISION	**RANGE OF NORMAL VISION**					
		20/10	20/13	20/16	20/20	20/25	
		2.0	1.6	1.25	1.0	0.8	
		NEAR-NORMAL VISION					
			20/30	20/40	20/50	20/60	
		0.7	0.6	0.5	0.4	0.3	
	LOW VISION	**MODERATE VISUAL IMPAIRMENT**					Moderate low vision
		20/70	20/80	20/100	20/125	20/160	
			0.25	0.20	0.16	0.12	
		SEVERE VISUAL IMPAIRMENT					Severe low vision, "legal" blindness
			20/200	20/250	20/320	20/400	
			0.10	0.08	0.06	0.05	
LEGAL BLINDNESS		Visual Field:	20 degrees or less				
	BLINDNESS	**PROFOUND VISUAL IMPAIRMENT**					Profound low vision, moderate blindness
			20/500	20/630	20/800	20/1000	
			0.04	0.03	0.025	0.02	
		Count Fingers at:	less than 3m (10 ft)				
		Visual Field:	10 degrees or less				
		NEAR-TOTAL VISUAL IMPAIRMENT					Severe blindness
		Visual Acuity:	less than 0.02 (20/1000)				
		Count Fingers at:	1m (3 ft) or less				
(USA) both eyes	(WHO) one or both eyes	Hand Movements:	5m (15 ft) or less				Near-total blindness
		Light projection, light perception					
		Visual Field:	5 degrees or less				
		TOTAL VISUAL IMPAIRMENT					Total blindness
		No light perception (NLP)					

Visual acuity refers to best achievable acuity with correction

Non-listed Snellen fractions may be classified by converting to the nearest decimal equivalent, e.g., 10/200=0.05, 6/30=0.20

CF (count fingers) without designation of distance, may be classified to profound impairment.

HM (hand motion) without designation of distance, may be classified to near-total impairment.

Visual field measurements refer to the largest field diameter for a 1/100 white test object.

369.75 One eye: moderate impairment; other eye: near-normal vision

369.76 One eye: moderate impairment; other eye: normal vision

369.8 **Unqualified visual loss, one eye**

369.9 **Unspecified visual loss**

    ● Code new to this edition   ▲ Revision of existing code   ④ ⑤ Fourth or fifth digit required

370 Keratitis

⑤ **370.0 Corneal ulcer**

> *Excludes:* *that due to vitamin A deficiency (264.3)*

> **370.00 Corneal ulcer, unspecified**
>
> **370.01 Marginal corneal ulcer**
>
> **370.02 Ring corneal ulcer**
>
> **370.03 Central corneal ulcer**
>
> **370.04 Hypopyon ulcer**
> Serpiginous ulcer
>
> **370.05 Mycotic corneal ulcer**
>
> **370.06 Perforated corneal ulcer**
>
> **370.07 Mooren's ulcer**

⑤ **370.2 Superficial keratitis without conjunctivitis**

> *Excludes:* *dendritic [herpes simplex] keratitis (054.42)*

> **370.20 Superficial keratitis, unspecified**
>
> **370.21 Punctate keratitis**
> Thygeson's superficial punctate keratitis
>
> **370.22 Macular keratitis**
>
> | Keratitis: | Keratitis: |
> |---|---|
> | areolar | stellate |
> | nummular | striate |
>
> **370.23 Filamentary keratitis**
>
> **370.24 Photokeratitis**
> Snow blindness   Welders' keratitis

⑤ **370.3 Certain types of keratoconjunctivitis**

> **370.31 Phlyctenular keratoconjunctivitis**
> Phlyctenulosis
> Use additional code for any associated tuberculosis (017.3)
>
> **370.32 Limbar and corneal involvement in vernal conjunctivitis**
> Use additional code for vernal conjunctivitis (372.13)
>
> **370.33 Keratoconjunctivitis sicca, not specified as Sjögren's**

> *Excludes:* *Sjögren's syndrome (710.2)*

> **370.34 Exposure keratoconjunctivitis**
>
> **370.35 Neurotrophic keratoconjunctivitis**

⑤ **370.4 Other and unspecified keratoconjunctivitis**

> **370.40 Keratoconjunctivitis, unspecified**
> Superficial keratitis with conjunctivitis NOS
>
> ***370.44 Keratitis or keratoconjunctivitis in exanthema***
> *Code first underlying condition (050.0-052.9)*

> *Excludes:* *herpes simplex (054.43)*
> *herpes zoster (053.21)*
> *measles (055.71)*

> **370.49 Other**

> *Excludes:* *epidemic keratoconjunctivitis (077.1)*

⑤ **370.5 Interstitial and deep keratitis**

> **370.50 Interstitial keratitis, unspecified**
>
> **370.52 Diffuse interstitial keratitis**
> Cogan's syndrome
>
> **370.54 Sclerosing keratitis**
>
> **370.55 Corneal abscess**
>
> **370.59 Other**

> *Excludes:* *disciform herpes simplex keratitis (054.43)*
> *syphilitic keratitis (090.3)*

⑤ **370.6 Corneal neovascularization**

> **370.60 Corneal neovascularization, unspecified**

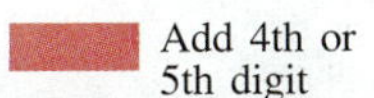

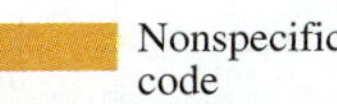

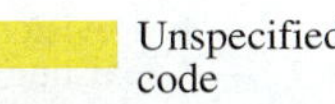

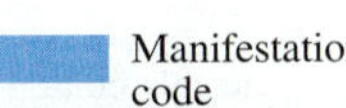

370.61 Localized vascularization of cornea

370.62 Pannus (corneal)

370.63 Deep vascularization of cornea

370.64 Ghost vessels (corneal)

370.8 Other forms of keratitis

370.9 Unspecified keratitis

371 Corneal opacity and other disorders of cornea

⑤ **371.0 Corneal scars and opacities**

Excludes: *that due to vitamin A deficiency (264.6)*

371.00 Corneal opacity, unspecified
Corneal scar NOS

371.01 Minor opacity of cornea
Corneal nebula

371.02 Peripheral opacity of cornea
Corneal macula not interfering with central vision

371.03 Central opacity of cornea
Corneal:
leucoma } interfering with central vision
macula

371.04 Adherent leucoma

371.05 *Phthisical cornea*
Code first underlying tuberculosis (017.3)

⑤ **371.1 Corneal pigmentations and deposits**

371.10 Corneal deposit, unspecified

371.11 Anterior pigmentations
Stähli's lines

371.12 Stromal pigmentations
Hematocornea

371.13 Posterior pigmentations
Krukenberg spindle

371.14 Kayser-Fleischer ring

371.15 Other deposits associated with metabolic disorders

371.16 Argentous deposits

⑤ **371.2 Corneal edema**

371.20 Corneal edema, unspecified

371.21 Idiopathic corneal edema

371.22 Secondary corneal edema

371.23 Bullous keratopathy

371.24 Corneal edema due to wearing of contact lenses

⑤ **371.3 Changes of corneal membranes**

371.30 Corneal membrane change, unspecified

371.31 Folds and rupture of Bowman's membrane

371.32 Folds in Descemet's membrane

371.33 Rupture in Descemet's membrane

⑤ **371.4 Corneal degenerations**

371.40 Corneal degeneration, unspecified

371.41 Senile corneal changes
Arcus senilis   Hassall-Henle bodies

371.42 Recurrent erosion of cornea

Excludes: *Mooren's ulcer (370.07)*

371.43 Band-shaped keratopathy

371.44 Other calcerous degenerations of cornea

371.45 Keratomalacia NOS

Excludes: *that due to vitamin A deficiency (264.4)*

● Code new
to this edition

▲ Revision of
existing code

④ ⑤ Fourth or fifth
digit required

371.46 **Nodular degeneration of cornea**
Salzmann's nodular dystrophy

371.48 **Peripheral degenerations of cornea**
Marginal degeneration of cornea [Terrien's]

`371.49` **Other**
Discrete colliquative keratopathy

⑤ 371.5 **Hereditary corneal dystrophies**

`371.50` **Corneal dystrophy, unspecified**

371.51 **Juvenile epithelial corneal dystrophy**

`371.52` **Other anterior corneal dystrophies**
Corneal dystrophy:
microscopic cystic
ring-like

371.53 **Granular corneal dystrophy**

371.54 **Lattice corneal dystrophy**

371.55 **Macular corneal dystrophy**

`371.56` **Other stromal corneal dystrophies**
Crystalline corneal dystrophy

371.57 **Endothelial corneal dystrophy**
Combined corneal dystrophy
Cornea guttata
Fuchs' endothelial dystrophy

`371.58` **Other posterior corneal dystrophies**
Polymorphous corneal dystrophy

⑤ 371.6 **Keratoconus**

`371.60` **Keratoconus, unspecified**

371.61 **Keratoconus, stable condition**

371.62 **Keratoconus, acute hydrops**

⑤ 371.7 **Other corneal deformities**

`371.70` **Corneal deformity, unspecified**

371.71 **Corneal ectasia**

371.72 **Descemetocele**

371.73 **Corneal staphyloma**

⑤ 371.8 **Other corneal disorders**

371.81 **Corneal anesthesia and hypoesthesia**

371.82 **Corneal disorder due to contact lens**

Excludes: *corneal edema due to contact lens (371.24)*

`371.89` **Other**

`371.9` **Unspecified corneal disorder**

`372` **Disorders of conjunctiva**

Excludes: *keratoconjunctivitis (370.3-370.4)*

⑤ 372.0 **Acute conjunctivitis**

`372.00` **Acute conjunctivitis, unspecified**

372.01 **Serous conjunctivitis, except viral**

Excludes: *viral conjunctivitis NOS (077.9)*

372.02 **Acute follicular conjunctivitis**
Conjunctival folliculosis NOS

Excludes: *conjunctivitis:*
adenoviral (acute follicular) (077.3)
epidemic hemorrhagic (077.4)
inclusion (077.0)
Newcastle (077.8)
epidemic keratoconjunctivitis (077.1)
pharyngoconjunctival fever (077.2)

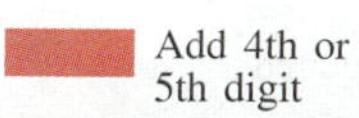

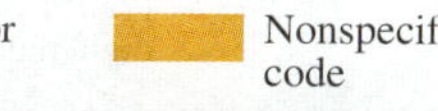

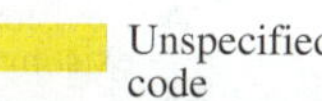

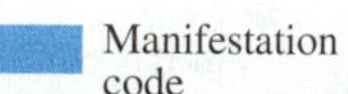

372.03 **Other mucopurulent conjunctivitis**
Catarrhal conjunctivitis

Excludes: *blennorrhea neonatorum (gonococcal) (098.40)*
neonatal conjunctivitis (771.6)
ophthalmia neonatorum NOS (771.6)

372.04 **Pseudomembranous conjunctivitis**
Membranous conjunctivitis

Excludes: *diphtheritic conjunctivitis (032.81)*

372.05 **Acute atopic conjunctivitis**

⑤ **372.1** **Chronic conjunctivitis**

372.10 **Chronic conjunctivitis, unspecified**

372.11 **Simple chronic conjunctivitis**

372.12 **Chronic follicular conjunctivitis**

372.13 **Vernal conjunctivitis**

372.14 **Other chronic allergic conjunctivitis**

372.15 *Parasitic conjunctivitis*
Code first underlying disease, as:
filariasis (125.0-125.9)
mucocutaneous leishmaniasis (085.5)

⑤ **372.2** **Blepharoconjunctivitis**

372.20 **Blepharoconjunctivitis, unspecified**

372.21 **Angular blepharoconjunctivitis**

372.22 **Contact blepharoconjunctivitis**

⑤ **372.3** **Other and unspecified conjunctivitis**

372.30 **Conjunctivitis, unspecified**

372.31 *Rosacea conjunctivitis*
Code first underlying rosacea dermatitis (695.3)

372.33 *Conjunctivitis in mucocutaneous disease*
Code first underlying disease, as:
erythema multiforme (695.1)
Reiter's disease (099.3)

Excludes: *ocular pemphigoid (694.61)*

372.39 **Other**

⑤ **372.4** **Pterygium**

Excludes: *pseudopterygium (372.52)*

372.40 **Pterygium, unspecified**

372.41 **Peripheral pterygium, stationary**

372.42 **Peripheral pterygium, progressive**

372.43 **Central pterygium**

372.44 **Double pterygium**

372.45 **Recurrent pterygium**

⑤ **372.5** **Conjunctival degenerations and deposits**

372.50 **Conjunctival degeneration, unspecified**

372.51 **Pinguecula**

372.52 **Pseudopterygium**

372.53 **Conjunctival xerosis**

Excludes: *conjunctival xerosis due to vitamin A deficiency (264.0, 264.1, 264.7)*

372.54 **Conjunctival concretions**

372.55 **Conjunctival pigmentations**
Conjunctival argyrosis

372.56 **Conjunctival deposits**

⑤ **372.6** **Conjunctival scars**

372.61 **Granuloma of conjunctiva**

372.62 **Localized adhesions and strands of conjunctiva**

  ● Code new
to this edition   ▲ Revision of
existing code   ④ ⑤ Fourth or fifth
digit required

372.63 Symblepharon
Extensive adhesions of conjunctiva

372.64 Scarring of conjunctiva
Contraction of eye socket (after enucleation)

⑤ **372.7 Conjunctival vascular disorders and cysts**

372.71 Hyperemia of conjunctiva

372.72 Conjunctival hemorrhage
Hyposphagma
Subconjunctival hemorrhage

372.73 Conjunctival edema
Chemosis of conjunctiva
Subconjunctival edema

372.74 Vascular abnormalities of conjunctiva
Aneurysm(ata) of conjunctiva

372.75 Conjunctival cysts

⑤ **372.8 Other disorders of conjunctiva**

372.81 Conjunctivochalasis

372.89 Other disorders of conjunctiva

372.9 Unspecified disorder of conjunctiva

373 Inflammation of eyelids

⑤ **373.0 Blepharitis**

Excludes: *blepharoconjunctivitis (372.20-372.22)*

373.00 Blepharitis, unspecified

373.01 Ulcerative blepharitis

373.02 Squamous blepharitis

⑤ **373.1 Hordeolum and other deep inflammation of eyelid**

373.11 Hordeolum externum
Hordeolum NOS
Stye

373.12 Hordeolum internum
Infection of meibomian gland

373.13 Abscess of eyelid
Furuncle of eyelid

373.2 Chalazion
Meibomian (gland) cyst

Excludes: *infected meibomian gland (373.12)*

⑤ **373.3 Noninfectious dermatoses of eyelid**

373.31 Eczematous dermatitis of eyelid

373.32 Contact and allergic dermatitis of eyelid

373.33 Xeroderma of eyelid

373.34 Discoid lupus erythematosus of eyelid

373.4 *Infective dermatitis of eyelid of types resulting in deformity*
Code first underlying disease, as:
leprosy (030.0-030.9)
lupus vulgaris (tuberculous) (017.0)
yaws (102.0-102.9)

373.5 *Other infective dermatitis of eyelid*
Code first underlying disease, as:
actinomycosis (039.3)
impetigo (684)
mycotic dermatitis (110.0-111.9)
vaccinia (051.0)
postvaccination (999.0)

Excludes: *herpes:*
simplex (054.41)
zoster (053.20)

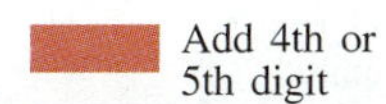

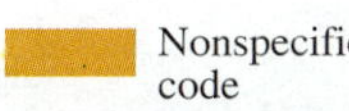

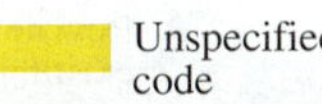

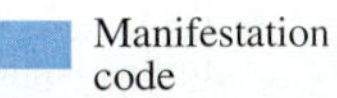

373.6 *Parasitic infestation of eyelid*
  Code first underlying disease, as:
    leishmaniasis (085.0-085.9)
    loiasis (125.2)
    onchocerciasis (125.3)
    pediculosis (132.0)

373.8 **Other inflammations of eyelids**

373.9 **Unspecified inflammation of eyelid**

374 **Other disorders of eyelids**

⑤ **374.0** **Entropion and trichiasis of eyelid**

  374.00 **Entropion, unspecified**

  374.01 **Senile entropion**

  374.02 **Mechanical entropion**

  374.03 **Spastic entropion**

  374.04 **Cicatricial entropion**

  374.05 **Trichiasis without entropion**

⑤ **374.1** **Ectropion**

  374.10 **Ectropion, unspecified**

  374.11 **Senile ectropion**

  374.12 **Mechanical ectropion**

  374.13 **Spastic ectropion**

  374.14 **Cicatricial ectropion**

⑤ **374.2** **Lagophthalmos**

  374.20 **Lagophthalmos, unspecified**

  374.21 **Paralytic lagophthalmos**

  374.22 **Mechanical lagophthalmos**

  374.23 **Cicatricial lagophthalmos**

⑤ **374.3** **Ptosis of eyelid**

  374.30 **Ptosis of eyelid, unspecified**

  374.31 **Paralytic ptosis**

  374.32 **Myogenic ptosis**

  374.33 **Mechanical ptosis**

  374.34 **Blepharochalasis**
    Pseudoptosis

⑤ **374.4** **Other disorders affecting eyelid function**

  | Excludes: | *blepharoclonus (333.81)* |

  blepharospasm (333.81)
  facial nerve palsy (351.0)
  third nerve palsy or paralysis (378.51-378.52)
  tic (psychogenic) (307.20-307.23)
    organic (333.3)

  374.41 **Lid retraction or lag**

  374.43 **Abnormal innervation syndrome**
    Jaw-blinking
    Paradoxical facial movements

  374.44 **Sensory disorders**

  374.45 **Other sensorimotor disorders**
    Deficient blink reflex

  374.46 **Blepharophimosis**
    Ankyloblepharon

⑤ **374.5** **Degenerative disorders of eyelid and periocular area**

  374.50 **Degenerative disorder of eyelid, unspecified**

  374.51 *Xanthelasma*
    Xanthoma (planum) (tuberosum) of eyelid
    Code first underlying condition (272.0-272.9)

  374.52 **Hyperpigmentation of eyelid**
    Chloasma   Dyspigmentation

● Code new
  to this edition

▲ Revision of
  existing code

④ ⑤ Fourth or fifth
  digit required

374.53 **Hypopigmentation of eyelid**
Vitiligo of eyelid

374.54 **Hypertrichosis of eyelid**

374.55 **Hypotrichosis of eyelid**
Madarosis of eyelid

374.56 **Other degenerative disorders of skin affecting eyelid**

⑤ **374.8 Other disorders of eyelid**

374.81 **Hemorrhage of eyelid**

| *Excludes:* | black eye (921.0) |

374.82 **Edema of eyelid**
Hyperemia of eyelid

374.83 **Elephantiasis of eyelid**

374.84 **Cysts of eyelids**
Sebaceous cyst of eyelid

374.85 **Vascular anomalies of eyelid**

374.86 **Retained foreign body of eyelid**

374.87 **Dermatochalasis**

374.89 **Other disorders of eyelid**

374.9 Unspecified disorder of eyelid

375 Disorders of lacrimal system

⑤ **375.0 Dacryoadenitis**

375.00 **Dacryoadenitis, unspecified**

375.01 **Acute dacryoadenitis**

375.02 **Chronic dacryoadenitis**

375.03 **Chronic enlargement of lacrimal gland**

⑤ **375.1 Other disorders of lacrimal gland**

375.11 **Dacryops**

375.12 **Other lacrimal cysts and cystic degeneration**

375.13 **Primary lacrimal atrophy**

375.14 **Secondary lacrimal atrophy**

375.15 **Tear film insufficiency, unspecified**
Dry eye syndrome

375.16 **Dislocation of lacrimal gland**

⑤ **375.2 Epiphora**

375.20 **Epiphora, unspecified as to cause**

375.21 **Epiphora due to excess lacrimation**

375.22 **Epiphora due to insufficient drainage**

⑤ **375.3 Acute and unspecified inflammation of lacrimal passages**

| *Excludes:* | neonatal dacryocystitis (771.6) |

375.30 **Dacryocystitis, unspecified**

375.31 **Acute canaliculitis, lacrimal**

375.32 **Acute dacryocystitis**
Acute peridacryocystitis

375.33 **Phlegmonous dacryocystitis**

⑤ **375.4 Chronic inflammation of lacrimal passages**

375.41 **Chronic canaliculitis**

375.42 **Chronic dacryocystitis**

375.43 **Lacrimal mucocele**

⑤ **375.5 Stenosis and insufficiency of lacrimal passages**

375.51 **Eversion of lacrimal punctum**

375.52 **Stenosis of lacrimal punctum**

375.53 **Stenosis of lacrimal canaliculi**

375.54 **Stenosis of lacrimal sac**

| ■ Add 4th or 5th digit | ■ Nonspecific code | ■ Unspecified code | ■ Manifestation code |

375.55 Obstruction of nasolacrimal duct, neonatal

Excludes: *congenital anomaly of nasolacrimal duct (743.65)*

375.56 Stenosis of nasolacrimal duct, acquired

375.57 Dacryolith

⑤ 375.6 Other changes of lacrimal passages

375.61 Lacrimal fistula

375.69 Other

⑤ 375.8 Other disorders of lacrimal system

375.81 Granuloma of lacrimal passages

375.89 Other

375.9 Unspecified disorder of lacrimal system

376 **Disorders of the orbit**

⑤ 376.0 Acute inflammation of orbit

376.00 Acute inflammation of orbit, unspecified

376.01 Orbital cellulitis
Abscess of orbit

376.02 Orbital periostitis

376.03 Orbital osteomyelitis

376.04 Tenonitis

⑤ 376.1 Chronic inflammatory disorders of orbit

376.10 Chronic inflammation of orbit, unspecified

376.11 Orbital granuloma
Pseudotumor (inflammatory) of orbit

376.12 Orbital myositis

376.13 *Parasitic infestation of orbit*
Code first underlying disease, as:
hydatid infestation of orbit (122.3, 122.6, 122.9)
myiasis of orbit (134.0)

⑤ 376.2 *Endocrine exophthalmos*
Code first underlying thyroid disorder (242.0-242.9)

376.21 *Thyrotoxic exophthalmos*

376.22 *Exophthalmic ophthalmoplegia*

⑤ 376.3 Other exophthalmic conditions

376.30 Exophthalmos, unspecified

376.31 Constant exophthalmos

376.32 Orbital hemorrhage

376.33 Orbital edema or congestion

376.34 Intermittent exophthalmos

376.35 Pulsating exophthalmos

376.36 Lateral displacement of globe

⑤ 376.4 Deformity of orbit

376.40 Deformity of orbit, unspecified

376.41 Hypertelorism of orbit

376.42 Exostosis of orbit

376.43 Local deformities due to bone disease

376.44 Orbital deformities associated with craniofacial deformities

376.45 Atrophy of orbit

376.46 Enlargement of orbit

376.47 Deformity due to trauma or surgery

⑤ 376.5 Enophthalmos

376.50 Enophthalmos, unspecified as to cause

376.51 Enophthalmos due to atrophy of orbital tissue

376.52 Enophthalmos due to trauma or surgery

● Code new to this edition   ▲ Revision of existing code   ④ ⑤ Fourth or fifth digit required

376.6 Retained (old) foreign body following penetrating wound of orbit
Retrobulbar foreign body

⑤ **376.8 Other orbital disorders**

376.81 Orbital cysts
Encephalocele of orbit

376.82 Myopathy of extraocular muscles

376.89 Other

376.9 Unspecified disorder of orbit

377 Disorders of optic nerve and visual pathways

⑤ **377.0 Papilledema**

377.00 Papilledema, unspecified

377.01 Papilledema associated with increased intracranial pressure

377.02 Papilledema associated with decreased ocular pressure

377.03 Papilledema associated with retinal disorder

377.04 Foster-Kennedy syndrome

⑤ **377.1 Optic atrophy**

377.10 Optic atrophy, unspecified

377.11 Primary optic atrophy

Excludes: neurosyphilitic optic atrophy (094.84)

377.12 Postinflammatory optic atrophy

377.13 Optic atrophy associated with retinal dystrophies

377.14 Glaucomatous atrophy [cupping] of optic disc

377.15 Partial optic atrophy
Temporal pallor of optic disc

377.16 Hereditary optic atrophy
Optic atrophy:
dominant hereditary
Leber's

⑤ **377.2 Other disorders of optic disc**

377.21 Drusen of optic disc

377.22 Crater-like holes of optic disc

377.23 Coloboma of optic disc

377.24 Pseudopapilledema

⑤ **377.3 Optic neuritis**

Excludes: meningococcal optic neuritis (036.81)

377.30 Optic neuritis, unspecified

377.31 Optic papillitis

377.32 Retrobulbar neuritis (acute)

Excludes: syphilitic retrobulbar neuritis (094.85)

377.33 Nutritional optic neuropathy

377.34 Toxic optic neuropathy
Toxic amblyopia

377.39 Other

Excludes: ischemic optic neuropathy (377.41)

⑤ **377.4 Other disorders of optic nerve**

377.41 Ischemic optic neuropathy

377.42 Hemorrhage in optic nerve sheaths

377.49 Other
Compression of optic nerve

⑤ **377.5 Disorders of optic chiasm**

377.51 Associated with pituitary neoplasms and disorders

377.52 Associated with other neoplasms

377.53 Associated with vascular disorders

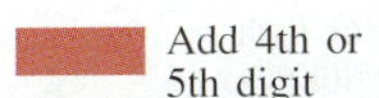

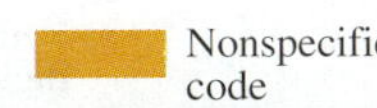

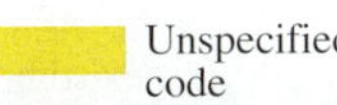

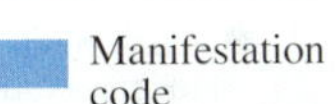

377.54 **Associated with inflammatory disorders**

⑤ **377.6 Disorders of other visual pathways**

377.61 **Associated with neoplasms**

377.62 **Associated with vascular disorders**

377.63 **Associated with inflammatory disorders**

⑤ **377.7 Disorders of visual cortex**

Excludes: *visual:*
>> *agnosia (368.16)*
>> *hallucinations (368.16)*
>> *halos (368.15)*

377.71 **Associated with neoplasms**

377.72 **Associated with vascular disorders**

377.73 **Associated with inflammatory disorders**

377.75 **Cortical blindness**

377.9 Unspecified disorder of optic nerve and visual pathways

378 Strabismus and other disorders of binocular eye movements

Excludes: *nystagmus and other irregular eye movements (379.50-379.59)*

⑤ **378.0 Esotropia**
Convergent concomitant strabismus

Excludes: *intermittent esotropia (378.20-378.22)*

378.00 Esotropia, unspecified

378.01 **Monocular esotropia**

378.02 **Monocular esotropia with A pattern**

378.03 **Monocular esotropia with V pattern**

378.04 **Monocular esotropia with other noncomitancies**
Monocular esotropia with X or Y pattern

378.05 **Alternating esotropia**

378.06 **Alternating esotropia with A pattern**

378.07 **Alternating esotropia with V pattern**

378.08 Alternating esotropia with other noncomitancies
Alternating esotropia with X or Y pattern

⑤ **378.1 Exotropia**
Divergent concomitant strabismus

Excludes: *intermittent exotropia (378.20, 378.23-378.24)*

378.10 Exotropia, unspecified

378.11 **Monocular exotropia**

378.12 **Monocular exotropia with A pattern**

378.13 **Monocular exotropia with V pattern**

378.14 Monocular exotropia with other noncomitancies
Monocular exotropia with X or Y pattern

378.15 **Alternating exotropia**

378.16 **Alternating exotropia with A pattern**

378.17 **Alternating exotropia with V pattern**

378.18 Alternating exotropia with other noncomitancies
Alternating exotropia with X or Y pattern

⑤ **378.2 Intermittent heterotropia**

Excludes: *vertical heterotropia (intermittent) (378.31)*

378.20 Intermittent heterotropia, unspecified
Intermittent:
> esotropia NOS
> exotropia NOS

378.21 **Intermittent esotropia, monocular**

378.22 **Intermittent esotropia, alternating**

378.23 **Intermittent exotropia, monocular**

● Code new to this edition　　　▲ Revision of existing code　　　④ ⑤ Fourth or fifth digit required

378.24 **Intermittent exotropia, alternating**

⑤ **378.3 Other and unspecified heterotropia**

378.30 **Heterotropia, unspecified**

378.31 **Hypertropia**
Vertical heterotropia (constant) (intermittent)

378.32 **Hypotropia**

378.33 **Cyclotropia**

378.34 **Monofixation syndrome**
Microtropia

378.35 **Accommodative component in esotropia**

⑤ **378.4 Heterophoria**

378.40 **Heterophoria, unspecified**

378.41 **Esophoria**

378.42 **Exophoria**

378.43 **Vertical heterophoria**

378.44 **Cyclophoria**

378.45 **Alternating hyperphoria**

⑤ **378.5 Paralytic strabismus**

378.50 **Paralytic strabismus, unspecified**

378.51 **Third or oculomotor nerve palsy, partial**

378.52 **Third or oculomotor nerve palsy, total**

378.53 **Fourth or trochlear nerve palsy**

378.54 **Sixth or abducens nerve palsy**

378.55 **External ophthalmoplegia**

378.56 **Total ophthalmoplegia**

⑤ **378.6 Mechanical strabismus**

378.60 **Mechanical strabismus, unspecified**

378.61 **Brown's (tendon) sheath syndrome**

378.62 **Mechanical strabismus from other musculofascial disorders**

378.63 **Limited duction associated with other conditions**

⑤ **378.7 Other specified strabismus**

378.71 **Duane's syndrome**

378.72 **Progressive external ophthalmoplegia**

378.73 **Strabismus in other neuromuscular disorders**

⑤ **378.8 Other disorders of binocular eye movements**

Excludes: *nystagmus (379.50-379.56)*

378.81 **Palsy of conjugate gaze**

378.82 **Spasm of conjugate gaze**

378.83 **Convergence insufficiency or palsy**

378.84 **Convergence excess or spasm**

378.85 **Anomalies of divergence**

378.86 **Internuclear ophthalmoplegia**

378.87 **Other dissociated deviation of eye movements**
Skew deviation

378.9 **Unspecified disorder of eye movements**
Ophthalmoplegia NOS   Strabismus NOS

379 **Other disorders of eye**

⑤ **379.0 Scleritis and episcleritis**

Excludes: *syphilitic episcleritis (095.0)*

379.00 **Scleritis, unspecified**
Episcleritis NOS

379.01 **Episcleritis periodica fugax**

379.02 **Nodular episcleritis**

379.03 Anterior scleritis

379.04 Scleromalacia perforans

379.05 Scleritis with corneal involvement
Scleroperikeratitis

379.06 Brawny scleritis

379.07 Posterior scleritis
Sclerotenonitis

379.09 Other
Scleral abscess

⑤ **379.1 Other disorders of sclera**

Excludes: blue sclera (743.47)

379.11 Scleral ectasia
Scleral staphyloma NOS

379.12 Staphyloma posticum

379.13 Equatorial staphyloma

379.14 Anterior staphyloma, localized

379.15 Ring staphyloma

379.16 Other degenerative disorders of sclera

379.19 Other

⑤ **379.2 Disorders of vitreous body**

379.21 Vitreous degeneration
Vitreous:
  cavitation
  detachment
  liquefaction

379.22 Crystalline deposits in vitreous
Asteroid hyalitis   Synchysis scintillans

379.23 Vitreous hemorrhage

379.24 Other vitreous opacities
Vitreous floaters

379.25 Vitreous membranes and strands

379.26 Vitreous prolapse

379.29 Other disorders of vitreous

Excludes: vitreous abscess (360.04)

⑤ **379.3 Aphakia and other disorders of lens**

Excludes: after-cataract (366.50-366.53)

379.31 Aphakia

Excludes: cataract extraction status (V45.61)

379.32 Subluxation of lens

379.33 Anterior dislocation of lens

379.34 Posterior dislocation of lens

379.39 Other disorders of lens

⑤ **379.4 Anomalies of pupillary function**

379.40 Abnormal pupillary function, unspecified

379.41 Anisocoria

379.42 Miosis (persistent), not due to miotics

379.43 Mydriasis (persistent) not due to mydriatics

379.45 Argyll Robertson pupil, atypical
Argyll Robertson phenomenon or pupil, nonsyphilitic

Excludes: Argyll Robertson pupil (syphilitic) (094.89)

379.46 Tonic pupillary reaction
Adie's pupil or syndrome

379.49 Other
Hippus
Pupillary paralysis

● Code new   ▲ Revision of   ④ ⑤ Fourth or fifth
  to this edition   existing code   digit required

⑤ **379.5 Nystagmus and other irregular eye movements**

379.50 Nystagmus, unspecified

379.51 Congenital nystagmus

379.52 Latent nystagmus

379.53 Visual deprivation nystagmus

379.54 Nystagmus associated with disorders of the vestibular system

379.55 Dissociated nystagmus

379.56 Other forms of nystagmus

379.57 Deficiencies of saccadic eye movements
Abnormal optokinetic response

379.58 Deficiencies of smooth pursuit movements

379.59 Other irregularities of eye movements
Opsoclonus

379.8 Other specified disorders of eye and adnexa

⑤ **379.9 Unspecified disorder of eye and adnexa**

379.90 Disorder of eye, unspecified

379.91 Pain in or around eye

379.92 Swelling or mass of eye

379.93 Redness or discharge of eye

379.99 Other ill-defined disorders of eye

| Excludes: | blurred vision NOS (368.8) |

DISEASES OF THE EAR AND MASTOID PROCESS (380-389)

380 Disorders of external ear

⑤ **380.0 Perichondritis of pinna**
Perichondritis of auricle

380.00 Perichondritis of pinna, unspecified

380.01 Acute perichondritis of pinna

380.02 Chronic perichondritis of pinna

⑤ **380.1 Infective otitis externa**

380.10 Infective otitis externa, unspecified
Otitis externa (acute):
NOS
circumscribed
diffuse
hemorrhagica
infective NOS

380.11 Acute infection of pinna

| Excludes: | furuncular otitis externa (680.0) |

380.12 Acute swimmers' ear
Beach ear   Tank ear

380.13 Other acute infections of external ear
Code first underlying disease, as:
erysipelas (035)
impetigo (684)
seborrheic dermatitis (690.10-690.18)

| Excludes: | herpes simplex (054.73) |
| | herpes zoster (053.71) |

380.14 Malignant otitis externa

380.15 Chronic mycotic otitis externa
Code first underlying disease, as:
aspergillosis (117.3)
otomycosis NOS (111.9)

| Excludes: | candidal otitis externa (112.82) |

380.16 Other chronic infective otitis externa
Chronic infective otitis externa NOS

⑤ **380.2 Other otitis externa**

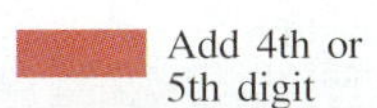

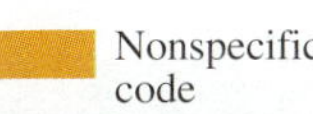

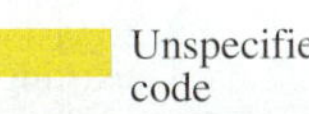

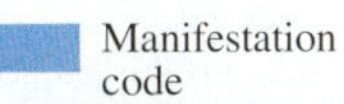

380.21 Cholesteatoma of external ear
  Keratosis obturans of external ear (canal)

Excludes: *cholesteatoma NOS (385.30-385.35)*
  postmastoidectomy (383.32)

380.22 Other acute otitis externa
  Acute otitis externa:
    actinic
    chemical
    contact
    eczematoid
    reactive

380.23 Other chronic otitis externa
  Chronic otitis externa NOS

⑤ **380.3 Noninfectious disorders of pinna**

380.30 Disorder of pinna, unspecified

380.31 Hematoma of auricle or pinna

380.32 Acquired deformities of auricle or pinna

Excludes: *cauliflower ear (738.7)*

380.39 Other

Excludes: *gouty tophi of ear (274.81)*

380.4 Impacted cerumen
  Wax in ear

⑤ **380.5 Acquired stenosis of external ear canal**
  Collapse of external ear canal

380.50 Acquired stenosis of external ear canal, unspecified as to cause

380.51 Secondary to trauma

380.52 Secondary to surgery

380.53 Secondary to inflammation

⑤ **380.8 Other disorders of external ear**

380.81 Exostosis of external ear canal

380.89 Other

380.9 Unspecified disorder of external ear

381 Nonsuppurative otitis media and Eustachian tube disorders

⑤ **381.0 Acute nonsuppurative otitis media**
  Acute tubotympanic catarrh
  Otitis media, acute or subacute:
    catarrhal
    exudative
    transudative
    with effusion

Excludes: *otitic barotrauma (993.0)*

381.00 Acute nonsuppurative otitis media, unspecified

381.01 Acute serous otitis media
  Acute or subacute secretory otitis media

381.02 Acute mucoid otitis media
  Acute or subacute seromucinous otitis media
  Blue drum syndrome

381.03 Acute sanguinous otitis media

381.04 Acute allergic serous otitis media

381.05 Acute allergic mucoid otitis media

381.06 Acute allergic sanguinous otitis media

⑤ **381.1 Chronic serous otitis media**
  Chronic tubotympanic catarrh

381.10 Chronic serous otitis media, simple or unspecified

381.19 Other
  Serosanguinous chronic otitis media

● Code new
  to this edition
▲ Revision of
  existing code
④ ⑤ Fourth or fifth
  digit required

⑤ **381.2   Chronic mucoid otitis media**
Glue ear

Excludes: adhesive middle ear disease (385.10-385.19)

381.20   Chronic mucoid otitis media, simple or unspecified

381.29   Other
Mucosanguinous chronic otitis media

381.3   Other and unspecified chronic nonsuppurative otitis media
Otitis media, chronic: Otitis media, chronic:
  allergic   seromucinous
  exudative   transudative
  secretory   with effusion

381.4   Nonsuppurative otitis media, not specified as acute or chronic
Otitis media: Otitis media:
  allergic   secretory
  catarrhal   seromucinous
  exudative   serous
  mucoid   transudative
                                  with effusion

⑤ **381.5   Eustachian salpingitis**

381.50   Eustachian salpingitis, unspecified

381.51   Acute Eustachian salpingitis

381.52   Chronic Eustachian salpingitis

⑤ **381.6   Obstruction of Eustachian tube**
Stenosis ⎫
Stricture ⎭ of Eustachian tube

381.60   Obstruction of Eustachian tube, unspecified

381.61   Osseous obstruction of Eustachian tube
Obstruction of Eustachian tube from cholesteatoma, polyp, or other osseous lesion

381.62   Intrinsic cartilagenous obstruction of Eustachian tube

381.63   Extrinsic cartilagenous obstruction of Eustachian tube
Compression of Eustachian tube

381.7   Patulous Eustachian tube

⑤ **381.8   Other disorders of Eustachian tube**

381.81   Dysfunction of Eustachian tube

381.89   Other

381.9   Unspecified Eustachian tube disorder

382   Suppurative and unspecified otitis media

⑤ **382.0   Acute suppurative otitis media**
Otitis media, acute:
  necrotizing NOS
  purulent

382.00   Acute suppurative otitis media without spontaneous rupture of ear drum

382.01   Acute suppurative otitis media with spontaneous rupture of ear drum

382.02   *Acute suppurative otitis media in diseases classified elsewhere*
Code first underlying disease, as:
  influenza (487.8)
  scarlet fever (034.1)

Excludes: postmeasles otitis (055.2)

382.1   Chronic tubotympanic suppurative otitis media
Benign chronic suppurative otitis media ⎫ (with anterior perforation of ear
Chronic tubotympanic disease   ⎭ drum)

382.2   Chronic atticoantral suppurative otitis media
Chronic atticoantral disease ⎫ (with posterior or superior
Persistent mucosal disease   ⎭ marginal perforation of ear drum)

382.3   Unspecified chronic suppurative otitis media
Chronic purulent otitis media

Excludes: tuberculous otitis media (017.4)

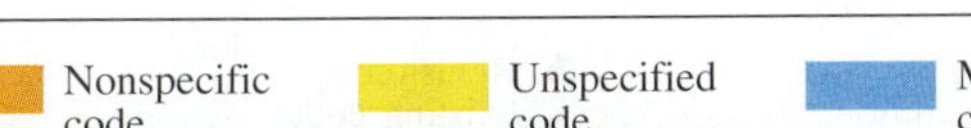

382.4 Unspecified suppurative otitis media
Purulent otitis media NOS

382.9 Unspecified otitis media
Otitis media:
NOS
acute NOS
chronic NOS

383 Mastoiditis and related conditions

⑤ **383.0 Acute mastoiditis**
Abscess of mastoid   Empyema of mastoid

383.00 Acute mastoiditis without complications

383.01 Subperiosteal abscess of mastoid

383.02 Acute mastoiditis with other complications
Gradenigo's syndrome

383.1 Chronic mastoiditis
Caries of mastoid   Fistula of mastoid

Excludes:	*tuberculous mastoiditis (015.6)*

⑤ **383.2 Petrositis**
Coalescing osteitis
Inflammation } of petrous bone
Osteomyelitis

383.20 Petrositis, unspecified

383.21 Acute petrositis

383.22 Chronic petrositis

⑤ **383.3 Complications following mastoidectomy**

383.30 Postmastoidectomy complication, unspecified

383.31 Mucosal cyst of postmastoidectomy cavity

383.32 Recurrent cholesteatoma of postmastoidectomy cavity

383.33 Granulations of postmastoidectomy cavity
Chronic inflammation of postmastoidectomy cavity

⑤ **383.8 Other disorders of mastoid**

383.81 Postauricular fistula

383.89 Other

383.9 Unspecified mastoiditis

384 Other disorders of tympanic membrane

⑤ **384.0 Acute myringitis without mention of otitis media**

384.00 Acute myringitis, unspecified
Acute tympanitis NOS

384.01 Bullous myringitis
Myringitis bullosa hemorrhagica

384.09 Other

384.1 Chronic myringitis without mention of otitis media
Chronic tympanitis

⑤ **384.2 Perforation of tympanic membrane**
Perforation of ear drum:
NOS
persistent posttraumatic
postinflammatory

Excludes:	*otitis media with perforation of tympanic membrane (382.00-382.9)*
	traumatic perforation [current injury] (872.61)

384.20 Perforation of tympanic membrane, unspecified

384.21 Central perforation of tympanic membrane

384.22 Attic perforation of tympanic membrane
Pars flaccida

384.23 Other marginal perforation of tympanic membrane

384.24 Multiple perforations of tympanic membrane

384.25 Total perforation of tympanic membrane

● Code new to this edition   ▲ Revision of existing code   ④ ⑤ Fourth or fifth digit required

⑤ **384.8 Other specified disorders of tympanic membrane**

    384.81 Atrophic flaccid tympanic membrane
       Healed perforation of ear drum

    384.82 Atrophic nonflaccid tympanic membrane

384.9 Unspecified disorder of tympanic membrane

385 Other disorders of middle ear and mastoid

    Excludes: mastoiditis (383.0-383.9)

⑤ **385.0 Tympanosclerosis**

    385.00 Tympanosclerosis, unspecified as to involvement

    385.01 Tympanosclerosis involving tympanic membrane only

    385.02 Tympanosclerosis involving tympanic membrane and ear ossicles

    385.03 Tympanosclerosis involving tympanic membrane, ear ossicles, and middle ear

    385.09 Tympanosclerosis involving other combination of structures

⑤ **385.1 Adhesive middle ear disease**
    Adhesive otitis   Otitis media:
                          chronic adhesive
                          fibrotic

    Excludes: glue ear (381.20-381.29)

    385.10 Adhesive middle ear disease, unspecified as to involvement

    385.11 Adhesions of drum head to incus

    385.12 Adhesions of drum head to stapes

    385.13 Adhesions of drum head to promontorium

    385.19 Other adhesions and combinations

⑤ **385.2 Other acquired abnormality of ear ossicles**

    385.21 Impaired mobility of malleus
       Ankylosis of malleus

    385.22 Impaired mobility of other ear ossicles
       Ankylosis of ear ossicles, except malleus

    385.23 Discontinuity or dislocation of ear ossicles

    385.24 Partial loss or necrosis of ear ossicles

⑤ **385.3 Cholesteatoma of middle ear and mastoid**
    Cholesterosis
    Epidermosis   } of (middle) ear
    Keratosis
    Polyp

    Excludes: cholesteatoma:
       external ear canal (380.21)
       recurrent of postmastoidectomy cavity (383.32)

    385.30 Cholesteatoma, unspecified

    385.31 Cholesteatoma of attic

    385.32 Cholesteatoma of middle ear

    385.33 Cholesteatoma of middle ear and mastoid

    385.35 Diffuse cholesteatosis

⑤ **385.8 Other disorders of middle ear and mastoid**

    385.82 Cholesterin granuloma

    385.83 Retained foreign body of middle ear

    385.89 Other

385.9 Unspecified disorder of middle ear and mastoid

386 Vertiginous syndromes and other disorders of vestibular system

    Excludes: vertigo NOS (780.4)

⑤ **386.0 Ménière's disease**
    Endolymphatic hydrops   Ménière's syndrome or vertigo
    Lermoyez's syndrome

    386.00 Ménière's disease, unspecified
       Ménière's disease (active)

Add 4th or 5th digit	Nonspecific code	Unspecified code	Manifestation code

386.01 Active Ménière's disease, cochleovestibular

386.02 Active Ménière's disease, cochlear

386.03 Active Ménière's disease, vestibular

386.04 Inactive Ménière's disease
Ménière's disease in remission

⑤ **386.1 Other and unspecified peripheral vertigo**

> Excludes: *epidemic vertigo (078.81)*

386.10 Peripheral vertigo, unspecified

386.11 Benign paroxysmal positional vertigo
Benign paroxysmal positional nystagmus

386.12 Vestibular neuronitis
Acute (and recurrent) peripheral vestibulopathy

386.19 Other
Aural vertigo   Otogenic vertigo

386.2 Vertigo of central origin
Central positional nystagmus
Malignant positional vertigo

⑤ **386.3 Labyrinthitis**

386.30 Labyrinthitis, unspecified

386.31 Serous labyrinthitis
Diffuse labyrinthitis

386.32 Circumscribed labyrinthitis
Focal labyrinthitis

386.33 Suppurative labyrinthitis
Purulent labyrinthitis

386.34 Toxic labyrinthitis

386.35 Viral labyrinthitis

⑤ **386.4 Labyrinthine fistula**

386.40 Labyrinthine fistula, unspecified

386.41 Round window fistula

386.42 Oval window fistula

386.43 Semicircular canal fistula

386.48 Labyrinthine fistula of combined sites

⑤ **386.5 Labyrinthine dysfunction**

386.50 Labyrinthine dysfunction, unspecified

386.51 Hyperactive labyrinth, unilateral

386.52 Hyperactive labyrinth, bilateral

386.53 Hypoactive labyrinth, unilateral

386.54 Hypoactive labyrinth, bilateral

386.55 Loss of labyrinthine reactivity, unilateral

386.56 Loss of labyrinthine reactivity, bilateral

386.58 Other forms and combinations

386.8 Other disorders of labyrinth

386.9 Unspecified vertiginous syndromes and labyrinthine disorders

387 Otosclerosis
Includes: otospongiosis

387.0 Otosclerosis involving oval window, nonobliterative

387.1 Otosclerosis involving oval window, obliterative

387.2 Cochlear otosclerosis
Otosclerosis involving:
otic capsule
round window

387.8 Other otosclerosis

387.9 Otosclerosis, unspecified

388 Other disorders of ear

● Code new   ▲ Revision of   ④ ⑤ Fourth or fifth
to this edition   existing code   digit required

⑤ **388.0 Degenerative and vascular disorders of ear**

388.00 Degenerative and vascular disorders, unspecified

388.01 Presbyacusis

388.02 Transient ischemic deafness

⑤ **388.1 Noise effects on inner ear**

388.10 Noise effects on inner ear, unspecified

388.11 Acoustic trauma (explosive) to ear
Otitic blast injury

388.12 Noise-induced hearing loss

388.2 Sudden hearing loss, unspecified

⑤ **388.3 Tinnitus**

388.30 Tinnitus, unspecified

388.31 Subjective tinnitus

388.32 Objective tinnitus

⑤ **388.4 Other abnormal auditory perception**

388.40 Abnormal auditory perception, unspecified

388.41 Diplacusis

388.42 Hyperacusis

388.43 Impairment of auditory discrimination

388.44 Recruitment

388.5 Disorders of acoustic nerve
Acoustic neuritis
Degeneration
Disorder } of acoustic or eighth nerve

Excludes: *acoustic neuroma (225.1)*
syphilitic acoustic neuritis (094.86)

⑤ **388.6 Otorrhea**

388.60 Otorrhea, unspecified
Discharging ear NOS

388.61 Cerebrospinal fluid otorrhea

Excludes: *cerebrospinal fluid rhinorrhea (349.81)*

388.69 Other
Otorrhagia

⑤ **388.7 Otalgia**

388.70 Otalgia, unspecified
Earache NOS

388.71 Otogenic pain

388.72 Referred pain

388.8 Other disorders of ear

388.9 Unspecified disorder of ear

389 Hearing loss

⑤ **389.0 Conductive hearing loss**
Conductive deafness

389.00 Conductive hearing loss, unspecified

389.01 Conductive hearing loss, external ear

389.02 Conductive hearing loss, tympanic membrane

389.03 Conductive hearing loss, middle ear

389.04 Conductive hearing loss, inner ear

389.08 Conductive hearing loss of combined types

⑤ **389.1 Sensorineural hearing loss**
Perceptive hearing loss or deafness

Excludes: *abnormal auditory perception (388.40-388.44)*
psychogenic deafness (306.7)

389.10 Sensorineural hearing loss, unspecified

Add 4th or 5th digit	Nonspecific code	Unspecified code	Manifestation code

389.11 Sensory hearing loss

389.12 Neural hearing loss

389.14 Central hearing loss

389.18 Sensorineural hearing loss of combined types

389.2 Mixed conductive and sensorineural hearing loss
Deafness or hearing loss of type classifiable to 389.0 with type classifiable to 389.1

389.7 Deaf mutism, not elsewhere classifiable
Deaf, nonspeaking

389.8 Other specified forms of hearing loss

389.9 Unspecified hearing loss
Deafness NOS

● Code new
  to this edition

▲ Revision of
  existing code

④ ⑤ Fourth or fifth
  digit required

7. DISEASES OF THE CIRCULATORY SYSTEM (390-459)

ACUTE RHEUMATIC FEVER (390-392)

390 Rheumatic fever without mention of heart involvement
Arthritis, rheumatic, acute or subacute
Rheumatic fever (active) (acute)
Rheumatism, articular, acute or subacute

> *Excludes:* *that with heart involvement (391.0-391.9)*

391 Rheumatic fever with heart involvement

> *Excludes:* *chronic heart diseases of rheumatic origin (393.0-398.9) unless rheumatic fever is also present or there is evidence of recrudescence or activity of the rheumatic process*

391.0 Acute rheumatic pericarditis
Rheumatic:
  fever (active) (acute) with pericarditis
  pericarditis (acute)
Any condition classifiable to 390 with pericarditis

> *Excludes:* *that not specified as rheumatic (420.0-420.9)*

391.1 Acute rheumatic endocarditis
Rheumatic:
  endocarditis, acute
  fever (active) (acute) with endocarditis or valvulitis
  valvulitis acute
Any condition classifiable to 390 with endocarditis or valvulitis

391.2 Acute rheumatic myocarditis
Rheumatic fever (active) (acute) with myocarditis
Any condition classifiable to 390 with myocarditis

391.8 Other acute rheumatic heart disease
Rheumatic:
  fever (active) (acute) with other or multiple types of heart involvement
  pancarditis, acute
Any condition classifiable to 390 with other or multiple types of heart involvement

391.9 Acute rheumatic heart disease, unspecified
Rheumatic:
  carditis, acute
  fever (active) (acute) with unspecified type of heart involvement
  heart disease, active or acute
Any condition classifiable to 390 with unspecified type of heart involvement

392 Rheumatic chorea
Includes: Sydenham's chorea

> *Excludes:* *chorea:*
>
>> *NOS (333.5)*
>> *Huntington's (333.4)*

392.0 With heart involvement
Rheumatic chorea with heart involvement of any type classifiable to 391

392.9 Without mention of heart involvement

CHRONIC RHEUMATIC HEART DISEASE (393-398)

393 Chronic rheumatic pericarditis
Adherent pericardium, rheumatic
Chronic rheumatic:
  mediastinopericarditis
  myopericarditis

> *Excludes:* *pericarditis NOS or not specified as rheumatic (423.0-423.9)*

394 Diseases of mitral valve

> *Excludes:* *that with aortic valve involvement (396.0-396.9)*

394.0 Mitral stenosis
Mitral (valve):
  obstruction (rheumatic)
  stenosis NOS

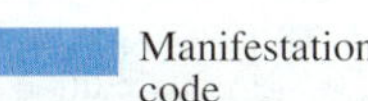

	Add 4th or 5th digit		Nonspecific code		Unspecified code		Manifestation code

394.1 Rheumatic mitral insufficiency
Rheumatic mitral:
  incompetence
  regurgitation

Excludes: *that not specified as rheumatic (424.0)*

394.2 Mitral stenosis with insufficiency
Mitral stenosis with incompetence or regurgitation

394.9 Other and unspecified mitral valve diseases
Mitral (valve):
  disease (chronic)
  failure

395 Diseases of aortic valve

Excludes: *that not specified as rheumatic (424.1)*
  that with mitral valve involvement (396.0-396.9)

395.0 Rheumatic aortic stenosis
Rheumatic aortic (valve) obstruction

395.1 Rheumatic aortic insufficiency
Rheumatic aortic:
  incompetence
  regurgitation

395.2 Rheumatic aortic stenosis with insufficiency
Rheumatic aortic stenosis with incompetence or regurgitation

395.9 Other and unspecified rheumatic aortic diseases
Rheumatic aortic (valve) disease

396 Diseases of mitral and aortic valves
Includes: involvement of both mitral and aortic valves, whether specified as rheumatic or not

396.0 Mitral valve stenosis and aortic valve stenosis
Atypical aortic (valve) stenosis
Mitral and aortic (valve) obstruction (rheumatic)

396.1 Mitral valve stenosis and aortic valve insufficiency

396.2 Mitral valve insufficiency and aortic valve stenosis

396.3 Mitral valve insufficiency and aortic valve insufficiency
Mitral and aortic (valve):
  incompetence
  regurgitation

396.8 Multiple involvement of mitral and aortic valves
Stenosis and insufficiency of mitral or aortic valve with stenosis or insufficiency, or both, of the other valve

396.9 Mitral and aortic valve diseases, unspecified

397 Diseases of other endocardial structures

397.0 Diseases of tricuspid valve
Tricuspid (valve) (rheumatic):
  disease
  insufficiency
  obstruction
  regurgitation
  stenosis

397.1 Rheumatic diseases of pulmonary valve

Excludes: *that not specified as rheumatic (424.3)*

397.9 Rheumatic diseases of endocardium, valve unspecified
Rheumatic:
  endocarditis (chronic)
  valvulitis (chronic)

Excludes: *that not specified as rheumatic (424.90-424.99)*

398 Other rheumatic heart disease

398.0 Rheumatic myocarditis
Rheumatic degeneration of myocardium

Excludes: *myocarditis not specified as rheumatic (429.0)*

⑤ **398.9 Other and unspecified rheumatic heart diseases**

● Code new
to this edition

▲ Revision of
existing code

④ ⑤ Fourth or fifth
digit required

398.90 Rheumatic heart disease, unspecified
Rheumatic:
  carditis
  heart disease NOS

Excludes: *carditis not specified as rheumatic (429.89)*
heart disease NOS not specified as rheumatic (429.9)

398.91 Rheumatic heart failure (congestive)
Rheumatic left ventricular failure

398.99 Other

HYPERTENSIVE DISEASE (401-405)

Excludes: *that complicating pregnancy, childbirth, or the puerperium (642.0-642.9)*
that involving coronary vessels (410.00-414.9)

401 Essential hypertension
Includes: high blood pressure
hyperpiesia
hyperpiesis
hypertension (arterial) (essential) (primary) (systemic)
hypertensive vascular:
  degeneration
  disease

Excludes: *elevated blood pressure without diagnosis of hypertension (796.2)*
pulmonary hypertension (416.0-416.9)
that involving vessels of:
  brain (430-438)
  eye (362.11)

401.0 Malignant

401.1 Benign

401.9 Unspecified

402 Hypertensive heart disease
Includes: hypertensive:
    cardiomegaly
    cardiopathy
    cardiovascular disease
    heart (disease) (failure)
any condition classifiable to 428, 429.0-429.3, 429.8, 429.9 due to hypertension
Use additional code to specify type of heart failure (428.0, 428.20-428.23, 428.30-428.33,
    428.40-428.43)

⑤ **402.0 Malignant**

▲ **402.00 Without heart failure**

▲ **402.01 With heart failure**

⑤ **402.1 Benign**

▲ **402.10 Without heart failure**

▲ **402.11 With heart failure**

⑤ **402.9 Unspecified**

▲ **402.90 Without heart failure**

▲ **402.91 With heart failure**

⑤ **403 Hypertensive renal disease**
The following fifth-digit subclassification is for use with category 403:

    0 without mention of renal failure

    1 with renal failure
Includes: arteriolar nephritis
        arteriosclerosis of:
          kidney
          renal arterioles
        arteriosclerotic nephritis (chronic) (interstitial)
        hypertensive:
          nephropathy
          renal failure
          uremia (chronic)
        nephrosclerosis
        renal sclerosis with hypertension
        any condition classifiable to 585, 586, or 587 with any condition classifiable to
          401

> *Excludes:* *acute renal failure (584.5-584.9)*
> *renal disease stated as not due to hypertension*
> *renovascular hypertension (405.0-405.9 with fifth-digit 1)*

⑤ **403.0 Malignant**

⑤ **403.1 Benign**

⑤ **403.9 Unspecified**

▲ **404 Hypertensive heart and renal disease**
Use additional code to specify type of heart failure (428.0, 428.20-428.23, 428.30-428.33,
   428.40-428.43)

The following fifth-digit subclassification is for use with category 404:

    0 without mention of heart failure or renal failure

    1 with heart failure

    2 with renal failure

    3 with heart failure and renal failure
Includes: disease:
        cardiornal
        cardiovascular renal
    any condition classifiable to 402 with any condition classifiable to 403

⑤ **404.0 Malignant**

⑤ **404.1 Benign**

⑤ **404.9 Unspecified**

405 Secondary hypertension

⑤ **405.0 Malignant**

    405.01 Renovascular

    405.09 Other

⑤ **405.1 Benign**

    405.11 Renovascular

    405.19 Other

⑤ **405.9 Unspecified**

    405.91 Renovascular

    405.99 Other

● Code new to this edition   ▲ Revision of existing code   ④ ⑤ Fourth or fifth digit required

ISCHEMIC HEART DISEASE (410-414)

Includes: that with mention of hypertension

Use additional code, if desired, to identify presence of hypertension (401.0-405.9)

⑤ **410 Acute myocardial infarction**
    Includes: cardiac infarction
      coronary (artery):
        embolism
        occlusion
        rupture
        thrombosis
      infarction of heart, myocardium, or ventricle
      rupture of heart, myocardium, or ventricle
      any condition classifiable to 414.1-414.9 specified as acute or with a stated duration of 8 weeks or less

The following fifth-digit subclassification is for use with category 410:

0 episode of care unspecified
    Use when the source document does not contain sufficient information for the assignment of fifth digit 1 or 2.

1 initial episode of care
    Use fifth digit 1 to designate the first episode of care (regardless of facility site) for a newly diagnosed myocardial infarction. The fifth digit 1 is assigned regardless of the number of times a patient may be transferred during the initial episode of care

2 subsequent episode of care
    Use fifth digit 2 to designate an episode of care following the initial episode when the patient is admitted for further observation, evaluation, or treatment for a myocardial infarction that has received initial treatment, but is still less than 8 weeks old.

⑤ **410.0 Of anterolateral wall**

⑤ **410.1 Of other anterior wall**
    Infarction:
        anterior (wall) NOS
        anteroapical   (with contiguous portion of intraventricular septum)
        anteroseptal

⑤ **410.2 Of inferolateral wall**

⑤ **410.3 Of inferoposterior wall**

⑤ **410.4 Of other inferior wall**
    Infarction:
        diaphragmatic wall
        inferior (wall) NOS   (with contiguous portion of intraventricular septum)

⑤ **410.5 Of other lateral wall**
    Infarction: Infarction:
        apical-lateral   high lateral
        basal-lateral   posterolateral

⑤ **410.6 True posterior wall infarction**
    Infarction:
        posterobasal
        strictly posterior

⑤ **410.7 Subendocardial infarction**
    Nontransmural infarction

⑤ **410.8 Of other specified sites**
    Infarction of:
        atrium
        papillary muscle
        septum alone

⑤ **410.9 Unspecified site**
    Acute myocardial infarction NOS
    Coronary occlusion NOS

411 Other acute and subacute forms of ischemic heart disease

411.0 Postmyocardial infarction syndrome
    Dressler's syndrome

411.1 Intermediate coronary syndrome
Impending infarction   Preinfarction syndrome
Preinfarction angina   Unstable angina

Excludes: angina (pectoris) (413.9)
decubitus (413.0)

⑤ **411.8 Other**

411.81 Acute coronary occlusion without myocardial infarction
Acute coronary (artery):
embolism
obstruction
occlusion   without or not resulting in myocardial infarction
thrombosis

Excludes: obstruction without infarction due to atherosclerosis (414.00-414.06)
occlusion without infarction due to atherosclerosis (414.00-414.06)

411.89 Other
Coronary insufficiency (acute)
Subendocardial ischemia

412 Old myocardial infarction
Healed myocardial infarction
Past myocardial infarction diagnosed on ECG [EKG] or other special investigation, but
currently presenting no symptoms

413 Angina pectoris

413.0 Angina decubitus
Nocturnal angina

413.1 Prinzmetal angina
Variant angina pectoris

413.9 Other and unspecified angina pectoris
Angina: Anginal syndrome
NOS   Status anginosus
cardiac   Stenocardia
of effort   Syncope anginosa

Excludes: preinfarction angina (411.1)

414 Other forms of chronic ischemic heart disease

Excludes: arteriosclerotic cardiovascular disease [ASCVD] (429.2)
cardiovascular:
arteriosclerosis or sclerosis (429.2)
degeneration or disease (429.2)

⑤ **414.0 Coronary atherosclerosis**
Arteriosclerotic heart disease [ASHD]
Atherosclerotic heart disease
Coronary (artery):
arteriosclerosis
arteritis or endarteritis
atheroma
sclerosis
stricture

Excludes: embolism of graft (996.72)
occlusion NOS of graft (996.72)
thrombus of graft (996.72)

414.00 Of unspecified type of vessel, native or graft

414.01 Of native coronary artery

414.02 Of autologous vein bypass graft

414.03 Of nonautologous biological bypass graft

414.04 Of artery bypass graft
Internal mammary artery

414.05 Of unspecified type of bypass graft
Bypass graft NOS

● **414.06 Of coronary artery of transplanted heart**

● Code new   ▲ Revision of   ④ ⑤ Fourth or fifth
to this edition   existing code   digit required

▲ **414.1** **Aneurysm and dissection of heart**

  ▲ **414.10** **Aneurysm of heart (wall)**
      Aneurysm (arteriovenous):
        mural
        ventricular

  ▲ **414.11** **Aneurysm of coronary vessels**
      Aneurysm (arteriovenous) of coronary vessels

  ● **414.12** **Dissection of coronary artery**

  ▲ **414.19** **Other aneurysm of heart**
      Arteriovenous fistula, acquired, of heart

414.8 **Other specified forms of chronic ischemic heart disease**
    Chronic coronary insufficiency
    Ischemia, myocardial (chronic)
    Any condition classifiable to 410 specified as chronic, or presenting with symptoms after
      8 weeks from date of infarction

    | *Excludes:* | *coronary insufficiency (acute) (411.89)* |

414.9 **Chronic ischemic heart disease, unspecified**
    Ischemic heart disease NOS

DISEASES OF PULMONARY CIRCULATION (415-417)

415 **Acute pulmonary heart disease**

415.0 **Acute cor pulmonale**

    | *Excludes:* | *cor pulmonale NOS (416.9)* |

⑤ **415.1** **Pulmonary embolism and infarction**
    Pulmonary (artery) (vein):
      apoplexy
      embolism
      infarction (hemorrhagic)
      thrombosis

    | *Excludes:* | *that complicating:* |

        abortion (634-638 with .6, 639.6)
        ectopic or molar pregnancy (639.6)
        pregnancy, childbirth, or the puerperium (673.0-673.8)

  415.11 **Iatrogenic pulmonary embolism and infarction**

  415.19 **Other**

416 **Chronic pulmonary heart disease**

416.0 **Primary pulmonary hypertension**
    Idiopathic pulmonary arteriosclerosis
    Pulmonary hypertension (essential) (idiopathic) (primary)

416.1 **Kyphoscoliotic heart disease**

416.8 **Other chronic pulmonary heart diseases**
    Pulmonary hypertension, secondary

416.9 **Chronic pulmonary heart disease, unspecified**
    Chronic cardiopulmonary disease
    Cor pulmonale (chronic) NOS

417 **Other diseases of pulmonary circulation**

417.0 **Arteriovenous fistula of pulmonary vessels**

    | *Excludes:* | *congenital arteriovenous fistula (747.3)* |

417.1 **Aneurysm of pulmonary artery**

    | *Excludes:* | *congenital aneurysm (747.3)* |

417.8 **Other specified diseases of pulmonary circulation**
    Pulmonary:
      arteritis
      endarteritis
    Rupture ⎫
    Stricture ⎭ of pulmonary vessel

417.9 **Unspecified disease of pulmonary circulation**

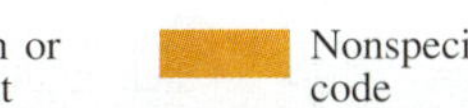

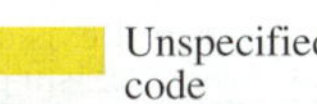

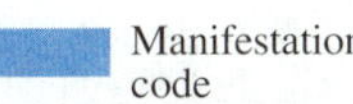

Manifestation
code

OTHER FORMS OF HEART DISEASE (420-429)

420 Acute pericarditis

Includes: acute:
mediastinopericarditis
myopericarditis
pericardial effusion
pleuropericarditis
pneumopericarditis

Excludes: *acute rheumatic pericarditis (391.0)*

postmyocardial infarction syndrome [Dressler's] (411.0)

420.0 Acute pericarditis in diseases classified elsewhere
Code first underlying disease, as:
actinomycosis (039.8)
amebiasis (006.8)
nocardiosis (039.8)
tuberculosis (017.9)
uremia (585)

Excludes: *pericarditis (acute) (in):*

Coxsackie (virus) (074.21)
gonococcal (098.83)
histoplasmosis (115.0-115.9 with fifth-digit 3)
meningococcal infection (036.41)
syphilitic (093.81)

⑤ **420.9 Other and unspecified acute pericarditis**

420.90 Acute pericarditis, unspecified
Pericarditis (acute):
NOS
infective NOS
sicca

420.91 Acute idiopathic pericarditis
Pericarditis, acute:
benign
nonspecific
viral

420.99 Other
Pericarditis (acute): | Pericarditis (acute):
pneumococcal | streptococcal
purulent | suppurative
staphylococcal | Pneumopyopericardium
| Pyopericardium

Excludes: *pericarditis in diseases classified elsewhere (420.0)*

421 Acute and subacute endocarditis

421.0 Acute and subacute bacterial endocarditis
Endocarditis (acute) | Endocarditis (acute) (chronic) (subacute):
(chronic) (subacute): | septic
bacterial | ulcerative
infective NOS | vegetative
lenta | Infective aneurysm
malignant | Subacute bacterial endocarditis [SBE]
purulent

Use additional code, if desired, to identify infectious organism [e.g., Streptococcus 041.0, Staphylococcus 041.1]

421.1 Acute and subacute infective endocarditis in diseases classified elsewhere
Code first underlying disease, as:
blastomycosis (116.0)
Q fever (083.0)
typhoid (fever) (002.0)

Excludes: *endocarditis (in):*

Coxsackie (virus) (074.22)
gonococcal (098.84)
histoplasmosis (115.0-115.9 with fifth-digit 4)
meningococcal infection (036.42)
monilial (112.81)

● Code new   ▲ Revision of   ④ ⑤ Fourth or fifth
to this edition   existing code   digit required

421.9 Acute endocarditis, unspecified

Endocarditis
Myoendocarditis } acute or subacute
Periendocarditis

Excludes: acute rheumatic endocarditis (391.1)

422 Acute myocarditis

Excludes: acute rheumatic myocarditis (391.2)

422.0 Acute myocarditis in diseases classified elsewhere

Code first underlying disease, as:
myocarditis (acute):
  influenzal (487.8)
  tuberculous (017.9)

Excludes: myocarditis (acute) (due to):

aseptic, of newborn (074.23)
Coxsackie (virus) (074.23)
diphtheritic (032.82)
meningococcal infection (036.43)
syphilitic (093.82)
toxoplasmosis (130.3)

⑤ **422.9 Other and unspecified acute myocarditis**

422.90 Acute myocarditis, unspecified

Acute or subacute (interstitial) myocarditis

422.91 Idiopathic myocarditis

Myocarditis (acute or subacute):
  Fiedler's
  giant cell
  isolated (diffuse) (granulomatous)
  nonspecific granulomatous

422.92 Septic myocarditis

Myocarditis, acute or subacute:
  pneumococcal
  staphylococcal

Use additional code, if desired, to identify infectious organism [e.g., Staphylococcus 041.1]

Excludes: myocarditis, acute or subacute:

in bacterial diseases classified elsewhere (422.0)
streptococcal (391.2)

422.93 Toxic myocarditis

422.99 Other

423 Other diseases of pericardium

Excludes: that specified as rheumatic (393)

423.0 Hemopericardium

423.1 Adhesive pericarditis

Adherent pericardium
Fibrosis of pericardium
Milk spots

Pericarditis:
  adhesive
  obliterative
Soldiers' patches

423.2 Constrictive pericarditis

Concato's disease
Pick's disease of heart (and liver)

423.8 Other specified diseases of pericardium

Calcification
Fistula } of pericardium

423.9 Unspecified disease of pericardium

424 Other diseases of endocardium

Excludes: bacterial endocarditis (421.0-421.9)

rheumatic endocarditis (391.1, 394.0-397.9)
syphilitic endocarditis (093.20-093.24)

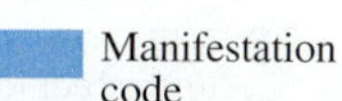

Add 4th or 5th digit	Nonspecific code	Unspecified code	Manifestation code

424.0 Mitral valve disorders
Mitral (valve):
  incompetence
  insufficiency } NOS of specified cause, except rheumatic
  regurgitation

Excludes: *mitral (valve):*
  disease (394.9)
  failure (394.9)
  stenosis (394.0)
  the listed conditions:
    specified as rheumatic (394.1)
    unspecified as to cause but with mention of:
      diseases of aortic valve (396.0-396.9)
      mitral stenosis or obstruction (394.2)

424.1 Aortic valve disorders
Aortic (valve):
  incompetence
  insufficiency } NOS of specified cause, except rheumatic
  regurgitation
  stenosis

Excludes: *hypertrophic subaortic stenosis (425.1)*
  that specified as rheumatic (395.0-395.9)
  that of unspecified cause but with mention of diseases of mitral valve
  (396.0-396.9)

424.2 Tricuspid valve disorders, specified as nonrheumatic
Tricuspid valve:
  incompetence
  insufficiency } of specified cause, except rheumatic
  regurgitation
  stenosis

Excludes: *rheumatic or of unspecified cause (397.0)*

424.3 Pulmonary valve disorders
Pulmonic: Pulmonic:
  incompetence NOS   regurgitation NOS
  insufficiency NOS   stenosis NOS

Excludes: *that specified as rheumatic (397.1)*

⑤ **424.9 Endocarditis, valve unspecified**

424.90 Endocarditis, valve unspecified, unspecified cause
Endocarditis (chronic):
  NOS
  nonbacterial thrombotic
Valvular:
  incompetence
  insufficiency
  regurgitation } of unspecified valve, unspecified
  stenosis   cause
Valvulitis (chronic)

424.91 *Endocarditis in diseases classified elsewhere*
Code first underlying disease, as:
  atypical verrucous endocarditis [Libman-Sacks] (710.0)
  disseminated lupus erythematosus (710.0)
  tuberculosis (017.9)

Excludes: *syphilitic (093.20-093.24)*

424.99 Other
Any condition classifiable to 424.90 with specified cause, except rheumatic

Excludes: *endocardial fibroelastosis (425.3)*
  that specified as rheumatic (397.9)

425 Cardiomyopathy
Includes: myocardiopathy

425.0 Endomyocardial fibrosis

425.1 Hypertrophic obstructive cardiomyopathy
Hypertrophic subaortic stenosis (idiopathic)

    ● Code new   ▲ Revision of   ④ ⑤ Fourth or fifth
        to this edition   existing code   digit required

425.2 Obscure cardiomyopathy of Africa
Becker's disease
Idiopathic mural endomyocardial disease

425.3 Endocardial fibroelastosis
Elastomyofibrosis

425.4 Other primary cardiomyopathies
Cardiomyopathy:	Cardiomyopathy:
NOS	idiopathic
congestive	nonobstructive
constrictive	obstructive
familial	restrictive
hypertrophic	Cardiovascular collagenosis

425.5 Alcoholic cardiomyopathy

425.7 *Nutritional and metabolic cardiomyopathy*
Code first underlying disease, as:
amyloidosis (277.3)
beriberi (265.0)
cardiac glycogenosis (271.0)
mucopolysaccharidosis (277.5)
thyrotoxicosis (242.0-242.9)

Excludes: gouty tophi of heart (274.82)

425.8 *Cardiomyopathy in other diseases classified elsewhere*
Code first underlying disease, as:
Friedreich's ataxia (334.0)
myotonia atrophica (359.2)
progressive muscular dystrophy (359.1)
sarcoidosis (135)

Excludes: cardiomyopathy in Chagas' disease (086.0)

425.9 Secondary cardiomyopathy, unspecified

426 Conduction disorders

426.0 Atrioventricular block, complete
Third degree atrioventricular block

⑤ **426.1 Atrioventricular block, other and unspecified**

426.10 Atrioventricular block, unspecified
Atrioventricular [AV] block (incomplete) (partial)

426.11 First degree atrioventricular block
Incomplete atrioventricular block, first degree
Prolonged P-R interval NOS

426.12 Mobitz (type) II atrioventricular block
Incomplete atrioventricular block:
Mobitz (type) II
second degree, Mobitz (type) II

426.13 Other second degree atrioventricular block
Incomplete atrioventricular block:
Mobitz (type) I [Wenckebach's]
second degree:
NOS
Mobitz (type) I
with 2:1 atrioventricular response [block]
Wenckebach's phenomenon

426.2 Left bundle branch hemiblock
Block:
left anterior fascicular
left posterior fascicular

426.3 Other left bundle branch block
Left bundle branch block:
NOS
anterior fascicular with posterior fascicular
complete
main stem

426.4 Right bundle branch block

⑤ **426.5 Bundle branch block, other and unspecified**

426.50 Bundle branch block, unspecified

Add 4th or 5th digit	Nonspecific code	Unspecified code	Manifestation code

426.51 Right bundle branch block and left posterior fascicular block

426.52 Right bundle branch block and left anterior fascicular block

426.53 Other bilateral bundle branch block
Bifascicular block NOS
Bilateral bundle branch block NOS
Right bundle branch with left bundle branch block (incomplete) (main stem)

426.54 Trifascicular block

426.6 Other heart block
Intraventricular block: Sinoatrial block
  NOS   Sinoauricular block
  diffuse
  myofibrillar

426.7 Anomalous atrioventricular excitation
Atrioventricular conduction:
  accelerated
  accessory
  pre-excitation
Ventricular pre-excitation
Wolff-Parkinson-White syndrome

⑤ **426.8 Other specified conduction disorders**

426.81 Lown-Ganong-Levine syndrome
Syndrome of short P-R interval, normal QRS complexes, and supraventricular
tachycardias

426.89 Other
Dissociation:
  atrioventricular [AV]
  interference
  isorhythmic
Nonparoxysmal AV nodal tachycardia

426.9 Conduction disorder, unspecified
Heart block NOS
Stokes-Adams syndrome

427 Cardiac dysrhythmias

Excludes:	*that complicating:*

abortion (634-638 with .7, 639.8)
ectopic or molar pregnancy (639.8)
labor or delivery (668.1, 669.4)

427.0 Paroxysmal supraventricular tachycardia
Paroxysmal tachycardia:
  atrial [PAT]
  atrioventricular [AV]
  junctional
  nodal

427.1 Paroxysmal ventricular tachycardia
Ventricular tachycardia (paroxysmal)

427.2 Paroxysmal tachycardia, unspecified
Bouveret-Hoffmann syndrome
Paroxysmal tachycardia:
  NOS
  essential

⑤ **427.3 Atrial fibrillation and flutter**

427.31 Atrial fibrillation

427.32 Atrial flutter

⑤ **427.4 Ventricular fibrillation and flutter**

427.41 Ventricular fibrillation

427.42 Ventricular flutter

427.5 Cardiac arrest
Cardiorespiratory arrest

⑤ **427.6 Premature beats**

● Code new   ▲ Revision of   ④ ⑤ Fourth or fifth
   to this edition   existing code   digit required

427.60 **Premature beats, unspecified**
 Ectopic beats
 Extrasystoles
 Extrasystolic arrhythmia
 Premature contractions or systoles NOS

427.61 **Supraventricular premature beats**
 Atrial premature beats, contractions, or systoles

427.69 **Other**
 Ventricular premature beats, contractions, or systoles

⑤ **427.8** **Other specified cardiac dysrhythmias**

427.81 **Sinoatrial node dysfunction**
 Sinus bradycardia: Syndrome:
  persistent   sick sinus
  severe   tachycardia-bradycardia

Excludes: *sinus bradycardia NOS (427.89)*

427.89 **Other**
 Rhythm disorder: Wandering (atrial) pacemaker
  coronary sinus
  ectopic
  nodal

Excludes: *carotid sinus syncope (337.0)*
   neonatal bradycardia (779.81)
   neonatal tachycardia (779.82)
   reflex bradycardia (337.0)
   tachycardia (785.0)

427.9 **Cardiac dysrhythmia, unspecified**
 Arrhythmia (cardiac) NOS

428 **Heart failure**

Excludes: *following cardiac surgery (429.4)*
   rheumatic (398.91)
   that complicating:
    abortion (634-638 with .7, 639.8)
    ectopic or molar pregnancy (639.8)
    labor or delivery (668.1, 669.4)

Code, if applicable, heart failure due to hypertension first (402.0-402.9, with fifth-digit 1 or 404.0-404.9 with fifth-digit 1 or 3)

428.0 **Congestive heart failure, unspecified**
 Congestive heart disease
 Right heart failure (secondary to left heart failure)

Excludes: *fluid overload NOS (276.6)*

428.1 **Left heart failure**
 Acute edema of lung
 Acute pulmonary edema } with heart disease NOS or heart failure
 Cardiac asthma
 Left ventricular failure

● **428.2** **Systolic heart failure**

Excludes: *combined systolic and diastolic heart failure (428.40-428.43)*

 ● **428.20** **Unspecified**
 ● **428.21** **Acute**
 ● **428.22** **Chronic**
 ● **428.23** **Acute on chronic**

● **428.3** **Diastolic heart failure**

Excludes: *combined systolic and diastolic heart failure (428.40-428.43)*

 ● **428.30** **Unspecified**
 ● **428.31** **Acute**
 ● **428.32** **Chronic**
 ● **428.33** **Acute on chronic**

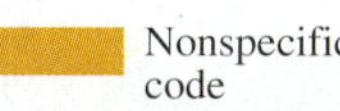

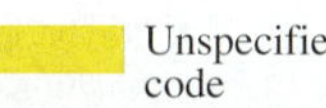

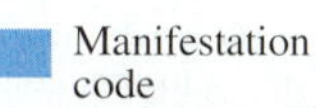

● **428.4 Combined systolic and diastolic heart failure**
  ● **428.40 Unspecified**
  ● **428.41 Acute**
  ● **428.42 Chronic**
  ● **428.43 Acute on chronic**

428.9 Heart failure, unspecified
  Cardiac failure NOS Myocardial failure NOS
  Heart failure NOS Weak heart

429 Ill-defined descriptions and complications of heart disease

429.0 Myocarditis, unspecified
  Myocarditis:
    NOS
    chronic (interstitial) } (with mention of arteriosclerosis)
    fibroid
    senile

Use additional code, if desired, to identify presence of arteriosclerosis

Excludes: *acute or subacute (422.0-422.9)*
          rheumatic (398.0)
            acute (391.2)
          that due to hypertension (402.0-402.9)

429.1 Myocardial degeneration
  Degeneration of heart or myocardium:
    fatty
    mural
    muscular } (with mention of arteriosclerosis)
  Myocardial:
    degeneration disease

Use additional code, if desired, to identify presence of arteriosclerosis

Excludes: *that due to hypertension (402.0-402.9)*

429.2 Cardiovascular disease, unspecified
  Arteriosclerotic cardiovascular disease [ASCVD]
  Cardiovascular arteriosclerosis
  Cardiovascular:
    degeneration
    disease } (with mention of arteriosclerosis)
    sclerosis

Use additional code, if desired, to identify presence of arteriosclerosis

Excludes: *that due to hypertension (402.0-402.9)*

429.3 Cardiomegaly
  Cardiac: Ventricular dilatation
    dilatation
    hypertrophy

Excludes: *that due to hypertension (402.0-402.9)*

429.4 Functional disturbances following cardiac surgery
  Cardiac insufficiency } following cardiac surgery or due to prosthesis
  Heart failure
  Postcardiotomy syndrome
  Postvalvulotomy syndrome

Excludes: *cardiac failure in the immediate postoperative period (997.1)*

429.5 Rupture of chordae tendineae

429.6 Rupture of papillary muscle

⑤ **429.7 Certain sequelae of myocardial infarction, not elsewhere classified**
Use additional code to identify the associated myocardial infarction:
    with onset of 8 weeks or less (410.00-410.92)
    with onset of more than 8 weeks (414.8)

Excludes: *congenital defects of heart (745, 746)*
          coronary aneurysm (414.11)
          disorders of papillary muscle (429.6, 429.81)
          postmyocardial infarction syndrome (411.0)
          rupture of chordae tendineae (429.5)

● Code new   ▲ Revision of   ④ ⑤ Fourth or fifth
  to this edition   existing code   digit required

429.71 **Acquired cardiac septal defect**

Excludes: acute septal infarction (410.00-410.92)

429.79 **Other**
Mural thrombus (atrial) (ventricular), acquired, following myocardial infarction

⑤ **429.8** **Other ill-defined heart diseases**

429.81 **Other disorders of papillary muscle**

Papillary muscle:
atrophy
degeneration
dysfunction

Papillary muscle:
incompetence
incoordination
scarring

429.82 **Hyperkinetic heart disease**

429.89 **Other**
Carditis

Excludes: that due to hypertension (402.0-402.9)

429.9 **Heart disease, unspecified**
Heart disease (organic) NOS
Morbus cordis NOS

Excludes: that due to hypertension (402.0-402.9)

CEREBROVASCULAR DISEASE (430-438)

Includes: with mention of hypertension (conditions classifiable to 401-405)

Use additional code, if desired, to identify presence of hypertension

Excludes: any condition classifiable to 430-434, 436, 437 occurring during pregnancy,
childbirth, or the puerperium, or specified as puerperal (674.0)
iatrogenic cerebrovascular infarction or hemorrhage (997.02)

430 **Subarachnoid hemorrhage**
Meningeal hemorrhage
Ruptured:
berry aneurysm
(congenital) cerebral aneurysm NOS

Excludes: syphilitic ruptured cerebral aneurysm (094.87)

431 **Intracerebral hemorrhage**

Hemorrhage (of):
basilar
bulbar
cerebellar
cerebral
cerebromeningeal
cortical
internal capsule

Hemorrhage (of):
intrapontine
pontine
subcortical
ventricular
Rupture of blood vessel in brain

432 **Other and unspecified intracranial hemorrhage**

432.0 **Nontraumatic extradural hemorrhage**
Nontraumatic epidural hemorrhage

432.1 **Subdural hemorrhage**
Subdural hematoma, nontraumatic

432.9 **Unspecified intracranial hemorrhage**
Intracranial hemorrhage NOS

⑤ **433** **Occlusion and stenosis of precerebral arteries**

The following fifth-digit subclassification is for use with category 433:

0 **without mention of cerebral infarction**

1 **with cerebral infarction**

Includes:

embolism
narrowing
obstruction
thrombosis
} of basilar, carotid, and vertebral arteries

Excludes: insufficiency NOS of precerebral arteries (435.0-435.9)

⑤ **433.0** **Basilar artery**

⑤ **433.1** **Carotid artery**

⑤ **433.2** **Vertebral artery**

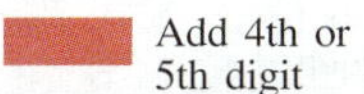

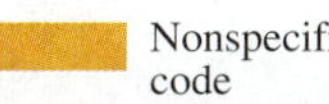

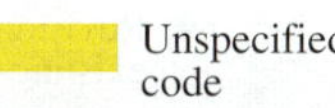

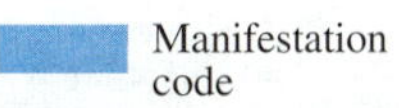

⑤ **433.3 Multiple and bilateral**

⑤ **433.8 Other specified precerebral artery**

⑤ **433.9 Unspecified precerebral artery**
   Precerebral artery NOS

⑤ **434 Occlusion of cerebral arteries**
   The following fifth-digit subclassification is for use with category 434:

   0 without mention of cerebral infarction

   1 with cerebral infarction

⑤ **434.0 Cerebral thrombosis**
   Thrombosis of cerebral arteries

⑤ **434.1 Cerebral embolism**

⑤ **434.9 Cerebral artery occlusion, unspecified**

435 Transient cerebral ischemia
   Includes: cerebrovascular insufficiency (acute) with transient focal neurological signs and
            symptoms
            insufficiency of basilar, carotid, and vertebral arteries
            spasm of cerebral arteries

   Excludes: *acute cerebrovascular insufficiency NOS (437.1)*
            that due to any condition classifiable to 433 (433.0-433.9)

   435.0 Basilar artery syndrome

   435.1 Vertebral artery syndrome

   435.2 Subclavian steal syndrome

   435.3 Vertebrobasilar artery syndrome

   435.8 Other specified transient cerebral ischemias

   435.9 Unspecified transient cerebral ischemia
      Impending cerebrovascular accident
      Intermittent cerebral ischemia
      Transient ischemic attack [TIA]

436 Acute, but ill-defined, cerebrovascular disease
   Apoplexy, apoplectic: Cerebral seizure
      NOS   Cerebrovascular accident [CVA] NOS
      attack   Stroke
      cerebral
      seizure

   Excludes: *any condition classifiable to categories 430-435*
            postoperative cerebrovascular accident (997.02)

437 Other and ill-defined cerebrovascular disease

   437.0 Cerebral atherosclerosis
      Atheroma of cerebral arteries
      Cerebral arteriosclerosis

   437.1 Other generalized ischemic cerebrovascular disease
      Acute cerebrovascular insufficiency NOS
      Cerebral ischemia (chronic)

   437.2 Hypertensive encephalopathy

   437.3 Cerebral aneurysm, nonruptured
      Internal carotid artery, intracranial portion
      Internal carotid artery NOS

      Excludes: *congenital cerebral aneurysm, nonruptured (747.81)*
               internal carotid artery, extracranial portion (442.81)

   437.4 Cerebral arteritis

   437.5 Moyamoya disease

   437.6 Nonpyogenic thrombosis of intracranial venous sinus

      Excludes: *pyogenic (325)*

   437.7 Transient global amnesia

   437.8 Other

   437.9 Unspecified
      Cerebrovascular disease or lesion NOS

● Code new   ▲ Revision of   ④ ⑤ Fourth or fifth
  to this edition   existing code   digit required

438 Late effects of cerebrovascular disease

Note: This category is to be used to indicate conditions in 430-437 as the cause of late effects. The "late effects" include conditions specified as such, as sequelae, which may occur at any time after the onset of the causal condition.

438.0 Cognitive deficits

⑤ **438.1 Speech and language deficits**

    438.10 Speech and language deficit, unspecified

    438.11 **Aphasia**

    438.12 **Dysphasia**

    438.19 Other speech and language deficits

⑤ **438.2 Hemiplegia/hemiparesis**

    438.20 Hemiplegia affecting unspecified side

    438.21 **Hemiplegia affecting dominant side**

    438.22 **Hemiplegia affecting nondominant side**

⑤ **438.3 Monoplegia of upper limb**

    438.30 Monoplegia of upper limb affecting unspecified side

    438.31 **Monoplegia of upper limb affecting dominant side**

    438.32 **Monoplegia of upper limb affecting nondominant side**

⑤ **438.4 Monoplegia of lower limb**

    438.40 Monoplegia of lower limb affecting unspecified side

    438.41 **Monoplegia of lower limb affecting dominant side**

    438.42 **Monoplegia of lower limb affecting nondominant side**

⑤ **438.5 Other paralytic syndrome**

Use additional code to identify type of paralytic syndrome, such as:
    locked-in state (344.81)
    quadriplegia (344.00-344.09)

    Excludes: *late effects of cerebrovascular accident with:*
        hemiplegia/hemiparesis (438.20-438.22)
        monoplegia of lower limb (438.40-438.42)
        monoplegia of upper limb (438.30-438.32)

    438.50 Other paralytic syndrome affecting unspecified side

    438.51 Other paralytic syndrome affecting dominant side

    438.52 Other paralytic syndrome affecting nondominant side

    438.53 Other paralytic syndrome, bilateral

● **438.6 Alterations of sensations**
    Use additional code to identify the altered sensation

● **438.7 Disturbances of vision**
    Use additional code to identify the visual disturbance

⑤ **438.8 Other late effects of cerebrovascular disease**

    438.81 **Apraxia**

    438.82 **Dysphagia**

    ● 438.83 **Facial weakness**
        Facial droop

    ● 438.84 **Ataxia**

    ● 438.85 **Vertigo**

    438.89 Other late effects of cerebrovascular disease
    Use additional code to identify the late effect

438.9 Unspecified late effects of cerebrovascular disease

DISEASES OF ARTERIES, ARTERIOLES, AND CAPILLARIES (440-448)

440 Atherosclerosis

Includes: arteriolosclerosis
arteriosclerosis (obliterans) (senile)
arteriosclerotic vascular disease
atheroma
degeneration:
arterial
arteriovascular
vascular
endarteritis deformans or obliterans
senile arteritis
senile endarteritis

Excludes: *atheroembolism (445.01-445.89)*

atherosclerosis of bypass graft of the extremities (440.30-440.32)

440.0 Of aorta

440.1 Of renal artery

Excludes: *atherosclerosis of renal arterioles (403.00-403.91)*

⑤ **440.2 Of native arteries of the extremities**

Excludes: *atherosclerosis of bypass graft of the extremities (440.30-440.32)*

440.20 Atherosclerosis of the extremities, unspecified

440.21 Atherosclerosis of the extremities with intermittent claudication

440.22 Atherosclerosis of the extremities with rest pain
Includes: any condition classifiable to 440.21

440.23 Atherosclerosis of the extremities with ulceration
Includes: any condition classifiable to 440.21 and 440.22
Use additional code for any associated ulceration (707.10-707.9)

440.24 Atherosclerosis of the extremities with gangrene
Includes: any condition classifiable to 440.21, 440.22, and 440.23
with ischemic gangrene 785.4

Excludes: *gas gangrene 040.0*

440.29 Other

⑤ **440.3 Of bypass graft of the extremities**

Excludes: *atherosclerosis of native artery of the extremity (440.21-440.24)*

embolism [occlusion NOS] [thrombus]
of graft (996.74)

440.30 Of unspecified graft

440.31 Of autologous vein bypass graft

440.32 Of nonautologous biological bypass graft

440.8 Of other specified arteries

Excludes: *basilar (433.0)*

carotid (433.1)
cerebral (437.0)
coronary (414.00-414.06)
mesenteric (557.1)
precerebral (433.0-433.9)
pulmonary (416.0)
vertebral (433.2)

440.9 Generalized and unspecified atherosclerosis
Arteriosclerotic vascular disease NOS

Excludes: *arteriosclerotic cardiovascular disease [ASCVD] (429.2)*

441 Aortic aneurysm and dissection

Excludes: *syphilitic aortic aneurysm (093.0)*

traumatic aortic aneurysm (901.0, 902.0)

⑤ **441.0 Dissection of aorta**

441.00 Unspecified site

441.01 Thoracic

441.02 Abdominal

● Code new
to this edition   ▲ Revision of
existing code   ④ ⑤ Fourth or fifth
digit required

441.03   Thoracoabdominal

441.1   Thoracic aneurysm, ruptured

441.2   Thoracic aneurysm without mention of rupture

441.3   Abdominal aneurysm, ruptured

441.4   Abdominal aneurysm without mention of rupture

441.5   Aortic aneurysm of unspecified site, ruptured
Rupture of aorta NOS

441.6   Thoracoabdominal aneurysm, ruptured

441.7   Thoracoabdominal aneurysm, without mention of rupture

441.9   Aortic aneurysm of unspecified site without mention of rupture
Aneurysm
Dilatation   } of aorta
Hyaline necrosis

442   Other aneurysm
Includes: aneurysm (ruptured) (cirsoid) (false) (varicose)
aneurysmal varix

Excludes: *arteriovenous aneurysm or fistula:*
acquired (447.0)
congenital (747.60-747.69)
traumatic (900.0-904.9)

442.0   Of artery of upper extremity

442.1   Of renal artery

442.2   Of iliac artery

442.3   Of artery of lower extremity
Aneurysm:
femoral   } artery
popliteal

⑤ **442.8   Of other specified artery**

442.81   Artery of neck
Aneurysm of carotid artery (common) (external) (internal, extracranial portion)

Excludes: *internal carotid artery, intracranial portion (437.3)*

442.82   Subclavian artery

442.83   Splenic artery

442.84   Other visceral artery
Aneurysm:
celiac
gastroduodenal
gastroepiploic
hepatic   } artery
pancreaticoduodenal
superior mesenteric

442.89   Other
Aneurysm:
mediastinal } artery
spinal

Excludes: *cerebral (nonruptured) (437.3)*
congenital (747.81)
ruptured (430)
coronary (414.11)
heart (414.10)
pulmonary (417.1)

442.9   Of unspecified site

443   Other peripheral vascular disease

443.0   Raynaud's syndrome
Raynaud's:
disease
phenomenon (secondary)

Use additional code, if desired, to identify gangrene (785.4)

443.1   Thromboangiitis obliterans [Buerger's disease]
Presenile gangrene

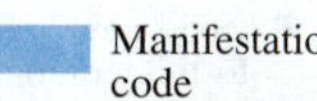

● **443.2 Other arterial dissection**

> *Excludes:* *dissection of aorta (441.00-441.03)*
> *dissection of coronary arteries (414.12)*

   ● **443.21 Dissection of carotid artery**

   ● **443.22 Dissection of iliac artery**

   ● **443.23 Dissection of renal artery**

   ● **443.24 Dissection of vertebral artery**

   ● **443.29 Dissection of other artery**

⑤ **443.8 Other specified peripheral vascular diseases**

   443.81 *Peripheral angiopathy in diseases classified elsewhere*
   Code first underlying disease, as:
   diabetes mellitus (250.7)

   443.89 Other
   Acrocyanosis
   Acroparesthesia:
     simple [Schultze's type]
     vasomotor [Nothnagel's type]
   Erythrocyanosis
   Erythromelalgia

> *Excludes:* *chilblains (991.5)*
> *frostbite (991.0-991.3)*
> *immersion foot (991.4)*

443.9 Peripheral vascular disease, unspecified
Intermittent claudication NOS
Peripheral:
  angiopathy NOS
  vascular disease NOS
Spasm of artery

> *Excludes:* *atherosclerosis of the arteries of the extremities (440.20-440.22)*
> *spasm of cerebral artery (435.0-435.9)*

444 Arterial embolism and thrombosis
Includes: infarction:
        embolic
        thrombotic
     occlusion

> *Excludes:* *atheroembolism (445.01-445.89)*
>
> *that complicating:*
> *abortion (634-638 with .6, 639.6)*
> *ectopic or molar pregnancy (639.6)*
> *pregnancy, childbirth, or the puerperium (673.0-673.8)*

444.0 Of abdominal aorta
Aortic bifurcation syndrome   Leriche's syndrome
Aortoiliac obstruction   Saddle embolus

444.1 Of thoracic aorta
Embolism or thrombosis of aorta (thoracic)

⑤ **444.2 Of arteries of the extremities**

   444.21 Upper extremity

   444.22 Lower extremity
   Arterial embolism or thrombosis:
     femoral
     peripheral NOS
     popliteal

> *Excludes:* *iliofemoral (444.81)*

⑤ **444.8 Of other specified artery**

   444.81 Iliac artery

● Code new to this edition   ▲ Revision of existing code   ④ ⑤ Fourth or fifth digit required

444.89 Other

Excludes: basilar (433.0)

carotid (433.1)
cerebral (434.0-434.9)
coronary (410.00-410.92)
mesenteric (557.0)
ophthalmic (362.30-362.34)
precerebral (433.0-433.9)
pulmonary (415.19)
renal (593.81)
retinal (362.30-362.34)
vertebral (433.2)

444.9 Of unspecified artery

● **445 Atheroembolism**

Includes: Atherothrombotic microembolism
Cholesterol embolism

● **445.0 Of extremities**

● **445.01 Upper extremity**

● **445.02 Lower extremity**

● **445.8 Of other sites**

● **445.81 Kidney**
Use additional code for any associated kidney failure (584, 585)

● **445.89 Other site**

446 Polyarteritis nodosa and allied conditions

446.0 Polyarteritis nodosa

Disseminated necrotizing   Panarteritis (nodosa)
  periarteritis   Periarteritis (nodosa)
Necrotizing angiitis

446.1 Acute febrile mucocutaneous lymph node syndrome [MCLS]
Kawasaki disease

⑤ **446.2 Hypersensitivity angiitis**

Excludes: antiglomerular basement membrane disease without pulmonary hemorrhage (583.89)

446.20 Hypersensitivity angiitis, unspecified

446.21 Goodpasture's syndrome
Antiglomerular basement membrane antibody-mediated nephritis with pulmonary
hemorrhage
Use additional code, if desired, to identify renal disease (583.81)

446.29 Other specified hypersensitivity angiitis

446.3 Lethal midline granuloma
Malignant granuloma of face

446.4 Wegener's granulomatosis
Necrotizing respiratory granulomatosis
Wegener's syndrome

446.5 Giant cell arteritis
Cranial arteritis   Temporal arteritis
Horton's disease

446.6 Thrombotic microangiopathy
Moschcowitz's syndrome
Thrombotic thrombocytopenic purpura

446.7 Takayasu's disease
Aortic arch arteritis   Pulseless disease

447 Other disorders of arteries and arterioles

447.0 Arteriovenous fistula, acquired
Arteriovenous aneurysm, acquired

Excludes: cerebrovascular (437.3)

coronary (414.19)
pulmonary (417.0)
surgically created arteriovenous shunt or fistula:
  complication (996.1, 996.61-996.62)
  status or presence (V45.1)
traumatic (900.0-904.9)

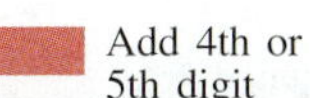

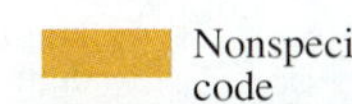

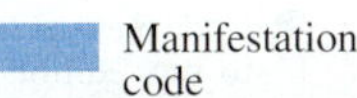

447.1 Stricture of artery

447.2 Rupture of artery
Erosion of artery
Fistula, except arteriovenous, of artery
Ulcer of artery

Excludes: *traumatic rupture of artery (900.0-904.9)*

447.3 Hyperplasia of renal artery
Fibromuscular hyperplasia of renal artery

447.4 Celiac artery compression syndrome
Celiac axis syndrome   Marable's syndrome

447.5 Necrosis of artery

447.6 Arteritis, unspecified
Aortitis NOS
Endarteritis NOS

Excludes: *arteritis, endarteritis:*
aortic arch (446.7)
cerebral (437.4)
coronary (414.00-414.06)
deformans (440.0-440.9)
obliterans (440.0-440.9)
pulmonary (417.8)
senile (440.0-440.9)
polyarteritis NOS (446.0)
syphilitic aortitis (093.1)

447.8 Other specified disorders of arteries and arterioles
Fibromuscular hyperplasia of arteries, except renal

447.9 Unspecified disorders of arteries and arterioles

448 Disease of capillaries

448.0 Hereditary hemorrhagic telangiectasia
Rendu-Osler-Weber disease

448.1 Nevus, non-neoplastic
Nevus: Nevus:
   araneus   spider
   senile   stellar

Excludes: *neoplastic (216.0-216.9)*
port wine (757.32)
strawberry (757.32)

448.9 Other and unspecified capillary diseases
Capillary:
   hemorrhage
   hyperpermeability
   thrombosis

Excludes: *capillary fragility (hereditary) (287.8)*

DISEASES OF VEINS AND LYMPHATICS, AND OTHER DISEASES OF CIRCULATORY SYSTEM (451-459)

451 Phlebitis and thrombophlebitis
Includes: endophlebitis
           inflammation, vein
           periphlebitis
           suppurative phlebitis

Use additional E Code, if desired, to identify drug, if drug-induced

Excludes: *that complicating:*
abortion (634-638 with .7, 639.8)
ectopic or molar pregnancy (639.8)
pregnancy, childbirth, or the puerperium (671.0-671.9)
that due to or following:
implant or catheter device (996.61-996.62)
infusion, perfusion, or transfusion (999.2)

451.0 Of superficial vessels of lower extremities
Saphenous vein (greater) (lesser)

⑤ **451.1 Of deep vessels of lower extremities**

● Code new to this edition   ▲ Revision of existing code   ④ ⑤ Fourth or fifth digit required

451.11 **Femoral vein (deep) (superficial)**

451.19 **Other**
Femoropopliteal vein
Popliteal vein
Tibial vein

451.2 **Of lower extremities, unspecified**

⑤ **451.8** **Of other sites**

Excludes: *intracranial venous sinus (325)*
nonpyogenic (437.6)
portal (vein) (572.1)

451.81 **Iliac vein**

451.82 **Of superficial veins of upper extremities**
Antecubital vein
Basilic vein
Cephalic vein

451.83 **Of deep veins of upper extremities**
Brachial vein
Radial vein
Ulnar vein

451.84 **Of upper extremities, unspecified**

451.89 **Other**
Axillary vein
Jugular vein
Subclavian vein
Thrombophlebitis of breast (Mondor's disease)

451.9 **Of unspecified site**

452 **Portal vein thrombosis**
Portal (vein) obstruction

Excludes: *hepatic vein thrombosis (453.0)*
phlebitis of portal vein (572.1)

453 **Other venous embolism and thrombosis**

Excludes: *that complicating:*
abortion (634-638 with .7, 639.8)
ectopic or molar pregnancy (639.8)
pregnancy, childbirth, or the puerperium (671.0-671.9)
that with inflammation, phlebitis, and thrombophlebitis (451.0-451.9)

453.0 **Budd-Chiari syndrome**
Hepatic vein thrombosis

453.1 **Thrombophlebitis migrans**

453.2 **Of vena cava**

453.3 **Of renal vein**

453.8 **Of other specified veins**

Excludes: *cerebral (434.0-434.9)*
coronary (410.00-410.92)
intracranial venous sinus (325)
nonpyogenic (437.6)
mesenteric (557.0)
portal (452)
precerebral (433.0-433.9)
pulmonary (415.19)

453.9 **Of unspecified site**
Embolism of vein   Thrombosis (vein)

454 **Varicose veins of the lower extremities**

Excludes: *that complicating pregnancy, childbirth, or the puerperium (671.0)*

454.0 **With ulcer**
Varicose ulcer (lower extremity, any part)
Varicose veins with ulcer of lower extremity [any part] or of unspecified site
Any condition classifiable to 454.9 with ulcer or specified as ulcerated

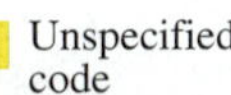

Add 4th or 5th digit   Nonspecific code   Unspecified code   Manifestation code

454.1 With inflammation
Stasis dermatitis
Varicose veins with inflammation of lower extremity [any part] or of unspecified site
Any condition classifiable to 454.9 with inflammation or specified as inflamed

454.2 With ulcer and inflammation
Varicose veins with ulcer and inflammation of lower extremity [any part] or of
    unspecified site
Any condition classifiable to 454.9 with ulcer and inflammation

● **454.8 With other complications**
Edema
Pain
Swelling

▲ **454.9 Asymptomatic varicose veins**
Phlebectasia of lower extremity [any part] or of unspecified site
Varicose veins of lower extremity [any part] or of unspecified site
Varicose veins NOS
Varix of lower extremity [any part] or of unspecified site

455 Hemorrhoids
Includes: hemorrhoids (anus) (rectum)
        piles
        varicose veins, anus or rectum

Excludes: *that complicating pregnancy, childbirth or the puerperium (671.8)*

455.0 Internal hemorrhoids without mention of complication

455.1 Internal thrombosed hemorrhoids

455.2 Internal hemorrhoids with other complication
Internal hemorrhoids: Internal hemorrhoids:
    bleeding   strangulated
    prolapsed   ulcerated

455.3 External hemorrhoids without mention of complication

455.4 External thrombosed hemorrhoids

455.5 External hemorrhoids with other complication
External hemorrhoids: External hemorrhoids:
    bleeding   strangulated
    prolapsed   ulcerated

455.6 Unspecified hemorrhoids without mention of complication
Hemorrhoids NOS

455.7 Unspecified thrombosed hemorrhoids
Thrombosed hemorrhoids, unspecified whether internal or external

455.8 Unspecified hemorrhoids with other complication
Hemorrhoids, unspecified whether internal or external:
    bleeding
    prolapsed
    strangulated
    ulcerated

455.9 Residual hemorrhoidal skin tags
Skin tags, anus or rectum

456 Varicose veins of other sites

456.0 Esophageal varices with bleeding

456.1 Esophageal varices without mention of bleeding

⑤ ***456.2 Esophageal varices in diseases classified elsewhere***
Code first underlying cause, as:
    cirrhosis of liver (571.0-571.9)
    portal hypertension (572.3)

456.20 *With bleeding*

456.21 *Without mention of bleeding*

456.3 Sublingual varices

456.4 Scrotal varices
Varicocele

456.5 Pelvic varices
Varices of broad ligament

● Code new   ▲ Revision of   ④ ⑤ Fourth or fifth
  to this edition   existing code   digit required

456.6 Vulval varices
Varices of perineum

Excludes: *that complicating pregnancy, childbirth, or the puerperium (671.1)*

456.8 Varices of other sites
Varicose veins of nasal septum (with ulcer)

Excludes: *placental varices (656.7)*
retinal varices (362.17)
varicose ulcer of unspecified site (454.0)
varicose veins of unspecified site (454.9)

457 Noninfectious disorders of lymphatic channels

457.0 Postmastectomy lymphedema syndrome
Elephantiasis
Obliteration of lymphatic vessel } due to mastectomy

457.1 Other lymphedema
Elephantiasis (nonfilarial) NOS
Lymphangiectasis
Lymphedema:
    acquired (chronic)
    praecox
    secondary
Obliteration, lymphatic vessel

Excludes: *elephantiasis (nonfilarial):*
congenital (757.0)
eyelid (374.83)
vulva (624.8)

457.2 Lymphangitis
Lymphangitis:
    NOS
    chronic
    subacute

Excludes: *acute lymphangitis (682.0-682.9)*

457.8 Other noninfectious disorders of lymphatic channels
Chylocele (nonfilarial)
Chylous:
    ascites
    cyst
Lymph node or vessel:
    fistula
    infarction
    rupture

Excludes: *chylocele:*
filarial (125.0-125.9)
tunica vaginalis (nonfilarial) (608.84)

457.9 Unspecified noninfectious disorder of lymphatic channels

458 Hypotension
Includes: hypopiesis

Excludes: *cardiovascular collapse (785.50)*
maternal hypotension syndrome (669.2)
shock (785.50-785.59)
Shy-Drager syndrome (333.0)

458.0 Orthostatic hypotension
Hypotension:
    orthostatic (chronic)
    postural

458.1 Chronic hypotension
Permanent idiopathic hypotension

458.2 Iatrogenic hypotension
Postoperative hypotension

458.8 Other specified hypotension

458.9 Hypotension, unspecified
Hypotension (arterial) NOS

459 Other disorders of circulatory system

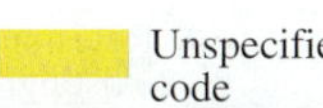

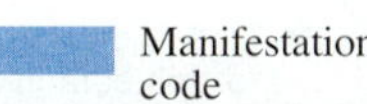

Manifestation
code

459.0 **Hemorrhage, unspecified**
Rupture of blood vessel NOS
Spontaneous hemorrhage NEC

Excludes: *hemorrhage:*
gastrointestinal NOS (578.9)
in newborn NOS (772.9)
secondary or recurrent following trauma (958.2)
traumatic rupture of blood vessel (900.0-904.9)

⑤ **459.1** **Postphlebitic syndrome**
Chronic venous hypertension due to deep vein thrombosis

Excludes: *chronic venous hypertension without deep vein thrombosis (459.30-459.39)*

● **459.10** **Postphlebetic syndrome without complications**
Asymptomatic postphlebetic syndrome
Postphlebetic syndrome NOS

● **459.11** **Postphlebetic syndrome with ulcer**

● **459.12** **Postphlebetic syndrome with inflammation**

● **459.13** **Postphlebetic syndrome with ulcer and inflammation**

● **459.19** **Postphlebetic syndrome with other complication**

459.2 **Compression of vein**
Stricture of vein
Vena cava syndrome (inferior) (superior)

● **459.3** **Chronic venous hypertension (idiopathic)**
Stasis edema

Excludes: *chronic venous hypertension due to deep vein thrombosis (459.10-459.19)*
varicose veins (454.0-454.9)

● **459.30** **Chronic venous hypertension without complications**
Asymptomatic chronic venous hypertension
Chronic venous hypertension NOS

● **459.31** **Chronic venous hypertension with ulcer**

● **459.32** **Chronic venous hypertension with inflammation**

● **459.33** **Chronic venous hypertension with ulcer and inflammation**

● **459.39** **Chronic venous hypertension with other complication**

⑤ **459.8** **Other specified disorders of circulatory system**

459.81 **Venous (peripheral) insufficiency, unspecified**
Chronic venous insufficiency NOS
Use additional code for any associated ulceration (707.10-707.9)

459.89 **Other**
Collateral circulation (venous), any site
Phlebosclerosis
Venofibrosis

459.9 **Unspecified circulatory system disorder**

● Code new
to this edition

▲ Revision of
existing code

④ ⑤ Fourth or fifth
digit required

8.   DISEASES OF THE RESPIRATORY SYSTEM (460-519)

Use additional code, if desired, to identify infectious organism

ACUTE RESPIRATORY INFECTIONS (460-466)

Excludes: *pneumonia and influenza (480.0-487.8)*

460   Acute nasopharyngitis [common cold]

Coryza (acute)
Nasal catarrh, acute
Nasopharyngitis:
  NOS
  acute
  infective NOS

Rhinitis:
  acute
  infective

Excludes: *nasopharyngitis, chronic (472.2)*

pharyngitis:
  acute or unspecified (462)
  chronic (472.1)
rhinitis:
  allergic (477.0-477.9)
  chronic or unspecified (472.0)
sore throat:
  acute or unspecified (462)
  chronic (472.1)

461   Acute sinusitis

Includes: abscess
        empyema
        infection   } acute, of sinus (accessory) (nasal)
        inflammation
        suppuration

Excludes: *chronic or unspecified sinusitis (473.0-473.9)*

461.0   Maxillary
Acute antritis

461.1   Frontal

461.2   Ethmoidal

461.3   Sphenoidal

461.8   Other acute sinusitis
Acute pansinusitis

461.9   Acute sinusitis, unspecified
Acute sinusitis NOS

462   Acute pharyngitis

Acute sore throat NOS
Pharyngitis (acute):
  NOS
  gangrenous
  infective
  phlegmonous
  pneumococcal

Pharyngitis (acute):
  staphylococcal
  suppurative
  ulcerative
Sore throat (viral) NOS
Viral pharyngitis

Excludes: *abscess:*

peritonsillar [quinsy] (475)
pharyngeal NOS (478.29)
retropharyngeal (478.24)
chronic pharyngitis (472.1)
infectious mononucleosis (075)
that specified as (due to):
  Coxsackie (virus) (074.0)
  gonococcus (098.6)
  herpes simplex (054.79)
  influenza (487.1)
  septic (034.0)
  streptococcal (034.0)

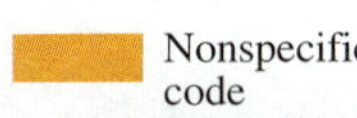

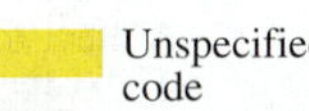

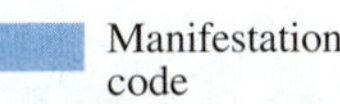

Manifestation
code

463 Acute tonsillitis

Tonsillitis (acute): Tonsillitis (acute):
 NOS   septic
 follicular   staphylococcal
 gangrenous   suppurative
 infective   ulcerative
 pneumococcal   viral

> *Excludes:* *chronic tonsillitis (474.0)*
> *hypertrophy of tonsils (474.1)*
> *peritonsillar abscess [quinsy] (475)*
> *sore throat:*
> *acute or NOS (462)*
> *septic (034.0)*
> *streptococcal tonsillitis (034.0)*

464 Acute laryngitis and tracheitis

> *Excludes:* *that associated with influenza (487.1)*
> *that due to Streptococcus (034.0)*

⑤ **464.0 Acute laryngitis**

Laryngitis (acute): Laryngitis (acute):
 NOS   pneumococcal
 edematous   septic
 Hemophilus influenza suppurative
 [H. influenzae] ulcerative

> *Excludes:* *chronic laryngitis (476.0-476.1)*
> *influenzal laryngitis (487.1)*

464.00 Without mention of obstruction

464.01 With obstruction

⑤ **464.1 Acute tracheitis**

Tracheitis (acute):
 NOS
 catarrhal
 viral

> *Excludes:* *chronic tracheitis (491.8)*

464.10 Without mention of obstruction

464.11 With obstruction

⑤ **464.2 Acute laryngotracheitis**
 Laryngotracheitis (acute)
 Tracheitis (acute) with laryngitis (acute)

> *Excludes:* *chronic laryngotracheitis (476.1)*

464.20 Without mention of obstruction

464.21 With obstruction

⑤ **464.3 Acute epiglottitis**
 Viral epiglottitis

> *Excludes:* *epiglottitis, chronic (476.1)*

464.30 Without mention of obstruction

464.31 With obstruction

464.4 Croup
 Croup syndrome

⑤ **464.5 Supraglottitis, unspecified**

464.50 Without mention of obstruction

464.51 With obstruction

465 Acute upper respiratory infections of multiple or unspecified sites

> *Excludes:* *upper respiratory infection due to:*
> *influenza (487.1)*
> *Streptococcus (034.0)*

465.0 Acute laryngopharyngitis

465.8 Other multiple sites
 Multiple URI

 ● Code new   ▲ Revision of   ④ ⑤ Fourth or fifth
  to this edition   existing code   digit required

465.9 Unspecified site
Acute URI NOS
Upper respiratory infection (acute)

466 Acute bronchitis and bronchiolitis
Includes: that with:
bronchospasm
obstruction

466.0 Acute bronchitis
Bronchitis, acute or subacute:
fibrinous
membranous
pneumococcal
purulent
septic
viral
with tracheitis
Croupous bronchitis
Tracheobronchitis, acute

Excludes: *acute bronchitis with:*
bronchiectasis (494.1)
chronic obstructive pulmonary disease (491.21)

⑤ **466.1 Acute bronchiolitis**
Bronchiolitis (acute)
Capillary pneumonia

466.11   Acute bronchiolitis due to respiratory syncytial virus (RSV)

466.19   Acute bronchiolitis due to other infectious organisms
Use additional code to identify organism

OTHER DISEASES OF THE UPPER RESPIRATORY TRACT (470-478)

470 Deviated nasal septum
Deflected septum (nasal) (acquired)

Excludes: *congenital (754.0)*

471 Nasal polyps

Excludes: *adenomatous polyps (212.0)*

471.0 Polyp of nasal cavity
Polyp:
choanal
nasopharyngeal

471.1 Polypoid sinus degeneration
Woakes' syndrome or ethmoiditis

471.8 Other polyp of sinus
Polyp of sinus: Polyp of sinus:
accessory   maxillary
ethmoidal   sphenoidal

471.9 Unspecified nasal polyp
Nasal polyp NOS

472 Chronic pharyngitis and nasopharyngitis

472.0 Chronic rhinitis
Ozena   Rhinitis:
Rhinitis: hypertrophic
NOS   obstructive
atrophic   purulent
granulomatous   ulcerative

Excludes: *allergic rhinitis (477.0-477.9)*

472.1 Chronic pharyngitis
Chronic sore throat
Pharyngitis:
atrophic
granular (chronic)
hypertrophic

472.2 Chronic nasopharyngitis

Excludes: *acute or unspecified nasopharyngitis (460)*

	Add 4th or 5th digit		Nonspecific code		Unspecified code		Manifestation code

473 Chronic sinusitis
Includes:

abscess
empyema
infection
suppuration
} (chronic) of sinus (accessory) (nasal)

| Excludes: | *acute sinusitis (461.0-461.9)*

473.0 Maxillary
Antritis (chronic)

473.1 Frontal

473.2 Ethmoidal

| Excludes: | *Woakes' ethmoiditis (471.1)*

473.3 Sphenoidal

473.8 Other chronic sinusitis
Pansinusitis (chronic)

473.9 Unspecified sinusitis (chronic)
Sinusitis (chronic) NOS

474 Chronic disease of tonsils and adenoids

⑤ **474.0 Chronic tonsillitis and adenoiditis**

| Excludes: | *acute or unspecified tonsillitis (463)*

474.00 Chronic tonsillitis

474.01 Chronic adenoiditis

474.02 Chronic tonsillitis and adenoiditis

⑤ **474.1 Hypertrophy of tonsils and adenoids**
Enlargement
Hyperplasia
Hypertrophy
} of tonsils or adenoids

| Excludes: | *that with adenoiditis (474.01)*
that with adenoiditis and tonsillitis (474.02)
that with tonsillitis (474.00)

474.10 Tonsils with adenoids

474.11 Tonsils alone

474.12 Adenoids alone

474.2 Adenoid vegetations

474.8 Other chronic disease of tonsils and adenoids
Amygdalolith
Calculus, tonsil
Cicatrix of tonsil (and adenoid)
Tonsillar tag
Ulcer, tonsil

474.9 Unspecified chronic disease of tonsils and adenoids
Disease (chronic) of tonsils (and adenoids)

475 Peritonsillar abscess
Abscess of tonsil   Quinsy
Peritonsillar cellulitis

| Excludes: | *tonsillitis:*
acute or NOS (463)
chronic (474.0)

476 Chronic laryngitis and laryngotracheitis

476.0 Chronic laryngitis
Laryngitis:
catarrhal
hypertrophic
sicca

● Code new
to this edition

▲ Revision of
existing code

④ ⑤ Fourth or fifth
digit required

476.1 Chronic laryngotracheitis
Laryngitis, chronic, with tracheitis (chronic)
Tracheitis, chronic, with laryngitis

Excludes: *chronic tracheitis (491.8)*
laryngitis and tracheitis, acute or unspecified (464.00-464.51)

477 Allergic rhinitis
Includes: allergic rhinitis (nonseasonal) (seasonal)
hay fever
spasmodic rhinorrhea

Excludes: *allergic rhinitis with asthma (bronchial) (493.0)*

477.0 Due to pollen
Pollinosis

477.1 Due to food

477.8 Due to other allergen

477.9 Cause unspecified

478 Other diseases of upper respiratory tract

478.0 Hypertrophy of nasal turbinates

478.1 Other diseases of nasal cavity and sinuses
Abscess
Necrosis } of nose (septum)
Ulcer
Cyst or mucocele of sinus (nasal)
Rhinolith

Excludes: *varicose ulcer of nasal septum (456.8)*

⑤ **478.2 Other diseases of pharynx, not elsewhere classified**

478.20 Unspecified disease of pharynx

478.21 Cellulitis of pharynx or nasopharynx

478.22 Parapharyngeal abscess

478.24 Retropharyngeal abscess

478.25 Edema of pharynx or nasopharynx

478.26 Cyst of pharynx or nasopharynx

478.29 Other
Abscess of pharynx or nasopharynx

Excludes: *ulcerative pharyngitis (462)*

⑤ **478.3 Paralysis of vocal cords or larynx**

478.30 Paralysis, unspecified
Laryngoplegia   Paralysis of glottis

478.31 Unilateral, partial

478.32 Unilateral, complete

478.33 Bilateral, partial

478.34 Bilateral, complete

478.4 Polyp of vocal cord or larynx

Excludes: *adenomatous polyps (212.1)*

478.5 Other diseases of vocal cords
Abscess
Cellulitis } of vocal cords
Granuloma
Leukoplakia
Chorditis (fibrinous) (nodosa) (tuberosa)
Singers' nodes

478.6 Edema of larynx
Edema (of):
glottis
subglottic
supraglottic

⑤ **478.7 Other diseases of larynx, not elsewhere classified**

478.70 Unspecified disease of larynx

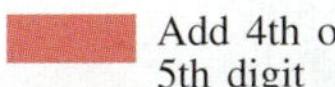

478.71 Cellulitis and perichondritis of larynx

478.74 Stenosis of larynx

478.75 Laryngeal spasm
Laryngismus (stridulus)

478.79 Other
Abscess
Necrosis
Obstruction   } of larynx
Pachyderma
Ulcer

Excludes: ulcerative laryngitis (464.00-464.01)

478.8 Upper respiratory tract hypersensitivity reaction, site unspecified

Excludes: hypersensitivity reaction of lower respiratory tract, as:
extrinsic allergic alveolitis (495.0-495.9)
pneumoconiosis (500-505)

478.9 Other and unspecified diseases of upper respiratory tract
Abscess   } of trachea
Cicatrix

PNEUMONIA AND INFLUENZA (480-487)

Excludes: pneumonia:
allergic or eosinophilic (518.3)
aspiration:
NOS (507.0)
newborn (770.1)
solids and liquids (507.0-507.8)
congenital (770.0)
lipoid (507.1)
passive (514)
rheumatic (390)

480 Viral pneumonia

480.0 Pneumonia due to adenovirus

480.1 Pneumonia due to respiratory syncytial virus

480.2 Pneumonia due to parainfluenza virus

480.8 Pneumonia due to other virus not elsewhere classified

Excludes: congenital rubella pneumonitis (771.0)
influenza with pneumonia, any form (487.0)
pneumonia complicating viral diseases classified elsewhere (484.1-484.8)

480.9 Viral pneumonia, unspecified

481 Pneumococcal pneumonia [Streptococcus pneumoniae pneumonia]
Lobar pneumonia, organism unspecified

482 Other bacterial pneumonia

482.0 Pneumonia due to Klebsiella pneumoniae

482.1 Pneumonia due to Pseudomonas

482.2 Pneumonia due to Hemophilus influenzae [H. influenzae]

⑤ **482.3 Pneumonia due to Streptococcus**

Excludes: Streptococcus pneumoniae pneumonia (481)

482.30 Streptococcus, unspecified

482.31 Group A

482.32 Group B

482.39 Other Streptococcus

⑤ **482.4 Pneumonia due to Staphylococcus**

482.40 Pneumonia due to Staphylococcus, unspecified

482.41 Pneumonia due to Staphylococcus aureus

482.49 Other Staphylococcus pneumonia

⑤ **482.8 Pneumonia due to other specified bacteria**

Excludes: pneumonia complicating infectious disease classified elsewhere (484.1-484.8)

● Code new
to this edition

▲ Revision of
existing code

④ ⑤ Fourth or fifth
digit required

482.81 Anaerobes
Bacteroides (melaninogenicus)
Gram-negative anaerobes

482.82 Escherichia coli [E. coli]

482.83 Other gram-negative bacteria
Gram-negative pneumonia NOS
Proteus
Serratia marcescens

Excludes: *Gram-negative anaerobes (482.81)*
Legionnaires' disease (482.84)

482.84 Legionnaires' disease

482.89 Other specified bacteria

482.9 Bacterial pneumonia unspecified

483 Pneumonia due to other specified organism

483.0 Mycoplasma pneumoniae
Eaton's agent
Pleuropneumonia-like organism [PPLO]

483.1 Chlamydia

483.8 Other specified organism

484 Pneumonia in infectious diseases classified elsewhere

Excludes: *influenza with pneumonia, any form (487.0)*

484.1 Pneumonia in cytomegalic inclusion disease
Code first underlying disease (078.5)

484.3 Pneumonia in whooping cough
Code first underlying disease (033.0-033.9)

484.5 Pneumonia in anthrax
Code first underlying disease (022.1)

484.6 Pneumonia in aspergillosis
Code first underlying disease (117.3)

484.7 Pneumonia in other systemic mycoses
Code first underlying disease

Excludes: *pneumonia in:*

candidiasis (112.4)
coccidioidomycosis (114.0)
histoplasmosis (115.0-115.9 with fifth-digit 5)

484.8 Pneumonia in other infectious diseases classified elsewhere
Code first underlying disease, as:
Q fever (083.0)
typhoid fever (002.0)

Excludes: *pneumonia in:*

actinomycosis (039.1)
measles (055.1)
nocardiosis (039.1)
ornithosis (073.0)
Pneumocystis carinii (136.3)
salmonellosis (003.22)
toxoplasmosis (130.4)
tuberculosis (011.6)
tularemia (021.2)
varicella (052.1)

485 Bronchopneumonia, organism unspecified

Bronchopneumonia:	Pneumonia:
hemorrhagic	lobular
terminal	segmental
Pleurobronchopneumonia	

Excludes: *bronchiolitis (acute) (466.11-466.19)*
chronic (491.8)
lipoid pneumonia (507.1)

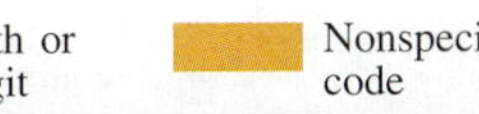

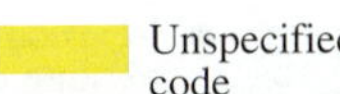

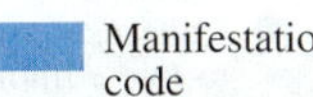

486 Pneumonia, organism unspecified

> *Excludes:* *hypostatic or passive pneumonia (514)*
> *influenza with pneumonia, any form (487.0)*
> *inhalation or aspiration pneumonia due to foreign materials (507.0-507.8)*
> *pneumonitis due to fumes and vapors (506.0)*

487 Influenza

> *Excludes:* *Hemophilus influenzae [H. influenzae]:*
> *infection NOS (041.5)*
> *laryngitis (464.00-464.01)*
> *meningitis (320.0)*
> *pneumonia (482.2)*

487.0 With pneumonia
Influenza with pneumonia, any form
Influenzal:
   bronchopneumonia
   pneumonia

487.1 With other respiratory manifestations
Influenza NOS
Influenzal:
   laryngitis
   pharyngitis
   respiratory infection (upper) (acute)

487.8 With other manifestations
Encephalopathy due to influenza
Influenza with involvement of gastrointestinal tract

> *Excludes:* *"intestinal flu" [viral gastroenteritis] (008.8)*

CHRONIC OBSTRUCTIVE PULMONARY DISEASE AND ALLIED CONDITIONS (490-496)

490 Bronchitis, not specified as acute or chronic
Bronchitis NOS: Tracheobronchitis NOS
   catarrhal
   with tracheitis NOS

> *Excludes:* *bronchitis:*
> *allergic NOS (493.9)*
> *asthmatic NOS (493.9)*
> *due to fumes and vapors (506.0)*

491 Chronic bronchitis

> *Excludes:* *chronic obstructive asthma (493.2)*

491.0 Simple chronic bronchitis
Catarrhal bronchitis, chronic
Smokers' cough

491.1 Mucopurulent chronic bronchitis
Bronchitis (chronic) (recurrent):
   fetid
   mucopurulent
   purulent

⑤ **491.2 Obstructive chronic bronchitis**
Bronchitis: Bronchitis with:
   emphysematous   chronic airway obstruction
   obstructive (chronic) (diffuse)   emphysema

> *Excludes:* *asthmatic bronchitis (acute) NOS (493.9)*
> *chronic obstructive asthma (493.2)*

491.20 Without mention of acute exacerbation
Emphysema with chronic bronchitis

491.21 With acute exacerbation
Acute bronchitis with chronic obstructive pulmonary disease [COPD]
Acute and chronic obstructive bronchitis
Acute exacerbation of chronic obstructive pulmonary disease [COPD]
Emphysema with both acute and chronic bronchitis

> *Excludes:* *chronic obstructive asthma with acute exacerbation (493.22)*

● Code new   ▲ Revision of   ④ ⑤ Fourth or fifth
to this edition   existing code   digit required

491.8 **Other chronic bronchitis**
Chronic:
tracheitis
tracheobronchitis

491.9 **Unspecified chronic bronchitis**

492 **Emphysema**

492.0 **Emphysematous bleb**
Giant bullous emphysema
Ruptured emphysematous bleb
Tension pneumatocele
Vanishing lung

492.8 **Other emphysema**
Emphysema (lung or pulmonary):
NOS
centriacinar
centrilobular
obstructive
panacinar
Emphysema (lung or pulmonary):
panlobular
unilateral
vesicular
MacLeod's syndrome
Swyer-James syndrome
Unilateral hyperlucent lung

Excludes: *emphysema:*
compensatory (518.2)
due to fumes and vapors (506.4)
interstitial (518.1)
newborn (770.2)
mediastinal (518.1)
surgical (subcutaneous) (998.81)
traumatic (958.7)
with chronic bronchitis (491.20)
with both acute and chronic bronchitis (491.21)

⑤ **493** **Asthma**

Excludes: *wheezing NOS (786.07)*

The following fifth-digit subclassification is for use with category 493:

0 **without mention of status asthmaticus or acute exacerbation or unspecified**

1 **with status asthmaticus**

2 **with acute exacerbation**

⑤ **493.0** **extrinsic asthma**
Asthma:
allergic with stated cause
atopic
childhood
hay
platinum
Hay fever with asthma

Excludes: *asthma:*
allergic NOS (493.9)
detergent (507.8)
miners' (500)
wood (495.8)

⑤ **493.1** **Intrinsic asthma**
Late-onset asthma

⑤ **493.2** **Chronic obstructive asthma**
Asthma with chronic obstructive pulmonary disease [COPD]
Chronic asthmatic bronchitis

Excludes: *chronic obstructive bronchitis (491.2)*
acute bronchitis (466.0)

⑤ **493.9** **Asthma, unspecified**
Asthma (bronchial) (allergic NOS)
Bronchitis:
allergic
asthmatic

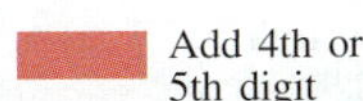

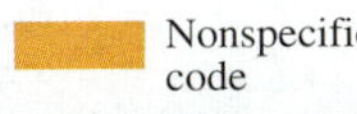

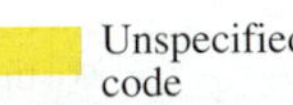

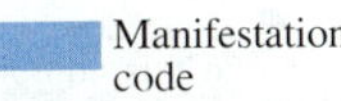

494 Bronchiectasis
Bronchiectasis (fusiform) (postinfectious) (recurrent)
Bronchiolectasis

> Excludes: *congenital (748.61)*
> *tuberculous bronchiectasis (current disease) (011.5)*

494.0 Bronchiectasis without acute exacerbation

494.1 Bronchiectasis with acute exacerbation
Acute bronchitis with bronchiectasis

495 Extrinsic allergic alveolitis
Includes: allergic alveolitis and pneumonitis due to inhaled organic dust particles of fungal, thermophilic actinomycete, or other origin

495.0 Farmers' lung

495.1 Bagassosis

495.2 Bird-fanciers' lung
Budgerigar-fanciers' disease or lung
Pigeon-fanciers' disease or lung

495.3 Suberosis
Cork-handlers' disease or lung

495.4 Malt workers' lung
Alveolitis due to Aspergillus clavatus

495.5 Mushroom workers' lung

495.6 Maple bark-strippers' lung
Alveolitis due to Cryptostroma corticale

495.7 "Ventilation" pneumonitis
Allergic alveolitis due to fungal, thermophilic actinomycete, and other organisms growing in ventilation [air conditioning] systems

495.8 Other specified allergic alveolitis and pneumonitis

Cheese-washers' lung   Pituitary snuff-takers' disease
Coffee workers' lung   Sequoiosis or red-cedar asthma
Fish-meal workers' lung   Wood asthma
Furriers' lung
Grain-handlers' disease or lung

495.9 Unspecified allergic alveolitis and pneumonitis
Alveolitis, allergic (extrinsic)
Hypersensitivity pneumonitis

496 Chronic airway obstruction, not elsewhere classified
Note: This code is not to be used with any code from categories 491-493
Chronic:
nonspecific lung disease
obstructive lung disease
obstructive pulmonary disease [COPD] NOS

> Excludes: *chronic obstructive lung disease [COPD] specified (as) (with):*
> *allergic alveolitis (495.0-495.9)*
> *asthma (493.2)*
> *bronchiectasis (494.0-494.1)*
> *bronchitis (491.20-491.21)*
> *with emphysema (491.20-491.21)*
> *emphysema (492.0-492.8)*

PNEUMOCONIOSES AND OTHER LUNG DISEASES DUE TO EXTERNAL AGENTS (500-508)

500 Coal workers' pneumoconiosis

Anthracosilicosis   Coal workers' lung
Anthracosis   Miner's asthma
Black lung disease

501 Asbestosis

502 Pneumoconiosis due to other silica or silicates
Pneumoconiosis due to talc
Silicotic fibrosis (massive) of lung
Silicosis (simple) (complicated)

● Code new   ▲ Revision of   ④ ⑤ Fourth or fifth
  to this edition   existing code   digit required

503 Pneumoconiosis due to other inorganic dust
Aluminosis (of lung)   Graphite fibrosis (of lung)
Bauxite fibrosis (of lung)   Siderosis
Berylliosis   Stannosis

504 Pneumonopathy due to inhalation of other dust
Byssinosis   Flax-dressers' disease
Cannabinosis

> *Excludes:* *allergic alveolitis (495.0-495.9)*
> *asbestosis (501)*
> *bagassosis (495.1)*
> *farmers' lung (495.0)*

505 Pneumoconiosis, unspecified

506 Respiratory conditions due to chemical fumes and vapors
Use additional E code, if desired, to identify cause

506.0 Bronchitis and pneumonitis due to fumes and vapors
Chemical bronchitis (acute)

506.1 Acute pulmonary edema due to fumes and vapors
Chemical pulmonary edema (acute)

> *Excludes:* *acute pulmonary edema NOS (518.4)*
> *chronic or unspecified pulmonary edema (514)*

506.2 Upper respiratory inflammation due to fumes and vapors

506.3 Other acute and subacute respiratory conditions due to fumes and vapors

506.4 Chronic respiratory conditions due to fumes and vapors
Emphysema (diffuse) (chronic)
Obliterative bronchiolitis (chronic) (subacute)   } due to inhalation of chemical
Pulmonary fibrosis (chronic)   fumes and vapors

506.9 Unspecified respiratory conditions due to fumes and vapors
Silo-fillers' disease

507 Pneumonitis due to solids and liquids

> *Excludes:* *fetal aspiration pneumonitis (770.1)*

507.0 Due to inhalation of food or vomitus
Aspiration pneumonia (due to):
NOS
food (regurgitated)
gastric secretions
milk
saliva
vomitus

507.1 Due to inhalation of oils and essences
Lipoid pneumonia (exogenous)

> *Excludes:* *endogenous lipoid pneumonia (516.8)*

507.8 Due to other solids and liquids
Detergent asthma

508 Respiratory conditions due to other and unspecified external agents
Use additional E code, if desired, to identify cause

508.0 Acute pulmonary manifestations due to radiation
Radiation pneumonitis

508.1 Chronic and other pulmonary manifestations due to radiation
Fibrosis of lung following radiation

508.8 Respiratory conditions due to other specified external agents

508.9 Respiratory conditions due to unspecified external agent

OTHER DISEASES OF RESPIRATORY SYSTEM (510-519)

510 Empyema
Use additional code, if desired, to identify infectious organism (041.0-041.9)

> *Excludes:* *abscess of lung (513.0)*

500

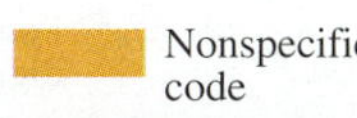

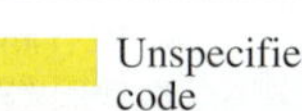

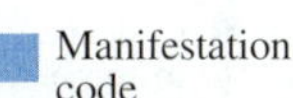

Manifestation
code

510.0 With fistula
Fistula:
    bronchocutaneous
    bronchopleural
    hepatopleural
Fistula:
    mediastinal
    pleural
    thoracic
Any condition classifiable to 510.9 with fistula

510.9 Without mention of fistula
Abscess:
    pleura
    thorax
Empyema (chest) (lung)
    (pleura)
Fibrinopurulent pleurisy
Pleurisy:
    purulent
    septic
    seropurulent
    suppurative
Pyopneumothorax
Pyothorax

511 Pleurisy

> |Excludes:| *malignant pleural effusion (197.2)*
> *pleurisy with mention of tuberculosis, current disease (012.0)*

511.0 Without mention of effusion or current tuberculosis
Adhesion, lung or pleura
Calcification of pleura
Pleurisy (acute) (sterile):
    diaphragmatic
    fibrinous
    interlobar
Pleurisy:
    NOS
    pneumococcal
    staphylococcal
    streptococcal
Thickening of pleura

511.1 With effusion, with mention of a bacterial cause other than tuberculosis
Pleurisy with effusion (exudative) (serous):
    pneumococcal
    staphylococcal
    streptococcal
    other specified nontuberculous bacterial cause

511.8 Other specified forms of effusion, except tuberculous
Encysted pleurisy
Hemopneumothorax
Hemothorax
Hydropneumothorax
Hydrothorax

> |Excludes:| *traumatic (860.2-860.5, 862.29, 862.39)*

511.9 Unspecified pleural effusion
Pleural effusion NOS
Pleurisy:
    exudative
    serofibrinous
Pleurisy:
    serous
    with effusion NOS

512 Pneumothorax

512.0 Spontaneous tension pneumothorax

512.1 Iatrogenic pneumothorax
Postoperative pneumothorax

512.8 Other spontaneous pneumothorax
Pneumothorax:
    NOS
    acute
    chronic

> |Excludes:| *pneumothorax:*
> *congenital (770.2)*
> *traumatic (860.0-860.1, 860.4-860.5)*
> *tuberculous, current disease (011.7)*

513 Abscess of lung and mediastinum

513.0 Abscess of lung
Abscess (multiple) of lung
Gangrenous or necrotic pneumonia
Pulmonary gangrene or necrosis

513.1 Abscess of mediastinum

● Code new
  to this edition

▲ Revision of
  existing code

④ ⑤ Fourth or fifth
    digit required

514 Pulmonary congestion and hypostasis
Hypostatic:
bronchopneumonia
pneumonia
Passive pneumonia
Pulmonary congestion (chronic) (passive)
Pulmonary edema:
NOS
chronic

> *Excludes:* *acute pulmonary edema:*
> *NOS (518.4)*
> *with mention of heart disease or failure (428.1)*

515 Postinflammatory pulmonary fibrosis
Cirrhosis of lung
Fibrosis of lung (atrophic)
(confluent) (massive)
(perialveolar) (peribronchial)
Induration of lung
} chronic or unspecified

516 Other alveolar and parietoalveolar pneumonopathy

516.0 Pulmonary alveolar proteinosis

516.1 *Idiopathic pulmonary hemosiderosis*
Essential brown induration of lung
Code first underlying disease (275.0)

516.2 Pulmonary alveolar microlithiasis

516.3 Idiopathic fibrosing alveolitis
Alveolar capillary block
Diffuse (idiopathic) (interstitial) pulmonary fibrosis
Hamman-Rich syndrome

516.8 Other specified alveolar and parietoalveolar pneumonopathies
Endogenous lipoid pneumonia
Interstitial pneumonia (desquamative) (lymphoid)

> *Excludes:* *lipoid pneumonia, exogenous or unspecified (507.1)*

516.9 Unspecified alveolar and parietoalveolar pneumonopathy

517 Lung involvement in conditions classified elsewhere

> *Excludes:* *rheumatoid lung (714.81)*

517.1 *Rheumatic pneumonia*
Code first underlying disease (390)

517.2 *Lung involvement in systemic sclerosis*
Code first underlying disease (710.1)

517.8 *Lung involvement in other diseases classified elsewhere*
Code first underlying disease, as:
amyloidosis (277.3)
polymyositis (710.4)
sarcoidosis (135)
Sjögren's disease (710.2)
systemic lupus erythematosus (710.0)

> *Excludes:* *syphilis (095.1)*

518 Other diseases of lung

518.0 Pulmonary collapse
Atelectasis
Collapse of lung
Middle lobe syndrome

> *Excludes:* *atelectasis:*
> *congenital (partial) (770.5)*
> *primary (770.4)*
> *tuberculous, current disease (011.8)*

518.1 Interstitial emphysema
Mediastinal emphysema

> *Excludes:* *surgical (subcutaneous) emphysema (998.81)*
> *that in fetus or newborn (770.2)*
> *traumatic emphysema (958.7)*

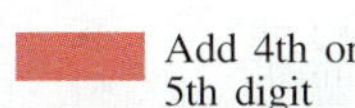

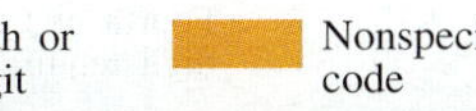

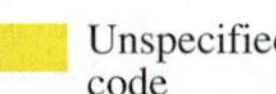

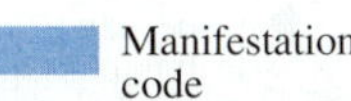

518.2 Compensatory emphysema

518.3 Pulmonary eosinophilia

Eosinophilic asthma

Löffler's syndrome

Pneumonia:

  allergic

  eosinophilic

Tropical eosinophilia

518.4 Acute edema of lung, unspecified

Acute pulmonary edema NOS

Pulmonary edema, postoperative

Excludes: *pulmonary edema:*

acute, with mention of heart disease or failure (428.1)

chronic or unspecified (514)

due to external agents (506.0-508.9)

518.5 Pulmonary insufficiency following trauma and surgery

Adult respiratory distress syndrome

Pulmonary insufficiency following:

  shock

  surgery

  trauma

Shock lung

Excludes: *adult respiratory distress syndrome associated with other conditions (518.82)*

pneumonia:

aspiration (507.0)

hypostatic (514)

respiratory failure in other conditions (518.81, 518.83-518.84)

518.6 Allergic bronchopulmonary aspergillosis

⑤ **518.8 Other diseases of lung**

518.81 Acute respiratory failure

Respiratory failure NOS

Excludes: *acute and chronic respiratory failure (518.84)*

acute respiratory distress (518.82)

chronic respiratory failure (518.83)

respiratory arrest (799.1)

respiratory failure, newborn (770.84)

518.82 Other pulmonary insufficiency, not elsewhere classified

Acute respiratory distress

Acute respiratory insufficiency

Adult respiratory distress syndrome NEC

Excludes: *adult respiratory distress syndrome associated with trauma and surgery (518.5)*

pulmonary insufficiency following trauma and surgery (518.5)

respiratory distress:

NOS (786.09)

newborn (770.89)

syndrome, newborn (769)

shock lung (518.5)

518.83 Chronic respiratory failure

518.84 Acute and chronic respiratory failure

Acute or chronic respiratory failure

518.89 Other diseases of lung, not elsewhere classified

Broncholithiasis

Calcification of lung

Lung disease NOS

Pulmolithiasis

519 Other diseases of respiratory system

⑤ **519.0 Tracheostomy complications**

519.00 Tracheostomy complication, unspecified

519.01 Infection of tracheostomy

Use additional code to identify type of infection, such as:

  abscess or cellulitis of neck (682.1)

  septicemia (038.0-038.9)

Use additional code to identify organism (041.00-041.9)

519.02 Mechanical complication of tracheostomy

Tracheal stenosis due to tracheostomy

● Code new to this edition ▲ Revision of existing code ④ ⑤ Fourth or fifth digit required

519.09 Other tracheostomy complications
Hemorrhage due to tracheostomy
Tracheoesophageal fistula due to tracheostomy

519.1 Other diseases of trachea and bronchus, not elsewhere classified
Calcification of bronchus or trachea
Stenosis of bronchus or trachea
Ulcer of bronchus or trachea

519.2 Mediastinitis

519.3 Other diseases of mediastinum, not elsewhere classified
Fibrosis of mediastinum
Hernia of mediastinum
Retraction of mediastinum

519.4 Disorders of diaphragm
Diaphragmitis
Paralysis of diaphragm
Relaxation of diaphragm

Excludes: *congenital defect of diaphragm (756.6)*
diaphragmatic hernia (551-553 with .3)
congenital (756.6)

519.8 Other diseases of respiratory system, not elsewhere classified

519.9 Unspecified disease of respiratory system
Respiratory disease (chronic) NOS

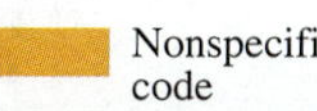

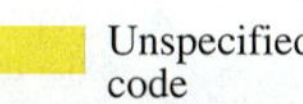

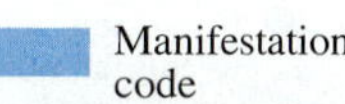

● Code new
  to this edition
▲ Revision of
  existing code
④ ⑤ Fourth or fifth
  digit required

9. DISEASES OF THE DIGESTIVE SYSTEM (520-579)

DISEASES OF ORAL CAVITY, SALIVARY GLANDS, AND JAWS (520-529)

520 **Disorders of tooth development and eruption**

520.0 Anodontia
Absence of teeth (complete) (congenital) (partial)
Hypodontia
Oligodontia

Excludes: *acquired absence of teeth (525.10-525.19)*

520.1 Supernumerary teeth
Distomolar   Paramolar
Fourth molar   Supplemental teeth
Mesiodens

Excludes: *supernumerary roots (520.2)*

520.2 Abnormalities of size and form
Concrescence ⎤   Macrodontia
Fusion   ⎥ of teeth   Microdontia
Gemination   ⎥   Peg-shaped [conical] teeth
Dens evaginatus ⎦   Supernumerary roots
Dens in dente   Taurodontism
Dens invaginatus   Tuberculum paramolare
Enamel pearls

Excludes: *that due to congenital syphilis (090.5)*
tuberculum Carabelli, which is regarded as a normal variation

520.3 Mottled teeth
Dental fluorosis
Mottling of enamel
Nonfluoride enamel opacities

520.4 Disturbances of tooth formation
Aplasia and hypoplasia of cementum   Horner's teeth
Dilaceration of tooth   Hypocalcification of teeth
Enamel hypoplasia (neonatal) (postnatal) (prenatal)   Regional odontodysplasia
                                         Turner's tooth

Excludes: *Hutchinson's teeth and mulberry molars in congenital syphilis (090.5)*
mottled teeth (520.3)

520.5 Hereditary disturbances in tooth structure, not elsewhere classified
Amelogenesis   ⎤
Dentinogenesis ⎥ imperfecta
Odontogenesis ⎦
Dentinal dysplasia
Shell teeth

520.6 Disturbances of tooth eruption
Teeth: Tooth eruption:
  embedded   late
  impacted   obstructed
  natal   premature
  neonatal
  primary [deciduous]:
    persistent
    shedding, premature

Excludes: *exfoliation of teeth (attributable to disease of surrounding tissues) (525.0-525.19)*
impacted or embedded teeth with abnormal position of such teeth or adjacent teeth
(524.3)

520.7 Teething syndrome

520.8 **Other specified disorders of tooth development and eruption**
Color changes during tooth formation
Pre-eruptive color changes

Excludes: *posteruptive color changes (521.7)*

520.9 **Unspecified disorder of tooth development and eruption**

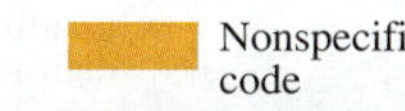

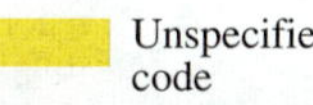

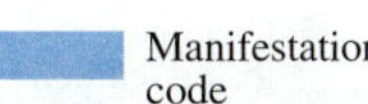

Manifestation
code

521 Diseases of hard tissues of teeth

⑤ **521.0 Dental caries**

521.00 Dental caries, unspecified

521.01 Dental caries limited to enamel
Initial caries
White spot lesion

521.02 Dental caries extending into dentine

521.03 Dental caries extending into pulp

521.04 Arrested dental caries

521.05 Odontoclasia
Infantile melanodontia
Melanodontoclasia

Excludes: *internal and external resorption of teeth (521.4)*

521.09 Other dental caries

521.1 Excessive attrition
Approximal wear   Occlusal wear

521.2 Abrasion
Abrasion:
  dentifrice
  habitual
  occupational   } of teeth
  ritual
  traditional
Wedge defect NOS

521.3 Erosion
Erosion of teeth: Erosion of teeth:
  NOS   idiopathic
  due to: occupational
    medicine
    persistent vomiting

521.4 Pathological resorption
Internal granuloma of pulp
Resorption of tooth or root (external) (internal)

521.5 Hypercementosis
Cementation hyperplasia

521.6 Ankylosis of teeth

521.7 Posteruptive color changes
Staining [discoloration] of teeth:
  NOS
  due to:
    drugs
    metals
    pulpal bleeding

Excludes: *accretions [deposits] on teeth (523.6)*
          pre-eruptive color changes (520.8)

521.8 Other specified diseases of hard tissues of teeth
Irradiated enamel   Sensitive dentin

521.9 Unspecified disease of hard tissues of teeth

522 Diseases of pulp and periapical tissues

522.0 Pulpitis
Pulpal: Pulpitis:
  abscess   acute
  polyp   chronic (hyperplastic) (ulcerative)
                              suppurative

● Code new   ▲ Revision of   ④ ⑤ Fourth or fifth
   to this edition   existing code   digit required

522.1 Necrosis of the pulp
Pulp gangrene

522.2 Pulp degeneration
Denticles   Pulp stones
  Pulp calcifications

522.3 Abnormal hard tissue formation in pulp
Secondary or irregular dentin

522.4 Acute apical periodontitis of pulpal origin

522.5 Periapical abscess without sinus
Abscess:
  dental
  dentoalveolar

Excludes: periapical abscess with sinus (522.7)

522.6 Chronic apical periodontitis
Apical or periapical granuloma
Apical periodontitis NOS

522.7 Periapical abscess with sinus
Fistula:
  alveolar process
  dental

522.8 Radicular cyst
Cyst:
  apical (periodontal)
  periapical
  radiculodental
  residual radicular

Excludes: lateral developmental or lateral periodontal cyst (526.0)

522.9 Other and unspecified diseases of pulp and periapical tissues

523 Gingival and periodontal diseases

523.0 Acute gingivitis

Excludes: acute necrotizing ulcerative gingivitis (101)
             herpetic gingivostomatitis (054.2)

523.1 Chronic gingivitis
Gingivitis (chronic):   Gingivitis (chronic):
  NOS   simple marginal
  desquamative   ulcerative
  hyperplastic   Gingivostomatitis

Excludes: herpetic gingivostomatitis (054.2)

523.2 Gingival recession
Gingival recession (generalized) (localized) (postinfective) (postoperative)

523.3 Acute periodontitis
Acute: Paradontal abscess
  pericementitis   Periodontal abscess
  pericoronitis

Excludes: acute apical periodontitis (522.4)
             periapical abscess (522.5, 522.7)

523.4 Chronic periodontitis
Alveolar pyorrhea   Periodontitis:
Chronic pericoronitis   NOS
Pericementitis (chronic)   complex
                                 simplex

Excludes: chronic apical periodontitis (522.6)

523.5 Periodontosis

523.6 Accretions on teeth
Dental calculus: Deposits on teeth:
  subgingival   betel
  supragingival   materia alba
                                 soft
                                 tartar
                                 tobacco

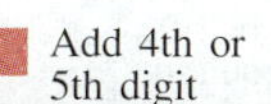

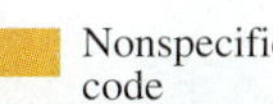

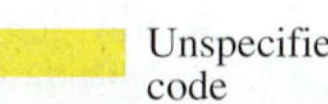

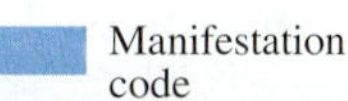

523.8 **Other specified periodontal diseases**

Giant cell:
  epulis
  peripheral granuloma
Gingival:
  cysts
  enlargement NOS
  fibromatosis

Gingival polyp
Periodontal lesions due to traumatic occlusion
Peripheral giant cell granuloma

Excludes: *leukoplakia of gingiva (528.6)*

523.9 **Unspecified gingival and periodontal disease**

524 **Dentofacial anomalies, including malocclusion**

⑤ **524.0** **Major anomalies of jaw size**

Excludes: *hemifacial atrophy or hypertrophy (754.0)*
    unilateral condylar hyperplasia or hypoplasia of mandible (526.89)

524.00 **Unspecified anomaly**

524.01 **Maxillary hyperplasia**

524.02 **Mandibular hyperplasia**

524.03 **Maxillary hypoplasia**

524.04 **Mandibular hypoplasia**

524.05 **Macrogenia**

524.06 **Microgenia**

524.09 **Other specified anomaly**

⑤ **524.1** **Anomalies of relationship of jaw to cranial base**

524.10 **Unspecified anomaly**
  prognathism
  retrognathism

524.11 **Maxillary asymmetry**

524.12 **Other jaw asymmetry**

524.19 **Other specified anomaly**

524.2 **Anomalies of dental arch relationship**

Crossbite (anterior) (posterior)
Disto-occlusion
Mesio-occlusion
Midline deviation
Open bite (anterior) (posterior)

Overbite (excessive)
  deep
  horizontal
  vertical
Overjet
Posterior lingual occlusion of mandibular teeth
Soft tissue impingement

Excludes: *hemifacial atrophy or hypertrophy (754.0)*
    unilateral condylar hyperplasia or hypoplasia of mandible (526.89)

524.3 **Anomalies of tooth position**

Crowding
Diastema
Displacement   } of tooth, teeth
Rotation
Spacing, abnormal
Transposition
Impacted or embedded teeth with abnormal position of such teeth or adjacent teeth

524.4 **Malocclusion, unspecified**

524.5 **Dentofacial functional abnormalities**

Abnormal jaw closure
Malocclusion due to:
  abnormal swallowing
  mouth breathing
  tongue, lip, or finger habits

⑤ **524.6** **Temporomandibular joint disorders**

Excludes: *current temporomandibular joint:*
  dislocation (830.0-830.1)
  strain (848.1)

524.60 **Temporomandibular joint disorders, unspecified**
Temporomandibular joint-pain-dysfunction syndrome [TMJ]

● Code new
to this edition

▲ Revision of
existing code

④ ⑤ Fourth or fifth
digit required

      524.61   Adhesions and ankylosis (bony or fibrous)

      524.62   Arthralgia of temporomandibular joint

      524.63   Articular disc disorder (reducing or non-reducing)

      524.69   Other specified temporomandibular joint disorders

⑤ **524.7 Dental alveolar anomalies**

      524.70   Unspecified alveolar anomaly

      524.71   Alveolar maxillary hyperplasia

      524.72   Alveolar mandibular hyperplasia

      524.73   Alveolar maxillary hypoplasia

      524.74   Alveolar mandibular hypoplasia

      524.79   Other specified alveolar anomaly

524.8 Other specified dentofacial anomalies

524.9 Unspecified dentofacial anomalies

525 Other diseases and conditions of the teeth and supporting structures

  525.0 Exfoliation of teeth due to systemic causes

⑤ **525.1 Loss of teeth due to trauma, extraction, or periodontal disease**

      525.10   Acquired absence of teeth, unspecified
            Edentulism
            Tooth extraction status, NOS

      525.11   Loss of teeth due to trauma

      525.12   Loss of teeth due to periodontal disease

      525.13   Loss of teeth due to caries

      525.19   Other loss of teeth

  525.2 Atrophy of edentulous alveolar ridge

  525.3 Retained dental root

  525.8 Other specified disorders of the teeth and supporting structures
      Enlargement of alveolar ridge NOS
      Irregular alveolar process

  525.9 Unspecified disorder of the teeth and supporting structures

526 Diseases of the jaws

  526.0 Developmental odontogenic cysts

Cyst: Cyst:
  dentigerous   lateral periodontal
  eruption   primordial
  follicular   Keratocyst
  lateral developmental

Excludes: *radicular cyst (522.8)*

  526.1 Fissural cysts of jaw
      Cyst:
        globulomaxillary
        incisor canal
        median anterior maxillary
        median palatal
        nasopalatine
        palatine of papilla

Excludes: *cysts of oral soft tissues (528.4)*

  526.2 Other cysts of jaws
Cyst of jaw: Cyst of jaw:
  NOS   hemorrhagic
  aneurysmal   traumatic

  526.3 Central giant cell (reparative) granuloma

Excludes: *peripheral giant cell granuloma (523.8)*

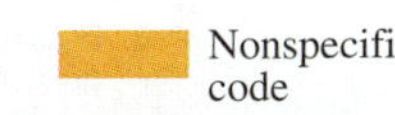

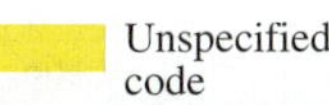

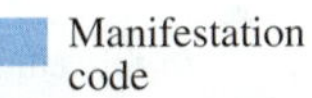

526.4 Inflammatory conditions
Abscess
Osteitis
Osteomyelitis (neonatal) } of jaw (acute) (chronic) (suppurative)
Periostitis
Sequestrum of jaw bone

Excludes: alveolar osteitis (526.5)

526.5 Alveolitis of jaw
Alveolar osteitis
Dry socket

⑤ **526.8 Other specified diseases of the jaws**

526.81 Exostosis of jaw
Torus mandibularis
Torus palatinus

526.89 Other
Cherubism
Fibrous dysplasia
Latent bone cyst } of jaw(s)
Osteoradionecrosis of jaw(s)
Unilateral condylar hyperplasia or hypoplasia of mandible

526.9 Unspecified disease of the jaws

527 Diseases of the salivary glands

527.0 Atrophy

527.1 Hypertrophy

527.2 Sialoadenitis
Parotitis: Sialoangitis
 NOS   Sialodochitis
 allergic
 toxic

Excludes: epidemic or infectious parotitis (072.0-072.9)
   uveoparotid fever (135)

527.3 Abscess

527.4 Fistula

Excludes: congenital fistula of salivary glands (750.24)

527.5 Sialolithiasis
Calculus
Stone } of salivary gland or duct
Sialodocholithiasis

527.6 Mucocele
Mucous:
 extravasation cyst of salivary gland
 retention cyst of salivary gland
Ranula

527.7 Disturbance of salivary secretion
Hyposecretion   Sialorrhea
Ptyalism   Xerostomia

527.8 Other specified diseases of the salivary glands
Benign lymphoepithelial lesion of salivary gland
Sialectasia
Sialosis
Stenosis
Stricture } of salivary duct

527.9 Unspecified disease of the salivary glands

● Code new   ▲ Revision of   ④ ⑤ Fourth or fifth
 to this edition   existing code   digit required

528 **Diseases of the oral soft tissues, excluding lesions specific for gingiva and tongue**

528.0 Stomatitis

Stomatitis:
 NOS
 ulcerative

Vesicular stomatitis

Excludes: *stomatitis:*

 acute necrotizing ulcerative (101)
 aphthous (528.2)
 gangrenous (528.1)
 herpetic (054.2)
 Vincent's (101)

528.1 Cancrum oris

Gangrenous stomatitis

Noma

528.2 Oral aphthae

Aphthous stomatitis
Canker sore
Periadenitis mucosa necrotica recurrens

Recurrent aphthous ulcer
Stomatitis herpetiformis

Excludes: *herpetic stomatitis (054.2)*

528.3 Cellulitis and abscess

Cellulitis of mouth (floor)
Ludwig's angina
Oral fistula

Excludes: *abscess of tongue (529.0)*

 cellulitis or abscess of lip (528.5)
 fistula (of):
  dental (522.7)
  lip (528.5)
 gingivitis (523.0-523.1)

528.4 Cysts

Dermoid cyst
Epidermoid cyst
Epstein's pearl
Lymphoepithelial cyst
Nasoalveolar cyst
Nasolabial cyst

} of mouth

Excludes: *cyst:*

 gingiva (523.8)
 tongue (529.8)

528.5 Diseases of lips

Abscess
Cellulitis
Fistula
Hypertrophy

} of lip(s)

Cheilitis:
 NOS
 angular
Cheilodynia
Cheilosis

Excludes: *actinic cheilitis (692.79)*

 congenital fistula of lip (750.25)
 leukoplakia of lips (528.6)

528.6 Leukoplakia of oral mucosa, including tongue

Leukokeratosis of oral mucosa
Leukoplakia of:
 gingiva
 lips
 tongue

Excludes: *carcinoma in situ (230.0, 232.0)*

 leukokeratosis nicotina palati (528.7)

528.7 Other disturbances of oral epithelium, including tongue

Erythroplakia
Focal epithelial
 hyperplasia
Leukoedema
Leukokeratosis
 nicotina palati

} of mouth or tongue

Excludes: *carcinoma in situ (230.0, 232.0)*

 leukokeratosis NOS (702)

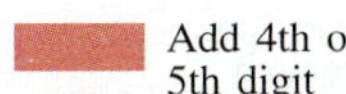

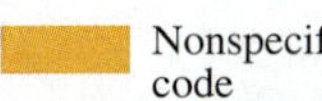

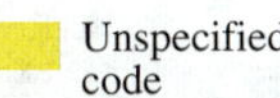

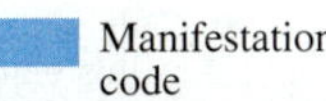

528.8 Oral submucosal fibrosis, including of tongue

528.9 Other and unspecified diseases of the oral soft tissues
Cheek and lip biting
Denture sore mouth
Denture stomatitis
Melanoplakia
Papillary hyperplasia of palate
Eosinophilic granuloma ⎫
Irritative hyperplasia   ⎬ of oral mucosa
Pyogenic granuloma   ⎪
Ulcer (traumatic) ⎭

529 Diseases and other conditions of the tongue

529.0 Glossitis
Abscess ⎫
Ulceration (traumatic) ⎬ of tongue

> Excludes: glossitis:
>
> benign migratory (529.1)
> Hunter's (529.4)
> median rhomboid (529.2)
> Moeller's (529.4)

529.1 Geographic tongue
Benign migratory glossitis
Glossitis areata exfoliativa

529.2 Median rhomboid glossitis

529.3 Hypertrophy of tongue papillae
Black hairy tongue
Coated tongue
Hypertrophy of foliate papillae
Lingua villosa nigra

529.4 Atrophy of tongue papillae
Bald tongue   Glossodynia exfoliativa
Glazed tongue   Smooth atrophic tongue
Glossitis:
  Hunter's
  Moeller's

529.5 Plicated tongue
Fissured ⎫
Furrowed ⎬ tongue
Scrotal ⎭

> Excludes: fissure of tongue, congenital (750.13)

529.6 Glossodynia
Glossopyrosis   Painful tongue

> Excludes: glossodynia exfoliativa (529.4)

529.8 Other specified conditions of the tongue
Atrophy ⎫
Crenated ⎪
Enlargement ⎬ (of) tongue
Hypertrophy ⎪
Glossocele ⎪
Glossoptosis ⎭

> Excludes: erythroplasia of tongue (528.7)
>
> leukoplakia of tongue (528.6)
> macroglossia (congenital) (750.15)
> microglossia (congenital) (750.16)
> oral submucosal fibrosis (528.8)

529.9 Unspecified condition of the tongue

DISEASES OF ESOPHAGUS, STOMACH, AND DUODENUM (530-537)

530 Diseases of esophagus

> Excludes: esophageal varices (456.0-456.2)

● Code new   ▲ Revision of   ④ ⑤ Fourth or fifth
  to this edition   existing code   digit required

530.0 Achalasia and cardiospasm
Achalasia (of cardia)
Aperistalsis of esophagus
Megaesophagus

Excludes: *congenital cardiospasm (750.7)*

⑤ **530.1 Esophagitis**
Abscess of esophagus
Esophagitis:
  NOS
  chemical
  peptic
Esophagitis:
  postoperative
  regurgitant

Use additional E code, if desired, to identify cause, if induced by chemical

Excludes: *tuberculous esophagitis (017.8)*

530.10 Esophagitis, unspecified

530.11 Reflux esophagitis

530.12 Acute esophagitis

530.19 Other esophagitis

530.2 Ulcer of esophagus
Ulcer of esophagus
  fungal
  peptic
Ulcer of esophagus due to ingestion of:
  aspirin
  chemicals
  medicines

Use additional E code, if desired, to identify cause, if induced by chemical or drug

530.3 Stricture and stenosis of esophagus
Compression of esophagus
Obstruction of esophagus

Excludes: *congenital stricture of esophagus (750.3)*

530.4 Perforation of esophagus
Rupture of esophagus

Excludes: *traumatic perforation of esophagus (862.22, 862.32, 874.4-874.5)*

530.5 Dyskinesia of esophagus
Corkscrew esophagus
Curling esophagus
Esophagospasm
Spasm of esophagus

Excludes: *cardiospasm (530.0)*

530.6 Diverticulum of esophagus, acquired
Diverticulum, acquired:
  epiphrenic
  pharyngoesophageal
  pulsion
  subdiaphragmatic
  traction
  Zenker's (hypopharyngeal)
Esophageal pouch, acquired
Esophagocele, acquired

Excludes: *congenital diverticulum of esophagus (750.4)*

530.7 Gastroesophageal laceration-hemorrhage syndrome
Mallory-Weiss syndrome

⑤ **530.8 Other specified disorders of esophagus**

530.81 Esophageal reflux
Gastroesophageal reflux

Excludes: *reflux esophagitis (530.11)*

530.82 Esophageal hemorrhage

Excludes: *hemorrhage due to esophageal varices (456.0-456.2)*

530.83 Esophageal leukoplakia

530.84 Tracheoesophageal fistula

Excludes: *congenital tracheoesophageal fistula (750.3)*

530.89 Other

Excludes: *Paterson-Kelly syndrome (280.8)*

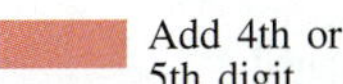
Add 4th or
5th digit

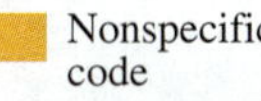
Nonspecific
code

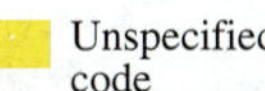
Unspecified
code

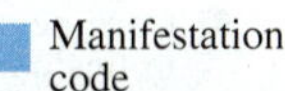
Manifestation
code

530.9 Unspecified disorder of esophagus

⑤ **531 Gastric ulcer**
Includes: ulcer (peptic):
             prepyloric
             pylorus
             stomach

Use additional E code, if desired, to identify drug, if drug-induced

| Excludes: | peptic ulcer NOS (533.0-533.9)

The following fifth-digit subclassification is for use with category 531:

0 without mention of obstruction

1 with obstruction

⑤ **531.0 Acute with hemorrhage**

⑤ **531.1 Acute with perforation**

⑤ **531.2 Acute with hemorrhage and perforation**

⑤ **531.3 Acute without mention of hemorrhage or perforation**

⑤ **531.4 Chronic or unspecified with hemorrhage**

⑤ **531.5 Chronic or unspecified with perforation**

⑤ **531.6 Chronic or unspecified with hemorrhage and perforation**

⑤ **531.7 Chronic without mention of hemorrhage or perforation**

⑤ **531.9 Unspecified as acute or chronic, without mention of hemorrhage or perforation**

⑤ **532 Duodenal ulcer**
Includes: erosion (acute) of duodenum
             ulcer (peptic):
               duodenum
               postpyloric

Use additional E code, if desired, to identify drug, if drug-induced

| Excludes: | peptic ulcer NOS (533.0-533.9)

The following fifth-digit subclassification is for use with category 532:

0 without mention of obstruction

1 with obstruction

⑤ **532.0 Acute with hemorrhage**

⑤ **532.1 Acute with perforation**

⑤ **532.2 Acute with hemorrhage and perforation**

⑤ **532.3 Acute without mention of hemorrhage or perforation**

⑤ **532.4 Chronic or unspecified with hemorrhage**

⑤ **532.5 Chronic or unspecified with perforation**

⑤ **532.6 Chronic or unspecified with hemorrhage and perforation**

⑤ **532.7 Chronic without mention of hemorrhage or perforation**

⑤ **532.9 Unspecified as acute or chronic, without mention of hemorrhage or perforation**

⑤ **533 Peptic ulcer, site unspecified**
Includes: gastroduodenal ulcer NOS
             peptic ulcer NOS
             stress ulcer NOS

Use additional E code, if desired, to identify drug, if drug-induced

| Excludes: | peptic ulcer:
               duodenal (532.0-532.9)
               gastric (531.0-531.9)

The following fifth-digit subclassification is for use with category 533:

0 without mention of obstruction

1 with obstruction

⑤ **533.0 Acute with hemorrhage**

⑤ **533.1 Acute with perforation**

⑤ **533.2 Acute with hemorrhage and perforation**

⑤ **533.3 Acute without mention of hemorrhage and perforation**

⑤ **533.4 Chronic or unspecified with hemorrhage**

⑤ **533.5 Chronic or unspecified with perforation**

● Code new   ▲ Revision of   ④ ⑤ Fourth or fifth
to this edition   existing code   digit required

⑤ **533.6 Chronic or unspecified with hemorrhage and perforation**

⑤ **533.7 Chronic without mention of hemorrhage or perforation**

⑤ **533.9 Unspecified as acute or chronic, without mention of hemorrhage or perforation**

⑤ **534 Gastrojejunal ulcer**

Includes: ulcer (peptic) or erosion:
      anastomotic
      gastrocolic
      gastrointestinal
      gastrojejunal
      jejunal
      marginal
      stomal

Excludes: primary ulcer of small intestine (569.82)

The following fifth-digit subclassification is for use with category 534:

   0   without mention of obstruction

   1   with obstruction

⑤ **534.0 Acute with hemorrhage**

⑤ **534.1 Acute with perforation**

⑤ **534.2 Acute with hemorrhage and perforation**

⑤ **534.3 Acute without mention of hemorrhage or perforation**

⑤ **534.4 Chronic or unspecified with hemorrhage**

⑤ **534.5 Chronic or unspecified with perforation**

⑤ **534.6 Chronic or unspecified with hemorrhage and perforation**

⑤ **534.7 Chronic without mention of hemorrhage or perforation**

⑤ **534.9 Unspecified as acute or chronic, without mention of hemorrhage or perforation**

⑤ **535 Gastritis and duodenitis**

The following fifth-digit subclassification is for use with category 535

   0   without mention of hemorrhage

   1   with hemorrhage

⑤ **535.0 Acute gastritis**

⑤ **535.1 Atrophic gastritis**

Gastritis:
  atrophic-hyperplastic
  chronic (atrophic)

⑤ **535.2 Gastric mucosal hypertrophy**

Hypertrophic gastritis

⑤ **535.3 Alcoholic gastritis**

⑤ **535.4 Other specified gastritis**

Gastritis: Gastritis:
  allergic   superficial
  bile induced   toxic
  irritant

⑤ **535.5 Unspecified gastritis and gastroduodenitis**

⑤ **535.6 Duodenitis**

536 Disorders of function of stomach

Excludes: functional disorders of stomach specified as psychogenic (306.4)

536.0 Achlorhydria

536.1 Acute dilatation of stomach

Acute distention of stomach

536.2 Persistent vomiting

Habit vomiting
Persistent vomiting [not of pregnancy]
Uncontrollable vomiting

Excludes: excessive vomiting in pregnancy (643.0-643.9)
         vomiting NOS (787.0)

536.3 Gastroparesis

⑤ **536.4 Gastrostomy complications**

536.40   Gastrostomy complications, unspecified

536.41 Infection of gastrostomy
Use additional code to specify type of infection, such as:
abscess or cellulitis of abdomen (682.2)
septicemia (038.0-038.9)
Use additional code to identify organism (041.00-041.9)

536.42 Mechanical complication of gastrostomy

536.49 Other gastrostomy complications

536.8 Dyspepsia and other specified disorders of function of stomach
Achylia gastrica   Hyperchlorhydria
Hourglass contraction of stomach   Hypochlorhydria
Hyperacidity   Indigestion

Excludes: achlorhydria (536.0)
heartburn (787.1)

536.9 Unspecified functional disorder of stomach
Functional gastrointestinal:
disorder
disturbance
irritation

537 **Other disorders of stomach and duodenum**

537.0 Acquired hypertrophic pyloric stenosis
Constriction
Obstruction   } of pylorus, acquired or adult
Stricture

Excludes: congenital or infantile pyloric stenosis (750.5)

537.1 Gastric diverticulum

Excludes: congenital diverticulum of stomach (750.7)

537.2 Chronic duodenal ileus

537.3 Other obstruction of duodenum
Cicatrix
Stenosis   } of duodenum
Stricture
Volvulus

Excludes: congenital obstruction of duodenum (751.1)

537.4 Fistula of stomach or duodenum
Gastrocolic fistula
Gastrojejunocolic fistula

537.5 Gastroptosis

537.6 Hourglass stricture or stenosis of stomach
Cascade stomach

Excludes: congenital hourglass stomach (750.7)
hourglass contraction of stomach (536.8)

⑤ **537.8 Other specified disorders of stomach and duodenum**

537.81 Pylorospasm

Excludes: congenital pylorospasm (750.5)

537.82 Angiodysplasia of stomach and duodenum without mention of hemorrhage

537.83 Angiodysplasia of stomach and duodenum with hemorrhage

● **537.84 Dieulafoy lesion (hemorrhagic) of stomach and duodenum**

537.89 Other
Gastric or duodenal:
prolapse
rupture
Intestinal metaplasia of gastric mucosa
Passive congestion of stomach

Excludes: diverticula of duodenum (562.00-562.01)
gastrointestinal hemorrhage (578.0-578.9)

537.9 Unspecified disorder of stomach and duodenum

● Code new   ▲ Revision of   ④ ⑤ Fourth or fifth
to this edition   existing code   digit required

APPENDICITIS (540-543)

540 **Acute appendicitis**

540.0 **With generalized peritonitis**

Appendicitis (acute):
  fulminating
  gangrenous
  obstructive
Cecitis (acute)
Rupture of appendix

} with: perforation peritonitis (generalized) rupture

Excludes: *acute appendicitis with peritoneal abscess (540.1)*

540.1 **With peritoneal abscess**

Abscess of appendix
With generalized peritonitis

540.9 **Without mention of peritonitis**

Acute:
  appendicitis:
    fulminating
    gangrenous
    inflamed
    obstructive
  cecitis

} without mention of perforation, peritonitis, or rupture

541 **Appendicitis, unqualified**

542 **Other appendicitis**

Appendicitis:
  chronic
  recurrent

Appendicitis:
  relapsing
  subacute

Excludes: *hyperplasia (lymphoid) of appendix (543.0)*

543 **Other diseases of appendix**

543.0 **Hyperplasia of appendix (lymphoid)**

543.9 **Other and unspecified diseases of appendix**

Appendicular or appendiceal:
  colic
  concretion
  fistula
Diverticulum
Fecalith
Intussusception
Mucocele
Stercolith

} of appendix

HERNIA OF ABDOMINAL CAVITY (550-553)

Includes: hernia:
    acquired
    congenital, except diaphragmatic or hiatal

⑤ **550** **Inguinal hernia**

Includes: bubonocele
    inguinal hernia (direct) (double) (indirect) (oblique) (sliding)
    scrotal hernia

The following fifth-digit subclassification is for use with category 550:

0 **unilateral or unspecified (not specified as recurrent)**
Unilateral NOS

1 **unilateral or unspecified, recurrent**

2 **bilateral (not specified as recurrent)**
Bilateral NOS

3 **bilateral, recurrent**

⑤ **550.0** **Inguinal hernia, with gangrene**
Inguinal hernia with gangrene (and obstruction)

⑤ **550.1** **Inguinal hernia, with obstruction, without mention of gangrene**
Inguinal hernia with mention of incarceration, irreducibility, or strangulation

⑤ **550.9** **Inguinal hernia, without mention of obstruction or gangrene**
Inguinal hernia NOS

551 **Other hernia of abdominal cavity, with gangrene**
Includes: that with gangrene (and obstruction)

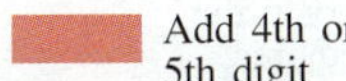

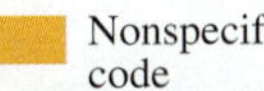

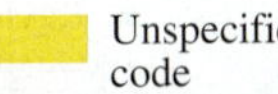

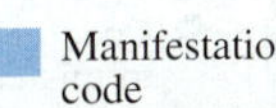

⑤ **551.0 Femoral hernia with gangrene**

    551.00 Unilateral or unspecified (not specified as recurrent)
        Femoral hernia NOS with gangrene

    551.01 Unilateral or unspecified, recurrent

    551.02 Bilateral (not specified as recurrent)

    551.03 Bilateral, recurrent

551.1 Umbilical hernia with gangrene
    Parumbilical hernia specified as gangrenous

⑤ **551.2 Ventral hernia with gangrene**

    551.20 Ventral, unspecified, with gangrene

    551.21 Incisional, with gangrene
        Hernia:
          postoperative   } specified as gangrenous
          recurrent, ventral

    551.29 Other
        Epigastric hernia specified as gangrenous

551.3 Diaphragmatic hernia with gangrene
    Hernia:
      hiatal (esophageal) (sliding)   } specified as gangrenous
      paraesophageal
    Thoracic stomach

    Excludes: *congenital diaphragmatic hernia (756.6)*

551.8 Hernia of other specified sites, with gangrene
    Any condition classifiable to 553.8 if specified as gangrenous

551.9 Hernia of unspecified site, with gangrene
    Any condition classifiable to 553.9 if specified as gangrenous

552 Other hernia of abdominal cavity, with obstruction, but without mention of gangrene

    Excludes: *that with mention of gangrene (551.0-551.9)*

⑤ **552.0 Femoral hernia with obstruction**
    Femoral hernia specified as incarcerated, irreducible, strangulated, or causing obstruction

    552.00 Unilateral or unspecified (not specified as recurrent)

    552.01 Unilateral or unspecified, recurrent

    552.02 Bilateral (not specified as recurrent)

    552.03 Bilateral, recurrent

552.1 Umbilical hernia with obstruction
    Parumbilical hernia specified as incarcerated, irreducible, strangulated, or causing
      obstruction

⑤ **552.2 Ventral hernia with obstruction**
    Ventral hernia specified as incarcerated, irreducible, strangulated, or causing obstruction

    552.20 Ventral, unspecified, with obstruction

    552.21 Incisional, with obstruction
        Hernia:
          postoperative   } specified as incarcerated, irreducible, strangulated, or
          recurrent, ventral   causing obstruction

    552.29 Other
        Epigastric hernia specified as incarcerated, irreducible, strangulated, or causing
        obstruction

552.3 Diaphragmatic hernia with obstruction
    Hernia:
      hiatal (esophageal) (sliding)   } specified as incarcerated,
      paraesophageal   irreducible, strangulated, or
    Thoracic stomach   causing obstruction

    Excludes: *congenital diaphragmatic hernia (756.6)*

552.8 Hernia of other specified sites, with obstruction
    Any condition classifiable to 553.8 if specified as incarcerated, irreducible, strangulated,
      or causing obstruction

552.9 Hernia of unspecified site, with obstruction
    Any condition classifiable to 553.9 if specified as incarcerated, irreducible, strangulated,
      or causing obstruction

● Code new   ▲ Revision of   ④ ⑤ Fourth or fifth
   to this edition   existing code   digit required

553 **Other hernia of abdominal cavity without mention of obstruction or gangrene**

Excludes: *the listed conditions with mention of:*
gangrene (and obstruction) (551.0-551.9)
obstruction (552.0-552.9)

⑤ **553.0** **Femoral hernia**

553.00 **Unilateral or unspecified (not specified as recurrent)**
Femoral hernia NOS

553.01 **Unilateral or unspecified, recurrent**

553.02 **Bilateral (not specified as recurrent)**

553.03 **Bilateral, recurrent**

553.1 **Umbilical hernia**
Parumbilical hernia

⑤ **553.2** **Ventral hernia**

553.20 **Ventral, unspecified**

553.21 **Incisional**
Hernia:
postoperative
recurrent, ventral

553.29 **Other**
Hernia:
epigastric
spigelian

553.3 **Diaphragmatic hernia**
Hernia:
hiatal (esophageal) (sliding)
paraesophageal
Thoracic stomach

Excludes: *congenital:*

diaphragmatic hernia (756.6)
hiatal hernia (750.6)
esophagocele (530.6)

553.8 **Hernia of other specified sites**
Hernia:
ischiatic
ischiorectal
lumbar
obturator
pudendal

Hernia:
retroperitoneal
sciatic
Other abdominal hernia of specified site

Excludes: *vaginal enterocele (618.6)*

553.9 **Hernia of unspecified site**
Enterocele
Epiplocele
Hernia:
NOS
interstitial

Hernia:
intestinal
intra-abdominal
Rupture (nontraumatic)
Sarcoepiplocele

NONINFECTIOUS ENTERITIS AND COLITIS (555-558)

555 **Regional enteritis**
Includes: Crohn's disease
Granulomatous enteritis

Excludes: *ulcerative colitis (556)*

555.0 **Small intestine**
Ileitis:
regional
segmental
terminal

Regional enteritis or Crohn's disease of:
duodenum
ileum
jejunum

555.1 **Large intestine**
Colitis:
granulomatous
regional
transmural

Regional enteritis or Crohn's disease of:
colon
large bowel
rectum

555.2 **Small intestine with large intestine**
Regional ileocolitis

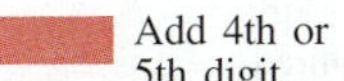

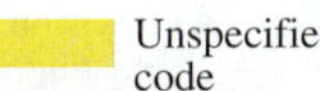

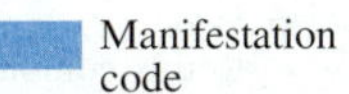

Manifestation
code

555.9 Unspecified site
  Crohn's disease NOS
  Regional enteritis NOS

556 Ulcerative colitis

556.0 Ulcerative (chronic) enterocolitis

556.1 Ulcerative (chronic) ileocolitis

556.2 Ulcerative (chronic) proctitis

556.3 Ulcerative (chronic) proctosigmoiditis

556.4 Pseudopolyposis of colon

556.5 Left-sided ulcerative (chronic) colitis

556.6 Universal ulcerative (chronic) colitis
  Pancolitis

556.8 Other ulcerative colitis

556.9 Ulcerative colitis, unspecified
  Ulcerative enteritis NOS

557 Vascular insufficiency of intestine

> **Excludes:** *necrotizing enterocolitis of the newborn (777.5)*

557.0 Acute vascular insufficiency of intestine
  Acute:
    hemorrhagic enterocolitis
    ischemic colitis, enteritis, or enterocolitis
    massive necrosis of intestine
  Bowel infarction
  Embolism of mesenteric artery
  Fulminant enterocolitis
  Hemorrhagic necrosis of intestine
  Infarction of appendices epiploicae
  Intestinal gangrene
  Intestinal infarction (acute) (agnogenic) (hemorrhagic) (nonocclusive)
  Mesenteric infarction (embolic) (thrombotic)
  Necrosis of intestine
  Terminal hemorrhagic enteropathy
  Thrombosis of mesenteric artery

557.1 Chronic vascular insufficiency of intestine
  Angina, abdominal
  Chronic ischemic colitis, enteritis, or enterocolitis
  Ischemic stricture of intestine
  Mesenteric:
    angina
    artery syndrome (superior)
    vascular insufficiency

557.9 Unspecified vascular insufficiency of intestine
  Alimentary pain due to vascular insufficiency
  Ischemic colitis, enteritis, or enterocolitis NOS

558 Other and unspecified noninfectious gastroenteritis and colitis

> **Excludes:** *infectious:*
>   *colitis, enteritis, or gastroenteritis (009.0-009.1)*
>   *diarrhea (009.2-009.3)*

558.1 Gastroenteritis and colitis due to radiation
  Radiation enterocolitis

558.2 Toxic gastroenteritis and colitis
Use additional E code, if desired, to identify cause

558.3 Allergic gastroenteritis and colitis

558.9 Other and unspecified noninfectious gastroenteritis and colitis
  Colitis NOS, dietetic, or noninfectious
  Enteritis NOS, dietetic, or noninfectious
  Gastroenteritis NOS, dietetic, or noninfectious
  Ileitis NOS, dietetic, or noninfectious
  Jejunitis NOS, dietetic, or noninfectious
  Sigmoiditis NOS, dietetic, or noninfectious

● Code new
  to this edition   ▲ Revision of
  existing code   ④ ⑤ Fourth or fifth
  digit required

OTHER DISEASES OF INTESTINES AND PERITONEUM (560-569)

560 Intestinal obstruction without mention of hernia

Excludes: duodenum (537.2-537.3)
inguinal hernia with obstruction (550.1)
intestinal obstruction complicating hernia (552.0-552.9)
mesenteric:
  embolism (557.0)
  infarction (557.0)
  thrombosis (557.0)
neonatal intestinal obstruction (277.01, 777.1-777.2, 777.4)

560.0 Intussusception
Intussusception (colon) (intestine) (rectum)
Invagination of intestine or colon

Excludes: intussusception of appendix (543.9)

560.1 Paralytic ileus
Adynamic ileus
Ileus (of intestine) (of bowel) (of colon)
Paralysis of intestine or colon

Excludes: gallstone ileus (560.31)

560.2 Volvulus
Knotting
Strangulation } of intestine, bowel, or colon
Torsion
Twist

⑤ **560.3 Impaction of intestine**

560.30 Impaction of intestine, unspecified
Impaction of colon

560.31 Gallstone ileus
Obstruction of intestine by gallstone

560.39 Other
Concretion of intestine
Enterolith
Fecal impaction

⑤ **560.8 Other specified intestinal obstruction**

560.81 Intestinal or peritoneal adhesions with obstruction (postoperative) (postinfection)

Excludes: adhesions without obstruction (568.0)

560.89 Other
Mural thickening causing obstruction

Excludes: ischemic stricture of intestine (557.1)

560.9 Unspecified intestinal obstruction
Enterostenosis
Obstruction
Occlusion } of intestine or colon
Stenosis
Stricture

Excludes: congenital stricture or stenosis of intestine (751.1-751.2)

562 Diverticula of intestine
Use additional code, if desired, to identify any associated:
peritonitis (567.0-567.9)

Excludes: congenital diverticulum of colon (751.5)
diverticulum of appendix (543.9)
Meckel's diverticulum (751.0)

⑤ **562.0 Small intestine**

562.00 Diverticulosis of small intestine (without mention of hemorrhage)
Diverticulosis:
  duodenum
  ileum } without mention of diverticulitis
  jejunum

562.01 Diverticulitis of small intestine (without mention of hemorrhage)
Diverticulitis (with diverticulosis):
duodenum
ileum
jejunum
small intestine

562.02 Diverticulosis of small intestine with hemorrhage

562.03 Diverticulitis of small intestine with hemorrhage

⑤ **562.1 Colon**

562.10 Diverticulosis of colon (without mention of hemorrhage)
Diverticulosis:
NOS
intestine (large) } without mention of diverticulitis
Diverticular disease (colon)

562.11 Diverticulitis of colon (without mention of hemorrhage)
Diverticulitis (with diverticulosis):
NOS
colon
intestine (large)

562.12 Diverticulosis of colon with hemorrhage

562.13 Diverticulitis of colon with hemorrhage

564 Functional digestive disorders, not elsewhere classified

Excludes: *functional disorders of stomach (536.0-536.9)*
those specified as psychogenic (306.4)

⑤ **564.0 Constipation**

564.00 Constipation, unspecified

564.01 Slow transit constipation

564.02 Outlet dysfunction constipation

564.09 Other constipation

564.1 Irritable bowel syndrome
Irritable colon   Spastic colon

564.2 Postgastric surgery syndromes
Dumping syndrome   Postgastrectomy syndrome
Jejunal syndrome   Postvagotomy syndrome

Excludes: *malnutrition following gastrointestinal surgery (579.3)*
postgastrojejunostomy ulcer (534.0-534.9)

564.3 Vomiting following gastrointestinal surgery
Vomiting (bilious) following gastrointestinal surgery

564.4 Other postoperative functional disorders
Diarrhea following gastrointestinal surgery

Excludes: *colostomy and enterostomy complications (569.60-569.69)*

564.5 Functional diarrhea

Excludes: *diarrhea:*
NOS (787.91)
psychogenic (306.4)

564.6 Anal spasm
Proctalgia fugax

564.7 Megacolon, other than Hirschsprung's
Dilatation of colon

Excludes: *megacolon:*
congenital [Hirschsprung's] (751.3)
toxic (556)

⑤ **564.8 Other specified functional disorders of intestine**

Excludes: *malabsorption (579.0-579.9)*

564.81 Neurogenic bowel

564.89 Other functional disorders of intestine
Atony of colon

564.9 Unspecified functional disorder of intestine

● Code new
to this edition

▲ Revision of
existing code

④ ⑤ Fourth or fifth
digit required

565 Anal fissure and fistula

565.0 Anal fissure
Tear of anus, nontraumatic

| Excludes: | traumatic (863.89, 863.99) |

565.1 Anal fistula
Fistula:
anorectal
rectal
rectum to skin

Excludes:	fistula of rectum to internal organs—see Alphabetic Index
	ischiorectal fistula (566)
	rectovaginal fistula (619.1)

566 Abscess of anal and rectal regions

Abscess:
ischiorectal
perianal
perirectal

Cellulitis:
anal
perirectal
rectal
Ischiorectal fistula

567 Peritonitis

| Excludes: | peritonitis: |

benign paroxysmal (277.3)
pelvic, female (614.5, 614.7)
periodic familial (277.3)
puerperal (670)
with or following:
abortion (634-638 with .0, 639.0)
appendicitis (540.0-540.1)
ectopic or molar pregnancy (639.0)

567.0 Peritonitis in infectious diseases classified elsewhere
Code first underlying disease

| Excludes: | peritonitis: |

gonococcal (098.86)
syphilitic (095.2)
tuberculous (014.0)

567.1 Pneumococcal peritonitis

567.2 Other suppurative peritonitis

Abscess (of):
abdominopelvic
mesenteric
omentum
peritoneum
retrocecal
retroperitoneal
subdiaphragmatic

Abscess (of):
subhepatic
subphrenic
Peritonitis (acute):
general
pelvic, male
subphrenic
suppurative

567.8 Other specified peritonitis
Chronic proliferative peritonitis
Fat necrosis of peritoneum
Mesenteric saponification
Peritonitis due to:
bile
urine

567.9 Unspecified peritonitis
Peritonitis:
NOS
of unspecified cause

| Add 4th or 5th digit | Nonspecific code | Unspecified code | Manifestation code |

568 **Other disorders of peritoneum**

    568.0 **Peritoneal adhesions (postoperative) (postinfection)**

Adhesions (of):	Adhesions (of):
abdominal (wall)	mesenteric
diaphragm	omentum
intestine	stomach
male pelvis	Adhesive bands

        | *Excludes:* | *adhesions:* |

           pelvic, female (614.6)
           with obstruction:
             duodenum (537.3)
             intestine (560.81)

⑤ **568.8** **Other specified disorders of peritoneum**

      568.81 **Hemoperitoneum (nontraumatic)**

      568.82 **Peritoneal effusion (chronic)**

    | *Excludes:* | *ascites NOS (789.5)* |

      568.89 **Other**

        Peritoneal:
          cyst
          granuloma

    568.9 **Unspecified disorder of peritoneum**

569 **Other disorders of intestine**

    569.0 **Anal and rectal polyp**

      Anal and rectal polyp NOS

    | *Excludes:* | *adenomatous anal and rectal polyp (211.4)* |

    569.1 **Rectal prolapse**

Procidentia:	Prolapse:
anus (sphincter)	anal canal
rectum (sphincter)	rectal mucosa
Proctoptosis	

    | *Excludes:* | *prolapsed hemorrhoids (455.2, 455.5)* |

    569.2 **Stenosis of rectum and anus**

      Stricture of anus (sphincter)

    569.3 **Hemorrhage of rectum and anus**

    | *Excludes:* | *gastrointestinal bleeding NOS (578.9)* |

          melena (578.1)

⑤ **569.4** **Other specified disorders of rectum and anus**

      569.41 **Ulcer of anus and rectum**

        Solitary ulcer ⎫
        Stercoral ulcer ⎬ of anus (sphincter) or rectum (sphincter)

      569.42 **Anal or rectal pain**

      569.49 **Other**

        Granuloma ⎫
        Rupture ⎬ of rectum (sphincter)

        Hypertrophy of anal papillae
        Proctitis NOS

    | *Excludes:* | *fistula of rectum to:* |

        internal organs—see Alphabetic Index
        skin (565.1)
        hemorrhoids (455.0-455.9)
        incontinence of sphincter ani (787.6)

    569.5 **Abscess of intestine**

    | *Excludes:* | *appendiceal abscess (540.1)* |

⑤ **569.6** **Colostomy and enterostomy complications**

      569.60 **Colostomy and enterostomy complication, unspecified**

● Code new   ▲ Revision of   ④ ⑤ Fourth or fifth
   to this edition   existing code   digit required

569.61 **Infection of colostomy or enterostomy**
Use additional code to specify type of infection, such as:
abscess or cellulitis of abdomen (682.2)
septicemia (038.0-038.9)
Use additional code to identify organism (041.00-041.9)

569.62 **Mechanical complication of colostomy and enterostomy**
Malfunction of colostomy and enterostomy

569.69 **Other complication**
Fistula
Hernia
Prolapse

⑤ **569.8** **Other specified disorders of intestine**

569.81 **Fistula of intestine, excluding rectum and anus**
Fistula: Fistula:
abdominal wall   enteroenteric
enterocolic   ileorectal

Excludes: *fistula of intestine to internal organs —see Alphabetic Index*
persistent postoperative fistula (998.6)

569.82 **Ulceration of intestine**
Primary ulcer of intestine
Ulceration of colon

Excludes: *that with perforation (569.83)*

569.83 **Perforation of intestine**

569.84 **Angiodysplasia of intestine (without mention of hemorrhage)**

569.85 **Angiodysplasia of intestine with hemorrhage**

● **569.86** **Dieulafoy lesion (hemorrhagic) of intestine**

569.89 **Other**
Enteroptosis
Granuloma
Prolapse   } of intestine
Pericolitis
Perisigmoiditis
Visceroptosis

Excludes: *gangrene of intestine, mesentery, or omentum (557.0)*
hemorrhage of intestine NOS (578.9)
obstruction of intestine (560.0-560.9)

569.9 **Unspecified disorder of intestine**

OTHER DISEASES OF DIGESTIVE SYSTEM (570-579)

570 **Acute and subacute necrosis of liver**
Acute hepatic failure
Acute or subacute hepatitis, not specified as infective
Necrosis of liver (acute) (diffuse) (massive) (subacute)
Parenchymatous degeneration of liver
Yellow atrophy (liver) (acute) (subacute)

Excludes: *icterus gravis of newborn (773.0-773.2)*
serum hepatitis (070.2-070.3)
that with:
abortion (634-638 with .7, 639.8)
ectopic or molar pregnancy (639.8)
pregnancy, childbirth, or the puerperium (646.7)
viral hepatitis (070.0-070.9)

571 **Chronic liver disease and cirrhosis**

571.0 **Alcoholic fatty liver**

571.1 **Acute alcoholic hepatitis**
Acute alcoholic liver disease

571.2 **Alcoholic cirrhosis of liver**
Florid cirrhosis
Laennec's cirrhosis (alcoholic)

571.3 **Alcoholic liver damage, unspecified**

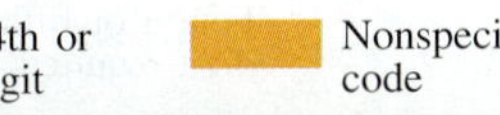

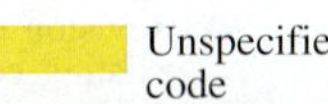

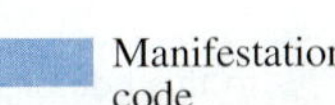

Manifestation
code

⑤ **571.4 Chronic hepatitis**

Excludes: *viral hepatitis (acute) (chronic) (070.0-070.9)*

571.40 Chronic hepatitis, unspecified

571.41 Chronic persistent hepatitis

571.49 Other
Chronic hepatitis:
active
aggressive
Recurrent hepatitis

571.5 Cirrhosis of liver without mention of alcohol
Cirrhosis of liver: Cirrhosis of liver:
NOS   posthepatitic
cryptogenic   postnecrotic
macronodular   Healed yellow atrophy (liver)
micronodular   Portal cirrhosis

571.6 Biliary cirrhosis
Chronic nonsuppurative destructive cholangitis
Cirrhosis:
cholangitic
cholestatic

571.8 Other chronic nonalcoholic liver disease
Chronic yellow atrophy (liver)
Fatty liver, without mention of alcohol

571.9 Unspecified chronic liver disease without mention of alcohol

572 Liver abscess and sequelae of chronic liver disease

572.0 Abscess of liver

Excludes: *amebic liver abscess (006.3)*

572.1 Portal pyemia
Phlebitis of portal vein   Pylephlebitis
Portal thrombophlebitis   Pylethrombophlebitis

572.2 Hepatic coma
Hepatic encephalopathy
Hepatocerebral intoxication
Portal-systemic encephalopathy

572.3 Portal hypertension

572.4 Hepatorenal syndrome

Excludes: *that following delivery (674.8)*

572.8 Other sequelae of chronic liver disease

573 Other disorders of liver

Excludes: *amyloid or lardaceous degeneration of liver (277.3)*
congenital cystic disease of liver (751.62)
glycogen infiltration of liver (271.0)
hepatomegaly NOS (789.1)
portal vein obstruction (452)

573.0 Chronic passive congestion of liver

573.1 *Hepatitis in viral diseases classified elsewhere*
Code first underlying disease as:
Coxsackie virus disease (074.8)
cytomegalic inclusion virus disease (078.5)
infectious mononucleosis (075)

Excludes: *hepatitis (in):*
mumps (072.71)
viral (070.0-070.9)
yellow fever (060.0-060.9)

● Code new   ▲ Revision of   ④ ⑤ Fourth or fifth
to this edition   existing code   digit required

573.2 *Hepatitis in other infectious diseases classified elsewhere*
Code first underlying disease, as:
malaria (084.9)

Excludes: *hepatitis in:*
late syphilis (095.3)
secondary syphilis (091.62)
toxoplasmosis (130.5)

573.3 Hepatitis, unspecified
Toxic (noninfectious) hepatitis

Use additional E code, if desired, to identify cause

573.4 Hepatic infarction

573.8 Other specified disorders of liver
Hepatoptosis

573.9 Unspecified disorder of liver

⑤ **574 Cholelithiasis**

The following fifth-digit subclassification is for use with category 574:

0 without mention of obstruction

1 with obstruction

⑤ **574.0 Calculus of gallbladder with acute cholecystitis**
Biliary calculus
Calculus of cystic } with acute cholecystitis
   duct
Cholelithiasis
Any condition classifiable to 574.2 with acute cholecystitis

⑤ **574.1 Calculus of gallbladder with other cholecystitis**
Biliary calculus
Calculus of cystic } with cholecystitis
   duct
Cholelithiasis
Cholecystitis with cholelithiasis NOS
Any condition classifiable to 574.2 with cholecystitis (chronic)

⑤ **574.2 Calculus of gallbladder without mention of cholecystitis**
Biliary: Cholelithiasis NOS
   calculus NOS   Colic (recurrent) of gallbladder
   colic NOS   Gallstone (impacted)
Calculus of cystic duct

⑤ **574.3 Calculus of bile duct with acute cholecystitis**
Calculus of bile } with acute cholecystitis
   duct [any]
Choledocholithiasis
Any condition classifiable to 574.5 with acute cholecystitis

⑤ **574.4 Calculus of bile duct with other cholecystitis**
Calculus of bile } with cholecystitis (chronic)
   duct [any]
Choledocholithiasis
Any condition classifiable to 574.5 with cholecystitis (chronic)

⑤ **574.5 Calculus of bile duct without mention of cholecystitis**
Calculus of: Choledocholithiasis
   bile duct [any]   Hepatic:
   common duct   colic (recurrent)
   hepatic duct   lithiasis

⑤ **574.6 Calculus of gallbladder and bile duct with acute cholecystitis**
Any condition classifiable to 574.0 and 574.3

⑥ **574.7 Calculus of gallbladder and bile duct with other cholecystitis**
Any condition classifiable to 574.1 and 574.4

⑤ **574.8 Calculus of gallbladder and bile duct with acute and chronic cholecystitis**
Any condition classifiable to 574.6 and 574.7

⑤ **574.9 Calculus of gallbladder and bile duct without cholecystitis**
Any condition classifiable to 574.2 and 574.5

Add 4th or 5th digit   Nonspecific code   Unspecified code   Manifestation code

575 **Other disorders of gallbladder**

575.0 **Acute cholecystitis**
Abscess of gallbladder
Angiocholecystitis
Cholecystitis:
  emphysematous (acute)
  gangrenous
  suppurative
Empyema of gallbladder
Gangrene of gallbladder
} without mention of calculus

Excludes: *that with:*
   acute and chronic cholecystitis (575.12)
   choledocholithiasis (574.3)
   choledocholithiasis and cholelithiasis (574.6)
   cholelithiasis (574.0)

⑤ **575.1** **Other cholecystitis**
Cholecystitis:
  NOS
  chronic
} without mention of calculus

Excludes: *that with:*
   choledocholithiasis (574.4)
   choledocholithiasis and cholelithiasis (574.8)
   cholelithiasis (574.1)

575.10 **Cholecystitis, unspecified**
Cholecystitis NOS

575.11 **Chronic cholecystitis**

575.12 **Acute and chronic cholecystits**

575.2 **Obstruction of gallbladder**
Occlusion
Stenosis
Stricture
} of cystic duct or gallbladder without mention of calculus

Excludes: *that with calculus (574.0-574.2 with fifth-digit 1)*

575.3 **Hydrops of gallbladder**
Mucocele of gallbladder

575.4 **Perforation of gallbladder**
Rupture of cystic duct or gallbladder

575.5 **Fistula of gallbladder**
Fistula:
  cholecystoduodenal
  cholecystoenteric

575.6 **Cholesterolosis of gallbladder**
Strawberry gallbladder

575.8 **Other specified disorders of gallbladder**
Adhesions
Atrophy
Cyst
Hypertrophy
Nonfunctioning
Ulcer
Biliary dyskinesia
} (of) { cystic duct / gallbladder

Excludes: *nonvisualization of gallbladder (793.3)*
   Hartmann's pouch of intestine (V44.3)

575.9 **Unspecified disorder of gallbladder**

576 **Other disorders of biliary tract**

Excludes: *that involving the:*
   cystic duct (575.0-575.9)
   gallbladder (575.0-575.9)

576.0 **Postcholecystectomy syndrome**

● Code new
  to this edition

▲ Revision of
  existing code

④ ⑤ Fourth or fifth
  digit required

576.1 Cholangitis

Cholangitis:
 NOS
 acute
 ascending
 chronic
 primary

Cholangitis:
 recurrent
 sclerosing
 secondary
 stenosing
 suppurative

576.2 Obstruction of bile duct

Occlusion
Stenosis
Stricture
} of bile duct, except cystic duct, without mention of calculus

Excludes: *congenital (751.61)*
 that with calculus (574.3-574.5 with fifth-digit 1)

576.3 Perforation of bile duct

Rupture of bile duct, except cystic duct

576.4 Fistula of bile duct

Choledochoduodenal fistula

576.5 Spasm of sphincter of Oddi

576.8 Other specified disorders of biliary tract

Adhesions
Atrophy
Cyst
Hypertrophy
Stasis
Ulcer
} of bile duct [any]

Excludes: *congenital choledochal cyst (751.69)*

576.9 Unspecified disorder of biliary tract

577 Diseases of pancreas

577.0 Acute pancreatitis

Abscess of pancreas
Necrosis of pancreas:
 acute
 infective

Pancreatitis:
 NOS
 acute (recurrent)
 apoplectic
 hemorrhagic
 subacute
 suppurative

Excludes: *mumps pancreatitis (072.3)*

577.1 Chronic pancreatitis

Chronic pancreatitis:
 NOS
 infectious
 interstitial

Pancreatitis:
 painless
 recurrent
 relapsing

577.2 Cyst and pseudocyst of pancreas

577.8 Other specified diseases of pancreas

Atrophy
Calculus
Cirrhosis
Fibrosis
} of pancreas

Pancreatic:
 infantilism
 necrosis:
  NOS
  aseptic
  fat
Pancreatolithiasis

Excludes: *fibrocystic disease of pancreas (277.00-277.09)*
 islet cell tumor of pancreas (211.7)
 pancreatic steatorrhea (579.4)

577.9 Unspecified disease of pancreas

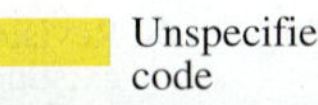

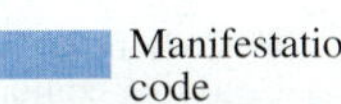

578 Gastrointestinal hemorrhage

Excludes: *that with mention of :*

angiodysplasia of stomach and duodenum (537.83)
angiodysplasia of intestine (569.85)
diverticulitis, intestine:
large (562.13)
small (562.03)
diverticulosis, intestine:
large (562.12)
small (562.02)
gastritis and duodenitis (535.0-535.6)
ulcer:
duodenal (532.0-532.9)
gastric (531.0-531.9)
gastrojejunal (534.0-534.9)
peptic (533.0-533.9)

578.0 Hematemesis
Vomiting of blood

578.1 Blood in stool
Melena

Excludes: *occult blood (792.1)*

578.9 Hemorrhage of gastrointestinal tract, unspecified
Gastric hemorrhage   Intestinal hemorrhage

579 Intestinal malabsorption

579.0 Celiac disease
Celiac: Gee (-Herter) disease
crisis   Gluten enteropathy
infantilism   Idiopathic steatorrhea
rickets   Nontropical sprue

579.1 Tropical sprue
Sprue: Tropical steatorrhea
NOS
tropical

579.2 Blind loop syndrome
Postoperative blind loop syndrome

579.3 Other and unspecified postsurgical nonabsorption
Hypoglycemia
Malnutrition   } following gastrointestinal surgery

579.4 Pancreatic steatorrhea

579.8 Other specified intestinal malabsorption
Enteropathy: Steatorrhea (chronic)
exudative
protein-losing

579.9 Unspecified intestinal malabsorption
Malabsorption syndrome NOS

● Code new
 to this edition

▲ Revision of
existing code

④ ⑤ Fourth or fifth
digit required

10. DISEASES OF THE GENITOURINARY SYSTEM (580-629)

NEPHRITIS, NEPHROTIC SYNDROME, AND NEPHROSIS (580-589)

> Excludes: hypertensive renal disease (403.00-403.91)

580 Acute glomerulonephritis
Includes: acute nephritis

580.0 With lesion of proliferative glomerulonephritis
Acute (diffuse) proliferative glomerulonephritis
Acute poststreptococcal glomerulonephritis

580.4 With lesion of rapidly progressive glomerulonephritis
Acute nephritis with lesion of necrotizing glomerulitis

⑤ **580.8 With other specified pathological lesion in kidney**

580.81 *Acute glomerulonephritis in diseases classified elsewhere*
Code first underlying disease, as:
infectious hepatitis (070.0-070.9)
mumps (072.79)
subacute bacterial endocarditis (421.0)
typhoid fever (002.0)

580.89 Other
Glomerulonephritis, acute, with lesion of:
exudative nephritis
interstitial (diffuse) (focal) nephritis

580.9 Acute glomerulonephritis with unspecified pathological lesion in kidney
Glomerulonephritis:
NOS
hemorrhagic ⎫ specified as acute
Nephritis
Nephropathy

581 Nephrotic syndrome

581.0 With lesion of proliferative glomerulonephritis

581.1 With lesion of membranous glomerulonephritis
Epimembranous nephritis
Idiopathic membranous glomerular disease
Nephrotic syndrome with lesion of:
focal glomerulosclerosis
sclerosing membranous glomerulonephritis
segmental hyalinosis

581.2 With lesion of membranoproliferative glomerulonephritis
Nephrotic syndrome with lesion (of):
endothelial
hypocomplementemic persistent
lobular ⎬ glomerulonephritis
mesangiocapillary
mixed membranous and proliferative

581.3 With lesion of minimal change glomerulonephritis
Foot process disease   Minimal change:
Lipoid nephrosis   glomerular disease
glomerulitis
nephrotic syndrome

⑤ **581.8 With other specified pathological lesion in kidney**

581.81 *Nephrotic syndrome in diseases classified elsewhere*
Code first underlying disease, as:
amyloidosis (277.3)
diabetes mellitus (250.4)
malaria (084.9)
polyarteritis (446.0)
systemic lupus erythematosus (710.0)

> Excludes: nephrosis in epidemic hemorrhagic fever (078.6)

581.89 Other
Glomerulonephritis with edema and lesion of:
exudative nephritis
interstitial (diffuse) (focal) nephritis

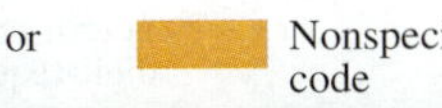

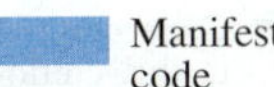

581.9 Nephrotic syndrome with unspecified pathological lesion in kidney
Glomerulonephritis with edema NOS
Nephritis:
  nephrotic NOS
  with edema NOS
Nephrosis NOS
Renal disease with edema NOS

582 Chronic glomerulonephritis
Includes: chronic nephritis

582.0 With lesion of proliferative glomerulonephritis
Chronic (diffuse) proliferative glomerulonephritis

582.1 With lesion of membranous glomerulonephritis
Chronic glomerulonephritis:
  membranous
  sclerosing
Focal glomerulosclerosis
Segmental hyalinosis

582.2 With lesion of membranoproliferative glomerulonephritis
Chronic glomerulonephritis:
  endothelial
  hypocomplementemic persistent
  lobular
  membranoproliferative
  mesangiocapillary
  mixed membranous and proliferative

582.4 With lesion of rapidly progressive glomerulonephritis
Chronic nephritis with lesion of necrotizing glomerulitis

⑤ **582.8 With other specified pathological lesion in kidney**

582.81 Chronic glomerulonephritis in diseases classified elsewhere
Code first underlying disease, as:
  amyloidosis (277.3)
  systemic lupus erythematosus (710.0)

582.89 Other
Chronic glomerulonephritis with lesion of:
  exudative nephritis
  interstitial (diffuse) (focal) nephritis

582.9 Chronic glomerulonephritis with unspecified pathological lesion in kidney
Glomerulonephritis:
  NOS
  hemorrhagic   } specified as chronic
Nephritis
Nephropathy

583 Nephritis and nephropathy, not specified as acute or chronic
Includes: "renal disease" so stated, not specified as acute or chronic but with stated pathology
  or cause

583.0 With lesion of proliferative glomerulonephritis
Proliferative:
  glomerulonephritis (diffuse) NOS
  nephritis NOS
  nephropathy NOS

583.1 With lesion of membranous glomerulonephritis
Membranous: Membranous nephropathy NOS
  glomerulonephritis NOS
  nephritis NOS

583.2 With lesion of membranoproliferative glomerulonephritis
Membranoproliferative:
  glomerulonephritis NOS
  nephritis NOS
  nephropathy NOS
Nephritis NOS, with lesion of:
  hypocomplementemic persistent
  lobular   } glomerulonephritis
  mesangiocapillary
  mixed membranous and proliferative

● Code new
  to this edition

▲ Revision of
  existing code

④ ⑤ Fourth or fifth
  digit required

583.4 With lesion of rapidly progressive glomerulonephritis
Necrotizing or rapidly progressive:
  glomerulitis NOS
  glomerulonephritis NOS
  nephritis NOS
  nephropathy NOS
Nephritis, unspecified, with lesion of necrotizing glomerulitis

583.6 With lesion of renal cortical necrosis
Nephritis NOS
Nephropathy NOS } with (renal) cortical necrosis
Renal cortical necrosis NOS

583.7 With lesion of renal medullary necrosis
Nephritis NOS
Nephropathy NOS } with (renal) medullary [papillary] necrosis

⑤ **583.8 With other specified pathological lesion in kidney**

583.81 *Nephritis and nephropathy, not specified as acute or chronic, in diseases classified elsewhere*
Code first underlying disease, as:
  amyloidosis (277.3)
  diabetes mellitus (250.4)
  gonococcal infection (098.19)
  Goodpasture's syndrome (446.21)
  systemic lupus erythematosus (710.0)
  tuberculosis (016.0)

Excludes: *gouty nephropathy (274.10)*
syphilitic nephritis (095.4)

583.89 Other
Glomerulitis
Glomerulo-
  nephritis   with lesion of:
Nephritis   exudative nephritis
Nephropathy   interstitial nephritis
Renal disease

583.9 With unspecified pathological lesion in kidney
Glomerulitis
Glomerulonephritis
Nephritis   } NOS
Nephropathy

Excludes: *nephropathy complicating pregnancy, labor, or the puerperium (642.0-642.9, 646.2)*
renal disease NOS with no stated cause (593.9)

584 Acute renal failure

Excludes: *following labor and delivery (669.3)*
posttraumatic (958.5)
that complicating:
abortion (634-638 with .3, 639.3)
ectopic or molar pregnancy (639.3)

584.5 With lesion of tubular necrosis
Lower nephron nephrosis
Renal failure with (acute) tubular necrosis
Tubular necrosis:
  NOS
  acute

584.6 With lesion of renal cortical necrosis

584.7 With lesion of renal medullary [papillary] necrosis
Necrotizing renal papillitis

584.8 With other specified pathological lesion in kidney

584.9 Acute renal failure, unspecified

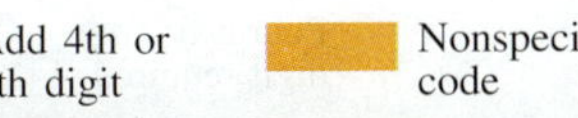

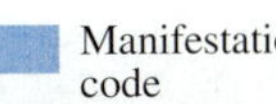

Manifestation
code

585 Chronic renal failure
Chronic uremia

Use additional code, if desired, to identify manifestation as:
uremic:
neuropathy (357.4)
pericarditis (420.0)

Excludes: *that with any condition classifiable to 401 (403.0-403.9 with fifth-digit 1)*

586 Renal failure, unspecified
Uremia NOS

Excludes: *following labor and delivery (669.3)*
posttraumatic renal failure (958.5)
that complicating:
abortion (634-638 with .3, 639.3)
ectopic or molar pregnancy (639.3)
uremia:
extrarenal (788.9)
prerenal (788.9)
with any condition classifiable to 401 (403.0-403.9 with fifth-digit 1)

587 Renal sclerosis, unspecified

Atrophy of kidney	Renal:
Contracted kidney	cirrhosis
	fibrosis

Excludes: *nephrosclerosis (arteriolar) (arteriosclerotic) (403.00-403.92)*
with hypertension (403.00-403.92)

588 Disorders resulting from impaired renal function

588.0 Renal osteodystrophy

Azotemic osteodystrophy	Renal:
Phosphate-losing tubular	dwarfism
disorders	infantilism
	rickets

588.1 Nephrogenic diabetes insipidus

Excludes: *diabetes insipidus NOS (253.5)*

588.8 Other specified disorders resulting from impaired renal function
Hypokalemic nephropathy
Secondary hyperparathyroidism (of renal origin)

Excludes: *secondary hypertension (405.0-405.9)*

588.9 Unspecified disorder resulting from impaired renal function

589 Small kidney of unknown cause

589.0 Unilateral small kidney

589.1 Bilateral small kidneys

589.9 Small kidney, unspecified

OTHER DISEASES OF URINARY SYSTEM (590-599)

590 Infections of kidney

Use additional code, if desired, to identify organism, such as Escherichia coli [E. coli] (041.4)

⑤ **590.0 Chronic pyelonephritis**
Chronic pyelitis
Chronic pyonephrosis
Code, if applicable, any causal condition first

590.00 Without lesion of renal medullary necrosis

590.01 With lesion of renal medullary necrosis

⑤ **590.1 Acute pyelonephritis**

Acute pyelitis	Acute pyonephrosis

590.10 Without lesion of renal medullary necrosis

590.11 With lesion of renal medullary necrosis

● Code new
to this edition   ▲ Revision of
existing code   ④ ⑤ Fourth or fifth
digit required

590.2 Renal and perinephric abscess
    Abscess: Carbuncle of kidney
      kidney
      nephritic
      perirenal

590.3 Pyeloureteritis cystica
    Infection of renal pelvis and ureter
    Ureteritis cystica

⑤ **590.8 Other pyelonephritis or pyonephrosis, not specified as acute or chronic**

    590.80 Pyelonephritis, unspecified
        Pyelitis NOS   Pyelonephritis NOS

    590.81 Pyelitis or pyelonephritis in diseases classified elsewhere
        Code first underlying disease, as:
          tuberculosis (016.0)

590.9 Infection of kidney, unspecified

    Excludes: *urinary tract infection NOS (599.0)*

591 Hydronephrosis
    Hydrocalycosis   Hydroureteronephrosis
    Hydronephrosis

    Excludes: *congenital hydronephrosis (753.29)*
        hydroureter (593.5)

592 Calculus of kidney and ureter

    Excludes: *nephrocalcinosis (275.4)*

592.0 Calculus of kidney
    Nephrolithiasis NOS   Staghorn calculus
    Renal calculus or stone   Stone in kidney

    Excludes: *uric acid nephrolithiasis (274.11)*

592.1 Calculus of ureter
    Ureteric stone   Ureterolithiasis

592.9 Urinary calculus, unspecified

593 Other disorders of kidney and ureter

593.0 Nephroptosis
    Floating kidney
    Mobile kidney

593.1 Hypertrophy of kidney

593.2 Cyst of kidney, acquired
    Cyst (multiple) (solitary) of kidney, not congenital
    Peripelvic (lymphatic) cyst

    Excludes: *calyceal or pyelogenic cyst of kidney (591)*
        congenital cyst of kidney (753.1)
        polycystic (disease of) kidney (753.1)

593.3 Stricture or kinking of ureter
    Angulation   ⎱
                  ⎰ of ureter (postoperative)
    Constriction   ⎰
    Stricture of pelviureteric junction

593.4 Other ureteric obstruction
    Idiopathic retroperitoneal fibrosis
    Occlusion NOS of ureter

    Excludes: *that due to calculus (592.1)*

593.5 Hydroureter

    Excludes: *congenital hydroureter (753.22)*
        hydroureteronephrosis (591)

593.6 Postural proteinuria
    Benign postural proteinuria
    Orthostatic proteinuria

    Excludes: *proteinuria NOS (791.0)*

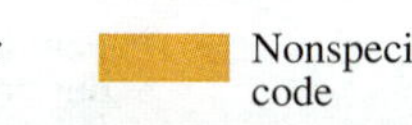

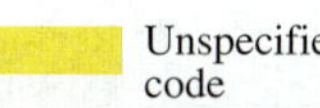

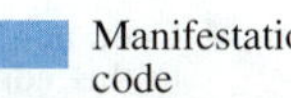

⑤ **593.7 Vesicoureteral reflux**

593.70 Unspecified or without reflux nephropathy

593.71 With reflux nephropathy, unilateral

593.72 With reflux nephropathy, bilateral

593.73 With reflux nephropathy NOS

⑤ **593.8 Other specified disorders of kidney and ureter**

593.81 Vascular disorders of kidney
Renal (artery):   Renal infarction
    embolism
    hemorrhage
    thrombosis

593.82 Ureteral fistula
Intestinoureteral fistula

Excludes: *fistula between ureter and female genital tract (619.0)*

593.89 Other
Adhesions, kidney or   Polyp of ureter
    ureter   Pyelectasia
Periureteritis   Ureterocele

Excludes: *tuberculosis of ureter (016.2)*
ureteritis cystica (590.3)

593.9 Unspecified disorder of kidney and ureter
Renal disease NOS
Salt-losing nephritis or syndrome

Excludes: *cystic kidney disease (753.1)*
nephropathy, so stated (583.0-583.9)
renal disease:
acute (580.0-580.9)
arising in pregnancy or the puerperium (642.1-642.2, 642.4-642.7, 646.2)
chronic (582.0-582.9)
not specified as acute or chronic, but with stated pathology or cause
(583.0-583.9)

594 Calculus of lower urinary tract

594.0 Calculus in diverticulum of bladder

594.1 Other calculus in bladder
Urinary bladder stone

Excludes: *staghorn calculus (592.0)*

594.2 Calculus in urethra

594.8 Other lower urinary tract calculus

594.9 Calculus of lower urinary tract, unspecified

Excludes: *calculus of urinary tract NOS (592.9)*

595 Cystitis

Excludes: *prostatocystitis (601.3)*

Use additional code, if desired, to identify organism, such as Escherichia coli [E. coli] (041.4)

595.0 Acute cystitis

Excludes: *trigonitis (595.3)*

595.1 Chronic interstitial cystitis
Hunner's ulcer   Submucous cystitis
Panmural fibrosis of bladder

595.2 Other chronic cystitis
Chronic cystitis NOS   Subacute cystitis

Excludes: *trigonitis (595.3)*

595.3 Trigonitis
Follicular cystitis
Trigonitis (acute) (chronic)
Urethrotrigonitis

● Code new
    to this edition

▲ Revision of
    existing code

④ ⑤ Fourth or fifth
        digit required

595.4 Cystitis in diseases classified elsewhere
Code first underlying disease, as:
actinomycosis (039.8)
amebiasis (006.8)
bilharziasis (120.0-120.9)
Echinococcus infestation (122.3, 122.6)

Excludes: cystitis:
diphtheritic (032.84)
gonococcal (098.11, 098.31)
monilial (112.2)
trichomonal (131.09)
tuberculous (016.1)

⑤ **595.8 Other specified types of cystitis**

595.81   Cystitis cystica

595.82   Irradiation cystitis
Use additional E code, if desired, to identify cause

595.89   Other
Abscess of bladder
Cystitis:
bullous
emphysematous
glandularis

595.9 Cystitis, unspecified

596 Other disorders of bladder
Use additional code, if desired, to identify urinary incontinence (625.6, 788.30-788.39)

596.0 Bladder neck obstruction
Contracture (acquired)
Obstruction (acquired) } of bladder neck or vesicourethral orifice
Stenosis (acquired)

Excludes: congenital (753.6)

596.1 Intestinovesical fistula

Fistula:
enterovesical
vesicocolic

Fistula:
vesicoenteric
vesicorectal

596.2 Vesical fistula, not elsewhere classified

Fistula:
bladder NOS
urethrovesical

Fistula:
vesicocutaneous
vesicoperineal

Excludes: fistula between bladder and female genital tract (619.0)

596.3 Diverticulum of bladder
Diverticulitis of bladder
Diverticulum (acquired) (false) of bladder

Excludes: that with calculus in diverticulum of bladder (594.0)

596.4 Atony of bladder
High compliance bladder
Hypotonicity of bladder
Inertia of bladder

Excludes: neurogenic bladder (596.54)

⑤ **596.5 Other functional disorders of bladder**

Excludes: cauda equina syndrome
with neurogenic bladder (344.61)

596.51   Hypertonicity of bladder
Hyperactivity
Overactive bladder

596.52   Low bladder compliance

596.53   Paralysis of bladder

596.54   Neurogenic bladder NOS

596.55   Detrusor sphincter dyssynergia

596.59   Other functional disorder of bladder
Detrusor instability

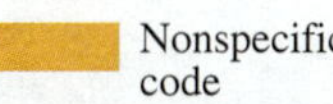

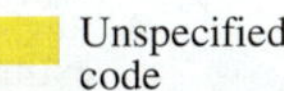

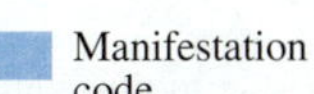

Manifestation
code

596.6 Rupture of bladder, nontraumatic

596.7 Hemorrhage into bladder wall
    Hyperemia of bladder

> *Excludes:* *acute hemorrhagic cystitis (595.0)*

596.8 Other specified disorders of bladder

Bladder:	Bladder:
calcified	hemorrhage
contracted	hypertrophy

> *Excludes:* *cystocele, female (618.0, 618.2-618.4)*
>   *hernia or prolapse of bladder, female (618.0, 618.2-618.4)*

596.9 Unspecified disorder of bladder

597 Urethritis, not sexually transmitted, and urethral syndrome

> *Excludes:* *nonspecific urethritis, so stated (099.4)*

597.0 Urethral abscess

Abscess of:	Abscess:
bulbourethral gland	periurethral
Cowper's gland	urethral (gland)
Littré's gland	Periurethral cellulitis

> *Excludes:* *urethral caruncle (599.3)*

⑤ **597.8 Other urethritis**

    597.80 Urethritis, unspecified

    597.81 Urethral syndrome NOS

    597.89 Other

Adenitis, Skene's	Meatitis, urethral
glands	Ulcer, urethra (meatus)
Cowperitis	Verumontanitis

> *Excludes:* *trichomonal (131.02)*

598 Urethral stricture
    Includes: pinhole meatus
              stricture of urinary meatus

> *Excludes:* *congenital stricture of urethra and urinary meatus (753.6)*

Use additional code to identify urinary incontinence (625.6, 788.30-788.39)

⑤ **598.0 Urethral stricture due to infection**

    598.00 Due to unspecified infection

    598.01 *Due to infective diseases classified elsewhere*
        Code first underlying disease, as:
          gonococcal infection (098.2)
          schistosomiasis (120.0-120.9)
          syphilis (095.8)

598.1 Traumatic urethral stricture
    Stricture of urethra:
      late effect of injury
      postobstetric

> *Excludes:* *postoperative following surgery on genitourinary tract (598.2)*

598.2 Postoperative urethral stricture
    Postcatheterization stricture of urethra

598.8 Other specified causes of urethral stricture

598.9 Urethral stricture, unspecified

599 Other disorders of urethra and urinary tract

599.0 Urinary tract infection, site not specified
    Pyuria

> *Excludes:* *Candidiasis of urinary tract (112.2)*
>   *urinary tract infection of newborn (771.82)*

Use additional code to identify organism, such as Escherichia coli [*E. coli*] (041.4)

● Code new   ▲ Revision of   ④ ⑤ Fourth or fifth
  to this edition   existing code   digit required

599.1 Urethral fistula
Fistula:
   urethroperineal
   urethrorectal

Urinary fistula NOS

> *Excludes:* *fistula:*
>   *urethroscrotal (608.89)*
>   *urethrovaginal (619.0)*
>   *urethrovesicovaginal (619.0)*

599.2 Urethral diverticulum

599.3 Urethral caruncle
Polyp of urethra

599.4 Urethral false passage

599.5 Prolapsed urethral mucosa
Prolapse of urethra   Urethrocele

> *Excludes:* *urethrocele, female (618.0, 618.2-618.4)*

599.6 Urinary obstruction, unspecified
Obstructive uropathy NOS
Urinary (tract) obstruction NOS

> *Excludes:* *obstructive nephropathy NOS (593.89)*

Use additional code, if desired, to identify urinary incontinence (625.6, 788.30-788.39)

599.7 Hematuria
Hematuria (benign) (essential)

> *Excludes:* *hemoglobinuria (791.2)*

⑤ **599.8 Other specified disorders of urethra and urinary tract**

> *Excludes:* *symptoms and other conditions classifiable to 788.0-788.9, 791.0-791.9*

Use additional code, if desired, to identify urinary incontinence (625.6, 788.30-788.39)

    599.81 Urethral hypermobility

    599.82 Intrinsic (urethral) sphincter deficiency [ISD]

    599.83 Urethral instability

    599.84 Other specified disorders of urethra
       Rupture of urethra (nontraumatic)
       Urethral:
          cyst
          granuloma

    599.89 Other specified disorders of urinary tract

599.9 Unspecified disorder of urethra and urinary tract

DISEASES OF MALE GENITAL ORGANS (600-608)

600 Hyperplasia of prostate
Use additional code, if desired, to identify urinary incontinence (788.30-788.39)

600.0 Hypertrophy (benign) of prostate
Benign prostatic hypertrophy
Enlargement of prostate
Smooth enlarged prostate
Soft enlarged prostate

600.1 Nodular prostate
Hard, firm prostate
Multinodular prostate

> *Excludes:* *malignant neoplasm of prostate (185)*

600.2 Benign localized hyperplasia of prostate
Adenofibromatous hypertrophy of prostate
Adenoma of prostate
Fibroadenoma of prostate
Fibroma of prostate
Myoma of prostate
Polyp of prostate

> *Excludes:* *benign neoplasms of prostate (222.2)*
>   *hypertrophy of prostate (600.0)*
>   *malignant neoplasm of prostate (185)*

600

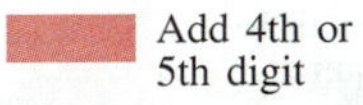

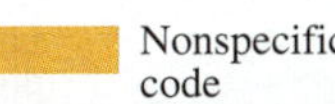

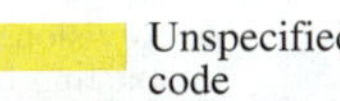

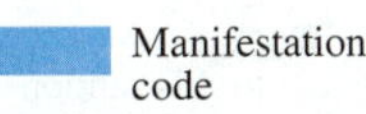

600.3 Cyst of prostate

600.9 Hyperplasia of prostate, unspecified
Median bar
Prostatic obstruction NOS

601 Inflammatory diseases of prostate
Use additional code, if desired, to identify organism, such as Staphylococcus (041.1), or Streptococcus (041.0)

601.0 Acute prostatitis

601.1 Chronic prostatitis

601.2 Abscess of prostate

601.3 Prostatocystitis

601.4 Prostatitis in diseases classified elsewhere
Code first underlying disease, as:
actinomycosis (039.8)
blastomycosis (116.0)
syphilis (095.8)
tuberculosis (016.5)

Excludes: *prostatitis:*
gonococcal (098.12, 098.32)
monilial (112.2)
trichomonal (131.03)

601.8 Other specified inflammatory diseases of prostate
Prostatitis:
cavitary
diverticular
granulomatous

601.9 Prostatitis, unspecified
Prostatitis NOS

602 Other disorders of prostate

602.0 Calculus of prostate
Prostatic stone

602.1 Congestion or hemorrhage of prostate

602.2 Atrophy of prostate

602.3 Dysplasia of prostate
Prostatic intraepithelial neoplasia I (PIN I)
Prostatic intraepithelial neoplasia II (PIN II)

Excludes: *Prostatic intraepithelial neoplasia III (PIN III) (233.4)*

602.8 Other specified disorders of prostate
Fistula
Infarction } of prostate   Periprostatic adhesions
Stricture

602.9 Unspecified disorder of prostate

603 Hydrocele
Includes: hydrocele of spermatic cord, testis, or tunica vaginalis

Excludes: *congenital (778.6)*

603.0 Encysted hydrocele

603.1 Infected hydrocele
Use additional code, if desired, to identify organism

603.8 Other specified types of hydrocele

603.9 Hydrocele, unspecified

604 Orchitis and epididymitis
Use additional code, if desired, to identify organism, such as Escherichia coli [E. coli] (041.4), Staphylococcus (041.1), or Streptococcus (041.0)

604.0 Orchitis, epididymitis, and epididymo-orchitis, with abscess
Abscess of epididymis or testis

⑤ **604.9 Other orchitis, epididymitis, and epididymo-orchitis, without mention of abscess**

604.90 Orchitis and epididymitis, unspecified

● Code new   ▲ Revision of   ④ ⑤ Fourth or fifth
  to this edition   existing code   digit required

604.91 *Orchitis and epididymitis in diseases classified elsewhere*
    Code first underlying disease, as:
        diphtheria (032.89)
        filariasis (125.0-125.9)
        syphilis (095.8)

    Excludes: *orchitis:*
        gonococcal (098.13, 098.33)
        mumps (072.0)
        tuberculous (016.5)
        tuberculous epididymitis (016.4)

604.99 **Other**

605 Redundant prepuce and phimosis

Adherent prepuce   Phimosis (congenital)
Paraphimosis   Tight foreskin

606 Infertility, male

606.0 **Azoospermia**
    Absolute infertility
    Infertility due to:
      germinal (cell) aplasia
      spermatogenic arrest (complete)

606.1 **Oligospermia**
    Infertility due to:
      germinal cell desquamation
      hypospermatogenesis
      incomplete spermatogenic arrest

606.8 **Infertility due to extratesticular causes**
    Infertility due to:
      drug therapy
      infection
      obstruction of efferent ducts
      radiation
      systemic disease

606.9 **Male infertility, unspecified**

607 Disorders of penis

    Excludes: *phimosis (605)*

607.0 **Leukoplakia of penis**
    Kraurosis of penis

    Excludes: *carcinoma in situ of penis (233.5)*
        erythroplasia of Queyrat (233.5)

607.1 **Balanoposthitis**
    Balanitis
Use additional code, if desired, to identify organism

607.2 **Other inflammatory disorders of penis**
    Abscess
    Boil
    Carbuncle   } of corpus cavernosum or penis
    Cellulitis
    Cavernitis (penis)

Use additional code, if desired, to identify organism

    Excludes: *herpetic infection (054.13)*

607.3 **Priapism**
    Painful erection

⑤ **607.8** **Other specified disorders of penis**

    607.81 **Balanitis xerotica obliterans**
        Induratio penis plastica

    607.82 **Vascular disorders of penis**
        Embolism
        Hematoma
          (nontraumatic) } of corpus cavernosum or penis
        Hemorrhage
        Thrombosis

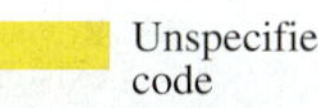

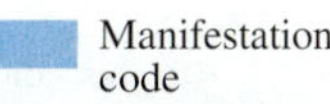

Manifestation
code

607.83 Edema of penis

607.84 Impotence of organic origin

Excludes: *nonorganic or unspecified (302.72)*

607.89 Other

Atrophy
Fibrosis
Hypertrophy
Ulcer (chronic)
} of corpus cavernosum or penis

607.9 Unspecified disorder of penis

608 Other disorders of male genital organs

608.0 Seminal vesiculitis

Abscess
Cellulitis
Vesiculitis (seminal)
} of seminal vesicle

Use additional code, if desired, to identify organism

Excludes: *gonococcal infection (098.14, 098.34)*

608.1 Spermatocele

608.2 Torsion of testis

Torsion of:
  epididymis
  spermatic cord
  testicle

608.3 Atrophy of testis

608.4 Other inflammatory disorders of male genital organs

Abscess
Boil
Carbuncle
Cellulitis
Vasitis
} of scrotum, spermatic cord, testis [except abscess], tunica vaginalis, or vas deferens

Use additional code, if desired, to identify organism

Excludes: *abscess of testis (604.0)*

⑤ **608.8 Other specified disorders of male genital organs**

608.81 Disorders of male genital organs in diseases classified elsewhere

Code first underlying disease, as:
  filariasis (125.0-125.9)
  tuberculosis (016.5)

608.82 Hematospermia

608.83 Vascular disorders

Hematoma (nontraumatic)
Hemorrhage
Thrombosis
} of seminal vesicle, spermatic cord, testis, scrotum, tunica vaginalis, or vas deferens

Hematocele NOS, male

608.84 Chylocele of tunica vaginalis

608.85 Stricture

Stricture of:
  spermatic cord
  tunica vaginalis
  vas deferens

608.86 Edema

608.87 Retrograde ejaculation

608.89 Other

Atrophy
Fibrosis
Hypertrophy
Ulcer
} of seminal vesicle, spermatic cord, testis, scrotum, tunica vaginalis, or vas deferens

Excludes: *atrophy of testis (608.3)*

608.9 Unspecified disorder of male genital organs

● Code new
  to this edition

▲ Revision of
  existing code

④ ⑤ Fourth or fifth
  digit required

DISORDERS OF BREAST (610-611)

610 Benign mammary dysplasias

610.0 Solitary cyst of breast
Cyst (solitary) of breast

610.1 Diffuse cystic mastopathy
Chronic cystic mastitis   Fibrocystic disease of breast
Cystic breast

610.2 Fibroadenosis of breast
Fibroadenosis of breast: Fibroadenosis of breast:
  NOS   diffuse
  chronic   periodic
  cystic   segmental

610.3 Fibrosclerosis of breast

610.4 Mammary duct ectasia
Comedomastitis   Mastitis:
Dust ectasia   periductal
                      plasma cell

610.8 Other specified benign mammary dysplasias
Mazoplasia   Sebaceous cyst of breast

610.9 Benign mammary dysplasia, unspecified

611 Other disorders of breast

Excludes: *that associated with lactation or the puerperium (675.0-676.9)*

611.0 Inflammatory disease of breast
Abscess (acute) (chronic) (nonpuerperal) of:
  areola
  breast
Mammillary fistula
Mastitis (acute) (subacute) (nonpuerperal):
  NOS
  infective
  retromammary
  submammary

Excludes: *carbuncle of breast (680.2)*
chronic cystic mastitis (610.1)
neonatal infective mastitis (771.5)
thrombophlebitis of breast [Mondor's disease] (451.89)

611.1 Hypertrophy of breast
Gynecomastia   Hypertrophy of breast:
                    NOS
                    massive pubertal

611.2 Fissure of nipple

611.3 Fat necrosis of breast
Fat necrosis (segmental) of breast

611.4 Atrophy of breast

611.5 Galactocele

611.6 Galactorrhea not associated with childbirth

⑤ **611.7 Signs and symptoms in breast**

611.71 Mastodynia
Pain in breast

611.72 Lump or mass in breast

611.79 Other
Induration of breast   Nipple discharge
Inversion of nipple   Retraction of nipple

611.8 Other specified disorders of breast
Hematoma (nontraumatic) ⎫
Infarction   ⎬ of breast
Occlusion of breast duct ⎭
Subinvolution of breast (postlactational) (postpartum)

611.9 Unspecified breast disorder

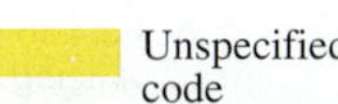

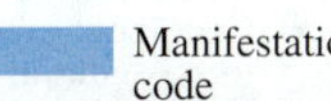

Manifestation
code

INFLAMMATORY DISEASE OF FEMALE PELVIC ORGANS (614-616)

Use additional code, if desired, to identify organism, such as Staphylococcus (041.1), or Streptococcus (041.0)

Excludes: *that associated with pregnancy, abortion, childbirth, or the puerperium (630-676.9)*

614 Inflammatory disease of ovary, fallopian tube, pelvic cellular tissue, and peritoneum

Excludes: *endometritis (615.0-615.9)*
major infection following delivery (670)
that complicating:
abortion (634-638 with .0, 639.0)
ectopic or molar pregnancy (639.0)
pregnancy or labor (646.6)

614.0 Acute salpingitis and oophoritis
Any condition classifiable to 614.2, specified as acute or subacute

614.1 Chronic salpingitis and oophoritis
Hydrosalpinx
Salpingitis:
follicularis
isthmica nodosa
Any condition classifiable to 614.2, specified as chronic

614.2 Salpingitis and oophoritis not specified as acute, subacute, or chronic
Abscess (of):   Perisalpingitis
  fallopian tube   Pyosalpinx
  ovary   Salpingitis
  tubo-ovarian   Salpingo-oophoritisRTubo-ovarian inflammatory disease
Oophoritis
Perioophoritis

Excludes: *gonococcal infection (chronic) (098.37)*
acute (098.17)
tuberculous (016.6)

614.3 Acute parametritis and pelvic cellulitis
Acute inflammatory pelvic disease
Any condition classifiable to 614.4, specified as acute

614.4 Chronic or unspecified parametritis and pelvic cellulitis
Abscess (of):
  broad ligament
  parametrium   } chronic or NOS
  pelvis, female
  pouch of Douglas
Chronic inflammatory pelvic disease
Pelvic cellulitis, female

Excludes: *tuberculous (016.7)*

614.5 Acute or unspecified pelvic peritonitis, female

614.6 Pelvic peritoneal adhesions, female (postoperative) (postinfection)
Adhesions:
peritubal
tubo-ovarian

Use additional code, if desired, to identify any associated infertility (628.2)

614.7 Other chronic pelvic peritonitis, female

Excludes: *tuberculous (016.7)*

614.8 Other specified inflammatory disease of female pelvic organs and tissues

614.9 Unspecified inflammatory disease of female pelvic organs and tissues
Pelvic infection or inflammation, female NOS
Pelvic inflammatory disease [PID]

 Code new
to this edition

▲ Revision of
existing code

④ ⑤ Fourth or fifth
digit required

615 Inflammatory diseases of uterus, except cervix

Excludes: *following delivery (670)*
hyperplastic endometritis (621.3)
that complicating:
abortion (634-638 with .0, 639.0)
ectopic or molar pregnancy (639.0)
pregnancy or labor (646.6)

615.0 Acute
Any condition classifiable to 615.9, specified as acute or subacute

615.1 Chronic
Any condition classifiable to 615.9, specified as chronic

615.9 Unspecified inflammatory disease of uterus
Endometritis   Perimetritis
Endomyometritis   Pyometra
Metritis   Uterine abscess
Myometritis

616 Inflammatory disease of cervix, vagina, and vulva

Excludes: *that complicating:*
abortion (634-638 with .0, 639.0)
ectopic or molar pregnancy (639.0)
pregnancy, childbirth, or the puerperium (646.6)

616.0 Cervicitis and endocervicitis
Cervicitis
Endocervicitis   } with or without mention of erosion or ectropion
Nabothian (gland) cyst or follicle

Excludes: *erosion or ectropion without mention of cervicitis (622.0)*

⑤ **616.1 Vaginitis and vulvovaginitis**

616.10 Vaginitis and vulvovaginitis, unspecified
Vaginitis: Vulvitis NOS
NOS   Vulvovaginitis NOS
postirradiation
Use additional code, if desired, to identify organism, such as Escherichia coli [E. coli]
(041.4), Staphylococcus (041.1), or Streptococcus (041.0)

Excludes: *noninfective leukorrhea (623.5)*
postmenopausal or senile vaginitis (627.3)

616.11 *Vaginitis and vulvovaginitis in diseases classified elsewhere*
Code first underlying disease, as:
pinworm vaginitis (127.4)

Excludes: *herpetic vulvovaginitis (054.11)*
monilial vulvovaginitis (112.1)
trichomonal vaginitis or vulvovaginitis (131.01)

616.2 Cyst of Bartholin's gland
Bartholin's duct cyst

616.3 Abscess of Bartholin's gland
Vulvovaginal gland abscess

616.4 Other abscess of vulva
Abscess
Carbuncle   } of vulva
Furuncle

⑤ **616.5 Ulceration of vulva**

616.50 Ulceration of vulva, unspecified
Ulcer NOS of vulva

616.51 *Ulceration of vulva in diseases classified elsewhere*
Code first underlying disease, as:
Behçet's syndrome (136.1)
tuberculosis (016.7)

Excludes: *vulvar ulcer (in):*
gonococcal (098.0)
herpes simplex (054.12)
syphilitic (091.0)

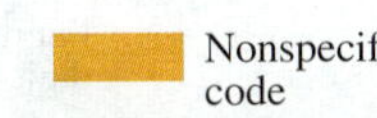

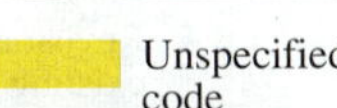

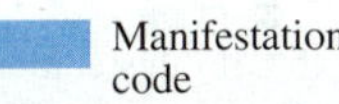

616.8 **Other specified inflammatory diseases of cervix, vagina, and vulva**
    Caruncle, vagina or labium
    Ulcer, vagina

    Excludes: *noninflammatory disorders of:*
        cervix (622.0-622.9)
        vagina (623.0-623.9)
        vulva (624.0-624.9)

616.9 **Unspecified inflammatory disease of cervix, vagina, and vulva**

OTHER DISORDERS OF FEMALE GENITAL TRACT (617-629)

617 **Endometriosis**

617.0 **Endometriosis of uterus**
    Adenomyosis   Endometriosis:
                          cervix
                          internal
                          myometrium

    Excludes: *stromal endometriosis (236.0)*

617.1 **Endometriosis of ovary**
    Chocolate cyst of ovary
    Endometrial cystoma of ovary

617.2 **Endometriosis of fallopian tube**

617.3 **Endometriosis of pelvic peritoneum**
    Endometriosis: Endometriosis:
      broad ligament   parametrium
      cul-de-sac (Douglas')   round ligament

617.4 **Endometriosis of rectovaginal septum and vagina**

617.5 **Endometriosis of intestine**
    Endometriosis:
      appendix
      colon
      rectum

617.6 **Endometriosis in scar of skin**

617.8 **Endometriosis of other specified sites**
    Endometriosis: Endometriosis:
      bladder   umbilicus
      lung   vulva

617.9 **Endometriosis, site unspecified**

618 **Genital prolapse**

Use additional code, if desired, to identify urinary incontinence (625.6, 788.31, 788.33-788.39)

    Excludes: *that complicating pregnancy, labor, or delivery (654.4)*

618.0 **Prolapse of vaginal walls without mention of uterine prolapse**
    Cystocele
    Cystourethrocele
    Proctocele, female
    Rectocele   } without mention of uterine prolapse
    Urethrocele, female
    Vaginal prolapse

    Excludes: *that with uterine prolapse (618.2-618.4)*
        enterocele (618.6)
        vaginal vault prolapse following hysterectomy (618.5)

618.1 **Uterine prolapse without mention of vaginal wall prolapse**
    Descensus uteri   Uterine prolapse:
    Uterine prolapse: first degree
      NOS   second degree
      complete   third degree

    Excludes: *that with mention of cystocele, urethrocele, or rectocele (618.2-618.4)*

618.2 **Uterovaginal prolapse, incomplete**

618.3 **Uterovaginal prolapse, complete**

618.4 **Uterovaginal prolapse, unspecified**

618.5 **Prolapse of vaginal vault after hysterectomy**

● Code new
to this edition
    ▲ Revision of
existing code
    ④ ⑤ Fourth or fifth
digit required

618.6 Vaginal enterocele, congenital or acquired
Pelvic enterocele, congenital or acquired

618.7 Old laceration of muscles of pelvic floor

618.8 Other specified genital prolapse
Incompetence or weakening of pelvic fundus
Relaxation of vaginal outlet or pelvis

618.9 Unspecified genital prolapse

619 Fistula involving female genital tract

> *Excludes:* vesicorectal and intestinovesical fistula (596.1)

619.0 Urinary-genital tract fistula, female

Fistula:
cervicovesical
ureterovaginal
urethrovaginal
urethrovesicovaginal

Fistula:
uteroureteric
uterovesical
vesicocervicovaginal
vesicovaginal

619.1 Digestive-genital tract fistula, female

Fistula:
intestinouterine
intestinovaginal
rectovaginal

Fistula:
rectovulval
sigmoidovaginal
uterorectal

619.2 Genital tract-skin fistula, female
Fistula:
uterus to abdominal wall
vaginoperineal

619.8 Other specified fistulas involving female genital tract

Fistula:
cervix
cul-de-sac (Douglas')

Fistula:
uterus
vagina

619.9 Unspecified fistula involving female genital tract

620 Noninflammatory disorders of ovary, fallopian tube, and broad ligament

> *Excludes:* hydrosalpinx (614.1)

620.0 Follicular cyst of ovary
Cyst of graafian follicle

620.1 Corpus luteum cyst or hematoma
Corpus luteum hemorrhage or rupture
Lutein cyst

620.2 Other and unspecified ovarian cyst
Cyst:
  NOS
  corpus albicans
  retention NOS   } of ovary
  serous
  theca-lutein
Simple cystoma of ovary

> *Excludes:* cystadenoma (benign) (serous) (220)
> developmental cysts (752.0)
> neoplastic cysts (220)
> polycystic ovaries (256.4)
> Stein-Leventhal syndrome (256.4)

620.3 Acquired atrophy of ovary and fallopian tube
Senile involution of ovary

620.4 Prolapse or hernia of ovary and fallopian tube
Displacement of ovary and fallopian tube
Salpingocele

620.5 Torsion of ovary, ovarian pedicle, or fallopian tube
Torsion:
accessory tube
hydatid of Morgagni

620.6 Broad ligament laceration syndrome
Masters-Allen syndrome

620.7 Hematoma of broad ligament
Hematocele, broad ligament

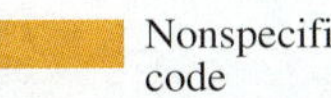

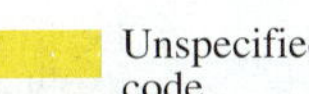

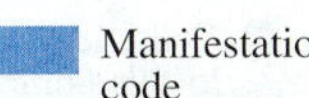

Manifestation
code

620.8 Other noninflammatory disorders of ovary, fallopian tube, and broad ligament

Cyst
Polyp } of broad ligament or fallopian tube
Infarction
Rupture } of ovary or fallopian tube
Hematosalpinx

Excludes: *hematosalpinx in ectopic pregnancy (639.2)*
peritubal adhesions (614.6)
torsion of ovary, ovarian pedicle, or fallopian tube (620.5)

620.9 Unspecified noninflammatory disorder of ovary, fallopian tube, and broad ligament

621 Disorders of uterus, not elsewhere classified

621.0 Polyp of corpus uteri
Polyp:
endometrium
uterus NOS

Excludes: *cervical polyp NOS (622.7)*

621.1 Chronic subinvolution of uterus

Excludes: *puerperal (674.8)*

621.2 Hypertrophy of uterus
Bulky or enlarged uterus

Excludes: *puerperal (674.8)*

621.3 Endometrial cystic hyperplasia
Hyperplasia (adenomatous) (cystic) (glandular) of endometrium
Hyperplastic endometritis

621.4 Hematometra
Hemometra

Excludes: *that in congenital anomaly (752.2-752.3)*

621.5 Intrauterine synechiae
Adhesions of uterus   Band(s) of uterus

621.6 Malposition of uterus
Anteversion
Retroflexion } of uterus
Retroversion

Excludes: *malposition complicating pregnancy, labor, or delivery (654.3-654.4)*
prolapse of uterus (618.1-618.4)

621.7 Chronic inversion of uterus

Excludes: *current obstetrical trauma (665.2)*
prolapse of uterus (618.1-618.4)

621.8 Other specified disorders of uterus, not elsewhere classified
Atrophy, acquired
Cyst
Fibrosis NOS } of uterus
Old laceration (postpartum)
Ulcer

Excludes: *bilharzial fibrosis (120.0-120.9)*
endometriosis (617.0)
fistulas (619.0-619.8)
inflammatory diseases (615.0-615.9)

621.9 Unspecified disorder of uterus

622 Noninflammatory disorders of cervix

Excludes: *abnormality of cervix complicating pregnancy, labor, or delivery (654.5-654.6)*
fistula (619.0-619.8)

622.0 Erosion and ectropion of cervix
Eversion
Ulcer } of cervix

Excludes: *that in chronic cervicitis (616.0)*

● Code new to this edition   ▲ Revision of existing code   ④ ⑤ Fourth or fifth digit required

622.1 Dysplasia of cervix (uteri)
Anaplasia of cervix
Cervical atypism
Cervical intraepithelial neoplasia I (CIN I)
Cervical intraepithelial neoplasia II (CIN II)
High grade squamous intraepithelial dysplasia (HGSIL)
Low grade squamous intraepithelial dysplasia (LGSIL)

Excludes: *carcinoma in situ of cervix (233.1)*
cervical intraepithelial neoplasia III [CIN III] (233.1)

622.2 Leukoplakia of cervix (uteri)

Excludes: *carcinoma in situ of cervix (233.1)*

622.3 Old laceration of cervix
Adhesions
Band(s) } of cervix
Cicatrix (postpartum)

Excludes: *current obstetrical trauma (665.3)*

622.4 Stricture and stenosis of cervix
Atresia (acquired)
Contracture } of cervix
Occlusion
Pinpoint os uteri

Excludes: *congenital (752.49)*
that complicating labor (654.6)

622.5 Incompetence of cervix

Excludes: *complicating pregnancy (654.5)*
that affecting fetus or newborn (761.0)

622.6 Hypertrophic elongation of cervix

622.7 Mucous polyp of cervix
Polyp NOS of cervix

Excludes: *adenomatous polyp of cervix (219.0)*

622.8 Other specified noninflammatory disorders of cervix
Atrophy (senile)
Cyst } of cervix
Fibrosis
Hemorrhage

Excludes: *endometriosis (617.0)*
fistula (619.0-619.8)
inflammatory diseases (616.0)

622.9 Unspecified noninflammatory disorder of cervix

623 Noninflammatory disorders of vagina

Excludes: *abnormality of vagina complicating pregnancy, labor, or delivery (654.7)*
congenital absence of vagina (752.49)
congenital diaphragm or bands (752.49)
fistulas involving vagina (619.0-619.8)

623.0 Dysplasia of vagina

Excludes: *carcinoma in situ of vagina (233.3)*

623.1 Leukoplakia of vagina

623.2 Stricture or atresia of vagina
Adhesions (postoperative) (postradiation) of vagina
Occlusion of vagina
Stenosis, vagina

Use additional E code, if desired, to identify any external cause

Excludes: *congenital atresia or stricture (752.49)*

623.3 Tight hymenal ring
Rigid hymen
Tight hymenal ring } acquired or congenital
Tight introitus

Excludes: *imperforate hymen (752.42)*

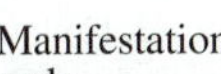

623.4 Old vaginal laceration

Excludes: *old laceration involving muscles of pelvic floor (618.7)*

623.5 Leukorrhea, not specified as infective
Leukorrhea NOS of vagina   Vaginal discharge NOS

Excludes: *trichomonal (131.00)*

623.6 Vaginal hematoma

Excludes: *current obstetrical trauma (665.7)*

623.7 Polyp of vagina

623.8 Other specified noninflammatory disorders of vagina
Cyst   }
Hemorrhage   } of vagina

623.9 Unspecified noninflammatory disorder of vagina

624 Noninflammatory disorders of vulva and perineum

Excludes: *abnormality of vulva and perineum complicating pregnancy, labor, or delivery (654.8)*
condyloma acuminatum (078.1)
fistulas involving:
  perineum—see Alphabetic Index
  vulva (619.0-619.8)
vulval varices (456.6)
vulvar involvement in skin conditions (690-709.9)

624.0 Dystrophy of vulva
Kraurosis   }
Leukoplakia   } of vulva

Excludes: *carcinoma in situ of vulva (233.3)*

624.1 Atrophy of vulva

624.2 Hypertrophy of clitoris

Excludes: *that in endocrine disorders (255.2, 256.1)*

624.3 Hypertrophy of labia
Hypertrophy of vulva NOS

624.4 Old laceration or scarring of vulva

624.5 Hematoma of vulva

Excludes: *that complicating delivery (664.5)*

624.6 Polyp of labia and vulva

624.8 Other specified noninflammatory disorders of vulva and perineum
Cyst   }
Edema   } of vulva
Stricture }

624.9 Unspecified noninflammatory disorder of vulva and perineum

625 Pain and other symptoms associated with female genital organs

625.0 Dyspareunia

Excludes: *psychogenic dyspareunia (302.76)*

625.1 Vaginismus
Colpospasm   Vulvismus

Excludes: *psychogenic vaginismus (306.51)*

625.2 Mittelschmerz
Intermenstrual pain   Ovulation pain

625.3 Dysmenorrhea
Painful menstruation

Excludes: *psychogenic dysmenorrhea (306.52)*

625.4 Premenstrual tension syndromes
Menstrual: Premenstrual syndrome
  migraine   Premenstrual tension NOS
  molimen

● Code new to this edition   ▲ Revision of existing code   ④ ⑤ Fourth or fifth digit required

625.5 Pelvic congestion syndrome
Congestion-fibrosis syndrome
Taylor's syndrome

625.6 Stress incontinence, female

Excludes: *mixed incontinence (788.33)*
stress incontinence, male (788.32)

625.8 Other specified symptoms associated with female genital organs

625.9 Unspecified symptom associated with female genital organs

626 Disorders of menstruation and other abnormal bleeding from female genital tract

Excludes: *menopausal and premenopausal bleeding (627.0)*
pain and other symptoms associated with menstrual cycle (625.2-625.4)
postmenopausal bleeding (627.1)

626.0 Absence of menstruation
Amenorrhea (primary) (secondary)

626.1 Scanty or infrequent menstruation
Hypomenorrhea   Oligomenorrhea

626.2 Excessive or frequent menstruation
Heavy periods   Menorrhagia
Menometrorrhagia   Polymenorrhea

Excludes: *premenopausal (627.0)*
that in puberty (626.3)

626.3 Puberty bleeding
Excessive bleeding associated with onset of menstrual periods
Pubertal menorrhagia

626.4 Irregular menstrual cycle
Irregular:
  bleeding NOS
  menstruation
  periods

626.5 Ovulation bleeding
Regular intermenstrual bleeding

626.6 Metrorrhagia
Bleeding unrelated to menstrual cycle
Irregular intermenstrual bleeding

626.7 Postcoital bleeding

626.8 Other
Dysfunctional or functional uterine hemorrhage NOS
Menstruation:
  retained
  suppression of

626.9 Unspecified

627 Menopausal and postmenopausal disorders

Excludes: *asymptomatic age-related (natural) postmenopausal status (V49.81)*

627.0 Premenopausal menorrhagia
Excessive bleeding associated   Menorrhagia:
  with onset of menopause   climacteric
                                    menopausal
                                    preclimacteric

627.1 Postmenopausal bleeding

▲ 627.2 Symptomatic menopausal or female climacteric states
Symptoms, such as flushing, sleeplessness, headache, lack of concentration, associated with the menopause

627.3 Postmenopausal atrophic vaginitis
Senile (atrophic) vaginitis

▲ 627.4 Symptomatic states associated with artificial menopause
Postartificial menopause syndromes
Any condition classifiable to 627.1, 627.2, or 627.3 which follows induced menopause

627.8 Other specified menopausal and postmenopausal disorders

Excludes: *premature menopause NOS (256.31)*

627.9 Unspecified menopausal and postmenopausal disorder

	Add 4th or 5th digit		Nonspecific code		Unspecified code		Manifestation code

628 Infertility, female
Includes: primary and secondary sterility

628.0 Associated with anovulation
Anovulatory cycle

Use additional code for any associated Stein-Leventhal syndrome (256.4)

628.1 *Of pituitary-hypothalamic origin*
Code first underlying cause, as:
adiposogenital dystrophy (253.8)
anterior pituitary disorder (253.0-253.4)

628.2 Of tubal origin
Infertility associated with congenital anomaly of tube
Tubal:
block
occlusion
stenosis

Use additional code for any associated peritubal adhesions (614.6)

628.3 Of uterine origin
Infertility associated with congenital anomaly of uterus
Nonimplantation

Use additional code for any associated tuberculous endometritis (016.7)

628.4 Of cervical or vaginal origin
Infertility associated with:
anomaly of cervical mucus
congenital structural anomaly
dysmucorrhea

628.8 Of other specified origin

628.9 Of unspecified origin

629 Other disorders of female genital organs

629.0 Hematocele, female, not elsewhere classified

Excludes: *hematocele or hematoma:*
broad ligament (620.7)
fallopian tube (620.8)
that associated with ectopic pregnancy (633.00-633.91)
uterus (621.4)
vagina (623.6)
vulva (624.5)

629.1 Hydrocele, canal of Nuck
Cyst of canal of Nuck (acquired)

Excludes: *congenital (752.41)*

629.8 Other specified disorders of female genital organs

629.9 Unspecified disorder of female genital organs
Habitual aborter without current pregnancy

● Code new to this edition   ▲ Revision of existing code   ④ ⑤ Fourth or fifth digit required

11. COMPLICATIONS OF PREGNANCY, CHILDBIRTH, AND THE PUERPERIUM (630-677)

ECTOPIC AND MOLAR PREGNANCY (630-633)

Use additional code from category 639 to identify any complications

630 Hydatidiform mole
Trophoblastic disease NOS
Vesicular mole

> | Excludes: | chorioadenoma (destruens) (236.1)
> chorionepithelioma (181)
> malignant hydatidiform mole (236.1)

631 Other abnormal product of conception

Blighted ovum
Mole:
 NOS
 carneous

Mole:
 fleshy
 stone

632 Missed abortion
Early fetal death before completion of 22 weeks' gestation with retention of dead fetus
Retained products of conception, not following spontaneous or induced abortion or delivery

> | Excludes: | failed induced abortion (638.0-638.9)
> fetal death (intrauterine) (late) (656.4)
> missed delivery (656.4)
> that with abnormal product of conception (630, 631)

633 Ectopic pregnancy
Includes: ruptured ectopic pregnancy

⑤ **633.0 Abdominal pregnancy**
Intraperitoneal pregnancy

● **633.00   Abdominal pregnancy without intrauterine pregnancy**

● **633.01   Abdominal pregnancy with intrauterine pregnancy**

⑤ **633.1 Tubal pregnancy**
Fallopian pregnancy
Rupture of (fallopian) tube due to pregnancy
Tubal abortion

● **633.10   Tubal pregnancy without intrauterine pregnancy**

● **633.11   Tubal pregnancy with intrauterine pregnancy**

⑤ **633.2 Ovarian pregnancy**

● **633.20   Ovarian pregnancy without intrauterine pregnancy**

● **633.21   Ovarian pregnancy with intrauterine pregnancy**

⑤ **633.8 Other ectopic pregnancy**

Pregnancy:
 cervical
 combined
 cornual

Pregnancy:
 intraligamentous
 mesometric
 mural

● **633.80   Other ectopic pregnancy without intrauterine pregnancy**

● **633.81   Other ectopic pregnancy with intrauterine pregnancy**

⑤ **633.9 Unspecified ectopic pregnancy**

● **633.90   Unspecified ectopic pregnancy without intrauterine pregnancy**

● **633.91   Unspecified ectopic pregnancy with intrauterine pregnancy**

OTHER PREGNANCY WITH ABORTIVE OUTCOME (634-639)

Note: Use the following fifth-digit subclassification with categories 634-637:

0 Unspecified

1 Incomplete

2 Complete

The following fourth-digit subdivisions are for use with categories 634-638:

.0 Complicated by genital tract and pelvic infection
Endometritis
Salpingo-oophoritis
Sepsis NOS
Septicemia NOS
Any condition classifiable to 639.0, with condition classifiable to 634-638

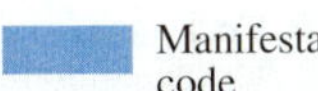

Excludes: *urinary tract infection (634-638 with .7)*

.1 Complicated by delayed or excessive hemorrhage
Afibrinogenemia
Defibrination syndrome
Intravascular hemolysis
Any condition classifiable to 639.1, with condition classifiable to 634-638

.2 Complicated by damage to pelvic organs and tissues
Laceration, perforation, or tear of:
bladder
uterus
Any condition classifiable to 639.2, with condition classifiable to 634-638

.3 Complicated by renal failure
Oliguria
Uremia
Any condition classifiable to 639.3, with condition classifiable to 634-638

.4 Complicated by metabolic disorder
Electrolyte imbalance with conditions classifiable to 634-638

.5 Complicated by shock
Circulatory collapse
Shock (postoperative) (septic)
Any condition classifiable to 639.5, with condition classifiable to 634-638

.6 Complicated by embolism
Embolism:
NOS
amniotic fluid
pulmonary
Any condition classifiable to 639.6, with condition classifiable to 634-638

.7 With other specified complications
Cardiac arrest or failure
Urinary tract infection
Any condition classifiable to 639.8, with condition classifiable to 634-638

.8 With unspecified complication

.9 Without mention of complication

⑤ **634 Abortion**
Includes: miscarriage
spontaneous abortion

⑤ **634.0 Complicated by genital tract and pelvic infection**

⑤ **634.1 Complicated by delayed or excessive hemorrhage**

⑤ **634.2 Complicated by damage to pelvic organs or tissues**

⑤ **634.3 Complicated by renal failure**

⑤ **634.4 Complicated by metabolic disorder**

⑤ **634.5 Complicated by shock**

⑤ **634.6 Complicated by embolism**

⑤ **634.7 With other specified complications**

⑤ **634.8 With unspecified complication**

⑤ **634.9 Without mention of complication**

⑤ **635 Legally induced abortion**
Includes: abortion or termination of pregnancy:
elective
legal
therapeutic

Excludes: *menstrual extraction or regulation (V25.3)*

⑤ **635.0 Complicated by genital tract and pelvic infection**

⑤ **635.1 Complicated by delayed or excessive hemorrhage**

⑤ **635.2 Complicated by damage to pelvic organs or tissues**

⑤ **635.3 Complicated by renal failure**

⑤ **635.4 Complicated by metabolic disorder**

⑤ **635.5 Complicated by shock**

⑤ **635.6 Complicated by embolism**

⑤ **635.7 With other specified complications**

● Code new
to this edition

▲ Revision of
existing code

④ ⑤ Fourth or fifth
digit required

⑤ **635.8 With unspecified complication**

⑤ **635.9 Without mention of complication**

⑤ **636 Illegally induced abortion**
Includes: abortion:
criminal
illegal
self-induced

⑤ **636.0 Complicated by genital tract and pelvic infection**

⑤ **636.1 Complicated by delayed or excessive hemorrhage**

⑤ **636.2 Complicated by damage to pelvic organs or tissues**

⑤ **636.3 Complicated by renal failure**

⑤ **636.4 Complicated by metabolic disorder**

⑤ **636.5 Complicated by shock**

⑤ **636.6 Complicated by embolism**

⑤ **636.7 With other specified complications**

⑤ **636.8 With unspecified complication**

⑤ **636.9 Without mention of complication**

⑤ **637 Unspecified abortion**
Includes: abortion NOS
retained products of conception following abortion, not classifiable elsewhere

⑤ **637.0 Complicated by genital tract and pelvic infection**

⑤ **637.1 Complicated by delayed or excessive hemorrhage**

⑤ **637.2 Complicated by damage to pelvic organs or tissues**

⑤ **637.3 Complicated by renal failure**

⑤ **637.4 Complicated by metabolic disorder**

⑤ **637.5 Complicated by shock**

⑤ **637.6 Complicated by embolism**

⑤ **637.7 With other specified complications**

⑤ **637.8 With unspecified complication**

⑤ **637.9 Without mention of complication**

638 Failed attempted abortion
Includes: failure of attempted induction of (legal) abortion

Excludes: *incomplete abortion (634.0-637.9)*

638.0 Complicated by genital tract and pelvic infection

638.1 Complicated by delayed or excessive hemorrhage

638.2 Complicated by damage to pelvic organs or tissues

638.3 Complicated by renal failure

638.4 Complicated by metabolic disorder

638.5 Complicated by shock

638.6 Complicated by embolism

638.7 With other specified complications

638.8 With unspecified complication

638.9 Without mention of complication

639 Complications following abortion and ectopic and molar pregnancies
Note: This category is provided for use when it is required to classify separately the
complications classifiable to the fourth-digit level in categories 634 638; for example:
   a) when the complication itself was responsible for an episode of medical care, the
abortion, ectopic or molar pregnancy itself having been dealt with at a previous
episode
   b) when these conditions are immediate complications of ectopic or molar pregnancies
classifiable to 630-633 where they cannot be identified at fourth-digit level.

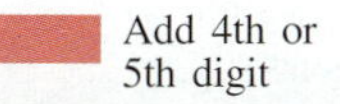

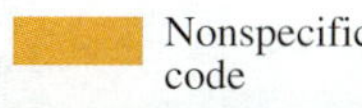

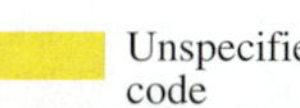

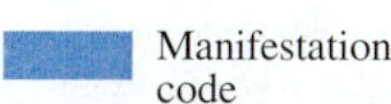

639.0 Genital tract and pelvic infection
Endometritis
Parametritis
Pelvic peritonitis
Salpingitis } following conditions classifiable to 630-638
Salpingo-oophoritis
Sepsis NOS
Septicemia NOS

Excludes: urinary tract infection (639.8)

639.1 Delayed or excessive hemorrhage
Afibrinogenemia
Defibrination syndrome } following conditions classifiable to 630-638
Intravascular hemolysis

639.2 Damage to pelvic organs and tissues
Laceration, perforation, or tear of:
 bladder
 bowel
 broad ligament } following conditions classifiable
 cervix   to 630-638
 periurethral tissue
 uterus
 vagina

639.3 Renal failure
Oliguria
Renal:
 failure (acute) } following conditions classifiable to 630-638
 shutdown
 tubular necrosis
Uremia

639.4 Metabolic disorders
Electrolyte imbalance following conditions classifiable to 630-638

639.5 Shock
Circulatory collapse } following conditions classifiable
Shock (postoperative) (septic)   to 630-638

639.6 Embolism
Embolism:
 NOS
 air
 amniotic fluid
 blood-clot
 fat } following conditions classifiable to 630-638
 pulmonary
 pyemic
 septic
 soap

639.8 Other specified complications following abortion or ectopic and molar pregnancy
Acute yellow atrophy or necrosis of liver
Cardiac arrest or failure } following conditions classifiable
Cerebral anoxia   to 630-638
Urinary tract infection

639.9 Unspecified complication following abortion or ectopic and molar pregnancy
Complication(s) not further specified following conditions classifiable to 630-638

COMPLICATIONS MAINLY RELATED TO PREGNANCY (640-648)

Includes: the listed conditions even if they arose or were present during labor, delivery, or the puerperium

The following fifth-digit subclassification is for use with categories 640-648 to denote the current episode of care:

 0 unspecified as to episode of care or not applicable

 1 delivered, with or without mention of antepartum condition
  Antepartum condition with delivery
  Delivery NOS } (with mention of antepartum
  Intrapartum obstetric condition   complication during current
  Pregnancy, delivered   episode of care)

 2 delivered, with mention of postpartum complication
  Delivery with mention of puerperal complication during current episode of care

● Code new
to this edition
▲ Revision of
existing code
④ ⑤ Fourth or fifth
digit required

> **3**   **antepartum condition or complication**
> Antepartum obstetric condition, not delivered during the current episode of care
>
> **4**   **postpartum condition or complication**
> Postpartum or puerperal obstetric condition or complication following delivery that occurred:
> during previous episode of care
> outside hospital, with subsequent admission for observation or care

⑤ **640** **Hemorrhage in early pregnancy**
Includes: hemorrhage before completion of 22 weeks' gestation

⑤ **640.0** **Threatened abortion**
[0,1,3]

⑤ **640.8** **Other specified hemorrhage in early pregnancy**
[0,1,3]

⑤ **640.9** **Unspecified hemorrhage in early pregnancy**
[0,1,3]

⑤ **641** **Antepartum hemorrhage, abruptio placentae, and placenta previa**

⑤ **641.0** **Placenta previa without hemorrhage**
[0,1,3]   Low implantation of placenta
Placenta previa noted:
during pregnancy
before labor (and delivered by cesarean delivery) } without hemorrhage

⑤ **641.1** **Hemorrhage from placenta previa**
[0,1,3]   Low-lying placenta
Placenta previa
incomplete
marginal } NOS or with hemorrhage (intrapartum)
partial
total

> | Excludes: | hemorrhage from vasa previa (663.5)

⑤ **641.2** **Premature separation of placenta**
[0,1,3]   Ablatio placentae
Abruptio placentae
Accidental antepartum hemorrhage
Couvelaire uterus
Detachment of placenta (premature)
Premature separation of normally implanted placenta

⑤ **641.3** **Antepartum hemorrhage associated with coagulation defects**
[0,1,3]   Antepartum or intrapartum hemorrhage associated with:
afibrinogenemia
hyperfibrinolysis
hypofibrinogenemia

⑤ **641.8** **Other antepartum hemorrhage**
[0,1,3]   Antepartum or intrapartum hemorrhage associated with:
trauma
uterine leiomyoma

⑤ **641.9** **Unspecified antepartum hemorrhage**
[0,1,3]   Hemorrhage:
antepartum NOS
intrapartum NOS
of pregnancy NOS

⑤ **642** **Hypertension complicating pregnancy, childbirth, and the puerperium**

⑤ **642.0** **Benign essential hypertension complicating pregnancy, childbirth, and the puerperium**
[0-4]   Hypertension:
benign essential
chronic NOS } specified as complicating, or as a reason for obstetric
essential   care during pregnancy, childbirth, or the puerperium
pre-existing NOS

⑤ **642.1** **Hypertension secondary to renal disease, complicating pregnancy, childbirth, and the puerperium**
[0-4]   Hypertension secondary to renal disease, specified as complicating, or as a reason for obstetric care during pregnancy, childbirth, or the puerperium

---

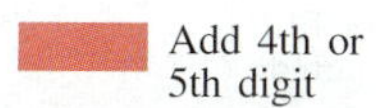

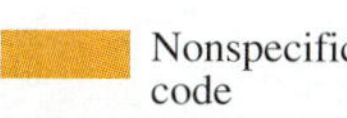

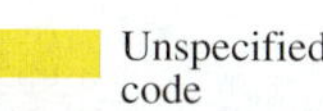

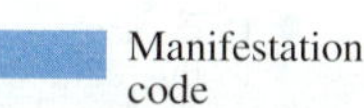

⑤ **642.2 Other pre-existing hypertension complicating pregnancy, childbirth, and the puerperium**

[0-4] Hypertensive:
heart and renal disease } specified as complicating, as a reason for obstetric care
heart disease during pregnancy, childbirth, or the puerperium
renal disease
Malignant hypertension

⑤ **642.3 Transient hypertension of pregnancy**

[0-4] Gestational hypertension
Transient hypertension, so described, in pregnancy, childbirth, or the puerperium

⑤ **642.4 Mild or unspecified pre-eclampsia**

[0-4] Hypertension in pregnancy, childbirth, or the puerperium, not specified as pre-existing, with either albuminuria or edema, or both; mild or unspecified
Pre-eclampsia: Toxemia (pre-eclamptic):
NOS NOS
mild mild

Excludes: *albuminuria in pregnancy, without mention of hypertension (646.2)*
edema in pregnancy, without mention of hypertension (646.1)

⑤ **642.5 Severe pre-eclampsia**

[0-4] Hypertension in pregnancy, childbirth, or the puerperium, not specified as pre-existing, with either albuminuria or edema, or both; specified as severe
Pre-eclampsia, severe
Toxemia (pre-eclamptic), severe

⑤ **642.6 Eclampsia**

[0-4] Toxemia:
eclamptic
with convulsions

⑤ **642.7 Pre-eclampsia or eclampsia superimposed on pre-existing hypertension**

[0-4] Conditions classifiable to 642.4-642.6, with conditions classifiable to 642.0-642.2

⑤ **642.9 Unspecified hypertension complicating pregnancy, childbirth, or the puerperium**

[0-4] Hypertension NOS, without mention of albuminuria or edema, complicating pregnancy, childbirth, or the puerperium

⑤ **643 Excessive vomiting in pregnancy**

Includes:
hyperemesis }
vomiting: } arising during pregnancy
persistent
vicious
hyperemesis gravidarum

⑤ **643.0 Mild hyperemesis gravidarum**

[0,1,3] Hyperemesis gravidarum, mild or unspecified, starting before the end of the 22nd week of gestation

⑤ **643.1 Hyperemesis gravidarum with metabolic disturbance**

[0,1,3] Hyperemesis gravidarum, starting before the end of the 22nd week of gestation, with metabolic disturbance, such as:
carbohydrate depletion
dehydration
electrolyte imbalance

⑤ **643.2 Late vomiting of pregnancy**

[0,1,3] Excessive vomiting starting after 22 completed weeks of gestation

⑤ **643.8 Other vomiting complicating pregnancy**

[0,1,3] Vomiting due to organic disease or other cause, specified as complicating pregnancy, or as a reason for obstetric care during pregnancy

Use additional code, if desired, to specify cause

⑤ **643.9 Unspecified vomiting of pregnancy**

[0,1,3] Vomiting as a reason for care during pregnancy, length of gestation unspecified

⑤ **644 Early or threatened labor**

⑤ **644.0 Threatened premature labor**

[0,3] Premature labor after 22 weeks, but before 37 completed weeks of gestation without delivery

Excludes: *that occurring before 22 completed weeks of gestation (640.0)*

● Code new ▲ Revision of ④ ⑤ Fourth or fifth
to this edition existing code digit required

⑤ **644.1 Other threatened labor**
[0,3]　　　False labor:
　　　　　　NOS
　　　　　　after 37 completed weeks of gestation　⎫
　　　　　Threatened labor NOS　　　　　　　　　⎬　without delivery
　　　　　　　　　　　　　　　　　　　　　　　⎭

⑤ **644.2 Early onset of delivery**
[0,1]　　　Onset (spontaneous) of delivery　　　⎫　before 37 completed weeks of
　　　　　Premature labor with onset of delivery　⎬　　gestation
　　　　　　　　　　　　　　　　　　　　　　⎭

⑤ **645 Late pregnancy**

⑤ **645.1 Post term pregnancy**
[0,1,3]　　Pregnancy over 40 completed weeks to 42 completed weeks gestation

⑤ **645.2 Prolonged pregnancy**
[0,1,3]　　Pregnancy which has advanced beyond 42 completed weeks gestation

⑤ **646 Other complications of pregnancy, not elsewhere classified**
　　　Use additional code(s) to further specify complication

⑤ **646.0 Papyraceous fetus**
[0,1,3]

⑤ **646.1 Edema or excessive weight gain in pregnancy, without mention of hypertension**
[0-4]　　　Gestational edema
　　　　　Maternal obesity syndrome

　　　　　| *Excludes:* | *that with mention of hypertension (642.0-642.9)* |

⑤ **646.2 Unspecified renal disease in pregnancy, without mention of hypertension**
[0-4]　　　Albuminuria　　　　　⎫
　　　　　Nephropathy NOS　　　 ⎪
　　　　　Renal disease NOS　　　⎬　in pregnancy or the puerperium, without mention of hypertension
　　　　　Uremia　　　　　　　　⎪
　　　　　Gestational proteinuria ⎭

　　　　　| *Excludes:* | *that with mention of hypertension (642.0-642.9)* |

⑤ **646.3 Habitual aborter**
[0,1,3]

　　　　　| *Excludes:* | *with current abortion (634.0-634.9)* |
　　　　　| | *without current pregnancy (629.9)* |

⑤ **646.4 Peripheral neuritis in pregnancy**
[0-4]

⑤ **646.5 Asymptomatic bacteriuria in pregnancy**
[0-4]

⑤ **646.6 Infections of genitourinary tract in pregnancy**
[0-4]　　　Conditions classifiable to 590, 595, 597, 599.0, 616 complicating pregnancy, childbirth,
　　　　　　or the puerperium
　　　　　Conditions classifiable to 614.0-614.5, 614.7-614.9, 615

　　　　　| *Excludes:* | *major puerperal infection (670)* |

⑤ **646.7 Liver disorders in pregnancy**
[0,1,3]　　Acute yellow atrophy of liver (obstetric) (true)　⎫
　　　　　Icterus gravis　　　　　　　　　　　　　　⎬　of pregnancy
　　　　　Necrosis of liver　　　　　　　　　　　　　⎭

　　　　　| *Excludes:* | *hepatorenal syndrome following delivery (674.8)* |
　　　　　| | *viral hepatitis (647.6)* |

⑤ **646.8 Other specified complications of pregnancy**
[0-4]　　　Fatigue during pregnancy　　　Insufficient weight gain of pregnancy
　　　　　Herpes gestationis　　　　　　Uterine size-date discrepancy

⑤ **646.9 Unspecified complication of pregnancy**
[0,1,3]

⑤ **647 Infectious and parasitic conditions in the mother classifiable elsewhere, but complicating pregnancy, childbirth, or the puerperium**
　　　Includes:　the listed conditions when complicating the pregnant state, aggravated by the
　　　　　　　　pregnancy, or when a main reason for obstetric care

　　　　　| *Excludes:* | *those conditions in the mother known or suspected to have affected the fetus* |
　　　　　| | *(655.0-655.9)* |

　　　Use additional code(s) to further specify complication

| ▮ Add 4th or 5th digit | ▮ Nonspecific code | ▮ Unspecified code | ▮ Manifestation code |

⑤ **647.0 Syphilis**
[0-4]   Conditions classifiable to 090-097

⑤ **647.1 Gonorrhea**
[0-4]   Conditions classifiable to 098

⑤ **647.2 Other venereal diseases**
[0-4]   Conditions classifiable to 099

⑤ **647.3 Tuberculosis**
[0-4]   Conditions classifiable to 010-018

⑤ **647.4 Malaria**
[0-4]   Conditions classifiable to 084

⑤ **647.5 Rubella**
[0-4]   Conditions classifiable to 056

⑤ **647.6 Other viral diseases**
[0-4]   Conditions classifiable to 042 and 050-079, except 056

⑤ **647.8 Other specified infectious and parasitic diseases**
[0-4]

⑤ **647.9 Unspecified infection or infestation**
[0-4]

⑤ **648 Other current conditions in the mother classifiable elsewhere, but complicating pregnancy, childbirth, or the puerperium**
Includes: the listed conditions when complicating the pregnant state, aggravated by the pregnancy, or when a main reason for obstetric care

Excludes: *those conditions in the mother known or suspected to have affected the fetus (655.0-655.9)*

Use additional code(s) to identify the condition

⑤ **648.0 Diabetes mellitus**
[0-4]   Conditions classifiable to 250

Excludes: *gestational diabetes (648.8)*

⑤ **648.1 Thyroid dysfunction**
[0-4]   Conditions classifiable to 240-246

⑤ **648.2 Anemia**
[0-4]   Conditions classifiable to 280-285

⑤ **648.3 Drug dependence**
[0-4]   Conditions classifiable to 304

⑤ **648.4 Mental disorders**
[0-4]   Conditions classifiable to 290-303, 305-316, 317-319

⑤ **648.5 Congenital cardiovascular disorders**
[0-4]   Conditions classifiable to 745-747

⑤ **648.6 Other cardiovascular diseases**
[0-4]   Conditions classifiable to 390-398, 410-429

Excludes: *cerebrovascular disorders in the puerperium (674.0)*
venous complications (671.0-671.9)

⑤ **648.7 Bone and joint disorders of back, pelvis, and lower limbs**
[0-4]   Conditions classifiable to 720-724, and those classifiable to 711-719 or 725-738, specified as affecting the lower limbs

⑤ **648.8 Abnormal glucose tolerance**
[0-4]   Conditions classifiable to 790.2
Gestational diabetes

⑤ **648.9 Other current conditions classifiable elsewhere**
[0-4]   Conditions classifiable to 440-459
Nutritional deficiencies [conditions classifiable to 260-269]

● Code new to this edition   ▲ Revision of existing code   ④ ⑤ Fourth or fifth digit required

NORMAL DELIVERY, AND OTHER INDICATIONS FOR CARE IN PREGNANCY, LABOR, AND DELIVERY (650-659)

650 Normal delivery

Delivery requiring minimal or no assistance, with or without episiotomy, without fetal manipulation [e.g., rotation version] or instrumentation [forceps] of spontaneous, cephalic, vaginal, full-term, single, live born infant. This code is for use as a single diagnosis code and is not to be used with any other code in the range 630-676.

> *Excludes:* breech delivery (assisted) (spontaneous) NOS (652.2)
>> delivery by vacuum extractor, forceps, cesarean section, or breech extraction, without specified complication (669.5-669.7)

Use additional code to indicate outcome of delivery (V27.0)

The following fifth-digit subclassification is for use with categories 651-659 to denote the current episode of care:

    0 unspecified as to episode of care or not applicable

    1 delivered, with or without mention of antepartum condition

    2 delivered, with mention of postpartum complication

    3 antepartum condition or complication

    4 postpartum condition or complication

651 Multiple gestation

651.0 Twin pregnancy
[0,1,3]

651.1 Triplet pregnancy
[0,1,3]

651.2 Quadruplet pregnancy
[0,1,3]

651.3 Twin pregnancy with fetal loss and retention of one fetus
[0,1,3]

651.4 Triplet pregnancy with fetal loss and retention of one or more fetus(es)
[0,1,3]

651.5 Quadruplet pregnancy with fetal loss and retention of one or more fetus(es)
[0,1,3]

651.6 Other multiple pregnancy with fetal loss and retention of one or more fetus(es)
[0,1,3]

651.8 Other specified multiple gestation
[0,1,3]

651.9 Unspecified multiple gestation
[0,1,3]

652 Malposition and malpresentation of fetus

Code first any associated obstructed labor (660.0)

652.0 Unstable lie
[0,1,3]

652.1 Breech or other malpresentation successfully converted to cephalic presentation
[0,1,3]   Cephalic version NOS

652.2 Breech presentation without mention of version
[0,1,3]   Breech delivery (assisted) (spontaneous) NOS
    Buttocks presentation
    Complete breech
    Frank breech

> *Excludes:* footling presentation (652.8)
>> incomplete breech (652.8)

652.3 Transverse or oblique presentation
[0,1,3]   Oblique lie   Transverse lie

> *Excludes:* transverse arrest of fetal head (660.3)

652.4 Face or brow presentation
[0,1,3]   Mentum presentation

652.5 High head at term
[0,1,3]   Failure of head to enter pelvic brim

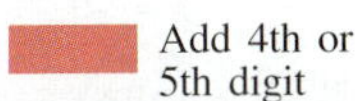

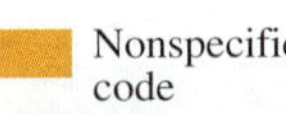

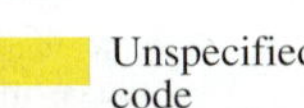

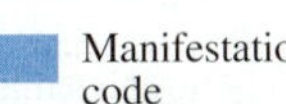

⑤ **652.6 Multiple gestation with malpresentation of one fetus or more**
[0,1,3]

⑤ **652.7 Prolapsed arm**
[0,1,3]

⑤ **652.8 Other specified malposition or malpresentation**
[0,1,3]   Compound presentation

⑤ **652.9 Unspecified malposition or malpresentation**
[0,1,3]

⑤ **653 Disproportion**
Code first any associated obstructed labor (660.1)

⑤ **653.0 Major abnormality of bony pelvis, not further specified**
[0,1,3]   Pelvic deformity NOS

⑤ **653.1 Generally contracted pelvis**
[0,1,3]   Contracted pelvis NOS

⑤ **653.2 Inlet contraction of pelvis**
[0,1,3]   Inlet contraction (pelvis)

⑤ **653.3 Outlet contraction of pelvis**
[0,1,3]   Outlet contraction (pelvis)

⑤ **653.4 Fetopelvic disproportion**
[0,1,3]   Cephalopelvic disproportion NOS
Disproportion of mixed maternal and fetal origin, with normally formed fetus

⑤ **653.5 Unusually large fetus causing disproportion**
[0,1,3]   Disproportion of fetal origin with normally formed fetus
Fetal disproportion NOS

> **Excludes:** *that when the reason for medical care was concern for the fetus (656.6)*

⑤ **653.6 Hydrocephalic fetus causing disproportion**
[0,1,3]

> **Excludes:** *that when the reason for medical care was concern for the fetus (655.0)*

⑤ **653.7 Other fetal abnormality causing disproportion**
[0,1,3]   Conjoined twins   Fetal:
Fetal: myelomeningocele
  ascites   sacral teratoma
  hydrops   tumor

⑤ **653.8 Disproportion of other origin**
[0,1,3]

> **Excludes:** *shoulder (girdle) dystocia (660.4)*

⑤ **653.9 Unspecified disproportion**
[0,1,3]

⑤ **654 Abnormality of organs and soft tissues of pelvis**
Includes: the listed conditions during pregnancy, childbirth, or the puerperium
Code first any associated obstructed labor (660.2)

⑤ **654.0 Congenital abnormalities of uterus**
[0-4]   Double uterus   Uterus bicornis

⑤ **654.1 Tumors of body of uterus**
[0-4]   Uterine fibroids

⑤ **654.2 Previous cesarean delivery NOS**
[0,1,3]   Uterine scar from previous cesarean delivery

⑤ **654.3 Retroverted and incarcerated gravid uterus**
[0-4]

⑤ **654.4 Other abnormalities in shape or position of gravid uterus and of neighboring structures**
[0-4]   Cystocele   Prolapse of gravid uterus
Pelvic floor repair   Rectocele
Pendulous abdomen   Rigid pelvic floor

⑤ **654.5 Cervical incompetence**
[0-4]   Presence of Shirodkar suture with or without mention of cervical incompetence

⑤ **654.6 Other congenital or acquired abnormality of cervix**
[0-4]   Cicatricial cervix   Stenosis or stricture of cervix
Polyp of cervix   Tumor of cervix
Previous surgery to cervix
Rigid cervix (uteri)

● Code new   ▲ Revision of   ④ ⑤ Fourth or fifth
  to this edition   existing code   digit required

⑤ **654.7 Congenital or acquired abnormality of vagina**
[0-4]   Previous surgery to vagina   Stricture of vagina
         Septate vagina   Tumor of vagina
         Stenosis of vagina (acquired)
             (congenital)

⑤ **654.8 Congenital or acquired abnormality of vulva**
[0-4]   Fibrosis of perineum
         Persistent hymen
         Previous surgery to perineum or vulva
         Rigid perineum
         Tumor of vulva

         | Excludes: | *varicose veins of vulva (671.1)*

⑤ **654.9 Other and unspecified**
[0-4]   Uterine scar NEC

⑤ **655 Known or suspected fetal abnormality affecting management of mother**
         Includes: the listed conditions in the fetus as a reason for observation or obstetrical care of the
                    mother, or for termination of pregnancy

⑤ **655.0 Central nervous system malformation in fetus**
[0,1,3] Fetal or suspected fetal:
             anencephaly
             hydrocephalus
             spina bifida (with myelomeningocele)

⑤ **655.1 Chromosomal abnormality in fetus**
[0,1,3]

⑤ **655.2 Hereditary disease in family possibly affecting fetus**
[0,1,3]

⑤ **655.3 Suspected damage to fetus from viral disease in the mother**
[0,1,3] Suspected damage to fetus from maternal rubella

⑤ **655.4 Suspected damage to fetus from other disease in the mother**
[0,1,3] Suspected damage to fetus from maternal:
             alcohol addiction
             listeriosis
             toxoplasmosis

⑤ **655.5 Suspected damage to fetus from drugs**
[0,1,3]

⑤ **655.6 Suspected damage to fetus from radiation**
[0,1,3]

⑤ **655.7 Decreased fetal movements**
[0,1,3]

⑤ **655.8 Other known or suspected fetal abnormality, not elsewhere classified**
[0,1,3] Suspected damage to fetus from:
             environmental toxins
             intrauterine contraceptive device

⑤ **655.9 Unspecified**
[0,1,3]

⑤ **656 Other fetal and placental problems affecting management of mother**

⑤ **656.0 Fetal-maternal hemorrhage**
[0,1,3] Leakage (microscopic) of fetal blood into maternal circulation

⑤ **656.1 Rhesus isoimmunization**
[0,1,3] Anti-D [Rh] antibodies
         Rh incompatibility

⑤ **656.2 Isoimmunization from other and unspecified blood-group incompatibility**
[0,1,3] ABO isoimmunization

⑤ **656.3 Fetal distress**
[0,1,3] Fetal metabolic acidemia

         | Excludes: | *abnormal fetal acid-base balance (656.8)*

                    abnormality in fetal heart rate or rhythm (659.7)
                    fetal bradycardia (659.7)
                    fetal tachycardia (659.7)
                    meconium in liquor (656.8)

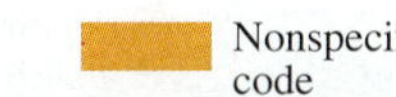

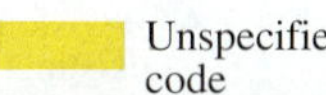

⑤ **656.4 Intrauterine death**
[0,1,3]   Fetal death:
          NOS
          after completion of 22 weeks' gestation
          late
      Missed delivery

> Excludes: *missed abortion (632)*

⑤ **656.5 Poor fetal growth**
[0,1,3]   "Light-for-dates"   "Small-for-dates"
      "Placental insufficiency"

⑤ **656.6 Excessive fetal growth**
[0,1,3]   "Large-for-dates"

⑤ **656.7 Other placental conditions**
[0,1,3]   Abnormal placenta   Placental infarct

> Excludes: *placental polyp (674.4)*
> *placentitis (658.4)*

⑤ **656.8 Other specified fetal and placental problems**
[0,1,3]   Abnormal acid-base balance
      Intrauterine acidosis
      Lithopedian
      Meconium in liquor

⑤ **656.9 Unspecified fetal and placental problem**
[0,1,3]

⑤ **657 Polyhydramnios**
[0,1,3]   Hydramnios
      Use 0 as fourth-digit for this category

⑤ **658 Other problems associated with amniotic cavity and membranes**

> Excludes: *amniotic fluid embolism (673.1)*

⑤ **658.0 Oligohydramnios**
[0,1,3]   Oligohydramnios without mention of rupture of membranes

⑤ **658.1 Premature rupture of membranes**
[0,1,3]   Rupture of amniotic sac less than 24 hours prior to the onset of labor

⑤ **658.2 Delayed delivery after spontaneous or unspecified rupture of membranes**
[0,1,3]   Prolonged rupture of membranes NOS
      Rupture of amniotic sac 24 hours or more prior to the onset of labor

⑤ **658.3 Delayed delivery after artificial rupture of membranes**
[0,1,3]

⑤ **658.4 Infection of amniotic cavity**
[0,1,3]   Amnionitis   Membranitis
      Chorioamnionitis   Placentitis

⑤ **658.8 Other**
[0,1,3]   Amnion nodosum   Amniotic cyst

⑤ **658.9 Unspecified**
[0,1,3]

⑤ **659 Other indications for care or intervention related to labor and delivery, not elsewhere classified**

⑤ **659.0 Failed mechanical induction**
[0,1,3]   Failure of induction of labor by surgical or other instrumental methods

⑤ **659.1 Failed medical or unspecified induction**
[0,1,3]   Failed induction NOS
      Failure of induction of labor by medical methods, such as oxytocic drugs

⑤ **659.2 Maternal pyrexia during labor, unspecified**
[0,1,3]

⑤ **659.3 Generalized infection during labor**
[0,1,3]   Septicemia during labor

⑤ **659.4 Grand multiparity**
[0,1,3]

> Excludes: *supervision only, in pregnancy (V23.3)*
> *without current pregnancy (V61.5)*

● Code new
  to this edition   ▲ Revision of
  existing code   ④ ⑤ Fourth or fifth
  digit required

⑤ **659.5 Elderly primigravida**
[0,1,3] First pregnancy in a woman who will be 35 years of age or older at expected date of delivery

Excludes: supervision only, in pregnancy (V23.81)

⑤ **659.6 Elderly multigravida**
[0,1,3] Second or more pregnancy in a woman who will be 35 years of age or older at expected date of delivery

Excludes: elderly primigravida 659.5
supervision only, in pregnancy (V23.82)

⑤ **659.7 Abnormality in fetal heart rate or rhythm**
[0,1,3] Depressed fetal heart tones
Fetal:
bradycardia
tachycardia
Fetal heart rate decelerations
Non-reassuring fetal heart rate or rhythm

⑤ **659.8 Other specified indications for care or intervention related to labor and delivery**
[0,1,3] Pregnancy in female less than 16 years old at expected date of delivery
Very young maternal age

⑤ **659.9 Unspecified indication for care or intervention related to labor and delivery**
[0,1,3]

COMPLICATIONS OCCURRING MAINLY IN THE COURSE OF LABOR AND DELIVERY (660-669)

The following fifth-digit subclassification is for use with categories 660-669 to denote the current episode of care:

0 unspecified as to episode of care or not applicable

1 delivered, with or without mention of antepartum condition

2 delivered, with mention of postpartum complication

3 antepartum condition or complication

4 postpartum condition or complication

⑤ **660 Obstructed labor**

⑤ **660.0 Obstruction caused by malposition of fetus at onset of labor**
[0,1,3] Any condition classifiable to 652, causing obstruction during labor
Use additional code from 652.0-652.9, if desired, to identify condition

⑤ **660.1 Obstruction by bony pelvis**
[0,1,3] Any condition classifiable to 653, causing obstruction during labor
Use additional code from 653.0-653.9, if desired, to identify condition

⑤ **660.2 Obstruction by abnormal pelvic soft tissues**
[0,1,3] Prolapse of anterior lip of cervix
Any condition classifiable to 654, causing obstruction during labor
Use additional code from 654.0-654.9, if desired, to identify condition

⑤ **660.3 Deep transverse arrest and persistent occipitoposterior position**
[0,1,3]

⑤ **660.4 Shoulder (girdle) dystocia**
[0,1,3] Impacted shoulders

⑤ **660.5 Locked twins**
[0,1,3]

⑤ **660.6 Failed trial of labor, unspecified**
[0,1,3] Failed trial of labor, without mention of condition or suspected condition

⑤ **660.7 Failed forceps or vacuum extractor, unspecified**
[0,1,3] Application of ventouse or forceps, without mention of condition

⑤ **660.8 Other causes of obstructed labor**
[0,1,3]

⑤ **660.9 Unspecified obstructed labor**
[0,1,3] Dystocia:
NOS
fetal NOS
maternal NOS

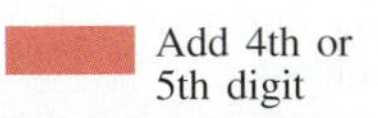

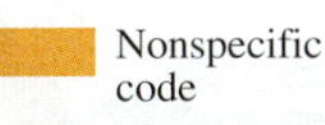

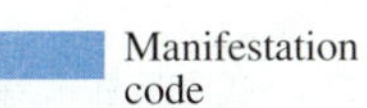

⑤ **661** **Abnormality of forces of labor**

  ⑤ **661.0** **Primary uterine inertia**
[0,1,3] Failure of cervical dilation
Hypotonic uterine dysfunction, primary
Prolonged latent phase of labor

  ⑤ **661.1** **Secondary uterine inertia**
[0,1,3] Arrested active phase of labor
Hypotonic uterine dysfunction, secondary

  ⑤ **661.2** **Other and unspecified uterine inertia**
[0,1,3] Desultory labor   Poor contractions
Irregular labor   Slow slope active phase of labor

  ⑤ **661.3** **Precipitate labor**
[0,1,3]

  ⑤ **661.4** **Hypertonic, incoordinate, or prolonged uterine contractions**
[0,1,3] Cervical spasm   Incoordinate uterine action
Contraction ring (dystocia)   Retraction ring (Bandl's) (pathological)
Dyscoordinate labor   Tetanic contractions
Hourglass contraction of   Uterine dystocia NOS
    uterus   Uterine spasm
Hypertonic uterine dysfunction

  ⑤ **661.9** **Unspecified abnormality of labor**
[0,1,3]

⑤ **662** **Long labor**

  ⑤ **662.0** **Prolonged first stage**
[0,1,3]

  ⑤ **662.1** **Prolonged labor, unspecified**
[0,1,3]

  ⑤ **662.2** **Prolonged second stage**
[0,1,3]

  ⑤ **662.3** **Delayed delivery of second twin, triplet, etc.**
[0,1,3]

⑤ **663** **Umbilical cord complications**

  ⑤ **663.0** **Prolapse of cord**
[0,1,3] Presentation of cord

  ⑤ **663.1** **Cord around neck, with compression**
[0,1,3] Cord tightly around neck

  ⑤ **663.2** **Other and unspecified cord entanglement, with compression**
[0,1,3] Entanglement of cords of twins in mono-amniotic sac
Knot in cord (with compression)

  ⑤ **663.3** **Other and unspecified cord entanglement, without mention of compression**
[0,1,3]

  ⑤ **663.4** **Short cord**
[0,1,3]

  ⑤ **663.5** **Vasa previa**
[0,1,3]

  ⑤ **663.6** **Vascular lesions of cord**
[0,1,3] Bruising of cord   Thrombosis of vessels of cord
Hematoma of cord

  ⑤ **663.8** **Other umbilical cord complications**
[0,1,3] Velamentous insertion of umbilical cord

  ⑤ **663.9** **Unspecified umbilical cord complication**
[0,1,3]

⑤ **664** **Trauma to perineum and vulva during delivery**
Includes: damage from instruments
that from extension of episiotomy

● Code new   ▲ Revision of   ④ ⑤ Fourth or fifth
to this edition   existing code   digit required

⑤ **664.0 First-degree perineal laceration**
[0,1,4]   Perineal laceration, rupture, or tear involving:
             fourchette
             hymen
             labia
             skin
             vagina
             vulva

⑤ **664.1 Second-degree perineal laceration**
[0,1,4]   Perineal laceration, rupture, or tear (following episiotomy) involving:
             pelvic floor
             perineal muscles
             vaginal muscles

> | Excludes: | that involving anal sphincter (664.2)

⑤ **664.2 Third-degree perineal laceration**
[0,1,4]   Perineal laceration, rupture, or tear (following episiotomy) involving:
             anal sphincter
             rectovaginal septum
             sphincter NOS

> | Excludes: | that with anal or rectal mucosal laceration (664.3)

⑤ **664.3 Fourth-degree perineal laceration**
[0,1,4]   Perineal laceration, rupture, or tear as classifiable to 664.2 and involving also:
             anal mucosa
             rectal mucosa

⑤ **664.4 Unspecified perineal laceration**
[0,1,4]   Central laceration

⑤ **664.5 Vulval and perineal hematoma**
[0,1,4]

⑤ **664.8 Other specified trauma to perineum and vulva**
[0,1,4]

⑤ **664.9 Unspecified trauma to perineum and vulva**
[0,1,4]

⑤ **665 Other obstetrical trauma**
             Includes: damage from instruments

⑤ **665.0 Rupture of uterus before onset of labor**
[0,1,3]

⑤ **665.1 Rupture of uterus during labor**
[0,1]   Rupture of uterus NOS

⑤ **665.2 Inversion of uterus**
[0,2,4]

⑤ **665.3 Laceration of cervix**
[0,1,4]

⑤ **665.4 High vaginal laceration**
[0,1,4]   Laceration of vaginal wall or sulcus without mention of perineal laceration

⑤ **665.5 Other injury to pelvic organs**
[0,1,4]   Injury to:
             bladder
             urethra

⑤ **665.6 Damage to pelvic joints and ligaments**
[0,1,4]   Avulsion of inner symphyseal cartilage
             Damage to coccyx
             Separation of symphysis (pubis)

⑤ **665.7 Pelvic hematoma**
[0,1,2,4]   Hematoma of vagina

⑤ **665.8 Other specified obstetrical trauma**
[0-4]

⑤ **665.9 Unspecified obstetrical trauma**
[0-4]

⑤ **666 Postpartum hemorrhage**

⑤ **666.0 Third-stage hemorrhage**
[0,2,4]   Hemorrhage associated with retained, trapped, or adherent placenta
             Retained placenta NOS

Add 4th or 5th digit	Nonspecific code	Unspecified code	Manifestation code

⑤ **666.1** **Other immediate postpartum hemorrhage**
[0,2,4]   Atony of uterus
    Hemorrhage within the first 24 hours following delivery of placenta
    Postpartum hemorrhage (atonic) NOS

⑤ **666.2** **Delayed and secondary postpartum hemorrhage**
[0,2,4]   Hemorrhage:
      after the first 24 hours following delivery
      associated with retained portions of placenta or membranes
    Postpartum hemorrhage specified as delayed or secondary
    Retained products of conception NOS, following delivery

⑤ **666.3** **Postpartum coagulation defects**
[0,2,4]   Postpartum afibrinogenemia
    Postpartum fibrinolysis

⑤ **667** **Retained placenta or membranes, without hemorrhage**

⑤ **667.0** **Retained placenta without hemorrhage**
[0,2,4]   Placenta accreta
    Retained placenta: } without hemorrhage
      NOS
      total

⑤ **667.1** **Retained portions of placenta or membranes, without hemorrhage**
[0,2,4]   Retained products of conception following delivery, without hemorrhage

⑤ **668** **Complications of the administration of anesthetic or other sedation in labor and delivery**
    Includes: complications arising from the administration of a general or local anesthetic,
      analgesic, or other sedation in labor and delivery

    Excludes: *reaction to spinal or lumbar puncture (349.0)*
      spinal headache (349.0)

  Use additional code(s) to further specify complication

⑤ **668.0** **Pulmonary complications**
[0-4]   Inhalation [aspiration] of stomach contents or
      secretions
    Mendelson's syndrome   } following anesthesia or other
    Pressure collapse of lung   } sedation in labor or delivery

⑤ **668.1** **Cardiac complications**
[0-4]   Cardiac arrest or failure following anesthesia or other sedation in labor and delivery

⑤ **668.2** **Central nervous system complications**
[0-4]   Cerebral anoxia following anesthesia or other sedation in labor and delivery

⑤ **668.8** **Other complications of anesthesia or other sedation in labor and delivery**
[0-4]

⑤ **668.9** **Unspecified complication of anesthesia and other sedation**
[0-4]

⑤ **669** **Other complications of labor and delivery, not elsewhere classified**

⑤ **669.0** **Maternal distress**
[0-4]   Metabolic disturbance in labor and delivery

⑤ **669.1** **Shock during or following labor and delivery**
[0-4]   Obstetric shock

⑤ **669.2** **Maternal hypotension syndrome**
[0-4]

⑤ **669.3** **Acute renal failure following labor and delivery**
[0,2,4]

⑤ **669.4** **Other complications of obstetrical surgery and procedures**
[0-4]   Cardiac:
      arrest   } following cesarean or other obstetrical surgery or
      failure   } procedure, including delivery NOS
    Cerebral anoxia

    Excludes: *complications of obstetrical surgical wounds (674.1-674.3)*

⑤ **669.5** **Forceps or vacuum extractor delivery without mention of indication**
[0,1]   Delivery by ventouse, without mention of indication

⑤ **669.6** **Breech extraction, without mention of indication**
[0,1]

    Excludes: *breech delivery NOS (652.2)*

   ● Code new   ▲ Revision of   ④ ⑤ Fourth or fifth
    to this edition   existing code   digit required

⑤ **669.7 Cesarean delivery, without mention of indication**
[0,1]

⑤ **669.8 Other complications of labor and delivery**
[0-4]

⑤ **669.9 Unspecified complication of labor and delivery**
[0-4]

COMPLICATIONS OF THE PUERPERIUM (670-677)

Note: Categories 671 and 673-676 include the listed conditions even if they occur during pregnancy or childbirth.

The following fifth-digit subclassification is for use with categories 670-676 to denote the current episode of care:

0 unspecified as to episode of care or not applicable

1 delivered, with or without mention of antepartum condition

2 delivered, with mention of postpartum complication

3 antepartum condition or complication

4 postpartum condition or complication

⑤ **670 Major puerperal infection**
[0,2,4]

Puerperal:	Puerperal:
endometritis	peritonitis
fever (septic)	pyemia
pelvic:	salpingitis
cellulitis	septicemia
sepsis	

Use 0 as fourth-digit for this category

> *Excludes:* *infection following abortion (639.0)*
> *minor genital tract infection following delivery (646.6)*
> *puerperal pyrexia NOS (672)*
> *puerperal fever NOS (672)*
> *puerperal pyrexia of unknown origin (672)*
> *urinary tract infection following delivery (646.6)*

⑤ **671 Venous complications in pregnancy and the puerperium**

  ⑤ **671.0 Varicose veins of legs**
[0-4]   Varicose veins NOS

  ⑤ **671.1 Varicose veins of vulva and perineum**
[0-4]

  ⑤ **671.2 Superficial thrombophlebitis**
[0-4]   Thrombophlebitis (superficial)

  ⑤ **671.3 Deep phlebothrombosis, antepartum**
[0,1,3]   Deep-vein thrombosis, antepartum

  ⑤ **671.4 Deep phlebothrombosis, postpartum**
[0,2,4]   Deep-vein thrombosis, postpartum
    Pelvic thrombophlebitis, postpartum
    Phlegmasia alba dolens (puerperal)

  ⑤ **671.5 Other phlebitis and thrombosis**
[0-4]   Cerebral venous thrombosis
    Thrombosis of intracranial venous sinus

  ⑤ **671.8 Other venous complications**
[0-4]   Hemorrhoids

  ⑤ **671.9 Unspecified venous complication**
[0-4]   Phlebitis NOS
    Thrombosis NOS

⑤ **672 Pyrexia of unknown origin during the puerperium**
[0,2,4]   Puerperal fever NOS
    Postpartum fever NOS

Use 0 as fourth-digit for this category

⑤ **673 Obstetrical pulmonary embolism**
Includes: pulmonary emboli in pregnancy, childbirth, or the puerperium, or specified as puerperal

> *Excludes:* *embolism following abortion (639.6)*

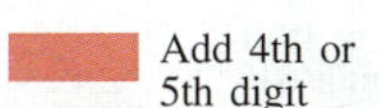
Add 4th or 5th digit

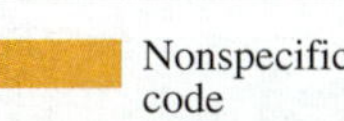
Nonspecific code

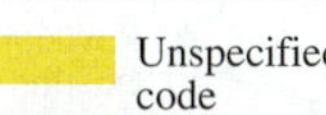
Unspecified code

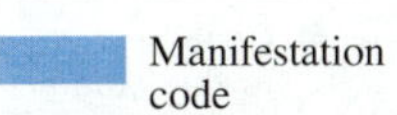
Manifestation code

⑤ **673.0 Obstetrical air embolism**
[0-4]

⑤ **673.1 Amniotic fluid embolism**
[0-4]

⑤ **673.2 Obstetrical blood-clot embolism**
[0-4]   Puerperal pulmonary embolism NOS

⑤ **673.3 Obstetrical pyemic and septic embolism**
[0-4]

⑤ **673.8 Other pulmonary embolism**
[0-4]   Fat embolism

⑤ **674 Other and unspecified complications of the puerperium, not elsewhere classified**

⑤ **674.0 Cerebrovascular disorders in the puerperium**
[0-4]   Any condition classifiable to 430-434, 436-437 occurring during pregnancy, childbirth, or the puerperium, or specified as puerperal

> Excludes: *intracranial venous sinus thrombosis (671.5)*

⑤ **674.1 Disruption of cesarean wound**
[0,2,4]   Dehiscence or disruption of uterine wound

> Excludes: *uterine rupture before onset of labor (665.0)*
> *uterine rupture during labor (665.1)*

⑤ **674.2 Disruption of perineal wound**
[0,2,4]   Breakdown of perineum   Secondary perineal tear
Disruption of wound of:
  episiotomy
  perineal laceration

⑤ **674.3 Other complications of obstetrical surgical wounds**
[0,2,4]   Hematoma of cesarean section or perineal wound
Hemorrhage of cesarean section or perineal wound
Infection of cesarean section or perineal wound

> Excludes: *damage from instruments in delivery (664.0-665.9)*

⑤ **674.4 Placental polyp**
[0,2,4]

⑤ **674.8 Other**
[0,2,4]   Hepatorenal syndrome, following delivery
Postpartum:
  cardiomyopathy
  subinvolution of uterus
  uterine hypertrophy

⑤ **674.9 Unspecified**
[0,2,4]   Sudden death of unknown cause during the puerperium

⑤ **675 Infections of the breast and nipple associated with childbirth**
    Includes: the listed conditions during pregnancy, childbirth, or the puerperium

⑤ **675.0 Infections of nipple**
[0-4]   Abscess of nipple

⑤ **675.1 Abscess of breast**
[0-4]   Abscess: Mastitis:
  mammary   purulent
  subareolar   retromammary
  submammary   submammary

⑤ **675.2 Nonpurulent mastitis**
[0-4]   Lymphangitis of breast   Mastitis:
                                      NOS
                                      interstitial
                                      parenchymatous

⑤ **675.8 Other specified infections of the breast and nipple**
[0-4]

⑤ **675.9 Unspecified infection of the breast and nipple**
[0-4]

⑤ **676 Other disorders of the breast associated with childbirth and disorders of lactation**
    Includes: the listed conditions during pregnancy, the puerperium, or lactation

● Code new   ▲ Revision of   ④ ⑤ Fourth or fifth
to this edition   existing code   digit required

⑤ **676.0 Retracted nipple**
[0-4]

⑤ **676.1 Cracked nipple**
[0-4]   Fissure of nipple

⑤ **676.2 Engorgement of breasts**
[0-4]

⑤ **676.3 Other and unspecified disorder of breast**
[0-4]

⑤ **676.4 Failure of lactation**
[0-4]   Agalactia

⑤ **676.5 Suppressed lactation**
[0-4]

⑤ **676.6 Galactorrhea**
[0-4]

> *Excludes:* galactorrhea not associated with childbirth (611.6)

⑤ **676.8 Other disorders of lactation**
[0-4]   Galactocele

⑤ **676.9 Unspecified disorder of lactation**
[0-4]

677 Late effect of complication of pregnancy, childbirth, and the puerperium

Note: This category is to be used to indicate conditions in 632-648.9 and 651-676.9 as the cause of the late effect, themselves classifiable elsewhere. The "late effects" include conditions specified as such, or as sequelae, which may occur at any time after the puerperium.
Code first any sequelae

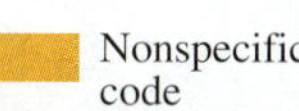

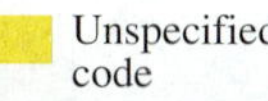

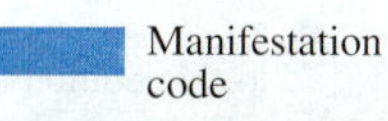

● Code new
to this edition

▲ Revision of
existing code

④ ⑤ Fourth or fifth
digit required

12. DISEASES OF THE SKIN AND SUBCUTANEOUS TISSUE (680-709)

INFECTIONS OF SKIN AND SUBCUTANEOUS TISSUE (680-686)

Excludes: certain infections of skin classified under "Infectious and Parasitic Diseases," such
as:
erysipelas (035)
erysipeloid of Rosenbach (027.1)
herpes:
simplex (054.0-054.9)
zoster (053.0-053.9)
molluscum contagiosum (078.0)
viral warts (078.1)

680 Carbuncle and furuncle
Includes: boil
furunculosis

680.0 Face
Ear [any part]
Face [any part, except eye]
Nose (septum)
Temple (region)

Excludes: eyelid (373.13)
lacrimal apparatus (375.31)
orbit (376.01)

680.1 Neck

680.2 Trunk

Abdominal wall	Flank
Back [any part, except	Groin
buttocks]	Pectoral region
Breast	Perineum
Chest wall	Umbilicus

Excludes: buttocks (680.5)
external genital organs:
female (616.4)
male (607.2, 608.4)

680.3 Upper arm and forearm
Arm [any part, except hand]
Axilla
Shoulder

680.4 Hand

Finger [any]	Wrist
Thumb	

680.5 Buttock

Anus	Gluteal region

680.6 Leg, except foot

Ankle	Knee
Hip	Thigh

680.7 Foot

Heel	Toe

680.8 Other specified sites
Head [any part, except face]
Scalp

Excludes: external genital organs:
female (616.4)
male (607.2, 608.4)

680.9 Unspecified site

Boil NOS	Furuncle NOS
Carbuncle NOS	

681 Cellulitis and abscess of finger and toe
Includes: that with lymphangitis
Use additional code, if desired, to identify organism, such as Staphylococcus (041.1)

⑤ **681.0 Finger**

681.00 Cellulitis and abscess, unspecified

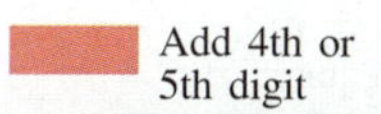

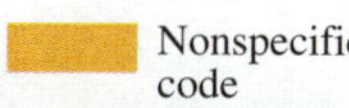

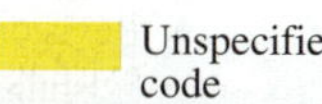

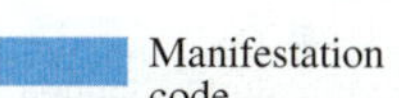

681.01 Felon
Pulp abscess   Whitlow

> *Excludes:* *herpetic whitlow (054.6)*

681.02 Onychia and paronychia of finger
Panaritium ⎫
Perionychia ⎬ of finger

⑤ **681.1 Toe**

681.10 Cellulitis and abscess, unspecified

681.11 Onychia and paronychia of toe
Panaritium ⎫
Perionychia ⎬ of toe

681.9 Cellulitis and abscess of unspecified digit
Infection of nail NOS

682 Other cellulitis and abscess
Includes:
abscess (acute) ⎫
cellulitis (diffuse) ⎬ (with lymphangitis) except of finger or toe
lymphangitis, acute ⎭

Use additional code, if desired, to identify organism, such as Staphylococcus (041.1)

> *Excludes:* *lymphangitis (chronic) (subacute) (457.2)*

682.0 Face
Cheek, external   Nose, external
Chin   Submandibular
Forehead   Temple (region)

> *Excludes:* *ear [any part] (380.10-380.16)*
> *eyelid (373.13)*
> *lacrimal apparatus (375.31)*
> *lip (528.5)*
> *mouth (528.3)*
> *nose (internal) (478.1)*
> *orbit (376.01)*

682.1 Neck

682.2 Trunk
Abdominal wall   Groin
Back [any part, except   Pectoral region
  buttock]   Perineum
Chest wall   Umbilicus, except newborn
Flank

> *Excludes:* *anal and rectal regions (566)*
> *breast:*
>   *NOS (611.0)*
>   *puerperal (675.1)*
> *external genital organs:*
>   *female (616.3-616.4)*
>   *male (604.0, 607.2, 608.4)*
> *umbilicus, newborn (771.4)*

682.3 Upper arm and forearm
Arm [any part, except hand]
Axilla
Shoulder

> *Excludes:* *hand (682.4)*

682.4 Hand, except fingers and thumb
Wrist

> *Excludes:* *finger and thumb (681.00-681.02)*

682.5 Buttock
Gluteal region

> *Excludes:* *anal and rectal regions (566)*

682.6 Leg, except foot
Ankle   Knee
Hip   Thigh

● Code new   ▲ Revision of   ④ ⑤ Fourth or fifth
  to this edition   existing code   digit required

682.7 **Foot, except toes**
Heel

> *Excludes:* toe (681.10-681.11)

682.8 **Other specified sites**
Head [except face]   Scalp

> *Excludes:* face (682.0)

682.9 **Unspecified site**
Abscess NOS   Lymphangitis, acute NOS
Cellulitis NOS

> *Excludes:* lymphangitis NOS (457.2)

683 **Acute lymphadenitis**
Abscess (acute)
Adenitis, acute   } lymph gland or node, except mesenteric
Lymphadenitis, acute

Use additional code, if desired, to identify organism, such as Staphylococcus (041.1)

> *Excludes:* enlarged glands NOS (785.6)
>
> lymphadenitis:
> chronic or subacute, except mesenteric (289.1)
> mesenteric (acute) (chronic) (subacute) (289.2)
> unspecified (289.3)

684 **Impetigo**
Impetiginization of other dermatoses
Impetigo (contagiosa) [any site] [any organism]:
bullous
circinate
neonatorum
simplex
Pemphigus neonatorum

> *Excludes:* impetigo herpetiformis (694.3)

685 **Pilonidal cyst**
Includes:
fistula
sinus   } coccygeal or pilonidal

685.0 **With abscess**

685.1 **Without mention of abscess**

686 **Other local infections of skin and subcutaneous tissue**
Use additional code, if desired, to identify any infectious organism (041.0-041.8)

⑤ **686.0** **Pyoderma**
Dermatitis:
purulent
septic
suppurative

686.00 **Pyoderma, unspecified**

686.01 **Pyoderma gangrenosum**

686.09 **Other pyoderma**

686.1 **Pyogenic granuloma**
Granuloma:
septic
suppurative
telangiectaticum

> *Excludes:* pyogenic granuloma of oral mucosa (528.9)

686.8 **Other specified local infections of skin and subcutaneous tissue**
Bacterid (pustular)   Ecthyma
Dermatitis vegetans   Perlèche

> *Excludes:* dermatitis infectiosa eczematoides (690.8)
>
> panniculitis (729.30-729.39)

686.9 **Unspecified local infection of skin and subcutaneous tissue**
Fistula of skin NOS   Skin infection NOS

> *Excludes:* fistula to skin from internal organs—see Alphabetic Index

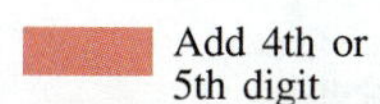

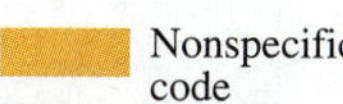

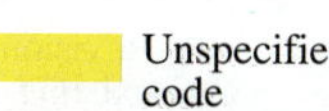

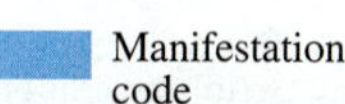

OTHER INFLAMMATORY CONDITIONS OF SKIN AND SUBCUTANEOUS TISSUE (690-698)

> *Excludes:* *panniculitis (729.30-729.39)*

690 Erythematosquamous dermatosis

> *Excludes:* *eczematous dermatitis of eyelid (373.31)*
> *parakeratosis variegata (696.2)*
> *psoriasis (696.0-696.1)*
> *seborrheic keratosis (702.11-702.19)*

⑤ **690.1 Seborrheic dermatitis**

690.10 Seborrheic dermatitis, unspecified
Seborrheic dermatitis NOS

690.11 Seborrhea capitis
Cradle cap

690.12 Seborrheic infantile dermatitis

690.18 Other seborrheic dermatitis

690.8 Other erythematosquamous dermatosis

691 Atopic dermatitis and related conditions

691.0 Diaper or napkin rash
Ammonia dermatitis
Diaper or napkin:
  dermatitis
  erythema
  rash
Psoriasiform napkin eruption

691.8 Other atopic dermatitis and related conditions

Atopic dermatitis
Besnier's prurigo
Eczema:
  atopic
  flexural
  intrinsic (allergic)

Neurodermatitis:
  atopic
  diffuse (of Brocq)

692 Contact dermatitis and other eczema
Includes:

dermatitis:
  NOS
  contact
  occupational
  venenata

eczema (acute) (chronic):
  NOS
  allergic
  erythematous
  occupational

> *Excludes:* *allergy NOS (995.3)*
> *contact dermatitis of eyelids (373.32)*
> *dermatitis due to substances taken internally (693.0-693.9)*
> *eczema of external ear (380.22)*
> *perioral dermatitis (695.3)*
> *urticarial reactions (708.0-708.9, 995.1)*

692.0 Due to detergents

692.1 Due to oils and greases

692.2 Due to solvents
Dermatitis due to solvents of:
  chlorocompound group
  cyclohexane group
  ester group
  glycol group
  hydrocarbon group
  ketone group

● Code new
to this edition

▲ Revision of
existing code

④ ⑤ Fourth or fifth
digit required

692.3 Due to drugs and medicines in contact with skin
Dermatitis (allergic) (contact) due to:
  arnica
  fungicides
  iodine
  keratolytics
  mercurials
  neomycin
  pediculocides
  phenols
  scabicides
  any drug applied to skin
Dermatitis medicamentosa due to drug applied to skin
Use additional E code, if desired, to identify drug

Excludes: *allergy NOS due to drugs (995.2)*
  dermatitis due to ingested drugs (693.0)
  dermatitis medicamentosa NOS (693.0)

692.4 Due to other chemical products
Dermatitis due to:
  acids
  adhesive plaster
  alkalis
  caustics
  dichromate

Dermatitis due to:
  insecticide
  nylon
  plastic
  rubber

692.5 Due to food in contact with skin
Dermatitis, contact, due to:
  cereals
  fish
  flour

Dermatitis, contact, due to:
  fruit
  meat
  milk

Excludes: *dermatitis due to:*
  dyes (692.89)
  ingested foods (693.1)
  preservatives (692.89)

692.6 Due to plants [except food]
Dermatitis due to:
  lacquer tree [Rhus verniciflua]
  poison ivy [Rhus toxicodendron]
  poison oak [Rhus diversiloba]
  poison sumac [Rhus venenata]
  poison vine [Rhus radicans]
  primrose [Primula]
  ragweed [Senecio jacobae]
  other plants in contact with the skin

Excludes: *allergy NOS due to pollen (477.0)*
  nettle rash (708.8)

⑤ **692.7 Due to solar radiation**

Excludes: *sunburn due to other ultraviolet radiation exposure (692.82)*

692.70 Unspecified dermatitis due to sun

692.71 Sunburn
First degree sunburn
Sunburn NOS

692.72 Acute dermatitis due to solar radiation
Berloque dermatitis
Photoallergic response
Phototoxic response
Polymorphus light eruption
Acute solar skin damage NOS

Excludes: *sunburn (692.71, 692.76-692.77)*
Use additional E code, if desired, to identify drug, if drug induced

692.73 Actinic reticuloid and actinic granuloma

692.74 Other chronic dermatitis due to solar radiation
solar elastosis
chronic solar skin damage NOS

Excludes: *actinic [solar] keratosis (702.0)*

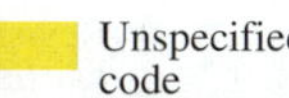

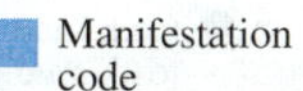

692.75 Disseminated superficial actinic porokeratosis (DSAP)

692.76 Sunburn of second degree

692.77 Sunburn of third degree

692.79 Other dermatitis due to solar radiation
Hydroa aestivale
Photodermatitis due to sun
Photosensitiveness due to sun
Solar skin damage NOS

⑤ **692.8 Due to other specified agents**

692.81 Dermatitis due to cosmetics

692.82 Dermatitis due to other radiation
Infrared rays
Light, except from sun
Radiation NOS
Ultraviolet rays, except from sun
X-rays
Tanning bed

Excludes: that due to solar radiation (692.70-692.79)

692.83 Dermatitis due to metals
jewelry

692.89 Other
Dermatitis due to:
cold weather
dyes
furs
hot weather
preservatives

Excludes: allergy NOS due to animal hair, dander (animal), or dust (477.8)
sunburn (692.71, 692.76-692.77)

692.9 Unspecified cause
Dermatitis: Eczema NOS
  NOS
  contact NOS
  venenata NOS

693 Dermatitis due to substances taken internally

Excludes: adverse effect NOS of drugs and medicines (995.2)
allergy NOS (995.3)
contact dermatitis (692.0-692.9)
urticarial reactions (708.0-708.9, 995.1)

693.0 Due to drugs and medicines
Dermatitis medicamentosa NOS
Use additional E code, if desired, to identify drug

Excludes: that due to drugs in contact with skin (692.3)

693.1 Due to food

693.8 Due to other specified substances taken internally

693.9 Due to unspecified substance taken internally

Excludes: dermatitis NOS (692.9)

694 Bullous dermatoses

694.0 Dermatitis herpetiformis
Dermatosis herpetiformis
Duhring's disease
Hydroa herpetiformis

Excludes: herpes gestationis (646.8)

dermatitis herpetiformis:
juvenile (694.2)
senile (694.5)

694.1 Subcorneal pustular dermatosis
Sneddon-Wilkinson disease or syndrome

694.2 Juvenile dermatitis herpetiformis
Juvenile pemphigoid

● Code new   ▲ Revision of   ④ ⑤ Fourth or fifth
to this edition   existing code   digit required

694.3 Impetigo herpetiformis

694.4 Pemphigus
Pemphigus:
  NOS
  erythematosus
  foliaceus

Pemphigus:
  malignant
  vegetans
  vulgaris

Excludes: *pemphigus neonatorum (684)*

694.5 Pemphigoid
Benign pemphigus NOS
Bullous pemphigoid
Herpes circinatus bullosus
Senile dermatitis herpetiformis

⑤ **694.6 Benign mucous membrane pemphigoid**
Cicatricial pemphigoid
Mucosynechial atrophic bullous dermatitis

694.60 Without mention of ocular involvement

694.61 With ocular involvement
Ocular pemphigus

694.8 Other specified bullous dermatoses

Excludes: *herpes gestationis (646.8)*

694.9 Unspecified bullous dermatoses

695 Erythematous conditions

695.0 Toxic erythema
Erythema venenatum

695.1 Erythema multiforme
Erythema iris
Herpes iris
Lyell's syndrome

Scalded skin syndrome
Stevens-Johnson syndrome
Toxic epidermal necrolysis

695.2 Erythema nodosum

Excludes: *tuberculous erythema nodosum (017.1)*

695.3 Rosacea
Acne:
  erythematosa
  rosacea

Perioral dermatitis
Rhinophyma

695.4 Lupus erythematosus
Lupus:
  erythematodes (discoid)
  erythematosus (discoid), not disseminated

Excludes: *lupus (vulgaris) NOS (017.0)*
systemic [disseminated] lupus erythematosus (710.0)

⑤ **695.8 Other specified erythematous conditions**

695.81 Ritter's disease
Dermatitis exfoliativa neonatorum

695.89 Other
Erythema intertrigo
Intertrigo
Pityriasis rubra (Hebra)

Excludes: *mycotic intertrigo (111.0-111.9)*

695.9 Unspecified erythematous condition
Erythema NOS

Erythroderma (secondary)

696 Psoriasis and similar disorders

696.0 Psoriatic arthropathy

696.1 Other psoriasis
Acrodermatitis continua
Dermatitis repens
Psoriasis:
  NOS
  any type, except arthropathic

Excludes: *psoriatic arthropathy (696.0)*

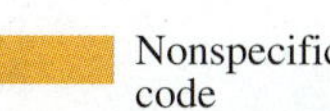

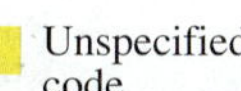

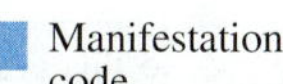

Manifestation
code

696.2 Parapsoriasis
    Parakeratosis variegata
    Parapsoriasis lichenoides chronica
    Pityriasis lichenoides et varioliformis

696.3 Pityriasis rosea
    Pityriasis circinata (et maculata)

696.4 Pityriasis rubra pilaris
    Devergie's disease
    Lichen ruber acuminatus

> *Excludes:* *pityriasis rubra (Hebra) (695.89)*

696.5 Other and unspecified pityriasis
    Pityriasis:
      NOS
      alba
      streptogenes

> *Excludes:* *pityriasis simplex (690.18)*
>   *pityriasis versicolor (111.0)*

696.8 Other

697 Lichen

> *Excludes:* *lichen:*
>
>   *obtusus corneus (698.3)*
>   *pilaris (congenital) (757.39)*
>   *ruber acuminatus (696.4)*
>   *sclerosus et atrophicus (701.0)*
>   *scrofulosus (017.0)*
>   *simplex chronicus (698.3)*
>   *spinulosus (congenital) (757.39)*
>   *urticatus (698.2)*

697.0 Lichen planus
    Lichen:
      planopilaris
      ruber planus

697.1 Lichen nitidus
    Pinkus' disease

697.8 Other lichen, not elsewhere classified
    Lichen:
      ruber moniliforme
      striata

697.9 Lichen, unspecified

698 Pruritus and related conditions

> *Excludes:* *pruritus specified as psychogenic (306.3)*

698.0 Pruritus ani
    Perianal itch

698.1 Pruritus of genital organs

698.2 Prurigo
    Lichen urticatus   Urticaria papulosa (Hebra)
    Prurigo:
      NOS
      Hebra's
      mitis
      simplex

> *Excludes:* *prurigo nodularis (698.3)*

698.3 Lichenification and lichen simplex chronicus
    Hyde's disease
    Neurodermatitis (circumscripta) (local)
    Prurigo nodularis

> *Excludes:* *neurodermatitis, diffuse (of Brocq) (691.8)*

698.4 Dermatitis factitia [artefacta]
    Dermatitis ficta
    Neurotic excoriation
Use additional code, if desired, to identify any associated mental disorder

● Code new
    to this edition

▲ Revision of
    existing code

④ ⑤ Fourth or fifth
       digit required

698.8 Other specified pruritic conditions
Pruritus: Winter itch
  hiemalis
  senilis

698.9 Unspecified pruritic disorder
Itch NOS   Pruritus NOS

OTHER DISEASES OF SKIN AND SUBCUTANEOUS TISSUE (700-709)

Excludes: *conditions confined to eyelids (373.0-374.9)*
congenital conditions of skin, hair, and nails (757.0-757.9)

700 Corns and callosities
Callus   Clavus

701 Other hypertrophic and atrophic conditions of skin

Excludes: *dermatomyositis (710.3)*
hereditary edema of legs (757.0)
scleroderma (generalized) (710.1)

701.0 Circumscribed scleroderma
Addison's keloid
Dermatosclerosis, localized
Lichen sclerosus et atrophicus
Morphea
Scleroderma, circumscribed or localized

701.1 Keratoderma, acquired
Acquired:
  ichthyosis
  keratoderma palmaris et plantaris
Elastosis perforans serpiginosa
Hyperkeratosis:
  NOS
  follicularis in cutem penetrans
  palmoplantaris climacterica
Keratoderma:
  climactericum
  tylodes, progressive
Keratosis (blennorrhagica)

Excludes: *Darier's disease [keratosis follicularis] (congenital) (757.39)*
keratosis:
arsenical (692.4)
gonococcal (098.81)

701.2 Acquired acanthosis nigricans
Keratosis nigricans

701.3 Striae atrophicae
Atrophic spots of skin
Atrophoderma maculatum
Atrophy blanche (of Milian)
Degenerative colloid atrophy
Senile degenerative atrophy
Striae distensae

701.4 Keloid scar
Cheloid   Keloid
Hypertrophic scar

701.5 Other abnormal granulation tissue
Excessive granulation

701.8 Other specified hypertrophic and atrophic conditions of skin
Acrodermatitis atrophicans chronica
Atrophia cutis senilis
Atrophoderma neuriticum
Confluent and reticulate papillomatosis
Cutis laxa senilis
Elastosis senilis
Folliculitis ulerythematosa reticulata
Gougerot-Carteaud syndrome or disease

701.9 Unspecified hypertrophic and atrophic conditions of skin
Atrophoderma

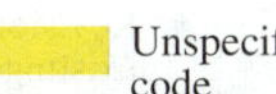

702 **Other dermatoses**

Excludes: carcinoma in situ (232.0-232.9)

702.0 **Actinic keratosis**

⑤ **702.1** **Seborrheic keratosis**

702.11 **Inflamed seborrheic keratosis**

702.19 **Other seborrheic keratosis**
Seborrheic keratosis NOS

702.8 **Other specified dermatoses**

703 **Diseases of nail**

Excludes: congenital anomalies (757.5)
onychia and paronychia (681.02, 681.11)

703.0 **Ingrowing nail**
Ingrowing nail with infection
Unguis incarnatus

Excludes: infection, nail NOS (681.9)

703.8 **Other specified diseases of nail**
Dystrophia unguium   Onychauxis
Hypertrophy of nail   Onychogryposis
Koilonychia   Onycholysis
Leukonychia (punctata) (striata)

703.9 **Unspecified disease of nail**

704 **Diseases of hair and hair follicles**

Excludes: congenital anomalies (757.4)

⑤ **704.0** **Alopecia**

Excludes: madarosis (374.55)
syphilitic alopecia (091.82)

704.00 **Alopecia, unspecified**
Baldness   Loss of hair

704.01 **Alopecia areata**
Ophiasis

704.02 **Telogen effluvim**

704.09 **Other**
Folliculitis decalvans
Hypotrichosis:
NOS
postinfectional NOS
Pseudopelade

704.1 **Hirsutism**
Hypertrichosis: Polytrichia
NOS
lanuginosa, acquired

Excludes: hypertrichosis of eyelid (374.54)

704.2 **Abnormalities of the hair**
Atrophic hair   Trichiasis:
Clastothrix   NOS
Fragilitas crinium   cicatrical
Trichorrhexis (nodosa)

Excludes: trichiasis of eyelid (374.05)

704.3 **Variations in hair color**
Canities (premature)   Poliosis:
Grayness, hair (premature)   NOS
Heterochromia of hair   circumscripta, acquired

● Code new
to this edition

▲ Revision of
existing code

④ ⑤ Fourth or fifth
digit required

704.8 Other specified diseases of hair and hair follicles

Folliculitis:
  NOS
  abscedens et suffodiens
  pustular
Perifolliculitis:
  NOS
  capitis abscedens et suffodiens
  scalp

Sycosis:
  NOS
  barbae [not parasitic]
  lupoid
  vulgaris

704.9 Unspecified disease of hair and hair follicles

705 Disorders of sweat glands

705.0 Anhidrosis
  Hypohidrosis   Oligohidrosis

705.1 Prickly heat
  Heat rash
  Miliaria rubra (tropicalis)
  Sudamina

⑤ **705.8 Other specified disorders of sweat glands**

   705.81 Dyshidrosis
     Cheiropompholyx   Pompholyx

   705.82 Fox-Fordyce disease

   705.83 Hidradenitis
     Hidradenitis suppurativa

   705.89 Other
     Bromhidrosis   Granulosis rubra nasi
     Chromhidrosis   Urhidrosis

Excludes: hidrocystoma (216.0-216.9)
        hyperhidrosis (780.8)

705.9 Unspecified disorder of sweat glands
  Disorder of sweat glands NOS

706 Diseases of sebaceous glands

706.0 Acne varioliformis
  Acne:
    frontalis
    necrotica

706.1 Other acne
  Acne: Blackhead
    NOS   Comedo
    conglobata
    cystic
    pustular
    vulgaris

Excludes: acne rosacea (695.3)

706.2 Sebaceous cyst
  Atheroma, skin   Wen
  Keratin cyst

706.3 Seborrhea

Excludes: seborrhea:
     capitis (690.11)
     sicca (690.18)
    seborrheic dermatitis (690.11)
    seborrheic keratosis (702.11-702.19)

706.8 Other specified diseases of sebaceous glands
  Asteatosis (cutis)   Xerosis cutis

706.9 Unspecified disease of sebaceous glands

707 Chronic ulcer of skin
  Includes: non-infected sinus of skin
             non-healing ulcer

Excludes: specific infections classified under "Infectious and Parasitic Diseases" (001.0-136.9)
    varicose ulcer (454.0, 454.2)

707.0 Decubitus ulcer
Bed sore
Decubitus ulcer [any site]
Plaster ulcer
Pressure ulcer

⑤ **707.1 Ulcer of lower limbs, except decubitus**
Ulcer, chronic, neurogenic, of lower limb
Ulcer, chronic, trophic, of lower limb

Code, if applicable, any causal condition first:
atherosclerosis of the extremities with ulceration (440.23)
chronic venous hypertension with ulcer (459.31)
chronic venous hypertension with ulcer and inflammation (459.33)
diabetes mellitus (250.80-250.83)
postphlebetic syndrome with ulcer (459.11)
postphlebetic syndrome with ulcer and inflammation (459.13)

707.10 Ulcer of lower limb, unspecified

707.11 Ulcer of thigh

707.12 Ulcer of calf

707.13 Ulcer of ankle

707.14 Ulcer of heel and midfoot
Plantar surface of midfoot

707.15 Ulcer of other part of foot
Toes

707.19 Ulcer of other part of lower limb

707.8 Chronic ulcer of other specified sites
Ulcer, chronic:
neurogenic } of other specified sites
trophic

707.9 Chronic ulcer of unspecified site
Chronic ulcer NOS
Trophic ulcer NOS
Tropical ulcer NOS
Ulcer of skin NOS

708 Urticaria

Excludes: *edema:*

angioneurotic (995.1)
Quincke's (995.1)
hereditary angioedema (277.6)
urticaria:
giant (995.1)
papulosa (Hebra) (698.2)
pigmentosa (juvenile) (congenital) (757.33)

708.0 Allergic urticaria

708.1 Idiopathic urticaria

708.2 Urticaria due to cold and heat
Thermal urticaria

708.3 Dermatographic urticaria
Dermatographia
Factitial urticaria

708.4 Vibratory urticaria

708.5 Cholinergic urticaria

708.8 Other specified urticaria
Nettle rash
Urticaria:
chronic
recurrent periodic

708.9 Urticaria, unspecified
Hives NOS

709 Other disorders of skin and subcutaneous tissue

⑤ **709.0 Dyschromia**

Excludes: *albinism (270.2)*

pigmented nevus (216.0-216.9)
that of eyelid (374.52-374.53)

709.00 Dyschromia, unspecified

709.01 Vitiligo

709.09 Other

● Code new to this edition   ▲ Revision of existing code   ④ ⑤ Fourth or fifth digit required

709.1 Vascular disorders of skin
Angioma serpiginosum
Purpura (primary) annularis telangiectodes

709.2 Scar conditions and fibrosis of skin
Adherent scar (skin)
Cicatrix
Disfigurement (due to scar)
Fibrosis, skin NOS
Scar NOS

> *Excludes:* *keloid scar (701.4)*

709.3 Degenerative skin disorders

Calcinosis:
  circumscripta
  cutis
Colloid milium

Degeneration, skin
Deposits, skin
Senile dermatosis NOS
Subcutaneous calcification

709.4 Foreign body granuloma of skin and subcutaneous tissue

> *Excludes:* *residual foreign body without granuloma of skin and subcutaneous tissue (729.6)*
> *that of muscle (728.82)*

709.8 Other specified disorders of skin
Epithelial hyperplasia   Vesicular eruption
Menstrual dermatosis

709.9 Unspecified disorder of skin and subcutaneous tissue
Dermatosis NOS

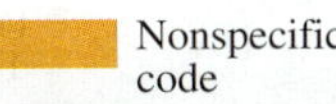

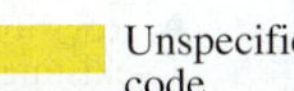

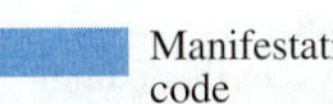

Manifestation
code

● Code new
to this edition

▲ Revision of
existing code

④ ⑤ Fourth or fifth
digit required

13. DISEASES OF THE MUSCULOSKELETAL SYSTEM AND CONNECTIVE TISSUE (710-739)

The following fifth-digit subclassification is for use with categories 711-712, 715-716, 718-719, and 730:

0   site unspecified

1   shoulder region
    Acromioclavicular
    Glenohumeral   } joint(s)
    Sternoclavicular
    Clavicle
    Scapula

2   upper arm
    Elbow joint   Humerus

3   forearm
    Radius   Wrist joint
    Ulna

4   hand
    Carpus   Phalanges [fingers]
    Metacarpus

5   pelvic region and thigh
    Buttock   Hip (joint)
    Femur

6   lower leg
    Fibula   Patella
    Knee joint   Tibia

7   ankle and foot
    Ankle joint   Phalanges, foot
    Digits [toes]   Tarsus
    Metatarsus   Other joints in foot

8   other specified sites
    Head   Skull
    Neck   Trunk
    Ribs   Vertebral column

9   multiple sites

ARTHROPATHIES AND RELATED DISORDERS (710-719)

> *Excludes:* *disorders of spine (720.0-724.9)*

710   **Diffuse diseases of connective tissue**
Includes: all collagen diseases whose effects are not mainly confined to a single system

> *Excludes:* *those affecting mainly the cardiovascular system, i.e., polyarteritis nodosa and allied conditions (446.0-446.7)*

710.0   **Systemic lupus erythematosus**
    Disseminated lupus erythematosus
    Libman-Sacks disease

Use additional code to identify manifestation, as:
    endocarditis (424.91)
    nephritis (583.81)
      chronic (582.81)
    nephrotic syndrome (581.81)

> *Excludes:* *lupus erythematosus (discoid) NOS (695.4)*

710.1   **Systemic sclerosis**
    Acrosclerosis
    CRST syndrome
    Progressive systemic sclerosis
    Scleroderma

Use additional code to identify manifestation, as:
    lung involvement (517.8)
    myopathy (359.6)

> *Excludes:* *circumscribed scleroderma (701.0)*

710.2   **Sicca syndrome**
    Keratoconjunctivitis sicca
    Sjögren's disease

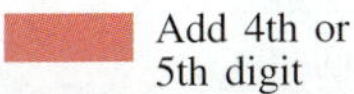

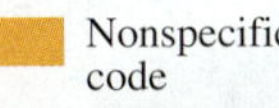

Unspecified
code

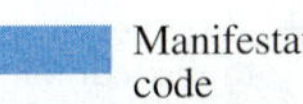

710.3 Dermatomyositis
Poikilodermatomyositis
Polymyositis with skin involvement

710.4 Polymyositis

710.5 Eosinophilia myalgia syndrome
Toxic oil syndrome

Use additional E code, if desired, to identify drug, if drug induced

710.8 Other specified diffuse diseases of connective tissue
Multifocal fibrosclerosis (idiopathic) NEC
Systemic fibrosclerosing syndrome

710.9 Unspecified diffuse connective tissue disease
Collagen disease NOS

⑤ **711 Arthropathy associated with infections**
Includes:

arthritis
arthropathy } associated with conditions classifiable below
polyarthritis
polyarthropathy

Excludes: *rheumatic fever (390)*

The following fifth-digit subclassification is for use with category 711; valid digits are in [brackets] under each code. For definitions, see the beginning of this chapter:

0 site unspecified

1 shoulder region

2 upper arm

3 forearm

4 hand

5 pelvic region and thigh

6 lower leg

7 ankle and foot

8 other specified sites

9 multiple sites

⑤ **711.0 Pyogenic arthritis**
[0-9]   Arthritis or polyarthritis (due to):
coliform [Escherichia coli]
Hemophilus influenzae [H. influenzae]
pneumococcal
Pseudomonas
staphylococcal
streptococcal
Pyarthrosis

Use additional code, if desired, to identify infectious organism (041.0-041.8)

⑤ ***711.1 Arthropathy associated with Reiter's disease and nonspecific urethritis***
[0-9]   *Code first underlying disease, as:*
nonspecific urethritis (099.4)
Reiter's disease (099.3)

⑤ ***711.2 Arthropathy in Behçet's syndrome***
[0-9]   *Code first underlying disease (136.1)*

⑤ ***711.3 Postdysenteric arthropathy***
[0-9]   *Code first underlying disease, as:*
dysentery (009.0)
enteritis, infectious (008.0-009.3)
paratyphoid fever (002.1-002.9)
typhoid fever (002.0)

Excludes: *salmonella arthritis (003.23)*

● Code new
to this edition

▲ Revision of
existing code

④ ⑤ Fourth or fifth
digit required

⑤ **711.4** ***Arthropathy associated with other bacterial diseases***
[0-9]   *Code first underlying disease, as:*
diseases classifiable to 010-040, 090-099, except as in 711.1, 711.3, and 713.5
leprosy (030.0-030.9)
tuberculosis (015.0-015.9)

Excludes: *gonococcal arthritis (098.50)*
meningococcal arthritis (036.82)

⑤ **711.5** ***Arthropathy associated with other viral diseases***
[0-9]   *Code first underlying disease, as:*
diseases classifiable to 045-049, 050-079, 480, 487
O'nyong nyong (066.3)

Excludes: *that due to rubella (056.71)*

⑤ **711.6** ***Arthropathy associated with mycoses***
[0-9]   *Code first underlying disease (110.0-118)*

⑤ **711.7** ***Arthropathy associated with helminthiasis***
[0-9]   *Code first underlying disease, as:*
filariasis (125.0-125.9)

⑤ **711.8** ***Arthropathy associated with other infectious and parasitic diseases***
[0-9]   *Code first underlying disease, as:*
diseases classifiable to 080-088, 100-104, 130-136

Excludes: *arthropathy associated with sarcoidosis (713.7)*

⑤ **711.9** **Unspecified infective arthritis**
[0-9]   Infective arthritis or polyarthritis (acute) (chronic) (subacute) NOS

⑤ **712** **Crystal arthropathies**
Includes: crystal-induced arthritis and synovitis

Excludes: *gouty arthropathy (274.0)*

The following fifth-digit subclassification is for use with category 712; valid digits are in
[brackets] under each code. See beginning of this chapter for definitions:

0 **site unspecified**
1 **shoulder region**
2 **upper arm**
3 **forearm**
4 **hand**
5 **pelvic region and thigh**
6 **lower leg**
7 **ankle and foot**
8 **other specified sites**
9 **multiple sites**

⑤ **712.1** ***Chondrocalcinosis due to dicalcium phosphate crystals***
[0-9]   Chondrocalcinosis due to dicalcium phosphate crystals (with other crystals)
Code first underlying disease (275.4)

⑤ **712.2** ***Chondrocalcinosis due to pyrophosphate crystals***
[0-9]   *Code first underlying disease (275.4)*

⑤ **712.3** ***Chondrocalcinosis, unspecified***
[0-9]   *Code first underlying disease (275.4)*

⑤ **712.8** **Other specified crystal arthropathies**
[0-9]

⑤ **712.9** **Unspecified crystal arthropathy**
[0-9]

<table>
<tr><td>Add 4th or 5th digit</td><td>Nonspecific code</td><td>Unspecified code</td><td>Manifestation code</td></tr>
</table>

713 Arthropathy associated with other disorders classified elsewhere
Includes:

arthritis
arthropathy
polyarthritis
polyarthropathy
} associated with conditions classifiable below

713.0 *Arthropathy associated with other endocrine and metabolic disorders*
Code first underlying disease, as:
acromegaly (253.0)
hemochromatosis (275.0)
hyperparathyroidism (252.0)
hypogammaglobulinemia (279.00-279.09)
hypothyroidism (243-244.9)
lipoid metabolism disorder (272.0-272.9)
ochronosis (270.2)

Excludes: *arthropathy associated with:*

amyloidosis (713.7)
crystal deposition disorders, except gout (712.1-712.9)
diabetic neuropathy (713.5)
gouty arthropathy (274.0)

713.1 *Arthropathy associated with gastrointestinal conditions other than infections*
Code first underlying disease, as:
regional enteritis (555.0-555.9)
ulcerative colitis (556)

713.2 *Arthropathy associated with hematological disorders*
Code first underlying disease, as:
hemoglobinopathy (282.4-282.7)
hemophilia (286.0-286.2)
leukemia (204.0-208.9)
malignant reticulosis (202.3)
multiple myelomatosis (203.0)

Excludes: *arthropathy associated with Henoch-Schönlein purpura (713.6)*

713.3 *Arthropathy associated with dermatological disorders*
Code first underlying disease, as:
erythema multiforme (695.1)
erythema nodosum (695.2)

Excludes: *psoriatic arthropathy (696.0)*

713.4 *Arthropathy associated with respiratory disorders*
Code first underlying disease, as:
diseases classifiable to 490-519

Excludes: *arthropathy associated with respiratory infections (711.0, 711.4-711.8)*

713.5 *Arthropathy associated with neurological disorders*
Charcot's arthropathy
Neuropathic arthritis
} associated with diseases classifiable elsewhere
Code first underlying disease, as:
neuropathic joint disease [Charcot's joints]:
NOS (094.0)
diabetic (250.6)
syringomyelic (336.0)
tabetic [syphilitic] (094.0)

713.6 *Arthropathy associated with hypersensitivity reaction*
Code first underlying disease, as:
Henoch (-Schönlein) purpura (287.0)
serum sickness (999.5)

Excludes: *allergic arthritis NOS (716.2)*

713.7 *Other general diseases with articular involvement*
Code first underlying disease, as:
amyloidosis (277.3)
familial Mediterranean fever (277.3)
sarcoidosis (135)

● Code new
to this edition
▲ Revision of
existing code
④ ⑤ Fourth or fifth
digit required

713.8 *Arthropathy associated with other conditions classifiable elsewhere*
Code first underlying disease, as:
conditions classifiable elsewhere except as in 711.1-711.8, 712, and 713.0-713.7

714 **Rheumatoid arthritis and other inflammatory polyarthropathies**

Excludes: *rheumatic fever (390)*
rheumatoid arthritis of spine NOS (720.0)

714.0 Rheumatoid arthritis
Arthritis or polyarthritis:
atrophic
rheumatic (chronic)
Use additional code, if desired, to identify manifestation, as:
myopathy (359.6)
polyneuropathy (357.1)

Excludes: *juvenile rheumatoid arthritis NOS (714.30)*

714.1 Felty's syndrome
Rheumatoid arthritis with splenoadenomegaly and leukopenia

714.2 Other rheumatoid arthritis with visceral or systemic involvement
Rheumatoid carditis

714.3 Juvenile chronic polyarthritis

714.30 Polyarticular juvenile rheumatoid arthritis, chronic or unspecified
Juvenile rheumatoid arthritis NOS
Still's disease

714.31 Polyarticular juvenile rheumatoid arthritis, acute

714.32 Pauciarticular juvenile rheumatoid arthritis

714.33 Monoarticular juvenile rheumatoid arthritis

714.4 Chronic postrheumatic arthropathy
Chronic rheumatoid nodular fibrositis
Jaccoud's syndrome

714.8 Other specified inflammatory polyarthropathies

714.81 Rheumatoid lung
Caplan's syndrome
Diffuse interstitial rheumatoid disease of lung
Fibrosing alveolitis, rheumatoid

714.89 Other

714.9 Unspecified inflammatory polyarthropathy
Inflammatory polyarthropathy or polyarthritis NOS

Excludes: *polyarthropathy NOS (716.5)*

715 Osteoarthrosis and allied disorders
Note: Localized, in the subcategories below, includes bilateral involvement of the same site.
Includes: arthritis or polyarthritis:
degenerative
hypertrophic
degenerative joint disease
osteoarthritis

Excludes: *Marie-Strümpell spondylitis (720.0)*
osteoarthrosis [osteoarthritis] of spine (721.0-721.9)

The following fifth-digit subclassification is for use with category 715; valid digits are in [brackets] under each code. See beginning of this chapter for definitions:

0   **site unspecified**

1   **shoulder region**

2   **upper arm**

3   **forearm**

4   **hand**

5   **pelvic region and thigh**

6   **lower leg**

7   **ankle and foot**

8   **other specified sites**

9   **multiple sites**

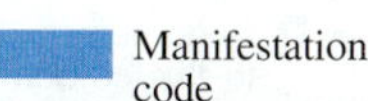

⑤ **715.0 Osteoarthrosis, generalized**
[0,4,9]   Degenerative joint disease, involving multiple joints
             Primary generalized hypertrophic osteoarthrosis

⑤ **715.1 Osteoarthrosis, localized, primary**
[0-8]   Localized osteoarthropathy, idiopathic

⑤ **715.2 Osteoarthrosis, localized, secondary**
[0-8]   Coxae malum senilis

⑤ **715.3 Osteoarthrosis, localized, not specified whether primary or secondary**
[0-8]   Otto's pelvis

⑤ **715.8 Osteoarthrosis involving, or with mention of more than one site, but not specified as generalized**
[0,9]

⑤ **715.9 Osteoarthrosis, unspecified whether generalized or localized**
[0-8]

⑤ **716 Other and unspecified arthropathies**

   Excludes: *cricoarytenoid arthropathy (478.79)*

   The following fifth-digit subclassification is for use with category 716; valid digits are in
   [brackets] under each code. See beginning of this chapter for definitions:

   0 site unspecified

   1 shoulder region

   2 upper arm

   3 forearm

   4 hand

   5 pelvic region and thigh

   6 lower leg

   7 ankle and foot

   8 other specified sites

   9 multiple sites

⑤ **716.0 Kaschin-Beck disease**
[0-9]   Endemic polyarthritis

⑤ **716.1 Traumatic arthropathy**
[0-9]

⑤ **716.2 Allergic arthritis**
[0-9]

   Excludes: *arthritis associated with Henoch-Schönlein purpura or serum sickness (713.6)*

⑤ **716.3 Climacteric arthritis**
[0-9]   Menopausal arthritis

⑤ **716.4 Transient arthropathy**
[0-9]

   Excludes: *palindromic rheumatism (719.3)*

⑤ **716.5 Unspecified polyarthropathy or polyarthritis**
[0-9]

⑤ **716.6 Unspecified monoarthritis**
[0-8]   Coxitis

⑤ **716.8 Other specified arthropathy**
[0-9]

⑤ **716.9 Arthropathy, unspecified**
[0-9]   Arthritis
             Arthropathy   } (acute) (chronic) (subacute)
             Articular rheumatism (chronic)
             Inflammation of joint NOS

● Code new   ▲ Revision of   ④ ⑤ Fourth or fifth
  to this edition   existing code   digit required

717 Internal derangement of knee

Includes:

degeneration
rupture, old } of articular cartilage or meniscus of knee
tear, old

Excludes: *acute derangement of knee (836.0-836.6)*
ankylosis (718.5)
contracture (718.4)
current injury (836.0-836.6)
deformity (736.4-736.6)
recurrent dislocation (718.3)

717.0 Old bucket handle tear of medial meniscus
Old bucket handle tear of unspecified cartilage

717.1 Derangement of anterior horn of medial meniscus

717.2 Derangement of posterior horn of medial meniscus

717.3 Other and unspecified derangement of medial meniscus
Degeneration of internal semilunar cartilage

⑤ **717.4 Derangement of lateral meniscus**

717.40 Derangement of lateral meniscus, unspecified

717.41 Bucket handle tear of lateral meniscus

717.42 Derangement of anterior horn of lateral meniscus

717.43 Derangement of posterior horn of lateral meniscus

717.49 Other

717.5 Derangement of meniscus, not elsewhere classified
Congenital discoid meniscus
Cyst of semilunar cartilage
Derangement of semilunar cartilage NOS

717.6 Loose body in knee
Joint mice, knee
Rice bodies, knee (joint)

717.7 Chondromalacia of patella
Chondromalacia patellae
Degeneration [softening] of articular cartilage of patella

⑤ **717.8 Other internal derangement of knee**

717.81 Old disruption of lateral collateral ligament

717.82 Old disruption of medial collateral ligament

717.83 Old disruption of anterior cruciate ligament

717.84 Old disruption of posterior cruciate ligament

717.85 Old disruption of other ligaments of knee
Capsular ligament of knee

717.89 Other
Old disruption of ligaments of knee NOS

717.9 Unspecified internal derangement of knee
Derangement NOS of knee

⑤ **718 Other derangement of joint**

Excludes: *current injury (830.0-848.9)*
jaw (524.6)

The following fifth-digit subclassification is for use with category 718; valid digits are in [brackets] under each code. See beginning of this chapter for definitions:

0 site unspecified

1 shoulder region

2 upper arm

3 forearm

4 hand

5 pelvic region and thigh

6 lower leg

7 ankle and foot

continued

Add 4th or 5th digit   Nonspecific code   Unspecified code   Manifestation code

    8   other specified sites

    9   multiple sites

⑤ **718.0 Articular cartilage disorder**
[0-5, 7-9] Meniscus:
        disorder
        rupture, old
        tear, old
    Old rupture of ligament(s) of joint NOS

> | *Excludes:* | *articular cartilage disorder:*
>   *in ochronosis (270.2)*
>   *knee (717.0-717.9)*
>   *chondrocalcinosis (275.4)*
>   *metastatic calcification (275.4)*

⑤ **718.1 Loose body in joint**
[0-5, 7-9] Joint mice

> | *Excludes:* | *knee (717.6)*

⑤ **718.2 Pathological dislocation**
[0-9]   Dislocation or displacement of joint, not recurrent and not current injury
      Spontaneous dislocation (joint)

⑤ **718.3 Recurrent dislocation of joint**
[0-9]

⑤ **718.4 Contracture of joint**
[0-9]

⑤ **718.5 Ankylosis of joint**
[0-9]   Ankylosis of joint (fibrous) (osseous)

> | *Excludes:* | *spine (724.9)*
>   *stiffness of joint without mention of ankylosis (719.5)*

⑤ **718.6 Unspecified intrapelvic protrusion of acetabulum**
[0, 5]   Protrusio acetabuli, unspecified

⑤ **718.7 Developmental dislocation of joint**
[0-9]

> | *Excludes:* | *congenital dislocation of joint (754.0-755.8)*
>   *traumatic dislocation of joint (830-839)*

⑤ **718.8 Other joint derangement, not elsewhere classified**
[0-9]   Flail joint (paralytic)   Instability of joint

> | *Excludes:* | *deformities classifiable to 736 (736.0-736.9)*

⑤ **718.9 Unspecified derangement of joint**
[0-5, 7-9]

> | *Excludes:* | *knee (717.9)*

⑤ **719 Other and unspecified disorders of joint**

> | *Excludes:* | *jaw (524.6)*

The following fifth-digit subclassification is for use with category 719; valid digits are in
    [brackets] under each code. See beginning of this chapter for definitions:

    0   site unspecified

    1   shoulder region

    2   upper arm

    3   forearm

    4   hand

    5   pelvic region and thigh

    6   lower leg

    7   ankle and foot

    8   other specified sites

    9   multiple sites

⑤ **719.0 Effusion of joint**
[0-9]   Hydrarthrosis
      Swelling of joint, with or without pain

> | *Excludes:* | *intermittent hydrarthrosis (719.3)*

● Code new   ▲ Revision of   ④ ⑤ Fourth or fifth
  to this edition   existing code   digit required

⑤ **719.1 Hemarthrosis**
[0-9]

> | Excludes: | current injury (840.0-848.9)

⑤ **719.2 Villonodular synovitis**
[0-9]

⑤ **719.3 Palindromic rheumatism**
[0-9]   Hench-Rosenberg syndrome
Intermittent hydrarthrosis

⑤ **719.4 Pain in joint**
[0-9]   Arthralgia

⑤ **719.5 Stiffness of joint, not elsewhere classified**
[0-9]

⑤ **719.6 Other symptoms referable to joint**
[0-9]   Joint crepitus   Snapping hip

⑤ **719.7 Difficulty in walking**
[0, 5-9]

> | Excludes: | abnormality of gait (781.2)

⑤ **719.8 Other specified disorders of joint**
[0-9]   Calcification of joint   Fistula of joint

> | Excludes: | temporomandibular joint-pain-dysfunction syndrome [Costen's syndrome] (524.6)

⑤ **719.9 Unspecified disorder of joint**
[0-9]

DORSOPATHIES (720-724)

> | Excludes: | curvature of spine (737.0-737.9)
>
> osteochondrosis of spine (juvenile) (732.0)
> adult (732.8)

720 Ankylosing spondylitis and other inflammatory spondylopathies

720.0 Ankylosing spondylitis
Rheumatoid arthritis of spine NOS
Spondylitis:
Marie-Strümpell
rheumatoid

720.1 Spinal enthesopathy
Disorder of peripheral ligamentous or muscular attachments of spine
Romanus lesion

720.2 Sacroiliitis, not elsewhere classified
Inflammation of sacroiliac joint NOS

⑤ **720.8 Other inflammatory spondylopathies**

720.81 Inflammatory spondylopathies in diseases classified elsewhere
Code first underlying disease, as:
tuberculosis (015.0)

720.89 Other

720.9 Unspecified inflammatory spondylopathy
Spondylitis NOS

721 Spondylosis and allied disorders

721.0 Cervical spondylosis without myelopathy
Cervical or cervicodorsal:
arthritis
osteoarthritis
spondylarthritis

721.1 Cervical spondylosis with myelopathy
Anterior spinal artery compression syndrome
Spondylogenic compression of cervical spinal cord
Vertebral artery compression syndrome

Add 4th or 5th digit	Nonspecific code	Unspecified code	Manifestation code

721.2 Thoracic spondylosis without myelopathy
Thoracic:
  arthritis
  osteoarthritis
  spondylarthritis

721.3 Lumbosacral spondylosis without myelopathy
Lumbar or lumbosacral:
  arthritis
  osteoarthritis
  spondylarthritis

⑤ **721.4 Thoracic or lumbar spondylosis with myelopathy**

    721.41 Thoracic region
       Spondylogenic compression of thoracic spinal cord

    721.42 Lumbar region
       Spondylogenic compression of lumbar spinal cord

721.5 Kissing spine
Baastrup's syndrome

721.6 Ankylosing vertebral hyperostosis

721.7 Traumatic spondylopathy
Kümmell's disease or spondylitis

721.8 Other allied disorders of spine

⑤ **721.9 Spondylosis of unspecified site**

    721.90 Without mention of myelopathy
       Spinal:
        arthritis (deformans) (degenerative) (hypertrophic)
        osteoarthritis NOS
       Spondylarthrosis NOS

    721.91 With myelopathy
       Spondylogenic compression of spinal cord NOS

722 Intervertebral disc disorders

722.0 Displacement of cervical intervertebral disc without myelopathy
Neuritis (brachial) or radiculitis due to displacement or rupture of cervical intervertebral
  disc
Any condition classifiable to 722.2 of the cervical or cervicothoracic intervertebral disc

⑤ **722.1 Displacement of thoracic or lumbar intervertebral disc without myelopathy**

    722.10 Lumbar intervertebral disc without myelopathy
       Lumbago or sciatica due to displacement of intervertebral disc
       Neuritis or radiculitis due to displacement or rupture of lumbar intervertebral
        disc
       Any condition classifiable to 722.2 of the lumbar or lumbosacral intervertebral
        disc

    722.11 Thoracic intervertebral disc without myelopathy
       Any condition classifiable to 722.2 of thoracic intervertebral disc

722.2 Displacement of intervertebral disc, site unspecified, without myelopathy
Discogenic syndrome NOS
Herniation of nucleus pulposus NOS
Intervertebral disc NOS:
  extrusion
  prolapse
  protrusion
  rupture
Neuritis or radiculitis due to displacement or rupture of intervertebral disc

⑤ **722.3 Schmorl's nodes**

    722.30 Unspecified region

    722.31 Thoracic region

    722.32 Lumbar region

    722.39 Other

722.4 Degeneration of cervical intervertebral disc
Degeneration of cervicothoracic intervertebral disc

⑤ **722.5 Degeneration of thoracic or lumbar intervertebral disc**

    722.51 Thoracic or thoracolumbar intervertebral disc

    722.52 Lumbar or lumbosacral intervertebral disc

● Code new to this edition   ▲ Revision of existing code   ④ ⑤ Fourth or fifth digit required

722.6 **Degeneration of intervertebral disc, site unspecified**
Degenerative disc disease NOS
Narrowing of intervertebral disc or space NOS

⑤ **722.7** **Intervertebral disc disorder with myelopathy**

    722.70 Unspecified region

    722.71 Cervical region

    722.72 Thoracic region

    722.73 Lumbar region

⑤ **722.8** **Postlaminectomy syndrome**

    722.80 Unspecified region

    722.81 Cervical region

    722.82 Thoracic region

    722.83 Lumbar region

⑤ **722.9** **Other and unspecified disc disorder**
Calcification of intervertebral cartilage or disc
Discitis

    722.90 Unspecified region

    722.91 Cervical region

    722.92 Thoracic region

    722.93 Lumbar region

723 **Other disorders of cervical region**

    Excludes: *conditions due to:*
        intervertebral disc disorders (722.0-722.9)
        spondylosis (721.0-721.9)

723.0 **Spinal stenosis in cervical region**

723.1 **Cervicalgia**
Pain in neck

723.2 **Cervicocranial syndrome**
Barré-Liéou syndrome
Posterior cervical sympathetic syndrome

723.3 **Cervicobrachial syndrome (diffuse)**

723.4 **Brachial neuritis or radiculitis NOS**
Cervical radiculitis
Radicular syndrome of upper limbs

723.5 **Torticollis, unspecified**
Contracture of neck

    Excludes: *congenital (754.1)*
        due to birth injury (767.8)
        hysterical (300.11)
        ocular torticollis (781.93)
        psychogenic (306.0)
        spasmodic (333.83)
        traumatic, current (847.0)

723.6 **Panniculitis specified as affecting neck**

723.7 **Ossification of posterior longitudinal ligament in cervical region**

723.8 **Other syndromes affecting cervical region**
Cervical syndrome NEC
Klippel's disease
Occipital neuralgia

723.9 **Unspecified musculoskeletal disorders and symptoms referable to neck**
Cervical (region) disorder NOS

724 **Other and unspecified disorders of back**

    Excludes: *collapsed vertebra (code to cause, e.g., osteoporosis, 733.00-733.09)*
        conditions due to:
          intervertebral disc disorders (722.0-722.9)
          spondylosis (721.0-721.9)

⑤ **724.0** **Spinal stenosis, other than cervical**

    724.00 **Spinal stenosis, unspecified region**

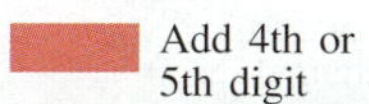 Add 4th or 5th digit	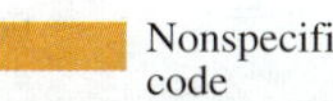 Nonspecific code	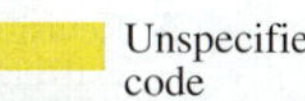 Unspecified code	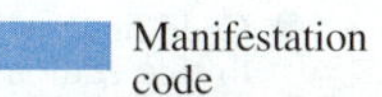 Manifestation code

  724.01 Thoracic region

  724.02 Lumbar region

  724.09 Other

 724.1 Pain in thoracic spine

 724.2 Lumbago
   Low back pain   Lumbalgia
   Low back syndrome

 724.3 Sciatica
   Neuralgia or neuritis of sciatic nerve

  Excludes: *specified lesion of sciatic nerve (355.0)*

 724.4 Thoracic or lumbosacral neuritis or radiculitis, unspecified
   Radicular syndrome of lower limbs

 724.5 Backache, unspecified
   Vertebrogenic (pain) syndrome NOS

 724.6 Disorders of sacrum
   Ankylosis
   Instability   lumbosacral or sacroiliac (joint)

 ⑤ **724.7 Disorders of coccyx**

  724.70 Unspecified disorder of coccyx

  724.71 Hypermobility of coccyx

  724.79 Other
    Coccygodynia

 724.8 Other symptoms referable to back
   Ossification of posterior longitudinal ligament NOS
   Panniculitis specified as sacral or affecting back

 724.9 Other unspecified back disorders
   Ankylosis of spine NOS
   Compression of spinal nerve root NEC
   Spinal disorder NOS

  Excludes: *sacroiliitis (720.2)*

RHEUMATISM, EXCLUDING THE BACK (725-729)

  Includes: disorders of muscles and tendons and their attachments, and of other soft tissues

725 Polymyalgia rheumatica

726 Peripheral enthesopathies and allied syndromes
 Note: Enthesopathies are disorders of peripheral ligamentous or muscular attachments.

  Excludes: *spinal enthesopathy (720.1)*

 726.0 Adhesive capsulitis of shoulder

 ⑤ **726.1 Rotator cuff syndrome of shoulder and allied disorders**

  726.10 Disorders of bursae and tendons in shoulder region, unspecified
    Rotator cuff syndrome NOS
    Supraspinatus syndrome NOS

  726.11 Calcifying tendinitis of shoulder

  726.12 Bicipital tenosynovitis

  726.19 Other specified disorders

  Excludes: *complete rupture of rotator cuff, nontraumatic (727.61)*

 726.2 Other affections of shoulder region, not elsewhere classified
   Periarthritis of shoulder
   Scapulohumeral fibrositis

 ⑤ **726.3 Enthesopathy of elbow region**

  726.30 Enthesopathy of elbow, unspecified

  726.31 Medial epicondylitis

  726.32 Lateral epicondylitis
    Epicondylitis NOS   Tennis elbow
    Golfers' elbow

  726.33 Olecranon bursitis
    Bursitis of elbow

  ● Code new   ▲ Revision of   ④ ⑤ Fourth or fifth
    to this edition   existing code   digit required

726.39 **Other**

726.4 **Enthesopathy of wrist and carpus**
Bursitis of hand or wrist
Periarthritis of wrist

726.5 **Enthesopathy of hip region**
Bursitis of hip   Psoas tendinitis
Gluteal tendinitis   Trochanteric tendinitis
Iliac crest spur

⑤ **726.6** **Enthesopathy of knee**

726.60 **Enthesopathy of knee, unspecified**
Bursitis of knee NOS

726.61 **Pes anserinus tendinitis or bursitis**

726.62 **Tibial collateral ligament bursitis**
Pellegrini-Stieda syndrome

726.63 **Fibular collateral ligament bursitis**

726.64 **Patellar tendinitis**

726.65 **Prepatellar bursitis**

726.69 **Other**
Bursitis:
infrapatellar
subpatellar

⑤ **726.7** **Enthesopathy of ankle and tarsus**

726.70 **Enthesopathy of ankle and tarsus, unspecified**
Metatarsalgia NOS

Excludes: *Morton's metatarsalgia (355.6)*

726.71 **Achilles bursitis or tendinitis**

726.72 **Tibialis tendinitis**
Tibialis (anterior) (posterior) tendinitis

726.73 **Calcaneal spur**

726.79 **Other**
Peroneal tendinitis

726.8 **Other peripheral enthesopathies**

⑤ **726.9** **Unspecified enthesopathy**

726.90 **Enthesopathy of unspecified site**
Capsulitis NOS   Tendinitis NOS
Periarthritis NOS

726.91 **Exostosis of unspecified site**
Bone spur NOS

727 **Other disorders of synovium, tendon, and bursa**

⑤ **727.0** **Synovitis and tenosynovitis**

727.00 **Synovitis and tenosynovitis, unspecified**
Synovitis NOS   Tenosynovitis NOS

727.01 *Synovitis and tenosynovitis in diseases classified elsewhere*
Code first underlying disease, as:
tuberculosis (015.0-015.9)

Excludes: *crystal-induced (275.4)*
gonococcal (098.51)
gouty (274.0)
syphilitic (095.7)

727.02 **Giant cell tumor of tendon sheath**

727.03 **Trigger finger (acquired)**

727.04 **Radial styloid tenosynovitis**
de Quervain's disease

727.05 **Other tenosynovitis of hand and wrist**

727.06 **Tenosynovitis of foot and ankle**

727.09 **Other**

727.1 **Bunion**

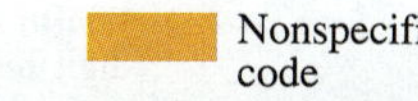

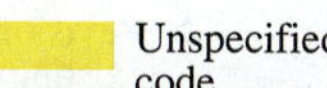

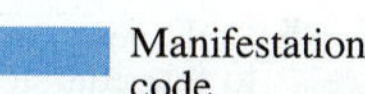

Manifestation
code

727.2 Specific bursitides often of occupational origin
   Beat: Chronic crepitant synovitis of wrist
     elbow   Miners':
     hand   elbow
     knee   knee

727.3 Other bursitis
   Bursitis NOS

   Excludes: *bursitis:*
        gonococcal (098.52)
        subacromial (726.19)
        subcoracoid (726.19)
        subdeltoid (726.19)
        syphilitic (095.7)
        "frozen shoulder" (726.0)

⑤ **727.4 Ganglion and cyst of synovium, tendon, and bursa**

    727.40 Synovial cyst, unspecified

   Excludes: *that of popliteal space (727.51)*

    727.41 Ganglion of joint

    727.42 Ganglion of tendon sheath

    727.43 Ganglion, unspecified

    727.49 Other
       Cyst of bursa

⑤ **727.5 Rupture of synovium**

    727.50 Rupture of synovium, unspecified

    727.51 Synovial cyst of popliteal space
       Baker's cyst (knee)

    727.59 Other

⑤ **727.6 Rupture of tendon, nontraumatic**

    727.60 Nontraumatic rupture of unspecified tendon

    727.61 Complete rupture of rotator cuff

    727.62 Tendons of biceps (long head)

    727.63 Extensor tendons of hand and wrist

    727.64 Flexor tendons of hand and wrist

    727.65 Quadriceps tendon

    727.66 Patellar tendon

    727.67 Achilles tendon

    727.68 Other tendons of foot and ankle

    727.69 Other

⑤ **727.8 Other disorders of synovium, tendon, and bursa**

    727.81 Contracture of tendon (sheath)
       Short Achilles tendon (acquired)

    727.82 Calcium deposits in tendon and bursa
       Calcification of tendon NOS
       Calcific tendinitis NOS

   Excludes: *peripheral ligamentous or muscular attachments (726.0-726.9)*

    727.83 Plica syndrome
       Plica knee

    727.89 Other
       Abscess of bursa or tendon

   Excludes: *xanthomatosis localized to tendons (272.7)*

727.9 Unspecified disorder of synovium, tendon, and bursa

728 Disorders of muscle, ligament, and fascia

   Excludes: *enthesopathies (726.0-726.9)*

        muscular dystrophies (359.0-359.1)
        myoneural disorders (358.0-358.9)
        myopathies (359.2-359.9)
        old disruption of ligaments of knee (717.81-717.89)

   ● Code new   ▲ Revision of   ④ ⑤ Fourth or fifth
      to this edition   existing code   digit required

728.0 Infective myositis
Myositis:
    purulent
    suppurative

Excludes: *myositis:*
    epidemic (074.1)
    interstitial (728.81)
    syphilitic (095.6)
    tropical (040.81)

⑤ **728.1 Muscular calcification and ossification**

    728.10 Calcification and ossification, unspecified
        Massive calcification (paraplegic)

    728.11 Progressive myositis ossificans

    728.12 Traumatic myositis ossificans
        Myositis ossificans (circumscripta)

    728.13 Postoperative heterotopic calcification

    728.19 Other
        Polymyositis ossificans

728.2 Muscular wasting and disuse atrophy, not elsewhere classified
Amyotrophia NOS   Myofibrosis

Excludes: *neuralgic amyotrophy (353.5)*
    progressive muscular atrophy (335.0-335.9)

728.3 Other specific muscle disorders
Arthrogryposis
Immobility syndrome (paraplegic)

Excludes: *arthrogryposis multiplex congenita (754.89)*
    stiff-man syndrome (333.91)

728.4 Laxity of ligament

728.5 Hypermobility syndrome

728.6 Contracture of palmar fascia
Dupuytren's contracture

⑤ **728.7 Other fibromatoses**

    728.71 Plantar fascial fibromatosis
        Contracture of plantar fascia
        Plantar fasciitis (traumatic)

    728.79 Other
        Garrod's or knuckle pads
        Nodular fasciitis
        Pseudosarcomatous fibromatosis (proliferative) (subcutaneous)

⑤ **728.8 Other disorders of muscle, ligament, and fascia**

    728.81 Interstitial myositis

    728.82 Foreign body granuloma of muscle
        Talc granuloma of muscle

    728.83 Rupture of muscle, nontraumatic

    728.84 Diastasis of muscle
        Diastasis recti (abdomen)

Excludes: *diastasis recti complicating pregnancy, labor, and delivery (665.8)*

    728.85 Spasm of muscle

    728.86 Necrotizing fasciitis
    Use additional code to identify:
        infectious organism (041.00 - 041.89)
        gangrene (785.4), if applicable

    728.89 Other
        Eosinophilic fasciitis
    Use additional E code, if desired, to identify drug, if drug induced

728.9 Unspecified disorder of muscle, ligament, and fascia

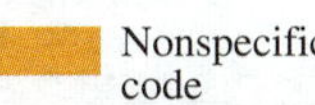

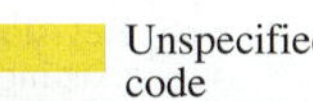

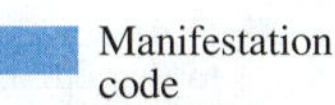

Manifestation
code

729 **Other disorders of soft tissues**

Excludes: acroparesthesia (443.89)
　　　　　carpal tunnel syndrome (354.0)
　　　　　disorders of the back (720.0-724.9)
　　　　　entrapment syndromes (354.0-355.9)
　　　　　palindromic rheumatism (719.3)
　　　　　periarthritis (726.0-726.9)
　　　　　psychogenic rheumatism (306.0)

729.0 **Rheumatism, unspecified and fibrositis**

729.1 **Myalgia and myositis, unspecified**
　　　　Fibromyositis NOS

729.2 **Neuralgia, neuritis, and radiculitis, unspecified**

Excludes: brachial radiculitis (723.4)
　　　　　cervical radiculitis (723.4)
　　　　　lumbosacral radiculitis (724.4)
　　　　　mononeuritis (354.0-355.9)
　　　　　radiculitis due to intervertebral disc involvement (722.0-722.2, 722.7)
　　　　　sciatica (724.3)

⑤ **729.3** **Panniculitis, unspecified**

　　729.30 **Panniculitis, unspecified site**
　　　　　Weber-Christian disease

　　729.31 **Hypertrophy of fat pad, knee**
　　　　　Hypertrophy of infrapatellar fat pad

　　729.39 **Other site**

Excludes: panniculitis specified as (affecting):
　　　　　back (724.8)
　　　　　neck (723.6)
　　　　　sacral (724.8)

729.4 **Fasciitis, unspecified**

Excludes: necrotizing fasciitis (728.86)
　　　　　nodular fasciitis (728.79)

729.5 **Pain in limb**

729.6 **Residual foreign body in soft tissue**

Excludes: foreign body granuloma:
　　　　　muscle (728.82)
　　　　　skin and subcutaneous tissue (709.4)

⑤ **729.8** **Other musculoskeletal symptoms referable to limbs**

　　729.81 **Swelling of limb**

　　729.82 **Cramp**

　　729.89 **Other**

Excludes: abnormality of gait (781.2)
　　　　　tetany (781.7)
　　　　　transient paralysis of limb (781.4)

729.9 **Other and unspecified disorders of soft tissue**
　　　　Polyalgia

OSTEOPATHIES, CHONDROPATHIES, AND ACQUIRED MUSCULOSKELETAL DEFORMITIES (730-739)

⑤ **730** **Osteomyelitis, periostitis, and other infections involving bone**

Excludes: jaw (526.4-526.5)
　　　　　petrous bone (383.2)

Use additional code, if desired, to identify organism, such as Staphylococcus (041.1)

The following fifth-digit subclassification is for use with category 730; valid digits are in [brackets] under each code. See beginning of this chapter for definitions:

　0 **site unspecified**

　1 **shoulder region**

　2 **upper arm**

　3 **forearm**

● Code new
　to this edition

▲ Revision of
　existing code

④ ⑤ Fourth or fifth
　　digit required

   4 **hand**

   5 **pelvic region and thigh**

   6 **lower leg**

   7 **ankle and foot**

   8 **other specified sites**

   9 **multiple sites**

⑤ **730.0 Acute osteomyelitis**
[0-9]
   Abscess of any bone except accessory sinus, jaw, or mastoid
   Acute or subacute osteomyelitis, with or without mention of periostitis

⑤ **730.1 Chronic osteomyelitis**
[0-9]
   Brodie's abscess
   Chronic or old osteomyelitis, with or without mention of periostitis
   Sequestrum of bone
   Sclerosing osteomyelitis of Garré

> *Excludes:* *aseptic necrosis of bone (733.40-733.49)*

⑤ **730.2 Unspecified osteomyelitis**
[0-9]
   Osteitis or osteomyelitis NOS, with or without mention of periostitis

⑤ **730.3 Periostitis without mention of osteomyelitis**
[0-9]

   Abscess of periosteum ⎫
   Periostosis   ⎬ without mention of osteomyelitis

> *Excludes:* *that in secondary syphilis (091.61)*

⑤ ***730.7 Osteopathy resulting from poliomyelitis***
[0-9]
   Code first underlying disease (045.0-045.9)

⑤ ***730.8 Other infections involving bone in diseases classified elsewhere***
[0-9]
   Code first underlying disease, as:
      tuberculosis (015.0-015.9)
      typhoid fever (002.0)

> *Excludes:* *syphilis of bone NOS (095.5)*

⑤ **730.9 Unspecified infection of bone**
[0-9]

731 Osteitis deformans and osteopathies associated with other disorders classified elsewhere

731.0 Osteitis deformans without mention of bone tumor
   Paget's disease of bone

731.1 Osteitis deformans in diseases classified elsewhere
   Code first underlying disease, as:
      malignant neoplasm of bone (170.0-170.9)

731.2 Hypertrophic pulmonary osteoarthropathy
   Bamberger-Marie disease

731.8 Other bone involvement in diseases classified elsewhere
   Code first underlying disease, as:
      diabetes mellitus (250.8)
   Use additional code to specify bone condition, such as:
      acute osteomyelitis (730.00-730.09)

732 Osteochondropathies

732.0 Juvenile osteochondrosis of spine
   Juvenile osteochondrosis (of):
      marginal or vertebral epiphysis (of Scheuermann)
      spine NOS
   Vertebral epiphysitis

> *Excludes:* *adolescent postural kyphosis (737.0)*

732.1 Juvenile osteochondrosis of hip and pelvis
   Coxa plana
   Ischiopubic synchondrosis (of van Neck)
   Osteochondrosis (juvenile) of:
      acetabulum
      head of femur (of Legg-Calvé-Perthes)
      iliac crest (of Buchanan)
      symphysis pubis (of Pierson)
   Pseudocoxalgia

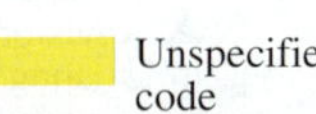

	Add 4th or 5th digit		Nonspecific code		Unspecified code		Manifestation code

732.2 Nontraumatic slipped upper femoral epiphysis
  Slipped upper femoral epiphysis NOS

732.3 Juvenile osteochondrosis of upper extremity
  Osteochondrosis (juvenile) of:
    capitulum of humerus (of Panner)
    carpal lunate (of Kienbock)
    hand NOS
    head of humerus (of Haas)
    heads of metacarpals (of Mauclaire)
    lower ulna (of Burns)
    radial head (of Brailsford)
    upper extremity NOS

732.4 Juvenile osteochondrosis of lower extremity, excluding foot
  Osteochondrosis (juvenile) of:
    lower extremity NOS
    primary patellar center (of Köhler)
    proximal tibia (of Blount)
    secondary patellar center (of Sinding-Larsen)
    tibial tubercle (of Osgood-Schlatter)
  Tibia vara

732.5 Juvenile osteochondrosis of foot
  Calcaneal apophysitis
  Epiphysitis, os calcis
  Osteochondrosis (juvenile) of:
    astragalus (of Diaz)
    calcaneum (of Sever)
    foot NOS
    metatarsal
      second (of Freiberg)
      fifth (of Iselin)
    os tibiale externum (Haglund)
    tarsal navicular (of Köhler)

`732.6` Other juvenile osteochondrosis
  Apophysitis
  Epiphysitis   } specified as juvenile, of other site, or site NOS
  Osteochondritis
  Osteochondrosis

732.7 Osteochondritis dissecans

`732.8` Other specified forms of osteochondropathy
  Adult osteochondrosis of spine

`732.9` Unspecified osteochondropathy
  Apophysitis
  Epiphysitis   NOS
  Osteochondritis   } Not specified as adult or juvenile, of unspecified site
  Osteochondrosis

`733` Other disorders of bone and cartilage

> *Excludes:* *bone spur (726.91)*
> *cartilage of, or loose body in, joint (717.0-717.9, 718.0-718.9)*
> *giant cell granuloma of jaw (526.3)*
> *osteitis fibrosa cystica generalisata (252.0)*
> *osteomalacia (268.2)*
> *polyostotic fibrous dysplasia of bone (756.54)*
> *prognathism, retrognathism (524.1)*
> *xanthomatosis localized to bone (272.7)*

⑤ **733.0 Osteoporosis**

  `733.00` Osteoporosis, unspecified
    Wedging of vertebra NOS

  733.01 Senile osteoporosis
    Postmenopausal osteoporosis

  733.02 Idiopathic osteoporosis

  733.03 Disuse osteoporosis

  `733.09` Other
    Drug-induced osteoporosis
    Use additional E code, if desired, to identify drug

● Code new
to this edition

▲ Revision of
existing code

④ ⑤ Fourth or fifth
digit required

⑤ **733.1 Pathologic fracture**
Spontaneous fracture

Excludes: traumatic fracture (800-829)
stress fracture (733.93-733.95)

733.10 Pathologic fracture, unspecified site

733.11 Pathologic fracture of humerus

733.12 Pathologic fracture of distal radius and ulna
Wrist NOS

733.13 Pathologic fracture of vertebrae
Collapse of vertebra NOS

733.14 Pathologic fracture of neck of femur
Femur NOS
Hip NOS

733.15 Pathologic fracture of other specified part of femur

733.16 Pathologic fracture of tibia or fibula
Ankle NOS

733.19 Pathologic fracture of other specified site

⑤ **733.2 Cyst of bone**

733.20 Cyst of bone (localized), unspecified

733.21 Solitary bone cyst
Unicameral bone cyst

733.22 Aneurysmal bone cyst

733.29 Other
Fibrous dysplasia (monostotic)

Excludes: cyst of jaw (526.0-526.2, 526.89)
osteitis fibrosa cystica (252.0)
polyostotic fibrous dysplasia of bone (756.54)

733.3 Hyperostosis of skull
Hyperostosis interna frontalis
Leontiasis ossium

⑤ **733.4 Aseptic necrosis of bone**

Excludes: osteochondropathies (732.0-732.9)

733.40 Aseptic necrosis of bone, site unspecified

733.41 Head of humerus

733.42 Head and neck of femur
Femur NOS

Excludes: Legg-Calvé-Perthes disease (732.1)

733.43 Medial femoral condyle

733.44 Talus

733.49 Other

733.5 Osteitis condensans
Piriform sclerosis of ilium

733.6 Tietze's disease
Costochondral junction syndrome
Costochondritis

733.7 Algoneurodystrophy
Disuse atrophy of bone   Sudeck's atrophy

⑤ **733.8 Malunion and nonunion of fracture**

733.81 Malunion of fracture

733.82 Nonunion of fracture
Pseudoarthrosis (bone)

⑤ **733.9 Other and unspecified disorders of bone and cartilage**

733.90 Disorder of bone and cartilage, unspecified

733.91 Arrest of bone development or growth
Epiphyseal arrest

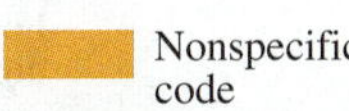

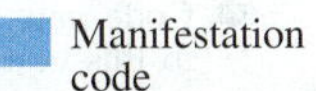

Manifestation
code

733.92 Chondromalacia
Chondromalacia:
NOS
localized, except patella
systemic
tibial plateau

Excludes: *chondromalacia of patella (717.7)*

733.93 Stress fracture of tibia or fibula
Stress reaction of tibia or fibula

733.94 Stress fracture of the metatarsals
Stress reaction of metatarsals

733.95 Stress fracture of other bone
Stress reaction of other bone

733.99 Other
Diaphysitis   Relapsing polychondritis
Hypertrophy of bone

734 Flat foot
Pes planus (acquired)
Talipes planus (acquired)

Excludes: *congenital (754.61)*
rigid flat foot (754.61)
spastic (everted) flat foot (754.61)

735 Acquired deformities of toe

Excludes: *congenital (754.60-754.69, 755.65-755.66)*

735.0 Hallux valgus (acquired)

735.1 Hallux varus (acquired)

735.2 Hallux rigidus

735.3 Hallux malleus

735.4 Other hammer toe (acquired)

735.5 Claw toe (acquired)

735.8 Other acquired deformities of toe

735.9 Unspecified acquired deformity of toe

736 Other acquired deformities of limbs

Excludes: *congenital (754.3-755.9)*

⑤ **736.0 Acquired deformities of forearm, excluding fingers**

736.00 Unspecified deformity
Deformity of elbow, forearm, hand, or wrist (acquired) NOS

736.01 Cubitus valgus (acquired)

736.02 Cubitus varus (acquired)

736.03 Valgus deformity of wrist (acquired)

736.04 Varus deformity of wrist (acquired)

736.05 Wrist drop (acquired)

736.06 Claw hand (acquired)

736.07 Club hand, acquired

736.09 Other

736.1 Mallet finger

⑤ **736.2 Other acquired deformities of finger**

736.20 Unspecified deformity
Deformity of finger (acquired) NOS

736.21 Boutonniere deformity

736.22 Swan-neck deformity

736.29 Other

Excludes: *trigger finger (727.03)*

⑤ **736.3 Acquired deformities of hip**

● Code new
to this edition   ▲ Revision of
existing code   ④ ⑤ Fourth or fifth
digit required

736.30 **Unspecified deformity**
Deformity of hip (acquired) NOS

736.31 **Coxa valga (acquired)**

736.32 **Coxa vara (acquired)**

736.39 **Other**

⑤ 736.4 **Genu valgum or varum (acquired)**

736.41 **Genu valgum (acquired)**

736.42 **Genu varum (acquired)**

736.5 **Genu recurvatum (acquired)**

736.6 **Other acquired deformities of knee**
Deformity of knee (acquired) NOS

⑤ 736.7 **Other acquired deformities of ankle and foot**

Excludes:	*deformities of toe (acquired) (735.0-735.9)*
	pes planus (acquired) (734)

736.70 **Unspecified deformity of ankle and foot, acquired**

736.71 **Acquired equinovarus deformity**
Clubfoot, acquired

Excludes:	*clubfoot not specified as acquired (754.5-754.7)*

736.72 **Equinus deformity of foot, acquired**

736.73 **Cavus deformity of foot**

Excludes:	*that with claw foot (736.74)*

736.74 **Claw foot, acquired**

736.75 **Cavovarus deformity of foot, acquired**

736.76 **Other calcaneus deformity**

736.79 **Other**
Acquired:
pes
talipes ⎫ not elsewhere classified

⑤ 736.8 **Acquired deformities of other parts of limbs**

736.81 **Unequal leg length (acquired)**

736.89 **Other**
Deformity (acquired):
arm or leg, not elsewhere classified
shoulder

736.9 **Acquired deformity of limb, site unspecified**

737 **Curvature of spine**

Excludes:	*congenital (754.2)*

737.0 **Adolescent postural kyphosis**

Excludes:	*osteochondrosis of spine (juvenile) (732.0)*
	adult (732.8)

⑤ 737.1 **Kyphosis (acquired)**

737.10 **Kyphosis (acquired) (postural)**

737.11 **Kyphosis due to radiation**

737.12 **Kyphosis, postlaminectomy**

737.19 **Other**

Excludes:	*that associated with conditions classifiable elsewhere (737.41)*

⑤ 737.2 **Lordosis (acquired)**

737.20 **Lordosis (acquired) (postural)**

737.21 **Lordosis, postlaminectomy**

737.22 **Other postsurgical lordosis**

737.29 **Other**

Excludes:	*that associated with conditions classifiable elsewhere (737.42)*

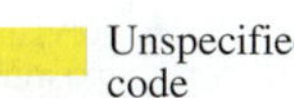

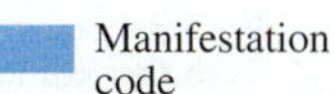

⑤ **737.3 Kyphoscoliosis and scoliosis**

    737.30 Scoliosis [and kyphoscoliosis], idiopathic

    737.31 Resolving infantile idiopathic scoliosis

    737.32 Progressive infantile idiopathic scoliosis

    737.33 Scoliosis due to radiation

    737.34 Thoracogenic scoliosis

    737.39 Other

    Excludes: *that associated with conditions classifiable elsewhere (737.43)*
    that in kyphoscoliotic heart disease (416.1)

⑤ **737.4 *Curvature of spine associated with other conditions***
    Code first associated condition, as:
    Charcot-Marie-Tooth disease (356.1)
    mucopolysaccharidosis (277.5)
    neurofibromatosis (237.7)
    osteitis deformans (731.0)
    osteitis fibrosa cystica (252.0)
    osteoporosis (733.00-733.09)
    poliomyelitis (138)
    tuberculosis [Pott's curvature] (015.0)

    737.40 *Curvature of spine, unspecified*

    737.41 *Kyphosis*

    737.42 *Lordosis*

    737.43 *Scoliosis*

737.8 Other curvatures of spine

737.9 Unspecified curvature of spine
    Curvature of spine (acquired) (idiopathic) NOS
    Hunchback, acquired

    Excludes: *deformity of spine NOS (738.5)*

738 Other acquired deformity

    Excludes: *congenital (754.0-756.9, 758.0-759.9)*
    dentofacial anomalies (524.0-524.9)

738.0 Acquired deformity of nose
    Deformity of nose (acquired)
    Overdevelopment of nasal bones

    Excludes: *deflected or deviated nasal septum (470)*

⑤ **738.1 Other acquired deformity of head**

    738.10 Unspecified deformity

    738.11 Zygomatic hyperplasia

    738.12 Zygomatic hypoplasia

    738.19 Other specified deformity

738.2 Acquired deformity of neck

738.3 Acquired deformity of chest and rib
    Deformity: Pectus:
    chest (acquired)   carinatum, acquired
    rib (acquired)   excavatum, acquired

738.4 Acquired spondylolisthesis
    Degenerative spondylolisthesis
    Spondylolysis, acquired

    Excludes: *congenital (756.12)*

738.5 Other acquired deformity of back or spine
    Deformity of spine NOS

    Excludes: *curvature of spine (737.0-737.9)*

738.6 Acquired deformity of pelvis
    Pelvic obliquity

    Excludes: *intrapelvic protrusion of acetabulum (718.6)*
    that in relation to labor and delivery (653.0-653.4, 653.8-653.9)

738.7 Cauliflower ear

  ● Code new
    to this edition
  ▲ Revision of
    existing code
  ④ ⑤ Fourth or fifth
       digit required

738.8 Acquired deformity of other specified site
Deformity of clavicle

738.9 Acquired deformity of unspecified site

739 Nonallopathic lesions, not elsewhere classified
Includes: segmental dysfunction
somatic dysfunction

739.0 Head region
Occipitocervical region

739.1 Cervical region
Cervicothoracic region

739.2 Thoracic region
Thoracolumbar region

739.3 Lumbar region
Lumbosacral region

739.4 Sacral region
Sacrococcygeal region   Sacroiliac region

739.5 Pelvic region
Hip region   Pubic region

739.6 Lower extremities

739.7 Upper extremities
Acromioclavicular region   Sternoclavicular region

739.8 Rib cage
Costochondral region   Sternochondral region
Costovertebral region

739.9 Abdomen and other

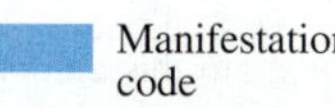

● Code new
to this edition

▲ Revision of
existing code

④ ⑤ Fourth or fifth
digit required

14. CONGENITAL ANOMALIES (740-759)

740 Anencephalus and similar anomalies

740.0 Anencephalus

Acrania
Amyelencephalus
Hemianencephaly
Hemicephaly

740.1 Craniorachischisis

740.2 Iniencephaly

741 Spina bifida

Excludes: spina bifida occulta (756.17)

The following fifth-digit subclassification is for use with category 741:

0 unspecified region

1 cervical region

2 dorsal [thoracic] region

3 lumbar region

741.0 With hydrocephalus
Arnold-Chiari syndrome, type II
Any condition classifiable to 741.9 with any condition classifiable to 742.3
Chiari malformation, type II

741.9 Without mention of hydrocephalus
Hydromeningocele (spinal)
Hydromyelocele
Meningocele (spinal)
Meningomyelocele
Myelocele
Myelocystocele
Rachischisis
Spina bifida (aperta)
Syringomyelocele

742 Other congenital anomalies of nervous system

742.0 Encephalocele
Encephalocystocele
Encephalomyelocele
Hydroencephalocele
Hydromeningocele, cranial
Meningocele, cerebral
Meningoencephalocele

742.1 Microcephalus
Hydromicrocephaly
Micrencephaly

742.2 Reduction deformities of brain
Absence
Agenesis
Aplasia
Hypoplasia
} of part of brain
Agyria
Arhinencephaly
Holoprosencephaly
Microgyria

742.3 Congenital hydrocephalus
Aqueduct of Sylvius:
anomaly
obstruction, congenital
stenosis
Atresia of foramina of Magendie and Luschka
Hydrocephalus in newborn

Excludes: hydrocephalus:
acquired (331.3-331.4)
due to congenital toxoplasmosis (771.2)
with any condition classifiable to 741.9 (741.0)

742.4 Other specified anomalies of brain
Congenital cerebral cyst
Macroencephaly
Macrogyria
Megalencephaly
Multiple anomalies of brain NOS
Porencephaly
Ulegyria

742.5 Other specified anomalies of spinal cord

742.51 Diastematomyelia

742.53 Hydromyelia
Hydrorhachis

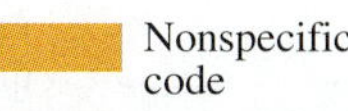

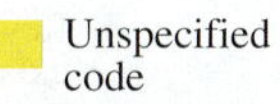

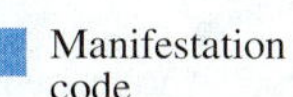

Manifestation
code

742.59 Other
     Amyelia
     Atelomyelia
     Congenital anomaly of spinal meninges
     Defective development of cauda equina
     Hypoplasia of spinal cord
     Myelatelia
     Myelodysplasia

742.8 Other specified anomalies of nervous system

Agenesis of nerve	Jaw-winking syndrome
Displacement of brachial	Marcus-Gunn syndrome
plexus	Riley-Day syndrome
Familial dysautonomia	

    Excludes: *neurofibromatosis (237.7)*

742.9 Unspecified anomaly of brain, spinal cord, and nervous system
    Anomaly
    Congenital:
      disease   } of { brain
      lesion   nervous system
    Deformity   spinal cord

743 Congenital anomalies of eye

⑤ **743.0 Anophthalmos**

    743.00 Clinical anophthalmos, unspecified
        Agenesis
        Congenital absence   } of eye
        Anophthalmos NOS

    743.03 Cystic eyeball, congenital

    743.06 Cryptophthalmos

⑤ **743.1 Microphthalmos**
    Dysplasia
    Hypoplasia   } of eye
    Rudimentary eye

    743.10 Microphthalmos, unspecified

    743.11 Simple microphthalmos

    743.12 Microphthalmos associated with other anomalies of eye and adnexa

⑤ **743.2 Buphthalmos**

Glaucoma:	Hydrophthalmos
congenital	
newborn	

    Excludes: *glaucoma of childhood (365.14)*
              traumatic glaucoma due to birth injury (767.8)

    743.20 Buphthalmos, unspecified

    743.21 Simple buphthalmos

    743.22 Buphthalmos associated with other ocular anomalies
        Keratoglobus, congenital
        Megalocornea   } associated with buphthalmos

⑤ **743.3 Congenital cataract and lens anomalies**

    Excludes: *infantile cataract (366.00-366.09)*

    743.30 Congenital cataract, unspecified

    743.31 Capsular and subcapsular cataract

    743.32 Cortical and zonular cataract

    743.33 Nuclear cataract

    743.34 Total and subtotal cataract, congenital

    743.35 Congenital aphakia
        Congenital absence of lens

    743.36 Anomalies of lens shape
        Microphakia   Spherophakia

    743.37 Congenital ectopic lens

    743.39 Other

● Code new   ▲ Revision of   ④ ⑤ Fourth or fifth
to this edition   existing code   digit required

⑤ **743.4 Coloboma and other anomalies of anterior segment**

    743.41 Anomalies of corneal size and shape
        Microcornea

    | *Excludes:* | *that associated with buphthalmos (743.22)* |

    743.42 Corneal opacities, interfering with vision, congenital

    743.43 Other corneal opacities, congenital

    743.44 Specified anomalies of anterior chamber, chamber angle, and related structures
        Anomaly:
          Axenfeld's
          Peters'
          Rieger's

    743.45 Aniridia

    743.46 Other specified anomalies of iris and ciliary body
        Anisocoria, congenital
        Atresia of pupil
        Coloboma of iris
        Corectopia

    743.47 Specified anomalies of sclera

    743.48 Multiple and combined anomalies of anterior segment

    743.49 Other

⑤ **743.5 Congenital anomalies of posterior segment**

    743.51 Vitreous anomalies
        Congenital vitreous opacity

    743.52 Fundus coloboma

    743.53 Chorioretinal degeneration, congenital

    743.54 Congenital folds and cysts of posterior segment

    743.55 Congenital macular changes

    743.56 Other retinal changes, congenital

    743.57 Specified anomalies of optic disc
        Coloboma of optic disc (congenital)

    743.58 Vascular anomalies
        Congenital retinal aneurysm

    743.59 Other

⑤ **743.6 Congenital anomalies of eyelids, lacrimal system, and orbit**

    743.61 Congenital ptosis

    743.62 Congenital deformities of eyelids
        Ablepharon   Congenital:
        Absence of eyelid   ectropion
        Accessory eyelid   entropion

    743.63 Other specified congenital anomalies of eyelid
        Absence, agenesis, of cilia

    743.64 Specified congenital anomalies of lacrimal gland

    743.65 Specified congenital anomalies of lacrimal passages
        Absence, agenesis of:
          lacrimal apparatus
          punctum lacrimale
        Accessory lacrimal canal

    743.66 Specified congenital anomalies of orbit

    743.69 Other
        Accessory eye muscles

743.8 Other specified anomalies of eye

    | *Excludes:* | *congenital nystagmus (379.51)* |
                ocular albinism (270.2)
                retinitis pigmentosa (362.74)

| ■ Add 4th or 5th digit | ■ Nonspecific code | ■ Unspecified code | ■ Manifestation code |

743.9 **Unspecified anomaly of eye**
Congenital:
anomaly NOS
deformity NOS } of eye [any part]

744 **Congenital anomalies of ear, face, and neck**
Excludes: *anomaly of:*
cervical spine (754.2, 756.10-756.19)
larynx (748.2-748.3)
nose (748.0-748.1)
parathyroid gland (759.2)
thyroid gland (759.2)
cleft lip (749.10-749.25)

⑤ **744.0** **Anomalies of ear causing impairment of hearing**
Excludes: *congenital deafness without mention of cause (389.0-389.9)*

744.00 **Unspecified anomaly of ear with impairment of hearing**

744.01 **Absence of external ear**
Absence of:
auditory canal (external)
auricle (ear) (with stenosis or atresia of auditory canal)

744.02 **Other anomalies of external ear with impairment of hearing**
Atresia or stricture of auditory canal (external)

744.03 **Anomaly of middle ear, except ossicles**
Atresia or stricture of osseous meatus (ear)

744.04 **Anomalies of ear ossicles**
Fusion of ear ossicles

744.05 **Anomalies of inner ear**
Congenital anomaly of:
membranous labyrinth
organ of Corti

744.09 **Other**
Absence of ear, congenital

744.1 **Accessory auricle**
Accessory tragus   Supernumerary:
Polyotia   ear
Preauricular appendage   lobule

⑤ **744.2** **Other specified anomalies of ear**
Excludes: *that with impairment of hearing (744.00-744.09)*

744.21 **Absence of ear lobe, congenital**

744.22 **Macrotia**

744.23 **Microtia**

744.24 **Specified anomalies of Eustachian tube**
Absence of Eustachian tube

744.29 **Other**
Bat ear   Prominence of auricle
Darwin's tubercle   Ridge ear
Pointed ear

Excludes: *preauricular sinus (744.46)*

744.3 **Unspecified anomaly of ear**
Congenital:
anomaly NOS
deformity NOS } of ear, not elsewhere classified

⑤ **744.4** **Branchial cleft cyst or fistula; preauricular sinus**

744.41 **Branchial cleft sinus or fistula**
Branchial:
sinus (external) (internal)
vestige

744.42 **Branchial cleft cyst**

744.43 **Cervical auricle**

744.46 **Preauricular sinus or fistula**

744.47 **Preauricular cyst**

● Code new   ▲ Revision of   ④ ⑤ Fourth or fifth
to this edition   existing code   digit required

744.49 **Other**
Fistula (of):
auricle, congenital
cervicoaural

744.5 **Webbing of neck**
Pterygium colli

⑤ **744.8** **Other specified anomalies of face and neck**

744.81 **Macrocheilia**
Hypertrophy of lip, congenital

744.82 **Microcheilia**

744.83 **Macrostomia**

744.84 **Microstomia**

744.89 **Other**

Excludes:	congenital fistula of lip (750.25)
	musculoskeletal anomalies (754.0-754.1, 756.0)

744.9 **Unspecified anomalies of face and neck**
Congenital:
anomaly NOS ⎫
deformity NOS ⎬ of face [any part] or neck [any part]

745 **Bulbus cordis anomalies and anomalies of cardiac septal closure**

745.0 **Common truncus**
Absent septum ⎫
Communication (abnormal) ⎬ between aorta and pulmonary artery
Aortic septal defect
Common aortopulmonary trunk
Persistent truncus arteriosus

⑤ **745.1** **Transposition of great vessels**

745.10 **Complete transposition of great vessels**
Transposition of great vessels:
NOS
classical

745.11 **Double outlet right ventricle**
Dextratransposition of aorta
Incomplete transposition of great vessels
Origin of both great vessels from right ventricle
Taussig-Bing syndrome or defect

745.12 **Corrected transposition of great vessels**

745.19 **Other**

745.2 **Tetralogy of Fallot**
Fallot's pentalogy
Ventricular septal defect with pulmonary stenosis or atresia, dextraposition of aorta, and
hypertrophy of right ventricle

Excludes:	Fallot's triad (746.09)

745.3 **Common ventricle**
Cor triloculare biatriatum   Single ventricle

745.4 **Ventricular septal defect**
Eisenmenger's defect or complex
Gerbode defect
Interventricular septal defect
Left ventricular-right atrial communication
Roger's disease

Excludes:	common atrioventricular canal type (745.69)
	single ventricle (745.3)

745.5 **Ostium secundum type atrial septal defect**
Defect: Patent or persistent:
atrium secundum   foramen ovale
fossa ovalis   ostium secundum
Lutembacher's syndrome

⑤ **745.6** **Endocardial cushion defects**

745.60 **Endocardial cushion defect, unspecified type**

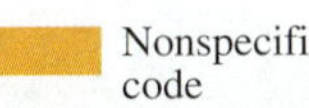

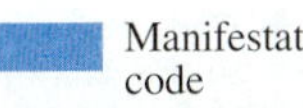

Manifestation
code

745.61 Ostium primum defect
Persistent ostium primum

745.69 Other
Absence of atrial septum
Atrioventricular canal type ventricular septal defect
Common atrioventricular canal
Common atrium

745.7 Cor biloculare
Absence of atrial and ventricular septa

745.8 Other

745.9 Unspecified defect of septal closure
Septal defect NOS

746 Other congenital anomalies of heart

Excludes: *endocardial fibroelastosis (425.3)*

⑤ **746.0 Anomalies of pulmonary valve**

Excludes: *infundibular or subvalvular pulmonic stenosis (746.83)*
tetralogy of Fallot (745.2)

746.00 Pulmonary valve anomaly, unspecified

746.01 Atresia, congenital
Congenital absence of pulmonary valve

746.02 Stenosis, congenital

746.09 Other
Congenital insufficiency of pulmonary valve
Fallot's triad or trilogy

746.1 Tricuspid atresia and stenosis, congenital
Absence of tricuspid valve

746.2 Ebstein's anomaly

746.3 Congenital stenosis of aortic valve
Congenital aortic stenosis

Excludes: *congenital:*
subaortic stenosis (746.81)
supravalvular aortic stenosis (747.22)

746.4 Congenital insufficiency of aortic valve
Bicuspid aortic valve
Congenital aortic insufficiency

746.5 Congenital mitral stenosis
Fused commissure
Parachute deformity } of mitral valve
Supernumerary cusps

746.6 Congenital mitral insufficiency

746.7 Hypoplastic left heart syndrome
Atresia, or marked hypoplasia, of aortic orifice or valve, with hypoplasia of ascending
aorta and defective development of left ventricle (with mitral valve atresia)

⑤ **746.8 Other specified anomalies of heart**

746.81 Subaortic stenosis

746.82 Cor triatriatum

746.83 Infundibular pulmonic stenosis
Subvalvular pulmonic stenosis

746.84 Obstructive anomalies of heart, not elsewhere classified
Uhl's disease

746.85 Coronary artery anomaly
Anomalous origin or communication of coronary artery
Arteriovenous malformation of coronary artery
Coronary artery:
absence
arising from aorta or pulmonary trunk
single

746.86 Congenital heart block
Complete or incomplete atrioventricular [AV] block

● Code new
to this edition

▲ Revision of
existing code

④ ⑤ Fourth or fifth
digit required

746.87   Malposition of heart and cardiac apex
Abdominal heart   Levocardia (isolated)
Dextrocardia   Mesocardia
Ectopia cordis

Excludes: *dextrocardia with complete transposition of viscera (759.3)*

746.89   Other
Atresia   } of cardiac vein
Hypoplasia
Congenital:
cardiomegaly
diverticulum, left ventricle
pericardial defect

746.9 Unspecified anomaly of heart
Congenital:
anomaly of heart NOS
heart disease NOS

747 Other congenital anomalies of circulatory system

747.0 Patent ductus arteriosus
Patent ductus Botalli
Persistent ductus arteriosus

⑤ **747.1 Coarctation of aorta**

747.10   Coarctation of aorta (preductal) (postductal)
Hypoplasia of aortic arch

747.11   Interruption of aortic arch

⑤ **747.2 Other anomalies of aorta**

747.20   Anomaly of aorta, unspecified

747.21   Anomalies of aortic arch
Anomalous origin, right subclavian artery
Dextraposition of aorta
Double aortic arch
Kommerell's diverticulum
Overriding aorta
Persistent:
convolutions, aortic arch
right aortic arch
Vascular ring

Excludes: *hypoplasia of aortic arch (747.10)*

747.22   Atresia and stenosis of aorta
Absence   }
Aplasia   } of aorta
Hypoplasia   }
Stricture   }
Supra (valvular)-aortic stenosis

Excludes: *congenital aortic (valvular) stenosis or stricture, so stated (746.3)*
hypoplasia of aorta in hypoplastic left heart syndrome (746.7)

747.29   Other
Aneurysm of sinus of Valsalva
Congenital:
aneurysm   } of aorta
dilation

747.3 Anomalies of pulmonary artery
Agenesis   }
Anomaly   }
Atresia   }
Coarctation   } of pulmonary artery
Hypoplasia   }
Stenosis   }
Pulmonary arteriovenous aneurysm

⑤ **747.4 Anomalies of great veins**

747.40   Anomaly of great veins, unspecified
Anomaly NOS of:
pulmonary veins
vena cava

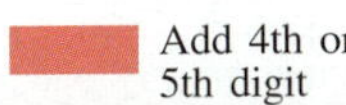

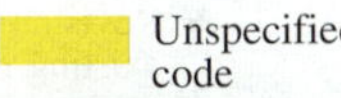

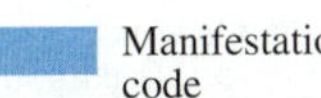

747.41 Total anomalous pulmonary venous connection
Total anomalous pulmonary venous return [TAPVR]:
subdiaphragmatic
supradiaphragmatic

747.42 Partial anomalous pulmonary venous connection
Partial anomalous pulmonary venous return

747.49 Other anomalies of great veins
Absence
Congenital stenosis } of vena cava (inferior) (superior)
Persistent:
left posterior cardinal vein
left superior vena cava
Scimitar syndrome
Transposition of pulmonary veins NOS

747.5 Absence or hypoplasia of umbilical artery
Single umbilical artery

⑤ **747.6 Other anomalies of peripheral vascular system**
Absence
Anomaly } of artery or vein, not elsewhere classified
Atresia
Arteriovenous aneurysm (peripheral)
Arteriovenous malformation of the peripheral vascular system
Congenital:
aneurysm (peripheral)
phlebectasia
stricture, artery
varix
Multiple renal arteries

Excludes: anomalies of:
cerebral vessels (747.81)
pulmonary artery (747.3)
congenital retinal aneurysm (743.58)
hemangioma (228.00-228.09)
lymphangioma (228.1)

747.60 Anomaly of the peripheral vascular system, unspecified site

747.61 Gastrointestinal vessel anomaly

747.62 Renal vessel anomaly

747.63 Upper limb vessel anomaly

747.64 Lower limb vessel anomaly

747.69 Anomalies of other specified sites of peripheral vascular system

⑤ **747.8 Other specified anomalies of circulatory system**

747.81 Anomalies of cerebrovascular system
Arteriovenous malformation of brain
Cerebral arteriovenous aneurysm, congenital
Congenital anomalies of cerebral vessels

Excludes: ruptured cerebral (arteriovenous) aneurysm (430)

747.82 Spinal vessel anomaly
Arteriovenous malformation of spinal vessel

● **747.83 Persistent fetal circulation**
Persistent pulmonary hypertension
Primary pulmonary hypertension of newborn

747.89 Other
Aneurysm, congenital, specified site not elsewhere classified

Excludes: congenital aneurysm:
coronary (746.85)
peripheral (747.6)
pulmonary (747.3)
retinal (743.58)

747.9 Unspecified anomaly of circulatory system

748 Congenital anomalies of respiratory system

Excludes: congenital defect of diaphragm (756.6)

● Code new   ▲ Revision of   ④ ⑤ Fourth or fifth
to this edition   existing code   digit required

748.0 Choanal atresia
Atresia
Congenital stenosis } of nares (anterior) (posterior)

748.1 Other anomalies of nose
Absent nose
Accessory nose
Cleft nose
Deformity of wall of nasal
  sinus

Congenital:
  deformity of nose
  notching of tip of nose
  perforation of wall of nasal sinus

Excludes: *congenital deviation of nasal septum (754.0)*

748.2 Web of larynx
Web of larynx:
  NOS
  glottic
  subglottic

748.3 Other anomalies of larynx, trachea, and bronchus
Absence or agenesis of:
  bronchus
  larynx
  trachea
Anomaly (of):
  cricoid cartilage
  epiglottis
  thyroid cartilage
  tracheal cartilage
Atresia (of):
  epiglottis
  glottis
  larynx
  trachea
Cleft thyroid, cartilage,
  congenital

Congenital:
  dilation, trachea
  stenosis:
    larynx
    trachea
  tracheocele
Diverticulum:
  bronchus
  trachea
Fissure of epiglottis
Laryngocele
Posterior cleft of cricoid cartilage (congenital)
Rudimentary tracheal bronchus
Stridor, laryngeal, congenital

748.4 Congenital cystic lung
Disease, lung:
  cystic, congenital
  polycystic, congenital

Honeycomb lung, congenital

Excludes: *acquired or unspecified cystic lung (518.89)*

748.5 Agenesis, hypoplasia, and dysplasia of lung
Absence of lung (fissures) (lobe)
Aplasia of lung
Hypoplasia of lung (lobe)
Sequestration of lung

⑤ **748.6 Other anomalies of lung**

748.60 Anomaly of lung, unspecified

748.61 **Congenital bronchiectasis**

748.69 Other
Accessory lung (lobe)
Azygos lobe (fissure), lung

748.8 Other specified anomalies of respiratory system
Abnormal communication between pericardial and pleural sacs
Anomaly, pleural folds
Atresia of nasopharynx
Congenital cyst of mediastinum

748.9 Unspecified anomaly of respiratory system
Anomaly of respiratory system NOS

749 **Cleft palate and cleft lip**

⑤ **749.0 Cleft palate**

749.00 Cleft palate, unspecified

749.01 **Unilateral, complete**

749.02 **Unilateral, incomplete**
Cleft uvula

749.03 **Bilateral, complete**

749.04 **Bilateral, incomplete**

Add 4th or 5th digit | Nonspecific code | Unspecified code | Manifestation code

⑤ **749.1 Cleft lip**
    Cheiloschisis   Harelip
    Congenital fissure of lip   Labium leporinum

    749.10 Cleft lip, unspecified

    749.11 Unilateral, complete

    749.12 Unilateral, incomplete

    749.13 Bilateral, complete

    749.14 Bilateral, incomplete

⑤ **749.2 Cleft palate with cleft lip**
    Cheilopalatoschisis

    749.20 Cleft palate with cleft lip, unspecified

    749.21 Unilateral, complete

    749.22 Unilateral, incomplete

    749.23 Bilateral, complete

    749.24 Bilateral, incomplete

    749.25 Other combinations

750 Other congenital anomalies of upper alimentary tract

    Excludes: *dentofacial anomalies (524.0-524.9)*

  750.0 Tongue tie
    Ankyloglossia

⑤ **750.1 Other anomalies of tongue**

    750.10 Anomaly of tongue, unspecified

    750.11 Aglossia

    750.12 Congenital adhesions of tongue

    750.13 Fissure of tongue
        Bifid tongue   Double tongue

    750.15 Macroglossia
        Congenital hypertrophy of tongue

    750.16 Microglossia
        Hypoplasia of tongue

    750.19 Other

⑤ **750.2 Other specified anomalies of mouth and pharynx**

    750.21 Absence of salivary gland

    750.22 Accessory salivary gland

    750.23 Atresia, salivary duct
        Imperforate salivary duct

    750.24 Congenital fistula of salivary gland

    750.25 Congenital fistula of lip
        Congenital (mucus) lip pits

    750.26 Other specified anomalies of mouth
        Absence of uvula

    750.27 Diverticulum of pharynx
        Pharyngeal pouch

    750.29 Other specified anomalies of pharynx
        Imperforate pharynx

  750.3 Tracheoesophageal fistula, esophageal atresia and stenosis
    Absent esophagus   Congenital fistula:
    Atresia of esophagus   esophagobronchial
    Congenital: esophagotracheal
      esophageal ring   Imperforate esophagus
      stenosis of esophagus Webbed esophagus
      stricture of esophagus

● Code new   ▲ Revision of   ④ ⑤ Fourth or fifth
  to this edition   existing code   digit required

750.4 Other specified anomalies of esophagus
Dilatation, congenital
Displacement, congenital
Diverticulum
Duplication } (of) esophagus
Giant
Esophageal pouch

Excludes: congenital hiatus hernia (750.6)

750.5 Congenital hypertrophic pyloric stenosis
Congenital or infantile:
  constriction
  hypertrophy
  spasm } of pylorus
  stenosis
  stricture

750.6 Congenital hiatus hernia
Displacement of cardia through esophageal hiatus

Excludes: congenital diaphragmatic hernia (756.6)

750.7 Other specified anomalies of stomach
Congenital: Duplication of stomach
  cardiospasm   Megalogastria
  hourglass stomach Microgastria
Displacement of stomach Transposition of stomach
Diverticulum of stomach,
  congenital

750.8 Other specified anomalies of upper alimentary tract

750.9 Unspecified anomaly of upper alimentary tract
Congenital:
  anomaly NOS
  deformity NOS } of upper alimentary tract [any part, except tongue]

751 Other congenital anomalies of digestive system

751.0 Meckel's diverticulum
Meckel's diverticulum (displaced) (hypertrophic)
Persistent:
  omphalomesenteric duct
  vitelline duct

751.1 Atresia and stenosis of small intestine
Atresia of:
  duodenum
  ileum
  intestine NOS
Congenital:
  absence
  obstruction
  stenosis } of small intestine or intestine NOS
  stricture
Imperforate jejunum

751.2 Atresia and stenosis of large intestine, rectum, and anal canal
Absence: Congenital or infantile:
  anus (congenital)   obstruction of large intestine
  appendix, congenital occlusion of anus
  large intestine, congenital stricture of anus
  rectum   Imperforate:
Atresia of: anus
  anus   rectum
  colon   Stricture of rectum, congenital
  rectum

751.3 Hirschsprung's disease and other congenital functional disorders of colon
Aganglionosis   Congenital megacolon
Congenital dilation of colon Macrocolon

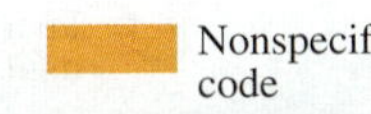

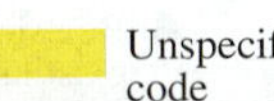

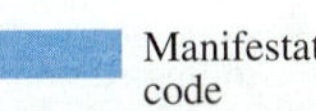

Manifestation
code

751.4 Anomalies of intestinal fixation

Congenital adhesions:
  omental, anomalous
  peritoneal
Jackson's membrane
Malrotation of colon

Rotation of cecum or colon:
  failure of
  incomplete
  insufficient
Universal mesentery

751.5 Other anomalies of intestine

Congenital diverticulum,
  colon
Dolichocolon
Duplication of:
  anus
  appendix
  cecum
  intestine
Ectopic anus

Megaloappendix
Megaloduodenum
Microcolon
Persistent cloaca
Transposition of:
  appendix
  colon
  intestine

⑤ **751.6 Anomalies of gallbladder, bile ducts, and liver**

751.60 Unspecified anomaly of gallbladder, bile ducts, and liver

751.61 Biliary atresia

Congenital:
  absence
  hypoplasia
  obstruction } of bile duct (common) or passage
  stricture

751.62 Congenital cystic disease of liver

Congenital polycystic disease of liver
Fibrocystic disease of liver

751.69 Other anomalies of gallbladder, bile ducts, and liver

Absence of:
  gallbladder, congenital
  liver (lobe)
Accessory:
  hepatic ducts
  liver
Congenital:
  choledochal cyst
  hepatomegaly

Duplication of:
  biliary duct
  cystic duct
  gallbladder
  liver
Floating:
  gallbladder
  liver
Intrahepatic gallbladder

751.7 Anomalies of pancreas

Absence
Agenesis } of pancreas
Hypoplasia
Accessory pancreas

Annular pancreas
Ectopic pancreatic tissue
Pancreatic heterotopia

Excludes: *diabetes mellitus:*
    congenital (250.0-250.9)
    neonatal (775.1)
  fibrocystic diseases of pancreas (277.00-277.09)

751.8 Other specified anomalies of digestive system

Absence (complete) (partial) of alimentary tract NOS
Duplication
Malposition, congenital } of digestive organs NOS

Excludes: *congenital diaphragmatic hernia (756.6)*
  congenital hiatus hernia (750.6)

751.9 Unspecified anomaly of digestive system

Congenital:
  anomaly NOS
  deformity NOS } of digestive system NOS

752 Congenital anomalies of genital organs

Excludes: *syndromes associated with anomalies in the number and form of chromosomes*
    (758.0-758.9)
  testicular feminization syndrome (257.8)

● Code new
to this edition

▲ Revision of
existing code

④ ⑤ Fourth or fifth
digit required

752.0 Anomalies of ovaries
Absence, congenital
Accessory
Ectopic ⎫ (of) ovary
Streak

⑤ **752.1 Anomalies of fallopian tubes and broad ligaments**

752.10 Unspecified anomaly of fallopian tubes and broad ligaments

752.11 Embryonic cyst of fallopian tubes and broad ligaments
Cyst: Cyst:
 epoophoron   Gartner's duct
 fimbrial   parovarian

752.19 Other
Absence
Accessory ⎬ (of) fallopian tube or broad ligament
Atresia

752.2 Doubling of uterus
Didelphic uterus
Doubling of uterus [any degree] (associated with doubling of cervix and vagina)

752.3 Other anomalies of uterus
Absence, congenital
Agenesis ⎬ of uterus
Aplasia
Bicornuate uterus
Uterus unicornis
Uterus with only one functioning horn

⑤ **752.4 Anomalies of cervix, vagina, and external female genitalia**

752.40 Unspecified anomaly of cervix, vagina, and external female genitalia

752.41 Embryonic cyst of cervix, vagina, and external female genitalia
Cyst of:
 canal of Nuck, congenital
 vagina, embryonal
 vulva, congenital

752.42 Imperforate hymen

752.49 Other anomalies of cervix, vagina, and external female genitalia
Absence ⎬ of cervix, clitoris, vagina, or vulva
Agenesis
Congenital stenosis or stricture of:
 cervical canal
 vagina

Excludes: *double vagina associated with total duplication (752.2)*

⑤ **752.5 Undescended and retractile testicle**

752.51 Undescended testis
Cryptorchism
Ectopic testis

752.52 Retractile testis

⑤ **752.6 Hypospadias and epispadias and other penile anomalies**

752.61 Hypospadias

752.62 Epispadias
Anaspadias

752.63 Congenital chordee

752.64 Micropenis

752.65 Hidden penis

752.69 Other penile anomalies

752.7 Indeterminate sex and pseudohermaphroditism

Gynandrism
Hermaphroditism
Ovotestis
Pseudohermaphroditism (male) (female)
Pure gonadal dysgenesis

Excludes: *pseudohermaphroditism:*

> *female, with adrenocortical disorder (255.2)*
> *male, with gonadal disorder (257.8)*
> *with specified chromosomal anomaly (758.0-758.9)*
> *testicular feminization syndrome (257.8)*

752.8 Other specified anomalies of genital organs

Absence of:
  prostate
  spermatic cord
  vas deferens
Anorchism
Aplasia (congenital) of:
  prostate
  round ligament
  testicle

Atresia of:
  ejaculatory duct
  vas deferens
Fusion of testes
Hypoplasia of testis
Monorchism
Polyorchism

Excludes: *congenital hydrocele (778.6)*

> *penile anomalies (752.61-752.69)*
> *phimosis or paraphimosis (605)*

752.9 Unspecified anomaly of genital organs

Congenital:
  anomaly NOS
  deformity NOS
} of genital organ, not elsewhere classified

753 Congenital anomalies of urinary system

753.0 Renal agenesis and dysgenesis

Atrophy of kidney:
  congenital
  infantile

Congenital absence of kidney(s)
Hypoplasia of kidney(s)

⑤ **753.1 Cystic kidney disease**

Excludes: *acquired cyst of kidney (593.2)*

753.10 Cystic kidney disease, unspecified

753.11 Congenital single renal cyst

753.12 Polycystic kidney, unspecified type

753.13 Polycystic kidney, autosomal dominant

753.14 Polycystic kidney, autosomal recessive

753.15 Renal dysplasia

753.16 Medullary cystic kidney
  Nephronopthisis

753.17 Medullary sponge kidney

753.19 Other specified cystic kidney disease
  Multicystic kidney

⑤ **753.2 Obstructive defects of renal pelvis and ureter**

753.20 Unspecified obstructive defect of renal pelvis and ureter

753.21 Congenital obstruction of ureteropelvic junction

753.22 Congenital obstruction of ureterovesical junction
  Adynamic ureter
  Congenital hydroureter

753.23 Congenital ureterocele

753.29 Other

● Code new
  to this edition

▲ Revision of
  existing code

④ ⑤ Fourth or fifth
  digit required

753.3 Other specified anomalies of kidney

Accessory kidney	Fusion of kidneys
Congenital:	Giant kidney
calculus of kidney	Horseshoe kidney
displaced kidney	Hyperplasia of kidney
Discoid kidney	Lobulation of kidney
Double kidney with double	Malrotation of kidney
pelvis	Trifid kidney (pelvis)
Ectopic kidney	

753.4 Other specified anomalies of ureter

Absent ureter	Double ureter
Accessory ureter	Ectopic ureter
Deviation of ureter	Implantation, anomalous of ureter
Displaced ureteric orifice	

753.5 Exstrophy of urinary bladder

Ectopia vesicae	Extroversion of bladder

753.6 Atresia and stenosis of urethra and bladder neck

Congenital obstruction:	Imperforate urinary meatus
bladder neck	Impervious urethra
urethra	Urethral valve formation
Congenital stricture of:	
urethra (valvular)	
urinary meatus	
vesicourethral orifice	

753.7 Anomalies of urachus

Cyst
Fistula } (of) urachus
Patent

Persistent umbilical sinus

753.8 Other specified anomalies of bladder and urethra

Absence, congenital of:	Congenital urethrorectal fistula
bladder	Congenital prolapse of:
urethra	bladder (mucosa)
Accessory:	urethra
bladder	Double:
urethra	urethra
Congenital:	urinary meatus
diverticulum of bladder	
hernia of bladder	

753.9 Unspecified anomaly of urinary system

Congenital:
anomaly NOS
deformity NOS } of urinary system [any part, except urachus]

754 Certain congenital musculoskeletal deformities

Includes: nonteratogenic deformities which are considered to be due to intrauterine malposition and pressure

754.0 Of skull, face, and jaw

Asymmetry of face	Dolichocephaly
Compression facies	Plagiocephaly
Depressions in skull	Potter's facies
Deviation of nasal	Squashed or bent nose, congenital
septum, congenital	

Excludes: dentofacial anomalies (524.0-524.9)
syphilitic saddle nose (090.5)

754.1 Of sternocleidomastoid muscle

Congenital sternomastoid torticollis
Congenital wryneck
Contracture of sternocleidomastoid (muscle)
Sternomastoid tumor

754.2 Of spine

Congenital postural:
lordosis
scoliosis

⑤ **754.3 Congenital dislocation of hip**

754.30 Congenital dislocation of hip, unilateral
Congenital dislocation of hip NOS

754.31 Congenital dislocation of hip, bilateral

Add 4th or 5th digit	Nonspecific code	Unspecified code	Manifestation code

754.32 Congenital subluxation of hip, unilateral
    Congenital flexion deformity, hip or thigh
    Predislocation status of hip at birth
    Preluxation of hip, congenital

754.33 Congenital subluxation of hip, bilateral

754.35 Congenital dislocation of one hip with subluxation of other hip

⑤ **754.4 Congenital genu recurvatum and bowing of long bones of leg**

754.40 Genu recurvatum

754.41 Congenital dislocation of knee (with genu recurvatum)

754.42 Congenital bowing of femur

754.43 Congenital bowing of tibia and fibula

754.44 Congenital bowing of unspecified long bones of leg

⑤ **754.5 Varus deformities of feet**

Excludes: acquired (736.71, 736.75, 736.79)

754.50 Talipes varus
    Congenital varus deformity of foot, unspecified
    Pes varus

754.51 Talipes equinovarus
    Equinovarus (congenital)

754.52 Metatarsus primus varus

754.53 Metatarsus varus

754.59 Other
    Talipes calcaneovarus

⑤ **754.6 Valgus deformities of feet**

Excludes: valgus deformity of foot (acquired) (736.79)

754.60 Talipes valgus
    Congenital valgus deformity of foot, unspecified

754.61 Congenital pes planus
    Congenital rocker bottom flat foot
    Flat foot, congenital

Excludes: pes planus (acquired) (734)

754.62 Talipes calcaneovalgus

754.69 Other
    Talipes:
       equinovalgus
       planovalgus

⑤ **754.7 Other deformities of feet**

Excludes: acquired (736.70-736.79)

754.70 Talipes, unspecified
    Congenital deformity of foot NOS

754.71 Talipes cavus
    Cavus foot (congenital)

754.79 Other
    Asymmetric talipes
    Talipes:
       calcaneus
       equinus

⑤ **754.8 Other specified nonteratogenic anomalies**

754.81 Pectus excavatum
    Congenital funnel chest

754.82 Pectus carinatum
    Congenital pigeon chest [breast]

754.89 Other
    Club hand (congenital)
    Congenital:
       deformity of chest wall
       dislocation of elbow
    Generalized flexion contractures of lower limb joints, congenital
    Spade-like hand (congenital)

● Code new
   to this edition
▲ Revision of
   existing code
④ ⑤ Fourth or fifth
   digit required

755 **Other congenital anomalies of limbs**

> Excludes: those deformities classifiable to 754.0-754.8

⑤ **755.0 Polydactyly**

755.00 **Polydactyly, unspecified digits**
Supernumerary digits

755.01 **Of fingers**
Accessory fingers

755.02 **Of toes**
Accessory toes

⑤ **755.1 Syndactyly**
Symphalangy   Webbing of digits

755.10 **Of multiple and unspecified sites**

755.11 **Of fingers without fusion of bone**

755.12 **Of fingers with fusion of bone**

755.13 **Of toes without fusion of bone**

755.14 **Of toes with fusion of bone**

⑤ **755.2 Reduction deformities of upper limb**

755.20 **Unspecified reduction deformity of upper limb**
Ectromelia NOS ⎤
Hemimelia NOS ⎦ of upper limb
Shortening of arm, congenital

755.21 **Transverse deficiency of upper limb**
Amelia of upper limb
Congenital absence of:
  fingers, all (complete or partial)
  forearm, including hand and fingers
  upper limb, complete
Congenital amputation of upper limb
Transverse hemimelia of upper limb

755.22 **Longitudinal deficiency of upper limb, not elsewhere classified**
Phocomelia NOS of upper limb
Rudimentary arm

755.23 **Longitudinal deficiency, combined, involving humerus, radius, and ulna (complete or incomplete)**
Congenital absence of arm and forearm (complete or incomplete) with or without metacarpal deficiency and/or phalangeal deficiency, incomplete
Phocomelia, complete, of upper limb

755.24 **Longitudinal deficiency, humeral, complete or partial (with or without distal deficiencies, incomplete)**
Congenital absence of humerus (with or without absence of some [but not all] distal elements)
Proximal phocomelia of upper limb

755.25 **Longitudinal deficiency, radioulnar, complete or partial (with or without distal deficiencies, incomplete)**
Congenital absence of radius and ulna (with or without absence of some [but not all] distal elements)
Distal phocomelia of upper limb

755.26 **Longitudinal deficiency, radial, complete or partial (with or without distal deficiencies, incomplete)**
Agenesis of radius
Congenital absence of radius (with or without absence of some [but not all] distal elements)

755.27 **Longitudinal deficiency, ulnar, complete or partial (with or without distal deficiencies, incomplete)**
Agenesis of ulna
Congenital absence of ulna (with or without absence of some [but not all] distal elements)

755.28 **Longitudinal deficiency, carpals or metacarpals, complete or partial (with or without incomplete phalangeal deficiency)**

Add 4th or 5th digit   Nonspecific code   Unspecified code   Manifestation code

755.29 Longitudinal deficiency, phalanges, complete or partial
Absence of finger, congenital
Aphalangia of upper limb, terminal, complete or partial

<u>Excludes:</u> *terminal deficiency of all five digits (755.21)*
transverse deficiency of phalanges (755.21)

⑤ **755.3 Reduction deformities of lower limb**

755.30 Unspecified reduction deformity of lower limb
Ectromelia NOS ⎫
Hemimelia NOS ⎬ of lower limb
Shortening of leg, congenital

755.31 Transverse deficiency of lower limb
Amelia of lower limb
Congenital absence of:
  foot
  leg, including foot and toes
  lower limb, complete
  toes, all, complete
Transverse hemimelia of lower limb

755.32 Longitudinal deficiency of lower limb, not elsewhere classified
Phocomelia NOS of lower limb

755.33 Longitudinal deficiency, combined, involving femur, tibia, and fibula (complete or incomplete)
Congenital absence of thigh and (lower) leg (complete or incomplete) with or without metacarpal deficiency and/or phalangeal deficiency, incomplete
Phocomelia, complete, of lower limb

755.34 Longitudinal deficiency, femoral, complete or partial (with or without distal deficiencies, incomplete)
Congenital absence of femur (with or without absence of some [but not all] distal elements)
Proximal phocomelia of lower limb

755.35 Longitudinal deficiency, tibiofibular, complete or partial (with or without distal deficiencies, incomplete)
Congenital absence of tibia and fibula (with or without absence of some [but not all] distal elements)
Distal phocomelia of lower limb

755.36 Longitudinal deficiency, tibia, complete or partial (with or without distal deficiencies, incomplete)
Agenesis of tibia
Congenital absence of tibia (with or without absence of some [but not all] distal elements)

755.37 Longitudinal deficiency, fibular, complete or partial (with or without distal deficiencies, incomplete)
Agenesis of fibula
Congenital absence of fibula (with or without absence of some [but not all] distal elements)

755.38 Longitudinal deficiency, tarsals or metatarsals, complete or partial (with or without incomplete phalangeal deficiency)

755.39 Longitudinal deficiency, phalanges, complete or partial
Absence of toe, congenital
Aphalangia of lower limb, terminal, complete or partial

<u>Excludes:</u> *terminal deficiency of all five digits (755.31)*
transverse deficiency of phalanges (755.31)

755.4 Reduction deformities, unspecified limb
Absence, congenital (complete or partial) of limb NOS
Amelia ⎫
Ectromelia ⎬ of unspecified limb
Hemimelia ⎪
Phocomelia ⎭

⑤ **755.5 Other anomalies of upper limb, including shoulder girdle**

755.50 Unspecified anomaly of upper limb

755.51 Congenital deformity of clavicle

755.52 Congenital elevation of scapula
Sprengel's deformity

755.53 Radioulnar synostosis

● Code new
to this edition

▲ Revision of
existing code

④ ⑤ Fourth or fifth
digit required

755.54 Madelung's deformity

755.55 Acrocephalosyndactyly
Apert's syndrome

755.56 Accessory carpal bones

755.57 Macrodactylia (fingers)

755.58 Cleft hand, congenital
Lobster-claw hand

755.59 Other
Cleidocranial dysostosis
Cubitus:
   valgus, congenital
   varus, congenital

Excludes: club hand (congenital) (754.89)
           congenital dislocation of elbow (754.89)

⑤ **755.6 Other anomalies of lower limb, including pelvic girdle**

755.60 Unspecified anomaly of lower limb

755.61 Coxa valga, congenital

755.62 Coxa vara, congenital

755.63 Other congenital deformity of hip (joint)
Congenital anteversion of femur (neck)

Excludes: congenital dislocation of hip (754.30-754.35)

755.64 Congenital deformity of knee (joint)
Congenital:
   absence of patella
   genu valgum [knock-knee]
   genu varum [bowleg]
Rudimentary patella

755.65 Macrodactylia of toes

755.66 Other anomalies of toes
Congenital:
   hallux valgus
   hallux varus
   hammer toe

755.67 Anomalies of foot, not elsewhere classified
Astragaloscaphoid synostosis
Calcaneonavicular bar
Coalition of calcaneus
Talonavicular synostosis
Tarsal coalitions

755.69 Other
Congenital:
   angulation of tibia
   deformity (of):
      ankle (joint)
      sacroiliac (joint)
   fusion of sacroiliac joint

755.8 Other specified anomalies of unspecified limb

755.9 Unspecified anomaly of unspecified limb
Congenital:
   anomaly NOS ⎫
   deformity NOS ⎭ of unspecified limb

Excludes: reduction deformity of unspecified limb (755.4)

756 Other congenital musculoskeletal anomalies

Excludes: those deformities classifiable to 754.0-754.8

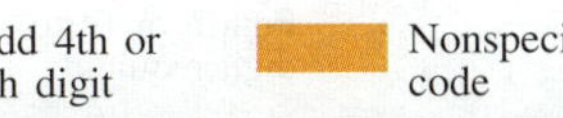

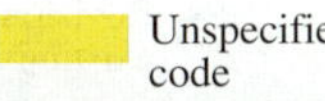

756.0 Anomalies of skull and face bones
Absence of skull bones
Acrocephaly
Congenital deformity of
forehead
Craniosynostosis
Crouzon's disease
Hypertelorism
Imperfect fusion of skull
Oxycephaly
Platybasia
Premature closure of cranial sutures
Tower skull
Trigonocephaly

Excludes: *acrocephalosyndactyly [Apert's syndrome] (755.55)*
dentofacial anomalies (524.0-524.9)
skull defects associated with brain anomalies, such as:
anencephalus (740.0)
encephalocele (742.0)
hydrocephalus (742.3)
microcephalus (742.1)

⑤ **756.1 Anomalies of spine**

756.10 Anomaly of spine, unspecified

756.11 Spondylolysis, lumbosacral region
Prespondylolisthesis (lumbosacral)

756.12 Spondylolisthesis

756.13 Absence of vertebra, congenital

756.14 Hemivertebra

756.15 Fusion of spine [vertebra], congenital

756.16 Klippel-Feil syndrome

756.17 Spina bifida occulta

Excludes: *spina bifida (aperta) (741.0-741.9)*

756.19 Other
Platyspondylia
Supernumerary vertebra

756.2 Cervical rib
Supernumerary rib in the cervical region

756.3 Other anomalies of ribs and sternum
Congenital absence of:
rib
sternum
Congenital:
fissure of sternum
fusion of ribs
Sternum bifidum

Excludes: *nonteratogenic deformity of chest wall (754.81-754.89)*

756.4 Chondrodystrophy
Achondroplasia
Chondrodystrophia (fetalis)
Dyschondroplasia
Enchondromatosis
Ollier's disease

Excludes: *lipochondrodystrophy [Hurler's syndrome] (277.5)*
Morquio's disease (277.5)

⑤ **756.5 Osteodystrophies**

756.50 Osteodystrophy, unspecified

756.51 Osteogenesis imperfecta
Fragilitas ossium
Osteopsathyrosis

756.52 Osteopetrosis

756.53 Osteopoikilosis

756.54 Polyostotic fibrous dysplasia of bone

756.55 Chondroectodermal dysplasia
Ellis-van Creveld syndrome

756.56 Multiple epiphyseal dysplasia

756.59 Other
Albright (-McCune)-Sternberg syndrome

● Code new
to this edition
▲ Revision of
existing code
④ ⑤ Fourth or fifth
digit required

756.6 Anomalies of diaphragm
Absence of diaphragm   Eventration of diaphragm
Congenital hernia:
  diaphragmatic
  foramen of Morgagni

Excludes: *congenital hiatus hernia (750.6)*

⑤ **756.7 Anomalies of abdominal wall**
Omphalocele
Exomphalos   Prune belly (syndrome)
Gastroschisis

756.70 Anomaly of abdominal wall, unspecified

756.71 Prune belly syndrome
Eagle-Barrett syndrome
Prolapse of bladder mucosa

756.79 Other congenital anomalies of abdominal wall
Exomphalos
Gastroschisis
Omphalocele

Excludes: *umbilical hernia (551-553 with .1)*

⑤ **756.8 Other specified anomalies of muscle, tendon, fascia, and connective tissue**

756.81 Absence of muscle and tendon
Absence of muscle (pectoral)

756.82 Accessory muscle

756.83 Ehlers-Danlos syndrome

756.89 Other
Amyotrophia congenita
Congenital shortening of tendon

756.9 Other and unspecified anomalies of musculoskeletal system
Congenital:
  anomaly NOS   ⎫
  deformity NOS   ⎬ of musculoskeletal system, not elsewhere classified

757 Congenital anomalies of the integument
Includes: anomalies of skin, subcutaneous tissue, hair, nails, and breast

Excludes: *hemangioma (228.00-228.09)*
pigmented nevus (216.0-216.9)

757.0 Hereditary edema of legs
Congenital lymphedema   Milroy's disease
Hereditary trophedema

757.1 Ichthyosis congenita
Congenital ichthyosis
Harlequin fetus
Ichthyosiform erythroderma

757.2 Dermatoglyphic anomalies
Abnormal palmar creases

⑤ **757.3 Other specified anomalies of skin**

757.31 Congenital ectodermal dysplasia

757.32 Vascular hamartomas
Birthmarks
Port-wine stain
Strawberry nevus

757.33 Congenital pigmentary anomalies of skin
Congenital poikiloderma
Urticaria pigmentosa
Xeroderma pigmentosum

Excludes: *albinism (270.2)*

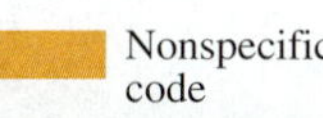

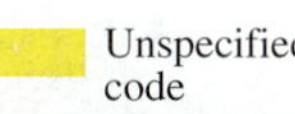

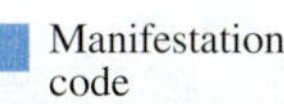

757.39 Other
>   Accessory skin tags, congenital
>   Congenital scar
>   Epidermolysis bullosa
>   Keratoderma (congenital)

Excludes: *pilonidal cyst (685.0-685.1)*

757.4 Specified anomalies of hair

Congenital:
  alopecia
  atrichosis
  beaded hair

Congenital:
  hypertrichosis
  monilethrix
Persistent lanugo

757.5 Specified anomalies of nails

Anonychia
Congenital:
  clubnail
  koilonychia

Congenital:
  leukonychia
  onychauxis
  pachyonychia

757.6 Specified anomalies of breast

Absent
Accessory   } breast or nipple
Supernumerary
Hypoplasia of breast

Excludes: *absence of pectoral muscle (756.81)*

757.8 Other specified anomalies of the integument

757.9 Unspecified anomaly of the integument

Congenital:
  anomaly NOS
  deformity NOS   } of integument

758 Chromosomal anomalies

Includes: syndromes associated with anomalies in the number and form of chromosomes

758.0 Down's syndrome

Mongolism
Translocation Down's
  syndrome

Trisomy:
  21 or 22
  G

758.1 Patau's syndrome

Trisomy:
  13
  D_1

758.2 Edwards' syndrome

Trisomy:
  18
  E_3

758.3 Autosomal deletion syndromes

Antimongolism syndrome   Cri-du-chat syndrome

758.4 Balanced autosomal translocation in normal individual

758.5 Other conditions due to autosomal anomalies

Accessory autosomes NEC

758.6 Gonadal dysgenesis

Ovarian dysgenesis   XO syndrome
Turner's syndrome

Excludes: *pure gonadal dysgenesis (752.7)*

758.7 Klinefelter's syndrome

XXY syndrome

⑤ **758.8 Other conditions due to chromosome anomalies**

758.81 Other conditions due to sex chromosome anomalies

758.89 Other

758.9 Conditions due to anomaly of unspecified chromosome

759 Other and unspecified congenital anomalies

759.0 Anomalies of spleen

Aberrant
Absent   } spleen
Accessory

Congenital splenomegaly
Ectopic spleen
Lobulation of spleen

● Code new
  to this edition

▲ Revision of
  existing code

④ ⑤ Fourth or fifth
  digit required

759.1 Anomalies of adrenal gland
Aberrant ⎫
Absent ⎬ adrenal gland
Accessory ⎭

Excludes: *adrenogenital disorders (255.2)*
congenital disorders of steroid metabolism (255.2)

759.2 Anomalies of other endocrine glands
Absent parathyroid gland
Accessory thyroid gland
Persistent thyroglossal or thyrolingual duct
Thyroglossal (duct) cyst

Excludes: *congenital:*
goiter (246.1)
hypothyroidism (243)

759.3 Situs inversus
Situs inversus or transversus: Transposition of viscera:
  abdominalis   abdominal
  thoracis   thoracic

Excludes: *dextrocardia without mention of complete transposition (746.87)*

759.4 Conjoined twins
Craniopagus   Thoracopagus
Dicephalus   Xiphopagus
Pygopagus

759.5 Tuberous sclerosis
Bourneville's disease   Epiloia

759.6 Other hamartoses, not elsewhere classified
Syndrome:
Peutz-Jeghers
Sturge-Weber (-Dimitri)
von Hippel-Lindau

Excludes: *neurofibromatosis (237.7)*

759.7 Multiple congenital anomalies, so described
Congenital:
anomaly, multiple NOS
deformity, multiple NOS

⑤ **759.8 Other specified anomalies**

759.81 Prader-Willi syndrome

759.82 Marfan syndrome

759.83 Fragile X syndrome

759.89 Other
Congenital malformation syndromes affecting multiple systems, not elsewhere
classified
Laurence-Moon-Biedl syndrome

759.9 Congenital anomaly, unspecified

	Add 4th or 5th digit		Nonspecific code		Unspecified code		Manifestation code

● Code new
to this edition

▲ Revision of
existing code

④ ⑤ Fourth or fifth
digit required

15.   CERTAIN CONDITIONS ORIGINATING IN THE PERINATAL PERIOD (760-779)

Includes: conditions which have their origin in the perinatal period even though death or morbidity occurs later

Use additional code(s) to further specify condition

MATERNAL CAUSES OF PERINATAL MORBIDITY AND MORTALITY (760-763)

760 **Fetus or newborn affected by maternal conditions which may be unrelated to present pregnancy**
Includes: the listed maternal conditions only when specified as a cause of mortality or morbidity of the fetus or newborn

Excludes: *maternal endocrine and metabolic disorders affecting fetus or newborn (775.0-775.9)*

760.0   Maternal hypertensive disorders
Fetus or newborn affected by maternal conditions classifiable to 642

760.1   Maternal renal and urinary tract diseases
Fetus or newborn affected by maternal conditions classifiable to 580-599

760.2   Maternal infections
Fetus or newborn affected by maternal infectious disease classifiable to 001-136 and 487, but fetus or newborn not manifesting that disease

Excludes: *congenital infectious diseases (771.0-771.8)*
maternal genital tract and other localized infections (760.8)

760.3   Other chronic maternal circulatory and respiratory diseases
Fetus or newborn affected by chronic maternal conditions classifiable to 390-459, 490-519, 745-748

760.4   Maternal nutritional disorders
Fetus or newborn affected by:
maternal disorders classifiable to 260-269
maternal malnutrition NOS

Excludes: *fetal malnutrition (764.10-764.29)*

760.5   Maternal injury
Fetus or newborn affected by maternal conditions classifiable to 800-995

760.6   Surgical operation on mother

Excludes: *cesarean section for present delivery (763.4)*
damage to placenta from amniocentesis, cesarean section, or surgical induction (762.1)
previous surgery to uterus or pelvic organs (763.89)

⑤ **760.7   Noxious influences affecting fetus via placenta or breast milk**
Fetus or newborn affected by noxious substance transmitted via placenta or breast milk

Excludes: *anesthetic and analgesic drugs administered during labor and delivery (763.5)*
drug withdrawal syndrome in newborn (779.5)

760.70   Unspecified noxious substance
Fetus or newborn affected by:
Drug NEC

760.71   Alcohol
Fetal alcohol syndrome

760.72   Narcotics

760.73   Hallucinogenic agents

760.74   Anti-infectives
Antibiotics

760.75   Cocaine

760.76   Diethylstilbestrol (DES)

760.79   Other
Fetus or newborn affected by:
immune sera transmitted via placenta or breast milk
medicinal agents NEC transmitted via placenta or breast milk
toxic substance NEC transmitted via placenta or breast milk

760.8   Other specified maternal conditions affecting fetus or newborn
Maternal genital tract and other localized infection affecting fetus or newborn, but fetus or newborn not manifesting that disease

Excludes: *maternal urinary tract infection affecting fetus or newborn (760.1)*

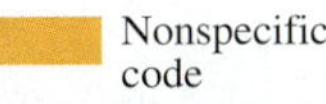

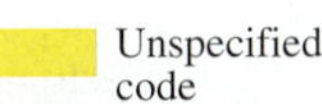

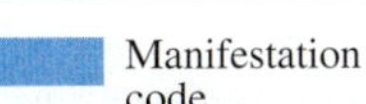

760.9 **Unspecified maternal condition affecting fetus or newborn**

761 **Fetus or newborn affected by maternal complications of pregnancy**
Includes: the listed maternal conditions only when specified as a cause of mortality or
morbidity of the fetus or newborn

761.0 **Incompetent cervix**

761.1 **Premature rupture of membranes**

761.2 **Oligohydramnios**

> Excludes: *that due to premature rupture of membranes (761.1)*

761.3 **Polyhydramnios**
Hydramnios (acute) (chronic)

761.4 **Ectopic pregnancy**
Pregnancy:
abdominal
intraperitoneal
tubal

761.5 **Multiple pregnancy**
Triplet (pregnancy)   Twin (pregnancy)

761.6 **Maternal death**

761.7 **Malpresentation before labor**
Breech presentation ⎤
External version   ⎥
Oblique lie   ⎬ before labor
Transverse lie   ⎥
Unstable lie   ⎦

761.8 **Other specified maternal complications of pregnancy affecting fetus or newborn**
Spontaneous abortion, fetus

761.9 **Unspecified maternal complication of pregnancy affecting fetus or newborn**

762 **Fetus or newborn affected by complications of placenta, cord, and membranes**
Includes: the listed maternal conditions only when specified as a cause of mortality or
morbidity in the fetus or newborn

762.0 **Placenta previa**

762.1 **Other forms of placental separation and hemorrhage**
Abruptio placentae
Antepartum hemorrhage
Damage to placenta from amniocentesis, cesarean section, or surgical induction
Maternal blood loss
Premature separation of placenta
Rupture of marginal sinus

762.2 **Other and unspecified morphological and functional abnormalities of placenta**
Placental:
dysfunction
infarction
insufficiency

762.3 **Placental transfusion syndromes**
Placental and cord abnormality resulting in twin-to-twin or other transplacental
transfusion

Use additional code, if desired, to indicate resultant condition in fetus or newborn:
fetal blood loss (772.0)
polycythemia neonatorum (776.4)

762.4 **Prolapsed cord**
Cord presentation

762.5 **Other compression of umbilical cord**
Cord around neck   Knot in cord
Entanglement of cord   Torsion of cord

762.6 **Other and unspecified conditions of umbilical cord**
Short cord   ⎤
Thrombosis   ⎥
Varices   ⎬ of umbilical cord
Velamentous insertion ⎥
Vasa previa   ⎦

> Excludes: *infection of umbilical cord (771.4)*
> *single umbilical artery (747.5)*

● Code new   ▲ Revision of   ④ ⑤ Fourth or fifth
to this edition   existing code   digit required

762.7 Chorioamnionitis
Amnionitis   Placentitis
Membranitis

762.8 Other specified abnormalities of chorion and amnion

762.9 Unspecified abnormality of chorion and amnion

763 Fetus or newborn affected by other complications of labor and delivery
Includes: the listed conditions only when specified as a cause of mortality or morbidity in the
fetus or newborn

763.0 Breech delivery and extraction

763.1 Other malpresentation, malposition, and disproportion during labor and delivery
Fetus or newborn affected by:
abnormality of bony pelvis
contracted pelvis
persistent occipitoposterior position
shoulder presentation
transverse lie
conditions classifiable to 652, 653, and 660

763.2 Forceps delivery
Fetus or newborn affected by forceps extraction

763.3 Delivery by vacuum extractor

763.4 Cesarean delivery

> *Excludes:* *placental separation or hemorrhage from cesarean section (762.1)*

763.5 Maternal anesthesia and analgesia
Reactions and intoxications from maternal opiates and tranquilizers during labor and
delivery

> *Excludes:* *drug withdrawal syndrome in newborn (779.5)*

763.6 Precipitate delivery
Rapid second stage

763.7 Abnormal uterine contractions
Fetus or newborn affected by:
contraction ring
hypertonic labor
hypotonic uterine dysfunction
uterine inertia or dysfunction
conditions classifiable to 661, except 661.3

⑤ **763.8 Other specified complications of labor and delivery affecting fetus or newborn**

763.81 Abnormality in fetal heart rate or rhythm before the onset of labor

763.82 Abnormality in fetal heart rate or rhythm during labor

763.83 Abnormality in fetal heart rate or rhythm, unspecified as to time of onset

763.89 Other specified complications of labor and delivery affecting fetus or newborn
Fetus or newborn affected by:
abnormality of maternal soft tissues
destructive operation on live fetus to facilitate delivery
induction of labor (medical)
previous surgery to uterus or pelvic organs
other conditions classifiable to 650-669
other procedures used in labor and delivery

763.9 Unspecified complication of labor and delivery affecting fetus or newborn

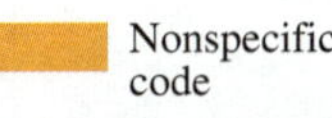

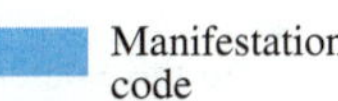

Manifestation
code

OTHER CONDITIONS ORIGINATING IN THE PERINATAL PERIOD (764-779)

The following fifth-digit subclassification is for use with category 764 and codes 765.0 and 765.1 to denote birthweight:

0 unspecified [weight]

1 less than 500 grams

2 500-749 grams

3 750-999 grams

4 1,000- 1,249 grams

5 1,250-1,499 grams

6 1,500-1,749 grams

7 1,750-1,999 grams

8 2,000-2,499 grams

9 2,500 grams and over

⑤ **764 Slow fetal growth and fetal malnutrition**

⑤ **764.0 "Light-for-dates" without mention of fetal malnutrition**
Infants underweight for gestational age
"Small-for-dates"

⑤ **764.1 "Light-for-dates" with signs of fetal malnutrition**
Infants "light-for-dates" classifiable to 764.0, who in addition show signs of fetal malnutrition, such as dry peeling skin and loss of subcutaneous tissue

⑤ **764.2 Fetal malnutrition without mention of "light-for-dates"**
Infants, not underweight for gestational age, showing signs of fetal malnutrition, such as dry peeling skin and loss of subcutaneous tissue
Intrauterine malnutrition

⑤ **764.9 Fetal growth retardation, unspecified**
Intrauterine growth retardation

▲ **765 Disorders relating to short gestation and low birthweight**
Includes: the listed conditions, without further specification, as causes of mortality, morbidity, or additional care, in fetus or newborn

⑤ **765.0 Extreme immaturity**
Note: Usually implies a birthweight of less than 1000 grams
Use additional code for weeks of gestation (765.20-765.29)

⑤ **765.1 Other preterm infants**
Prematurity NOS
Prematurity or small size, not classifiable to 765.0 or as "light-for-dates" in 764
Note: Usually implies a birthweight of 1000-2499 grams
Use additional code for weeks of gestation (765.20-765.29)

● **765.2 Weeks of gestation**

● **765.20 Unspecified weeks of gestation**

● 765.21 Less than 24 completed weeks of gestation

● 765.22 24 completed weeks of gestation

● 765.23 25-26 completed weeks of gestation

● 765.24 27-28 completed weeks of gestation

● 765.25 29-30 completed weeks of gestation

● 765.26 31-32 completed weeks of gestation

● 765.27 33-34 completed weeks of gestation

● 765.28 35-36 completed weeks of gestation

● 765.29 37 or more completed weeks of gestation

766 Disorders relating to long gestation and high birthweight
Includes: the listed conditions, without further specification, as causes of mortality, morbidity, or additional care, in fetus or newborn

766.0 Exceptionally large baby
Note: Usually implies a birthweight of 4500 grams or more.

766.1 Other "heavy-for-dates" infants
Other fetus or infant "heavy-" or "large-for-dates" regardless of period of gestation

---

766.2 **Post-term infant, not "heavy-for-dates"**
Fetus or infant with gestation period of 294 days or more [42 or more completed weeks], not "heavy-" or "large-for-dates"
Postmaturity NOS

767 **Birth trauma**

767.0 **Subdural and cerebral hemorrhage**
Subdural and cerebral hemorrhage, whether described as due to birth trauma or to intrapartum anoxia or hypoxia
Subdural hematoma (localized)
Tentorial tear

Use additional code, if desired, to identify cause

Excludes: *intraventricular hemorrhage (772.10-772.14)*
subarachnoid hemorrhage (772.2)

767.1 **Injuries to scalp**
Caput succedaneum
Cephalhematoma
Chignon (from vacuum extraction)
Massive epicranial subaponeurotic hemorrhage

767.2 **Fracture of clavicle**

767.3 **Other injuries to skeleton**
Fracture of:
long bones
skull

Excludes: *congenital dislocation of hip (754.30-754.35)*
fracture of spine, congenital (767.4)

767.4 **Injury to spine and spinal cord**
Dislocation
Fracture   } of spine or spinal cord due to birth trauma
Laceration
Rupture

767.5 **Facial nerve injury**
Facial palsy

767.6 **Injury to brachial plexus**
Palsy or paralysis:
brachial
Erb (-Duchenne)
Klumpke (-Déjérine)

767.7 **Other cranial and peripheral nerve injuries**
Phrenic nerve paralysis

767.8 **Other specified birth trauma**

Eye damage	Rupture of:
Hematoma of:	liver
liver (subcapsular)	spleen
testes	Scalpel wound
vulva	Traumatic glaucoma

Excludes: *hemorrhage classifiable to 772.0-772.9*

767.9 **Birth trauma, unspecified**
Birth injury NOS

768 **Intrauterine hypoxia and birth asphyxia**
Use only when associated with newborn morbidity classifiable elsewhere

768.0 **Fetal death from asphyxia or anoxia before onset of labor or at unspecified time**

768.1 **Fetal death from asphyxia or anoxia during labor**

768.2 **Fetal distress before onset of labor, in liveborn infant**
Fetal metabolic acidemia before onset of labor, in liveborn infant

768.3 **Fetal distress first noted during labor, in liveborn infant**
Fetal metabolic acidemia first noted during labor, in liveborn infant

768.4 **Fetal distress, unspecified as to time of onset, in liveborn infant**
Fetal metabolic acidemia unspecified as to time of onset, in liveborn infant

768.5 **Severe birth asphyxia**
Birth asphyxia with neurologic involvement

768.6 **Mild or moderate birth asphyxia**
Other specified birth asphyxia (without mention of neurologic involvement)

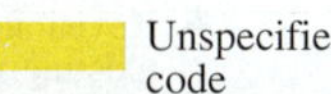
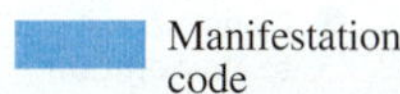

	Add 4th or 5th digit		Nonspecific code		Unspecified code		Manifestation code

768.9 Unspecified birth asphyxia in liveborn infant
    Anoxia
    Asphyxia   } NOS, in liveborn infant
    Hypoxia

769 Respiratory distress syndrome
    Cardiorespiratory distress syndrome of newborn
    Hyaline membrane disease (pulmonary)
    Idiopathic respiratory distress syndrome [IRDS or RDS] of newborn
    Pulmonary hypoperfusion syndrome

    Excludes: *transient tachypnea of newborn (770.6)*

770 Other respiratory conditions of fetus and newborn

770.0 Congenital pneumonia
    Infective pneumonia acquired prenatally

    Excludes: *pneumonia from infection acquired after birth (480.0-486)*

770.1 Meconium aspiration syndrome
    Aspiration of contents of birth canal NOS
    Meconium aspiration below vocal cords
    Pneumonitis:
      fetal aspiration
      meconium

770.2 Interstitial emphysema and related conditions
    Pneumomediastinum
    Pneumopericardium } originating in the perinatal period
    Pneumothorax

770.3 Pulmonary hemorrhage
    Hemorrhage:
      alveolar (lung)
      intra-alveolar (lung) } originating in the perinatal period
      massive pulmonary

770.4 Primary atelectasis
    Pulmonary immaturity NOS

770.5 Other and unspecified atelectasis
    Atelectasis:
      NOS
      partial } originating in the perinatal period
      secondary
    Pulmonary collapse

770.6 Transitory tachypnea of newborn
    Idiopathic tachypnea of newborn
    Wet lung syndrome

    Excludes: *respiratory distress syndrome (769)*

770.7 Chronic respiratory disease arising in the perinatal period
    Bronchopulmonary dysplasia
    Interstitial pulmonary fibrosis of prematurity
    Wilson-Mikity syndrome

⑤ **770.8 Other respiratory problems after birth**

● **770.81 Primary apnea of newborn**
    Apneic spells of newborn NOS
    Essential apnea of newborn
    Sleep apnea of newborn

● **770.82 Other apnea of newborn**
    Obstructive apnea of newborn

● **770.83 Cyanotic attacks of newborn**

● **770.84 Respiratory failure of newborn**
    Excludes: *respiratory distress syndrome (769)*

● **770.89 Other respiratory problems after birth**

770.9 Unspecified respiratory condition of fetus and newborn

    ● Code new
      to this edition
    ▲ Revision of
      existing code
    ④ ⑤ Fourth or fifth
      digit required

771 Infections specific to the perinatal period
Includes: infections acquired before or during birth or via the umbilicus

Excludes: *congenital pneumonia (770.0)*
congenital syphilis (090.0-090.9)
maternal infectious disease as a cause of mortality or morbidity in fetus or newborn, but fetus or newborn not manifesting the disease (760.2)
ophthalmia neonatorum due to gonococcus (098.40)
other infections not specifically classified to this category

771.0 Congenital rubella
Congenital rubella pneumonitis

771.1 Congenital cytomegalovirus infection
Congenital cytomegalic inclusion disease

771.2 Other congenital infections
Congenital:
  herpes simplex
  listeriosis
  malaria

Congenital:
  toxoplasmosis
  tuberculosis

771.3 Tetanus neonatorum
Tetanus omphalitis

Excludes: *hypocalcemic tetany (775.4)*

771.4 Omphalitis of the newborn
Infection:
  navel cord
  umbilical stump

Excludes: *tetanus omphalitis (771.3)*

771.5 Neonatal infective mastitis

Excludes: *noninfective neonatal mastitis (778.7)*

771.6 Neonatal conjunctivitis and dacryocystitis
Ophthalmia neonatorum NOS

Excludes: *ophthalmia neonatorum due to gonococcus (098.40)*

771.7 Neonatal Candida infection
Neonatal moniliasis
Thrush in newborn

⑤ **771.8 Other infections specific to the perinatal period**
Use additional code to identify organism

● **771.81 Septicemia [sepsis] of newborn**

● **771.82 Urinary tract infection of newborn**

● **771.83 Bacteremia of newborn**

● **771.89 Other infections specific to the perinatal period**
Intra-amniotic infection of fetus NOS
Infection of newborn NOS

772 Fetal and neonatal hemorrhage

Excludes: *hematological disorders of fetus and newborn (776.0-776.9)*

772.0 Fetal blood loss
Fetal blood loss from:
  cut end of co-twin's cord
  placenta
  ruptured cord
  vasa previa

Fetal exsanguination
Fetal hemorrhage into:
  co-twin
  mother's circulation

⑤ **772.1 Intraventricular hemorrhage**
Intraventricular hemorrhage from any perinatal cause

772.10 Unspecified grade

772.11 Grade I
Bleeding into germinal matrix

772.12 Grade II
Bleeding into ventricle

772.13 Grade III
Bleeding with enlargement of ventricle

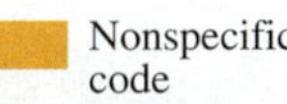

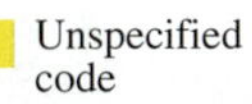

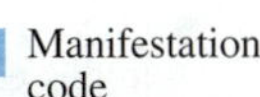

Manifestation
code

772.14 Grade IV
  Bleeding into cerebral cortex
772.2 Subarachnoid hemorrhage
  Subarachnoid hemorrhage from any perinatal cause

  Excludes: subdural and cerebral hemorrhage (767.0)

772.3 Umbilical hemorrhage after birth
  Slipped umbilical ligature
772.4 Gastrointestinal hemorrhage

  Excludes: swallowed maternal blood (777.3)

772.5 Adrenal hemorrhage
772.6 Cutaneous hemorrhage
  Bruising
  Ecchymoses
  Petechiae   } in fetus or newborn
  Superficial hematoma

772.8 Other specified hemorrhage of fetus or newborn

  Excludes: hemorrhagic disease of newborn (776.0)
            pulmonary hemorrhage (770.3)

772.9 Unspecified hemorrhage of newborn

773 Hemolytic disease of fetus or newborn, due to isoimmunization

773.0 Hemolytic disease due to Rh isoimmunization
  Anemia
  Erythroblastosis (fetalis)
  Hemolytic disease (fetus) (newborn)   due to RH:
  Jaundice   antibodies
  Rh hemolytic disease   isoimmunization
  Rh isoimmunization   maternal/fetal incompatibility

773.1 Hemolytic disease due to ABO isoimmunization
  ABO hemolytic disease
  ABO isoimmunization
  Anemia   due to ABO:
  Erythroblastosis (fetalis)   antibodies
  Hemolytic disease (fetus) (newborn)   isoimmunization
  Jaundice   maternal/fetal incompatibility

773.2 Hemolytic disease due to other and unspecified isoimmunization
  Erythroblastosis (fetalis) (neonatorum) NOS
  Hemolytic disease (fetus) (newborn) NOS
  Jaundice or anemia due to other and unspecified blood-group incompatibility

773.3 Hydrops fetalis due to isoimmunization
Use additional code, if desired, to identify type of isoimmunization (773.0-773.2)

773.4 Kernicterus due to isoimmunization
Use additional code, if desired, to identify type of isoimmunization (773.0-773.2)

773.5 Late anemia due to isoimmunization

774 Other perinatal jaundice

774.0 *Perinatal jaundice from hereditary hemolytic anemias*
  Code first underlying disease (282.0-282.9)

774.1 Perinatal jaundice from other excessive hemolysis
  Fetal or neonatal jaundice from:
    bruising
    drugs or toxins transmitted from mother
    infection
    polycythemia
    swallowed maternal blood
Use additional code, if desired, to identify cause

  Excludes: jaundice due to isoimmunization (773.0-773.2)

774.2 Neonatal jaundice associated with preterm delivery
  Hyperbilirubinemia of prematurity
  Jaundice due to delayed conjugation associated with preterm delivery
⑤ **774.3 Neonatal jaundice due to delayed conjugation from other causes**
  774.30 Neonatal jaundice due to delayed conjugation, cause unspecified

● Code new   ▲ Revision of   ④ ⑤ Fourth or fifth
  to this edition   existing code   digit required

774.31 *Neonatal jaundice due to delayed conjugation in diseases classified elsewhere*
Code first underlying diseases, as:
congenital hypothyroidism (243)
Crigler-Najjar syndrome (277.4)
Gilbert's syndrome (277.4)

774.39 **Other**
Jaundice due to delayed conjugation from causes, such as:
breast milk inhibitors
delayed development of conjugating system

774.4 **Perinatal jaundice due to hepatocellular damage**
Fetal or neonatal hepatitis
Giant cell hepatitis
Inspissated bile syndrome

774.5 *Perinatal jaundice from other causes*
Code first underlying cause, as:
congenital obstruction of bile duct (751.61)
galactosemia (271.1)
mucoviscidosis (277.00-277.09)

774.6 **Unspecified fetal and neonatal jaundice**
Icterus neonatorum
Neonatal hyperbilirubinemia (transient)
Physiologic jaundice NOS in newborn

Excludes: *that in preterm infants (774.2)*

774.7 **Kernicterus not due to isoimmunization**
Bilirubin encephalopathy
Kernicterus of newborn NOS

Excludes: *kernicterus due to isoimmunization (773.4)*

775 **Endocrine and metabolic disturbances specific to the fetus and newborn**
Includes: transitory endocrine and metabolic disturbances caused by the infant's response to maternal endocrine and metabolic factors, its removal from them, or its adjustment to extrauterine existence

775.0 **Syndrome of "infant of a diabetic mother"**
Maternal diabetes mellitus affecting fetus or newborn (with hypoglycemia)

775.1 **Neonatal diabetes mellitus**
Diabetes mellitus syndrome in newborn infant

775.2 **Neonatal myasthenia gravis**

775.3 **Neonatal thyrotoxicosis**
Neonatal hyperthyroidism (transient)

775.4 **Hypocalcemia and hypomagnesemia of newborn**
Cow's milk hypocalcemia
Hypocalcemic tetany, neonatal
Neonatal hypoparathyroidism
Phosphate-loading hypocalcemia

775.5 **Other transitory neonatal electrolyte disturbances**
Dehydration, neonatal

775.6 **Neonatal hypoglycemia**

Excludes: *infant of mother with diabetes mellitus (775.0)*

775.7 **Late metabolic acidosis of newborn**

775.8 **Other transitory neonatal endocrine and metabolic disturbances**
Amino-acid metabolic disorders described as transitory

775.9 **Unspecified endocrine and metabolic disturbances specific to the fetus and newborn**

776 **Hematological disorders of fetus and newborn**
Includes: disorders specific to the fetus or newborn

776.0 **Hemorrhagic disease of newborn**
Hemorrhagic diathesis of newborn
Vitamin K deficiency of newborn

Excludes: *fetal or neonatal hemorrhage (772.0-772.9)*

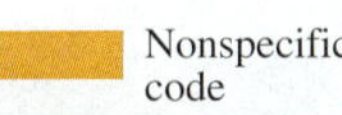

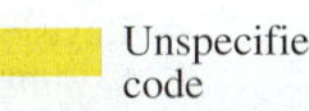

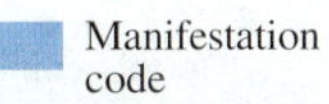

776.1 Transient neonatal thrombocytopenia
Neonatal thrombocytopenia due to:
   exchange transfusion
   idiopathic maternal thrombocytopenia
   isoimmunization

776.2 Disseminated intravascular coagulation in newborn

776.3 Other transient neonatal disorders of coagulation
Transient coagulation defect, newborn

776.4 Polycythemia neonatorum
Plethora of newborn
Polycythemia due to:
   donor twin transfusion
   maternal-fetal transfusion

776.5 Congenital anemia
Anemia following fetal blood loss

> *Excludes:* *anemia due to isoimmunization (773.0-773.2, 773.5)*
> *hereditary hemolytic anemias (282.0-282.9)*

776.6 Anemia of prematurity

776.7 Transient neonatal neutropenia
Isoimmune neutropenia
Maternal transfer neutropenia

> *Excludes:* *congenital neutropenia (nontransient) (288.0)*

776.8 Other specified transient hematological disorders

776.9 Unspecified hematological disorder specific to fetus or newborn

777 Perinatal disorders of digestive system
Includes: disorders specific to the fetus and newborn

> *Excludes:* *intestinal obstruction classifiable to 560.0-560.9*

777.1 Meconium obstruction
Congenital fecaliths
Delayed passage of meconium
Meconium ileus NOS
Meconium plug syndrome

> *Excludes:* *meconium ileus in cystic fibrosis (277.01)*

777.2 Intestinal obstruction due to inspissated milk

777.3 Hematemesis and melena due to swallowed maternal blood
Swallowed blood syndrome in newborn

> *Excludes:* *that not due to swallowed maternal blood (772.4)*

777.4 Transitory ileus of newborn

> *Excludes:* *Hirschsprung's disease (751.3)*

777.5 Necrotizing enterocolitis in fetus or newborn
Pseudomembranous enterocolitis in newborn

777.6 Perinatal intestinal perforation
Meconium peritonitis

777.8 Other specified perinatal disorders of digestive system

777.9 Unspecified perinatal disorder of digestive system

778 Conditions involving the integument and temperature regulation of fetus and newborn

778.0 Hydrops fetalis not due to isoimmunization
Idiopathic hydrops

> *Excludes:* *hydrops fetalis due to isoimmunization (773.3)*

778.1 Sclerema neonatorum
Subcutaneous fat necrosis

778.2 Cold injury syndrome of newborn

778.3 Other hypothermia of newborn

778.4 Other disturbances of temperature regulation of newborn
Dehydration fever in newborn
Environmentally-induced pyrexia
Hyperthermia in newborn
Transitory fever of newborn

● Code new to this edition   ▲ Revision of existing code   ④ ⑤ Fourth or fifth digit required

778.5 Other and unspecified edema of newborn
Edema neonatorum

778.6 Congenital hydrocele
Congenital hydrocele of tunica vaginalis

778.7 Breast engorgement in newborn
Noninfective mastitis of newborn

> *Excludes:* *infective mastitis of newborn (771.5)*

778.8 Other specified conditions involving the integument of fetus and newborn
Urticaria neonatorum

> *Excludes:* *impetigo neonatorum (684)*
> *pemphigus neonatorum (684)*

778.9 Unspecified condition involving the integument and temperature regulation of fetus and newborn

779 Other and ill-defined conditions originating in the perinatal period

779.0 Convulsions in newborn
Fits
Seizures } in newborn

779.1 Other and unspecified cerebral irritability in newborn

779.2 Cerebral depression, coma, and other abnormal cerebral signs
CNS dysfunction in newborn NOS

779.3 Feeding problems in newborn
Regurgitation of food
Slow feeding } in newborn
Vomiting

779.4 Drug reactions and intoxications specific to newborn
Gray syndrome from chloramphenicol administration in newborn

> *Excludes:* *fetal alcohol syndrome (760.71)*
> *reactions and intoxications from maternal opiates and tranquilizers (763.5)*

779.5 Drug withdrawal syndrome in newborn
Drug withdrawal syndrome in infant of dependent mother

> *Excludes:* *fetal alcohol syndrome (760.71)*

779.6 Termination of pregnancy (fetus)
Fetus death due to:
induced abortion
termination of pregnancy

> *Excludes:* *spontaneous abortion (fetus) (761.8)*

779.7 Periventricular leukomalacia

⑤ **779.8 Other specified conditions originating in the perinatal period**

● **779.81 Neonatal bradycardia**

> *Excludes:* *abnormality in fetal heart rate or rhythm complicating labor and delivery (763.81-763.83)*
> *bradycardia due to birth asphyxia (768.5-768.9)*

● **779.82 Neonatal tachycardia**

> *Excludes:* *abnormality in fetal heart rate or rhythm complicating labor and delivery (763.81-763.83)*

● **779.89 Other specified conditions originating in the perinatal period**

779.9 Unspecified condition originating in the perinatal period
Congenital debility NOS
Stillbirth NEC

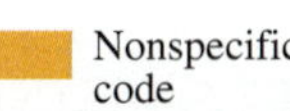

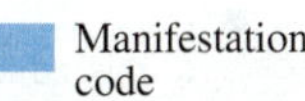

Manifestation
code

16.   SYMPTOMS, SIGNS, AND ILL-DEFINED CONDITIONS (780-799)

This section includes symptoms, signs, abnormal results of laboratory or other investigative procedures, and ill-defined conditions regarding which no diagnosis classifiable elsewhere is recorded.

Signs and symptoms that point rather definitely to a given diagnosis are assigned to some category in the preceding part of the classification. In general, categories 780-796 include the more ill-defined conditions and symptoms that point with perhaps equal suspicion to two or more diseases or to two or more systems of the body, and without the necessary study of the case to make a final diagnosis. Practically all categories in this group could be designated as "not otherwise specified," or as "unknown etiology," or as "transient." The Alphabetic Index should be consulted to determine which symptoms and signs are to be allocated here and which to more specific sections of the classification; the residual subcategories numbered .9 are provided for other relevant symptoms which cannot be allocated elsewhere in the classification.

The conditions and signs or symptoms included in categories 780-796 consist of: (a) cases for which no more specific diagnosis can be made even after all facts bearing on the case have been investigated; (b) signs or symptoms existing at the time of initial encounter that proved to be transient and whose causes could not be determined; (c) provisional diagnoses in a patient who failed to return for further investigation or care; (d) cases referred elsewhere for investigation or treatment before the diagnosis was made; (e) cases in which a more precise diagnosis was not available for any other reason; (f) certain symptoms which represent important problems in medical care and which it might be desired to classify in addition to a known cause.

SYMPTOMS (780-789)

780   General symptoms

⑤ **780.0   Alteration of consciousness**

> *Excludes:* *coma:*
>> *diabetic (250.2-250.3)*
>> *hepatic (572.2)*
>> *originating in the perinatal period (779.2)*

780.01   Coma

780.02   Transient alteration of awareness

780.03   Persistent vegetative state

780.09   Other

Drowsiness	Somnolence
Semicoma	Stupor
Unconsciousness	

780.1   Hallucinations

Hallucinations:	Hallucinations:
NOS	olfactory
auditory	tactile
gustatory	

> *Excludes:* *those associated with mental disorders, as functional psychoses (295.0-298.9)*
>> *organic brain syndromes (290.0-294.9, 310.0-310.9)*
>> *visual hallucinations (368.16)*

780.2   Syncope and collapse

Blackout	(Near) (Pre) syncope
Fainting	Vasovagal attack

> *Excludes:* *carotid sinus syncope (337.0)*
>> *heat syncope (992.1)*
>> *neurocirculatory asthenia (306.2)*
>> *orthostatic hypotension (458.0)*
>> *shock NOS (785.50)*

⑤ **780.3   Convulsions**

> *Excludes:* *convulsions:*
>> *epileptic (345.10-345.91)*
>> *in newborn (779.0)*

780.31   Febrile convulsions
> Febrile seizure

780.39   Other convulsions
> Convulsive disorder NOS
> Fit NOS
> Seizure NOS

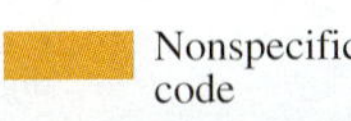

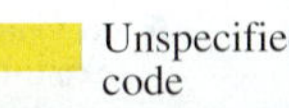

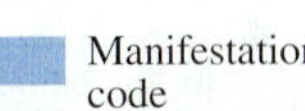

780.4 Dizziness and giddiness
Light-headedness   Vertigo NOS

Excludes: *Ménière's disease and other specified vertiginous syndromes (386.0-386.9)*

⑤ **780.5 Sleep disturbances**

Excludes: *that of nonorganic origin (307.40-307.49)*

780.50 Sleep disturbance, unspecified

780.51 Insomnia with sleep apnea

780.52 Other insomnia
Insomnia NOS

780.53 Hypersomnia with sleep apnea

780.54 Other hypersomnia
Hypersomnia NOS

780.55 Disruptions of 24-hour sleep-wake cycle
Inversion of sleep rhythm
Irregular sleep-wake rhythm NOS
Non-24-hour sleep-wake rhythm

780.56 Dysfunctions associated with sleep stages or arousal from sleep

780.57 Other and unspecified sleep apnea

780.59 Other

780.6 Fever
Chills with fever   Hyperpyrexia NOS
Fever NOS   Pyrexia NOS
Fever of unknown origin   Pyrexia of unknown origin
  (FUO)

Excludes: *pyrexia of unknown origin (during):*
   in newborn (778.4)
   labor (659.2)
   the puerperium (672)

⑤ **780.7 Malaise and fatigue**

Excludes: *debility, unspecified (799.3)*
   fatigue (during):
     combat (308.0-308.9)
     heat (992.6)
     pregnancy (646.8)
   neurasthenia (300.5)
   senile asthenia (797.5)

780.71 Chronic fatigue syndrome

780.79 Other malaise and fatigue
Asthenia NOS
Lethargy
Postviral (asthenic) syndrome
Tiredness

780.8 Hyperhidrosis
Diaphoresis
Excessive sweating

⑤ **780.9 Other general symptoms**

Excludes: *hypothermia:*
   NOS (accidental) (991.6)
   due to anesthesia (995.89)
   of newborn (778.2-778.3)
   memory disturbance as part of a pattern of mental disorder

● **780.91 Fussy infant (baby)**

● **780.92 Excessive crying of infant (baby)**

● **780.99 Other general symptoms**
Amnesia (retrograde)
Chill(s) NOS
Generalized pain
Hypothermia, not associated with low environmental temperature

● Code new to this edition   ▲ Revision of existing code   ④ ⑤ Fourth or fifth digit required

781 Symptoms involving nervous and musculoskeletal systems

> *Excludes:* *depression NOS (311)*
>
> *disorders specifically relating to:*
> *back (724.0-724.9)*
> *hearing (388.0-389.9)*
> *joint (718.0-719.9)*
> *limb (729.0-729.9)*
> *neck (723.0-723.9)*
> *vision (368.0-369.9)*
> *pain in limb (729.5)*

781.0 Abnormal involuntary movements
Abnormal head movements
Fasciculation
Spasms NOS
Tremor NOS

> *Excludes:* *abnormal reflex (796.1)*
>
> *chorea NOS (333.5)*
> *infantile spasms (345.60-345.61)*
> *spastic paralysis (342.1, 343.0-344.9)*
> *specified movement disorders classifiable to 333 (333.0-333.9)*
> *that of nonorganic origin (307.2-307.3)*

781.1 Disturbances of sensation of smell and taste

Anosmia	Parosmia
Parageusia	

781.2 Abnormality of gait

Gait:	Gait:
ataxic	spastic
paralytic	staggering

> *Excludes:* *ataxia:*
>
> *NOS (781.3)*
> *locomotor (progressive) (094.0)*
> *difficulty in walking (719.7)*

781.3 Lack of coordination

Ataxia NOS	Muscular incoordination

> *Excludes:* *ataxic gait (781.2)*
>
> *cerebellar ataxia (334.0-334.9)*
> *difficulty in walking (719.7)*
> *vertigo NOS (780.4)*

781.4 Transient paralysis of limb
Monoplegia, transient NOS

> *Excludes:* *paralysis (342.0-344.9)*

781.5 Clubbing of fingers

781.6 Meningismus
Dupré's syndrome
Meningism

781.7 Tetany
Carpopedal spasm

> *Excludes:* *tetanus neonatorum (771.3)*
>
> *tetany:*
> *hysterical (300.11)*
> *newborn (hypocalcemic) (775.4)*
> *parathyroid (252.1)*
> *psychogenic (306.0)*

781.8 Neurologic neglect syndrome

Asomatognosia	Left-sided neglect
Hemi-akinesia	Sensory extinction
Hemi-inattention	Sensory neglect
Hemispatial neglect	Visuospatial neglect

⑤ **781.9 Other symptoms involving nervous and musculoskeletal systems**

781.91 Loss of height

> *Excludes:* *osteoporosis (733.00-733.09)*

| Add 4th or 5th digit | Nonspecific code | Unspecified code | Manifestation code |

781.92 Abnormal posture

● **781.93 Ocular torticollis**

781.99 **Other symptoms involving nervous and musculoskeletal systems**

782 **Symptoms involving skin and other integumentary tissue**

Excludes: *symptoms relating to breast (611.71-611.79)*

782.0 Disturbance of skin sensation

Anesthesia of skin	Hypoesthesia
Burning or prickling	Numbness
sensation	Paresthesia
Hyperesthesia	Tingling

782.1 **Rash and other nonspecific skin eruption**
Exanthem

Excludes: *vesicular eruption (709.8)*

782.2 Localized superficial swelling, mass, or lump
Subcutaneous nodules

Excludes: *localized adiposity (278.1)*

782.3 Edema

Anasarca	Localized edema NOS
Dropsy	

Excludes: *ascites (789.5)*
      edema of:
        newborn NOS (778.5)
        pregnancy (642.0-642.9, 646.1)
      fluid retention (276.6)
      hydrops fetalis (773.3, 778.0)
      hydrothorax (511.8)
      nutritional edema (260, 262)

782.4 **Jaundice, unspecified, not of newborn**

Cholemia NOS	Icterus NOS

Excludes: *jaundice in newborn (774.0-774.7)*
      due to isoimmunization (773.0-773.2, 773.4)

782.5 Cyanosis

Excludes: *newborn (770.83)*

⑤ **782.6 Pallor and flushing**

782.61 Pallor

782.62 Flushing
Excessive blushing

782.7 Spontaneous ecchymoses
Petechiae

Excludes: *ecchymosis in fetus or newborn (772.6)*
      purpura (287.0-287.9)

782.8 Changes in skin texture
Induration of skin
Thickening of skin

782.9 **Other symptoms involving skin and integumentary tissues**

783 **Symptoms concerning nutrition, metabolism, and development**

783.0 Anorexia
Loss of appetite

Excludes: *anorexia nervosa (307.1)*
      loss of appetite of nonorganic origin (307.59)

783.1 Abnormal weight gain

Excludes: *excessive weight gain in pregnancy (646.1)*
      obesity (278.00)
      morbid (278.01)

⑤ **783.2 Abnormal loss of weight and underweight**

783.21 Loss of weight

783.22 Underweight

● Code new
to this edition

▲ Revision of
existing code

④ ⑤ Fourth or fifth
digit required

783.3 Feeding difficulties and mismanagement
Feeding problem (elderly) (infant)

Excludes: feeding disturbance or problems:
    in newborn (779.3)
    of nonorganic origin (307.50-307.59)

⑤ **783.4 Lack of expected normal physiological development in childhood**

Excludes: delay in sexual development and puberty (259.0)
    gonadal dysgenesis (758.6)
    pituitary dwarfism (253.3)
    slow fetal growth and fetal malnutrition (764.00-764.99)
    specific delays in mental development (315.0-315.9)

    783.40 Lack of normal physiological development, unspecified
        Inadequate development
        Lack of development

    783.41 Failure to thrive
        Failure to gain weight

    783.42 Delayed milestones
        Late talker
        Late walker

    783.43 Short stature
        Growth failure
        Growth retardation
        Lack of growth
        Physical retardation

783.5 Polydipsia
Excessive thirst

783.6 Polyphagia
Excessive eating
Hyperalimentation NOS

Excludes: disorders of eating of nonorganic origin (307.50-307.59)

783.7 Adult failure to thrive

783.9 Other symptoms concerning nutrition, metabolism, and development
Hypometabolism

Excludes: abnormal basal metabolic rate (794.7)
    dehydration (276.5)
    other disorders of fluid, electrolyte, and acid-base balance (276.0-276.9)

784 Symptoms involving head and neck

Excludes: encephalopathy NOS (348.3)
    specific symptoms involving neck classifiable to 723 (723.0-723.9)

784.0 Headache
Facial pain   Pain in head NOS

Excludes: atypical face pain (350.2)
    migraine (346.0-346.9)
    tension headache (307.81)

784.1 Throat pain

Excludes: dysphagia (787.2)
    neck pain (723.1)
    sore throat (462)
      chronic (472.1)

784.2 Swelling, mass, or lump in head and neck
Space-occupying lesion, intracranial NOS

784.3 Aphasia

Excludes: developmental aphasia (315.31)

⑤ **784.4 Voice disturbance**

    784.40 Voice disturbance, unspecified
    784.41 Aphonia
        Loss of voice

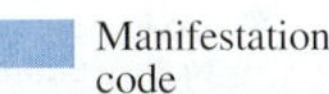

| Add 4th or 5th digit | Nonspecific code | Unspecified code | Manifestation code |

784.49 Other
Change in voice
Dysphonia
Hoarseness
Hypernasality
Hyponasality

784.5 Other speech disturbance
Dysarthria
Dysphasia
Slurred speech

Excludes: *stammering and stuttering (307.0)*
that of nonorganic origin (307.0, 307.9)

⑤ **784.6 Other symbolic dysfunction**

Excludes: *developmental learning delays (315.0-315.9)*

784.60 Symbolic dysfunction, unspecified

784.61 Alexia and dyslexia
Alexia (with agraphia)

784.69 Other
Acalculia
Agnosia
Agraphia NOS
Apraxia

784.7 Epistaxis
Hemorrhage from nose
Nosebleed

784.8 Hemorrhage from throat

Excludes: *hemoptysis (786.3)*

784.9 Other symptoms involving head and neck
Choking sensation
Halitosis
Mouth breathing
Sneezing

785 Symptoms involving cardiovascular system

Excludes: *heart failure NOS (428.9)*

785.0 Tachycardia, unspecified
Rapid heart beat

Excludes: *neonatal tachycardia (779.82)*
paroxysmal tachycardia (427.0-427.2)

785.1 Palpitations
Awareness of heart beat

Excludes: *specified dysrhythmias (427.0-427.9)*

785.2 Undiagnosed cardiac murmurs
Heart murmur NOS

785.3 Other abnormal heart sounds
Cardiac dullness, increased or decreased
Friction fremitus, cardiac
Precordial friction

785.4 Gangrene
Gangrenous cellulitis
Gangrene NOS
Gangrene spreading cutaneous
Phagedena

Code first any associated underlying condition, as:
diabetes (250.7)
Raynaud's syndrome (443.0)

Excludes: *gangrene of certain sites—see Alphabetic Index*
gangrene with atherosclerosis of the extremities (440.24)
gas gangrene (040.0)

⑤ **785.5 Shock without mention of trauma**

785.50 Shock, unspecified
Failure of peripheral circulation

785.51 Cardiogenic shock

● Code new
to this edition

▲ Revision of
existing code

④ ⑤ Fourth or fifth
digit required

785.59 Other

Shock:
  endotoxic
  gram-negative

Shock:
  hypovolemic
  septic

Excludes: *shock (due to):*
  anesthetic (995.4)
  anaphylactic (995.0)
   due to serum (999.4)
  electric (994.8)
  following abortion (639.5)
  lightning (994.0)
  obstetrical (669.1)
  postoperative (998.0)
  traumatic (958.4)

785.6 Enlargement of lymph nodes

Lymphadenopathy   "Swollen glands"

Excludes: *lymphadenitis (chronic) (289.1-289.3)*
  acute (683)

785.9 Other symptoms involving cardiovascular system

Bruit (arterial)   Weak pulse

786 Symptoms involving respiratory system and other chest symptoms

⑤ **786.0 Dyspnea and respiratory abnormalities**

786.00 Respiratory abnormality, unspecified

786.01 Hyperventilation

Excludes: *hyperventilation, psychogenic (306.1)*

786.02 Orthopnea

786.03 Apnea

Excludes: *apnea of newborn (770.81, 770.82)*
  sleep apnea (780.51, 780.53, 780.57)

786.04 Cheyne-Stokes respiration

786.05 Shortness of breath

786.06 Tachypnea

Excludes: *transitory tachypnea of newborn (770.6)*

786.07 Wheezing

Excludes: *asthma (493.00-493.92)*

786.09 Other

Respiratory:
  distress
  insufficiency

Excludes: *respiratory distress:*
  following trauma and surgery (518.5)
  newborn (770.89)
  syndrome (newborn) (769)
   adult (518.5)
  respiratory failure (518.81, 518.83-518.84)
  newborn (770.84)

786.1 Stridor

Excludes: *congenital laryngeal stridor (748.3)*

786.2 Cough

Excludes: *cough:*
  psychogenic (306.1)
  smokers' (491.0)
  with hemorrhage (786.3)

786.3 Hemoptysis

Cough with hemorrhage
Pulmonary hemorrhage NOS

Excludes: *pulmonary hemorrhage of newborn (770.3)*

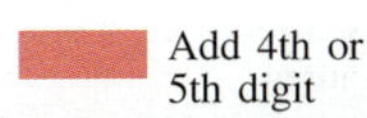

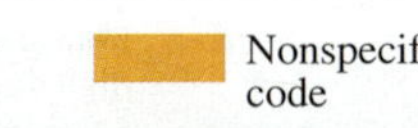

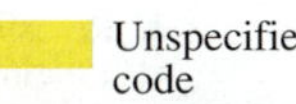

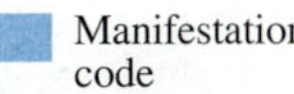

786.4 Abnormal sputum
Abnormal:
amount
color } (of) sputum
odor
Excessive

⑤ **786.5 Chest pain**

786.50 Chest pain, unspecified

786.51 Precordial pain

786.52 Painful respiration
Pain:
anterior chest wall
pleuritic
Pleurodynia

Excludes: *epidemic pleurodynia (074.1)*

786.59 Other
Discomfort
Pressure } in chest
Tightness

Excludes: *pain in breast (611.71)*

786.6 Swelling, mass, or lump in chest

Excludes: *lump in breast (611.72)*

786.7 Abnormal chest sounds
Abnormal percussion, chest   Rales
Friction sounds, chest   Tympany, chest

Excludes: *wheezing (786.07)*

786.8 Hiccough

Excludes: *psychogenic hiccough (306.1)*

786.9 Other symptoms involving respiratory system and chest
Breath-holding spell

787 Symptoms involving digestive system

Excludes: *constipation (564.00-564.09)*
pylorospasm (537.81)
congenital (750.5)

⑤ **787.0 Nausea and vomiting**
Emesis

Excludes: *hematemesis NOS (578.0)*

vomiting:
bilious, following gastrointestinal surgery (564.3)
cyclical (536.2)
psychogenic (306.4)
excessive, in pregnancy (643.0-643.9)
habit (536.2)
of newborn (779.3)
psychogenic NOS (307.54)

787.01 Nausea with vomiting

787.02 Nausea alone

787.03 Vomiting alone

787.1 Heartburn
Pyrosis
Waterbrash

Excludes: *dyspepsia or indigestion (536.8)*

787.2 Dysphagia
Difficulty in swallowing

787.3 Flatulence, eructation, and gas pain
Abdominal distention (gaseous)
Bloating
Tympanites (abdominal) (intestinal)

Excludes: *aerophagy (306.4)*

● Code new   ▲ Revision of   ④ ⑤ Fourth or fifth
to this edition   existing code   digit required

787.4 Visible peristalsis
Hyperperistalsis

787.5 Abnormal bowel sounds
Absent bowel sounds
Hyperactive bowel sounds

787.6 Incontinence of feces
Encopresis NOS
Incontinence of sphincter ani

Excludes: *that of nonorganic origin (307.7)*

787.7 Abnormal feces
Bulky stools

Excludes: *abnormal stool content (792.1)*
melena:
NOS (578.1)
newborn (772.4, 777.3)

⑤ **787.9 Other symptoms involving digestive system**

Excludes: *gastrointestinal hemorrhage (578.0-578.9)*
intestinal obstruction (560.0-560.9)
specific functional digestive disorders:
esophagus (530.0-530.9)
stomach and duodenum (536.0-536.9)
those not elsewhere classified (564.00-564.9)

787.91 Diarrhea
Diarrhea NOS

787.99 Other
Change in bowel habits
Tenesmus (rectal)

788 Symptoms involving urinary system

Excludes: *hematuria (599.7)*
nonspecific findings on examination of the urine (791.0-791.9)
small kidney of unknown cause (589.0-589.9)
uremia NOS (586)

788.0 Renal colic
Colic (recurrent) of:
kidney
ureter

788.1 Dysuria
Painful urination
Strangury

⑤ **788.2 Retention of urine**

788.20 Retention of urine, unspecified

788.21 Incomplete bladder emptying

788.29 Other specified retention of urine

⑤ **788.3 Incontinence of urine**

Excludes: *that of nonorganic origin (307.6)*
Code, if applicable, any causal condition first, such as:
congenital ureterocele (753.23)
genital prolapse (618.0-618.9)

788.30 Urinary incontinence, unspecified
Enuresis NOS

788.31 Urge incontinence

788.32 Stress incontinence, male

Excludes: *stress incontinence (female) (625.6)*

788.33 Mixed incontinence (male) (female)
Urge and stress

788.34 Incontinence without sensory awareness

788.35 Post-void dribbling

788.36 Nocturnal enuresis

788.37 Continuous leakage

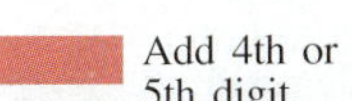

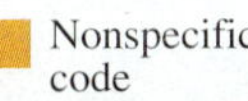

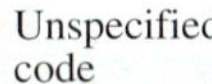

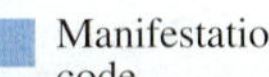

788.39 **Other urinary incontinence**

⑤ **788.4** **Frequency of urination and polyuria**

788.41 **Urinary frequency**
Frequency of micturition

788.42 **Polyuria**

788.43 **Nocturia**

788.5 **Oliguria and anuria**
Deficient secretion of urine
Suppression of urinary secretion

Excludes: *that complicating:*
abortion (634-638 with .3, 639.3)
ectopic or molar pregnancy (639.3)
pregnancy, childbirth, or the puerperium (642.0-642.9, 646.2)

⑤ **788.6** **Other abnormality of urination**

788.61 **Splitting of urinary stream**
Intermittent urinary stream

788.62 **Slowing of urinary stream**
Weak stream

788.69 **Other**

788.7 **Urethral discharge**
Penile discharge   Urethrorrhea

788.8 **Extravasation of urine**

788.9 **Other symptoms involving urinary system**
Extrarenal uremia
Vesical:
pain
tenesmus

789 **Other symptoms involving abdomen and pelvis**
The following fifth-digit subclassification is to be used for codes 789.0, 789.3, 789.4, 789.6

0 **unspecified site**

1 **right upper quadrant**

2 **left upper quadrant**

3 **right lower quadrant**

4 **left lower quadrant**

5 **periumbilic**

6 **epigastric**

7 **generalized**

9 **other specified site**
multiple sites

Excludes: *symptoms referable to genital organs:*
female (625.0-625.9)
male (607.0-608.9)
psychogenic (302.70-302.79)

⑤ **789.0** **Abdominal pain**
Colic:
NOS
infantile
Cramps, abdominal

Excludes: *renal colic (788.0)*

789.1 **Hepatomegaly**
Enlargement of liver

789.2 **Splenomegaly**
Enlargement of spleen

⑤ **789.3** **Abdominal or pelvic swelling, mass, or lump**
Diffuse or generalized swelling or mass:
abdominal NOS
umbilical

Excludes: *abdominal distention (gaseous) (787.3)*
ascites (789.5)

● Code new
to this edition   ▲ Revision of
existing code   ④ ⑤ Fourth or fifth
digit required

⑤ **789.4 Abdominal rigidity**

789.5 Ascites
Fluid in peritoneal cavity

⑤ **789.6 Abdominal tenderness**
Rebound tenderness

789.9 Other symptoms involving abdomen and pelvis
Umbilical:
  bleeding
  discharge

NONSPECIFIC ABNORMAL FINDINGS (790-796)

790 Nonspecific findings on examination of blood

Excludes: *abnormality of:*
  platelets (287.0-287.9)
  thrombocytes (287.0-287.9)
  white blood cells (288.0-288.9)

⑤ **790.0 Abnormality of red blood cells**

Excludes: *anemia:*
  congenital (776.5)
  newborn, due to isoimmunization (773.0-773.2, 773.5)
  of premature infant (776.6)
  other specified types (280.0-285.9)
  hemoglobin disorders (282.5-282.7)
  polycythemia:
  familial (289.6)
  neonatorum (776.4)
  secondary (289.0)
  vera (238.4)

790.01 Precipitous drop in hematocrit
Drop in hematocrit

790.09 Other abnormality of red blood cells
Abnormal red cell morphology NOS
Abnormal red cell volume NOS
Anisocytosis
Poikilocytosis

790.1 Elevated sedimentation rate

790.2 Abnormal glucose tolerance test

Excludes: *that complicating pregnancy, childbirth, or the puerperium (648.8)*

790.3 Excessive blood level of alcohol
Elevated blood-alcohol

790.4 Nonspecific elevation of levels of transaminase or lactic acid dehydrogenase [LDH]

790.5 Other nonspecific abnormal serum enzyme levels
Abnormal serum level of: Abnormal serum level of:
  acid phosphatase   amylase
  alkaline phosphatase   lipase

Excludes: *deficiency of circulating enzymes (277.6)*

790.6 Other abnormal blood chemistry
Abnormal blood level of: Abnormal blood level of:
  cobalt   magnesium
  copper   mineral
  iron   zinc
  lithium

Excludes: *abnormality of electrolyte or acid-base balance (276.0-276.9)*
  hypoglycemia NOS (251.2)
  specific finding indicating abnormality of:
  amino-acid transport and metabolism (270.0-270.9)
  carbohydrate transport and metabolism (271.0-271.9)
  lipid metabolism (272.0-272.9)
  uremia NOS (586)

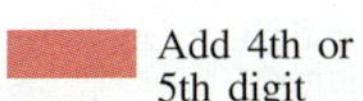

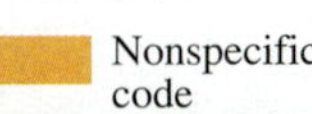

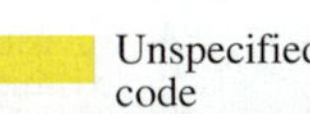

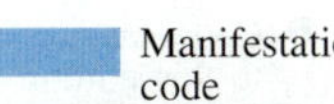

790.7 Bacteremia

> *Excludes:* *bacteremia of newborn (771.83)*
> *septicemia (038)*

Use additional code, if desired, to identify organism (041)

790.8 Viremia, unspecified

⑤ **790.9 Other nonspecific findings on examination of blood**

790.91 Abnormal arterial blood gases

790.92 Abnormal coagulation profile
Abnormal or prolonged:
bleeding time
coagulation time
partial thromboplastin time [PTT]
prothrombin time [PT]

> *Excludes:* *coagulation (hemorrhagic) disorders (286.0-286.9)*

790.93 Elevated prostate specific antigen (PSA)

790.94 Euthyroid sick syndrome

790.99 Other

791 Nonspecific findings on examination of urine

> *Excludes:* *hematuria NOS (599.7)*
> *specific findings indicating abnormality of:*
> *amino-acid transport and metabolism (270.0-270.9)*
> *carbohydrate transport and metabolism (271.0-271.9)*

791.0 Proteinuria
Albuminuria   Bence-Jones proteinuria

> *Excludes:* *postural proteinuria (593.6)*
> *that arising during pregnancy or the puerperium (642.0-642.9, 646.2)*

791.1 Chyluria

> *Excludes:* *filarial (125.0-125.9)*

791.2 Hemoglobinuria

791.3 Myoglobinuria

791.4 Biliuria

791.5 Glycosuria

> *Excludes:* *renal glycosuria (271.4)*

791.6 Acetonuria
Ketonuria

791.7 Other cells and casts in urine

791.9 Other nonspecific findings on examination of urine
Crystalluria
Elevated urine levels of:
17-ketosteroids
catecholamines
indolacetic acid
vanillylmandelic acid [VMA]
Melanuria

792 Nonspecific abnormal findings in other body substances

> *Excludes:* *that in chromosomal analysis (795.2)*

792.0 Cerebrospinal fluid

792.1 Stool contents
Abnormal stool color
Fat in stool   Occult blood
Mucus in stool   Pus in stool

> *Excludes:* *blood in stool [melena] (578.1)*
> *newborn (772.4, 777.3)*

792.2 Semen
Abnormal spermatozoa

> *Excludes:* *azoospermia (606.0)*
> *oligospermia (606.1)*

● Code new to this edition   ▲ Revision of existing code   ④ ⑤ Fourth or fifth digit required

792.3 Amniotic fluid

792.4 Saliva

> *Excludes:* *that in chromosomal analysis (795.2)*

792.5 Cloudy (hemodialysis) (peritoneal) dialysis effluent

792.9 Other nonspecific abnormal findings in body substances
Peritoneal fluid   Synovial fluid
Pleural fluid   Vaginal fluids

793 Nonspecific abnormal findings on radiological and other examinations of body structure
Includes: nonspecific abnormal findings of:
thermography
ultrasound examination [echogram]
x-ray examination

> *Excludes:* *abnormal results of function studies and radioisotope scans (794.0-794.9)*

793.0 Skull and head

> *Excludes:* *nonspecific abnormal echoencephalogram (794.01)*

793.1 Lung field
Coin lesion   ⎫
Shadow   ⎬ (of) lung

793.2 Other intrathoracic organ
Abnormal: Mediastinal shift
echocardiogram
heart shadow
ultrasound cardiogram

793.3 Biliary tract
Nonvisualization of gallbladder

793.4 Gastrointestinal tract

793.5 Genitourinary organs
Filling defect:
bladder
kidney
ureter

793.6 Abdominal area, including retroperitoneum

793.7 Musculoskeletal system

⑤ **793.8 Breast**

793.80 Abnormal mammogram, unspecified

793.81 Mammographic microcalcification

793.89 Other abnormal findings on radiological examination of breast

793.9 Other
Abnormal:
placental finding by x-ray or ultrasound method
radiological findings in skin and subcutaneous tissue

> *Excludes:* *abnormal finding by radioisotope localization of placenta (794.9)*

794 Nonspecific abnormal results of function studies
Includes: radioisotope:
scans
uptake studies
scintiphotography

⑤ **794.0 Brain and central nervous system**

794.00 Abnormal function study, unspecified

794.01 Abnormal echoencephalogram

794.02 Abnormal electroencephalogram [EEG]

794.09 Other
Abnormal brain scan

⑤ **794.1 Peripheral nervous system and special senses**

794.10 Abnormal response to nerve stimulation, unspecified

794.11 Abnormal retinal function studies
Abnormal electroretinogram [ERG]

794.12 Abnormal electro-oculogram [EOG]

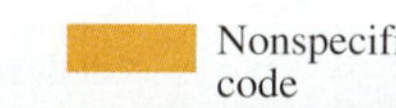

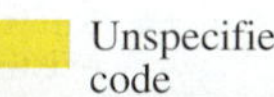

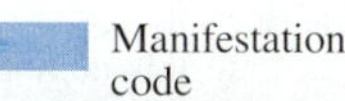

Manifestation
code

794.13 Abnormal visually evoked potential

794.14 Abnormal oculomotor studies

794.15 Abnormal auditory function studies

794.16 Abnormal vestibular function studies

794.17 Abnormal electromyogram [EMG]

Excludes: *that of eye (794.14)*

794.19 Other

794.2 Pulmonary
Abnormal lung scan
Reduced:
   ventilatory capacity
   vital capacity

⑤ **794.3 Cardiovascular**

794.30 Abnormal function study, unspecified

794.31 Abnormal electrocardiogram [ECG] [EKG]

794.39 Other
Abnormal:
   ballistocardiogram
   phonocardiogram
   vectorcardiogram

794.4 Kidney
Abnormal renal function test

794.5 Thyroid
Abnormal thyroid:
   scan
   uptake

794.6 Other endocrine function study

794.7 Basal metabolism
Abnormal basal metabolic rate [BMR]

794.8 Liver
Abnormal liver scan

794.9 Other
Bladder
Pancreas
Placenta
Spleen

795 Nonspecific abnormal histological and immunological findings

Excludes: *nonspecific abnormalities of red blood cells (790.01-790.09)*

⑤ **795.0 Nonspecific abnormal Papanicolaou smear of cervix**

Excludes: *carcinoma in-situ of cervix (233.1)*
   cervical intraepithelial neoplasia I (CIN I) (622.1)
   cervical intraepithelial neoplasia II (CIN II) (622.1)
   cervical intraepithelial neoplasia III (CIN III) (233.1)
   dysplasia of cervix (uteri) (622.1)
   high grade squamous intraepithelial dysplasia (HGSIL) (622.1)
   low grade squamous intraepithelial dysplasia (LGSIL) (622.1)

● **795.00 Nonspecific abnormal Papanicolaou smear of cervix, unspecified**

● **795.01 Atypical squamous cell changes of undetermined significance favor benign (ASCUS favor benign)**
Atypical glandular cell changes of undetermined significance favor benign
   (AGCUS favor benign)

● **795.02 Atypical squamous cell changes of undetermined significance favor dysplasia (ASCUS favor dysplasia)**
Atypical glandular cell changes of undetermined significance favor dysplasia
   (AGCUS favor dysplasia)

● **795.09 Other nonspecific abnormal Papanicolaou smear of cervix**
Benign cellular changes
Unsatisfactory smear

795.1 Nonspecific abnormal Papanicolaou smear of other site

● Code new
to this edition   ▲ Revision of
existing code   ④ ⑤ Fourth or fifth
digit required

795.2 Nonspecific abnormal findings on chromosomal analysis
Abnormal karyotype

⑤ **795.3 Nonspecific positive culture findings**
Positive culture findings in:
nose
sputum
throat
wound

Excludes: *that of:*
blood (790.7-790.8)
urine (791.9)

● **795.31 Nonspecific positive findings for anthrax**
Positive findings by nasal swab

● **795.39 Other nonspecific positive culture findings**

795.4 Other nonspecific abnormal histological findings

795.5 Nonspecific reaction to tuberculin skin test without active tuberculosis
Abnormal result of Mantoux test
PPD positive
Tuberculin (skin test):
positive
reactor

795.6 False positive serological test for syphilis
False positive Wassermann reaction

⑤ **795.7 Other nonspecific immunological findings**

Excludes: *isoimmunization, in pregnancy (656.1-656.2)*
affecting fetus or newborn (773.0-773.2)

795.71 Nonspecific serologic evidence of human immunodeficiency virus [HIV]
Inconclusive human immunodeficiency virus [HIV] test (adult) (infant)

Note: This code is ONLY to be used when a test finding is reported as nonspecific. Asymptomatic positive findings are coded to V08. If any HIV infection symptom or condition is present, see code 042. Negative findings are not coded.

Excludes: *acquired immunodeficiency syndrome [AIDS] (042)*
asymptomatic human immunodeficiency virus, [HIV] infection status (V08)
HIV infection, symptomatic (042)
human immunodeficiency virus [HIV] disease (042)
positive (status) NOS (V08)

795.79 Other and unspecified nonspecific immunological findings
Raised antibody titer
Raised level of immunoglobulins

796 Other nonspecific abnormal findings

796.0 Nonspecific abnormal toxicological findings
Abnormal levels of heavy metals or drugs in blood, urine, or other tissue

Excludes: *excessive blood level of alcohol (790.3)*

796.1 Abnormal reflex

796.2 Elevated blood pressure reading without diagnosis of hypertension
Note: This category is to be used to record an episode of elevated blood pressure in a patient in whom no formal diagnosis of hypertension has been made, or as an incidental finding.

796.3 Nonspecific low blood pressure reading

796.4 Other abnormal clinical findings

796.5 Abnormal finding on antenatal screening

796.9 Other

ILL-DEFINED AND UNKNOWN CAUSES OF MORBIDITY AND MORTALITY (797-799)

797 Senility without mention of psychosis
Old age
Senescence
Senile asthenia
Senile debility
Senile exhaustion

Excludes: *senile psychoses (290.0-290.9)*

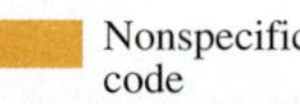

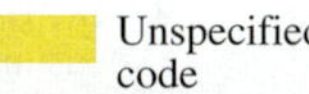

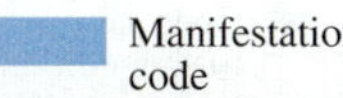

Manifestation
code

798 **Sudden death, cause unknown**

798.0 **Sudden infant death syndrome**
Cot death
Crib death
Sudden death of nonspecific cause in infancy

798.1 **Instantaneous death**

798.2 **Death occurring in less than 24 hours from onset of symptoms, not otherwise explained**
Death known not to be violent or instantaneous, for which no cause could be discovered
Died without sign of disease

798.9 **Unattended death**
Death in circumstances where the body of the deceased was found and no cause could
be discovered
Found dead

799 **Other ill-defined and unknown causes of morbidity and mortality**

799.0 **Asphyxia**

> *Excludes:* *asphyxia (due to):*
>
> *carbon monoxide (986)*
> *inhalation of food or foreign body (932-934.9)*
> *newborn (768.0-768.9)*
> *traumatic (994.7)*

799.1 **Respiratory arrest**
Cardiorespiratory failure

> *Excludes:* *cardiac arrest (427.5)*
>
> *failure of peripheral circulation (785.50)*
> *respiratory distress:*
> *NOS (786.09)*
> *acute (518.82)*
> *following trauma and surgery (518.5)*
> *newborn (770.89)*
> *syndrome (newborn) (769)*
>   *adult (following trauma and surgery) (518.5)*
>   *other (518.82)*
> *respiratory failure (518.81, 518.83-518.84)*
> *newborn (770.84)*
> *respiratory insufficiency (786.09)*
> *acute (518.82)*

799.2 **Nervousness**
"Nerves"

799.3 **Debility, unspecified**

> *Excludes:* *asthenia (780.79)*
>
> *nervous debility (300.5)*
> *neurasthenia (300.5)*
> *senile asthenia (797)*

799.4 **Cachexia**
Wasting disease

> *Excludes:* *nutritional marasmus (261)*

799.8 **Other ill-defined conditions**

799.9 **Other unknown and unspecified cause**
Undiagnosed disease, not specified as to site or system involved
Unknown cause of morbidity or mortality

● Code new to this edition   ▲ Revision of existing code   ④ ⑤ Fourth or fifth digit required

17. INJURY AND POISONING (800-999)

Use E code(s) to identify the cause and intent of the injury or poisoning (E800-E999)

Note:

1. The principle of multiple coding of injuries should be followed wherever possible. Combination categories for multiple injuries are provided for use when there is insufficient detail as to the nature of the individual conditions, or for primary tabulation purposes when it is more convenient to record a single code; otherwise, the component injuries should be coded separately.

   Where multiple sites of injury are specified in the titles, the word "with" indicates involvement of both sites, and the word "and" indicates involvement of either or both sites. The word "finger" includes thumb.

2. Categories for "late effect" of injuries are to be found at 905-909.

FRACTURES (800-829)

> *Excludes:* malunion (733.81)
>
> > nonunion (733.82)
> > pathologic or spontaneous fracture (733.10-733.19)
> > stress fractures (733.93-733.95)

The terms "condyle," "coronoid process," "ramus," and "symphysis" indicate the portion of the bone fractured, not the name of the bone involved.

The descriptions "closed" and "open" used in the fourth-digit subdivisions include the following terms:

closed (with or without delayed healing):

comminuted	impacted
depressed	linear
elevated	simple
fissured	slipped epiphysis
fracture NOS	spiral
greenstick	

open (with or without delayed healing):

compound	puncture
infected	with foreign body
missile	

A fracture not indicated as closed or open should be classified as closed.

FRACTURE OF SKULL (800-804)

The following fifth-digit subclassification is for use with the appropriate codes in categories 800, 801, 803, and 804:

0 **unspecified state of consciousness**

1 **with no loss of consciousness**

2 **with brief [less than one hour] loss of consciousness**

3 **with moderate [1-24 hours] loss of consciousness and return to pre-existing conscious level**

4 **with prolonged [more than 24 hours] loss of consciousness and return to pre-existing conscious level**

5 **with prolonged [more than 24 hours] loss of consciousness, without return to pre-existing conscious level**
Use fifth-digit 5 to designate when a patient is unconscious and dies before regaining consciousness, regardless of the duration of the loss of consciousness

6 **with loss of consciousness of unspecified duration**

9 **with concussion, unspecified**

⑤ **800** **Fracture of vault of skull**
Includes: frontal bone
parietal bone

⑤ **800.0** **Closed without mention of intracranial injury**

⑤ **800.1** **Closed with cerebral laceration and contusion**

⑤ **800.2** **Closed with subarachnoid, subdural, and extradural hemorrhage**

⑤ **800.3** **Closed with other and unspecified intracranial hemorrhage**

⑤ **800.4** **Closed with intracranial injury of other and unspecified nature**

⑤ **800.5** **Open without mention of intracranial injury**

⑤ **800.6** **Open with cerebral laceration and contusion**

⑤ **800.7** **Open with subarachnoid, subdural, and extradural hemorrhage**

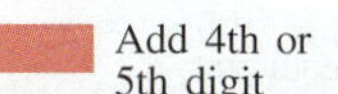

Add 4th or 5th digit	Nonspecific code	Unspecified code	Medicare secondary payer(MSP) alert

⑤ **800.8** **Open with other and unspecified intracranial hemorrhage**

⑤ **800.9** **Open with intracranial injury of other and unspecified nature**

⑤ **801** **Fracture of base of skull**
    Includes:

fossa:	sinus:
anterior	ethmoid
middle	frontal
posterior	sphenoid bone
occiput bone	temporal bone
orbital roof	

⑤ **801.0** **Closed without mention of intracranial injury**

⑤ **801.1** **Closed with cerebral laceration and contusion**

⑤ **801.2** **Closed with subarachnoid, subdural, and extradural hemorrhage**

⑤ **801.3** **Closed with other and unspecified intracranial hemorrhage**

⑤ **801.4** **Closed with intracranial injury of other and unspecified nature**

⑤ **801.5** **Open without mention of intracranial injury**

⑤ **801.6** **Open with cerebral laceration and contusion**

⑤ **801.7** **Open with subarachnoid, subdural, and extradural hemorrhage**

⑤ **801.8** **Open with other and unspecified intracranial hemorrhage**

⑤ **801.9** **Open with intracranial injury of other and unspecified nature**

802 **Fracture of face bones**

802.0 **Nasal bones, closed**

802.1 **Nasal bones, open**

⑤ **802.2** **Mandible, closed**
    Inferior maxilla   Lower jaw (bone)

    802.20 **Unspecified site**

    802.21 **Condylar process**

    802.22 **Subcondylar**

    802.23 **Coronoid process**

    802.24 **Ramus, unspecified**

    802.25 **Angle of jaw**

    802.26 **Symphysis of body**

    802.27 **Alveolar border of body**

    802.28 **Body, other and unspecified**

    802.29 **Multiple sites**

⑤ **802.3** **Mandible, open**

    802.30 **Unspecified site**

    802.31 **Condylar process**

    802.32 **Subcondylar**

    802.33 **Coronoid process**

    802.34 **Ramus, unspecified**

    802.35 **Angle of jaw**

    802.36 **Symphysis of body**

    802.37 **Alveolar border of body**

    802.38 **Body, other and unspecified**

    802.39 **Multiple sites**

802.4 **Malar and maxillary bones, closed**
    Superior maxilla   Zygoma
    Upper jaw (bone)   Zygomatic arch

802.5 **Malar and maxillary bones, open**

802.6 **Orbital floor (blow-out), closed**

802.7 **Orbital floor (blow-out), open**

● Code new
  to this edition   ▲ Revision of
        existing code   ④ ⑤ Fourth or fifth
          digit required

802.8 **Other facial bones, closed**
    Alveolus
    Orbit:
     NOS
     part other than roof or floor
    Palate

    Excludes: *orbital:*
        floor (802.6)
        roof (801.0-801.9)

802.9 **Other facial bones, open**

⑤ **803** **Other and unqualified skull fractures**
    Includes: skull NOS
             skull multiple NOS

⑤ **803.0** **Closed without mention of intracranial injury**

⑤ **803.1** **Closed with cerebral laceration and contusion**

⑤ **803.2** **Closed with subarachnoid, subdural, and extradural hemorrhage**

⑤ **803.3** **Closed with other and unspecified intracranial hemorrhage**

⑤ **803.4** **Closed with intracranial injury of other and unspecified nature**

⑤ **803.5** **Open without mention of intracranial injury**

⑤ **803.6** **Open with cerebral laceration and contusion**

⑤ **803.7** **Open with subarachnoid, subdural, and extradural hemorrhage**

⑤ **803.8** **Open with other and unspecified intracranial hemorrhage**

⑤ **803.9** **Open with intracranial injury of other and unspecified nature**

⑤ **804** **Multiple fractures involving skull or face with other bones**

⑤ **804.0** **Closed without mention of intracranial injury**

⑤ **804.1** **Closed with cerebral laceration and contusion**

⑤ **804.2** **Closed with subarachnoid, subdural, and extradural hemorrhage**

⑤ **804.3** **Closed with other and unspecified intracranial hemorrhage**

⑤ **804.4** **Closed with intracranial injury of other and unspecified nature**

⑤ **804.5** **Open without mention of intracranial injury**

⑤ **804.6** **Open with cerebral laceration and contusion**

⑤ **804.7** **Open with subarachnoid, subdural, and extradural hemorrhage**

⑤ **804.8** **Open with other and unspecified intracranial hemorrhage**

⑤ **804.9** **Open with intracranial injury of other and unspecified nature**

FRACTURE OF NECK AND TRUNK (805-809)

805 **Fracture of vertebral column without mention of spinal cord injury**
    Includes:

        neural arch   transverse process
        spine   vertebra
        spinous process

    The following fifth-digit subclassification is for use with codes 805.0-805.1:

    0 **cervical vertebra, unspecified level**

    1 **first cervical vertebra**

    2 **second cervical vertebra**

    3 **third cervical vertebra**

    4 **fourth cervical vertebra**

    5 **fifth cervical vertebra**

    6 **sixth cervical vertebra**

    7 **seventh cervical vertebra**

    8 **multiple cervical vertebrae**

⑤ **805.0** **Cervical, closed**
    Atlas   Axis

⑤ **805.1** **Cervical, open**

805.2 **Dorsal [thoracic], closed**

805.3 **Dorsal [thoracic], open**

	Add 4th or 5th digit		Nonspecific code		Unspecified code		Medicare secondary payer(MSP) alert

805.4 Lumbar, closed

805.5 Lumbar, open

805.6 Sacrum and coccyx, closed

805.7 Sacrum and coccyx, open

805.8 Unspecified, closed

805.9 Unspecified, open

806 Fracture of vertebral column with spinal cord injury
      Includes: any condition classifiable to 805 with:
            complete or incomplete transverse lesion (of cord)
            hematomyelia
        injury to:
            cauda equina
            nerve
        paralysis
        paraplegia
        quadriplegia
        spinal concussion

⑤ **806.0 Cervical, closed**

    806.00 C_1-C_4 level with unspecified spinal cord injury
        Cervical region NOS with spinal cord injury NOS

    806.01 C_1-C_4 level with complete lesion of cord

    806.02 C_1-C_4 level with anterior cord syndrome

    806.03 C_1-C_4 level with central cord syndrome

    806.04 C_1-C_4 level with other specified spinal cord injury
        C_1-C_4 level with:
          incomplete spinal cord lesion NOS
          posterior cord syndrome

    806.05 C_5-C_7 level with unspecified spinal cord injury

    806.06 C_5-C_7 level with complete lesion of cord

    806.07 C_5-C_7 level with anterior cord syndrome

    806.08 C_5-C_7 level with central cord syndrome

    806.09 C_5-C_7 level with other specified spinal cord injury
        C_5-C_7 level with:
          incomplete spinal cord lesion NOS
          posterior cord syndrome

⑤ **806.1 Cervical, open**

    806.10 C_1-C_4 level with unspecified spinal cord injury

    806.11 C_1-C_4 level with complete lesion of cord

    806.12 C_1-C_4 level with anterior cord syndrome

    806.13 C_1-C_4 level with central cord syndrome

    806.14 C_1-C_4 level with other specified spinal cord injury
        C_1-C_4 level with:
          incomplete spinal cord lesion NOS
          posterior cord syndrome

    806.15 C_5-C_7 level with unspecified spinal cord injury

    806.16 C_5-C_7 level with complete lesion of cord

    806.17 C_5-C_7 level with anterior cord syndrome

    806.18 C_5-C_7 level with central cord syndrome

    806.19 C_5-C_7 level with other specified spinal cord injury
        C_5-C_7 level with:
          incomplete spinal cord lesion NOS
          posterior cord syndrome

⑤ **806.2 Dorsal [thoracic], closed**

    806.20 T_1-T_6 level with unspecified spinal cord injury
        Thoracic region NOS with spinal cord injury NOS

    806.21 T_1-T_6 level with complete lesion of cord

    806.22 T_1-T_6 level with anterior cord syndrome

    806.23 T_1-T_6 level with central cord syndrome

● Code new   ▲ Revision of   ④ ⑤ Fourth or fifth
to this edition   existing code   digit required

806.24 T_1-T_6 level with other specified spinal cord injury
    T_1-T_6 level with:
        incomplete spinal cord lesion NOS
        posterior cord syndrome

806.25 T_7-T_{12} level with unspecified spinal cord injury

806.26 T_7-T_{12} level with complete lesion of cord

806.27 T_7-T_{12} level with anterior cord syndrome

806.28 T_7-T_{12} level with central cord syndrome

806.29 T_7-T_{12} level with other specified spinal cord injury
    T_7-T_{12} level with:
        incomplete spinal cord lesion NOS
        posterior cord syndrome

⑤ **806.3 Dorsal [thoracic], open**

806.30 T_1-T_6 level with unspecified spinal cord injury

806.31 T_1-T_6 level with complete lesion of cord

806.32 T_1-T_6 level with anterior cord syndrome

806.33 T_1-T_6 level with central cord syndrome

806.34 T_1-T_6 level with other specified spinal cord injury
    T_1-T_6 level with:
        incomplete spinal cord lesion NOS
        posterior cord syndrome

806.35 T_7-T_{12} level with unspecified spinal cord injury

806.36 T_7-T_{12} level with complete lesion of cord

806.37 T_7-$T1_2$ level with anterior cord syndrome

806.38 T_7-T_{12} level with central cord syndrome

806.39 T_7-T_{12} level with other specified spinal cord injury
    T_7-T_{12} level with:
        incomplete spinal cord lesion NOS
        posterior cord syndrome

806.4 Lumbar, closed

806.5 Lumbar, open

⑤ **806.6 Sacrum and coccyx, closed**

806.60 With unspecified spinal cord injury

806.61 With complete cauda equina lesion

806.62 With other cauda equina injury

806.69 With other spinal cord injury

⑤ **806.7 Sacrum and coccyx, open**

806.70 With unspecified spinal cord injury

806.71 With complete cauda equina lesion

806.72 With other cauda equina injury

806.79 With other spinal cord injury

806.8 Unspecified, closed

806.9 Unspecified, open

807 **Fracture of rib(s), sternum, larynx, and trachea**
The following fifth-digit subclassification is for use with codes 807.0-807.1:

0 rib(s), unspecified

1 one rib

2 two ribs

3 three ribs

4 four ribs

5 five ribs

6 six ribs

7 seven ribs

8 eight or more ribs

9 multiple ribs, unspecified

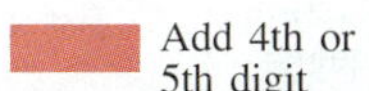
Add 4th or
5th digit

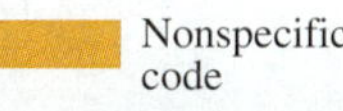
Nonspecific
code

Unspecified
code

Medicare secondary
payer(MSP) alert

⑤ **807.0** **Rib(s), closed**

⑤ **807.1** **Rib(s), open**

807.2 **Sternum, closed**

807.3 **Sternum, open**

807.4 **Flail chest**

807.5 **Larynx and trachea, closed**
      Hyoid bone   Trachea
      Thyroid cartilage

807.6 **Larynx and trachea, open**

808 **Fracture of pelvis**

808.0 **Acetabulum, closed**

808.1 **Acetabulum, open**

808.2 **Pubis, closed**

808.3 **Pubis, open**

⑤ **808.4** **Other specified part, closed**

    808.41 **Ilium**

    808.42 **Ischium**

    808.43 **Multiple pelvic fractures with disruption of pelvic circle**

    808.49 **Other**
          Innominate bone   Pelvic rim

⑤ **808.5** **Other specified part, open**

    808.51 **Ilium**

    808.52 **Ischium**

    808.53 **Multiple pelvic fractures with disruption of pelvic circle**

    808.59 **Other**

808.8 **Unspecified, closed**

808.9 **Unspecified, open**

809 **Ill-defined fractures of bones of trunk**
    Includes: bones of trunk with other bones except those of skull and face
               multiple bones of trunk

      | Excludes: | *multiple fractures of:* |

           pelvic bones alone (808.0-808.9)
           ribs alone (807.0-807.1, 807.4)
           ribs or sternum with limb bones (819.0-819.1, 828.0-828.1)
           skull or face with other bones (804.0-804.9)

809.0 **Fracture of bones of trunk, closed**

809.1 **Fracture of bones of trunk, open**

FRACTURE OF UPPER LIMB (810-819)

⑤ **810** **Fracture of clavicle**
    Includes: collar bone
               interligamentous part of clavicle

The following fifth-digit subclassification is for use with category 810:

    0 **unspecified part**
          Clavicle NOS

    1 **sternal end of clavicle**

    2 **shaft of clavicle**

    3 **acromial end of clavicle**

⑤ **810.0** **Closed**

⑤ **810.1** **Open**

⑤ **811** **Fracture of scapula**
    Includes: shoulder blade

The following fifth-digit subclassification is for use with category 811:

    0 **unspecified part**

    1 **acromial process**
          Acromion (process)

continued

● Code new   ▲ Revision of   ④ ⑤ Fourth or fifth
  to this edition   existing code   digit required

    2 **coracoid process**

    3 **glenoid cavity and neck of scapula**

    9 **other**
       Scapula body

⑤ **811.0** **Closed**

⑤ **811.1** **Open**

812 **Fracture of humerus**

⑤ **812.0** **Upper end, closed**

   812.00 **Upper end, unspecified part**
      Proximal end
      Shoulder

   812.01 **Surgical neck**
      Neck of humerus NOS

   812.02 **Anatomical neck**

   812.03 **Greater tuberosity**

   812.09 **Other**
      Head   Upper epiphysis

⑤ **812.1** **Upper end, open**

   812.10 **Upper end, unspecified part**

   812.11 **Surgical neck**

   812.12 **Anatomical neck**

   812.13 **Greater tuberosity**

   812.19 **Other**

⑤ **812.2** **Shaft or unspecified part, closed**

   812.20 **Unspecified part of humerus**
      Humerus NOS   Upper arm NOS

   812.21 **Shaft of humerus**

⑤ **812.3** **Shaft or unspecified part, open**

   812.30 **Unspecified part of humerus**

   812.31 **Shaft of humerus**

⑤ **812.4** **Lower end, closed**
    Distal end of humerus   Elbow

   812.40 **Lower end, unspecified part**

   812.41 **Supracondylar fracture of humerus**

   812.42 **Lateral condyle**
      External condyle

   812.43 **Medial condyle**
      Internal epicondyle

   812.44 **Condyle(s), unspecified**
      Articular process NOS
      Lower epiphysis NOS

   812.49 **Other**
      Multiple fractures of lower end
      Trochlea

⑤ **812.5** **Lower end, open**

   812.50 **Lower end, unspecified part**

   812.51 **Supracondylar fracture of humerus**

   812.52 **Lateral condyle**

   812.53 **Medial condyle**

   812.54 **Condyle(s), unspecified**

   812.59 **Other**

813 **Fracture of radius and ulna**

⑤ **813.0** **Upper end, closed**
    Proximal end

   813.00 **Upper end of forearm, unspecified**

   813.01 **Olecranon process of ulna**

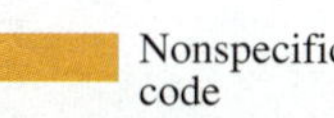

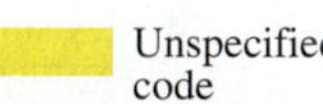

813.02 Coronoid process of ulna

813.03 Monteggia's fracture

813.04 **Other and unspecified fractures of proximal end of ulna (alone)**
Multiple fractures of ulna, upper end

813.05 Head of radius

813.06 Neck of radius

813.07 **Other and unspecified fractures of proximal end of radius (alone)**
Multiple fractures of radius, upper end

813.08 Radius with ulna, upper end [any part]

⑤ **813.1 Upper end, open**

813.10 **Upper end of forearm, unspecified**

813.11 Olecranon process of ulna

813.12 Coronoid process of ulna

813.13 Monteggia's fracture

813.14 **Other and unspecified fractures of proximal end of ulna (alone)**

813.15 Head of radius

813.16 Neck of radius

813.17 **Other and unspecified fractures of proximal end of radius (alone)**

813.18 Radius with ulna, upper end [any part]

⑤ **813.2 Shaft, closed**

813.20 **Shaft, unspecified**

813.21 Radius (alone)

813.22 Ulna (alone)

813.23 Radius with ulna

⑤ **813.3 Shaft, open**

813.30 **Shaft, unspecified**

813.31 Radius (alone)

813.32 Ulna (alone)

813.33 Radius with ulna

⑤ **813.4 Lower end, closed**
Distal end

813.40 **Lower end of forearm, unspecified**

813.41 Colles' fracture
Smith's fracture

813.42 **Other fractures of distal end of radius (alone)**
Dupuytren's fracture, radius
Radius, lower end

813.43 Distal end of ulna (alone)
Ulna: Ulna:
  head   lower epiphysis
  lower end   styloid process

813.44 Radius with ulna, lower end

● 813.45 Torus fracture of radius

⑤ **813.5 Lower end, open**

813.50 **Lower end of forearm, unspecified**

813.51 Colles' fracture

813.52 **Other fractures of distal end of radius (alone)**

813.53 Distal end of ulna (alone)

813.54 Radius with ulna, lower end

⑤ **813.8 Unspecified part, closed**

813.80 **Forearm, unspecified**

813.81 Radius (alone)

813.82 Ulna (alone)

813.83 Radius with ulna

● Code new
to this edition

▲ Revision of
existing code

④ ⑤ Fourth or fifth
digit required

⑤ **813.9　Unspecified part, open**

　　　`813.90`　**Forearm, unspecified**

　　　813.91　**Radius (alone)**

　　　813.92　**Ulna (alone)**

　　　813.93　**Radius with ulna**

⑤ `814`　**Fracture of carpal bone(s)**

The following fifth-digit subclassification is for use with category 814:

　　`0`　**carpal bone, unspecified**
　　　　Wrist NOS

　　1　**navicular [scaphoid] of wrist**

　　2　**lunate [semilunar] bone of wrist**

　　3　**triquetral [cuneiform] bone of wrist**

　　4　**pisiform**

　　5　**trapezium bone [larger multangular]**

　　6　**trapezoid bone [smaller multangular]**

　　7　**capitate bone [os magnum]**

　　8　**hamate [unciform] bone**

　　`9`　**other**

⑤ **814.0　Closed**

⑤ **814.1　Open**

⑤ `815`　**Fracture of metacarpal bone(s)**
Includes:hand [except finger]
　　　　　metacarpus

The following fifth-digit subclassification is for use with category 815:

　　`0`　**metacarpal bone(s), site unspecified**

　　1　**base of thumb [first] metacarpal**
　　　　Bennett's fracture

　　2　**base of other metacarpal bone(s)**

　　3　**shaft of metacarpal bone(s)**

　　4　**neck of metacarpal bone(s)**

　　`9`　**multiple sites of metacarpus**

⑤ **815.0　Closed**

⑤ **815.1　Open**

⑤ `816`　**Fracture of one or more phalanges of hand**
Includes:　finger(s)
　　　　　　thumb

The following fifth-digit subclassification is for use with category 816:

　　`0`　**phalanx or phalanges, unspecified**

　　1　**middle or proximal phalanx or phalanges**

　　2　**distal phalanx or phalanges**

　　`3`　**multiple sites**

⑤ **816.0　Closed**

⑤ **816.1　Open**

`817`　**Multiple fractures of hand bones**
Includes:　metacarpal bone(s) with phalanx or phalanges of same hand

`817.0`　**Closed**

`817.1`　**Open**

`818`　**Ill-defined fractures of upper limb**
Includes:　arm NOS
　　　　　　multiple bones of same upper limb

　　|Excludes:| *multiple fractures of:*
　　　　　　metacarpal bone(s) with phalanx or phalanges (817.0-817.1)
　　　　　　phalanges of hand alone (816.0-816.1)
　　　　　　radius with ulna (813.0-813.9)

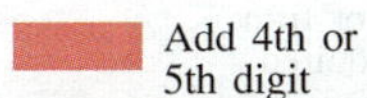 Add 4th or 5th digit

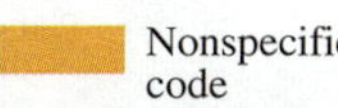 Nonspecific code

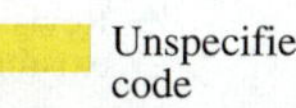 Unspecified code

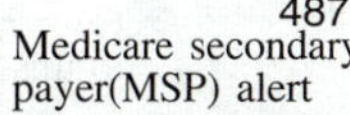 Medicare secondary payer(MSP) alert

818.0 Closed

818.1 Open

819 Multiple fractures involving both upper limbs, and upper limb with rib(s) and sternum
Includes: arm(s) with rib(s) or sternum
both arms [any bones]

819.0 Closed

819.1 Open

FRACTURE OF LOWER LIMB (820-829)

820 Fracture of neck of femur

⑤ **820.0 Transcervical fracture, closed**

820.00 Intracapsular section, unspecified

820.01 Epiphysis (separation) (upper)
Transepiphyseal

820.02 Midcervical section
Transcervical NOS

820.03 Base of neck
Cervicotrochanteric section

820.09 Other
Head of femur
Subcapital

⑤ **820.1 Transcervical fracture, open**

820.10 Intracapsular section, unspecified

820.11 Epiphysis (separation) (upper)

820.12 Midcervical section

820.13 Base of neck

820.19 Other

⑤ **820.2 Pertrochanteric fracture, closed**

820.20 Trochanteric section, unspecified
Trochanter:
NOS
greater
lesser

820.21 Intertrochanteric section

820.22 Subtrochanteric section

⑤ **820.3 Pertrochanteric fracture, open**

820.30 Trochanteric section, unspecified

820.31 Intertrochanteric section

820.32 Subtrochanteric section

820.8 Unspecified part of neck of femur, closed
Hip NOS   Neck of femur NOS

820.9 Unspecified part of neck of femur, open

821 Fracture of other and unspecified parts of femur

⑤ **821.0 Shaft or unspecified part, closed**

821.00 Unspecified part of femur
Thigh   Upper leg

Excludes: hip NOS (820.8)

821.01 Shaft

⑤ **821.1 Shaft or unspecified part, open**

821.10 Unspecified part of femur

821.11 Shaft

⑤ **821.2 Lower end, closed**
Distal end

821.20 Lower end, unspecified part

821.21 Condyle, femoral

821.22 Epiphysis, lower (separation)

● Code new
  to this edition
▲ Revision of
  existing code
④ ⑤ Fourth or fifth
  digit required

821.23   **Supracondylar fracture of femur**

821.29   **Other**
Multiple fractures of lower end

⑤ **821.3**   **Lower end, open**

821.30   **Lower end, unspecified part**

821.31   **Condyle, femoral**

821.32   **Epiphysis, lower (separation)**

821.33   **Supracondylar fracture of femur**

821.39   **Other**

822   **Fracture of patella**

822.0   **Closed**

822.1   **Open**

⑤ **823**   **Fracture of tibia and fibula**

> |Excludes:| *Dupuytren's fracture (824.4-824.5)*
> *ankle (824.4-824.5)*
> *radius (813.42, 813.52)*
> *Pott's fracture (824.4-824.5)*
> *that involving ankle (824.0-824.9)*

The following fifth-digit subclassification is for use with category 823:

0   **tibia alone**

1   **fibula alone**

2   **fibula with tibia**

⑤ **823.0**   **Upper end, closed**
Head   Tibia:
Proximal end   condyles
                              tuberosity

⑤ **823.1**   **Upper end, open**

⑤ **823.2**   **Shaft, closed**

⑤ **823.3**   **Shaft, open**

● **823.4**   **Torus fracture**

⑤ **823.8**   **Unspecified part, closed**
Lower leg NOS

⑤ **823.9**   **Unspecified part, open**

824   **Fracture of ankle**

824.0   **Medial malleolus, closed**
Tibia involving:
    ankle
    malleolus

824.1   **Medial malleolus, open**

824.2   **Lateral malleolus, closed**
Fibula involving:
    ankle
    malleolus

824.3   **Lateral malleolus, open**

824.4   **Bimalleolar, closed**
Dupuytren's fracture, fibula
Pott's fracture

824.5   **Bimalleolar, open**

824.6   **Trimalleolar, closed**
Lateral and medial malleolus with anterior or posterior lip of tibia

824.7   **Trimalleolar, open**

824.8   **Unspecified, closed**
Ankle NOS

824.9   **Unspecified, open**

825   **Fracture of one or more tarsal and metatarsal bones**

825.0   **Fracture of calcaneus, closed**
Heel bone   Os calcis

	Add 4th or 5th digit		Nonspecific code		Unspecified code		Medicare secondary payer(MSP) alert

825.1 **Fracture of calcaneus, open**

⑤ 825.2 **Fracture of other tarsal and metatarsal bones, closed**

825.20 **Unspecified bone(s) of foot [except toes]**
Instep

825.21 **Astragalus**
Talus

825.22 **Navicular [scaphoid], foot**

825.23 **Cuboid**

825.24 **Cuneiform, foot**

825.25 **Metatarsal bone(s)**

825.29 **Other**
Tarsal with metatarsal bone(s) only

Excludes: *calcaneus (825.0)*

⑤ 825.3 **Fracture of other tarsal and metatarsal bones, open**

825.30 **Unspecified bone(s) of foot [except toes]**

825.31 **Astragalus**

825.32 **Navicular [scaphoid], foot**

825.33 **Cuboid**

825.34 **Cuneiform, foot**

825.35 **Metatarsal bone(s)**

825.39 **Other**

826 **Fracture of one or more phalanges of foot**
Includes: toe(s)

826.0 **Closed**

826.1 **Open**

827 **Other, multiple, and ill-defined fractures of lower limb**
Includes: leg NOS
multiple bones of same lower limb

Excludes: *multiple fractures of:*
ankle bones alone (824.4-824.9)
phalanges of foot alone (826.0-826.1)
tarsal with metatarsal bones (825.29, 825.39)
tibia with fibula (823.0-823.9 with fifth-digit 2)

827.0 **Closed**

827.1 **Open**

828 **Multiple fractures involving both lower limbs, lower with upper limb, and lower limb(s) with rib(s) and sternum**
Includes: arm(s) with leg(s) [any bones]
both legs [any bones]
leg(s) with rib(s) or sternum

828.0 **Closed**

828.1 **Open**

829 **Fracture of unspecified bones**

829.0 **Unspecified bone, closed**

829.1 **Unspecified bone, open**

● Code new
to this edition

▲ Revision of
existing code

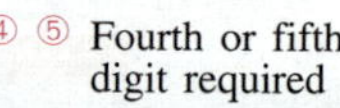
④ ⑤ Fourth or fifth
digit required

DISLOCATION (830-839)

Includes: displacement
subluxation

Excludes: *congenital dislocation (754.0-755.8)*
pathological dislocation (718.2)
recurrent dislocation (718.3)

The descriptions "closed" and "open", used in the fourth-digit subdivisions, include the following terms:

closed:	open:
complete	compound
dislocation NOS	infected
partial	with foreign body
simple	
uncomplicated	

A dislocation not indicated as closed or open should be classified as closed.

830 Dislocation of jaw

Includes: jaw (cartilage) (meniscus)
mandible
maxilla (inferior)
temporomandibular (joint)

830.0 Closed dislocation

830.1 Open dislocation

831 Dislocation of shoulder

Excludes: *sternoclavicular joint (839.61, 839.71)*
sternum (839.61, 839.71)

The following fifth-digit subclassification is for use with category 831:

0 shoulder, unspecified
Humerus NOS

1 anterior dislocation of humerus

2 posterior dislocation of humerus

3 inferior dislocation of humerus

4 acromioclavicular (joint)
Clavicle

9 other
Scapula

831.0 Closed dislocation

831.1 Open dislocation

832 Dislocation of elbow

The following fifth-digit subclassification is for use with category 832:

0 elbow unspecified

1 anterior dislocation of elbow

2 posterior dislocation of elbow

3 medial dislocation of elbow

4 lateral dislocation of elbow

9 other

832.0 Closed dislocation

832.1 Open dislocation

833 Dislocation of wrist

The following fifth-digit subclassification is for use with category 833:

0 wrist, unspecified part
Carpal (bone)   Radius, distal end

1 radioulnar (joint), distal

2 radiocarpal (joint)

3 midcarpal (joint)

4 carpometacarpal (joint)

5 metacarpal (bone), proximal end

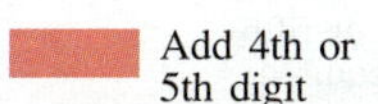 Add 4th or 5th digit

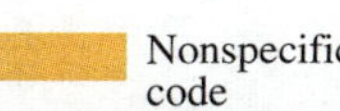 Nonspecific code

 Unspecified code

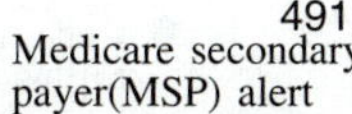 Medicare secondary payer(MSP) alert

9 other
   Ulna, distal end

⑤ **833.0 Closed dislocation**

⑤ **833.1 Open dislocation**

⑤ **834 Dislocation of finger**
   Includes: finger(s)
           phalanx of hand
           thumb

The following fifth-digit subclassification is for use with category 834:

   0 finger, unspecified part

   1 metacarpophalangeal (joint)
      Metacarpal (bone), distal end

   2 interphalangeal (joint), hand

⑤ **834.0 Closed dislocation**

⑤ **834.1 Open dislocation**

⑤ **835 Dislocation of hip**

The following fifth-digit subclassification is for use with category 835:

   0 dislocation of hip, unspecified

   1 posterior dislocation

   2 obturator dislocation

   3 other anterior dislocation

⑤ **835.0 Closed dislocation**

⑤ **835.1 Open dislocation**

836 Dislocation of knee

   Excludes: *dislocation of knee:*
      old or pathological (718.2)
      recurrent (718.3)
      internal derangement of knee joint (717.0-717.5, 717.8-717.9)
      old tear of cartilage or meniscus of knee (717.0-717.5, 717.8-717.9)

836.0 Tear of medial cartilage or meniscus of knee, current
   Bucket handle tear:
      NOS
      medial meniscus } current injury

836.1 Tear of lateral cartilage or meniscus of knee, current

836.2 Other tear of cartilage or meniscus of knee, current
   Tear of:
      cartilage (semilunar) } current injury, not specified as medial or lateral
      meniscus

836.3 Dislocation of patella, closed

836.4 Dislocation of patella, open

⑤ **836.5 Other dislocation of knee, closed**

   836.50 Dislocation of knee, unspecified

   836.51 Anterior dislocation of tibia, proximal end
      Posterior dislocation of femur, distal end

   836.52 Posterior dislocation of tibia, proximal end
      Anterior dislocation of femur, distal end

   836.53 Medial dislocation of tibia, proximal end

   836.54 Lateral dislocation of tibia, proximal end

   836.59 Other

⑤ **836.6 Other dislocation of knee, open**

   836.60 Dislocation of knee, unspecified

   836.61 Anterior dislocation of tibia, proximal end

   836.62 Posterior dislocation of tibia, proximal end

   836.63 Medial dislocation of tibia, proximal end

   836.64 Lateral dislocation of tibia, proximal end

   836.69 Other

● Code new to this edition   ▲ Revision of existing code   ④ ⑤ Fourth or fifth digit required

837 Dislocation of ankle

Includes:

astragalus	navicular, foot
fibula, distal end	scaphoid, foot
	tibia, distal end

837.0 Closed dislocation

837.1 Open dislocation

838 Dislocation of foot

The following fifth-digit subclassification is for use with category 838:

0 foot, unspecified

1 tarsal (bone), joint unspecified

2 midtarsal (joint)

3 tarsometatarsal (joint)

4 metatarsal (bone), joint unspecified

5 metatarsophalangeal (joint)

6 interphalangeal (joint), foot

9 other

Phalanx of foot	Toe(s)

838.0 Closed dislocation

838.1 Open dislocation

839 Other, multiple, and ill-defined dislocations

839.0 Cervical vertebra, closed

Cervical spine	Neck

839.00 Cervical vertebra, unspecified

839.01 First cervical vertebra

839.02 Second cervical vertebra

839.03 Third cervical vertebra

839.04 Fourth cervical vertebra

839.05 Fifth cervical vertebra

839.06 Sixth cervical vertebra

839.07 Seventh cervical vertebra

839.08 Multiple cervical vertebrae

839.1 Cervical vertebra, open

839.10 Cervical vertebra, unspecified

839.11 First cervical vertebra

839.12 Second cervical vertebra

839.13 Third cervical vertebra

839.14 Fourth cervical vertebra

839.15 Fifth cervical vertebra

839.16 Sixth cervical vertebra

839.17 Seventh cervical vertebra

839.18 Multiple cervical vertebrae

839.2 Thoracic and lumbar vertebra, closed

839.20 Lumbar vertebra

839.21 Thoracic vertebra

Dorsal [thoracic] vertebra

839.3 Thoracic and lumbar vertebra, open

839.30 Lumbar vertebra

839.31 Thoracic vertebra

839.4 Other vertebra, closed

839.40 Vertebra, unspecified site

Spine NOS

839.41 Coccyx

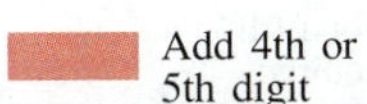

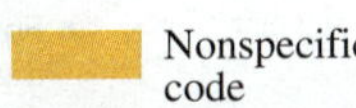

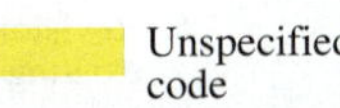

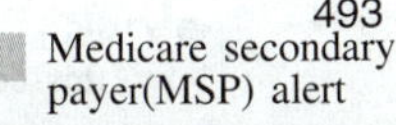

839.42 Sacrum
Sacroiliac (joint)

839.49 Other

⑤ **839.5 Other vertebra, open**

839.50 Vertebra, unspecified site

839.51 Coccyx

839.52 Sacrum

839.59 Other

⑤ **839.6 Other location, closed**

839.61 Sternum
Sternoclavicular joint

839.69 Other
Pelvis

⑤ **839.7 Other location, open**

839.71 Sternum

839.79 Other

839.8 Multiple and ill-defined, closed
Arm
Back
Hand
Multiple locations, except fingers or toes alone
Other ill-defined locations
Unspecified location

839.9 Multiple and ill-defined, open

SPRAINS AND STRAINS OF JOINTS AND ADJACENT MUSCLES (840-848)

Includes:

avulsion	
hemarthrosis	joint capsule
laceration	ligament
rupture	of: muscle
sprain	tendon
strain	
tear	

Excludes: *laceration of tendon in open wounds (880-884 and 890-894 with .2)*

840 Sprains and strains of shoulder and upper arm

840.0 Acromioclavicular (joint) (ligament)

840.1 Coracoclavicular (ligament)

840.2 Coracohumeral (ligament)

840.3 Infraspinatus (muscle) (tendon)

840.4 Rotator cuff (capsule)

Excludes: *complete rupture of rotator cuff, nontraumatic (727.61)*

840.5 Subscapularis (muscle)

840.6 Supraspinatus (muscle) (tendon)

840.7 Superior glenoid labrum lesion
SLAP lesion

840.8 Other specified sites of shoulder and upper arm

840.9 Unspecified site of shoulder and upper arm
Arm NOS   Shoulder NOS

841 Sprains and strains of elbow and forearm

841.0 Radial collateral ligament

841.1 Ulnar collateral ligament

841.2 Radiohumeral (joint)

841.3 Ulnohumeral (joint)

841.8 Other specified sites of elbow and forearm

841.9 Unspecified site of elbow and forearm
Elbow NOS

● Code new
to this edition

▲ Revision of
existing code

④ ⑤ Fourth or fifth
digit required

842 Sprains and strains of wrist and hand

⑤ **842.0 Wrist**

    842.00 Unspecified site

    842.01 Carpal (joint)

    842.02 Radiocarpal (joint) (ligament)

    842.09 Other
        Radioulnar joint, distal

⑤ **842.1 Hand**

    842.10 Unspecified site

    842.11 Carpometacarpal (joint)

    842.12 Metacarpophalangeal (joint)

    842.13 Interphalangeal (joint)

    842.19 Other
        Midcarpal (joint)

843 Sprains and strains of hip and thigh

    843.0 Iliofemoral (ligament)

    843.1 Ischiocapsular (ligament)

    843.8 Other specified sites of hip and thigh

    843.9 Unspecified site of hip and thigh
        Hip NOS   Thigh NOS

844 Sprains and strains of knee and leg

    844.0 Lateral collateral ligament of knee

    844.1 Medial collateral ligament of knee

    844.2 Cruciate ligament of knee

    844.3 Tibiofibular (joint) (ligament), superior

    844.8 Other specified sites of knee and leg

    844.9 Unspecified site of knee and leg
        Knee NOS   Leg NOS

845 Sprains and strains of ankle and foot

⑤ **845.0 Ankle**

    845.00 Unspecified site

    845.01 Deltoid (ligament), ankle
        Internal collateral (ligament), ankle

    845.02 Calcaneofibular (ligament)

    845.03 Tibiofibular (ligament), distal

    845.09 Other
        Achilles tendon

⑤ **845.1 Foot**

    845.10 Unspecified site

    845.11 Tarsometatarsal (joint) (ligament)

    845.12 Metatarsophalangeal (joint)

    845.13 Interphalangeal (joint), toe

    845.19 Other

846 Sprains and strains of sacroiliac region

    846.0 Lumbosacral (joint) (ligament)

    846.1 Sacroiliac ligament

    846.2 Sacrospinatus (ligament)

    846.3 Sacrotuberous (ligament)

    846.8 Other specified sites of sacroiliac region

    846.9 Unspecified site of sacroiliac region

847 Sprains and strains of other and unspecified parts of back

    Excludes: lumbosacral (846.0)

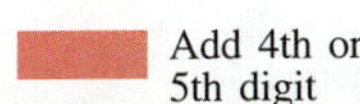 Add 4th or 5th digit    Nonspecific code   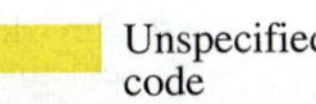 Unspecified code   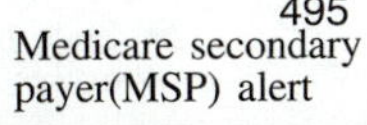 Medicare secondary payer(MSP) alert

847.0 **Neck**
      Anterior longitudinal (ligament), cervical
      Atlanto-axial (joints)
      Atlanto-occipital (joints)
      Whiplash injury
    Excludes: *neck injury NOS (959.0)*
          thyroid region (848.2)

847.1 **Thoracic**

847.2 **Lumbar**

847.3 **Sacrum**
      Sacrococcygeal (ligament)

847.4 **Coccyx**

847.9 **Unspecified site of back**
      Back NOS

848 **Other and ill-defined sprains and strains**

848.0 **Septal cartilage of nose**

848.1 **Jaw**
      Temporomandibular (joint) (ligament)

848.2 **Thyroid region**
      Cricoarytenoid (joint) (ligament)
      Cricothyroid (joint) (ligament)
      Thyroid cartilage

848.3 **Ribs**
      Chondrocostal (joint) ⎫
      Costal cartilage ⎬ without mention of injury to sternum

⑤ **848.4** **Sternum**

    848.40 **Unspecified site**

    848.41 **Sternoclavicular (joint) (ligament)**

    848.42 **Chondrosternal (joint)**

    848.49 **Other**
        Xiphoid cartilage

848.5 **Pelvis**
      Symphysis pubis
    Excludes: *that in childbirth (665.6)*

848.8 **Other specified sites of sprains and strains**

848.9 **Unspecified site of sprain and strain**

INTRACRANIAL INJURY, EXCLUDING THOSE WITH SKULL FRACTURE (850-854)

    Excludes: *intracranial injury with skull fracture (800-801 and 803-804, except .0 and .5)*
        open wound of head without intracranial injury (870.0-873.9)
        skull fracture alone (800-801 and 803-804 with .0, .5)

The description "with open intracranial wound," used in the fourth-digit subdivisions, includes those specified as open or with mention of infection or foreign body.

The following fifth-digit subclassification is for use with categories 851-854:

  0   **unspecified state of consciousness**

  1   **with no loss of consciousness**

  2   **with brief [less than one hour] loss of consciousness**

  3   **with moderate [1-24 hours] loss of consciousness**

  4   **with prolonged [more than 24 hours] loss of consciousness and return to pre-existing conscious level**

  5   **with prolonged [more than 24 hours] loss of consciousness, without return to pre-existing conscious level**

      Use fifth-digit 5 to designate when a patient is unconscious and dies before regaining consciousness, regardless of the duration of the loss of consciousness

  6   **with loss of consciousness of unspecified duration**

  9   **with concussion, unspecified**

  ● Code new to this edition   ▲ Revision of existing code   ④ ⑤ Fourth or fifth digit required

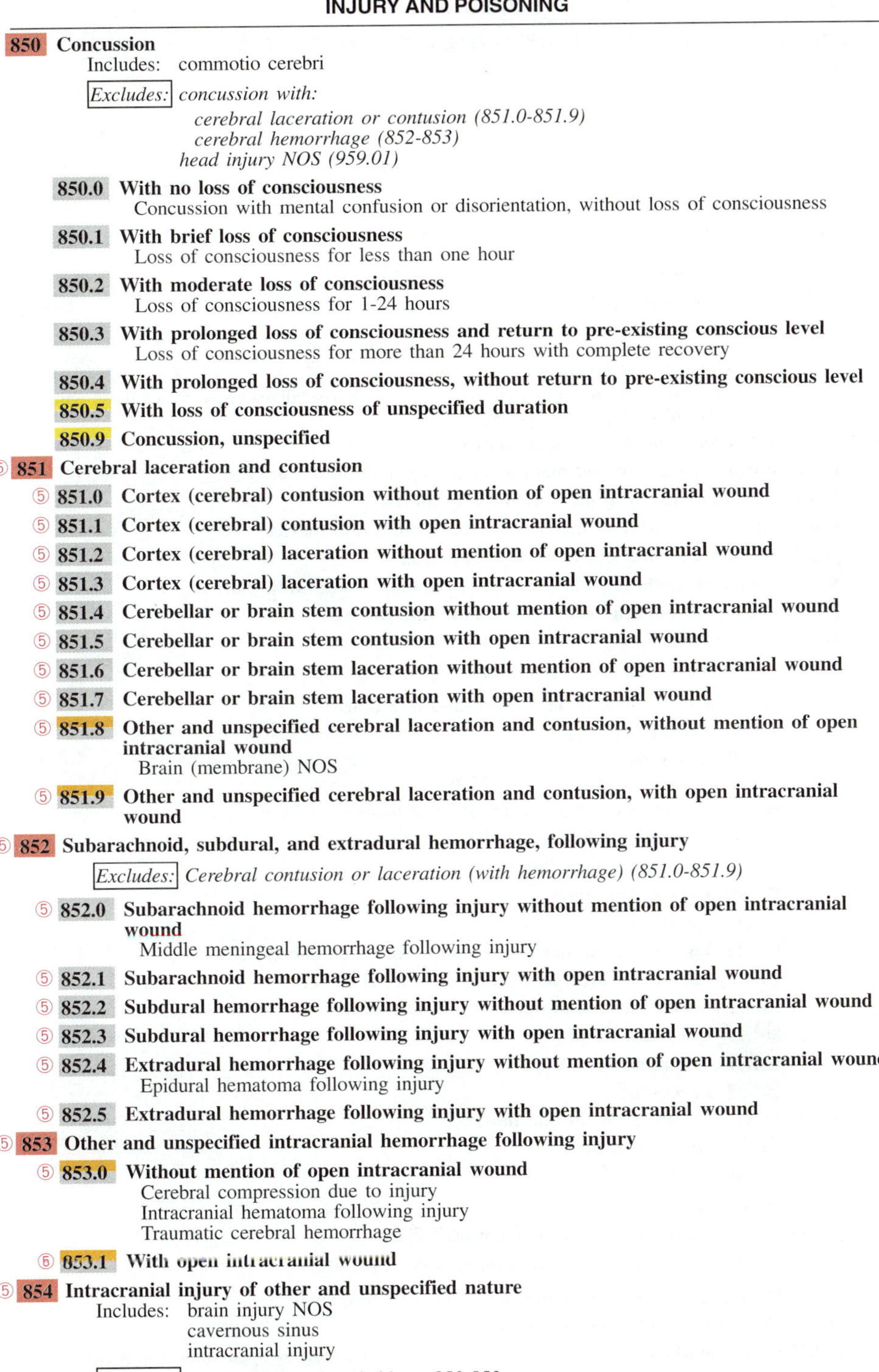

850 Concussion
Includes: commotio cerebri

Excludes: concussion with:
cerebral laceration or contusion (851.0-851.9)
cerebral hemorrhage (852-853)
head injury NOS (959.01)

850.0 With no loss of consciousness
Concussion with mental confusion or disorientation, without loss of consciousness

850.1 With brief loss of consciousness
Loss of consciousness for less than one hour

850.2 With moderate loss of consciousness
Loss of consciousness for 1-24 hours

850.3 With prolonged loss of consciousness and return to pre-existing conscious level
Loss of consciousness for more than 24 hours with complete recovery

850.4 With prolonged loss of consciousness, without return to pre-existing conscious level

850.5 With loss of consciousness of unspecified duration

850.9 Concussion, unspecified

851 Cerebral laceration and contusion

851.0 Cortex (cerebral) contusion without mention of open intracranial wound

851.1 Cortex (cerebral) contusion with open intracranial wound

851.2 Cortex (cerebral) laceration without mention of open intracranial wound

851.3 Cortex (cerebral) laceration with open intracranial wound

851.4 Cerebellar or brain stem contusion without mention of open intracranial wound

851.5 Cerebellar or brain stem contusion with open intracranial wound

851.6 Cerebellar or brain stem laceration without mention of open intracranial wound

851.7 Cerebellar or brain stem laceration with open intracranial wound

851.8 Other and unspecified cerebral laceration and contusion, without mention of open intracranial wound
Brain (membrane) NOS

851.9 Other and unspecified cerebral laceration and contusion, with open intracranial wound

852 Subarachnoid, subdural, and extradural hemorrhage, following injury

Excludes: *Cerebral contusion or laceration (with hemorrhage) (851.0-851.9)*

852.0 Subarachnoid hemorrhage following injury without mention of open intracranial wound
Middle meningeal hemorrhage following injury

852.1 Subarachnoid hemorrhage following injury with open intracranial wound

852.2 Subdural hemorrhage following injury without mention of open intracranial wound

852.3 Subdural hemorrhage following injury with open intracranial wound

852.4 Extradural hemorrhage following injury without mention of open intracranial wound
Epidural hematoma following injury

852.5 Extradural hemorrhage following injury with open intracranial wound

853 Other and unspecified intracranial hemorrhage following injury

853.0 Without mention of open intracranial wound
Cerebral compression due to injury
Intracranial hematoma following injury
Traumatic cerebral hemorrhage

853.1 With open intracranial wound

854 Intracranial injury of other and unspecified nature
Includes: brain injury NOS
cavernous sinus
intracranial injury

Excludes: *any condition classifiable to 850-853*
head injury NOS (959.01)

854.0 Without mention of open intracranial wound

854.1 With open intracranial wound

INTERNAL INJURY OF THORAX, ABDOMEN, AND PELVIS (860-869)

Includes:

> blast injuries
> blunt trauma
> bruise
> concussion injuries (except cerebral)
> crushing
> hematoma   } of internal organs
> laceration
> puncture
> tear
> traumatic rupture

Excludes: *concussion NOS (850.0-850.9)*
flail chest (807.4)
foreign body entering through orifice (930.0-939.9)
injury to blood vessels (901.0-902.9)

The description "with open wound," used in the fourth-digit subdivisions, includes those with mention of infection or foreign body.

860 Traumatic pneumothorax and hemothorax

860.0 Pneumothorax without mention of open wound into thorax

860.1 Pneumothorax with open wound into thorax

860.2 Hemothorax without mention of open wound into thorax

860.3 Hemothorax with open wound into thorax

860.4 Pneumohemothorax without mention of open wound into thorax

860.5 Pneumohemothorax with open wound into thorax

861 Injury to heart and lung

Excludes: *injury to blood vessels of thorax (901.0-901.9)*

⑤ **861.0 Heart, without mention of open wound into thorax**

861.00 Unspecified injury

861.01 Contusion

Cardiac contusion   Myocardial contusion

861.02 Laceration without penetration of heart chambers

861.03 Laceration with penetration of heart chambers

⑤ **861.1 Heart, with open wound into thorax**

861.10 Unspecified injury

861.11 Contusion

861.12 Laceration without penetration of heart chambers

861.13 Laceration with penetration of heart chambers

⑤ **861.2 Lung, without mention of open wound into thorax**

861.20 Unspecified injury

861.21 Contusion

861.22 Laceration

⑤ **861.3 Lung, with open wound into thorax**

861.30 Unspecified injury

861.31 Contusion

861.32 Laceration

862 Injury to other and unspecified intrathoracic organs

Excludes: *injury to blood vessels of thorax (901.0-901.9)*

862.0 Diaphragm, without mention of open wound into cavity

862.1 Diaphragm, with open wound into cavity

⑤ **862.2 Other specified intrathoracic organs, without mention of open wound into cavity**

862.21 Bronchus

862.22 Esophagus

862.29 Other

Pleura   Thymus gland

● Code new
to this edition

▲ Revision of
existing code

④ ⑤ Fourth or fifth
digit required

⑤ **862.3 Other specified intrathoracic organs, with open wound into cavity**

    862.31 Bronchus

    862.32 Esophagus

    862.39 Other

862.8 Multiple and unspecified intrathoracic organs, without mention of open wound into cavity
Crushed chest
Multiple intrathoracic organs

862.9 Multiple and unspecified intrathoracic organs, with open wound into cavity

863 Injury to gastrointestinal tract

    Excludes: anal sphincter laceration during delivery (664.2)
              bile duct (868.0-868.1 with fifth-digit 2)
              gallbladder (868.0-868.1 with fifth-digit 2)

863.0 Stomach, without mention of open wound into cavity

863.1 Stomach, with open wound into cavity

⑤ **863.2 Small intestine, without mention of open wound into cavity**

    863.20 Small intestine, unspecified site

    863.21 Duodenum

    863.29 Other

⑤ **863.3 Small intestine, with open wound into cavity**

    863.30 Small intestine, unspecified site

    863.31 Duodenum

    863.39 Other

⑤ **863.4 Colon or rectum, without mention of open wound into cavity**

    863.40 Colon, unspecified site

    863.41 Ascending [right] colon

    863.42 Transverse colon

    863.43 Descending [left] colon

    863.44 Sigmoid colon

    863.45 Rectum

    863.46 Multiple sites in colon and rectum

    863.49 Other

⑤ **863.5 Colon or rectum, with open wound into cavity**

    863.50 Colon, unspecified site

    863.51 Ascending [right] colon

    863.52 Transverse colon

    863.53 Descending [left] colon

    863.54 Sigmoid colon

    863.55 Rectum

    863.56 Multiple sites in colon and rectum

    863.59 Other

⑤ **863.8 Other and unspecified gastrointestinal sites, without mention of open wound into cavity**

    863.80 Gastrointestinal tract, unspecified site

    863.81 Pancreas, head

    863.82 Pancreas, body

    863.83 Pancreas, tail

    863.84 Pancreas, multiple and unspecified sites

    863.85 Appendix

    863.89 Other
        Intestine NOS

⑤ **863.9 Other and unspecified gastrointestinal sites, with open wound into cavity**

    863.90 Gastrointestinal tract, unspecified site

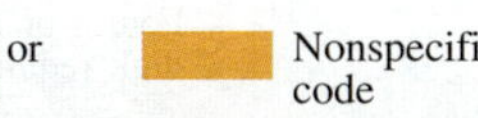

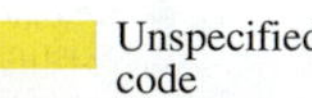

863.91 **Pancreas, head**

863.92 **Pancreas, body**

863.93 **Pancreas, tail**

863.94 **Pancreas, multiple and unspecified sites**

863.95 **Appendix**

863.99 **Other**

⑤ **864 Injury to liver**

The following fifth-digit subclassification is for use with category 864:

  0 **unspecified injury**

  1 **hematoma and contusion**

  2 **laceration, minor**
Laceration involving capsule only, or without significant involvement of hepatic parenchyma [i.e., less than 1 cm deep]

  3 **laceration, moderate**
Laceration involving parenchyma but without major disruption of parenchyma [i.e., less than 10 cm long and less than 3 cm deep]

  4 **laceration, major**
Laceration with significant disruption of hepatic parenchyma [i.e., 10 cm long and 3 cm deep]
Multiple moderate lacerations, with or without hematoma
Stellate lacerations of liver

  5 **laceration, unspecified**

  9 **other**

⑤ **864.0** **Without mention of open wound into cavity**

⑤ **864.1** **With open wound into cavity**

⑤ **865 Injury to spleen**

The following fifth-digit subclassification is for use with category 865:

  0 **unspecified injury**

  1 **hematoma without rupture of capsule**

  2 **capsular tears, without major disruption of parenchyma**

  3 **laceration extending into parenchyma**

  4 **massive parenchymal disruption**

  9 **other**

⑤ **865.0** **Without mention of open wound into cavity**

⑤ **865.1** **With open wound into cavity**

⑤ **866 Injury to kidney**

The following fifth-digit subclassification is for use with category 866:

  0 **unspecified injury**

  1 **hematoma without rupture of capsule**

  2 **laceration**

  3 **complete disruption of kidney parenchyma**

⑤ **866.0** **Without mention of open wound into cavity**

⑤ **866.1** **With open wound into cavity**

867 Injury to pelvic organs

> *Excludes:* *injury during delivery (664.0-665.9)*

867.0 **Bladder and urethra, without mention of open wound into cavity**

867.1 **Bladder and urethra, with open wound into cavity**

867.2 **Ureter, without mention of open wound into cavity**

867.3 **Ureter, with open wound into cavity**

867.4 **Uterus, without mention of open wound into cavity**

867.5 **Uterus, with open wound into cavity**

867.6 **Other specified pelvic organs, without mention of open wound into cavity**
Fallopian tube   Seminal vesicle
Ovary   Vas deferens
Prostate

● Code new to this edition   ▲ Revision of existing code   ④ ⑤ Fourth or fifth digit required

867.7 Other specified pelvic organs, with open wound into cavity

867.8 Unspecified pelvic organs, without mention of open wound into cavity

867.9 Unspecified pelvic organ, with open wound into cavity

⑤ **868** **Injury to other intra-abdominal organs**

The following fifth-digit subclassification is for use with category 868:

0 unspecified intra-abdominal organ

1 adrenal gland

2 bile duct and gallbladder

3 peritoneum

4 retroperitoneum

9 other and multiple intra-abdominal organs

⑤ **868.0** Without mention of open wound into cavity

⑤ **868.1** With open wound into cavity

869 **Internal injury to unspecified or ill-defined organs**

Includes: internal injury NOS
multiple internal injury NOS

869.0 Without mention of open wound into cavity

869.1 With open wound into cavity

OPEN WOUND (870-897)

Includes:

animal bite	laceration
avulsion	puncture wound
cut	traumatic amputation

Excludes: *burn (940.0-949.5)*
crushing (925-929.9)
puncture of internal organs (860.0-869.1)
superficial injury (910.0-919.9)
that incidental to:
dislocation (830.0-839.9)
fracture (800.0-829.1)
internal injury (860.0-869.1)
intracranial injury (851.0-854.1)

Note: The description "complicated" used in the fourth-digit subdivisions includes those with mention of delayed healing, delayed treatment, foreign body, or infection.

Use additional code to identify infection.

OPEN WOUND OF HEAD, NECK, AND TRUNK (870-879)

870 **Open wound of ocular adnexa**

870.0 Laceration of skin of eyelid and periocular area

870.1 Laceration of eyelid, full-thickness, not involving lacrimal passages

870.2 Laceration of eyelid involving lacrimal passages

870.3 Penetrating wound of orbit, without mention of foreign body

870.4 Penetrating wound of orbit with foreign body

Excludes: *retained (old) foreign body in orbit (376.6)*

870.8 Other specified open wounds of ocular adnexa

870.9 Unspecified open wound of ocular adnexa

871 **Open wound of eyeball**

Excludes: *2nd cranial nerve [optic] injury (950.0-950.9)*
3rd cranial nerve [oculomotor] injury (951.0)

871.0 Ocular laceration without prolapse of intraocular tissue

871.1 Ocular laceration with prolapse or exposure of intraocular tissue

871.2 Rupture of eye with partial loss of intraocular tissue

871.3 Avulsion of eye
Traumatic enucleation

871.4 Unspecified laceration of eye

871.5 Penetration of eyeball with magnetic foreign body

> *Excludes:* *retained (old) magnetic foreign body in globe (360.50-360.59)*

871.6 Penetration of eyeball with (nonmagnetic) foreign body

> *Excludes:* *retained (old) (nonmagnetic) foreign body in globe (360.60-360.69)*

871.7 Unspecified ocular penetration

871.9 Unspecified open wound of eyeball

872 Open wound of ear

⑤ **872.0 External ear, without mention of complication**

    872.00 External ear, unspecified site

    872.01 Auricle, ear
        Pinna

    872.02 Auditory canal

⑤ **872.1 External ear, complicated**

    872.10 External ear, unspecified site

    872.11 Auricle, ear

    872.12 Auditory canal

⑤ **872.6 Other specified parts of ear, without mention of complication**

    872.61 Ear drum
        Drumhead   Tympanic membrane

    872.62 Ossicles

    872.63 Eustachian tube

    872.64 Cochlea

    872.69 Other and multiple sites

⑤ **872.7 Other specified parts of ear, complicated**

    872.71 Ear drum

    872.72 Ossicles

    872.73 Eustachian tube

    872.74 Cochlea

    872.79 Other and multiple sites

872.8 Ear, part unspecified, without mention of complication
    Ear NOS

872.9 Ear, part unspecified, complicated

873 Other open wound of head

873.0 Scalp, without mention of complication

873.1 Scalp, complicated

⑤ **873.2 Nose, without mention of complication**

    873.20 Nose, unspecified site

    873.21 Nasal septum

    873.22 Nasal cavity

    873.23 Nasal sinus

    873.29 Multiple sites

⑤ **873.3 Nose, complicated**

    873.30 Nose, unspecified site

    873.31 Nasal septum

    873.32 Nasal cavity

    873.33 Nasal sinus

    873.39 Multiple sites

⑤ **873.4 Face, without mention of complication**

    873.40 Face, unspecified site

    873.41 Cheek

    873.42 Forehead
        Eyebrow

    873.43 Lip

● Code new to this edition   ▲ Revision of existing code   ④ ⑤ Fourth or fifth digit required

    873.44   **Jaw**

    873.49   **Other and multiple sites**

⑤ 873.5 **Face, complicated**

    873.50   **Face, unspecified site**

    873.51   **Cheek**

    873.52   **Forehead**

    873.53   **Lip**

    873.54   **Jaw**

    873.59   **Other and multiple sites**

⑤ 873.6 **Internal structures of mouth, without mention of complication**

    873.60   **Mouth, unspecified site**

    873.61   **Buccal mucosa**

    873.62   **Gum (alveolar process)**

    873.63   **Tooth (broken)**

    873.64   **Tongue and floor of mouth**

    873.65   **Palate**

    873.69   **Other and multiple sites**

⑤ 873.7 **Internal structures of mouth, complicated**

    873.70   **Mouth, unspecified site**

    873.71   **Buccal mucosa**

    873.72   **Gum (alveolar process)**

    873.73   **Tooth (broken)**

    873.74   **Tongue and floor of mouth**

    873.75   **Palate**

    873.79   **Other and multiple sites**

  873.8 **Other and unspecified open wound of head without mention of complication**
     Head NOS

  873.9 **Other and unspecified open wound of head, complicated**

874 **Open wound of neck**

⑤ 874.0 **Larynx and trachea, without mention of complication**

    874.00   **Larynx with trachea**

    874.01   **Larynx**

    874.02   **Trachea**

⑤ 874.1 **Larynx and trachea, complicated**

    874.10   **Larynx with trachea**

    874.11   **Larynx**

    874.12   **Trachea**

  874.2 **Thyroid gland, without mention of complication**

  874.3 **Thyroid gland, complicated**

  874.4 **Pharynx, without mention of complication**
     Cervical esophagus

  874.5 **Pharynx, complicated**

  874.8 **Other and unspecified parts, without mention of complication**
     Nape of neck   Throat NOS
     Supraclavicular region

  874.9 **Other and unspecified parts, complicated**

875 **Open wound of chest (wall)**

      | Excludes: | *open wound into thoracic cavity (860.0-862.9)* |
      traumatic pneumothorax and hemothorax (860.1, 860.3, 860.5)

  875.0 **Without mention of complication**

  875.1 **Complicated**

| Add 4th or 5th digit | Nonspecific code | Unspecified code | Medicare secondary payer(MSP) alert |

876 Open wound of back
Includes: loin   lumbar region

> *Excludes:*   *open wound into thoracic cavity (860.0-862.9)*
> *traumatic pneumothorax and hemothorax (860.1, 860.3, 860.5)*

876.0 Without mention of complication

876.1 Complicated

877 Open wound of buttock
Includes: sacroiliac region

877.0 Without mention of complication

877.1 Complicated

878 Open wound of genital organs (external), including traumatic amputation

> *Excludes:*   *injury during delivery (664.0-665.9)*
> *internal genital organs (867.0-867.9)*

878.0 Penis, without mention of complication

878.1 Penis, complicated

878.2 Scrotum and testes, without mention of complication

878.3 Scrotum and testes, complicated

878.4 Vulva, without mention of complication
Labium (majus) (minus)

878.5 Vulva, complicated

878.6 Vagina, without mention of complication

878.7 Vagina, complicated

878.8 Other and unspecified parts, without mention of complication

878.9 Other and unspecified parts, complicated

879 Open wound of other and unspecified sites, except limbs

879.0 Breast, without mention of complication

879.1 Breast, complicated

879.2 Abdominal wall, anterior, without mention of complication
Abdominal wall NOS   Pubic region
Epigastric region   Umbilical region
Hypogastric region

879.3 Abdominal wall, anterior, complicated

879.4 Abdominal wall, lateral, without mention of complication
Flank   Iliac (region)
Groin   Inguinal region
Hypochondrium

879.5 Abdominal wall, lateral, complicated

879.6 Other and unspecified parts of trunk, without mention of complication
Pelvic region   Trunk NOS
Perineum

879.7 Other and unspecified parts of trunk, complicated

879.8 Open wound(s) (multiple) of unspecified site(s) without mention of complication
Multiple open wounds NOS
Open wound NOS

879.9 Open wound(s) (multiple) of unspecified site(s), complicated

OPEN WOUND OF UPPER LIMB (880-887)

⑤ **880 Open wound of shoulder and upper arm**
The following fifth-digit subclassification is for use with category 880:

     0   **shoulder region**

     1   **scapular region**

     2   **axillary region**

     3   **upper arm**

     9   **multiple sites**

⑤ **880.0 Without mention of complication**

⑤ **880.1 Complicated**

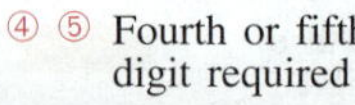

● Code new   ▲ Revision of   ④ ⑤ Fourth or fifth
   to this edition   existing code   digit required

⑤ **880.2 With tendon involvement**

⑤ **881 Open wound of elbow, forearm, and wrist**
The following fifth-digit subclassification is for use with category 881:

      0 forearm

      1 elbow

      2 wrist

⑤ **881.0 Without mention of complication**

⑤ **881.1 Complicated**

⑤ **881.2 With tendon involvement**

882 Open wound of hand except finger(s) alone

  882.0 Without mention of complication

  882.1 Complicated

  882.2 With tendon involvement

883 Open wound of finger(s)
Includes: fingernail   thumb (nail)

  883.0 Without mention of complication

  883.1 Complicated

  883.2 With tendon involvement

884 Multiple and unspecified open wound of upper limb
Includes: arm NOS
         multiple sites of one upper limb
         upper limb NOS

  884.0 Without mention of complication

  884.1 Complicated

  884.2 With tendon involvement

885 Traumatic amputation of thumb (complete) (partial)
Includes: thumb(s) (with finger(s) of either hand)

  885.0 Without mention of complication

  885.1 Complicated

886 Traumatic amputation of other finger(s) (complete) (partial)
Includes: finger(s) of one or both hands, without mention of thumb(s)

  886.0 Without mention of complication

  886.1 Complicated

887 Traumatic amputation of arm and hand (complete) (partial)

  887.0 Unilateral, below elbow, without mention of complication

  887.1 Unilateral, below elbow, complicated

  887.2 Unilateral, at or above elbow, without mention of complication

  887.3 Unilateral, at or above elbow, complicated

  887.4 Unilateral, level not specified, without mention of complication

  887.5 Unilateral, level not specified, complicated

  887.6 Bilateral [any level], without mention of complication
     One hand and other arm

  887.7 Bilateral [any level], complicated

OPEN WOUND OF LOWER LIMB (890-897)

890 Open wound of hip and thigh

  890.0 Without mention of complication

  890.1 Complicated

  890.2 With tendon involvement

891 Open wound of knee, leg [except thigh], and ankle
Includes: leg NOS
         multiple sites of leg, except thigh

    Excludes: *that of thigh (890.0-890.2)*
           with multiple sites of lower limb (894.0-894.2)

  891.0 Without mention of complication

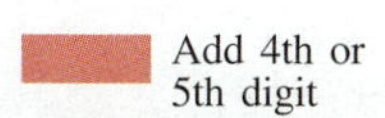

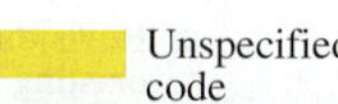

Medicare secondary
payer(MSP) alert

891.1 Complicated

891.2 With tendon involvement

892 Open wound of foot except toe(s) alone
    Includes: heel

892.0 Without mention of complication

892.1 Complicated

892.2 With tendon involvement

893 Open wound of toe(s)
    Includes: toenail

893.0 Without mention of complication

893.1 Complicated

893.2 With tendon involvement

894 Multiple and unspecified open wound of lower limb
    Includes: lower limb NOS
                multiple sites of one lower limb, with thigh

894.0 Without mention of complication

894.1 Complicated

894.2 With tendon involvement

895 Traumatic amputation of toe(s) (complete) (partial)
    Includes: toe(s) of one or both feet

895.0 Without mention of complication

895.1 Complicated

896 Traumatic amputation of foot (complete) (partial)

896.0 Unilateral, without mention of complication

896.1 Unilateral, complicated

896.2 Bilateral, without mention of complication

> *Excludes:* one foot and other leg (897.6-897.7)

896.3 Bilateral, complicated

897 Traumatic amputation of leg(s) (complete) (partial)

897.0 Unilateral, below knee, without mention of complication

897.1 Unilateral, below knee, complicated

897.2 Unilateral, at or above knee, without mention of complication

897.3 Unilateral, at or above knee, complicated

897.4 Unilateral, level not specified, without mention of complication

897.5 Unilateral, level not specified, complicated

897.6 Bilateral [any level], without mention of complication
        One foot and other leg

897.7 Bilateral [any level], complicated

INJURY TO BLOOD VESSELS (900-904)

    Includes:

<table>
<tr><td>arterial hematoma
avulsion
cut
laceration
rupture
traumatic aneurysm or fistula (arteriovenous)</td><td>of blood vessel, secondary to
other injuries e.g., fracture or
open wound</td></tr>
</table>

> *Excludes:* accidental puncture or laceration during medical procedure (998.2)
>   intracranial hemorrhage following injury (851.0-854.1)

900 Injury to blood vessels of head and neck

⑤ **900.0 Carotid artery**

900.00 Carotid artery, unspecified

900.01 Common carotid artery

900.02 External carotid artery

900.03 Internal carotid artery

● Code new
   to this edition

▲ Revision of
   existing code

④ ⑤ Fourth or fifth
      digit required

900.1 Internal jugular vein

⑤ **900.8** Other specified blood vessels of head and neck

    900.81 External jugular vein
       Jugular vein NOS

    900.82 Multiple blood vessels of head and neck

    900.89 Other

900.9 Unspecified blood vessel of head and neck

901 Injury to blood vessels of thorax

    Excludes: traumatic hemothorax (860.2-860.5)

901.0 Thoracic aorta

901.1 Innominate and subclavian arteries

901.2 Superior vena cava

901.3 Innominate and subclavian veins

⑤ **901.4** Pulmonary blood vessels

    901.40 Pulmonary vessel(s), unspecified

    901.41 Pulmonary artery

    901.42 Pulmonary vein

⑤ **901.8** Other specified blood vessels of thorax

    901.81 Intercostal artery or vein

    901.82 Internal mammary artery or vein

    901.83 Multiple blood vessels of thorax

    901.89 Other
       Azygos vein   Hemiazygos vein

901.9 Unspecified blood vessel of thorax

902 Injury to blood vessels of abdomen and pelvis

902.0 Abdominal aorta

⑤ **902.1** Inferior vena cava

    902.10 Inferior vena cava, unspecified

    902.11 Hepatic veins

    902.19 Other

⑤ **902.2** Celiac and mesenteric arteries

    902.20 Celiac and mesenteric arteries, unspecified

    902.21 Gastric artery

    902.22 Hepatic artery

    902.23 Splenic artery

    902.24 Other specified branches of celiac axis

    902.25 Superior mesenteric artery (trunk)

    902.26 Primary branches of superior mesenteric artery
       Ileo-colic artery

    902.27 Inferior mesenteric artery

    902.29 Other

⑤ **902.3** Portal and splenic veins

    902.31 Superior mesenteric vein and primary subdivisions
       Ileo-colic vein

    902.32 Inferior mesenteric vein

    902.33 Portal vein

    902.34 Splenic vein

    902.39 Other
       Cystic vein   Gastric vein

⑤ **902.4** Renal blood vessels

    902.40 Renal vessel(s), unspecified

    902.41 Renal artery

    902.42 Renal vein

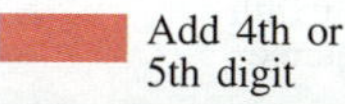

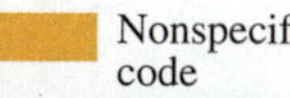

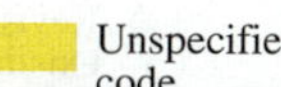

Medicare secondary
payer(MSP) alert

902.49 **Other**
Suprarenal arteries

⑤ **902.5 Iliac blood vessels**

902.50 **Iliac vessel(s), unspecified**

902.51 **Hypogastric artery**

902.52 **Hypogastric vein**

902.53 **Iliac artery**

902.54 **Iliac vein**

902.55 **Uterine artery**

902.56 **Uterine vein**

902.59 **Other**

⑤ **902.8 Other specified blood vessels of abdomen and pelvis**

902.81 **Ovarian artery**

902.82 **Ovarian vein**

902.87 **Multiple blood vessels of abdomen and pelvis**

902.89 **Other**

902.9 **Unspecified blood vessel of abdomen and pelvis**

903 Injury to blood vessels of upper extremity

⑤ **903.0 Axillary blood vessels**

903.00 **Axillary vessel(s), unspecified**

903.01 **Axillary artery**

903.02 **Axillary vein**

903.1 **Brachial blood vessels**

903.2 **Radial blood vessels**

903.3 **Ulnar blood vessels**

903.4 **Palmar artery**

903.5 **Digital blood vessels**

903.8 **Other specified blood vessels of upper extremity**
Multiple blood vessels of upper extremity

903.9 **Unspecified blood vessel of upper extremity**

904 Injury to blood vessels of lower extremity and unspecified sites

904.0 **Common femoral artery**
Femoral artery above profunda origin

904.1 **Superficial femoral artery**

904.2 **Femoral veins**

904.3 **Saphenous veins**
Saphenous vein (greater) (lesser)

⑤ **904.4 Popliteal blood vessels**

904.40 **Popliteal vessel(s), unspecified**

904.41 **Popliteal artery**

904.42 **Popliteal vein**

⑤ **904.5 Tibial blood vessels**

904.50 **Tibial vessel(s), unspecified**

904.51 **Anterior tibial artery**

904.52 **Anterior tibial vein**

904.53 **Posterior tibial artery**

904.54 **Posterior tibial vein**

904.6 **Deep plantar blood vessels**

904.7 **Other specified blood vessels of lower extremity**
Multiple blood vessels of lower extremity

904.8 **Unspecified blood vessel of lower extremity**

904.9 **Unspecified site**
Injury to blood vessel NOS

● Code new
to this edition

▲ Revision of
existing code

④ ⑤ Fourth or fifth
digit required

LATE EFFECTS OF INJURIES, POISONINGS, TOXIC EFFECTS, AND OTHER EXTERNAL CAUSES (905-909)

> Note: These categories are to be used to indicate conditions classifiable to 800-999 as the cause of late effects, which are themselves classified elsewhere. The "late effects" include those specified as such, or as sequelae, which may occur at any time after the acute injury.

905 Late effects of musculoskeletal and connective tissue injuries

905.0 Late effect of fracture of skull and face bones
Late effect of injury classifiable to 800-804

905.1 Late effect of fracture of spine and trunk without mention of spinal cord lesion
Late effect of injury classifiable to 805, 807-809

905.2 Late effect of fracture of upper extremities
Late effect of injury classifiable to 810-819

905.3 Late effect of fracture of neck of femur
Late effect of injury classifiable to 820

905.4 Late effect of fracture of lower extremities
Late effect of injury classifiable to 821-827

905.5 Late effect of fracture of multiple and unspecified bones
Late effect of injury classifiable to 828-829

905.6 Late effect of dislocation
Late effect of injury classifiable to 830-839

905.7 Late effect of sprain and strain without mention of tendon injury
Late effect of injury classifiable to 840-848, except tendon injury

905.8 Late effect of tendon injury
Late effect of tendon injury due to:
open wound [injury classifiable to 880-884 with .2, 890-894 with .2]
sprain and strain [injury classifiable to 840-848]

905.9 Late effect of traumatic amputation
Late effect of injury classifiable to 885-887, 895-897

> *Excludes:* *late amputation stump complication (997.60-997.69)*

906 Late effects of injuries to skin and subcutaneous tissues

906.0 Late effect of open wound of head, neck, and trunk
Late effect of injury classifiable to 870-879

906.1 Late effect of open wound of extremities without mention of tendon injury
Late effect of injury classifiable to 880-884, 890-894 except .2

906.2 Late effect of superficial injury
Late effect of injury classifiable to 910-919

906.3 Late effect of contusion
Late effect of injury classifiable to 920-924

906.4 Late effect of crushing
Late effect of injury classifiable to 925-929

906.5 Late effect of burn of eye, face, head, and neck
Late effect of injury classifiable to 940-941

906.6 Late effect of burn of wrist and hand
Late effect of injury classifiable to 944

906.7 Late effect of burn of other extremities
Late effect of injury classifiable to 943 or 945

906.8 Late effect of burns of other specified sites
Late effect of injury classifiable to 942, 946-947

906.9 Late effect of burn of unspecified site
Late effect of injury classifiable to 948-949

907 Late effects of injuries to the nervous system

907.0 Late effect of intracranial injury without mention of skull fracture
Late effect of injury classifiable to 850-854

907.1 Late effect of injury to cranial nerve
Late effect of injury classifiable to 950-951

907.2 Late effect of spinal cord injury
Late effect of injury classifiable to 806, 952

907.3 Late effect of injury to nerve root(s), spinal plexus(es), and other nerves of trunk
Late effect of injury classifiable to 953-954

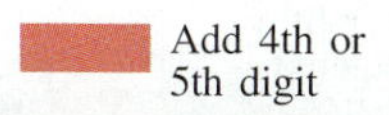
Add 4th or
5th digit

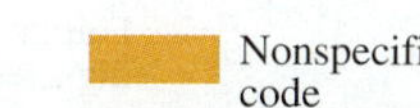
Nonspecific
code

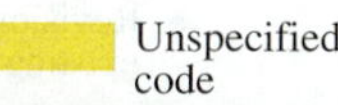
Unspecified
code

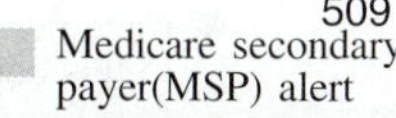
Medicare secondary
payer(MSP) alert

907.4 **Late effect of injury to peripheral nerve of shoulder girdle and upper limb**
Late effect of injury classifiable to 955

907.5 **Late effect of injury to peripheral nerve of pelvic girdle and lower limb**
Late effect of injury classifiable to 956

907.9 **Late effect of injury to other and unspecified nerve**
Late effect of injury classifiable to 957

908 **Late effects of other and unspecified injuries**

908.0 **Late effect of internal injury to chest**
Late effect of injury classifiable to 860-862

908.1 **Late effect of internal injury to intra-abdominal organs**
Late effect of injury classifiable to 863-866, 868

908.2 **Late effect of internal injury to other internal organs**
Late effect of injury classifiable to 867 or 869

908.3 **Late effect of injury to blood vessel of head, neck, and extremities**
Late effect of injury classifiable to 900, 903-904

908.4 **Late effect of injury to blood vessel of thorax, abdomen, and pelvis**
Late effect of injury classifiable to 901-902

908.5 **Late effect of foreign body in orifice**
Late effect of injury classifiable to 930-939

908.6 **Late effect of certain complications of trauma**
Late effect of complications classifiable to 958

908.9 **Late effect of unspecified injury**
Late effect of injury classifiable to 959

909 **Late effects of other and unspecified external causes**

909.0 **Late effect of poisoning due to drug, medicinal or biological substance**
Late effect of conditions classifiable to 960-979

Excludes: *late effect of adverse effect of drug, medicinal or biological substance (909.5)*

909.1 **Late effect of toxic effects of nonmedical substances**
Late effect of conditions classifiable to 980-989

909.2 **Late effect of radiation**
Late effect of conditions classifiable to 990

909.3 **Late effect of complications of surgical and medical care**
Late effect of conditions classifiable to 996-999

909.4 **Late effect of certain other external causes**
Late effect of conditions classifiable to 991-994

909.5 **Late effect of adverse effect of drug, medicinal or biological substance**

Excludes: *late effect of poisoning due to drug, medicinal or biological substance (909.0)*

909.9 **Late effect of other and unspecified external causes**

SUPERFICIAL INJURY (910-919)

Excludes: *burn (blisters) (940.0-949.5)*
contusion (920-924.9)
foreign body:
granuloma (728.82)
inadvertently left in operative wound (998.4)
residual, in soft tissue (729.6)
insect bite, venomous (989.5)
open wound with incidental foreign body (870.0-897.7)

910 **Superficial injury of face, neck, and scalp except eye**
Includes:

cheek	lip
ear	nose
gum	throat

Excludes: *eye and adnexa (918.0-918.9)*

910.0 **Abrasion or friction burn without mention of infection**

910.1 **Abrasion or friction burn, infected**

910.2 **Blister without mention of infection**

910.3 **Blister, infected**

910.4 **Insect bite, nonvenomous, without mention of infection**

● Code new to this edition   ▲ Revision of existing code   ④ ⑤ Fourth or fifth digit required

910.5 Insect bite, nonvenomous, infected

910.6 Superficial foreign body (splinter) without major open wound and without mention of infection

910.7 Superficial foreign body (splinter) without major open wound, infected

910.8 Other and unspecified superficial injury of face, neck, and scalp without mention of infection

910.9 Other and unspecified superficial injury of face, neck, and scalp, infected

911 Superficial injury of trunk

Includes:

abdominal wall	interscapular region
anus	labium (majus) (minus)
back	penis
breast	perineum
buttock	scrotum
chest wall	testis
flank	vagina
groin	vulva

Excludes: *hip (916.0-916.9)*
scapular region (912.0-912.9)

911.0 Abrasion or friction burn without mention of infection

911.1 Abrasion or friction burn, infected

911.2 Blister without mention of infection

911.3 Blister, infected

911.4 Insect bite, nonvenomous, without mention of infection

911.5 Insect bite, nonvenomous, infected

911.6 Superficial foreign body (splinter) without major open wound and without mention of infection

911.7 Superficial foreign body (splinter) without major open wound, infected

911.8 Other and unspecified superficial injury of trunk without mention of infection

911.9 Other and unspecified superficial injury of trunk, infected

912 Superficial injury of shoulder and upper arm

Includes: axilla   scapular region

912.0 Abrasion or friction burn without mention of infection

912.1 Abrasion or friction burn, infected

912.2 Blister without mention of infection

912.3 Blister, infected

912.4 Insect bite, nonvenomous, without mention of infection

912.5 Insect bite, nonvenomous, infected

912.6 Superficial foreign body (splinter) without major open wound and without mention of infection

912.7 Superficial foreign body (splinter) without major open wound, infected

912.8 Other and unspecified superficial injury of shoulder and upper arm without mention of infection

912.9 Other and unspecified superficial injury of shoulder and upper arm, infected

913 Superficial injury of elbow, forearm, and wrist

913.0 Abrasion or friction burn without mention of infection

913.1 Abrasion or friction burn, infected

913.2 Blister without mention of infection

913.3 Blister, infected

913.4 Insect bite, nonvenomous, without mention of infection

913.5 Insect bite, nonvenomous, infected

913.6 Superficial foreign body (splinter) without major open wound and without mention of infection

913.7 Superficial foreign body (splinter) without major open wound, infected

913.8 Other and unspecified superficial injury of elbow, forearm, and wrist without mention of infection

913.9 Other and unspecified superficial injury of elbow, forearm, and wrist, infected

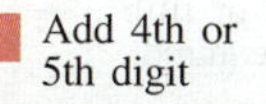

Nonspecific
code

Unspecified
code

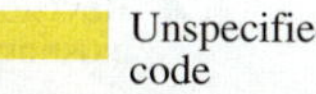

914 Superficial injury of hand(s) except finger(s) alone

914.0 Abrasion or friction burn without mention of infection

914.1 Abrasion or friction burn, infected

914.2 Blister without mention of infection

914.3 Blister, infected

914.4 Insect bite, nonvenomous, without mention of infection

914.5 Insect bite, nonvenomous, infected

914.6 Superficial foreign body (splinter) without major open wound and without mention of
infection

914.7 Superficial foreign body (splinter) without major open wound, infected

914.8 Other and unspecified superficial injury of hand without mention of infection

914.9 Other and unspecified superficial injury of hand, infected

915 Superficial injury of finger(s)

Includes: fingernail   thumb (nail)

915.0 Abrasion or friction burn without mention of infection

915.1 Abrasion or friction burn, infected

915.2 Blister without mention of infection

915.3 Blister, infected

915.4 Insect bite, nonvenomous, without mention of infection

915.5 Insect bite, nonvenomous, infected

915.6 Superficial foreign body (splinter) without major open wound and without mention
of infection

915.7 Superficial foreign body (splinter) without major open wound, infected

915.8 Other and unspecified superficial injury of fingers without mention of infection

915.9 Other and unspecified superficial injury of fingers, infected

916 Superficial injury of hip, thigh, leg, and ankle

916.0 Abrasion or friction burn without mention of infection

916.1 Abrasion or friction burn, infected

916.2 Blister without mention of infection

916.3 Blister, infected

916.4 Insect bite, nonvenomous, without mention of infection

916.5 Insect bite, nonvenomous, infected

916.6 Superficial foreign body (splinter) without major open wound and without mention
of infection

916.7 Superficial foreign body (splinter) without major open wound, infected

916.8 Other and unspecified superficial injury of hip, thigh, leg, and ankle without
mention of infection

916.9 Other and unspecified superficial injury of hip, thigh, leg, and ankle, infected

917 Superficial injury of foot and toe(s)

Includes: heel   toenail

917.0 Abrasion or friction burn without mention of infection

917.1 Abrasion or friction burn, infected

917.2 Blister without mention of infection

917.3 Blister, infected

917.4 Insect bite, nonvenomous, without mention of infection

917.5 Insect bite, nonvenomous, infected

917.6 Superficial foreign body (splinter) without major open wound and without mention
of infection

917.7 Superficial foreign body (splinter) without major open wound, infected

917.8 Other and unspecified superficial injury of foot and toes without mention of
infection

917.9 Other and unspecified superficial injury of foot and toes, infected

● Code new
to this edition   ▲ Revision of
existing code   ④ ⑤ Fourth or fifth
digit required

918 **Superficial injury of eye and adnexa**

> *Excludes:* *burn (940.0-940.9)*
> *foreign body on external eye (930.0-930.9)*

918.0 **Eyelids and periocular area**
Abrasion
Insect bite
Superficial foreign body (splinter)

918.1 **Cornea**
Corneal abrasion
Superficial laceration

> *Excludes:* *corneal injury due to contact lens (371.82)*

918.2 **Conjunctiva**

918.9 **Other and unspecified superficial injuries of eye**
Eye (ball) NOS

919 **Superficial injury of other, multiple, and unspecified sites**

> *Excludes:* *multiple sites classifiable to the same three-digit category (910.0-918.9)*

919.0 **Abrasion or friction burn without mention of infection**

919.1 **Abrasion or friction burn, infected**

919.2 **Blister without mention of infection**

919.3 **Blister, infected**

919.4 **Insect bite, nonvenomous, without mention of infection**

919.5 **Insect bite, nonvenomous, infected**

919.6 **Superficial foreign body (splinter) without major open wound and without mention of infection**

919.7 **Superficial foreign body (splinter) without major open wound, infected**

919.8 **Other and unspecified superficial injury without mention of infection**

919.9 **Other and unspecified superficial injury, infected**

CONTUSION WITH INTACT SKIN SURFACE (920-924)

Includes:
bruise
hematoma } without fracture or open wound

> *Excludes:* *concussion (850.0-850.9)*
> *hemarthrosis (840.0-848.9)*
> *internal organs (860.0-869.1)*
> *that incidental to:*
> *crushing injury (925-929.9)*
> *dislocation (830.0-839.9)*
> *fracture (800.0-829.1)*
> *internal injury (860.0-869.1)*
> *intracranial injury (850.0-854.1)*
> *nerve injury (950.0-957.9)*
> *open wound (870.0-897.7)*

920 **Contusion of face, scalp, and neck except eye(s)**
Cheek
Ear (auricle)
Gum
Lip
Mandibular joint area
Nose
Throat

921 **Contusion of eye and adnexa**

921.0 **Black eye, not otherwise specified**

921.1 **Contusion of eyelids and periocular area**

921.2 **Contusion of orbital tissues**

921.3 **Contusion of eyeball**

921.9 **Unspecified contusion of eye**
Injury of eye NOS

922 **Contusion of trunk**

922.0 **Breast**

922.1 **Chest wall**

922.2 **Abdominal wall**
Flank
Groin

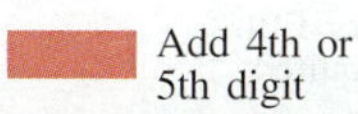 Add 4th or 5th digit 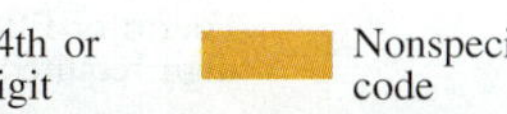 Nonspecific code 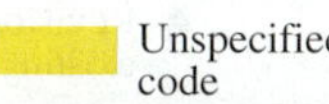 Unspecified code Medicare secondary payer(MSP) alert

⑤ **922.3 Back**

Excludes: scapular region (923.01)

    922.31 Back

    Excludes: interscapular region (922.33)

    922.32 Buttock

    922.33 Interscapular region

922.4 Genital organs

Labium (majus) (minus)	Testis
Penis	Vagina
Perineum	Vulva
Scrotum	

922.8 Multiple sites of trunk

922.9 Unspecified part
   Trunk NOS

923 Contusion of upper limb

⑤ **923.0 Shoulder and upper arm**

    923.00 Shoulder region

    923.01 Scapular region

    923.02 Axillary region

    923.03 Upper arm

    923.09 Multiple sites

⑤ **923.1 Elbow and forearm**

    923.10 Forearm

    923.11 Elbow

⑤ **923.2 Wrist and hand(s), except finger(s) alone**

    923.20 Hand(s)

    923.21 Wrist

923.3 Finger
   Fingernail   Thumb (nail)

923.8 Multiple sites of upper limb

923.9 Unspecified part of upper limb
   Arm NOS

924 Contusion of lower limb and of other and unspecified sites

⑤ **924.0 Hip and thigh**

    924.00 Thigh

    924.01 Hip

⑤ **924.1 Knee and lower leg**

    924.10 Lower leg

    924.11 Knee

⑤ **924.2 Ankle and foot, excluding toe(s)**

    924.20 Foot
       Heel

    924.21 Ankle

924.3 Toe
   Toenail

924.4 Multiple sites of lower limb

924.5 Unspecified part of lower limb
   Leg NOS

924.8 Multiple sites, not elsewhere classified

924.9 Unspecified site

● Code new to this edition   ▲ Revision of existing code   ④ ⑤ Fourth or fifth digit required

CRUSHING INJURY (925-929)

> *Excludes:* concussion (850.0-850.9)
>> fractures (800-829)
>> internal organs (860.0-869.1)
>> that incidental to:
>>> internal injury (860.0-869.1)
>>> intracranial injury (850.0-854.1)

925 Crushing injury of face, scalp, and neck

Cheek	Pharynx
Ear	Throat
Larynx	

925.1 Crushing injury of face and scalp

Cheek	Ear

925.2 Crushing injury of neck

Larynx	Throat
Pharynx	

926 Crushing injury of trunk

> *Excludes:* crush injury of internal organs (860.0-869.1)

926.0 External genitalia

Labium (majus) (minus)	Testis
Penis	Vulva
Scrotum	

926.1 Other specified sites

    926.11 Back

    926.12 Buttock

    926.19 Other
       Breast

> *Excludes:* crushing of chest (860.0-862.9)

926.8 Multiple sites of trunk

926.9 Unspecified site
    Trunk NOS

927 Crushing injury of upper limb

927.0 Shoulder and upper arm

    927.00 Shoulder region

    927.01 Scapular region

    927.02 Axillary region

    927.03 Upper arm

    927.09 Multiple sites

927.1 Elbow and forearm

    927.10 Forearm

    927.11 Elbow

927.2 Wrist and hand(s), except finger(s) alone

    927.20 Hand(s)

    927.21 Wrist

927.3 Finger(s)

927.8 Multiple sites of upper limb

927.9 Unspecified site
    Arm NOS

928 Crushing injury of lower limb

928.0 Hip and thigh

    928.00 Thigh

    928.01 Hip

928.1 Knee and lower leg

    928.10 Lower leg

    928.11 Knee

928.2 Ankle and foot, excluding toe(s) alone

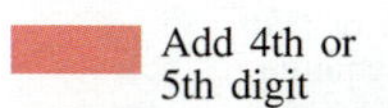

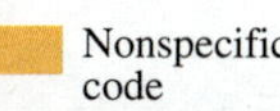

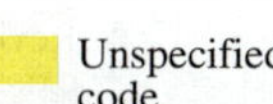

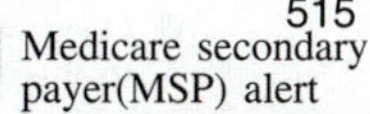

928.20 Foot
Heel

928.21 Ankle

928.3 Toe(s)

928.8 Multiple sites of lower limb

928.9 Unspecified site
Leg NOS

929 Crushing injury of multiple and unspecified sites

Excludes: *multiple internal injury NOS (869.0-869.1)*

929.0 Multiple sites, not elsewhere classified

929.9 Unspecified site

EFFECTS OF FOREIGN BODY ENTERING THROUGH ORIFICE (930-939)

Excludes: *foreign body:*
granuloma (728.82)
inadvertently left in operative wound (998.4, 998.7)
in open wound (800-839, 851-897)
residual, in soft tissues (729.6)
superficial without major open wound (910-919 with .6 or .7)

930 Foreign body on external eye

Excludes: *foreign body in penetrating wound of:*
eyeball (871.5-871.6)
retained (old) (360.5-360.6)
ocular adnexa (870.4)
retained (old) (376.6)

930.0 Corneal foreign body

930.1 Foreign body in conjunctival sac

930.2 Foreign body in lacrimal punctum

930.8 Other and combined sites

930.9 Unspecified site
External eye NOS

931 Foreign body in ear
Auditory canal   Auricle

932 Foreign body in nose
Nasal sinus   Nostril

933 Foreign body in pharynx and larynx

933.0 Pharynx
Nasopharynx   Throat NOS

933.1 Larynx
Asphyxia due to   Choking due to:
  foreign body   food (regurgitated)
                                          phlegm

934 Foreign body in trachea, bronchus, and lung

934.0 Trachea

934.1 Main bronchus

934.8 Other specified parts
Bronchioles   Lung

934.9 Respiratory tree, unspecified
Inhalation of liquid or vomitus, lower respiratory tract NOS

935 Foreign body in mouth, esophagus, and stomach

935.0 Mouth

935.1 Esophagus

935.2 Stomach

936 Foreign body in intestine and colon

937 Foreign body in anus and rectum
Rectosigmoid (junction)

938 Foreign body in digestive system, unspecified
Alimentary tract NOS   Swallowed foreign body

    ● Code new   ▲ Revision of   ④ ⑤ Fourth or fifth
       to this edition   existing code   digit required

939 Foreign body in genitourinary tract

939.0 Bladder and urethra

939.1 Uterus, any part

> Excludes: intrauterine contraceptive device:
> complications from (996.32, 996.65)
> presence of (V45.51)

939.2 Vulva and vagina

939.3 Penis

939.9 Unspecified site

BURNS (940-949)

> Includes: burns from:
> electrical heating appliance
> electricity
> flame
> hot object
> lightning
> radiation
> chemical burns (external) (internal)
> scalds

> Excludes: friction burns (910-919 with .0, .1)
> sunburn (692.71, 692.76-692.77)

940 Burn confined to eye and adnexa

940.0 Chemical burn of eyelids and periocular area

940.1 Other burns of eyelids and periocular area

940.2 Alkaline chemical burn of cornea and conjunctival sac

940.3 Acid chemical burn of cornea and conjunctival sac

940.4 Other burn of cornea and conjunctival sac

940.5 Burn with resulting rupture and destruction of eyeball

940.9 Unspecified burn of eye and adnexa

⑤ **941** Burn of face, head, and neck

> Excludes: mouth (947.0)

The following fifth-digit subclassification is for use with category 941:

  0 face and head, unspecified site

  1 ear [any part]

  2 eye (with other parts of face, head, and neck)

  3 lip(s)

  4 chin

  5 nose (septum)

  6 scalp [any part]
      Temple (region)

  7 forehead and cheek

  8 neck

  9 multiple sites [except with eye] of face, head, and neck

⑤ 941.0 Unspecified degree

⑤ 941.1 Erythema [first degree]

⑤ 941.2 Blisters, epidermal loss [second degree]

⑤ 941.3 Full-thickness skin loss [third degree NOS]

⑤ 941.4 Deep necrosis of underlying tissues [deep third degree] without mention of loss of a body part

⑤ 941.5 Deep necrosis of underlying tissues [deep third degree] with loss of a body part

⑤ **942** Burn of trunk

> Excludes: scapular region (943.0-943.5 with fifth-digit 6)

The following fifth-digit subclassification is for use with category 942:

  0 trunk, unspecified site

  1 breast

▮ Add 4th or 5th digit	▮ Nonspecific code	▮ Unspecified code	▮ Medicare secondary payer(MSP) alert

   2 **chest wall, excluding breast and nipple**

   3 **abdominal wall**
      Flank   Groin

   4 **back [any part]**
      Buttock   Interscapular region

   5 **genitalia**
      Labium (majus) (minus)   Scrotum
      Penis   Testis
      Perineum   Vulva

   9 **other and multiple sites of trunk**

⑤ **942.0** **Unspecified degree**

⑤ **942.1** **Erythema [first degree]**

⑤ **942.2** **Blisters, epidermal loss [second degree]**

⑤ **942.3** **Full-thickness skin loss [third degree NOS]**

⑤ **942.4** **Deep necrosis of underlying tissues [deep third degree] without mention of loss of a body part**

⑤ **942.5** **Deep necrosis of underlying tissues [deep third degree] with loss of a body part**

⑤ **943** **Burn of upper limb, except wrist and hand**

The following fifth-digit subclassification is for use with category 943:

   0 **upper limb, unspecified site**

   1 **forearm**

   2 **elbow**

   3 **upper arm**

   4 **axilla**

   5 **shoulder**

   6 **scapular region**

   9 **multiple sites of upper limb, except wrist and hand**

⑤ **943.0** **Unspecified degree**

⑤ **943.1** **Erythema [first degree]**

⑤ **943.2** **Blisters, epidermal loss [second degree]**

⑤ **943.3** **Full-thickness skin loss [third degree NOS]**

⑤ **943.4** **Deep necrosis of underlying tissues [deep third degree] without mention of loss of a body part**

⑤ **943.5** **Deep necrosis of underlying tissues [deep third degree] with loss of a body part**

⑤ **944** **Burn of wrist(s) and hand(s)**

The following fifth-digit subclassification is for use with category 944:

   0 **hand, unspecified site**

   1 **single digit [finger (nail)] other than thumb**

   2 **thumb (nail)**

   3 **two or more digits, not including thumb**

   4 **two or more digits including thumb**

   5 **palm**

   6 **back of hand**

   7 **wrist**

   8 **multiple sites of wrist(s) and hand(s)**

⑤ **944.0** **Unspecified degree**

⑤ **944.1** **Erythema [first degree]**

⑤ **944.2** **Blisters, epidermal loss [second degree]**

⑤ **944.3** **Full-thickness skin loss [third degree NOS]**

⑤ **944.4** **Deep necrosis of underlying tissues [deep third degree] without mention of loss of a body part**

⑤ **944.5** **Deep necrosis of underlying tissues [deep third degree] with loss of a body part**

● Code new to this edition   ▲ Revision of existing code   ④ ⑤ Fourth or fifth digit required

⑤ **945** **Burn of lower limb(s)**
The following fifth-digit subclassification is for use with category 945:

    0 **lower limb [leg], unspecified site**
    1 toe(s) (nail)
    2 foot
    3 ankle
    4 lower leg
    5 knee
    6 thigh [any part]
    9 **multiple sites of lower limb(s)**

⑤ **945.0** **Unspecified degree**

⑤ **945.1** **Erythema [first degree]**

⑤ **945.2** **Blisters, epidermal loss [second degree]**

⑤ **945.3** **Full-thickness skin loss [third degree NOS]**

⑤ **945.4** **Deep necrosis of underlying tissues [deep third degree] without mention of loss of a body part**

⑤ **945.5** **Deep necrosis of underlying tissues [deep third degree] with loss of a body part**

946 **Burns of multiple specified sites**
Includes: burns of sites classifiable to more than one three-digit category in 940-945

Excludes: *multiple burns NOS (949.0-949.5)*

946.0 **Unspecified degree**

946.1 **Erythema [first degree]**

946.2 **Blisters, epidermal loss [second degree]**

946.3 **Full-thickness skin loss [third degree NOS]**

946.4 **Deep necrosis of underlying tissues [deep third degree] without mention of loss of a body part**

946.5 **Deep necrosis of underlying tissues [deep third degree] with loss of a body part**

947 **Burn of internal organs**
Includes: burns from chemical agents (ingested)

947.0 **Mouth and pharynx**
    Gum
    Tongue

947.1 **Larynx, trachea, and lung**

947.2 **Esophagus**

947.3 **Gastrointestinal tract**
    Colon
    Rectum
    Small intestine
    Stomach

947.4 **Vagina and uterus**

947.8 **Other specified sites**

947.9 **Unspecified site**

⑤ **948** **Burns classified according to extent of body surface involved**

Excludes: *sunburn (692.71, 692.76-692.77)*

Note: This category is to be used when the site of the burn is unspecified, or with categories 940-947 when the site is specified.

The following fifth-digit subclassification is for use with category 948 to indicate the percent of *body surface* with *third degree* burn; valid digits are in [brackets] under each code:

    0 **less than 10 percent or unspecified**
    1 **10-19%**
    2 **20-29%**
    3 **30-39%**
    4 **40-49%**
    5 **50-59%**
    6 **60-69%**

	Add 4th or 5th digit		Nonspecific code		Unspecified code		Medicare secondary payer(MSP) alert

    7 **70-79%**

    8 **80-89%**

    9 **90% or more of body surface**

⑤ **948.0** **Burn [any degree] involving less than 10 percent of body surface**
[0]

⑤ **948.1** **10-19 percent of body surface**
[0-1]

⑤ **948.2** **20-29 percent of body surface**
[0-2]

⑤ **948.3** **30-39 percent of body surface**
[0-3]

⑤ **948.4** **40-49 percent of body surface**
[0-4]

⑤ **948.5** **50-59 percent of body surface**
[0-5]

⑤ **948.6** **60-69 percent of body surface**
[0-6]

⑤ **948.7** **70-79 percent of body surface**
[0-7]

⑤ **948.8** **80-89 percent of body surface**
[0-8]

⑤ **948.9** **90 percent or more of body surface**
[0-9]

949 **Burn, unspecified**

    Includes:

        burn NOS
        multiple burns NOS

    Excludes: *burn of unspecified site but with statement of the extent of body surface involved (948.0-948.9)*

949.0 **Unspecified degree**

949.1 **Erythema [first degree]**

949.2 **Blisters, epidermal loss [second degree]**

949.3 **Full-thickness skin loss [third degree NOS]**

949.4 **Deep necrosis of underlying tissues [deep third degree] without mention of loss of a body part**

949.5 **Deep necrosis of underlying tissues [deep third degree] with loss of a body part**

INJURY TO NERVES AND SPINAL CORD (950-957)

    Includes:

        division of nerve
        lesion in continuity
        traumatic neuroma   (with open wound)
        traumatic transient paralysis

    Excludes: *accidental puncture or laceration during medical procedure (998.2)*

950 **Injury to optic nerve and pathways**

950.0 **Optic nerve injury**
    Second cranial nerve

950.1 **Injury to optic chiasm**

950.2 **Injury to optic pathways**

950.3 **Injury to visual cortex**

950.9 **Unspecified**
    Traumatic blindness NOS

951 **Injury to other cranial nerve(s)**

951.0 **Injury to oculomotor nerve**
    Third cranial nerve

951.1 **Injury to trochlear nerve**
    Fourth cranial nerve

951.2 **Injury to trigeminal nerve**
    Fifth cranial nerve

● Code new to this edition   ▲ Revision of existing code   ④ ⑤ Fourth or fifth digit required

951.3 Injury to abducens nerve
Sixth cranial nerve

951.4 Injury to facial nerve
Seventh cranial nerve

951.5 Injury to acoustic nerve
Auditory nerve   Traumatic deafness NOS
Eighth cranial nerve

951.6 Injury to accessory nerve
Eleventh cranial nerve

951.7 Injury to hypoglossal nerve
Twelfth cranial nerve

951.8 Injury to other specified cranial nerves
Glossopharyngeal [9th cranial] nerve
Olfactory [1st cranial] nerve
Pneumogastric [10th cranial] nerve
Traumatic anosmia NOS
Vagus [10th cranial] nerve

951.9 Injury to unspecified cranial nerve

952 Spinal cord injury without evidence of spinal bone injury

⑤ **952.0 Cervical**

952.00 C_1-C_4 level with unspecified spinal cord injury
Spinal cord injury, cervical region NOS

952.01 C_1-C_4 level with complete lesion of spinal cord

952.02 C_1-C_4 level with anterior cord syndrome

952.03 C_1-C_4 level with central cord syndrome

952.04 C_1-C_4 level with other specified spinal cord injury
Incomplete spinal cord lesion at C_1-C_4 level:
NOS
with posterior cord syndrome

952.05 C_5-C_7 level with unspecified spinal cord injury

952.06 C_5-C_7 level with complete lesion of spinal cord

952.07 C_5-C_7 level with anterior cord syndrome

952.08 C_5-C_7 level with central cord syndrome

952.09 C_5-C_7 level with other specified spinal cord injury
Incomplete spinal cord lesion at C_5-C_7 level:
NOS
with posterior cord syndrome

⑤ **952.1 Dorsal [thoracic]**

952.10 T_1-T_6 level with unspecified spinal cord injury
Spinal cord injury, thoracic region NOS

952.11 T_1-T_6 level with complete lesion of spinal cord

952.12 T_1-T_6 level with anterior cord syndrome

952.13 T_1-T_6 level with central cord syndrome

952.14 T_1-T_6 level with other specified spinal cord injury
Incomplete spinal cord lesion at T_1-T_6 level:
NOS
with posterior cord syndrome

952.15 T_7-T_{12} level with unspecified spinal cord injury

952.16 T_7-T_{12} level with complete lesion of spinal cord

952.17 T_7-T_{12} level with anterior cord syndrome

952.18 T_7-T_{12} level with central cord syndrome

952.19 T_7-T_{12} level with other specified spinal cord injury
Incomplete spinal cord lesion at T_7-T_{12} level:
NOS
with posterior cord syndrome

952.2 Lumbar

952.3 Sacral

952.4 Cauda equina

952.8 Multiple sites of spinal cord

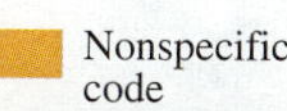
Add 4th or
5th digit

Nonspecific
code

Unspecified
code

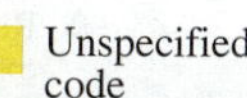
Medicare secondary
payer(MSP) alert

952.9 Unspecified site of spinal cord

953 Injury to nerve roots and spinal plexus

953.0 Cervical root

953.1 Dorsal root

953.2 Lumbar root

953.3 Sacral root

953.4 Brachial plexus

953.5 Lumbosacral plexus

953.8 Multiple sites

953.9 Unspecified site

954 Injury to other nerve(s) of trunk, excluding shoulder and pelvic girdles

954.0 Cervical sympathetic

954.1 Other sympathetic
Celiac ganglion or plexus   Splanchnic nerve(s)
Inferior mesenteric plexus   Stellate ganglion

954.8 Other specified nerve(s) of trunk

954.9 Unspecified nerve of trunk

955 Injury to peripheral nerve(s) of shoulder girdle and upper limb

955.0 Axillary nerve

955.1 Median nerve

955.2 Ulnar nerve

955.3 Radial nerve

955.4 Musculocutaneous nerve

955.5 Cutaneous sensory nerve, upper limb

955.6 Digital nerve

955.7 Other specified nerve(s) of shoulder girdle and upper limb

955.8 Multiple nerves of shoulder girdle and upper limb

955.9 Unspecified nerve of shoulder girdle and upper limb

956 Injury to peripheral nerve(s) of pelvic girdle and lower limb

956.0 Sciatic nerve

956.1 Femoral nerve

956.2 Posterior tibial nerve

956.3 Peroneal nerve

956.4 Cutaneous sensory nerve, lower limb

956.5 Other specified nerve(s) of pelvic girdle and lower limb

956.8 Multiple nerves of pelvic girdle and lower limb

956.9 Unspecified nerve of pelvic girdle and lower limb

957 Injury to other and unspecified nerves

957.0 Superficial nerves of head and neck

957.1 Other specified nerve(s)

957.8 Multiple nerves in several parts
Multiple nerve injury NOS

957.9 Unspecified site
Nerve injury NOS

CERTAIN TRAUMATIC COMPLICATIONS AND UNSPECIFIED INJURIES (958-959)

958 Certain early complications of trauma

> *Excludes:* *adult respiratory distress syndrome (518.5)*
> *flail chest (807.4)*
> *shock lung (518.5)*
> *that occurring during or following medical procedures (996.0-999.9)*

● Code new
to this edition

▲ Revision of
existing code

④ ⑤ Fourth or fifth
digit required

958.0 Air embolism
Pneumathemia

| *Excludes:* | *that complicating:* |

abortion (634-638 with .6, 639.6)
ectopic or molar pregnancy (639.6)
pregnancy, childbirth, or the puerperium (673.0)

958.1 Fat embolism

| *Excludes:* | *that complicating:* |

abortion (634-638 with .6, 639.6)
pregnancy, childbirth, or the puerperium (673.8)

958.2 Secondary and recurrent hemorrhage

958.3 Posttraumatic wound infection, not elsewhere classified

| *Excludes:* | *infected open wounds—code to complicated open wound of site* |

958.4 Traumatic shock
Shock (immediate) (delayed) following injury

| *Excludes:* | *shock:* |

anaphylactic (995.0)
  due to serum (999.4)
anesthetic (995.4)
electric (994.8)
following abortion (639.5)
lightning (994.0)
nontraumatic NOS (785.50)
obstetric (669.1)
postoperative (998.0)

958.5 Traumatic anuria
Crush syndrome
Renal failure following crushing

| *Excludes:* | *that due to a medical procedure (997.5)* |

958.6 Volkmann's ischemic contracture
Posttraumatic muscle contracture

958.7 Traumatic subcutaneous emphysema

| *Excludes:* | *subcutaneous emphysema resulting from a procedure (998.81)* |

958.8 Other early complications of trauma

959 Injury, other and unspecified
Includes: injury NOS

| *Excludes:* | *injury NOS of:* |

blood vessels (900.0-904.9)
eye (921.0-921.9)
internal organs (860.0-869.1)
intracranial sites (854.0-854.1)
nerves (950.0-951.9, 953.0-957.9)
spinal cord (952.0-952.9)

⑤ **959.0 Head, face and neck**

Cheek	Mouth
Ear	Nose
Eyebrow	Throat
Lip	

959.01 Head injury, unspecified

| *Excludes:* | *concussion (850.1-850.9)* |

with head injury NOS (850.1-850.9)
head injury NOS with loss of consciousness (850.1-850.5)
specified intracranial injuries (850.0-854.1)

959.09 Injury of face and neck

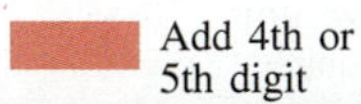
Add 4th or
5th digit

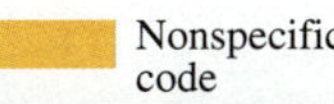
Nonspecific
code

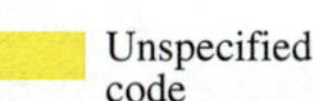
Unspecified
code

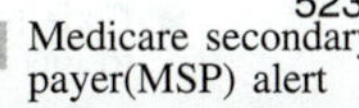
Medicare secondary
payer(MSP) alert

959.1 Trunk

Abdominal wall	External genital organs
Back	Flank
Breast	Groin
Buttock	Interscapular region
Chest wall	Perineum

Excludes: scapular region (959.2)

959.2 Shoulder and upper arm

Axilla	Scapular region

959.3 Elbow, forearm, and wrist

959.4 Hand, except finger

959.5 Finger

Fingernail	Thumb (nail)

959.6 Hip and thigh
Upper leg

959.7 Knee, leg, ankle, and foot

959.8 Other specified sites, including multiple

Excludes: multiple sites classifiable to the same four-digit category (959.0-959.7)

959.9 Unspecified site

POISONING BY DRUGS, MEDICINAL AND BIOLOGICAL SUBSTANCES (960-979)

Includes: overdose of these substances
wrong substances given or taken in error

Excludes: adverse effects ["hypersensitivity," "reaction," etc.] of correct substance properly
administered. Such cases are to be classified according to the nature of the
adverse effect, such as:
adverse effect NOS (995.2)
allergic lymphadenitis (289.3)
aspirin gastritis (535.4)
blood disorders (280.0-289.9)
dermatitis:
contact (692.0-692.9)
due to ingestion (693.0-693.9)
nephropathy (583.9)
[The drug giving rise to the adverse effect may be identified by use of
categories E930-E949]
drug dependence (304.0-304.9)
drug reaction and poisoning affecting the newborn (760.0-779.9)
nondependent abuse of drugs (305.0-305.9)
pathological drug intoxication (292.2)

Use additional code to specify the effects of the poisoning

960 Poisoning by antibiotics

Excludes: antibiotics:
ear, nose, and throat (976.6)
eye (976.5)
local (976.0)

960.0 Penicillins

Ampicillin	Cloxacillin
Carbenicillin	Penicillin G

960.1 Antifungal antibiotics

Amphotericin B	Nystatin
Griseofulvin	Trichomycin

Excludes: preparations intended for topical use (976.0-976.9)

960.2 Chloramphenicol group

Chloramphenicol	Thiamphenicol

960.3 Erythromycin and other macrolides

Oleandomycin	Spiramycin

960.4 Tetracycline group

Doxycycline	Oxytetracycline
Minocycline	

● Code new
to this edition

▲ Revision of
existing code

④ ⑤ Fourth or fifth
digit required

960.5 Cephalosporin group
Cephalexin   Cephaloridine
Cephaloglycin   Cephalothin

960.6 Antimycobacterial antibiotics
Cycloserine   Rifampin
Kanamycin   Streptomycin

960.7 Antineoplastic antibiotics
Actinomycin such as: Bleomycin
  Cactinomycin   Daunorubicin
  Dactinomycin   Mitomycin

960.8 Other specified antibiotics

960.9 Unspecified antibiotic

961 Poisoning by other anti-infectives

Excludes: *anti-infectives:*

ear, nose, and throat (976.6)
eye (976.5)
local (976.0)

961.0 Sulfonamides
Sulfadiazine   Sulfamethoxazole
Sulfafurazole

961.1 Arsenical anti-infectives

961.2 Heavy metal anti-infectives
Compounds of: Compounds of:
  antimony   lead
  bismuth   mercury

Excludes: *mercurial diuretics (974.0)*

961.3 Quinoline and hydroxyquinoline derivatives
Chiniofon   Diiodohydroxyquin

Excludes: *antimalarial drugs (961.4)*

961.4 Antimalarials and drugs acting on other blood protozoa
Chloroquine   Proguanil [chloroguanide]
Cycloguanil   Pyrimethamine
Primaquine   Quinine

961.5 Other antiprotozoal drugs
Emetine

961.6 Anthelmintics
Hexylresorcinol   Thiabendazole
Piperazine

961.7 Antiviral drugs
Methisazone

Excludes: *amantadine (966.4)*
cytarabine (963.1)
idoxuridine (976.5)

961.8 Other antimycobacterial drugs
Ethambutol   Para-aminosalicylic acid derivatives
Ethionamide   Sulfones
Isoniazid

961.9 Other and unspecified anti-infectives
Flucytosine   Nitrofuran derivatives

962 Poisoning by hormones and synthetic substitutes

Excludes: *oxytocic hormones (975.0)*

962.0 Adrenal cortical steroids
Cortisone derivatives
Desoxycorticosterone derivatives
Fluorinated corticosteroids

962.1 Androgens and anabolic congeners
Methandriol   Oxymetholone
Nandrolone   Testosterone

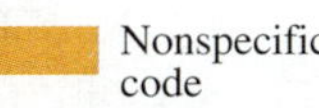

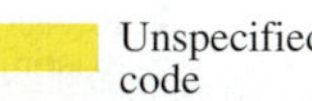

962.2 Ovarian hormones and synthetic substitutes
Contraceptives, oral
Estrogens
Estrogens and progestogens, combined
Progestogens

962.3 Insulins and antidiabetic agents
Acetohexamide
Biguanide derivatives, oral
Chlorpropamide
Glucagon
Insulin
Phenformin
Sulfonylurea derivatives, oral
Tolbutamide

962.4 Anterior pituitary hormones
Corticotropin
Gonadotropin
Somatotropin [growth hormone]

962.5 Posterior pituitary hormones
Vasopressin

> *Excludes:* *oxytocic hormones (975.0)*

962.6 Parathyroid and parathyroid derivatives

962.7 Thyroid and thyroid derivatives
Dextrothyroxin
Levothyroxine sodium
Liothyronine
Thyroglobulin

962.8 Antithyroid agents
Iodides
Thiouracil
Thiourea

962.9 Other and unspecified hormones and synthetic substitutes

963 Poisoning by primarily systemic agents

963.0 Antiallergic and antiemetic drugs
Antihistamines
Chlorpheniramine
Diphenhydramine
Diphenylpyraline
Thonzylamine
Tripelennamine

> *Excludes:* *phenothiazine-based tranquilizers (969.1)*

963.1 Antineoplastic and immunosuppressive drugs
Azathioprine
Busulfan
Chlorambucil
Cyclophosphamide
Cytarabine
Fluorouracil
Mercaptopurine
thio-TEPA

> *Excludes:* *antineoplastic antibiotics (960.7)*

963.2 Acidifying agents

963.3 Alkalizing agents

963.4 Enzymes, not elsewhere classified
Penicillinase

963.5 Vitamins, not elsewhere classified
Vitamin A
Vitamin D

> *Excludes:* *nicotinic acid (972.2)*
> *vitamin K (964.3)*

963.8 Other specified systemic agents
Heavy metal antagonists

963.9 Unspecified systemic agent

964 Poisoning by agents primarily affecting blood constituents

964.0 Iron and its compounds
Ferric salts
Ferrous sulfate and other ferrous salts

964.1 Liver preparations and other antianemic agents
Folic acid

964.2 Anticoagulants
Coumarin
Heparin
Phenindione
Warfarin sodium

964.3 Vitamin K [phytonadione]

● Code new
to this edition

▲ Revision of
existing code

④ ⑤ Fourth or fifth
digit required

964.4 Fibrinolysis-affecting drugs
Aminocaproic acid Streptokinase
Streptodornase Urokinase

964.5 Anticoagulant antagonists and other coagulants
Hexadimethrine Protamine sulfate

964.6 Gamma globulin

964.7 Natural blood and blood products
Blood plasma Packed red cells
Human fibrinogen Whole blood

Excludes: transfusion reactions (999.4-999.8)

964.8 Other specified agents affecting blood constituents
Macromolecular blood substitutes
Plasma expanders

964.9 Unspecified agent affecting blood constituents

965 Poisoning by analgesics, antipyretics, and antirheumatics

Excludes: drug dependence (304.0-304.9)
nondependent abuse (305.0-305.9)

⑤ **965.0 Opiates and related narcotics**

965.00 Opium (alkaloids), unspecified

965.01 Heroin
Diacetylmorphine

965.02 Methadone

965.09 Other
Codeine [methylmorphine]
Meperidine [pethidine]
Morphine

965.1 Salicylates
Acetylsalicylic acid [aspirin]
Salicylic acid salts

965.4 Aromatic analgesics, not elsewhere classified
Acetanilid
Paracetamol [acetaminophen]
Phenacetin [acetophenetidin]

965.5 Pyrazole derivatives
Aminophenazone [aminopyrine]
Phenylbutazone

⑤ **965.6 Antirheumatics [antiphlogistics]**

Excludes: salicylates (965.1)
steroids (962.0-962.9)

965.61 Propionic acid derivatives
Fenoprofen Ketoprofen
Flurbiprofen Naproxen
Ibuprofen Oxaprozin

965.69 Other antirheumatics
Gold salts
Indomethacin

965.7 Other non-narcotic analgesics
Pyrabital

965.8 Other specified analgesics and antipyretics
Pentazocine

965.9 Unspecified analgesic and antipyretic

966 Poisoning by anticonvulsants and anti-Parkinsonism drugs

966.0 Oxazolidine derivatives
Paramethadione Trimethadione

966.1 Hydantoin derivatives
Phenytoin

966.2 Succinimides
Ethosuximide Phensuximide

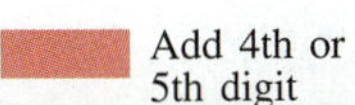

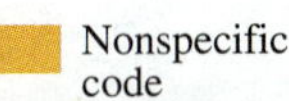

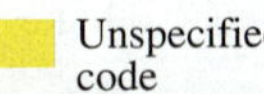

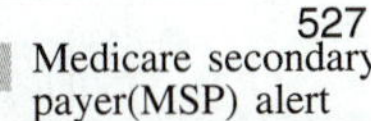

966.3 Other and unspecified anticonvulsants
Primidone

Excludes: *barbiturates (967.0)*
sulfonamides (961.0)

966.4 Anti-Parkinsonism drugs
Amantadine
Ethopropazine [profenamine]
Levodopa [L-dopa]

967 Poisoning by sedatives and hypnotics

Excludes: *drug dependence (304.0-304.9)*
nondependent abuse (305.0-305.9)

967.0 Barbiturates
Amobarbital [amylobarbitone]
Barbital [barbitone]
Butabarbital [butabarbitone]
Pentobarbital [pentobarbitone]
Phenobarbital [phenobarbitone]
Secobarbital [quinalbarbitone]

Excludes: *thiobarbiturate anesthetics (968.3)*

967.1 Chloral hydrate group

967.2 Paraldehyde

967.3 Bromine compounds
Bromide   Carbromal (derivatives)

967.4 Methaqualone compounds

967.5 Glutethimide group

967.6 Mixed sedatives, not elsewhere classified

967.8 Other sedatives and hypnotics

967.9 Unspecified sedative or hypnotic
Sleeping:
drug
pill   } NOS
tablet

968 Poisoning by other central nervous system depressants and anesthetics

Excludes: *drug dependence (304.0-304.9)*
nondependent abuse (305.0-305.9)

968.0 Central nervous system muscle-tone depressants
Chlorphenesin (carbamate)   Methocarbamol
Mephenesin

968.1 Halothane

968.2 Other gaseous anesthetics
Ether
Halogenated hydrocarbon derivatives, except halothane
Nitrous oxide

968.3 Intravenous anesthetics

Excludes: *Methohexital [methohexitone]*
Thiobarbiturates, such as thiopental sodium

968.4 Other and unspecified general anesthetics

968.5 Surface [topical] and infiltration anesthetics
Cocaine   Procaine
Lidocaine [lignocaine]   Tetracaine

968.6 Peripheral nerve and plexus-blocking anesthetics

968.7 Spinal anesthetics

968.9 Other and unspecified local anesthetics

969 Poisoning by psychotropic agents

Excludes: *drug dependence (304.0-304.9)*
nondependent abuse (305.0-305.9)

● Code new
to this edition

▲ Revision of
existing code

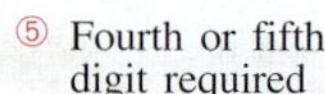

④ ⑤ Fourth or fifth
digit required

969.0 Antidepressants
Amitriptyline
Imipramine
Monoamine oxidase [MAO] inhibitors

969.1 Phenothiazine-based tranquilizers
Chlorpromazine
Fluphenazine
Prochlorperazine
Promazine

969.2 Butyrophenone-based tranquilizers
Haloperidol
Spiperone
Trifluperidol

969.3 Other antipsychotics, neuroleptics, and major tranquilizers

969.4 Benzodiazepine-based tranquilizers
Chlordiazepoxide
Diazepam
Flurazepam
Lorazepam
Medazepam
Nitrazepam

969.5 Other tranquilizers
Hydroxyzine
Meprobamate

969.6 Psychodysleptics [hallucinogens]
Cannabis (derivatives)
Lysergide [LSD]
Marihuana (derivatives)
Mescaline
Psilocin
Psilocybin

969.7 Psychostimulants
Amphetamine
Caffeine

Excludes: central appetite depressants (977.0)

969.8 Other specified psychotropic agents

969.9 Unspecified psychotropic agent

970 Poisoning by central nervous system stimulants

970.0 Analeptics
Lobeline
Nikethamide

970.1 Opiate antagonists
Levallorphan
Nalorphine
Naloxone

970.8 Other specified central nervous system stimulants

970.9 Unspecified central nervous system stimulant

971 Poisoning by drugs primarily affecting the autonomic nervous system

971.0 Parasympathomimetics [cholinergics]
Acetylcholine
Anticholinesterase:
  organophosphorus
  reversible
Pilocarpine

971.1 Parasympatholytics [anticholinergics and antimuscarinics] and spasmolytics
Atropine
Homatropine
Hyoscine [scopolamine]
Quaternary ammonium derivatives

Excludes: papaverine (972.5)

971.2 Sympathomimetics [adrenergics]
Epinephrine [adrenalin]
Levarterenol [noradrenalin]

971.3 Sympatholytics [antiadrenergics]
Phenoxybenzamine
Tolazoline hydrochloride

971.9 Unspecified drug primarily affecting autonomic nervous system

972 Poisoning by agents primarily affecting the cardiovascular system

972.0 Cardiac rhythm regulators
Practolol
Procainamide
Propranolol
Quinidine

Excludes: lidocaine (968.5)

972.1 Cardiotonic glycosides and drugs of similar action
Digitalis glycosides
Digoxin
Strophanthins

972.2 Antilipemic and antiarteriosclerotic drugs
Clofibrate
Nicotinic acid derivatives

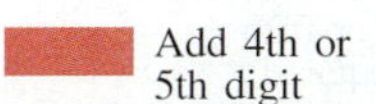

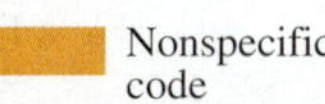

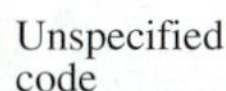

Medicare secondary
payer(MSP) alert

972.3 Ganglion-blocking agents
Pentamethonium bromide

972.4 Coronary vasodilators
Dipyridamole   Nitrites
Nitrates [nitroglycerin]

972.5 Other vasodilators
Cyclandelate   Papaverine
Diazoxide

> Excludes: nicotinic acid (972.2)

972.6 Other antihypertensive agents
Clonidine   Rauwolfia alkaloids
Guanethidine   Reserpine

972.7 Antivaricose drugs, including sclerosing agents
Sodium morrhuate   Zinc salts

972.8 Capillary-active drugs
Adrenochrome derivatives
Metaraminol

972.9 Other and unspecified agents primarily affecting the cardiovascular system

973 Poisoning by agents primarily affecting the gastrointestinal system

973.0 Antacids and antigastric secretion drugs
Aluminum hydroxide   Magnesium trisilicate

973.1 Irritant cathartics
Bisacodyl   Phenolphthalein
Castor oil

973.2 Emollient cathartics
Dioctyl sulfosuccinates

973.3 Other cathartics, including intestinal atonia drugs
Magnesium sulfate

973.4 Digestants
Pancreatin   Pepsin
Papain

973.5 Antidiarrheal drugs
Kaolin   Pectin

> Excludes: anti-infectives (960.0-961.9)

973.6 Emetics

973.8 Other specified agents primarily affecting the gastrointestinal system

973.9 Unspecified agent primarily affecting the gastrointestinal system

974 Poisoning by water, mineral, and uric acid metabolism drugs

974.0 Mercurial diuretics
Chlormerodrin   Mersalyl
Mercaptomerin

974.1 Purine derivative diuretics
Theobromine   Theophylline

> Excludes: aminophylline [theophylline ethylenediamine] (975.7)
> caffeine (969.7)

974.2 Carbonic acid anhydrase inhibitors
Acetazolamide

974.3 Saluretics
Benzothiadiazides   Chlorothiazide group

974.4 Other diuretics
Ethacrynic acid   Furosemide

974.5 Electrolytic, caloric, and water-balance agents

974.6 Other mineral salts, not elsewhere classified

974.7 Uric acid metabolism drugs
Allopurinol   Probenecid
Colchicine

975 Poisoning by agents primarily acting on the smooth and skeletal muscles and respiratory system

● Code new to this edition   ▲ Revision of existing code   ④ ⑤ Fourth or fifth digit required

975.0 Oxytocic agents
Ergot alkaloids   Prostaglandins
Oxytocin

975.1 Smooth muscle relaxants
Adiphenine
Metaproterenol [orciprenaline]

Excludes: papaverine (972.5)

975.2 Skeletal muscle relaxants

975.3 Other and unspecified drugs acting on muscles

975.4 Antitussives
Dextromethorphan   Pipazethate

975.5 Expectorants
Acetylcysteine   Terpin hydrate
Guaifenesin

975.6 Anti-common cold drugs

975.7 Antiasthmatics
Aminophylline [theophylline ethylenediamine]

975.8 Other and unspecified respiratory drugs

976 Poisoning by agents primarily affecting skin and mucous membrane, ophthalmological, otorhinolaryngological, and dental drugs

976.0 Local anti-infectives and anti-inflammatory drugs

976.1 Antipruritics

976.2 Local astringents and local detergents

976.3 Emollients, demulcents, and protectants

976.4 Keratolytics, keratoplastics, other hair treatment drugs and preparations

976.5 Eye anti-infectives and other eye drugs
Idoxuridine

976.6 Anti-infectives and other drugs and preparations for ear, nose, and throat

976.7 Dental drugs topically applied

Excludes: anti-infectives (976.0)
local anesthetics (968.5)

976.8 Other agents primarily affecting skin and mucous membrane
Spermicides [vaginal contraceptives]

976.9 Unspecified agent primarily affecting skin and mucous membrane

977 Poisoning by other and unspecified drugs and medicinal substances

977.0 Dietetics
Central appetite depressants

977.1 Lipotropic drugs

977.2 Antidotes and chelating agents, not elsewhere classified

977.3 Alcohol deterrents

977.4 Pharmaceutical excipients
Pharmaceutical adjuncts

977.8 Other specified drugs and medicinal substances
Contrast media used for diagnostic x-ray procedures
Diagnostic agents and kits

977.9 Unspecified drug or medicinal substance

978 Poisoning by bacterial vaccines

978.0 BCG

978.1 Typhoid and paratyphoid

978.2 Cholera

978.3 Plague

978.4 Tetanus

978.5 Diphtheria

978.6 Pertussis vaccine, including combinations with a pertussis component

978.8 Other and unspecified bacterial vaccines

978.9 Mixed bacterial vaccines, except combinations with a pertussis component

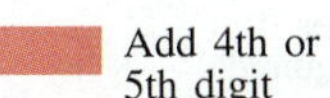

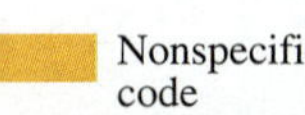

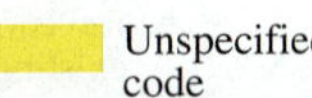

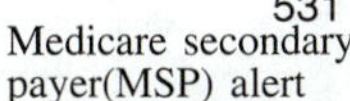

979 **Poisoning by other vaccines and biological substances**

> Excludes: *gamma globulin (964.6)*

979.0 **Smallpox vaccine**

979.1 **Rabies vaccine**

979.2 **Typhus vaccine**

979.3 **Yellow fever vaccine**

979.4 **Measles vaccine**

979.5 **Poliomyelitis vaccine**

979.6 **Other and unspecified viral and rickettsial vaccines**
Mumps vaccine

979.7 **Mixed viral-rickettsial and bacterial vaccines, except combinations with a pertussis component**

> Excludes: *combinations with a pertussis component (978.6)*

979.9 **Other and unspecified vaccines and biological substances**

TOXIC EFFECTS OF SUBSTANCES CHIEFLY NONMEDICINAL AS TO SOURCE (980-989)

> Excludes: *burns from chemical agents (ingested) (947.0-947.9)*
> *localized toxic effects indexed elsewhere (001.0-799.9)*
> *respiratory conditions due to external agents (506.0-508.9)*

Use additional code to specify the nature of the toxic effect

980 **Toxic effect of alcohol**

980.0 **Ethyl alcohol**
Denatured alcohol
Ethanol
Grain alcohol
Use additional code to identify any associated:
acute alcohol intoxication (305.0)
in alcoholism (303.0)
drunkenness (simple) (305.0)
pathological (291.4)

980.1 **Methyl alcohol**
Methanol   Wood alcohol

980.2 **Isopropyl alcohol**
Dimethyl carbinol   Rubbing alcohol
Isopropanol

980.3 **Fusel oil**
Alcohol:
amyl
butyl
propyl

980.8 **Other specified alcohols**

980.9 **Unspecified alcohol**

981 **Toxic effect of petroleum products**
Benzine   Petroleum:
Gasoline   ether
Kerosene   naphtha
Paraffin wax   spirit

982 **Toxic effect of solvents other than petroleum-based**

982.0 **Benzene and homologues**

982.1 **Carbon tetrachloride**

982.2 **Carbon disulfide**
Carbon bisulfide

982.3 **Other chlorinated hydrocarbon solvents**
Tetrachloroethylene   Trichloroethylene

> Excludes: *chlorinated hydrocarbon preparations other than solvents (989.2)*

982.4 **Nitroglycol**

982.8 **Other nonpetroleum-based solvents**
Acetone

● Code new
to this edition

▲ Revision of
existing code

④ ⑤ Fourth or fifth
digit required

983 **Toxic effect of corrosive aromatics, acids, and caustic alkalis**

983.0 **Corrosive aromatics**
Carbolic acid or phenol   Cresol

983.1 **Acids**
Acid:
  hydrochloric
  nitric
  sulfuric

983.2 **Caustic alkalis**
Lye   Sodium hydroxide
Potassium hydroxide

983.9 **Caustic, unspecified**

984 **Toxic effect of lead and its compounds (including fumes)**
Includes: that from all sources except medicinal substances

984.0 **Inorganic lead compounds**
Lead dioxide   Lead salts

984.1 **Organic lead compounds**
Lead acetate   Tetraethyl lead

984.8 **Other lead compounds**

984.9 **Unspecified lead compound**

985 **Toxic effect of other metals**
Includes: that from all sources except medicinal substances

985.0 **Mercury and its compounds**
Minamata disease

985.1 **Arsenic and its compounds**

985.2 **Manganese and its compounds**

985.3 **Beryllium and its compounds**

985.4 **Antimony and its compounds**

985.5 **Cadmium and its compounds**

985.6 **Chromium**

985.8 **Other specified metals**
Brass fumes   Iron compounds
Copper salts   Nickel compounds

985.9 **Unspecified metal**

986 **Toxic effect of carbon monoxide**
Carbon monoxide from any source

987 **Toxic effect of other gases, fumes, or vapors**

987.0 **Liquefied petroleum gases**
Butane   Propane

987.1 **Other hydrocarbon gas**

987.2 **Nitrogen oxides**
Nitrogen dioxide   Nitrous fumes

987.3 **Sulfur dioxide**

987.4 **Freon**
Dichloromonofluoromethane

987.5 **Lacrimogenic gas**
Bromobenzyl cyanide   Ethyliodoacetate
Chloroacetophenone

987.6 **Chlorine gas**

987.7 **Hydrocyanic acid gas**

987.8 **Other specified gases, fumes, or vapors**
Phosgene   Polyester fumes

987.9 **Unspecified gas, fume, or vapor**

988 Toxic effect of noxious substances eaten as food

Excludes: *allergic reaction to food, such as:*
gastroenteritis (558.3)
rash (692.5, 693.1)
food poisoning (bacterial) (005.0-005.9)
toxic effects of food contaminants, such as:
aflatoxin and other mycotoxin (989.7)
mercury (985.0)

988.0 Fish and shellfish

988.1 Mushrooms

988.2 Berries and other plants

988.8 Other specified noxious substances eaten as food

988.9 Unspecified noxious substance eaten as food

989 Toxic effect of other substances, chiefly nonmedicinal as to source

989.0 Hydrocyanic acid and cyanides
Potassium cyanide   Sodium cyanide

Excludes: *gas and fumes (987.7)*

989.1 Strychnine and salts

989.2 Chlorinated hydrocarbons
Aldrin   DDT
Chlordane   Dieldrin

Excludes: *chlorinated hydrocarbon solvents (982.0-982.3)*

989.3 Organophosphate and carbamate
Carbaryl   Parathion
Dichlorvos   Phorate
Malathion   Phosdrin

989.4 Other pesticides, not elsewhere classified
Mixtures of insecticides

989.5 Venom
Bites of venomous snakes, lizards, and spiders
Tick paralysis

989.6 Soaps and detergents

989.7 Aflatoxin and other mycotoxin [food contaminants]

⑤ **989.8 Other substances, chiefly nonmedicinal as to source**

989.81 Asbestos

Excludes: *asbestosis (501)*
exposure to asbestos (V15.84)

989.82 Latex

989.83 Silicone

Excludes: *silicone used in medical devices, implants and grafts (996.00-996.79)*

989.84 Tobacco

989.89 Other

989.9 Unspecified substance, chiefly nonmedicinal as to source

OTHER AND UNSPECIFIED EFFECTS OF EXTERNAL CAUSES (990-995)

990 Effects of radiation, unspecified
Complication of phototherapy   Radiation sickness
Complication of radiation therapy

Excludes: *specified adverse effects of radiation*
Such conditions are to be classified according to the nature of the adverse
effect, as:
burns (940.0-949.5)
dermatitis (692.7-692.8)
leukemia (204.0-208.9)
pneumonia (508.0)
sunburn (692.71, 692.76-692.77)
[The type of radiation giving rise to the adverse effect may be identified by use
of the E codes.]

     ● Code new   ▲ Revision of   ④ ⑤ Fourth or fifth
      to this edition   existing code   digit required

991 Effects of reduced temperature

991.0 Frostbite of face

991.1 Frostbite of hand

991.2 Frostbite of foot

991.3 Frostbite of other and unspecified sites

991.4 Immersion foot
Trench foot

991.5 Chilblains
Erythema pernio   Perniosis

991.6 Hypothermia
Hypothermia (accidental)

> *Excludes:*   *hypothermia following anesthesia (995.89)*
> *hypothermia not associated with low environmental temperature (780.99)*

991.8 Other specified effects of reduced temperature

991.9 Unspecified effect of reduced temperature
Effects of freezing or excessive cold NOS

992 Effects of heat and light

> *Excludes:*   *burns (940.0-949.5)*
> *diseases of sweat glands due to heat (705.0-705.9)*
> *malignant hyperpyrexia following anesthesia (995.86)*
> *sunburn (692.71, 692.76-692.77)*

992.0 Heat stroke and sunstroke
Heat apoplexy   Siriasis
Heat pyrexia   Thermoplegia
Ictus solaris

992.1 Heat syncope
Heat collapse

992.2 Heat cramps

992.3 Heat exhaustion, anhydrotic
Heat prostration due to water depletion

> *Excludes:*   *that associated with salt depletion (992.4)*

992.4 Heat exhaustion due to salt depletion
Heat prostration due to salt (and water) depletion

992.5 Heat exhaustion, unspecified
Heat prostration NOS

992.6 Heat fatigue, transient

992.7 Heat edema

992.8 Other specified heat effects

992.9 Unspecified

993 Effects of air pressure

993.0 Barotrauma, otitic
Aero-otitis media
Effects of high altitude on ears

993.1 Barotrauma, sinus
Aerosinusitis
Effects of high altitude on sinuses

993.2 Other and unspecified effects of high altitude
Alpine sickness   Hypobaropathy
Andes disease   Mountain sickness
Anoxia due to high altitude

993.3 Caisson disease
Bends   Decompression sickness
Compressed-air disease   Divers' palsy or paralysis

993.4 Effects of air pressure caused by explosion

993.8 Other specified effects of air pressure

993.9 Unspecified effect of air pressure

994 Effects of other external causes

> *Excludes:*   *certain adverse effects not elsewhere classified (995.0-995.8)*

Add 4th or 5th digit   Nonspecific code   Unspecified code   Medicare secondary payer(MSP) alert

994.0 Effects of lightning
Shock from lightning   Struck by lightning NOS

Excludes: *burns (940.0-949.5)*

994.1 Drowning and nonfatal submersion
Bathing cramp   Immersion

994.2 Effects of hunger
Deprivation of food   Starvation

994.3 Effects of thirst
Deprivation of water

994.4 Exhaustion due to exposure

994.5 Exhaustion due to excessive exertion
Overexertion

994.6 Motion sickness
Air sickness   Travel sickness
Seasickness

994.7 Asphyxiation and strangulation
Suffocation (by):   Suffocation (by):
  bedclothes   plastic bag
  cave-in   pressure
  constriction   strangulation
  mechanical

Excludes: *asphyxia from:*
carbon monoxide (986)
inhalation of food or foreign body (932-934.9)
other gases, fumes, and vapors (987.0-987.9)

994.8 Electrocution and nonfatal effects of electric current
Shock from electric current

Excludes: *electric burns (940.0-949.5)*

994.9 Other effects of external causes
Effects of:
  abnormal gravitational [G] forces or states
  weightlessness

995 Certain adverse effects not elsewhere classified

Excludes: *complications of surgical and medical care (996.0-999.9)*

995.0 Other anaphylactic shock
Allergic shock
Anaphylactic reaction   } NOS or due to adverse effect of correct medicinal
Anaphylaxis   substance properly administered

Excludes: *anaphylactic reaction to serum (999.4)*
anaphylactic shock due to adverse food reaction (995.60-995.69)

Use additional E code, if desired, to identify external cause, such as:
  adverse effects of correct medicinal substance properly administered (E930-E949)

995.1 Angioneurotic edema
Giant urticaria

Excludes: *Urticaria:*
due to serum (999.5)
other specified (698.2, 708.0-708.9, 757.33)

995.2 Unspecified adverse effect of drug, medicinal and biological substance
Adverse effect
Allergic reaction
Hypersensitivity   } (due) to correct medicinal substance properly administered
Idiosyncrasy

Drug:
  hypersensitivity NOS
  reaction NOS

Excludes: *pathological drug intoxication (292.2)*

● Code new   ▲ Revision of   ④ ⑤ Fourth or fifth
to this edition   existing code   digit required

995.3 Allergy, unspecified
Allergic reaction NOS   Idiosyncrasy NOS
Hypersensitivity NOS

Excludes: *allergic reaction NOS to correct medicinal substance properly administered (995.2)*
specific types of allergic reaction, such as:
allergic diarrhea (558.3)
dermatitis (691.0-693.9)
hay fever (477.0-477.9)

995.4 Shock due to anesthesia
Shock due to anesthesia in which the correct substance was properly administered

Excludes: *complications of anesthesia in labor or delivery (668.0-668.9)*
overdose or wrong substance given (968.0-969.9)
postoperative shock NOS (998.0)
specified adverse effects of anesthesia classified elsewhere, such as:
anoxic brain damage (348.1)
hepatitis (070.0-070.9), etc.
unspecified adverse effect of anesthesia (995.2)

⑤ **995.5 Child maltreatment syndrome**
Use additional code(s), if applicable, to identify any associated injuries
Use additional E code to identify:
nature of abuse (E960-E968)
perpetrator (E967.0-E967.9)

995.50   Child abuse, unspecified

995.51   Child emotional/psychological abuse

995.52   Child neglect (nutritional)

995.53   Child sexual abuse

995.54   Child physical abuse
Battered baby or child syndrome

Excludes: *Shaken infant syndrome (995.55)*

995.55   Shaken infant syndrome
Use additional code(s) to identify any associated injuries

995.59   Other child abuse and neglect
Multiple forms of abuse

⑤ **995.6 Anaphylactic shock due to adverse food reaction**
Anaphylactic shock due to nonpoisonous foods

995.60   Due to unspecified food

995.61   Due to peanuts

995.62   Due to crustaceans

995.63   Due to fruits and vegetables

995.64   Due to tree nuts and seeds

995.65   Due to fish

995.66   Due to food additives

995.67   Due to milk products

995.68   Due to eggs

995.69   Due to other specified food

995.7 Other adverse food reactions, not elsewhere classified
Use additional code to identify the type of reaction, such as:
hives (708.0)
wheezing (786.07)

Excludes: *unaphylactic shock due to adverse food reaction (995.60-995.69)*
asthma (493.0, 493.9)
dermatitis due to food (693.1)
in contact with the skin (692.5)
gastroenteritis and colitis due to food (558.3)
rhinitis due to food (477.1)

⑤ **995.8 Other specified adverse effects, not elsewhere classified**

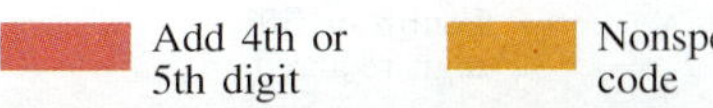

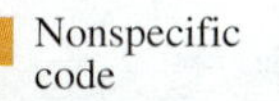

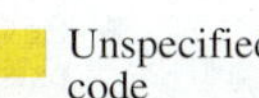

Medicare secondary
payer(MSP) alert

995.80 Adult maltreatment, unspecified
Abused person NOS
Use additional code to identify:
any associated injury
perpetrator (E967.0-E967.9)

995.81 Adult physical abuse
Battered:
person syndrome NEC
man
spouse
woman
Use additional code to identify:
any associated injury
nature of abuse (E960-E968)
perpetrator (E967.0-E967.9)

995.82 Adult emotional/psychological abuse
Use additional E code to identify perpetrator (E967.0-E967.9)

995.83 Adult sexual abuse
Use additional code to identify:
any associated injury
perpetrator (E967.0-E967.9)

995.84 Adult neglect (nutritional)
Use additional code to identify:
intent of neglect (E904.0, E968.4)
perpetrator (E967.0-967.9)

995.85 Other adult abuse and neglect
Multiple forms of abuse and neglect
Use additional code to identify:
any associated injury
intent of neglect (E904.0, E968.4)
nature of abuse (E960-E968)
perpetrator (E967.0-E967.9)

995.86 Malignant hyperthermia
Malignant hyperpyrexia due to anesthesia

995.89 Other
Hypothermia due to anesthesia

● **995.9 Systemic inflammatory response syndrome (SIRS)**

● **995.90 Systemic inflammatory response syndrome, unspecified**
SIRS NOS

● **995.91 Systemic inflammatory response syndrome due to infectious process without organ dysfunction**

● **995.92 Systemic inflammatory response syndrome due to infectious process with organ dysfunction**
Severe sepsis
Use additional code to specify organ dysfunction, such as:
encephalopathy (348.3)
heart failure (428.0-428.9)
kidney failure (584.5-584.9, 585, 586)

● **995.93 Systemic inflammatory response syndrome due to non-infectious process without organ dysfunction**

● **995.94 Systemic inflammatory response syndrome due to non-infectious process with organ dysfunction**
Use additional code to specify organ dysfunction, such as:
encephalopathy (348.3)
heart failure (428.0-428.9)
kidney failure (584.5-584.9, 585, 586)

● Code new to this edition   ▲ Revision of existing code   ④ ⑤ Fourth or fifth digit required

COMPLICATIONS OF SURGICAL AND MEDICAL CARE, NOT ELSEWHERE CLASSIFIED (996-999)

Excludes: *adverse effects of medicinal agents (001.0-799.9, 995.0-995.8)*
burns from local applications and irradiation (940.0-949.5)
complications of:
   conditions for which the procedure was performed
   surgical procedures during abortion, labor, and delivery (630-676.9)
poisoning and toxic effects of drugs and chemicals (960.0-989.9)
postoperative conditions in which no complications are present, such as:
   artificial opening status (V44.0-V44.9)
   closure of external stoma (V55.0-V55.9)
   fitting of prosthetic device (V52.0-V52.9)
specified complications classified elsewhere
   anesthetic shock (995.4)
   electrolyte imbalance (276.0-276.9)
   postlaminectomy syndrome (772.80-722.83)
   postmastectomy lymphedema syndrome (457.0)
   postoperative psychosis (293.0-293.9)
   any other condition classified elsewhere in the Alphabetic Index when described as due to a procedure

996 Complications peculiar to certain specified procedures
Includes: complications, not elsewhere classified, in the use of artificial substitutes [e.g., Dacron, metal, Silastic, Teflon] or natural sources [e.g., bone] involving:
   anastomosis (internal)
   graft (bypass) (patch)
   implant
   internal device:
      catheter
      electronic
      fixation
      prosthetic
   reimplant
   transplant

Excludes: *accidental puncture or laceration during procedure (998.2)*
complications of internal anastomosis of:
   gastrointestinal tract (997.4)
   urinary tract (997.5)
other specified complications classified elsewhere, such as:
   hemolytic anemia (283.1)
   functional cardiac disturbances (429.4)
   serum hepatitis (070.2-070.3)

⑤ **996.0 Mechanical complication of cardiac device, implant, and graft**
Breakdown (mechanical)   Obstruction, mechanical
Displacement   Perforation
Leakage   Protrusion

996.00 Unspecified device, implant, and graft

996.01 Due to cardiac pacemaker (electrode)

996.02 Due to heart valve prosthesis

996.03 Due to coronary bypass graft

Excludes: *atherosclerosis of graft (414.02, 414.03)*
embolism [occlusion NOS] [thrombus] of graft (996.72)

996.04 Due to automatic implantable cardiac defibrillator

996.09 Other

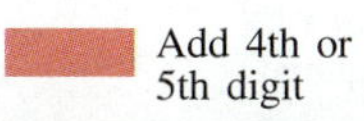

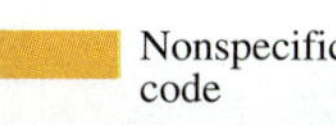

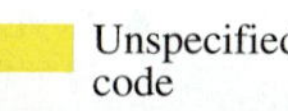

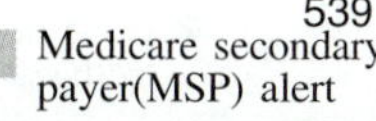

996.1 Mechanical complication of other vascular device, implant, and graft
Mechanical complications involving:
aortic (bifurcation) graft (replacement)
arteriovenous:
dialysis catheter
fistula surgically created
shunt surgicall created
balloon (counterpulsation) device, intra-aortic
carotid artery bypass graft
femoral-popliteal bypass graft
umbrella device, vena cava

Excludes: *atherosclerosis of biological graft (440.30-440.32)*
embolism [occlusion NOS] [thrombus] of (biological) (synthetic) graft (996.74)
peritoneal dialysis catheter (996.56)

996.2 Mechanical complication of nervous system device, implant, and graft
Mechanical complications involving:
dorsal column stimulator
electrodes implanted in brain [brain "pacemaker"]
peripheral nerve graft
ventricular (communicating) shunt

⑤ **996.3 Mechanical complication of genitourinary device, implant, and graft**

996.30 Unspecified device, implant, and graft

996.31 Due to urethral [indwelling] catheter

996.32 Due to intrauterine contraceptive device

996.39 Other
Cystostomy catheter
Prosthetic reconstruction of vas deferens
Repair (graft) of ureter without mention of resection

Excludes: *complications due to:*
external stoma of urinary tract (997.5)
internal anastomosis of urinary tract (997.5)

996.4 Mechanical complication of internal orthopedic device, implant, and graft
Mechanical complications involving:
external (fixation) device utilizing internal screw(s), pin(s) or other methods of fixation
grafts of bone, cartilage, muscle, or tendon
internal (fixation) device such as nail, plate, rod, etc.

Excludes: *complications of external orthopedic device, such as:*
pressure ulcer due to cast (707.0)

⑤ **996.5 Mechanical complication of other specified prosthetic device, implant, and graft**
Mechanical complications involving:
prosthetic implant in:
bile duct
breast
chin
orbit of eye
nonabsorbable surgical material NOS
other graft, implant, and internal device, not elsewhere classified

996.51 Due to corneal graft

996.52 Due to graft of other tissue, not elsewhere classified
Skin graft failure or rejection

Excludes: *failure of artificial skin graft (996.55)*
failure of decellularized allodermis (996.55)
sloughing of temporary skin allografts or xenografts (pigskin)—omit code

996.53 Due to ocular lens prosthesis

Excludes: *contact lenses—code to condition*

996.54 Due to breast prosthesis
Breast capsule (prosthesis)
Mammary implant

● Code new
to this edition
▲ Revision of
existing code
④ ⑤ Fourth or fifth
digit required

996.55   **Due to artificial skin graft and decellularized allodermis**
      Dislodgement
      Displacement
      Failure
      Non-adherence
      Poor incorporation
      Shearing

996.56   **Due to peritoneal dialysis catheter**

    Excludes: *mechanical complication of arteriovenous dialysis catheter (996.1)*

    996.59   **Due to other implant and internal device, not elsewhere classified**
      Nonabsorbable surgical material NOS
      Prosthetic implant in:
        bile duct
        chin
        orbit of eye

⑤ **996.6** **Infection and inflammatory reaction due to internal prosthetic device, implant, and graft**
    Infection (causing obstruction) due to (presence of) any device, implant and graft classifiable to 996.0-996.5
    Inflammation due to (presence of) any device, implant and graft classifiable to 996.0-996.5

Use additional code to identify specified infections

    996.60   **Due to unspecified device, implant, and graft**

    996.61   **Due to cardiac device, implant, and graft**
      Cardiac pacemaker or defibrillator:
        electrode(s), lead(s)
        pulse generator
        subcutaneous pocket
      Coronary artery bypass graft
      Heart valve prosthesis

    996.62   **Due to other vascular device, implant, and graft**
      Arterial graft
      Arteriovenous fistula or shunt
      Infusion pump
      Vascular catheter (arterial) (dialysis) (venous)

    996.63   **Due to nervous system device, implant, and graft**
      Electrodes implanted in brain
      Peripheral nerve graft
      Spinal canal catheter
      Ventricular (communicating) shunt (catheter)

    996.64   **Due to indwelling urinary catheter**
    Use additional code to identify specified infections, such as:
      Cystitis (595.0-595.9)
      Sepsis (038.0-038.9)

    996.65   **Due to other genitourinary device, implant, and graft**
      Intrauterine contraceptive device

    996.66   **Due to internal joint prosthesis**

    996.67   **Due to other internal orthopedic device, implant, and graft**
      Bone growth stimulator (electrode)
      Internal fixation device (pin) (rod) (screw)

    996.68   **Due to peritoneal dialysis catheter**
      Exit-site infection or inflammation

    996.69   **Due to other internal prosthetic device, implant, and graft**
      Breast prosthesis
      Ocular lens prosthesis
      Prosthetic orbital implant

Add 4th or 5th digit	Nonspecific code	Unspecified code	Medicare secondary payer(MSP) alert

⑤ **996.7** **Other complications of internal (biological) (synthetic) prosthetic device, implant, and graft**

Complication NOS
  occlusion NOS
Embolism
Fibrosis
Hemorrhage } due to (presence of) any device, implant, and graft
Pain   classifiable to 996.0-996.5
Stenosis
Thrombus

Excludes: *transplant rejection (996.8)*

996.70 **Due to unspecified device, implant, and graft**

996.71 **Due to heart valve prosthesis**

996.72 **Due to other cardiac device, implant, and graft**
Cardiac pacemaker or defibrillator:
  electrode(s), lead(s)
  subcutaneous pocket
Coronary artery bypass (graft)

Excludes: *occlusion due to atherosclerosis (414.00-414.06)*

996.73 **Due to renal dialysis device, implant, and graft**

996.74 **Due to other vascular device, implant, and graft**

Excludes: *occlusion of biological graft due to atherosclerosis (440.30-440.32)*

996.75 **Due to nervous system device, implant, and graft**

996.76 **Due to genitourinary device, implant, and graft**

996.77 **Due to internal joint prosthesis**

996.78 **Due to other internal orthopedic device, implant, and graft**

996.79 **Due to other internal prosthetic device, implant, and graft**

⑤ **996.8** **Complications of transplanted organ**
Use additional code, if desired, to identify nature of complication, such as:
  Cytomegalovirus (CMV) infection (078.5)
  Transplant failure or rejection

996.80 **Transplanted organ, unspecified**

996.81 **Kidney**

996.82 **Liver**

996.83 **Heart**

996.84 **Lung**

996.85 **Bone Marrow**
Graft-versus-host disease (acute) (chronic)

996.86 **Pancreas**

996.87 **Intestine**

996.89 **Other specified transplanted organ**

⑤ **996.9** **Complications of reattached extremity or body part**

996.90 **Unspecified extremity**

996.91 **Forearm**

996.92 **Hand**

996.93 **Finger(s)**

996.94 **Upper extremity, other and unspecified**

996.95 **Foot and toe(s)**

996.96 **Lower extremity, other and unspecified**

996.99 **Other specified body part**

● Code new   ▲ Revision of   ④ ⑤ Fourth or fifth
   to this edition   existing code   digit required

997 Complications affecting specified body systems, not elsewhere classified

Use additional code to identify complication

Excludes: *the listed conditions when specified as:*
> *causing shock (998.0)*
> *complications of:*
> > *anesthesia:*
> > > *adverse effect (001.0-799.9, 995.0-995.8)*
> > > *in labor or delivery (668.0-668.9)*
> > > *poisoning (968.0-969.9)*
> > *implanted device or graft (996.0-996.9)*
> > *obstetrical procedures (669.0-669.4)*
> > *reattached extremity (996.90-996.96)*
> > *transplanted organic (996.80-996.89)*

⑤ **997.0 Nervous system complications**

997.00 Nervous system complication, unspecified

997.01 Central nervous system complication
Anoxic brain damage
Cerebral hypoxia

Excludes: *cerebrovascular hemorrhage or infarction (997.02)*

997.02 Iatrogenic cerebrovascular infarction or hemorrhage
Postoperative stroke

997.09 Other nervous system complications

997.1 Cardiac complications
Cardiac arrest during or resulting from a procedure
Cardiac insufficiency during or resulting from a procedure
Cardiorespiratory failure during or resulting from a procedure
Heart failure during or resulting from a procedure

Excludes: *the listed conditions as long-term effects of cardiac surgery or due to the presence of cardiac prosthetic device (429.4)*

997.2 Peripheral vascular complications
Phlebitis or thrombophlebitis during or resulting from a procedure

Excludes: *the listed conditions due to:*
> *implant or catheter device (996.62)*
> *infusion, perfusion, or transfusion (999.2)*
> *complications affecting blood vessels (997.71-997.79)*

997.3 Respiratory complications
Mendelson's syndrome ⎫
Pneumonia (aspiration) ⎰ resulting from a procedure

Excludes: *iatrogenic [postoperative] pneumothorax (512.1)*
> *iatrogenic pulmonary embolism (415.11)*
> *Mendelson's syndrome in labor and delivery (668.0)*
> *specified complications classified elsewhere, such as:*
> > *adult respiratory distress syndrome (518.5)*
> > *pulmonary edema, postoperative (518.4)*
> > *respiratory insufficiency, acute, postoperative (518.5)*
> > *shock lung (518.5)*
> > *tracheostomy complications (519.00-519.09)*

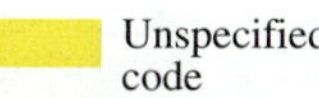

Add 4th or 5th digit   Nonspecific code   Unspecified code   Medicare secondary payer(MSP) alert

997.4 Digestive system complications
Complications of intestinal (internal) anastomosis and bypass, not elsewhere classified, except that involving urinary tract
Hepatic failure
Hepatorenal syndrome } specified as due to a procedure
Intestinal obstruction NOS

| Excludes: | *specified gastrointestinal complications classified elsewhere, such as:* |

blind loop syndrome (579.2)
colostomy or enterostomy complications (569.60-569.69)
gastrostomy complications (536.40-536.49)
gastrojejunal ulcer (534.0-534.9)
infection of external stoma (569.61)
pelvic peritoneal adhesions, female (614.6)
peritoneal adhesions (568.0)
peritoneal adhesions with obstruction (560.81)
postcholecystectomy syndrome (576.0)
postgastric surgery syndromes (564.2)

997.5 Urinary complications
Complications of:
external stoma of urinary tract
internal anastomosis and bypass of urinary tract, including that involving intestinal tract
Oliguria or anuria
Renal:
failure (acute)
insufficiency (acute) } specified as due to procedure
Tubular necrosis (acute)

| Excludes: | *specified complications classified elsewhere, such as:* |

postoperative stricture of:
ureter (593.3)
urethra (598.2)

⑤ **997.6 Amputation stump complication**

| Excludes: | *admission for treatment for a current traumatic amputation; code to complicated traumatic amputation* |

phantom limb (syndrome) (353.6)

997.60 Unspecified complication

997.61 Neuroma of amputation stump

997.62 Infection (chronic)
Use additional code to identify the organism

997.69 Other

⑤ **997.7 Vascular complications of other vessels**

| Excludes: | *peripheral vascular complications (997.2)* |

997.71 Vascular complications of mesenteric artery

997.72 Vascular complications of renal artery

997.79 Vascular complications of other vessels

⑤ **997.9 Complications affecting other specified body systems, not elsewhere classified**

| Excludes: | *specified complications classified elsewhere, such as:* |

broad ligament laceration syndrome (620.6)
postartificial menopause syndrome (627.4)
postoperative stricture of vagina (623.2)

997.91 Hypertension

| Excludes: | *essential hypertension (401.0-401.9)* |

997.99 Other
Vitreous touch syndrome

998 Other complications of procedures, NEC

● Code new to this edition　　▲ Revision of existing code　　④ ⑤ Fourth or fifth digit required

998.0   **Postoperative shock**
      Collapse NOS
      Shock (endotoxic) (hypo-   } during or resulting from a surgical procedure
        volemic) (septic)

      Excludes: *shock:*
           anaphylactic due to serum (999.4)
           anesthetic (995.4)
           electric (994.8)
           following abortion (639.5)
           obstetric (669.1)
           traumatic (958.4)

⑤ **998.1**   **Hemorrhage or hematoma or seroma complicating a procedure**

      Excludes: *hemorrhage due to implanted device or graft (996.70-996.79)*
           hemorrhage, hematoma or seroma complicating cesarean section or puerperal
              perineal wound (674.3)

        998.11   **Hemorrhage complicating a procedure**

        998.12   **Hematoma complicating a procedure**

        998.13   **Seroma complicating a procedure**

998.2   **Accidental puncture or laceration during a procedure**
      Accidental perforation by catheter or other instrument during a procedure on:
        blood vessel
        nerve
        organ

      Excludes: *iatrogenic [postoperative] pneumothorax (512.1)*
           puncture or laceration caused by implanted device intentionally left in operation
              wound (996.0-996.5)
           specified complications classified elsewhere, such as:
             broad ligament laceration syndrome (620.6)
           trauma from instruments during delivery (664.0-665.9)

⑤ **998.3**   **Disruption of operation wound**
      Dehiscence   }
      Rupture   } of operation wound

      Excludes: *disruption of:*
           cesarean wound (674.1)
           perineal wound, puerperal (674.2)

    ● **998.31**   **Disruption of internal operation wound**

    ● **998.32**   **Disruption of external operation wound**
        Disruption of operation wound NOS

998.4   **Foreign body accidentally left during a procedure**
      Adhesions   }
      Obstruction   } due to foreign body accidentally left in operative wound
      Perforation   }   or body cavity during a procedure

      Excludes: *obstruction or perforation caused by implanted device intentionally left in body*
           (996.0-996.5)

⑤ **998.5**   **Postoperative infection**

      Excludes: *infection due to:*
           implanted device (996.60-996.69)
           infusion, perfusion, or transfusion (999.3)
           postoperative obstetrical wound infection (674.3)

        998.51   **Infected postoperative seroma**
Use additional code to identify organism

        998.59   **Other postoperative infection**
          Abscess: postoperative
            intra-abdominal postoperative
            stitch postoperative
            subphrenic postoperative
            wound postoperative
          Septicemia postoperative
Use additional code to identify infection

998.6   **Persistent postoperative fistula**

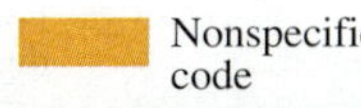

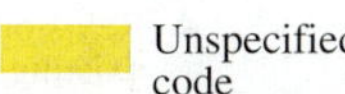

Unspecified
code

Medicare secondary
payer(MSP) alert

998.7 Acute reaction to foreign substance accidentally left during a procedure
Peritonitis:
aseptic
chemical

⑤ **998.8 Other specified complications of procedures, not elsewhere classified**

998.81 Emphysema (subcutaneous) (surgical) resulting from a procedure

998.82 Cataract fragments in eye following cataract surgery

998.83 Non-healing surgical wound

998.89 Other specified complications

998.9 Unspecified complication of procedure, not elsewhere classified
Postoperative complication NOS

| Excludes: | complication NOS of obstetrical surgery or procedure (669.4) |

999 Complications of medical care, not elsewhere classified
Includes: complications, not elsewhere classified, of:
dialysis (hemodialysis) (peritoneal) (renal)
extracorporeal circulation
hyperalimentation therapy
immunization
infusion
inhalation therapy
injection
inoculation
perfusion
transfusion
vaccination
ventilation therapy

| Excludes: | specified complications classified elsewhere such as:
complications of implanted device (996.0-996.9)
contact dermatitis due to drugs (692.3)
dementia dialysis (294.8)
transient (293.9)
dialysis disequilibrium syndrome (276.0-276.9)
poisoning and toxic effects of drugs and chemicals (960.0-989.9)
postvaccinal encephalitis (323.5)
water and electrolyte imbalance (276.0-276.9) |

999.0 Generalized vaccinia

999.1 Air embolism
Air embolism to any site following infusion, perfusion, or transfusion

| Excludes: | embolism specified as:
complicating:
abortion (634-638 with .6, 639.6)
ectopic or molar pregnancy (639.6)
pregnancy, childbirth, or the puerperium (673.0)
due to implanted device (996.7)
traumatic (958.0) |

999.2 Other vascular complications
Phlebitis
Thromboembolism   } following infusion, perfusion, or transfusion
Thrombophlebitis

| Excludes: | the listed conditions when specified as:
due to implanted device (996.61-996.62, 996.72-996.74)
postoperative NOS (997.2, 997.71-997.79) |

999.3 Other infection
Infection
Sepsis   } following infusion, injection, transfusion, or vaccination
Septicemia

| Excludes: | the listed conditions when specified as:
due to implanted device (996.60-996.69)
postoperative NOS (998.51-998.59) |

● Code new   ▲ Revision of   ④ ⑤ Fourth or fifth
   to this edition   existing code   digit required

999.4 Anaphylactic shock due to serum

Excludes: *shock:*
> *allergic NOS (995.0)*
> *anaphylactic:*
>> *NOS (995.0)*
>> *due to drugs and chemicals (995.0)*

999.5 Other serum reaction

Intoxication by serum   Serum sickness
Protein sickness   Urticaria due to serum
Serum rash

Excludes: *serum hepatitis (070.2-070.3)*

999.6 ABO incompatibility reaction

Incompatible blood transfusion
Reaction to blood group incompatibility in infusion or transfusion

999.7 Rh incompatibility reaction

Reactions due to Rh factor in infusion or transfusion

999.8 Other transfusion reaction

Septic shock due to transfusion
Transfusion reaction NOS

Excludes: *postoperative shock (998.0)*

999.9 Other and unspecified complications of medical care, not elsewhere classified

Complications, not elsewhere classified, of:
> electroshock
> inhalation
> ultrasound   } therapy
> ventilation
Unspecified misadventure of medical care

Excludes: *unspecified complication of:*
> *phototherapy (990)*
> *radiation therapy (990)*

Add 4th or 5th digit   Nonspecific code   Unspecified code   Medicare secondary payer(MSP) alert

● Code new
to this edition

▲ Revision of
existing code

④ ⑤ Fourth or fifth
digit required

SUPPLEMENTARY CLASSIFICATION OF FACTORS INFLUENCING HEALTH STATUS AND CONTACT WITH HEALTH SERVICES (V01-V82)

This classification is provided to deal with occasions when circumstances other than a disease or injury classifiable to categories 001-999 (the main part of ICD)are recorded as "diagnoses" or "problems." This can arise mainly in three ways:

a) When a person who is not currently sick encounters the health services for some specific purpose, such as to act as a donor of an organ or tissue, to receive prophylactic vaccination, or to discuss a problem which is in itself not a disease or injury. This will be a fairly rare occurrence among hospital inpatients, but will be relatively more common among hospital outpatients and patients of family practitioners, health clinics, etc.

b) When a person with a known disease or injury, whether it is current or resolving, encounters the health care system for a specific treatment of that disease or injury (e.g., dialysis for renal disease; chemotherapy for malignancy; cast change).

c) When some circumstance or problem is present which influences the person's health status but is not in itself a current illness or injury. Such factors may be elicited during population surveys, when the person may or may not be currently sick, or be recorded as an additional factor to be borne in mind when the person is receiving care for some current illness or injury classifiable to categories 001-999.

In the latter circumstances the V code should be used only as a supplementary code and should not be the one selected for use in primary, single cause tabulations. Examples of these circumstances are a personal history of certain diseases, or a person with an artificial heart valve in situ.

PERSONS WITH POTENTIAL HEALTH HAZARDS RELATED TO COMMUNICABLE DISEASES (V01-V06)

> Excludes: family history of infectious and parasitic diseases (V18.8)
> personal history of infectious and parasitic diseases (V12.0)

V01 Contact with or exposure to communicable diseases

V01.0 Cholera
Conditions classifiable to 001

V01.1 Tuberculosis
Conditions classifiable to 010-018

V01.2 Poliomyelitis
Conditions classifiable to 045

V01.3 Smallpox
Conditions classifiable to 050

V01.4 Rubella
Conditions classifiable to 056

V01.5 Rabies
Conditions classifiable to 071

V01.6 Venereal diseases
Conditions classifiable to 090-099

V01.7 Other viral diseases
Conditions classifiable to 042-078 and V08, except as above

⑤ **V01.8 Other communicable diseases**
Conditions classifiable to 001-136, except as above

● **V01.81 Anthrax**

● **V01.89 Other communicable diseases**

V01.9 Unspecified communicable disease

V02 Carrier or suspected carrier of infectious diseases

V02.0 Cholera

V02.1 Typhoid

V02.2 Amebiasis

V02.3 Other gastrointestinal pathogens

V02.4 Diphtheria

⑤ **V02.5 Other specified bacterial diseases**

V02.51 Group B streptococcus

V02.52 Other streptococcus

V02.59 Other specified bacterial diseases
Meningococcal
Staphylococcal

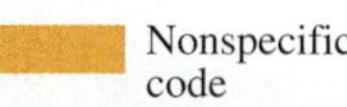

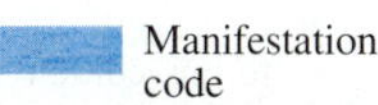

⑤ **V02.6 Viral hepatitis**
   Hepatitis Australian-antigen [HAA] [SH] carrier
   Serum hepatitis carrier

   V02.60 Viral hepatitis carrier, unspecified
   V02.61 Hepatitis B carrier
   V02.62 Hepatitis C carrier
   V02.69 Other viral hepatitis carrier
V02.7 Gonorrhea
V02.8 Other venereal diseases
V02.9 Other specified infectious organism

V03 Need for prophylactic vaccination and inoculation against bacterial diseases
   Excludes: *vaccination not carried out because of contraindication (V64.0)*
            vaccines against combinations of diseases (V06.0-V06.9)

V03.0 Cholera alone
V03.1 Typhoid-paratyphoid alone [TAB]
V03.2 Tuberculosis [BCG]
V03.3 Plague
V03.4 Tularemia
V03.5 Diphtheria alone
V03.6 Pertussis alone
V03.7 Tetanus toxoid alone
⑤ **V03.8 Other specified vaccinations against single bacterial diseases**
   V03.81 Hemophilus influenza, type B [Hib]
   V03.82 Streptococcus pneumoniae [pneumococcus]
   V03.89 Other specified vaccination
V03.9 Unspecified single bacterial disease

V04 Need for prophylactic vaccination and inoculation against certain viral diseases
   Excludes: *vaccines against combinations of diseases (V06.0-V06.9)*

V04.0 Poliomyelitis
V04.1 Smallpox
V04.2 Measles alone
V04.3 Rubella alone
V04.4 Yellow fever
V04.5 Rabies
V04.6 Mumps alone
V04.7 Common cold
V04.8 Influenza

V05 Need for other prophylactic vaccination and inoculation against single diseases
   Excludes: *vaccines against combinations of diseases (V06.0-V06.9)*

V05.0 Arthropod-borne viral encephalitis
V05.1 Other arthropod-borne viral diseases
V05.2 Leishmaniasis
V05.3 Viral hepatitis
V05.4 Varicella
   Chickenpox
V05.8 Other specified disease
V05.9 Unspecified single disease

V06 Need for prophylactic vaccination and inoculation against combinations of diseases
   Note: Use additional single vaccination codes from categories V03-V05 to identify any
   vaccinations not included in a combination code.

V06.0 Cholera with typhoid-paratyphoid [cholera + TAB]
V06.1 Diphtheria-tetanus-pertussis, combined [DTP]
V06.2 Diphtheria-tetanus-pertussis with typhoid-paratyphoid [DTP + TAB]

   ● Code new   ▲ Revision of   ④ ⑤ Fourth or fifth
      to this edition   existing code   digit required

V06.3 Diphtheria-tetanus-pertussis with poliomyelitis [DTP + polio]

V06.4 Measles-mumps-rubella [MMR]

V06.5 Tetanus-diphtheria [Td]

V06.6 Streptococcus pneumoniae [pneumococcus] and influenza

V06.8 Other combinations

> *Excludes:* *multiple single vaccination codes (V03.0-V05.9)*

V06.9 Unspecified combined vaccine

PERSONS WITH NEED FOR ISOLATION, OTHER POTENTIAL HEALTH HAZARDS AND PROPHYLACTIC MEASURES (V07-V09)

V07 Need for isolation and other prophylactic measures

> *Excludes:* *prophylactic organ removal (V50.41-V50.49)*

V07.0 Isolation
Admission to protect the individual from his surroundings or for isolation of individual after contact with infectious diseases

V07.1 Desensitization to allergens

V07.2 Prophylactic immunotherapy
Administration of:
antivenin
immune sera [gamma globulin]
RhoGAM
tetanus antitoxin

⑤ **V07.3 Other prophylactic chemotherapy**

V07.31 Prophylactic fluoride administration

V07.39 Other prophylactic chemotherapy

> *Excludes:* *maintenance chemotherapy following disease (V58.1)*

V07.4 Postmenopausal hormone replacement therapy

V07.8 Other specified prophylactic measure

V07.9 Unspecified prophylactic measure

V08 Asymptomatic human immunodeficiency virus [HIV] infection status
HIV positive NOS
Note: This code is ONLY to be used when NO HIV infection symptoms or conditions are present. If any HIV infection symptoms or conditions are present, see code 042.

> *Excludes:* *AIDS (042)*
> *human immunodeficiency virus [HIV] disease (042)*
> *exposure to HIV (V01.7)*
> *nonspecific serologic evidence of HIV (795.71)*
> *symptomatic human immunodeficiency virus [HIV] infection (042)*

V09 Infection with drug-resistant microorganisms
Note: This category is intended for use as an additional code for infectious conditions classified elsewhere to indicate the presence of drug-resistance of the infectious organism.

V09.0 Infection with microorganisms resistant to penicillins

V09.1 Infection with microorganisms resistant to cephalosporins and other B-lactam antibiotics

V09.2 Infection with microorganisms resistant to macrolides

V09.3 Infection with microorganisms resistant to tetracyclines

V09.4 Infection with microorganisms resistant to aminoglycosides

V09.5 Infection with microorganisms resistant to quinolones and fluoroquinolones

V09.50 Without mention of resistance to multiple quinolones and fluoroquinolones

V09.51 With resistance to multiple quinolones and fluoroquinolones

V09.6 Infection with microorganisms resistant to sulfonamides

⑤ **V09.7 Infection with microorganisms resistant to other specified antimycobacterial agents**

> *Excludes:* *Amikacin (V09.4)*
> *Kanamycin (V09.4)*
> *Streptomycin [SM] (V09.4)*

V09.70 Without mention of resistance to multiple antimycobacterial agents

V09.71 With resistance to multiple antimycobacterial agents

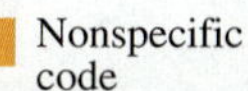
Add 4th or 5th digit

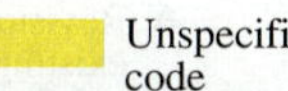
Nonspecific code

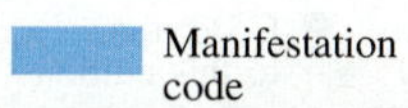
Unspecified code

Manifestation code

⑤ **V09.8 Infection with microorganisms resistant to other specified drugs**

    V09.80 Without mention of resistance to multiple drugs

    V09.81 With resistance to multiple drugs

⑤ **V09.9 Infection with drug-resistant microorganisms, unspecified**
    Drug resistance NOS

    V09.90 Without mention of multiple drug resistance

    V09.91 With multiple drug resistance
        Multiple drug resistance NOS

PERSONS WITH POTENTIAL HEALTH HAZARDS RELATED TO PERSONAL AND FAMILY HISTORY (V10-V19)

    Excludes: *obstetric patients where the possibility that the fetus might be affected is the reason for observation or management during pregnancy (655.0-655.9)*

V10 Personal history of malignant neoplasm

⑤ **V10.0 Gastrointestinal tract**
    History of conditions classifiable to 140-159

    V10.00 Gastrointestinal tract, unspecified

    V10.01 Tongue

    V10.02 Other and unspecified oral cavity and pharynx

    V10.03 Esophagus

    V10.04 Stomach

    V10.05 Large intestine

    V10.06 Rectum, rectosigmoid junction, and anus

    V10.07 Liver

    V10.09 Other

⑤ **V10.1 Trachea, bronchus, and lung**
    History of conditions classifiable to 162

    V10.11 Bronchus and lung

    V10.12 Trachea

⑤ **V10.2 Other respiratory and intrathoracic organs**
    History of conditions classifiable to 160, 161, 163-165

    V10.20 Respiratory organ, unspecified

    V10.21 Larynx

    V10.22 Nasal cavities, middle ear, and accessory sinuses

    V10.29 Other

V10.3 Breast
    History of conditions classifiable to 174 and 175

⑤ **V10.4 Genital organs**
    History of conditions classifiable to 179-187

    V10.40 Female genital organ, unspecified

    V10.41 Cervix uteri

    V10.42 Other parts of uterus

    V10.43 Ovary

    V10.44 Other female genital organs

    V10.45 Male genital organ, unspecified

    V10.46 Prostate

    V10.47 Testis

    V10.48 Epididymis

    V10.49 Other male genital organs

⑤ **V10.5 Urinary organs**
    History of conditions classifiable to 188 and 189

    V10.50 Urinary organ, unspecified

    V10.51 Bladder

● Code new to this edition   ▲ Revision of existing code   ④ ⑤ Fourth or fifth digit required

V10.52 Kidney

> *Excludes:* renal pelvis (V10.53)

V10.53 Renal pelvis

V10.59 Other

⑤ **V10.6 Leukemia**
Conditions classifiable to 204-208

> *Excludes:* leukemia in remission (204-208)

V10.60 Leukemia, unspecified

V10.61 Lymphoid leukemia

V10.62 Myeloid leukemia

V10.63 Monocytic leukemia

V10.69 Other

⑤ **V10.7 Other lymphatic and hematopoietic neoplasms**
Conditions classifiable to 200-203

> *Excludes:* listed conditions in 200-203 in remission

V10.71 Lymphosarcoma and reticulosarcoma

V10.72 Hodgkin's disease

V10.79 Other

⑤ **V10.8 Personal history of malignant neoplasm of other sites**
History of conditions classifiable to 170-173, 190-195

V10.81 Bone

V10.82 Malignant melanoma of skin

V10.83 Other malignant neoplasm of skin

V10.84 Eye

V10.85 Brain

V10.86 Other parts of nervous system

> *Excludes:* peripheral, sympathetic, and parasympathetic nerves (V10.89)

V10.87 Thyroid

V10.88 Other endocrine glands and related structures

V10.89 Other

V10.9 Unspecified personal history of malignant neoplasm

V11 Personal history of mental disorder

V11.0 Schizophrenia

> *Excludes:* that in remission (295.0-295.9 with fifth-digit 5)

V11.1 Affective disorders
Personal history of manic-depressive psychosis

> *Excludes:* that in remission (296.0-296.6 with fifth-digit
> 5, 6)

V11.2 Neurosis

V11.3 Alcoholism

V11.8 Other mental disorders

V11.9 Unspecified mental disorder

V12 Personal history of certain other diseases

⑥ **V12.0 Infectious and parasitic diseases**

V12.00 Unspecified infectious and parasitic disease

V12.01 Tuberculosis

V12.02 Poliomyelitis

V12.03 Malaria

V12.09 Other

V12.1 Nutritional deficiency

V12.2 Endocrine, metabolic, and immunity disorders

> *Excludes:* history of allergy (V14.0-V14.9, V15.01-V15.09)

	Add 4th or 5th digit		Nonspecific code		Unspecified code		Manifestation code

V12.3 **Diseases of blood and blood-forming organs**
⑤ V12.4 **Disorders of nervous system and sense organs**

    V12.40 **Unspecified disorder of nervous system and sense organs**

    V12.41 **Benign neoplasm of the brain**

    V12.49 **Other disorders of nervous system and sense organs**

⑤ V12.5 **Diseases of circulatory system**

    Excludes: *old myocardial infarction (412)*
                      postmyocardial infarction syndrome (411.0)

    V12.50 **Unspecified circulatory disease**

    V12.51 **Venous thrombosis and embolism**
            Pulmonary embolism

    V12.52 **Thrombophlebitis**

    V12.59 **Other**
        Note: Assign code V12.59 (and not a code from category 438) as an additional code
            for history of cerebrovascular disease when no neurologic deficits are present.

V12.6 **Diseases of respiratory system**
⑤ V12.7 **Diseases of digestive system**

    V12.70 **Unspecified digestive disease**

    V12.71 **Peptic ulcer disease**

    V12.72 **Colonic polyps**

    V12.79 **Other**

V13 **Personal history of other diseases**
⑤ V13.0 **Disorders of urinary system**

    V13.00 **Unspecified urinary disorder**

    V13.01 **Urinary calculi**

    V13.09 **Other**

V13.1 **Trophoblastic disease**

    Excludes: *supervision during a current pregnancy (V23.1)*

⑤ V13.2 **Other genital system and obstetric disorders**

    Excludes: *supervision during a current pregnancy of a woman with poor obstetric history*
              (V23.0-V23.9)
            habitual aborter (646.3)
             without current history (629.9)

    ● **V13.21 Personal history of pre-term labor**

    Excludes: *current pregnancy with history of pre-term labor (V23.41)*

    ● V13.29 **Other genital system and obstetric disorders**

V13.3 **Diseases of skin and subcutaneous tissue**

V13.4 **Arthritis**

V13.5 **Other musculoskeletal disorders**

⑤ V13.6 **Congenital malformations**

    V13.61 **Hypospadias**

    V13.69 **Other congenital malformations**

V13.7 **Perinatal problems**

    Excludes: *low birth weight status (V21.30-V21.35)*

V13.8 **Other specified diseases**

V13.9 **Unspecified disease**

V14 **Personal history of allergy to medicinal agents**

V14.0 **Penicillin**

V14.1 **Other antibiotic agent**

V14.2 **Sulfonamides**

V14.3 **Other anti-infective agent**

V14.4 **Anesthetic agent**

V14.5 **Narcotic agent**

● Code new to this edition   ▲ Revision of existing code   ④ ⑤ Fourth or fifth digit required

V14.6 Analgesic agent

V14.7 Serum or vaccine

V14.8 Other specified medicinal agents

V14.9 Unspecified medicinal agent

V15 Other personal history presenting hazards to health

⑤ **V15.0 Allergy, other than to medicinal agents**

> Excludes: *allergy to food substance used as base for medicinal agent (V14.0-V14.9)*

V15.01 Allergy to peanuts

V15.02 Allergy to milk products

> Excludes: *lactose intolerance (271.3)*

V15.03 Allergy to eggs

V15.04 Allergy to seafood
Seafood (octopus) (squid) ink
Shellfish

V15.05 Allergy to other foods
Food additives
Nuts other than peanuts

V15.06 Allergy to insects
Bugs
Insect bites and stings
Spiders

V15.07 Allergy to latex
Latex sensitivity

V15.08 Allergy to radiographic dye
Contrast media used for diagnostic x-ray procedures

V15.09 Other allergy, other than to medicinal agents

V15.1 Surgery to heart and great vessels

> Excludes: *replacement by transplant or other means (V42.1-V42.2, V43.2-V43.4)*

V15.2 Surgery to other major organs

> Excludes: *replacement by transplant or other means (V42.0-V43.8)*

V15.3 Irradiation
Previous exposure to therapeutic or other ionizing radiation

⑤ **V15.4 Psychological trauma**

> Excludes: *history of condition classifiable to 290-316 (V11.0-V11.9)*

V15.41 History of physical abuse
Rape

V15.42 History of emotional abuse
Neglect

V15.49 Other

V15.5 Injury

V15.6 Poisoning

V15.7 Contraception

> Excludes: *current contraceptive management (V25.0-V25.4)*
> *presence of intrauterine contraceptive device as incidental finding (V45.5)*

⑤ **V15.8 Other specified personal history presenting hazards to health**

V15.81 Noncompliance with medical treatment

V15.82 History of tobacco use

> Excludes: *tobacco dependence (305.1)*

V15.84 Exposure to asbestos

V15.85 Exposure to potentially hazardous body fluids

V15.86 Exposure to lead

V15.89 Other

V15.9 Unspecified personal history presenting hazards to health

V16 Family history of malignant neoplasm

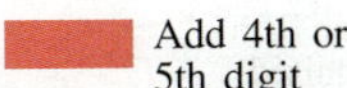

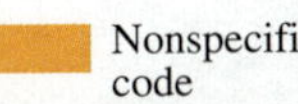

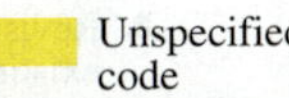

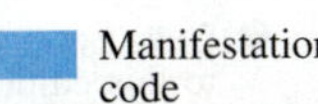

V16.0 Gastrointestinal tract
Family history of condition classifiable to 140-159

V16.1 Trachea, bronchus, and lung
Family history of condition classifiable to 162

V16.2 Other respiratory and intrathoracic organs
Family history of condition classifiable to 160-161, 163-165

V16.3 Breast
Family history of condition classifiable to 174

⑤ **V16.4 Genital organs**
Family history of condition classifiable to 179-187

V16.40 Genital organ, unspecified

V16.41 Ovary

V16.42 Prostate

V16.43 Testis

V16.49 Other

⑤ **V16.5 Urinary organs**
Family history of condition classifiable to 189

V16.51 Kidney

V16.59 Other

V16.6 Leukemia
Family history of condition classifiable to 204-208

V16.7 Other lymphatic and hematopoietic neoplasms
Family history of condition classifiable to 200-203

V16.8 Other specified malignant neoplasm
Family history of other condition classifiable to 140-199

V16.9 Unspecified malignant neoplasm

V17 Family history of certain chronic disabling diseases

V17.0 Psychiatric condition

> Excludes: family history of mental retardation (V18.4)

V17.1 Stroke (cerebrovascular)

V17.2 Other neurological diseases
Epilepsy   Huntington's chorea

V17.3 Ischemic heart disease

V17.4 Other cardiovascular diseases

V17.5 Asthma

V17.6 Other chronic respiratory conditions

V17.7 Arthritis

V17.8 Other musculoskeletal diseases

V18 Family history of certain other specific conditions

V18.0 Diabetes mellitus

V18.1 Other endocrine and metabolic diseases

V18.2 Anemia

V18.3 Other blood disorders

V18.4 Mental retardation

V18.5 Digestive disorders

⑤ **V18.6 Kidney diseases**

V18.61 Polycystic kidney

V18.69 Other kidney diseases

V18.7 Other genitourinary diseases

V18.8 Infectious and parasitic diseases

V19 Family history of other conditions

V19.0 Blindness or visual loss

V19.1 Other eye disorders

V19.2 Deafness or hearing loss

● Code new to this edition   ▲ Revision of existing code   ④ ⑤ Fourth or fifth digit required

V19.3 Other ear disorders

V19.4 Skin conditions

V19.5 Congenital anomalies

V19.6 Allergic disorders

V19.7 Consanguinity

V19.8 Other condition

PERSONS ENCOUNTERING HEALTH SERVICES IN CIRCUMSTANCES RELATED TO REPRODUCTION AND DEVELOPMENT (V20-V29)

V20 Health supervision of infant or child

V20.0 Foundling

V20.1 Other healthy infant or child receiving care

Medical or nursing care supervision of healthy infant in cases of:
maternal illness, physical or psychiatric
socioeconomic adverse condition at home
too many children at home preventing or interfering with normal care

V20.2 Routine infant or child health check

Developmental testing of infant or child
Immunizations appropriate for age
Routine vision and hearing testing

|Excludes:| special screening for developmental handicaps (V79.3)

Use additional code(s) to identify:
Special screening examination(s) performed (V73.0-V82.9)

V21 Constitutional states in development

V21.0 Period of rapid growth in childhood

V21.1 Puberty

V21.2 Other adolescence

⑤ **V21.3** Low birth weight status

|Excludes:| history of perinatal problems (V13.7)

V21.30 Low birth weight status, unspecified

V21.31 Low birth weight status, less than 500 grams

V21.32 Low birth weight status, 500-999 grams

V21.33 Low birth weight status, 1000-1499 grams

V21.34 Low birth weight status, 1500-1999 grams

V21.35 Low birth weight status, 2000-2500 grams

V21.8 Other specified constitutional states in development

V21.9 Unspecified constitutional state in development

V22 Normal pregnancy

|Excludes:| pregnancy examination or test, pregnancy unconfirmed (V72.4)

V22.0 Supervision of normal first pregnancy

V22.1 Supervision of other normal pregnancy

V22.2 Pregnant state, incidental

Pregnant state NOS

V23 Supervision of high-risk pregnancy

V23.0 Pregnancy with history of infertility

V23.1 Pregnancy with history of trophoblastic disease

Pregnancy with history of:
hydatidiform mole
vesicular mole

|Excludes:| that without current pregnancy (V13.1)

V23.2 Pregnancy with history of abortion

Pregnancy with history of conditions classifiable to 634-638

|Excludes:| habitual aborter:

care during pregnancy (646.3)
that without current pregnancy (629.9)

	Add 4th or 5th digit		Nonspecific code		Unspecified code		Manifestation code

V23.3 Grand multiparity

> *Excludes:* *care in relation to labor and delivery (659.4)*
> *that without current pregnancy (V61.5)*

⑤ **V23.4 Pregnancy with other poor obstetric history**
Pregnancy with history of other conditions classifiable to 630-676

- **V23.41 Pregnancy with history of pre-term labor**
- **V23.49 Pregnancy with other poor obstetric history**

V23.5 Pregnancy with other poor reproductive history
Pregnancy with history of stillbirth or neonatal death

V23.7 Insufficient prenatal care
History of little or no prenatal care

⑤ **V23.8 Other high-risk pregnancy**

V23.81 Elderly primigravida
First pregnancy in a woman who will be 35 years of age or older at expected date of delivery

> *Excludes:* *elderly primigravida complicating pregnancy (659.5)*

V23.82 Elderly multigravida
Second or more pregnancy in a woman who will be 35 years of age or older at expected date of delivery

> *Excludes:* *elderly multigravida complicating pregnancy (659.6)*

V23.83 Young primigravida
First pregnancy in a female less than 16 years old at expected date of delivery

> *Excludes:* *young primigravida complicating pregnancy (659.8)*

V23.84 Young multigravida
Second or more pregnancy in a female less than 16 years old at expected date of delivery

> *Excludes:* *young multigravida complicating pregnancy (659.8)*

V23.89 Other high-risk pregnancy

V23.9 Unspecified high-risk pregnancy

V24 Postpartum care and examination

V24.0 Immediately after delivery
Care and observation in uncomplicated cases

V24.1 Lactating mother
Supervision of lactation

V24.2 Routine postpartum follow-up

V25 Encounter for contraceptive management

⑤ **V25.0 General counseling and advice**

V25.01 Prescription of oral contraceptives

V25.02 Initiation of other contraceptive measures
Fitting of diaphragm
Prescription of foams, creams, or other agents

V25.09 Other
Family planning advice

V25.1 Insertion of intrauterine contraceptive device

V25.2 Sterilization
Admission for interruption of fallopian tubes or vas deferens

V25.3 Menstrual extraction
Menstrual regulation

⑤ **V25.4 Surveillance of previously prescribed contraceptive methods**
Checking, reinsertion, or removal of contraceptive device
Repeat prescription for contraceptive method
Routine examination in connection with contraceptive maintenance

> *Excludes:* *presence of intrauterine contraceptive device as incidental finding (V45.5)*

V25.40 Contraceptive surveillance, unspecified

V25.41 Contraceptive pill

V25.42 Intrauterine contraceptive device
Checking, reinsertion, or removal of intrauterine device

● Code new to this edition   ▲ Revision of existing code   ④ ⑤ Fourth or fifth digit required

V25.43 Implantable subdermal contraceptive

V25.49 Other contraceptive method

V25.5 Insertion of implantable subdermal contraceptive

V25.8 Other specified contraceptive management
Postvasectomy sperm count

Excludes: *sperm count following sterilization reversal (V26.22)*
sperm count for fertility testing (V26.21)

V25.9 Unspecified contraceptive management

V26 Procreative management

V26.0 Tuboplasty or vasoplasty after previous sterilization

V26.1 Artificial insemination

⑤ **V26.2 Investigation and testing**

Excludes: *postvasectomy sperm count (V25.8)*

V26.21 Fertility testing
Fallopian insufflation
Sperm count for fertility testing

Excludes: *Genetic counseling and testing (V26.3)*

V26.22 Aftercare following sterilization reversal
Fallopian insufflation following sterilization reversal
Sperm count following sterilization reversal

V26.29 Other investigation and testing

V26.3 Genetic counseling and testing

Excludes: *fertility testing (V26.21)*

V26.4 General counseling and advice

⑤ **V26.5 Sterilization status**

V26.51 Tubal ligation status

Excludes: *infertility not due to previous tubal ligation (628.0-628.9)*

V26.52 Vasectomy status

V26.8 Other specified procreative management

V26.9 Unspecified procreative management

V27 Outcome of delivery

Note: This category is intended for the coding of the outcome of delivery on the mother's record.

V27.0 Single liveborn

V27.1 Single stillborn

V27.2 Twins, both liveborn

V27.3 Twins, one liveborn and one stillborn

V27.4 Twins, both stillborn

V27.5 Other multiple birth, all liveborn

V27.6 Other multiple birth, some liveborn

V27.7 Other multiple birth, all stillborn

V27.9 Unspecified outcome of delivery
Single birth, outcome to infant unspecified
Multiple birth, outcome to infant unspecified

V28 Antenatal screening

Excludes: *abnormal findings on screening—code to findings*
routine prenatal care (V22.0-V23.9)

V28.0 Screening for chromosomal anomalies by amniocentesis

V28.1 Screening for raised alpha-fetoprotein levels in amniotic fluid

V28.2 Other screening based on amniocentesis

V28.3 Screening for malformation using ultrasonics

V28.4 Screening for fetal growth retardation using ultrasonics

V28.5 Screening for isoimmunization

V28.6 Screening for Streptococcus B

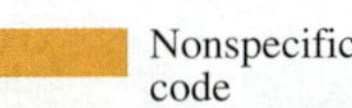
Add 4th or 5th digit

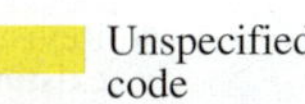
Nonspecific code

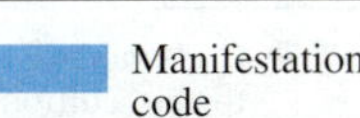
Unspecified code

Manifestation code

V28.8 Other specified antenatal screening

V28.9 Unspecified antenatal screening

V29 **Observation and evaluation of newborns for suspected condition not found**

Note: This category is to be used for newborns, within the neonatal period, (the first 28 days of life) who are suspected of having an abnormal condition resulting from exposure from the mother or the birth process, but without signs or symptoms, and, which after examination and observation, is found not to exist.

V29.0 Observation for suspected infectious condition

V29.1 Observation for suspected neurological condition

V29.2 Observation for suspected respiratory condition

V29.3 Observation for suspected genetic or metabolic condition

V29.8 Observation for other specified suspected condition

V29.9 Observation for unspecified suspected condition

LIVEBORN INFANTS ACCORDING TO TYPE OF BIRTH (V30-V39)

Note: These categories are intended for the coding of liveborn infants who are consuming health care [e.g., crib or bassinet occupancy].

The following fourth-digit subdivisions are for use with categories V30-V39:

　　.0　Born in hospital

　　.1　Born before admission to hospital

　　.2　Born outside hospital and not hospitalized

The following two fifth-digits are for use with the fourth-digit .0, Born in hospital:

　　0　delivered without mention of cesarean delivery

　　1　delivered by cesarean delivery

④ **V30** **Single liveborn**

④ **V31** **Twin, mate liveborn**

④ **V32** **Twin, mate stillborn**

④ **V33** **Twin, unspecified**

④ **V34** **Other multiple, mates all liveborn**

④ **V35** **Other multiple, mates all stillborn**

④ **V36** **Other multiple, mates live- and stillborn**

④ **V37** **Other multiple, unspecified**

④ **V39** **Unspecified**

PERSONS WITH A CONDITION INFLUENCING THEIR HEALTH STATUS (V40-V49)

Note: These categories are intended for use when these conditions are recorded as "diagnoses" or "problems."

V40 **Mental and behavioral problems**

V40.0 Problems with learning

V40.1 Problems with communication [including speech]

V40.2 Other mental problems

V40.3 Other behavioral problems

V40.9 Unspecified mental or behavioral problem

V41 **Problems with special senses and other special functions**

V41.0 Problems with sight

V41.1 Other eye problems

V41.2 Problems with hearing

V41.3 Other ear problems

V41.4 Problems with voice production

V41.5 Problems with smell and taste

V41.6 Problems with swallowing and mastication

V41.7 Problems with sexual function

> *Excludes:* *marital problems (V61.10)*
> *psychosexual disorders (302.0-302.9)*

V41.8 Other problems with special functions

● Code new to this edition　　▲ Revision of existing code　　④ ⑤ Fourth or fifth digit required

V41.9 Unspecified problem with special functions

V42 **Organ or tissue replaced by transplant**
　　Includes:　homologous or heterologous (animal) (human) transplant organ status

V42.0 Kidney

V42.1 Heart

V42.2 Heart valve

V42.3 Skin

V42.4 Bone

V42.5 Cornea

V42.6 Lung

V42.7 Liver

⑤ **V42.8** Other specified organ or tissue

　　V42.81 Bone marrow

　　V42.82 Peripheral stem cells

　　V42.83 Pancreas

　　V42.84 Intestines

　　V42.89 Other

V42.9 Unspecified organ or tissue

V43 **Organ or tissue replaced by other means**
　　Includes:　replacement of organ by:
　　　　　　　artificial device
　　　　　　　mechanical device
　　　　　　　prosthesis

　　Excludes: *cardiac pacemaker in situ (V45.01)*
　　　　　　　fitting and adjustment of prosthetic device (V52.0-V52.9)
　　　　　　　renal dialysis status (V45.1)

V43.0 Eye globe

V43.1 Lens
　　　Pseudophakos

V43.2 Heart

V43.3 Heart valve

V43.4 Blood vessel

V43.5 Bladder

⑤ **V43.6** Joint

　　V43.60 Unspecified joint

　　V43.61 Shoulder

　　V43.62 Elbow

　　V43.63 Wrist

　　V43.64 Hip

　　V43.65 Knee

　　V43.66 Ankle

　　V43.69 Other

V43.7 Limb

⑤ **V43.8** Other organ or tissue

　　V43.81 Larynx

　　V43.82 Breast

　　V43.83 Artificial skin

　　V43.89 Other

V44 **Artificial opening status**
　　Excludes: *artificial openings requiring attention or management (V55.0-V55.9)*

V44.0 Tracheostomy

V44.1 Gastrostomy

V44.2 Ileostomy

V44.3 Colostomy

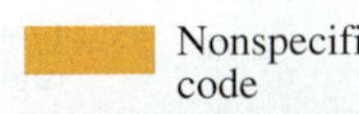

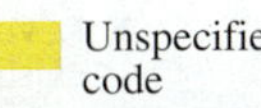

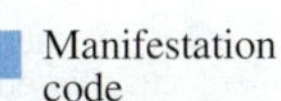

V44.4 Other artificial opening of gastrointestinal tract

⑤ **V44.5 Cystostomy**

    V44.50 Cystostomy, unspecified

    V44.51 Cutaneous-vesicostomy

    V44.52 Appendico-vesicostomy

    V44.59 Other cystostomy

V44.6 Other artificial opening of urinary tract
    Nephrostomy
    Ureterostomy
    Urethrostomy

V44.7 Artificial vagina

V44.8 Other artificial opening status

V44.9 Unspecified artificial opening status

V45 Other postsurgical states

    Excludes: *aftercare management (V51-V58.9)*

             malfunction or other complication—code to condition

⑤ **V45.0 Cardiac device in situ**

    V45.00 Unspecified cardiac device

    V45.01 Cardiac pacemaker

    V45.02 Automatic implantable cardiac defibrillator

    V45.09 Other specified cardiac device
        Carotid sinus pacemaker in situ

V45.1 Renal dialysis status
    Patient requiring intermittent renal dialysis
    Presence of arterial-venous shunt (for dialysis)

    Excludes: *admission for dialysis treatment, or session (V56.0)*

V45.2 Presence of cerebrospinal fluid drainage device
    Cerebral ventricle (communicating) shunt, valve, or device in situ

    Excludes: *malfunction (996.2)*

V45.3 Intestinal bypass or anastomosis status

V45.4 Arthrodesis status

⑤ **V45.5 Presence of contraceptive device**

    Excludes: *checking, reinsertion, or removal of device (V25.42)*

             complication from device (996.32)
             insertion of device (V25.1)

    V45.51 Intrauterine contraceptive device

    V45.52 Subdermal contraceptive implant

    V45.59 Other

⑤ **V45.6 States following surgery of eye and adnexa**
    Cataract extraction
    Filtering bleb   } state following eye surgery
    Surgical eyelid adhesion

    Excludes: *aphakia (379.31)*

             artificial eye globe (V43.0)

    V45.61 Cataract extraction status
Use additional code for associated artificial lens status (V43.1)

    V45.69 Other states following surgery of eye and adnexa

⑤ **V45.7 Acquired absence of organ**

    V45.71 Acquired absence of breast

    V45.72 Acquired absence of intestine (large) (small)

    V45.73 Acquired absence of kidney

    V45.74 Other parts of urinary tract
        Bladder

    V45.75 Stomach

    V45.76 Lung

● Code new to this edition   ▲ Revision of existing code   ④ ⑤ Fourth or fifth digit required

  V45.77 Genital organs

  V45.78 Eye

  V45.79 Other acquired absence of organ

⑤ **V45.8 Other postsurgical status**

  V45.81 Aortocoronary bypass status

  V45.82 Percutaneous transluminal coronary angioplasty status

  V45.83 Breast implant removal status

  V45.84 Dental restoration status
   Dental crowns status
   Dental fillings status

  V45.89 Other
   Presence of neuropacemaker or other electronic device

   | Excludes: | *artificial heart valve in situ (V43.3)*
    vascular prosthesis in situ (V43.4)

V46 Other dependence on machines

V46.0 Aspirator

V46.1 Respirator
 Iron lung

● **V46.2 Supplemental oxygen**
 Long-term oxygen therapy

V46.8 Other enabling machines
 Hyperbaric chamber
 Possum [Patient-Operated-Selector-Mechanism]

 | Excludes: | *cardiac pacemaker (V45.0)*
  kidney dialysis machine (V45.1)

V46.9 Unspecified machine dependence

V47 Other problems with internal organs

V47.0 Deficiencies of internal organs

V47.1 Mechanical and motor problems with internal organs

V47.2 Other cardiorespiratory problems
 Cardiovascular exercise intolerance with pain (with):
  at rest
  less than ordinary activity
  ordinary activity

V47.3 Other digestive problems

V47.4 Other urinary problems

V47.5 Other genital problems

V47.9 Unspecified

V48 Problems with head, neck, and trunk

V48.0 Deficiencies of head

 | Excludes: | *deficiencies of ears, eyelids, and nose (V48.8)*

V48.1 Deficiencies of neck and trunk

V48.2 Mechanical and motor problems with head

V48.3 Mechanical and motor problems with neck and trunk

V48.4 Sensory problem with head

V48.5 Sensory problem with neck and trunk

V48.6 Disfigurements of head

V48.7 Disfigurements of neck and trunk

V48.8 Other problems with head, neck, and trunk

V48.9 Unspecified problem with head, neck, or trunk

V49 Other conditions influencing health status

V49.0 Deficiencies of limbs

V49.1 Mechanical problems with limbs

V49.2 Motor problems with limbs

V49.3 Sensory problems with limbs

| Add 4th or 5th digit | Nonspecific code | Unspecified code | Manifestation code |

V49.4 Disfigurements of limbs

V49.5 Other problems of limbs

⑤ **V49.6 Upper limb amputation status**

V49.60 Unspecified level

V49.61 Thumb

V49.62 Other finger(s)

V49.63 Hand

V49.64 Wrist
    Disarticulation of wrist

V49.65 Below elbow

V49.66 Above elbow
    Disarticulation of elbow

V49.67 Shoulder
    Disarticulation of shoulder

⑤ **V49.7 Lower limb amputation status**

V49.70 Unspecified level

V49.71 Great toe

V49.72 Other toe(s)

V49.73 Foot

V49.74 Ankle
    Disarticulation of ankle

V49.75 Below knee

V49.76 Above knee
    Disarticulation of knee

V49.77 Hip
    Disarticulation of hip

⑤ **V49.8 Other specified conditions influencing health status**

▲ **V49.81 Asymptomatic postmenopausal status (age-related) (natural)**

Excludes: *menopausal and premenopausal disorders (627.0-627.9)*
postsurgical menopause (256.2)
premature menopause (256.31)
symptomatic menopause (627.0-627.9)

V49.82 Dental sealant status

V49.89 Other specified conditions influencing health status

V49.9 Unspecified

PERSONS ENCOUNTERING HEALTH SERVICES FOR SPECIFIC PROCEDURES AND AFTERCARE (V50-V59)

Note: Categories V51-V58 are intended for use to indicate a reason for care in patients who may have already been treated for some disease or injury not now present, but who are receiving care to consolidate the treatment, to deal with residual states, or to prevent recurrence.

Excludes: *follow-up examination for medical surveillance following treatment (V67.0-V67.9)*

V50 Elective surgery for purposes other than remedying health states

V50.0 Hair transplant

V50.1 Other plastic surgery for unacceptable cosmetic appearance
    Breast augmentation or reduction
    Face-lift

Excludes: *plastic surgery following healed injury or operation (V51)*

V50.2 Routine or ritual circumcision
    Circumcision in the absence of significant medical indication

V50.3 Ear piercing

⑤ **V50.4 Prophylactic organ removal**

Excludes: *organ donations (V59.0-V59.9)*
therapeutic organ removal—code to condition

V50.41 Breast

● Code new to this edition   ▲ Revision of existing code   ④ ⑤ Fourth or fifth digit required

V50.42 **Ovary**

V50.49 **Other**

V50.8 **Other**

V50.9 **Unspecified**

V51 **Aftercare involving the use of plastic surgery**
Plastic surgery following healed injury or operation

> *Excludes:* *cosmetic plastic surgery (V50.1)*
> *plastic surgery as treatment for current injury—code to condition*
> *repair of scarred tissue—code to scar*

V52 **Fitting and adjustment of prosthetic device and implant**
Includes: removal of device

> *Excludes:* *malfunction or complication of prosthetic device (996.0-996.7)*
> *status only, without need for care (V43.0-V43.8)*

V52.0 **Artificial arm (complete) (partial)**

V52.1 **Artificial leg (complete) (partial)**

V52.2 **Artificial eye**

V52.3 **Dental prosthetic device**

V52.4 **Breast prosthesis and implant**

> *Excludes:* *admission for implant insertion (V50.1)*

V52.8 **Other specified prosthetic device**

V52.9 **Unspecified prosthetic device**

V53 **Fitting and adjustment of other device**
Includes: removal of device
replacement of device

> *Excludes:* *status only, without need for care (V45.0-V45.8)*

⑤ **V53.0** **Devices related to nervous system and special senses**

V53.01 **Fitting and adjustment of cerebral ventricular (communicating) shunt**

V53.02 **Neuropacemaker (brain) (peripheral nerve) (spinal cord)**

V53.09 **Fitting and adjustment of other devices related to nervous system and special senses**
Auditory substitution device
Visual substitution device

V53.1 **Spectacles and contact lenses**

V53.2 **Hearing aid**

⑤ **V53.3** **Cardiac device**
Reprogramming

V53.31 **Cardiac pacemaker**

> *Excludes:* *mechanical complication of cardiac pacemaker (996.01)*

V53.32 **Automatic implantable cardiac defibrillator**

V53.39 **Other cardiac device**

V53.4 **Orthodontic devices**

V53.5 **Other intestinal appliance**

> *Excludes:* *colostomy (V55.3)*
> *ileostomy (V55.2)*
> *other artificial opening of digestive tract (V55.4)*

V53.6 **Urinary devices**
Urinary catheter

> *Excludes:* *cystostomy (V55.5)*
> *nephrostomy (V55.6)*
> *ureterostomy (V55.6)*
> *urethrostomy (V55.6)*

V53.7 **Orthopedic devices**
Orthopedic: Orthopedic:
brace   corset
cast   shoes

> *Excludes:* *other orthopedic aftercare (V54)*

	Add 4th or 5th digit		Nonspecific code		Unspecified code		Manifestation code

V53.8 Wheelchair

V53.9 Other and unspecified device

V54 Other orthopedic aftercare

> Excludes: *fitting and adjustment of orthopedic devices (V53.7)*
> *malfunction of internal orthopedic device (996.4)*
> *other complication of nonmechanical nature (996.60-996.79)*

V54.0 Aftercare involving removal of fracture plate or other internal fixation device

Removal of:	Removal of:
pins	rods
plates	screws

> Excludes: *removal of external fixation device (V54.89)*

- **V54.1 Aftercare for healing traumatic fracture**
  - **V54.10 Aftercare for healing traumatic fracture of arm, unspecified**
  - **V54.11 Aftercare for healing traumatic fracture of upper arm**
  - **V54.12 Aftercare for healing traumatic fracture of lower arm**
  - **V54.13 Aftercare for healing traumatic fracture of hip**
  - **V54.14 Aftercare for healing traumatic fracture of leg, unspecified**
  - **V54.15 Aftercare for healing traumatic fracture of upper leg**

    > Excludes: *aftercare for healing traumatic fracture of hip (V54.13)*

  - **V54.16 Aftercare for healing traumatic fracture of lower leg**
  - **V54.17 Aftercare for healing traumatic fracture of vertebrae**
  - **V54.19 Aftercare for healing traumatic fracture of other bone**
- **V54.2 Aftercare for healing pathologic fracture**
  - **V54.20 Aftercare for healing pathologic fracture of arm, unspecified**
  - **V54.21 Aftercare for healing pathologic fracture of upper arm**
  - **V54.22 Aftercare for healing pathologic fracture of lower arm**
  - **V54.23 Aftercare for healing pathologic fracture of hip**
  - **V54.24 Aftercare for healing pathologic fracture of leg, unspecified**
  - **V54.25 Aftercare for healing pathologic fracture of upper leg**

    > Excludes: *aftercare for healing traumatic fracture of hip (V54.23)*

  - **V54.26 Aftercare for healing pathologic fracture of lower leg**
  - **V54.27 Aftercare for healing pathologic fracture of vertebrae**
  - **V54.29 Aftercare for healing pathologic fracture of other bone**

⑤ **V54.8 Other orthopedic aftercare**

- **V54.81 Aftercare following joint replacement**
  Use additional code to identify joint replacement site (V43.60-V43.69)

- **V54.89 Other orthopedic aftercare**
  Aftercare for healing fracture NOS

V54.9 Unspecified orthopedic aftercare

V55 Attention to artificial openings

> Includes: adjustment or repositioning of catheter
> closure
> passage of sounds or bougies
> reforming
> removal or replacement of catheter
> toilet or cleansing

> Excludes: *complications of external stoma (519.00-519.09, 569.60-569.69, 997.4, 997.5)*
> *status only, without need for care (V44.0-V44.9)*

V55.0 Tracheostomy

V55.1 Gastrostomy

V55.2 Ileostomy

V55.3 Colostomy

V55.4 Other artificial opening of digestive tract

V55.5 Cystostomy

● Code new to this edition   ▲ Revision of existing code   ④ ⑤ Fourth or fifth digit required

V55.6 Other artificial opening of urinary tract
    Nephrostomy   Urethrostomy
    Ureterostomy

V55.7 Artificial vagina

V55.8 Other specified artificial opening

V55.9 Unspecified artificial opening

V56 Encounter for dialysis and dialysis catheter care
Use additional code to identify the associated condition

> *Excludes:* *dialysis preparation—code to condition*

V56.0 Extracorporeal dialysis
    Dialysis (renal) NOS

> *Excludes:* *dialysis status (V45.1)*

V56.1 Fitting and adjustment of extracorporeal dialysis catheter
    Removal or replacement of catheter
    Toilet or cleansing

Use additional code for any concurrent extracorporeal dialysis (V56.0)

V56.2 Fitting and adjustment of peritoneal dialysis catheter

Use additional code for any concurrent peritoneal dialysis (V56.8)

⑤ **V56.3 Encounter for adequacy testing for dialysis**

    V56.31 Encounter for adequacy testing for hemodialysis

    V56.32 Encounter for adequacy testing for peritoneal dialysis
        Peritoneal equilibration test

V56.8 Other dialysis
    Peritoneal dialysis

V57 Care involving use of rehabilitation procedures
Use additional code to identify underlying condition

V57.0 Breathing exercises

V57.1 Other physical therapy
    Therapeutic and remedial exercises, except breathing

⑤ **V57.2 Occupational therapy and vocational rehabilitation**

    V57.21 Encounter for occupational therapy

    V57.22 Encounter for vocational therapy

V57.3 Speech therapy

V57.4 Orthoptic training

⑤ **V57.8 Other specified rehabilitation procedure**

    V57.81 Orthotic training
        Gait training in the use of artificial limbs

    V57.89 Other
        Multiple training or therapy

V57.9 Unspecified rehabilitation procedure

V58 Encounter for other and unspecified procedures and aftercare

> *Excludes:* *convalescence and palliative care (V66)*

V58.0 Radiotherapy
    Encounter or admission for radiotherapy

> *Excludes:* *encounter for radioactive implant—code to condition*
> *radioactive iodine therapy—code to condition*

V58.1 Chemotherapy
    Encounter or admission for chemotherapy

> *Excludes:* *prophylactic chemotherapy against disease which has never been present (V03.0-V07.9)*

V58.2 Blood transfusion, without reported diagnosis

V58.3 Attention to surgical dressings and sutures
    Change of dressings
    Removal of sutures

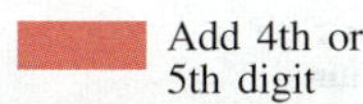

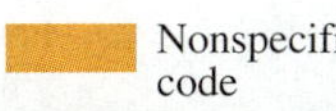

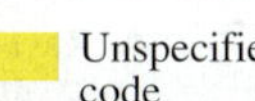

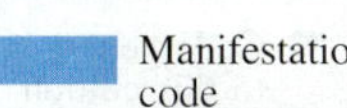

⑤ **V58.4 Other aftercare following surgery**

Note: Codes from this subcategory should be used in conjunction with other aftercare codes to fully identify the reason for the aftercare encounter

Excludes: *aftercare following sterilization reversal surgery (V26.22)*
attention to artificial openings (V55.0-V55.9)
orthopedic aftercare (V54.0-V54.9)

V58.41 Encounter for planned postoperative wound closure

Excludes: *disruption of operative wound (998.3)*

● **V58.42 Aftercare following surgery for neoplasm**
Conditions classifiable to 140-239

● **V58.43 Aftercare following surgery for injury and trauma**
Conditions classifiable to 800-999

Excludes: *aftercare for healing traumatic fracture (V54.10-V54.19)*

V58.49 Other specified aftercare following surgery

V58.5 Orthodontics

Excludes: *fitting and adjustment of orthodontic device (V53.4)*

⑤ **V58.6 Long-term (current) drug use**

Excludes: *drug abuse (305.00-305.93)*
drug dependence (304.00-304.93)

V58.61 Long-term (current) use of anticoagulants

V58.62 Long-term (current) use of antibiotics

V58.69 Long-term (current) use of other medications
High-risk medications

● **V58.7 Aftercare following surgery to specified body systems, not elsewhere classified**

Note: Codes from this subcategory should be used in conjunction with other aftercare codes to fully identify the reason for the aftercare encounter

● **V58.71 Aftercare following surgery of the sense organs, NEC**
Conditions classifiable to 360-379, 380-389

● **V58.72 Aftercare following surgery of the nervous system, NEC**
Conditions classifiable to 320-359

Excludes: *aftercare following surgery of the sense organs, NEC (V58.71)*

● **V58.73 Aftercare following surgery of the circulatory system, NEC**
Conditions classifiable to 390-459

● **V58.74 Aftercare following surgery of the respiratory system, NEC**
Conditions classifiable to 460-519

● **V58.75 Aftercare following surgery of the teeth, oral cavity and digestive system, NEC**
Conditions classifiable to 520-579

● **V58.76 Aftercare following surgery of the genitourinary system, NEC**
Conditions classifiable to 580-629

Excludes: *aftercare following sterilization reversal (V26.22)*

● **V58.77 Aftercare following surgery of the skin and subcutaneous tissue, NEC**
Conditions classifiable to 680-709

● **V58.78 Aftercare following surgery of the musculoskeletal system, NEC**
Conditions classifiable to 710-739

⑤ **V58.8 Other specified procedures and aftercare**

V58.81 Fitting and adjustment of vascular catheter
Removal or replacement of catheter
Toilet or cleansing

Excludes: *complication of renal dialysis catheter (996.73)*
complication of vascular catheter (996.74)
dialysis preparation -- code to condition
encounter for dialysis (V56.0-V56.8)
fitting and adjustment of dialysis catheter (V56.1)

● Code new
to this edition

▲ Revision of
existing code

④ ⑤ Fourth or fifth
digit required

V58.82 Fitting and adjustment of non-vascular catheter NEC
Removal or replacement of catheter
Toilet or cleansing

Excludes: *fitting and adjustment of peritoneal dialysis catheter (V56.2)*
fitting and adjustment of urinary catheter (V53.6)

V58.83 Encounter for therapeutic drug monitoring
Use additional code for any associated long-term (current) drug use (V58.61-V58.69)

Excludes: *blood-drug testing for medicolegal reasons (V70.4)*

V58.89 Other specified aftercare

V58.9 Unspecified aftercare

V59 Donors

Excludes: *examination of potential donor (V70.8)*
self-donation of organ or tissue -- code to condition

⑤ **V59.0 Blood**

V59.01 Whole blood

V59.02 Stem cells

V59.09 Other

V59.1 Skin

V59.2 Bone

V59.3 Bone marrow

V59.4 Kidney

V59.5 Cornea

V59.6 Liver

V59.8 Other specified organ or tissue

V59.9 Unspecified organ or tissue

PERSONS ENCOUNTERING HEALTH SERVICES IN OTHER CIRCUMSTANCES (V60-V69)

V60 Housing, household, and economic circumstances

V60.0 Lack of housing
Hobos   Transients
Social migrants   Vagabonds
Tramps

V60.1 Inadequate housing
Lack of heating
Restriction of space
Technical defects in home preventing adequate care

V60.2 Inadequate material resources
Economic problem   Poverty NOS

V60.3 Person living alone

V60.4 No other household member able to render care
Person requiring care (has) (is):
family member too handicapped, ill, or otherwise unsuited to render care
partner temporarily away from home
temporarily away from usual place of abode

Excludes: *holiday relief care (V60.5)*

V60.5 Holiday relief care
Provision of health care facilities to a person normally cared for at home, to enable
relatives to take a vacation

V60.6 Person living in residential institution
Boarding school resident

V60.8 Other specified housing or economic circumstances

V60.9 Unspecified housing or economic circumstance

V61 Other family circumstances
Includes: when these circumstances or fear of them, affecting the person directly involved or
others, are mentioned as the reason, justified or not, for seeking or receiving
medical advice or care

V61.0 Family disruption
Divorce   Estrangement

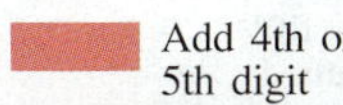

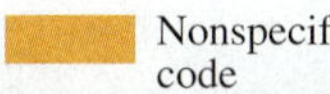

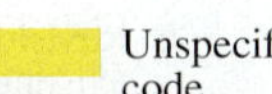

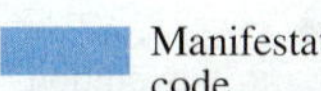

⑤ **V61.1 Counseling for marital and partner problems**

Excludes: *problems related to:*
    psychosexual disorders (302.0-302.9)
    sexual function (V41.7)

  V61.10 Counseling for marital and partner problems, unspecified
    Marital conflict
    Partner conflict

  V61.11 Counseling for victim of spousal and partner abuse

Excludes: *encounter for treatment of current injuries due to abuse (995.80-995.85)*

  V61.12 Counseling for perpetrator of spousal and partner abuse

⑤ **V61.2 Parent-child problems**

  V61.20 Counseling for parent-child problem, unspecified
    Concern about behavior of child
    Parent-child conflict

  V61.21 Counseling for victim of child abuse
    Child battering
    Child neglect

Excludes: *current injuries due to abuse (995.50-995.59)*

  V61.22 Counseling for perpetrator of parental child abuse

Excludes: *counseling for non-parental abuser (V62.83)*

  V61.29 Other
    Problem concerning adopted or foster child

V61.3 Problems with aged parents or in-laws

⑤ **V61.4 Health problems within family**

  V61.41 Alcoholism in family

  V61.49 Other
    Care of
    Presence of } sick or handicapped person in family or household

V61.5 Multiparity

V61.6 Illegitimacy or illegitimate pregnancy

V61.7 Other unwanted pregnancy

V61.8 Other specified family circumstances
  Problems with family members NEC

V61.9 Unspecified family circumstance

V62 Other psychosocial circumstances
  Includes: those circumstances or fear of them, affecting the person directly involved or others, mentioned as the reason, justified or not, for seeking or receiving medical advice or care

Excludes: *previous psychological trauma (V15.41-V15.49)*

V62.0 Unemployment

Excludes: *circumstances when main problem is economic inadequacy or poverty (V60.2)*

V62.1 Adverse effects of work environment

V62.2 Other occupational circumstances or maladjustment
  Career choice problem
  Dissatisfaction with employment

V62.3 Educational circumstances
  Dissatisfaction with school environment
  Educational handicap

V62.4 Social maladjustment
  Cultural deprivation
  Political, religious, or sex
    discrimination
  Social:
    isolation
    persecution

V62.5 Legal circumstances
  Imprisonment
  Legal investigation
  Litigation
  Prosecution

V62.6 Refusal of treatment for reasons of religion or conscience

⑤ **V62.8 Other psychological or physical stress, not elsewhere classified**

● Code new
to this edition
  ▲ Revision of
existing code
  ④ ⑤ Fourth or fifth
digit required

V62.81 Interpersonal problems, not elsewhere classified

V62.82 Bereavement, uncomplicated

Excludes: *bereavement as adjustment reaction (309.0)*

V62.83 Counseling for perpetrator of physical/sexual abuse

Excludes: *counseling for perpetrator of parental child abuse (V61.22)*
counseling for perpetrator of spousal and partner abuse (V61.12)

V62.89 Other
Life circumstance problems
Phase of life problems

V62.9 Unspecified psychosocial circumstance

V63 Unavailability of other medical facilities for care

V63.0 Residence remote from hospital or other health care facility

V63.1 Medical services in home not available

Excludes: *no other household member able to render care (V60.4)*

V63.2 Person awaiting admission to adequate facility elsewhere

V63.8 Other specified reasons for unavailability of medical facilities
Person on waiting list undergoing social agency investigation

V63.9 Unspecified reason for unavailability of medical facilities

V64 Persons encountering health services for specific procedures, not carried out

V64.0 Vaccination not carried out because of contraindication

V64.1 Surgical or other procedure not carried out because of contraindication

V64.2 Surgical or other procedure not carried out because of patient's decision

V64.3 Procedure not carried out for other reasons

V64.4 Laparoscopic surgical procedure converted to open procedure

V65 Other persons seeking consultation without complaint or sickness

V65.0 Healthy person accompanying sick person
Boarder

V65.1 Person consulting on behalf of another person
Advice or treatment for nonattending third party

Excludes: *concern (normal) about sick person in family (V61.41-V61.49)*

V65.2 Person feigning illness
Malingerer   Peregrinating patient

V65.3 Dietary surveillance and counseling
Dietary surveillance and counseling (in):
NOS
colitis
diabetes mellitus
food allergies or intolerance
gastritis
hypercholesterolemia
hypoglycemia
obesity

⑤ **V65.4 Other counseling, not elsewhere classified**
Health:
advice
education
instruction

Excludes: *counseling (for):*
contraception (V25.40-V25.49)
genetic (V26.3)
on behalf of third party (V65.1)
procreative management (V26.4)

V65.40 Counseling NOS

V65.41 Exercise counseling

V65.42 Counseling on substance use and abuse

V65.43 Counseling on injury prevention

V65.44 Human immunodeficiency virus [HIV] counseling

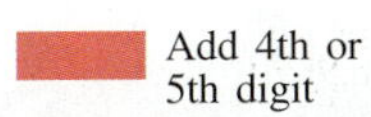

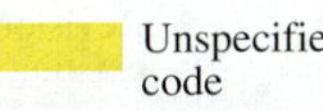

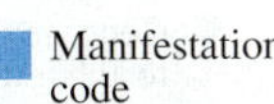

V65.45 Counseling on other sexually transmitted diseases

V65.49 Other specified counseling

V65.5 Person with feared complaint in whom no diagnosis was made
Feared condition not demonstrated
Problem was normal state
"Worried well"

V65.8 Other reasons for seeking consultation

Excludes: specified symptoms

V65.9 Unspecified reason for consultation

V66 Convalescence and palliative care

V66.0 Following surgery

V66.1 Following radiotherapy

V66.2 Following chemotherapy

V66.3 Following psychotherapy and other treatment for mental disorder

V66.4 Following treatment of fracture

V66.5 Following other treatment

V66.6 Following combined treatment

V66.7 *Encounter for palliative care*
End-of-life care
Hospice care
Terminal care

Code first underlying disease

V66.9 Unspecified convalescence

V67 Follow-up examination
Includes: surveillance only following completed treatment

Excludes: surveillance of contraception (V25.40-V25.49)

⑤ **V67.0 Following surgery**

V67.00 Following surgery, unspecified

V67.01 Follow-up vaginal pap smear
Vaginal pap smear, status-post hysterectomy for malignant condition
Use additional code to identify:
acquired absence of uterus (V45.77)
personal history of malignant neoplasm (V10.40-V10.44)

Excludes: vaginal pap smear status-post hysterectomy for non-malignant condition (V76.47)

V67.09 Following other surgery

Excludes: sperm count following sterilization reversal (V26.22)
sperm count for fertility testing (V26.21)

V67.1 Following radiotherapy

V67.2 Following chemotherapy
Cancer chemotherapy follow-up

V67.3 Following psychotherapy and other treatment for mental disorder

V67.4 Following treatment of healed fracture

Excludes: current (healing) fracture aftercare (V54.0-V54.9)

⑤ **V67.5 Following other treatment**

V67.51 Following completed treatment with high-risk medication, NEC

Excludes: long-term (current) drug use (V58.61-V58.69)

V67.59 Other

V67.6 Following combined treatment

V67.9 Unspecified follow-up examination

V68 Encounters for administrative purposes

V68.0 Issue of medical certificates
Issue of medical certificate of: cause of death
fitness
incapacity

Excludes: encounter for general medical examination (V70.0-V70.9)

● Code new
to this edition

▲ Revision of
existing code

④ ⑤ Fourth or fifth
digit required

V68.1 Issue of repeat prescriptions
Issue of repeat prescription for: appliance
glasses
medications

Excludes: *repeat prescription for contraceptives (V25.41-V25.49)*

V68.2 Request for expert evidence

⑤ **V68.8 Other specified administrative purpose**

V68.81 Referral of patient without examination or treatment

V68.89 Other

V68.9 Unspecified administrative purpose

V69 Problems related to lifestyle

V69.0 Lack of physical exercise

V69.1 Inappropriate diet and eating habits

Excludes: *anorexia nervosa (307.1)*
bulimia (783.6)
malnutrition and other nutritional deficiencies (260-269.9)
other and unspecified eating disorders (307.50-307.59)

V69.2 High-risk sexual behavior

V69.3 Gambling and betting

Excludes: *pathological gambling (312.31)*

V69.8 Other problems related to lifestyle
Self-damaging behavior

V69.9 Problem related to lifestyle, unspecified

PERSONS WITHOUT REPORTED DIAGNOSIS ENCOUNTERED DURING EXAMINATION AND INVESTIGATION OF INDIVIDUALS AND POPULATIONS (V70-V83)

Note: Nonspecific abnormal findings disclosed at the time of these examinations are classifiable to categories 790-796.

V70 General medical examination

Use additional code(s) to identify any special screening examination(s) performed (V73.0-V82.9)

V70.0 Routine general medical examination at a health care facility
Health checkup

Excludes: *health checkup of infant or child (V20.2)*

V70.1 General psychiatric examination, requested by the authority

V70.2 General psychiatric examination, other and unspecified

V70.3 Other medical examination for administrative purposes
General medical examination for:
admission to old age home   marriage
adoption   prison
camp   school admission
driving license   sports competition
immigration and naturalization
insurance certification

Excludes: *attendance for issue of medical certificates (V68.0)*
pre-employment screening (V70.5)

V70.4 Examination for medicolegal reasons
Blood-alcohol tests
Blood-drug tests
Paternity testing

Excludes: *examination and observation following:*
accidents (V71.3, V71.4)
assault (V71.6)
rape (V71.5)

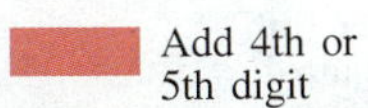

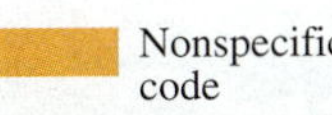

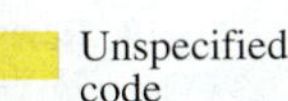

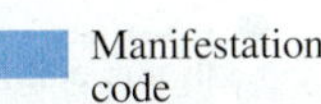

V70.5 Health examination of defined subpopulations

Armed forces personnel	Preschool children
Inhabitants of institutions	Prisoners
Occupational health	Prostitutes
examinations	Refugees
Pre-employment screening	School children
	Students

V70.6 Health examination in population surveys

Excludes: special screening (V73.0-V82.9)

V70.7 Examination of participant in clinical trial
Examination of participant or control in clinical research

V70.8 Other specified general medical examinations
Examination of potential donor of organ or tissue

V70.9 Unspecified general medical examination

V71 Observation and evaluation for suspected conditions not found

Note: This category is to be used when persons without a diagnosis are suspected of having an abnormal condition, without signs or symptoms, which requires study, but after examination and observation, is found not to exist. This category is also for use for administrative and legal observation status.

⑤ **V71.0 Observation for suspected mental condition**

V71.01 Adult antisocial behavior
Dyssocial behavior or gang activity in adult without manifest psychiatric disorder

V71.02 Childhood or adolescent antisocial behavior
Dyssocial behavior or gang activity in child or adolescent without manifest psychiatric disorder

V71.09 Other suspected mental condition

V71.1 Observation for suspected malignant neoplasm

V71.2 Observation for suspected tuberculosis

V71.3 Observation following accident at work

V71.4 Observation following other accident
Examination of individual involved in motor vehicle traffic accident

V71.5 Observation following alleged rape or seduction
Examination of victim or culprit

V71.6 Observation following other inflicted injury
Examination of victim or culprit

V71.7 Observation for suspected cardiovascular disease

▲ **V71.8 Observation and evaluation for other specified suspected conditions**

V71.81 Abuse and neglect

Excludes: adult abuse and neglect (995.80-995.85)
child abuse and neglect (995.50-995.59)

● **V71.82 Observation and evaluation for suspected exposure to anthrax**

● **V71.83 Observation and evaluation for suspected exposure to other biological agent**

V71.89 Other specified suspected conditions

V71.9 Observation for unspecified suspected condition

V72 Special investigations and examinations
Includes: routine examination of specific system

Excludes: general medical examination (V70.0-V70.4)
general screening examination of defined population groups (V70.5, V70.6, V70.7)
routine examination of infant or child (V20.2)

Use additional code(s) to identify any special screening examination(s) performed (V73.0-V82.9)

V72.0 Examination of eyes and vision

V72.1 Examination of ears and hearing

V72.2 Dental examination

● Code new to this edition	▲ Revision of existing code	④ ⑤ Fourth or fifth digit required

V72.3 Gynecological examination
   Papanicolaou cervical smear as part of general gynecological examination
   Pelvic examination (annual) (periodic)

Use additional code to identify routine vaginal Papanicolaou smear (V76.47)

> *Excludes:* *cervical Papanicolaou smear without general gynecological examination (V76.2)*
> *routine examination in contraceptive management (V25.40-V25.49)*

V72.4 Pregnancy examination or test, pregnancy unconfirmed
   Possible pregnancy, not (yet) confirmed

> *Excludes:* *pregnancy examination with immediate confirmation (V22.0-V22.1)*

V72.5 Radiological examination, not elsewhere classified
   Routine chest x-ray

> *Excludes:* *examination for suspected tuberculosis (V71.2)*

V72.6 Laboratory examination

> *Excludes:* *that for suspected disorder (V71.0-V71.9)*

V72.7 Diagnostic skin and sensitization tests
   Allergy tests
   Skin tests for hypersensitivity

> *Excludes:* *diagnostic skin tests for bacterial diseases (V74.0-V74.9)*

⑤ **V72.8 Other specified examinations**

   V72.81 Pre-operative cardiovascular examination

   V72.82 Pre-operative respiratory examination

   V72.83 Other specified pre-operative examination

   V72.84 Pre-operative examination, unspecified

   V72.85 Other specified examination

V72.9 Unspecified examination

V73 Special screening examination for viral and chlamydial diseases

V73.0 Poliomyelitis

V73.1 Smallpox

V73.2 Measles

V73.3 Rubella

V73.4 Yellow fever

V73.5 Other arthropod-borne viral diseases
   Dengue fever   Viral encephalitis:
   Hemorrhagic fever   mosquito-borne
                                       tick-borne

V73.6 Trachoma

⑤ **V73.8 Other specified viral and chlamydial diseases**

   V73.88 Other specified chlamydial diseases

   V73.89 Other specified viral diseases

⑤ **V73.9 Unspecified viral and chlamydial disease**

   V73.98 Unspecified chlamydial disease

   V73.99 Unspecified viral disease

V74 Special screening examination for bacterial and spirochetal diseases
   Includes: diagnostic skin tests for these diseases

V74.0 Cholera

V74.1 Pulmonary tuberculosis

V74.2 Leprosy [Hansen's disease]

V74.3 Diphtheria

V74.4 Bacterial conjunctivitis

V74.5 Venereal disease

V74.6 Yaws

V74.8 Other specified bacterial and spirochetal diseases
   Brucellosis   Tetanus
   Leptospirosis   Whooping cough
   Plague

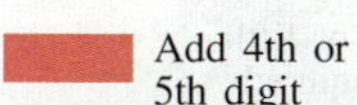

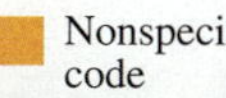

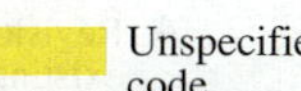

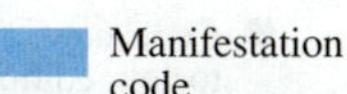

V74.9 Unspecified bacterial and spirochetal disease

V75 Special screening examination for other infectious diseases

V75.0 Rickettsial diseases

V75.1 Malaria

V75.2 Leishmaniasis

V75.3 Trypanosomiasis
    Chagas' disease   Sleeping sickness

V75.4 Mycotic infections

V75.5 Schistosomiasis

V75.6 Filariasis

V75.7 Intestinal helminthiasis

V75.8 Other specified parasitic infections

V75.9 Unspecified infectious disease

V76 Special screening for malignant neoplasms

V76.0 Respiratory organs

⑤ **V76.1** Breast

    V76.10 Breast screening, unspecified

    V76.11 Screening mammogram for high-risk patient

    V76.12 Other screening mammogram

    V76.19 Other screening breast examination

V76.2 Cervix
    Routine cervical Papanicolaou smear

    Excludes: *that as part of a general gynecological examination (V72.3)*

V76.3 Bladder

⑤ **V76.4** Other sites

    V76.41 Rectum

    V76.42 Oral cavity

    V76.43 Skin

    V76.44 Prostate

    V76.45 Testis

    V76.46 Ovary

    V76.47 Vagina
        Vaginal pap smear status-post hysterectomy for non-malignant condition
Use additional code to identify acquired absence of uterus (V45.77)

    Excludes: *vaginal pap smear status-post hysterectomy for malignant condition (V67.01)*

    V76.49 Other sites

⑤ **V76.5** Intestine

    V76.50 Intestine, unspecified

    V76.51 Colon

    Excludes: *rectum (V76.41)*

    V76.52 Small intestine

⑤ **V76.8** Other neoplasm

    V76.81 Nervous system

    V76.89 Other neoplasm

V76.9 Unspecified

V77 Special screening for endocrine, nutritional, metabolic, and immunity disorders

V77.0 Thyroid disorders

V77.1 Diabetes mellitus

V77.2 Malnutrition

V77.3 Phenylketonuria [PKU]

V77.4 Galactosemia

V77.5 Gout

● Code new to this edition   ▲ Revision of existing code   ④ ⑤ Fourth or fifth digit required

V77.6 Cystic fibrosis
Screening for mucoviscidosis

V77.7 Other inborn errors of metabolism

V77.8 Obesity

⑤ **V77.9 Other and unspecified endocrine, nutritional, metabolic, and immunity disorders**

    V77.91 Screening for lipoid disorders
Screening cholesterol level
Screening for hypercholesterolemia
Screening for hyperlipidemia

    V77.99 Other and unspecified endocrine, nutritional, metabolic, and immunity disorders

V78 Special screening for disorders of blood and blood-forming organs

V78.0 Iron deficiency anemia

V78.1 Other and unspecified deficiency anemia

V78.2 Sickle-cell disease or trait

V78.3 Other hemoglobinopathies

V78.8 Other disorders of blood and blood-forming organs

V78.9 Unspecified disorder of blood and blood-forming organs

V79 Special screening for mental disorders and developmental handicaps

V79.0 Depression

V79.1 Alcoholism

V79.2 Mental retardation

V79.3 Developmental handicaps in early childhood

V79.8 Other specified mental disorders and developmental handicaps

V79.9 Unspecified mental disorder and developmental handicap

V80 Special screening for neurological, eye, and ear diseases

V80.0 Neurological conditions

V80.1 Glaucoma

V80.2 Other eye conditions
Screening for:
cataract
congenital anomaly of eye
senile macular lesions

> *Excludes:* *general vision examination (V72.0)*

V80.3 Ear diseases

> *Excludes:* *general hearing examination (V72.1)*

V81 Special screening for cardiovascular, respiratory, and genitourinary diseases

V81.0 Ischemic heart disease

V81.1 Hypertension

V81.2 Other and unspecified cardiovascular conditions

V81.3 Chronic bronchitis and emphysema

V81.4 Other and unspecified respiratory conditions

> *Excludes:* *screening for:*
> *lung neoplasm (V76.0)*
> *pulmonary tuberculosis (V74.1)*

V81.5 Nephropathy
Screening for asymptomatic bacteriuria

V81.6 Other and unspecified genitourinary conditions

V82 Special screening for other conditions

V82.0 Skin conditions

V82.1 Rheumatoid arthritis

V82.2 Other rheumatic disorders

V82.3 Congenital dislocation of hip

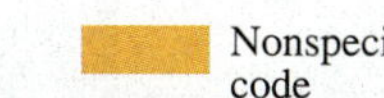

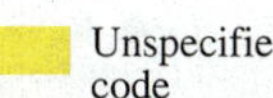

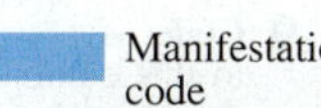

Manifestation
code

V82.4 Maternal postnatal screening for chromosomal anomalies

> *Excludes:* *antenatal screening by amniocentesis (V28.0)*

V82.5 Chemical poisoning and other contamination
Screening for:
heavy metal poisoning
ingestion of radioactive substance
poisoning from contaminated water supply
radiation exposure

V82.6 Multiphasic screening

⑤ **V82.8 Other specified conditions**

V82.81 Osteoporosis

Use additional code to identify:
postmenopausal hormone replacement therapy status (V07.4)
postmenopausal (natural) status (V49.81)

V82.89 Other specified conditions

V82.9 Unspecified condition

V83 Genetic carrier status

⑤ **V83.0 Hemophilia A carrier**

V83.01 Asymptomatic hemophilia A carrier

V83.02 Symptomatic hemophilia A carrier

● **V83.8 Other genetic carrier status**

● **V83.81 Cystic fibrosis gene carrier**

● **V83.89 Other genetic carrier status**

SUPPLEMENTARY CLASSIFICATION OF EXTERNAL CAUSES OF INJURY AND POISONING (E800-E999)

This section is provided to permit the classification of environmental events, circumstances, and conditions as the cause of injury, poisoning, and other adverse effects. Where a code from this section is applicable, it is intended that it shall be used in addition to a code from one of the main chapters of *ICD-9-CM* indicating the nature of the condition. Certain other conditions which may be stated to be due to external causes are classified in Chapters 1 to 16 of *ICD-9-CM*. For these, the "E" code classification should be used for more detailed analysis.

Machinery accidents [other than those connected with transport] are classifiable to category E919, in which the fourth-digit allows a broad classification of the type of machinery involved. If a more detailed classification of type of machinery is required, it is suggested that the "Classification of Industrial Accidents according to Agency," prepared by the International Labor Office, be used in addition. This is reproduced on page 571, for optional use.

Categories for "late effects" of accidents and other external causes are to be found at E929, E959, E969, E977, E989, and E999.

Definitions and examples related to transport accidents

    (a) A **transport accident** (E800-E848) is any accident involving a device designed primarily for, or being used at the time primarily for, conveying persons or goods from one place to another.

        Includes: accidents involving:
                aircraft and spacecraft (E840-E845)
                watercraft (E830-E838)
                motor vehicle (E810-E825)
                railway (E800-E807)
                other road vehicles (E826-E829)

    In classifying accidents which involve more than one kind of transport, the above order of precedence of transport accidents should be used.

    Accidents involving agriculture and construction machines, such as tractors, cranes, and bulldozers, are regarded as transport accidents only when these vehicles are under their own power on a highway [otherwise the vehicles are regarded as machinery]. Vehicles which can travel on land or water, such as hovercraft and other amphibious vehicles, are regarded as watercraft when on the water, as motor vehicles when on the highway, and as off-road motor vehicles when on land, but off the highway.

        | *Excludes:* | *accidents:*
in sports which involve the use of transport but where the transport vehicle itself was not involved in the accident
involving vehicles which are part of industrial equipment used entirely on industrial premises
occurring during transportation but unrelated to the hazards associated with the means of transportation [e.g., injuries received in a fight on board ship; transport vehicle involved in a cataclysm such as an earthquake]
to persons engaged in the maintenance or repair of transport equipment or vehicle not in motion, unless injured by another vehicle in motion

    (b) A **railway accident** is a transport accident involving a railway train or other railway vehicle operated on rails, whether in motion or not.

        | *Excludes:* | *accidents:*
in repair shops
in roundhouse or on turntable
on railway premises but not involving a train or other railway vehicle

    (c) A **railway train** or **railway vehicle** is any device with or without cars coupled to it, designed for traffic on a railway.

        Includes: interurban:
                electric car   } (operated chiefly on its own right-of-way, not open to
                streetcar   } other traffic)
                railway train, any power [diesel] [electric] [steam]
                  funicular
                  monorail or two-rail
                  subterranean or elevated
                other vehicle designed to run on a railway track

        | *Excludes:* | *interurban electric cars [streetcars] specified to be operating on a right-of-way that forms part of the public street or highway [definition (n)]*

    (d) A **railway** or **railroad** is a right-of-way designed for traffic on rails, which is used by carriages or wagons transporting passengers or freight, and by other rolling stock, and which is not open to other public vehicular traffic.

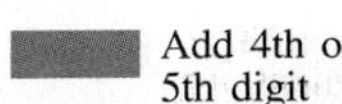
Add 4th or 5th digit

Nonspecific code

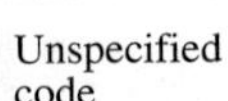
Unspecified code

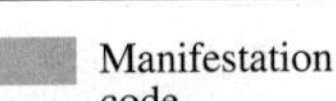
Manifestation code

(e) A **motor vehicle accident** is a transport accident involving a motor vehicle. It is defined as a motor vehicle traffic accident or as a motor vehicle nontraffic accident according to whether the accident occurs on a public highway or elsewhere.

> *Excludes:* *injury or damage due to cataclysm*
>
> *injury or damage while a motor vehicle, not under its own power, is being loaded on, or unloaded from, another conveyance*

(f) A **motor vehicle traffic accident** is any motor vehicle accident occurring on a public highway [i.e., originating, terminating, or involving a vehicle partially on the highway]. A motor vehicle accident is assumed to have occurred on the highway unless another place is specified, except in the case of accidents involving only off-road motor vehicles which are classified as nontraffic accidents unless the contrary is stated.

(g) A **motor vehicle nontraffic accident** is any motor vehicle accident which occurs entirely in any place other than a public highway.

(h) A **public highway [trafficway]** or **street** is the entire width between property lines [or other boundary lines] of every way or place, of which any part is open to the use of the public for purposes of vehicular traffic as a matter of right or custom. A roadway is that part of the public highway designed, improved, and ordinarily used, for vehicular travel.

Includes: approaches (public) to:
docks
public building
station

> *Excludes:* *driveway (private)*
>
> *parking lot*
> *ramp*
> *roads in:*
> *airfield*
> *farm*
> *industrial premises*
> *mine*
> *private grounds*
> *quarry*

(i) A **motor vehicle** is any mechanically or electrically powered device, not operated on rails, upon which any person or property may be transported or drawn upon a highway. Any object such as a trailer, coaster, sled, or wagon being towed by a motor vehicle is considered a part of the motor vehicle.

Includes: automobile [any type]
bus
construction machinery, farm and industrial machinery, steam roller, tractor, army tank, highway grader, or similar vehicle on wheels or treads, while in transport under own power
fire engine (motorized)
motorcycle
motorized bicycle [moped] or scooter
trolley bus not operating on rails
truck
van

> *Excludes:* *devices used solely to move persons or materials within the confines of a building and its premises, such as:*
> *building elevator*
> *coal car in mine*
> *electric baggage or mail truck used solely within a railroad station*
> *electric truck used solely within an industrial plant*
> *moving overhead crane*

(j) A **motorcycle** is a two-wheeled motor vehicle having one or two riding saddles and sometimes having a third wheel for the support of a sidecar. The sidecar is considered part of the motorcycle.

Includes: motorized:
bicycle [moped]
scooter
tricycle

(k) An **off-road motor vehicle** is a motor vehicle of special design, to enable it to negotiate rough or soft terrain or snow. Examples of special design are high construction, special wheels and tires, driven by treads, or support on a cushion of air.

Includes: all terrain vehicle [ATV]
army tank
hovercraft, on land or swamp
snowmobile

● Code new to this edition   ▲ Revision of existing code   ④ ⑤ Fourth or fifth digit required

(l) A **driver** of a motor vehicle is the occupant of the motor vehicle operating it or intending to operate it. A **motorcyclist** is the driver of a motorcycle. Other authorized occupants of a motor vehicle are **passengers**.

(m) An **other road vehicle** is any device, except a motor vehicle, in, on, or by which any person or property may be transported on a highway.

Includes: animal carrying a person or goods
animal-drawn vehicle
animal harnessed to conveyance
bicycle [pedal cycle]
streetcar
tricycle (pedal)

Excludes: *pedestrian conveyance [definition (q)]*

(n) A **streetcar** is a device designed and used primarily for transporting persons within a municipality, running on rails, usually subject to normal traffic control signals, and operated principally on a right-of-way that forms part of the traffic way. A trailer being towed by a streetcar is considered a part of the streetcar.

Includes: interurban or intraurban electric or streetcar, when specified to be operating on a street or public highway
tram (car)
trolley (car)

(o) A **pedal cycle** is any road transport vehicle operated solely by pedals.

Includes: bicycle
pedal cycle
tricycle

Excludes: *motorized bicycle [definition (i)]*

(p) A **pedal cyclist** is any person riding on a pedal cycle or in a sidecar attached to such a vehicle.

(q) A **pedestrian conveyance** is any human powered device by which a pedestrian may move other than by walking or by which a walking person may move another pedestrian.

Includes:

baby carriage	roller skates
coaster wagon	scooter
ice skates	skateboard
perambulator	skis
pushcart	sled
pushchair	wheelchair

(r) A **pedestrian** is any person involved in an accident who was not at the time of the accident riding in or on a motor vehicle, railroad train, streetcar, animal-drawn or other vehicle, or on a bicycle or animal.

Includes: person:
changing tire of vehicle
in or operating a pedestrian conveyance
making adjustment to motor of vehicle
on foot

(s) A **watercraft** is any device for transporting passengers or goods on the water.

(t) A **small boat** is any watercraft propelled by paddle, oars, or small motor, with a passenger capacity of less than ten.

Includes:

boat NOS	rowboat
canoe	rowing shell
coble	scull
dinghy	skiff
punt	small motorboat
raft	

Excludes: *barge*
lifeboat (used after abandoning ship)
raft (anchored) being used as diving platform
yacht

(u) An **aircraft** is any device for transporting passengers or goods in the air.

Includes: airplane [any type]
balloon
bomber
dirigible
glider (hang)
military aircraft
parachute

Add 4th or 5th digit   Nonspecific code   Unspecified code   Manifestation code

(v) A **commercial transport aircraft** is any device for collective passenger or freight transportation by air, whether run on commercial lines for profit or by government authorities, with the exception of military craft.

RAILWAY ACCIDENTS (E800-E807)

Note: For definitions of railway accident and related terms see definitions (a) to (d).

> *Excludes:* *accidents involving railway train and:*
> *aircraft (E840.0-E845.9)*
> *motor vehicle (E810.0-E825.9)*
> *watercraft (E830.0-E838.9)*

The following fourth-digit subdivisions are for use with categories E800-E807 to identify the injured person:

.0 Railway employee
Any person who by virtue of his employment in connection with a railway, whether by the railway company or not, is at increased risk of involvement in a railway accident, such as:
catering staff of train
driver
guard
porter
postal staff on train
railway fireman
shunter
sleeping car attendant

.1 Passenger on railway
Any authorized person traveling on a train, except a railway employee.

> *Excludes:* *intending passenger waiting at station (.8)*
> *unauthorized rider on railway vehicle (.8)*

.2 Pedestrian
See definition (r)

.3 Pedal cyclist
See definition (p)

.8 Other specified person
Intending passenger or bystander waiting at station
Unauthorized rider on railway vehicle

.9 Unspecified person

④ **E800 Railway accident involving collision with rolling stock**
Includes: collision between railway trains or railway vehicles, any kind
collision NOS on railway
derailment with antecedent collision with rolling stock or NOS

④ **E801 Railway accident involving collision with other object**
Includes: collision of railway train with:
buffers
fallen tree on railway
gates
platform
rock on railway
streetcar
other nonmotor vehicle
other object

> *Excludes:* *collision with:*
> *aircraft (E840.0-E842.9)*
> *motor vehicle (E810.0-E810.9, E820.0-E822.9)*

④ **E802 Railway accident involving derailment without antecedent collision**

④ **E803 Railway accident involving explosion, fire, or burning**

> *Excludes:* *explosion or fire, with antecedent derailment (E802.0-E802.9)*
> *explosion or fire, with mention of antecedent collision (E800.0-E801.9)*

④ **E804 Fall in, on, or from railway train**
Includes: fall while alighting from or boarding railway train

> *Excludes:* *fall related to collision, derailment, or explosion of railway train (E800.0-E803.9)*

● Code new
to this edition
▲ Revision of
existing code
④ ⑤ Fourth or fifth
digit required

④ **E805** **Hit by rolling stock**
      Includes:

crushed
injured
killed   } by railway train or part
knocked down
run over

      Excludes: *pedestrian hit by object set in motion by railway train (E806.0-E806.9)*

④ **E806** **Other specified railway accident**
      Includes: hit by object falling in railway train
injured by door or window on railway train
nonmotor road vehicle or pedestrian hit by object set in motion by railway train
railway train hit by falling:
earth NOS
rock
tree
other object

      Excludes: *railway accident due to cataclysm (E908-E909)*

④ **E807** **Railway accident of unspecified nature**
      Includes:

found dead   } on railway right-of-way NOS
injured

railway accident NOS

MOTOR VEHICLE TRAFFIC ACCIDENTS (E810-E819)

    Note: For definitions of motor vehicle traffic accident, and related terms, see definitions (e) to (k).

    Excludes: *accidents involving motor vehicle and aircraft (E840.0-E845.9)*

The following fourth-digit subdivisions are for use with categories E810-E819 to identify the injured person:

.0 **Driver of motor vehicle other than motorcycle**
    See definition (l)

.1 **Passenger in motor vehicle other than motorcycle**
    See definition (l)

.2 **Motorcyclist**
    See definition (l)

.3 **Passenger on motorcycle**
    See definition (l)

.4 **Occupant of streetcar**

.5 **Rider of animal; occupant of animal-drawn vehicle**

.6 **Pedal cyclist**
    See definition (p)

.7 **Pedestrian**
    See definition (r)

.8 **Other specified person**
    Occupant of vehicle other than above
    Person in railway train involved in accident
    Unauthorized rider of motor vehicle

.9 **Unspecified person**

④ **E810** **Motor vehicle traffic accident involving collision with train**

      Excludes: *motor vehicle collision with object set in motion by railway train (E815.0-E815.9)*
              railway train hit by object set in motion by motor vehicle (E818.0-E818.9)

④ **E811** **Motor vehicle traffic accident involving re-entrant collision with another motor vehicle**
      Includes: collision between motor vehicle which accidentally leaves the roadway then re-enters the same roadway, or the opposite roadway on a divided highway, and another motor vehicle

      Excludes: *collision on the same roadway when none of the motor vehicles involved have left and re-entered the roadway (E812.0-E812.9)*

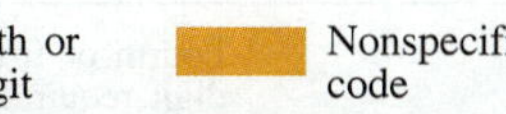

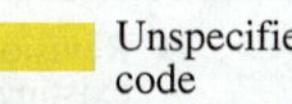

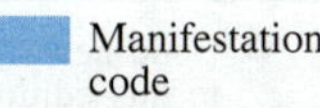

Manifestation
code

④ **E812** **Other motor vehicle traffic accident involving collision with motor vehicle**
    Includes: collision with another motor vehicle parked, stopped, stalled, disabled, or abandoned
              on the highway
          motor vehicle collision NOS

    | Excludes: | *collision with object set in motion by another motor vehicle (E815.0-E815.9)*
          re-entrant collision with another motor vehicle (E811.0-E811.9)

④ **E813** **Motor vehicle traffic accident involving collision with other vehicle**
    Includes: collision between motor vehicle, any kind, and:
          other road (nonmotor transport) vehicle, such as:
              animal carrying a person
              animal-drawn vehicle
              pedal cycle
              streetcar

    | Excludes: | *collision with:*

          object set in motion by nonmotor road vehicle (E815.0-E815.9)
          pedestrian (E814.0-E814.9)
        nonmotor road vehicle hit by object set in motion by motor vehicle
          (E818.0-E818.9)

④ **E814** **Motor vehicle traffic accident involving collision with pedestrian**
    Includes: collision between motor vehicle, any kind, and pedestrian
          pedestrian dragged, hit, or run over by motor vehicle, any kind

    | Excludes: | *pedestrian hit by object set in motion by motor vehicle (E818.0-E818.9)*

④ **E815** **Other motor vehicle traffic accident involving collision on the highway**
    Includes: collision (due to loss of control) (on highway) between motor vehicle, any kind, and:
          abutment (bridge) (overpass)
           animal (herded) (unattended)
           fallen stone, traffic sign, tree, utility pole
           guard rail or boundary fence
           interhighway divider
           landslide (not moving)
           object set in motion by railway train or road vehicle (motor) (nonmotor)
           object thrown in front of motor vehicle
           safety island
           temporary traffic sign or marker
           wall of cut made for road
           other object, fixed, movable, or moving

    | Excludes: | *collision with:*

          any object off the highway (resulting from loss of control) (E816.0-E816.9)
          any object which normally would have been off the highway and is not stated to
            have been on it (E816.0-E816.9)
          motor vehicle parked, stopped, stalled, disabled, or abandoned on highway
            (E812.0-E812.9)
          moving landslide (E909)
        motor vehicle hit by object:
          set in motion by railway train or road vehicle (motor) (nonmotor)
            (E818.0-E818.9)
          thrown into or on vehicle (E818.0-E818.9)

④ **E816** **Motor vehicle traffic accident due to loss of control, without collision on the highway**
    Includes: motor vehicle:
          failing to make curve
          going out of control (due to):
           blowout
           burst tire   and:
           driver falling asleep   colliding with object off the
           driver inattention   highway
           excessive speed   overturning
           failure of mechanical part stopping abruptly off the highway

    | Excludes: | *collision on highway following loss of control (E810.0-E815.9)*
          loss of control of motor vehicle following collision on the highway
            (E810.0-E815.9)

④ **E817** **Noncollision motor vehicle traffic accident while boarding or alighting**
    Includes:
          fall down stairs of motor bus
          fall from car in street
          injured by moving part of the vehicle while boarding or alighting
          trapped by door of motor bus

● Code new   ▲ Revision of   ④ ⑤ Fourth or fifth
  to this edition   existing code   digit required

④ **E818** **Other noncollision motor vehicle traffic accident**

Includes:

accidental poisoning from exhaust gas generated by
breakage of any part of
explosion of any part of
fall, jump, or being accidentally pushed from
fire starting in
hit by object thrown into or on
injured by being thrown against some part of,
    or object in
injury from moving part of
object falling in or on
object thrown on

} motor vehicle while in motion

collision of railway train or road vehicle except motor vehicle, with object set in
    motion by motor vehicle
motor vehicle hit by object set in motion by railway train or road vehicle (motor)
    (nonmotor)
pedestrian, railway train, or road vehicle (motor) (nonmotor) hit by object set in
    motion by motor vehicle

Excludes: *collision between motor vehicle and:*

object set in motion by railway train or road vehicle (motor) (nonmotor)
*   (E815.0-E815.9)*
object thrown towards the motor vehicle (E815.0-E815.9)
person overcome by carbon monoxide generated by stationary motor vehicle off the
*   roadway with motor running (E868.2)*

④ **E819** **Motor vehicle traffic accident of unspecified nature**

Includes: motor vehicle traffic accident NOS
             traffic accident NOS

MOTOR VEHICLE NONTRAFFIC ACCIDENTS (E820-E825)

Note: For definitions of motor vehicle nontraffic accident and related terms see definitions (a) to
    (k).

Includes: accidents involving motor vehicles being used in recreational or sporting activities off
         the highway
         collision and noncollision motor vehicle accidents occurring entirely off the highway

Excludes: *accidents involving motor vehicle and:*

aircraft (E840.0-E845.9)
watercraft (E830.0-E838.9)
accidents, not on the public highway, involving agricultural and construction
*   machinery but not involving another motor vehicle (E919.0, E919.2, E919.7)*

The following fourth-digit subdivisions are for use with categories E820-E825 to identify the
    injured person:

.0 **Driver of motor vehicle other than motorcycle**
See definition (l)

.1 **Passenger in motor vehicle other than motorcycle**
See definition (l)

.2 **Motorcyclist**
See definition (l)

.3 **Passenger on motorcycle**
See definition (l)

.4 **Occupant of streetcar**

.5 **Rider of animal; occupant of animal-drawn vehicle**

.6 **Pedal cyclist**
See definition (p)

.7 **Pedestrian**
See definition (r)

.8 **Other specified person**
Occupant of vehicle other than above
Person on railway train involved in accident
Unauthorized rider of motor vehicle

.9 **Unspecified person**

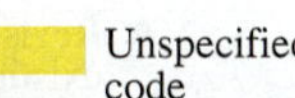

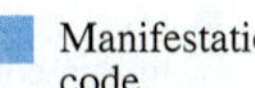

④ **E820 Nontraffic accident involving motor-driven snow vehicle**
    Includes:

breakage of part of
fall from
hit by ⎫ motor-driven snow vehicle (not
overturning of ⎬   on public highway)
run over or dragged by ⎭
collision of motor-driven snow vehicle with:
  animal (being ridden) (-drawn vehicle)
  another off-road motor vehicle
  other motor vehicle, not on public highway
  railway train
  other object, fixed or movable
injury caused by rough landing of motor-driven snow vehicle (after leaving
  ground on rough terrain)

Excludes: | *accident on the public highway involving motor driven snow vehicle*
(E810.0-E819.9)

④ **E821 Nontraffic accident involving other off-road motor vehicle**
    Includes:

breakage of part of
fall from
hit by ⎫ off-road motor vehicle, except
overturning of ⎬   snow vehicle (not on public
run over or dragged by ⎭   highway)
thrown against some part of or object in
collision with:
  animal (being ridden) (-drawn vehicle)
  another off-road motor vehicle, except snow vehicle
  other motor vehicle, not on public highway
  other object, fixed or movable

Excludes: | *accident on public highway involving off-road motor vehicle (E810.0-E819.9)*
collision between motor driven snow vehicle and other off-road motor vehicle
(E820.0-E820.9)
hovercraft accident on water (E830.0-E838.9)

④ **E822 Other motor vehicle nontraffic accident involving collision with moving object**
    Includes: collision, not on public highway, between motor vehicle, except off-road motor
        vehicle and:
      animal
      nonmotor vehicle
      other motor vehicle, except off-road motor vehicle
      pedestrian
      railway train
      other moving object

Excludes: | *collision with:*
  motor-driven snow vehicle (E820.0-E820.9)
  other off-road motor vehicle (E821.0-E821.9)

④ **E823 Other motor vehicle nontraffic accident involving collision with stationary object**
    Includes: collision, not on public highway, between motor vehicle, except off-road motor
        vehicle, and any object, fixed or movable, but not in motion

④ **E824 Other motor vehicle nontraffic accident while boarding and alighting**
    Includes:

fall ⎫ while boarding or alighting from
injury from moving part of motor vehicle ⎬   motor vehicle, except off-road
trapped by door of motor vehicle ⎭   motor vehicle, not on public
  highway

● Code new   ▲ Revision of   ④ ⑤ Fourth or fifth
  to this edition   existing code   digit required

④ **E825** **Other motor vehicle nontraffic accident of other and unspecified nature**

Includes:

accidental poisoning from carbon monoxide generated by
breakage of any part of
explosion of any part of
fall, jump, or being accidentally pushed from
fire starting in
hit by object thrown into, towards, or on
injured by being thrown against some part of, or object in
injury from moving part of
object falling in or on
motor vehicle nontraffic accident NOS

} motor vehicle while in motion, not on public highway

Excludes: *fall from or in stationary motor vehicle (E884.9, E885.9)*

overcome by carbon monoxide or exhaust gas generated by stationary motor vehicle off the roadway with motor running (E868.2)
struck by falling object from or in stationary motor vehicle (E916)

OTHER ROAD VEHICLE ACCIDENTS (E826-E829)

Note: Other road vehicle accidents are transport accidents involving road vehicles other than motor vehicles. For definitions of other road vehicle and related terms see definitions (m) to (o).

Includes: accidents involving other road vehicles being used in recreational or sporting activities

Excludes: *collision of other road vehicle [any] with:*

aircraft (E840.0-E845.9)
motor vehicle (E813.0-E813.9, E820.0-E822.9)
railway train (E801.0-E801.9)

The following fourth-digit subdivisions are for use with categories E826-E829 to identify the injured person:

.0 Pedestrian
See definition (r)

.1 Pedal cyclist
See definition (p)

.2 Rider of animal

.3 Occupant of animal-drawn vehicle

.4 Occupant of streetcar

.8 Other specified person

.9 Unspecified person

④ **E826** **Pedal cycle accident**

[0-9]

Includes: breakage of any part of pedal cycle
collision between pedal cycle and:
animal (being ridden) (herded) (unattended)
another pedal cycle
nonmotor road vehicle, any
pedestrian
other object, fixed, movable, or moving, not set in motion by motor vehicle, railway train, or aircraft
entanglement in wheel of pedal cycle
fall from pedal cycle
hit by object falling or thrown on the pedal cycle
pedal cycle accident NOS
pedal cycle overturned

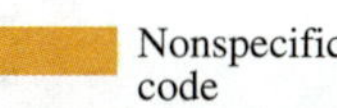

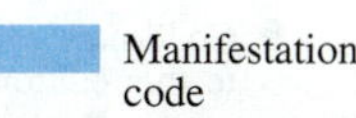

Manifestation code

④ **E827** **Animal-drawn vehicle accident**
[0,2-4,8,9]
> Includes   breakage of any part of vehicle
> collision between animal-drawn vehicle and:
>   animal (being ridden) (herded) (unattended)
>   nonmotor road vehicle, except pedal cycle
>   pedestrian, pedestrian conveyance, or pedestrian vehicle
>   other object, fixed, movable, or moving, not set in motion by motor vehicle,
>   railway train, or aircraft
> fall from
> knocked down by
> overturning of   } animal-drawn vehicle
> run over by
> thrown from

| Excludes: | collision of animal-drawn vehicle with pedal cycle (E826.0-E826.9) |

④ **E828** **Accident involving animal being ridden**
[0,2,4,8,9]
> Includes: collision between animal being ridden and:
>   another animal
>   nonmotor road vehicle, except pedal cycle, and animal-drawn vehicle
>   pedestrian, pedestrian conveyance, or pedestrian vehicle
>   other object, fixed, movable, or moving, not set in motion by motor vehicle,
>   railway train, or aircraft
> fall from
> knocked down by
> thrown from   } animal being ridden
> trampled by
>
> ridden animal stumbled and fell

Excludes:	collision of animal being ridden with:
	animal-drawn vehicle (E827.0-E827.9)
	pedal cycle (E826.0-E826.9)

④ **E829** **Other road vehicle accidents**
[0,4,8,9]
> Includes:
>   accident while boarding or alighting from
>   blow from object in
>   breakage of any part of   } streetcar nonmotor road vehicle
>   caught in door of   not classifiable to E826-E828
>   derailment of
>   fall in, on, or from
>   fire in
>   collision between streetcar or nonmotor road vehicle, except as in E826-E828, and:
>   animal (not being ridden)
>   another nonmotor road vehicle not classifiable to E826-E828
>   pedestrian
>   other object, fixed, movable, or moving, not set in motion by motor vehicle,
>   railway train, or aircraft
>   nonmotor road vehicle accident NOS
>   streetcar accident NOS

Excludes:	collision with:
	animal being ridden (E828.0-E828.9)
	animal-drawn vehicle (E827.0-E827.9)
	pedal cycle (E826.0-E826.9)

WATER TRANSPORT ACCIDENTS (E830-E838)

> Note: For definitions of water transport accident and related terms see definitions (a), (s), and (t).

> Includes: watercraft accidents in the course of recreational activities

| Excludes: | accidents involving both aircraft, including objects set in motion by aircraft, and watercraft (E840.0-E845.9) |

The following fourth-digit subdivisions are for use with categories E830-E838 to identify the injured person:

.0 Occupant of small boat, unpowered

.1 Occupant of small boat, powered
> See definition (t)

continued

● Code new to this edition   ▲ Revision of existing code   ④ ⑤ Fourth or fifth digit required

| *Excludes:* | *water skier (.4)* |

.2 Occupant of other watercraft—crew
    Persons:
        engaged in operation of watercraft
        providing passenger services [cabin attendants, ship's physician, catering personnel]
        working on ship during voyage in other capacity [musician in band, operators of
            shops and beauty parlors]

.3 Occupant of other watercraft—other than crew
    Passenger
    Occupant of lifeboat, other than crew, after abandoning ship

.4 Water skier

.5 Swimmer

.6 Dockers, stevedores
    Longshoreman employed on the dock in loading and unloading ships

.8 Other specified person
    Immigration and custom officials on board ship
    Person:
        accompanying passenger or member of crew
        visiting boat
    Pilot (guiding ship into port)

.9 Unspecified person

④ E830 Accident to watercraft causing submersion
    Includes: submersion and drowning due to:
          boat overturning
          boat submerging
          falling or jumping from burning ship
          falling or jumping from crushed watercraft
          ship sinking
          other accident to watercraft

④ E831 Accident to watercraft causing other injury
    Includes: any injury, except submersion and drowning, as a result of an accident to watercraft
          burned while ship on fire
          crushed between ships in collision
          crushed by lifeboat after abandoning ship
          fall due to collision or other accident to watercraft
          hit by falling object due to accident to watercraft
          injured in watercraft accident involving collision
          struck by boat or part thereof after fall or jump from damaged boat

| *Excludes:* | *burns from localized fire or explosion on board ship (E837.0-E837.9)* |

④ E832 Other accidental submersion or drowning in water transport accident
    Includes: submersion or drowning as a result of an accident other than accident to the
          watercraft, such as:
          fall:
            from gangplank
            from ship
            overboard
          thrown overboard by motion of ship
          washed overboard

| *Excludes:* | *submersion or drowning of swimmer or diver who voluntarily jumps from boat not involved in an accident (E910.0-E910.9)* |

④ E833 Fall on stairs or ladders in water transport

| *Excludes:* | *fall due to accident to watercraft (E831.0-E831.9)* |

④ E834 Other fall from one level to another in water transport

| *Excludes:* | *fall due to accident to watercraft (E831.0-E831.9)* |

④ E835 Other and unspecified fall in water transport

| *Excludes:* | *fall due to accident to watercraft (E831.0-E831.9)* |

| | Add 4th or 5th digit | | Nonspecific code | | Unspecified code | | Manifestation code |

④ **E836** **Machinery accident in water transport**
Includes: injuries in water transport caused by:
deck
engine room
galley   } machinery
laundry
loading

④ **E837** **Explosion, fire, or burning in watercraft**
Includes: explosion of boiler on steamship
localized fire on ship

Excludes: *burning ship (due to collision or explosion) resulting in:*
submersion or drowning (E830.0-E830.9)
other injury (E831.0-E831.9)

④ **E838** **Other and unspecified water transport accident**
Includes: accidental poisoning by gases or fumes on ship
atomic power plant malfunction in watercraft
crushed between ship and stationary object [wharf]
crushed between ships without accident to watercraft
crushed by falling object on ship or while loading or unloading
hit by boat while water skiing
struck by boat or part thereof (after fall from boat)
watercraft accident NOS

AIR AND SPACE TRANSPORT ACCIDENTS (E840-E845)

Note: For definition of aircraft and related terms see definitions (u) and (v).

The following fourth-digit subdivisions are for use with categories E840-E845 to identify the
injured person:

.0 Occupant of spacecraft

.1 Occupant of military aircraft, any
Crew
Passenger (civilian)
(military)   } in military aircraft [air force]
Troops   [army] [national guard] [navy]

Excludes: *occupants of aircraft operated under jurisdiction of police departments (.5)*
parachutist (.7)

.2 Crew of commercial aircraft (powered) in surface to surface transport

.3 Other occupant of commercial aircraft (powered) in surface to surface transport
Flight personnel:
not part of crew
on familiarization flight
Passenger on aircraft (powered) NOS

.4 Occupant of commercial aircraft (powered) in surface to air transport
Occupant [crew] [passenger] of aircraft (powered) engaged in activities, such as:
aerial spraying (crops) (fire retardants)
air drops of emergency supplies
air drops of parachutists, except from military craft
crop dusting
lowering of construction material [bridge or telephone pole]
sky writing

.5 Occupant of other powered aircraft
Occupant [crew] [passenger] of aircraft [powered] engaged in activities, such as:
aerobatic flying
aircraft racing
rescue operation
storm surveillance
traffic surveillance
Occupant of private plane NOS

.6 Occupant of unpowered aircraft, except parachutist
Occupant of aircraft classifiable to E842

.7 Parachutist (military) (other)
Person making voluntary descent

Excludes: *person making descent after accident to aircraft (.1-.6)*

   ● Code new   ▲ Revision of   ④ ⑤ Fourth or fifth
to this edition   existing code   digit required

 .8 Ground crew, airline employee
   Persons employed at airfields (civil) (military) or launching pads, not occupants of aircraft

 .9 Other person

④ **E840 Accident to powered aircraft at takeoff or landing**
  Includes:

    collision of aircraft with any object, fixed,
     movable, or moving
    crash
    explosion on aircraft   } while taking off or landing
    fire on aircraft
    forced landing

④ **E841 Accident to powered aircraft, other and unspecified**
  Includes: aircraft accident NOS
      aircraft crash or wreck NOS
      any accident to powered aircraft while in transit or when not specified whether in
       transit, taking off, or landing
      collision of aircraft with another aircraft, bird, or any object, while in transit
      explosion on aircraft while in transit
      fire on aircraft while in transit

④ **E842 Accident to unpowered aircraft**
  [6-9]
   Includes: any accident, except collision with powered aircraft, to:
      balloon
      glider
      hang glider
      kite carrying a person
     hit by object falling from unpowered aircraft

④ **E843 Fall in, on, or from aircraft**
  [0-9]
   Includes: accident in boarding or alighting from aircraft, any kind
      fall in, on, or from aircraft [any kind], while in transit, taking off, or landing,
       except when as a result of an accident to aircraft

④ **E844 Other specified air transport accidents**
  [0-9]
   Includes:

    hit by:
     aircraft
     object falling from aircraft
    injury by or from:
     machinery on aircraft
     rotating propeller   } without accident to aircraft
     voluntary parachute descent
    poisoning by carbon monoxide from aircraft
     while in transit
    sucked into jet
    any accident involving other transport vehicle (motor) (nonmotor) due to being hit
     by object set in motion by aircraft (powered)

   | *Excludes:* | *air sickness (E903)* |

     effects of:
      high altitude (E902.0-E902.1)
      pressure change (E902.0-E902.1)
     injury in parachute descent due to accident to aircraft (840.0-E842.9)

④ **E845 Accident involving spacecraft**
  [0,8,9]
   Includes: launching pad accident

   | *Excludes:* | *effects of weightlessness in spacecraft (E928.0)* |

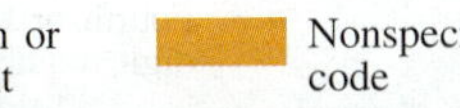

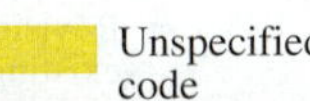

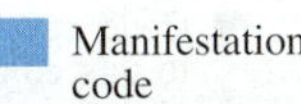

Manifestation
code

VEHICLE ACCIDENTS NOT ELSEWHERE CLASSIFIABLE (E846-E848)

E846 Accidents involving powered vehicles used solely within the buildings and premises of industrial or commercial establishment

Accident to, on, or involving:
  battery powered airport passenger vehicle
  battery powered trucks (baggage) (mail)
  coal car in mine
  logging car
  self propelled truck, industrial
  station baggage truck (powered)
  tram, truck, or tub (powered) in mine or quarry
Breakage of any part of vehicle
Collision with:
  pedestrian
  other vehicle or object within premises
Explosion of ⎫
Fall from ⎬ powered vehicle, industrial or commercial
Overturning of ⎪
Struck by ⎭

> Excludes: accidental poisoning by exhaust gas from vehicle not elsewhere classifiable (E868.2)
>   injury by crane, lift (fork), or elevator (E919.2)

E847 Accidents involving cable cars not running on rails

Accident to, on, or involving:
  cable car, not on rails
  ski chair-lift
  ski-lift with gondola
  téléférique
Breakage of cable ⎫
Caught or dragged by ⎪
Fall or jump from ⎬ cable car, not on rails
Object thrown from or in ⎭

E848 Accidents involving other vehicles, not elsewhere classifiable

Accident to, on, or involving:
  ice yacht
  land yacht
  nonmotor, nonroad vehicle NOS

E849 *Place of occurrence*

The following category is for use to denote the place where the injury or poisoning occurred.

E849.0 *Home*

Apartment	*Private:*
Boarding house	*driveway*
Farm house	*garage*
Home premises	*garden*
House (residential)	*home*
Noninstitutional place	*walk*
of residence	*Swimming pool in private house or garden*
	Yard of home

> *Excludes: home under construction but not yet occupied (E849.3)*
>   *institutional place of residence (E849.7)*

E849.1 *Farm*

Farm:
  buildings
  land under cultivation

> *Excludes: farm house and home premises of farm (E849.0)*

E849.2 *Mine and quarry*

Gravel pit	*Tunnel under construction*
Sand pit	

● Code new to this edition   ▲ Revision of existing code   ④ ⑤ Fourth or fifth digit required

E849.3 **Industrial place and premises**

Building under construction	Industrial yard
Dockyard	Loading platform (factory) (store)
Dry dock	Plant, industrial
Factory	Railway yard
building	Shop (place of work)
premises	Warehouse
Garage (place of work)	Workhouse

E849.4 **Place for recreation and sport**

Amusement park	Public park
Baseball field	Racecourse
Basketball court	Resort NOS
Beach resort	Riding school
Cricket ground	Rifle range
Fives court	Seashore resort
Football field	Skating rink
Golf course	Sports ground
Gymnasium	Sports palace
Hockey field	Stadium
Holiday camp	Swimming pool, public
Ice palace	Tennis court
Lake resort	Vacation resort
Mountain resort	
Playground, including	
school playground	

Excludes: that in private house or garden (E849.0)

E849.5 **Street and highway**

E849.6 **Public building**

Building (including adjacent grounds) used by the general public or by a particular group of the public, such as:

airport	nightclub
bank	office
café	office building
casino	opera house
church	post office
cinema	public hall
clubhouse	radio broadcasting station
courthouse	restaurant
dance hall	school (state) (public) (private)
garage building (for car	shop, commercial
storage)	station (bus) (railway)
hotel	store
market (grocery or other	theater
commodity)	
movie house	
music hall	

Excludes: home garage (E849.0)

        industrial building or workplace (E849.3)

E849.7 **Residential institution**

Children's home	Old people's home
Dormitory	Orphanage
Hospital	Prison
Jail	Reform school

E849.8 **Other specified places**

Beach NOS	Pond or pool (natural)
Canal	Prairie
Caravan site NOS	Public place NOS
Derelict house	Railway line
Desert	Reservoir
Dock	River
Forest	Sea
Harbor	Seashore NOS
Hill	Stream
Lake NOS	Swamp
Mountain	Trailer court
Parking lot	Woods
Parking place	

E849.9 **Unspecified place**

ACCIDENTAL POISONING BY DRUGS, MEDICINAL SUBSTANCES, AND BIOLOGICALS (E850-E858)

Includes: accidental overdose of drug, wrong drug given or taken in error, and drug taken inadvertently

accidents in the use of drugs and biologicals in medical and surgical procedures

Excludes: *administration with suicidal or homicidal intent or intent to harm, or in circumstances classifiable to E980-E989 (E950.0-E950.5, E962.0, E980.0-E980.5)*

correct drug properly administered in therapeutic or prophylactic dosage, as the cause of adverse effect (E930.0-E949.9)

See Alphabetic Index for more complete list of specific drugs to be classified under the fourth-digit subdivisions. The American Hospital Formulary numbers can be used to classify new drugs listed by the American Hospital Formulary Service (AHFS). See appendix C.

E850 Accidental poisoning by analgesics, antipyretics, and antirheumatics

E850.0 Heroin
Diacetylmorphine

E850.1 Methadone

E850.2 Other opiates and related narcotics
Codeine [methylmorphine]   Morphine
Meperidine [pethidine]   Opium (alkaloids)

E850.3 Salicylates
Acetylsalicylic acid [aspirin]
Amino derivatives of salicylic acid
Salicylic acid salts

E850.4 Aromatic analgesics, not elsewhere classified
Acetanilid
Paracetamol [acetaminophen]
Phenacetin [acetophenetidin]

E850.5 Pyrazole derivatives
Aminophenazone [amidopyrine]
Phenylbutazone

E850.6 Antirheumatics [antiphlogistics]
Gold salts   Indomethacin

Excludes: *salicylates (E850.3)*
steroids (E858.0)

E850.7 Other non-narcotic analgesics
Pyrabital

E850.8 Other specified analgesics and antipyretics
Pentazocine

E850.9 Unspecified analgesic or antipyretic

E851 Accidental poisoning by barbiturates
Amobarbital [amylobarbitone]
Barbital [barbitone]
Butabarbital [butabarbitone]
Pentobarbital [pentobarbitone]
Phenobarbital [phenobarbitone]
Secobarbital [quinalbarbitone]

Excludes: *thiobarbiturates (E855.1)*

E852 Accidental poisoning by other sedatives and hypnotics

E852.0 Chloral hydrate group

E852.1 Paraldehyde

E852.2 Bromine compounds
Bromides   Carbromal (derivatives)

E852.3 Methaqualone compounds

E852.4 Glutethimide group

E852.5 Mixed sedatives, not elsewhere classified

E852.8 Other specified sedatives and hypnotics

● Code new to this edition   ▲ Revision of existing code   ④ ⑤ Fourth or fifth digit required

E852.9 **Unspecified sedative or hypnotic**
Sleeping:
drug
pill } NOS
tablet

E853 **Accidental poisoning by tranquilizers**

E853.0 **Phenothiazine-based tranquilizers**
Chlorpromazine   Prochlorperazine
Fluphenazine   Promazine

E853.1 **Butyrophenone-based tranquilizers**
Haloperidol   Trifluperidol
Spiperone

E853.2 **Benzodiazepine-based tranquilizers**
Chlordiazepoxide   Lorazepam
Diazepam   Medazepam
Flurazepam   Nitrazepam

E853.8 **Other specified tranquilizers**
Hydroxyzine   Meprobamate

E853.9 **Unspecified tranquilizer**

E854 **Accidental poisoning by other psychotropic agents**

E854.0 **Antidepressants**
Amitriptyline   Monoamine oxidase [MAO] inhibitors
Imipramine

E854.1 **Psychodysleptics [hallucinogens]**
Cannabis derivatives   Mescaline
Lysergide [LSD]   Psilocin
Marihuana (derivatives) Psilocybin

E854.2 **Psychostimulants**
Amphetamine   Caffeine

Excludes: *central appetite depressants (E858.8)*

E854.3 **Central nervous system stimulants**
Analeptics   Opiate antagonists

E854.8 **Other psychotropic agents**

E855 **Accidental poisoning by other drugs acting on central and autonomic nervous system**

E855.0 **Anticonvulsant and anti-Parkinsonism drugs**
Amantadine
Hydantoin derivatives
Levodopa [L-dopa]
Oxazolidine derivatives [paramethadione] [trimethadione]
Succinimides

E855.1 **Other central nervous system depressants**
Ether   Intravenous anesthetics
Gaseous anesthetics   Thiobarbiturates, such as thiopental sodium
Halogenated hydrocarbon
    derivatives

E855.2 **Local anesthetics**
Cocaine   Procaine
Lidocaine [lignocaine] Tetracaine

E855.3 **Parasympathomimetics [cholinergics]**
Acetylcholine   Pilocarpine
Anticholinesterase:
    organophosphorus
    reversible

E855.4 **Parasympatholytics [anticholinergics and antimuscarinics] and spasmolytics**
Atropine   Hyoscine [scopolamine]
Homatropine   Quaternary ammonium derivatives

E855.5 **Sympathomimetics [adrenergics]**
Epinephrine [adrenalin]
Levarterenol [noradrenalin]

E855.6 **Sympatholytics [antiadrenergics]**
Phenoxybenzamine   Tolazoline hydrochloride

E855.8 **Other specified drugs acting on central and autonomic nervous systems**

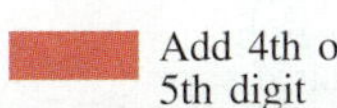

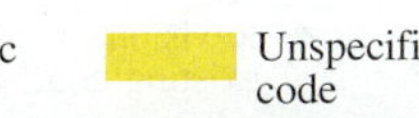

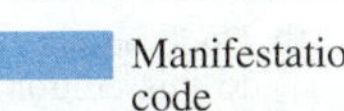

E855.9 Unspecified drug acting on central and autonomic nervous systems

E856 Accidental poisoning by antibiotics

E857 Accidental poisoning by other anti-infectives

E858 Accidental poisoning by other drugs

E858.0 Hormones and synthetic substitutes

E858.1 Primarily systemic agents

E858.2 Agents primarily affecting blood constituents

E858.3 Agents primarily affecting cardiovascular system

E858.4 Agents primarily affecting gastrointestinal system

E858.5 Water, mineral, and uric acid metabolism drugs

E858.6 Agents primarily acting on the smooth and skeletal muscles and respiratory system

E858.7 Agents primarily affecting skin and mucous membrane, ophthalmological,
otorhinolaryngological, and dental drugs

E858.8 Other specified drugs
Central appetite depressants

E858.9 Unspecified drug

ACCIDENTAL POISONING BY OTHER SOLID AND LIQUID SUBSTANCES, GASES, AND VAPORS (E860-E869)

Note: Categories in this section are intended primarily to indicate the external cause of poisoning
states classifiable to 980-989. They may also be used to indicate external causes of
localized effects classifiable to 001-799.

E860 Accidental poisoning by alcohol, not elsewhere classified

E860.0 Alcoholic beverages
Alcohol in preparations intended for consumption

E860.1 Other and unspecified ethyl alcohol and its products
Denatured alcohol   Grain alcohol NOS
Ethanol NOS   Methylated spirit

E860.2 Methyl alcohol
Methanol   Wood alcohol

E860.3 Isopropyl alcohol
Dimethyl carbinol   Secondary propyl alcohol
Isopropanol
Rubbing alcohol substitute

E860.4 Fusel oil
Alcohol:
amyl
butyl
propyl

E860.8 Other specified alcohols

E860.9 Unspecified alcohol

E861 Accidental poisoning by cleansing and polishing agents, disinfectants, paints, and varnishes

E861.0 Synthetic detergents and shampoos

E861.1 Soap products

E861.2 Polishes

E861.3 Other cleansing and polishing agents
Scouring powders

E861.4 Disinfectants
Household and other disinfectants not ordinarily used on the person

Excludes: carbolic acid or phenol (E864.0)

E861.5 Lead paints

E861.6 Other paints and varnishes
Lacquers   Paints, other than lead
Oil colors   White washes

E861.9 Unspecified

● Code new
to this edition

▲ Revision of
existing code

④ ⑤ Fourth or fifth
digit required

E862 **Accidental poisoning by petroleum products, other solvents and their vapors, not elsewhere classified**

E862.0 Petroleum solvents
Petroleum:
ether
benzine
naphtha

E862.1 Petroleum fuels and cleaners
Antiknock additives to petroleum fuels
Gas oils
Gasoline or petrol
Kerosene

Excludes: kerosene insecticides (E863.4)

E862.2 Lubricating oils

E862.3 Petroleum solids
Paraffin wax

E862.4 Other specified solvents
Benzene

E862.9 Unspecified solvent

E863 **Accidental poisoning by agricultural and horticultural chemical and pharmaceutical preparations other than plant foods and fertilizers**

Excludes: plant foods and fertilizers (E866.5)

E863.0 Insecticides of organochlorine compounds
Benzene hexachloride   Dieldrin
Chlordane   Endrine
DDT   Toxaphene

E863.1 Insecticides of organophosphorus compounds
Demeton   Parathion
Diazinon   Phenylsulphthion
Dichlorvos   Phorate
Malathion   Phosdrin
Methyl parathion

E863.2 Carbamates
Aldicarb   Propoxur
Carbaryl

E863.3 Mixtures of insecticides

E863.4 Other and unspecified insecticides
Kerosene insecticides

E863.5 Herbicides
2, 4-Dichlorophenoxyacetic acid [2, 4-D]
2, 4, 5-Trichlorophenoxyacetic acid [2, 4, 5-T]
Chlorates
Diquat
Mixtures of plant food and fertilizers with herbicides
Paraquat

E863.6 Fungicides
Organic mercurials (used in seed dressing)
Pentachlorophenols

E863.7 Rodenticides
Fluoroacetates   Warfarin
Squill and derivatives   Zinc phosphide
Thallium

E863.8 Fumigants
Cyanides   Phosphine
Methyl bromide

E863.9 Other and unspecified

E864 **Accidental poisoning by corrosives and caustics, not elsewhere classified**

Excludes: those as components of disinfectants (E861.4)

E864.0 Corrosive aromatics
Carbolic acid or phenol

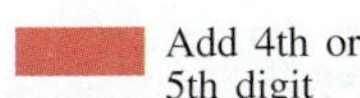

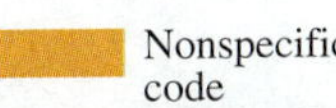

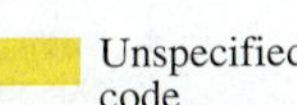

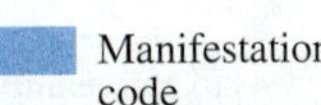

E864.1 Acids
Acid:
hydrochloric
nitric
sulfuric

E864.2 Caustic alkalis
Lye

E864.3 Other specified corrosives and caustics

E864.4 Unspecified corrosives and caustics

E865 Accidental poisoning from poisonous foodstuffs and poisonous plants
Includes: any meat, fish, or shellfish
plants, berries, and fungi eaten as, or in mistake for, food, or by a child

Excludes: *anaphylactic shock due to adverse food reaction (995.6)*
food poisoning (bacterial) (005.0-005.9)
poisoning and toxic reactions to venomous plants (E905.6-E905.7)

E865.0 Meat

E865.1 Shellfish

E865.2 Other fish

E865.3 Berries and seeds

E865.4 Other specified plants

E865.5 Mushrooms and other fungi

E865.8 Other specified foods

E865.9 Unspecified foodstuff or poisonous plant

E866 Accidental poisoning by other and unspecified solid and liquid substances

Excludes: *these substances as a component of:*
medicines (E850.0-E858.9)
paints (E861.5-E861.6)
pesticides (E863.0-E863.9)
petroleum fuels (E862.1)

E866.0 Lead and its compounds and fumes

E866.1 Mercury and its compounds and fumes

E866.2 Antimony and its compounds and fumes

E866.3 Arsenic and its compounds and fumes

E866.4 Other metals and their compounds and fumes

Beryllium (compounds)	Iron (compounds)
Brass fumes	Manganese (compounds)
Cadmium (compounds)	Nickel (compounds)
Copper salts	Thallium (compounds)

E866.5 Plant foods and fertilizers

Excludes: *mixtures with herbicides (E863.5)*

E866.6 Glues and adhesives

E866.7 Cosmetics

E866.8 Other specified solid or liquid substances

E866.9 Unspecified solid or liquid substance

E867 Accidental poisoning by gas distributed by pipeline
Carbon monoxide from incomplete combustion of piped gas
Coal gas NOS
Liquefied petroleum gas distributed through pipes (pure or mixed with air)
Piped gas (natural) (manufactured)

E868 Accidental poisoning by other utility gas and other carbon monoxide

E868.0 Liquefied petroleum gas distributed in mobile containers
Butane
Liquefied hydrocarbon gas NOS
Propane
} or carbon monoxide from incomplete combustion of these gases

● Code new
to this edition

▲ Revision of
existing code

④ ⑤ Fourth or fifth
digit required

E868.1 Other and unspecified utility gas

Acetylene
Gas NOS used for
  lighting,
  heating, or } or carbon monoxide from incomplete combustion of these gases
  cooking
Water gas

E868.2 Motor vehicle exhaust gas

Exhaust gas from:
  farm tractor, not in transit
  gas engine
  motor pump
  motor vehicle, not in transit
  any type of combustion engine not in watercraft

Excludes: *poisoning by carbon monoxide from:*
    aircraft while in transit (E844.0-E844.9)
    motor vehicle while in transit (E818.0-E818.9)
    watercraft whether or not in transit (E838.0-E838.9)

E868.3 Carbon monoxide from incomplete combustion of other domestic fuels

Carbon monoxide from incomplete combustion of:
  coal
  coke
  kerosene } in domestic stove or fireplace
  wood

Excludes: *carbon monoxide from smoke and fumes due to conflagration (E890.0-E893.9)*

E868.8 Carbon monoxide from other sources

Carbon monoxide from:
  blast furnace gas
  incomplete combustion of fuels in industrial use
  kiln vapor

E868.9 Unspecified carbon monoxide

E869 Accidental poisoning by other gases and vapors

Excludes: *effects of gases used as anesthetics (E855.1, E938.2)*
    fumes from heavy metals (E866.0-E866.4)
    smoke and fumes due to conflagration or explosion (E890.0-E899)

E869.0 Nitrogen oxides

E869.1 Sulfur dioxide

E869.2 Freon

E869.3 Lacrimogenic gas [tear gas]

Bromobenzyl cyanide   Ethyliodoacetate
Chloroacetophenone

E869.4 Second-hand tobacco smoke

E869.8 Other specified gases and vapors

Chlorine   Hydrocyanic acid gas

E869.9 Unspecified gases and vapors

MISADVENTURES TO PATIENTS DURING SURGICAL AND MEDICAL CARE (E870-E876)

Excludes: *accidental overdose of drug and wrong drug given in error (E850.0-E858.9)*
    surgical and medical procedures as the cause of abnormal reaction by the patient,
    without mention of misadventure at the time of procedure (E878.0-E879.9)

E870 Accidental cut, puncture, perforation, or hemorrhage during medical care

E870.0 Surgical operation

E870.1 Infusion or transfusion

E870.2 Kidney dialysis or other perfusion

E870.3 Injection or vaccination

E870.4 Endoscopic examination

E870.5 Aspiration of fluid or tissue, puncture, and catheterization

Abdominal paracentesis   Lumbar puncture
Aspirating needle biopsy   Thoracentesis
Blood sampling

Excludes: *heart catheterization (E870.6)*

Add 4th or 5th digit	Nonspecific code	Unspecified code	Manifestation code

E870.6 Heart catheterization

E870.7 Administration of enema

E870.8 Other specified medical care

E870.9 Unspecified medical care

E871 Foreign object left in body during procedure

E871.0 Surgical operation

E871.1 Infusion or transfusion

E871.2 Kidney dialysis or other perfusion

E871.3 Injection or vaccination

E871.4 Endoscopic examination

E871.5 Aspiration of fluid or tissue, puncture, and catheterization

 Abdominal paracentesis   Lumbar puncture
 Aspiration needle biopsy   Thoracentesis
 Blood sampling

> *Excludes:* *heart catheterization (E871.6)*

E871.6 Heart catheterization

E871.7 Removal of catheter or packing

E871.8 Other specified procedures

E871.9 Unspecified procedure

E872 Failure of sterile precautions during procedure

E872.0 Surgical operation

E872.1 Infusion or transfusion

E872.2 Kidney dialysis and other perfusion

E872.3 Injection or vaccination

E872.4 Endoscopic examination

E872.5 Aspiration of fluid or tissue, puncture, and catheterization

 Abdominal paracentesis   Lumbar puncture
 Aspirating needle biopsy   Thoracentesis
 Blood sampling

> *Excludes:* *heart catheterization (E872.6)*

E872.6 Heart catheterization

E872.8 Other specified procedures

E872.9 Unspecified procedure

E873 Failure in dosage

> *Excludes:* *accidental overdose of drug, medicinal or biological substance (E850.0-E858.9)*

E873.0 Excessive amount of blood or other fluid during transfusion or infusion

E873.1 Incorrect dilution of fluid during infusion

E873.2 Overdose of radiation in therapy

E873.3 Inadvertent exposure of patient to radiation during medical care

E873.4 Failure in dosage in electroshock or insulin-shock therapy

E873.5 Inappropriate [too hot or too cold] temperature in local application and packing

E873.6 Nonadministration of necessary drug or medicinal substance

E873.8 Other specified failure in dosage

E873.9 Unspecified failure in dosage

E874 Mechanical failure of instrument or apparatus during procedure

E874.0 Surgical operation

E874.1 Infusion and transfusion

 Air in system

E874.2 Kidney dialysis and other perfusion

E874.3 Endoscopic examination

● Code new to this edition   ▲ Revision of existing code   ④ ⑤ Fourth or fifth digit required

E874.4 Aspiration of fluid or tissue, puncture, and catheterization
Abdominal paracentesis
Aspirating needle biopsy
Blood sampling
Lumbar puncture
Thoracentesis

Excludes: heart catheterization (E874.5)

E874.5 Heart catheterization

E874.8 Other specified procedures

E874.9 Unspecified procedure

E875 Contaminated or infected blood, other fluid, drug, or biological substance
Includes: presence of:
bacterial pyrogens
endotoxin-producing bacteria
serum hepatitis-producing agent

E875.0 Contaminated substance transfused or infused

E875.1 Contaminated substance injected or used for vaccination

E875.2 Contaminated drug or biological substance administered by other means

E875.8 Other

E875.9 Unspecified

E876 Other and unspecified misadventures during medical care

E876.0 Mismatched blood in transfusion

E876.1 Wrong fluid in infusion

E876.2 Failure in suture and ligature during surgical operation

E876.3 Endotracheal tube wrongly placed during anesthetic procedure

E876.4 Failure to introduce or to remove other tube or instrument

Excludes: foreign object left in body during procedure (E871.0-E871.9)

E876.5 Performance of inappropriate operation

E876.8 Other specified misadventures during medical care
Performance of inappropriate treatment NEC

E876.9 Unspecified misadventure during medical care

SURGICAL AND MEDICAL PROCEDURES AS THE CAUSE OF ABNORMAL REACTION OF PATIENT OR LATER COMPLICATION, WITHOUT MENTION OF MISADVENTURE AT THE TIME OF PROCEDURE (E878-E879)

Includes: procedures as the cause of abnormal reaction, such as:
displacement or malfunction of prosthetic device
hepatorenal failure, postoperative
malfunction of external stoma
postoperative intestinal obstruction
rejection of transplanted organ

Excludes: anesthetic management properly carried out as the cause of adverse effect (E937.0-E938.9)
infusion and transfusion, without mention of misadventure in the technique of procedure (E930.0-E949.9)

E878 Surgical operation and other surgical procedures as the cause of abnormal reaction of patient, or of later complication, without mention of misadventure at the time of operation

E878.0 Surgical operation with transplant of whole organ
Transplantation of:
heart
kidney
liver

E878.1 Surgical operation with implant of artificial internal device
Cardiac pacemaker
Electrodes implanted in brain
Heart valve prosthesis
Internal orthopedic device

E878.2 Surgical operation with anastomosis, bypass, or graft, with natural or artificial tissues used as implant
Anastomosis:
arteriovenous
gastrojejunal
Graft of blood vessel, tendon, or skin

Excludes: external stoma (E878.3)

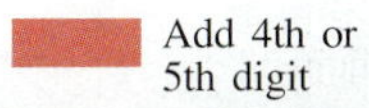

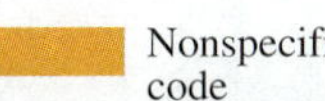

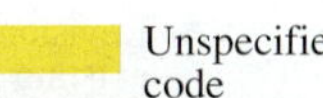

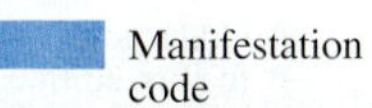

E878.3 Surgical operation with formation of external stoma
  Colostomy   Gastrostomy
  Cystostomy   Ureterostomy
  Duodenostomy

E878.4 Other restorative surgery

E878.5 Amputation of limb(s)

E878.6 Removal of other organ (partial) (total)

E878.8 Other specified surgical operations and procedures

E878.9 Unspecified surgical operations and procedures

E879 Other procedures, without mention of misadventure at the time of procedure, as the cause of abnormal reaction of patient, or of later complication

E879.0 Cardiac catheterization

E879.1 Kidney dialysis

E879.2 Radiological procedure and radiotherapy

  Excludes: radio-opaque dyes for diagnostic x-ray procedures (E947.8)

E879.3 Shock therapy
  Electroshock therapy   Insulin-shock therapy

E879.4 Aspiration of fluid
  Lumbar puncture   Thoracentesis

E879.5 Insertion of gastric or duodenal sound

E879.6 Urinary catheterization

E879.7 Blood sampling

E879.8 Other specified procedures
  Blood transfusion

E879.9 Unspecified procedure

ACCIDENTAL FALLS (E880-E888)

  Excludes: falls (in or from):
    burning building (E890.8, E891.8)
    into fire (E890.0-E899)
    into water (with submersion or drowning) (E910.0-E910.9)
    machinery (in operation) (E919.0-E919.9)
    on edged, pointed, or sharp object (E920.0-E920.9)
    transport vehicle (E800.0-E845.9)
    vehicle not elsewhere classifiable (E846-E848)

E880 Fall on or from stairs or steps

E880.0 Escalator

E880.1 Fall on or from sidewalk curb

  Excludes: fall from moving sidewalk (E885.9)

E880.9 Other stairs or steps

E881 Fall on or from ladders or scaffolding

E881.0 Fall from ladder

E881.1 Fall from scaffolding

E882 Fall from or out of building or other structure
  Fall from: Fall from:
  balcony   turret
  bridge   viaduct
  building   wall
  flagpole   window
  tower   Fall through roof

  Excludes: collapse of a building or structure (E916)
      fall or jump from burning building (E890.8, E891.8)

● Code new to this edition ▲ Revision of existing code ④ ⑤ Fourth or fifth digit required

E883   **Fall into hole or other opening in surface**
       Includes:

fall into:	fall into:
cavity	shaft
dock	swimming pool
hole	tank
pit	well
quarry	

       Excludes: *fall into water NOS (E910.9)*
              that resulting in drowning or submersion without mention of injury (E910.0-E910.9)

    E883.0   **Accident from diving or jumping into water [swimming pool]**
       Strike or hit:
         against bottom when jumping or diving into water
         wall or board of swimming pool
         water surface

       Excludes: *diving with insufficient air supply (E913.2)*
              effects of air pressure from diving (E902.2)

    E883.1   **Accidental fall into well**

    E883.2   **Accidental fall into storm drain or manhole**

    E883.9   **Fall into other hole or other opening in surface**

E884   **Other fall from one level to another**

    E884.0   **Fall from playground equipment**

       Excludes: *recreational machinery (E919.8)*

    E884.1   **Fall from cliff**

    E884.2   **Fall from chair**

    E884.3   **Fall from wheelchair**

    E884.4   **Fall from bed**

    E884.5   **Fall from other furniture**

    E884.6   **Fall from commode**
       Toilet

    E884.9   **Other fall from one level to another**

Fall from:	Fall from:
embankment	stationary vehicle
haystack	tree

E885   **Fall on same level from slipping, tripping, or stumbling**

   ● **E885.0**   **Fall from (nonmotorized) scooter**

    E885.1   **Fall from roller skates**
       In-line skates

    E885.2   **Fall from skateboard**

    E885.3   **Fall from skis**

    E885.4   **Fall from snowboard**

    E885.9   **Fall from other slipping, tripping or stumbling**
       Fall on moving sidewalk

E886   **Fall on same level from collision, pushing, or shoving, by or with other person**

       Excludes: *crushed or pushed by a crowd or human stampede (E917.1, E917.6)*

    E886.0   **In sports**
       Tackles in sports

       Excludes: *kicked, stepped on, struck by object, in sports (E917.0, E917.5)*

    E886.9   **Other and unspecified**
       Fall from collision of pedestrian (conveyance) with another pedestrian (conveyance)

E887   **Fracture, cause unspecified**

E888   **Other and unspecified fall**
    Accidental fall NOS
    Fall on same level NOS

    E888.0   **Fall resulting in striking against sharp object**
       Use additional external cause code to identify object (E920)

    E888.1   **Fall resulting in striking against other object**

E888.8 **Other fall**

E888.9 **Unspecified fall**
    Fall NOS

ACCIDENTS CAUSED BY FIRE AND FLAMES (E890-E899)

    Includes: asphyxia or poisoning due to conflagration or ignition
                  burning by fire
                  secondary fires resulting from explosion

    Excludes: *arson (E968.0)*

         fire in or on:
           machinery (in operation) (E919.0-E919.9)
           transport vehicle other than stationary vehicle (E800.0-E845.9)
           vehicle not elsewhere classifiable (E846-E848)

E890 **Conflagration in private dwelling**
    Includes: conflagration in:
            apartment
            boarding house
            camping place
            caravan
            farmhouse
            house
            lodging house
            mobile home
            private garage
            rooming house
            tenement
        conflagration originating from sources classifiable to E893-E898 in the above
            buildings

E890.0 **Explosion caused by conflagration**

E890.1 **Fumes from combustion of polyvinylchloride [PVC] and similar material in conflagration**

E890.2 **Other smoke and fumes from conflagration**
    Carbon monoxide
    Fumes NOS   } from conflagration in private building
    Smoke NOS

E890.3 **Burning caused by conflagration**

E890.8 **Other accident resulting from conflagration**
    Collapse of
    Fall from
    Hit by object falling from } burning private building
    Jump from

E890.9 **Unspecified accident resulting from conflagration in private dwelling**

E891 **Conflagration in other and unspecified building or structure**

Conflagration in:	Conflagration in:
barn	farm outbuildings
church	hospital
convalescent and other	hotel
residential home	school
dormitory of educational	store
institution	theater
factory	

  Conflagration originating from sources classifiable to E893-E898, in the above buildings

E891.0 **Explosion caused by conflagration**

E891.1 **Fumes from combustion of polyvinylchloride [PVC] and similar material in conflagration**

E891.2 **Other smoke and fumes from conflagration**
    Carbon monoxide
    Fumes NOS   } from conflagration in building or structure
    Smoke NOS

E891.3 **Burning caused by conflagration**

● Code new
  to this edition
▲ Revision of
  existing code
④ ⑤ Fourth or fifth
    digit required

E891.8 Other accident resulting from conflagration
    Collapse of
    Fall from
    Hit by object falling from   } burning building or structure
    Jump from

E891.9 Unspecified accident resulting from conflagration of other and unspecified building or structure

E892 Conflagration not in building or structure
    Fire (uncontrolled) (in) (of):
      forest
      grass
      hay
      lumber
      mine
      prairie
      transport vehicle [any], except while in transit
      tunnel

E893 Accident caused by ignition of clothing

    Excludes: *ignition of clothing:*
        from highly inflammable material (E894)
        with conflagration (E890.0-E892)

E893.0 From controlled fire in private dwelling
    Ignition of clothing from:
      normal fire (charcoal) (coal) (electric) (gas)
        (wood) in:
        brazier
        fireplace   } in private dwelling (as listed in
        furnace   E890)
        stove

E893.1 From controlled fire in other building or structure
    Ignition of clothing from:
      normal fire (charcoal) (coal) (electric)
        (gas) (wood) in:
        brazier
        fireplace   } in other building or structure (as
        furnace   listed in E891)
        stove

E893.2 From controlled fire not in building or structure
    Ignition of clothing from:
      bonfire (controlled)
      brazier fire (controlled), not in building or structure
      trash fire (controlled)

    Excludes: *conflagration not in building (E892)*
        trash fire out of control (E892)

E893.8 From other specified sources
    Ignition of clothing from: Ignition of clothing from:
      blowlamp   cigarette
      blowtorch   lighter
      burning bedspread   matches
      candle   pipe
      cigar   welding torch

E893.9 Unspecified source
    Ignition of clothing (from controlled fire NOS) (in building NOS) NOS

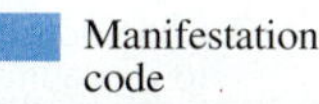

E894 Ignition of highly inflammable material
Ignition of:
  benzine
  gasoline
  fat
  kerosene   } (with ignition of clothing)
  paraffin
  petrol

    Excludes: *ignition of highly inflammable material with:*
        conflagration (E890.0-E892)
        explosion (E923.0-E923.9)

E895 Accident caused by controlled fire in private dwelling
Burning by (flame of) normal fire (charcoal) (coal)
  (electric) (gas) (wood) in:
  brazier
  fireplace   } in private dwelling (as listed in
  furnace   E890)
  stove

    Excludes: *burning by hot objects not producing fire or flames (E924.0-E924.9)*
        ignition of clothing from these sources (E893.0)
        poisoning by carbon monoxide from incomplete combustion of fuel (E867-E868.9)
        that with conflagration (E890.0-E890.9)

E896 Accident caused by controlled fire in other and unspecified building or structure
Burning by (flame of) normal fire (charcoal) (coal)
  (electric) (gas) (wood) in:
  brazier
  fireplace   } in other building or structure (as
  furnace   listed in E891)
  stove

    Excludes: *burning by hot objects not producing fire or flames (E924.0-E924.9)*
        ignition of clothing from these sources (E893.1)
        poisoning by carbon monoxide from incomplete combustion of fuel (E867-E868.9)
        that with conflagration (E891.0-E891.9)

E897 Accident caused by controlled fire not in building or structure
Burns from flame of:
  bonfire (controlled)
  brazier fire (controlled), not in building or structure
  trash fire (controlled)

    Excludes: *ignition of clothing from these sources (E893.2)*
        trash fire out of control (E892)
        that with conflagration (E892)

E898 Accident caused by other specified fire and flames

    Excludes: *conflagration (E890.0-E892)*
        that with ignition of:
          clothing (E893.0-E893.9)
          highly inflammable material (E894)

E898.0 Burning bedclothes
Bed set on fire NOS

E898.1 Other

Burning by: Burning by:
  blowlamp   lamp
  blowtorch   lighter
  candle   matches
  cigar   pipe
  cigarette   welding torch
  fire in room NOS

E899 Accident caused by unspecified fire
Burning NOS

● Code new   ▲ Revision of   ④ ⑤ Fourth or fifth
  to this edition   existing code   digit required

ACCIDENTS DUE TO NATURAL AND ENVIRONMENTAL FACTORS (E900-E909)

E900   Excessive heat

E900.0   Due to weather conditions
Excessive heat as the external cause of:
ictus solaris
siriasis
sunstroke

E900.1   Of man-made origin

Heat (in):	Heat (in):
boiler room	generated in transport vehicle
drying room	kitchen
factory	
furnace room	

E900.9   Of unspecified origin

E901   Excessive cold

E901.0   Due to weather conditions
Excessive cold as the cause of:
chilblains NOS
immersion foot

E901.1   Of man-made origin
Contact with or inhalation of:
dry ice
liquid air
liquid hydrogen
liquid nitrogen
Prolonged exposure in:
deep freeze unit
refrigerator

E901.8   Other specified origin

E901.9   Of unspecified origin

E902   High and low air pressure and changes in air pressure

E902.0   Residence or prolonged visit at high altitude
Residence or prolonged visit at high altitude as the cause of:
Acosta syndrome
Alpine sickness
altitude sickness
Andes disease
anoxia, hypoxia
barotitis, barodontalgia, barosinusitis, otitic barotrauma
hypobarism, hypobaropathy
mountain sickness
range disease

E902.1   In aircraft
Sudden change in air pressure in aircraft during ascent or descent as the cause of:
aeroneurosis
aviators' disease

E902.2   Due to diving
High air pressure from rapid descent in water ⎫ as the cause of:
Reduction in atmospheric pressure while ⎬ caisson disease
surfacing from deep water diving ⎭ divers' disease
divers' palsy or paralysis

E902.8   Due to other specified causes
Reduction in atmospheric pressure while surfacing from underground

E902.9   Unspecified cause

E903   Travel and motion

E904   Hunger, thirst, exposure, and neglect

Excludes: any condition resulting from homicidal intent (E968.0-E968.9)
hunger, thirst, and exposure resulting from accidents connected with transport
(E800.0-E848)

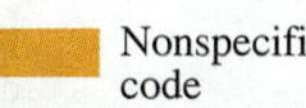

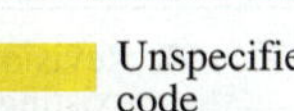

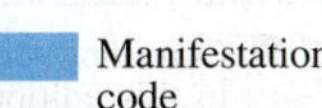

E904.0 Abandonment or neglect of infants and helpless persons

Exposure to weather conditions
Hunger or thirst } resulting from abandonment or neglect

Desertion of newborn
Inattention at or after birth
Lack of care (helpless person) (infant)

Excludes: criminal [purposeful] neglect (E968.4)

E904.1 Lack of food

Lack of food as the cause of:
  inanition
  insufficient nourishment
  starvation

Excludes: hunger resulting from abandonment or neglect (E904.0)

E904.2 Lack of water

Lack of water as the cause of:
  dehydration
  inanition

Excludes: dehydration due to acute fluid loss (276.5)

E904.3 Exposure (to weather conditions), not elsewhere classifiable

Exposure NOS   Struck by hailstones
Humidity

Excludes: struck by lightning (E907)

E904.9 Privation, unqualified

Destitution

E905 Venomous animals and plants as the cause of poisoning and toxic reactions

Includes: chemical released by animal
             insects
             release of venom through fangs, hairs, spines, tentacles, and other venom apparatus

Excludes: eating of poisonous animals or plants (E865.0-E865.9)

E905.0 Venomous snakes and lizards

Cobra   Mamba
Copperhead snake   Rattlesnake
Coral snake   Sea snake
Fer de lance   Snake (venomous)
Gila monster   Viper
Krait   Water moccasin

Excludes: bites of snakes and lizards known to be nonvenomous (E906.2)

E905.1 Venomous spiders

Black widow spider   Tarantula (venomous)
Brown spider

E905.2 Scorpion

E905.3 Hornets, wasps, and bees

Yellow jacket

E905.4 Centipede and venomous millipede (tropical)

E905.5 Other venomous arthropods

Sting of:
  ant
  caterpillar

E905.6 Venomous marine animals and plants

Puncture by sea urchin spine   Sting of:
Sting of: nematocysts
  coral   sea anemone
  jelly fish   sea cucumber
                     other marine animal or plant

Excludes: bites and other injuries caused by nonvenomous marine animal (E906.2-E906.8)
          bite of sea snake (venomous) (E905.0)

● Code new   ▲ Revision of   ④ ⑤ Fourth or fifth
   to this edition   existing code   digit required

E905.7 **Poisoning and toxic reactions caused by other plants**
Injection of poisons or toxins into or through skin by plant thorns, spines, or other mechanisms

Excludes: *puncture wound NOS by plant thorns or spines (E920.8)*

E905.8 **Other specified**

E905.9 **Unspecified**
Sting NOS   Venomous bite NOS

E906 **Other injury caused by animals**

Excludes: *poisoning and toxic reactions caused by venomous animals and insects (E905.0-E905.9)*
road vehicle accident involving animals (E827.0-E828.9)
tripping or falling over an animal (E885.9)

E906.0 **Dog bite**

E906.1 **Rat bite**

E906.2 **Bite of nonvenomous snakes and lizards**

E906.3 **Bite of other animal except arthropod**
Cats   Rodents, except rats
Moray eel   Shark

E906.4 **Bite of nonvenomous arthropod**
Insect bite NOS

E906.5 **Bite by unspecified animal**
Animal bite NOS

E906.8 **Other specified injury caused by animal**
Butted by animal
Fallen on by horse or other animal, not being ridden
Gored by animal
Implantation of quills of porcupine
Pecked by bird
Run over by animal, not being ridden
Stepped on by animal, not being ridden

Excludes: *injury by animal being ridden (E828.0-E828.9)*

E906.9 **Unspecified injury caused by animal**

E907 **Lightning**

Excludes: *injury from:*
fall of tree or other object caused by lightning (E916)
fire caused by lightning (E890.0-E892)

E908 **Cataclysmic storms, and floods resulting from storms**

Excludes: *collapse of dam or man-made structure causing flood (E909.3)*

E908.0 **Hurricane**
Storm surge
"Tidal wave" caused by storm action
Typhoon

E908.1 **Tornado**
Cyclone
Twisters

E908.2 **Floods**
Torrential rainfall
Flash flood

Excludes: *collapse of dam or man-made structure causing flood (909.3)*

E908.3 **Blizzard (snow) (ice)**

E908.4 **Dust storm**

E908.8 **Other cataclysmic storms**

E908.9 **Unspecified cataclysmic storms, and floods resulting from storms**
Storm NOS

E909 **Cataclysmic earth surface movements and eruptions**

Excludes: *"tidal wave" caused by storm action (E908.0)*
transport accident involving collision with avalanche or landslide not in motion (E800.0-E848)

	Add 4th or 5th digit		Nonspecific code		Unspecified code		Manifestation code

E909.0 Earthquakes

E909.1 Volcanic eruptions
Burns from lava
Ash inhalation

E909.2 Avalanche, landslide, or mudslide

E909.3 Collapse of dam or man-made structure

E909.4 Tidal wave caused by earthquake
Tidal wave NOS
Tsunami

> Excludes: *tidal wave caused by tropical storm (E908.0)*

E909.8 Other cataclysmic earth surface movements and eruptions

E909.9 Unspecified cataclysmic earth surface movements and eruptions

ACCIDENTS CAUSED BY SUBMERSION, SUFFOCATION, AND FOREIGN BODIES (E910-E915)

E910 Accidental drowning and submersion
Includes: immersion
swimmers' cramp

> Excludes: *diving accident (NOS) (resulting in injury except drowning) (E883.0)*
> *diving with insufficient air supply (E913.2)*
> *drowning and submersion due to:*
>   *cataclysm (E908-E909)*
>   *machinery accident (E919.0-E919.9)*
>   *transport accident (E800.0-E845.9)*
> *effect of high and low air pressure (E902.2)*
> *injury from striking against objects while in running water (E917.2)*

E910.0 While water-skiing
Fall from water skis with submersion or drowning

> Excludes: *accident to water-skier involving a watercraft and resulting in submersion or other injury (E830.4, E831.4)*

E910.1 While engaged in other sport or recreational activity with diving equipment
Scuba diving NOS
Skin diving NOS
Underwater spear fishing NOS

E910.2 While engaged in other sport or recreational activity without diving equipment
Fishing or hunting, except from boat or with diving equipment
Ice skating
Playing in water
Surfboarding
Swimming NOS
Voluntarily jumping from boat, not involved in accident, for swim NOS
Wading in water

> Excludes: *jumping into water to rescue another person (E910.3)*

E910.3 While swimming or diving for purposes other than recreation or sport
Marine salvage
Pearl diving
Placement of fishing nets   } (with diving equipment)
Rescue (attempt) of another person
Underwater construction or repairs

E910.4 In bathtub

E910.8 Other accidental drowning or submersion
Drowning in:
quenching tank
swimming pool

E910.9 Unspecified accidental drowning or submersion
Accidental fall into water NOS
Drowning NOS

● Code new to this edition   ▲ Revision of existing code   ④ ⑤ Fourth or fifth digit required

E911 Inhalation and ingestion of food causing obstruction of respiratory tract or suffocation

Aspiration and inhalation of food [any] (into respiratory tract) NOS

Asphyxia by
Choked on ⎫ food [including bone, seed in food, regurgitated food]
Suffocation by ⎭

Compression of trachea ⎫
Interruption of respiration ⎬ by food lodged in esophagus
Obstruction of respiration ⎭

Obstruction of pharynx by food (bolus)

Excludes: *injury, except asphyxia and obstruction of respiratory passage, caused by food*
(E915)
obstruction of esophagus by food without mention of asphyxia or obstruction of
respiratory passage (E915)

E912 Inhalation and ingestion of other object causing obstruction of respiratory tract or suffocation

Aspiration and inhalation of foreign body except food (into respiratory tract) NOS
Foreign object [bean] [marble] in nose
Obstruction of pharynx by foreign body
Compression ⎫
Interruption of respiration ⎬ by foreign body in esophagus
Obstruction of respiration ⎭

Excludes: *injury, except asphyxia and obstruction of respiratory passage, caused by foreign*
body (E915)
obstruction of esophagus by foreign body without mention of asphyxia or
obstruction in respiratory passage (E915)

E913 Accidental mechanical suffocation

Excludes: *mechanical suffocation from or by:*
accidental inhalation or ingestion of:
food (E911)
foreign object (E912)
cataclysm (E908-E909)
explosion (E921.0-E921.9, E923.0-E923.9)
machinery accident (E919.0-E919.9)

E913.0 In bed or cradle

Excludes: *suffocation by plastic bag (E913.1)*

E913.1 By plastic bag

E913.2 Due to lack of air (in closed place)
Accidentally closed up in refrigerator or other airtight enclosed space
Diving with insufficient air supply

Excludes: *suffocation by plastic bag (E913.1)*

E913.3 By falling earth or other substance
Cave-in NOS

Excludes: *cave-in caused by cataclysmic earth surface movements and eruptions (E909)*
struck by cave-in without asphyxiation or suffocation (E916)

E913.8 Other specified means
Accidental hanging, except in bed or cradle

E913.9 Unspecified means
Asphyxia, mechanical NOS
Strangulation NOS
Suffocation NOS

E914 Foreign body accidentally entering eye and adnexa

Excludes: *corrosive liquid (E924.1)*

E915 Foreign body accidentally entering other orifice

Excludes: *aspiration and inhalation of foreign body, any, (into respiratory tract) NOS*
(E911-E912)

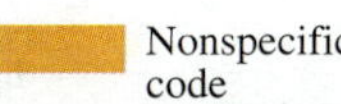

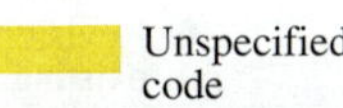

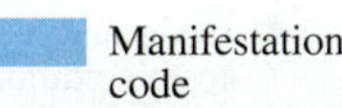

OTHER ACCIDENTS (E916-E928)

E916 Struck accidentally by falling object

Collapse of building, except on fire
Falling:
  rock
  snowslide NOS
  stone
  tree

Object falling from:
  machine, not in operation
  stationary vehicle

Code first: collapse of building on fire (E890.0-E891.9)
        falling object in:
            cataclysm (E908-E909)
            machinery accidents (E919.0-E919.9)
            transport accidents (E800.0-E845.9)
            vehicle accidents not elsewhere classifiable (E846-E848)
        object set in motion by:
            explosion (E921.0-E921.9, E923.0-E923.9)
            firearm (E922.0-E922.9)
        projected object (E917.0-E917.9)

E917 Striking against or struck accidentally by objects or persons

Includes:

bumping into or
    against
colliding with
kicking against
stepping on
struck by

object (moving) (projected)
    (stationary)
pedestrian conveyance
person

Excludes: *fall from:*

   collision with another person, except when caused by a crowd (E886.0-E886.9)
   stumbling over object (E885.9)
Fall resulting in striking against object (E888.0, E888.1)
injury caused by:
   assault (E960.0-E960.1, E967.0-E967.9)
   cutting or piercing instrument (E920.0-E920.9)
   explosion (E921.0-E921.9, E923.0-E923.9)
   firearm (E922.0-E922.9)
   machinery (E919.0-E919.9)
   transport vehicle (E800.0-E845.9)
   vehicle not elsewhere classifiable (E846-E848)

E917.0 In sports without subsequent fall
Kicked or stepped on during game (football) (rugby)
Struck by hit or thrown ball
Struck by hockey stick or puck

E917.1 Caused by a crowd, by collective fear or panic without subsequent fall
Crushed
Pushed
Stepped on
} by crown or human stampede

E917.2 In running water without subsequent fall

Excludes: *drowning or submersion (E910.0-E910.9)*
       that in sports (E917.0, E917.5)

E917.3 Furniture without subsequent fall

Excludes: *fall from furniture (E884.2, E884.4-E884.5)*

E917.4 Other stationary object without subsequent fall
Bath tub
Fence
Lamp-post

E917.5 Object in sports with subsequent fall
Knocked down while boxing

E917.6 Caused by a crowd, by collective fear or panic with subsequent fall

E917.7 Furniture with subsequent fall

Excludes: *fall from furniture (E884.2, E884.4-E884.5)*

E917.8 Other stationary object with subsequent fall
Bath tub
Fence
Lamp-post

● Code new
  to this edition

▲ Revision of
  existing code

④ ⑤ Fourth or fifth
    digit required

E917.9 Other striking against with or without subsequent fall

E918 Caught accidentally in or between objects
Caught, crushed, jammed, or pinched in or between moving or stationary objects, such as:
escalator
folding object
hand tools, appliances, or implements
sliding door and door frame
under packing crate
washing machine wringer

Excludes: *injury caused by:*
cutting or piercing instrument (E920.0-E920.9)
machinery (E919.0-E919.9)
transport vehicle (E800.0-E845.9)
vehicle not elsewhere classifiable (E846-E848)
struck accidentally by:
falling object (E916)
object (moving) (projected) (E917.0-E917.9)

E919 Accidents caused by machinery
Includes:
burned by
caught in (moving parts of)
collapse of
crushed by
cut or pierced by
drowning or submersion caused by
explosion of, on, in
fall from or into moving part of   } machinery (accident)
fire starting in or on
mechanical suffocation caused by
object falling from, on, in motion by
overturning of
pinned under
run over by
struck by
thrown from
caught between machinery and other object
machinery accident NOS

Excludes: *accidents involving machinery, not in operation (E884.9, E916-E918)*
injury caused by:
electric current in connection with machinery (E925.0-E925.9)
escalator (E880.0, E918)
explosion of pressure vessel in connection with machinery (E921.0-E921.9)
moving sidewalk (E885.9)
powered hand tools, appliances, and implements (E916-E918, E920.0-E921.9, E923.0-E926.9)
transport vehicle accidents involving machinery (E800.0-E848.9)
poisoning by carbon monoxide generated by machine (E868.8)

E919.0 Agriculture machines
Animal-powered   Farm tractor
   agricultural machine   Harvester
Combine   Hay mower or rake
Derrick, hay   Reaper
Farm machinery NOS   Thresher

Excludes: *that in transport under own power on the highway (E810.0-E819.9)*
that being towed by another vehicle on the highway (E810.0-E819.9, E827.0-E827.9, E829.0-E829.9)
that involved in accident classifiable to E820-E829 (E820.0-E829.9)

E919.1 Mining and earth-drilling machinery
Bore or drill (land) (seabed)   Shaft lift
Shaft hoist   Under-cutter

Excludes: *coal car, tram, truck, and tub in mine (E846)*

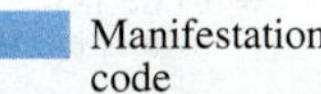

E919.2 Lifting machines and appliances

Chain hoist
Crane
Derrick
Elevator (building) (grain) } except in agricultural or mining operations
Forklift truck
Lift
Pulley block
Winch

Excludes: *that being towed by another vehicle on the highway (E810.0-E819.9,*
E827.0-E827.9, E829.0-E829.9)
that in transport under own power on the highway (E810.0-E819.9)
that involved in accident classifiable to E820-E829 (E820.0-E829.9)

E919.3 Metalworking machines

Abrasive wheel
Forging machine
Lathe
Mechanical shears

Metal:
drilling machine
milling machine
power press
rolling-mill
sawing machine

E919.4 Woodworking and forming machines

Band saw
Bench saw
Circular saw
Molding machine
Overhead plane

Powered saw
Radial saw
Sander

Excludes: *hand saw (E920.1)*

E919.5 Prime movers, except electrical motors

Gas turbine
Internal combustion engine

Steam engine
Water driven turbine

Excludes: *that being towed by other vehicle on the highway (E810.0-E819.9, E827.0-E827.9,*
E829.0-E829.9)
that in transport under own power on the highway (E810.0-E819.9)

E919.6 Transmission machinery

Transmission:
 belt
 cable
 chain
 gear

Transmission:
 pinion
 pulley
 shaft

E919.7 Earth moving, scraping, and other excavating machines

Bulldozer
Road scraper

Steam shovel

Excludes: *that being towed by other vehicle on the highway (E810.0-E819.9, E827.0-E827.9,*
E829.0-E829.9)
that in transport under own power on the highway (E810.0-E819.9)

E919.8 Other specified machinery

Machines for manufacture
of:
 clothing
 foodstuffs and beverages
 paper

Printing machine
Recreational machinery
Spinning, weaving, and textile machines

E919.9 Unspecified machinery

E920 Accidents caused by cutting and piercing instruments or objects

Includes: accidental injury (by) object:
 edged
 pointed
 sharp

E920.0 Powered lawn mower

● Code new
   to this edition

▲ Revision of
   existing code

④ ⑤ Fourth or fifth
   digit required

E920.1 Other powered hand tools
Any powered hand tool [compressed air] [electric] [explosive cartridge] [hydraulic power], such as:

drill	rivet gun
hand saw	snow blower
hedge clipper	staple gun

Excludes: band saw (E919.4)
bench saw (E919.4)

E920.2 Powered household appliances and implements

Blender	Electric:
Electric:	knife
beater or mixer	sewing machine
can opener	Garbage disposal appliance
fan	

E920.3 Knives, swords, and daggers

E920.4 Other hand tools and implements

Axe	Paper cutter
Can opener NOS	Pitchfork
Chisel	Rake
Fork	Scissors
Hand saw	Screwdriver
Hoe	Sewing machine, not powered
Ice pick	Shovel
Needle (sewing)	

E920.5 Hypodermic needle
Contaminated needle
Needle stick

E920.8 Other specified cutting and piercing instruments or objects

Arrow	Nail
Broken glass	Plant thorn
Dart	Splinter
Edge of stiff paper	Tin can lid
Lathe turnings	

Excludes: animal spines or quills (E906.8)
flying glass due to explosion (E921.0-E923.9)

E920.9 Unspecified cutting and piercing instrument or object

E921 Accident caused by explosion of pressure vessel
Includes: accidental explosion of pressure vessels, whether or not part of machinery

Excludes: explosion of pressure vessel on transport vehicle (E800.0-E845.9)

E921.0 Boilers

E921.1 Gas cylinders

Air tank	Pressure gas tank

E921.8 Other specified pressure vessels

Aerosol can	Pressure cooker
Automobile tire	

E921.9 Unspecified pressure vessel

E922 Accident caused by firearm and air gun missile

E922.0 Handgun

Pistol	Revolver

Excludes: Verey pistol (E922.8)

E922.1 Shotgun (automatic)

E922.2 Hunting rifle

E922.3 Military firearms

Army rifle	Machine gun

E922.4 Air gun

BB gun	Pellet gun

● **E922.5 Paintball gun**

E922.8 Other specified firearm missile
Verey pistol [flare]

E922.9 Unspecified firearm missile

Gunshot wound NOS	Shot NOS

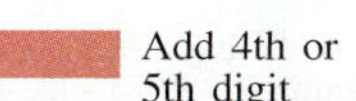

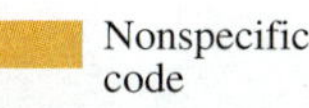

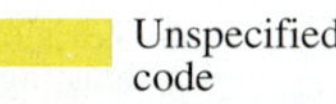

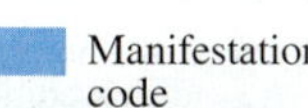

E923 **Accident caused by explosive material**
Includes: flash burns and other injuries resulting from explosion of explosive material
ignition of highly explosive material with explosion

Excludes: *explosion:*
in or on machinery (E919.0-E919.9)
on any transport vehicle, except stationary motor vehicle (E800.0-E848)
with conflagration (E890.0, E891.0, E892)
secondary fires resulting from explosion (E890.0-E899)

E923.0 **Fireworks**

E923.1 **Blasting materials**
Blasting cap
Detonator
Dynamite

Explosive [any] used in blasting operations

E923.2 **Explosive gases**
Acetylene
Butane
Coal gas
Explosion in mine NOS

Fire damp
Gasoline fumes
Methane
Propane

E923.8 **Other explosive materials**
Bomb
Explosive missile
Grenade
Mine
Shell

Torpedo
Explosion in munitions:
dump
factory

E923.9 **Unspecified explosive material**
Explosion NOS

E924 **Accident caused by hot substance or object, caustic or corrosive material, and steam**

Excludes: *burning NOS (E899)*
chemical burn resulting from swallowing a corrosive substance (E860.0-E864.4)
fire caused by these substances and objects (E890.0-E894)
radiation burns (E926.0-E926.9)
therapeutic misadventures (E870.0-E876.9)

E924.0 **Hot liquids and vapors, including steam**
Burning or scalding by:
boiling water
hot or boiling liquids not primarily caustic or corrosive
liquid metal
steam
other hot vapor

Excludes: *hot (boiling) tap water (E924.2)*

E924.1 **Caustic and corrosive substances**
Burning by:
acid [any kind]
ammonia
caustic oven cleaner or other substance
corrosive substance
lye
vitriol

E924.2 **Hot (boiling) tap water**

E924.8 **Other**
Burning by:
heat from electric heating appliance
hot object NOS
light bulb
steam pipe

E924.9 **Unspecified**

● Code new
to this edition

▲ Revision of
existing code

④ ⑤ Fourth or fifth
digit required

E925 Accident caused by electric current
Includes: electric current from exposed wire, faulty appliance, high voltage cable, live rail, or open electric socket as the cause of:

      burn
      cardiac fibrillation
      convulsion
      electric shock
      electrocution
      puncture wound
      respiratory paralysis

Excludes: *burn by heat from electrical appliance (E924.8)*
      lightning (E907)

E925.0 Domestic wiring and appliances

E925.1 Electric power generating plants, distribution stations, transmission lines
    Broken power line

E925.2 Industrial wiring, appliances, and electrical machinery
    Conductors   Electrical equipment and machinery
    Control apparatus   Transformers

E925.8 Other electric current
    Wiring and appliances in   Wiring and appliances in or on:
      or on: residential institutions
      farm [not farmhouse]   schools
      outdoors
      public building

E925.9 Unspecified electric current
    Burns or other injury from electric current NOS
    Electric shock NOS
    Electrocution NOS

E926 Exposure to radiation

Excludes: *abnormal reaction to or complication of treatment without mention of misadventure (E879.2)*
    atomic power plant malfunction in water transport (E838.0-E838.9)
    misadventure to patient in surgical and medical procedures (E873.2-E873.3)
    use of radiation in war operations (E996-E997.9)

E926.0 Radiofrequency radiation
    Overexposure to: from:
      microwave radiation   high-powered radio and
      radar radiation   television transmitters
      radiofrequency   industrial radiofrequency induction
      radiofrequency radiation [any]   heaters
                           radar installations

E926.1 Infra-red heaters and lamps
    Exposure to infra-red radiation from heaters and lamps as the cause of:
      blistering
      burning
      charring
      inflammatory change

Excludes: *physical contact with heater or lamp (E924.8)*

E926.2 Visible and ultraviolet light sources
    Arc lamps   Oxygas welding torch
    Black light sources   Sun rays
    Electrical welding arc   Tanning bed

Excludes: *excessive heat from these sources (E900.1-E900.9)*

E926.3 X-rays and other electromagnetic ionizing radiation
    Gamma rays   X-rays (hard) (soft)

E926.4 Lasers

E926.5 Radioactive isotopes
    Radiobiologicals   Radiopharmaceuticals

E926.8 Other specified radiation
    Artificially accelerated beams of ionized particles generated by:
      betatrons
      synchrotrons

E926.9 Unspecified radiation
    Radiation NOS

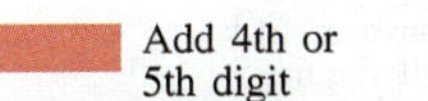

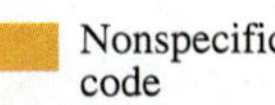

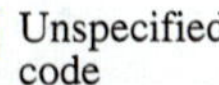

Manifestation
code

E927 Overexertion and strenuous movements
Excessive physical exercise
Overexertion (from):
  lifting
  pulling
  pushing

Strenuous movements in:
  recreational activities
  other activities

E928 Other and unspecified environmental and accidental causes

E928.0 Prolonged stay in weightless environment
Weightlessness in spacecraft (simulator)

E928.1 Exposure to noise
Noise (pollution)
Sound waves

Supersonic waves

E928.2 Vibration

E928.3 Human bite

E928.8 Other

E928.9 Unspecified accident
Accident NOS
Blow NOS
Casualty (not due to war)
Decapitation
Injury [any part of body, or unspecified] | stated as accidentally inflicted,
Killed | but not otherwise specified
Knocked down
Mangled
Wound

Excludes: *fracture, cause unspecified (E887)*
injuries undetermined whether accidentally or purposely inflicted (E980.0-E989)

LATE EFFECTS OF ACCIDENTAL INJURY (E929)

Note: This category is to be used to indicate accidental injury as the cause of death or disability from late effects, which are themselves classifiable elsewhere. The "late effects" include conditions reported as such or as sequelae which may occur at any time after the acute injury.

E929 Late effects of accidental injury
Excludes: *late effects of:*
  surgical and medical procedures (E870.0-E879.9)
  therapeutic use of drugs and medicines (E930.0-E949.9)

E929.0 Late effects of motor vehicle accident
Late effects of accidents classifiable to E810-E825

E929.1 Late effects of other transport accident
Late effects of accidents classifiable to E800-E807, E826-E838, E840-E848

E929.2 Late effects of accidental poisoning
Late effects of accidents classifiable to E850-E858, E860-E869

E929.3 Late effects of accidental fall
Late effects of accidents classifiable to E880-E888

E929.4 Late effects of accident caused by fire
Late effects of accidents classifiable to E890-E899

E929.5 Late effects of accident due to natural and environmental factors
Late effects of accidents classifiable to E900-E909

E929.8 Late effects of other accidents
Late effects of accidents classifiable to E910-E928.8

E929.9 Late effects of unspecified accident
Late effects of accidents classifiable to E928.9

● Code new to this edition   ▲ Revision of existing code   ④ ⑤ Fourth or fifth digit required

DRUGS, MEDICINAL AND BIOLOGICAL SUBSTANCES CAUSING ADVERSE EFFECTS IN THERAPEUTIC USE (E930-E949)

Includes: correct drug properly administered in therapeutic or prophylactic dosage, as the cause of any adverse effect including allergic or hypersensitivity reactions

Excludes: accidental overdose of drug and wrong drug given or taken in error (E850.0-E858.9)

accidents in the technique of administration of drug or biological substance, such as accidental puncture during injection, or contamination of drug (E870.0-E876.9)

administration with suicidal or homicidal intent or intent to harm, or in circumstances classifiable to E980-E989 (E950.0-E950.5, E962.0, E980.0-E980.5)

See Alphabetic Index for more complete list of specific drugs to be classified under the fourth-digit subdivisions. The American Hospital Formulary numbers can be used to classify new drugs listed by the American Hospital Formulary Service (AHFS). See appendix C.

E930 Antibiotics

Excludes: that used as eye, ear, nose, and throat [ENT], and local anti-infectives (E946.0-E946.9)

E930.0 Penicillins

Natural
Synthetic

Semisynthetic, such as:
 ampicillin
 cloxacillin
 nafcillin
 oxacillin

E930.1 Antifungal antibiotics

Amphotericin B
Griseofulvin

Hachimycin [trichomycin]
Nystatin

E930.2 Chloramphenicol group

Chloramphenicol

Thiamphenicol

E930.3 Erythromycin and other macrolides

Oleandomycin

Spiramycin

E930.4 Tetracycline group

Doxycycline
Minocycline
Oxytetracycline

E930.5 Cephalosporin group

Cephalexin
Cephaloglycin

Cephaloridine
Cephalothin

E930.6 Antimycobacterial antibiotics

Cycloserine
Kanamycin

Rifampin
Streptomycin

E930.7 Antineoplastic antibiotics

Actinomycins, such as:
 Cactinomycin
 Dactinomycin

Bleomycin
Daunorubicin
Mitomycin

Excludes: other antineoplastic drugs (E933.1)

E930.8 Other specified antibiotics

E930.9 Unspecified antibiotic

E931 Other anti-infectives

Excludes: ENT, and local anti-infectives (E946.0-E946.9)

E931.0 Sulfonamides

Sulfadiazine
Sulfafurazole

Sulfamethoxazole

E931.1 Arsenical anti infectives

E931.2 Heavy metal anti-infectives

Compounds of:
 antimony
 bismuth

Compounds of:
 lead
 mercury

Excludes: mercurial diuretics (E944.0)

E931.3 Quinoline and hydroxyquinoline derivatives

Chiniofon

Diiodohydroxyquin

Excludes: antimalarial drugs (E931.4)

Add 4th or 5th digit	Nonspecific code	Unspecified code	Manifestation code

E931.4 Antimalarials and drugs acting on other blood protozoa
    Chloroquine phosphate   Proguanil [chloroguanide]
    Cycloguanil   Pyrimethamine
    Primaquine   Quinine (sulphate)

E931.5 Other antiprotozoal drugs
    Emetine

E931.6 Anthelmintics
    Hexylresorcinol   Piperazine
    Male fern oleoresin   Thiabendazole

E931.7 Antiviral drugs
    Methisazone

> *Excludes:* *amantadine (E936.4)*
>
>   *cytarabine (E933.1)*
>   *idoxuridine (E946.5)*

E931.8 Other antimycobacterial drugs
    Ethambutol   Para-aminosalicylic acid derivatives
    Ethionamide   Sulfones
    Isoniazid

E931.9 Other and unspecified anti-infectives
    Flucytosine   Nitrofuran derivatives

E932 Hormones and synthetic substitutes

E932.0 Adrenal cortical steroids
    Cortisone derivatives
    Desoxycorticosterone derivatives
    Fluorinated corticosteroids

E932.1 Androgens and anabolic congeners
    Nandrolone phenpropionate
    Oxymetholone
    Testosterone and preparations

E932.2 Ovarian hormones and synthetic substitutes
    Contraceptives, oral
    Estrogens
    Estrogens and progestogens combined
    Progestogens

E932.3 Insulins and antidiabetic agents
    Acetohexamide   Insulin
    Biguanide derivatives, oral Phenformin
    Chlorpropamide   Sulfonylurea derivatives, oral
    Glucagon   Tolbutamide

> *Excludes:* *adverse effect of insulin administered for shock therapy (E879.3)*

E932.4 Anterior pituitary hormones
    Corticotropin   Somatotropin [growth hormone]
    Gonadotropin

E932.5 Posterior pituitary hormones
    Vasopressin

> *Excludes:* *oxytocic agents (E945.0)*

E932.6 Parathyroid and parathyroid derivatives

E932.7 Thyroid and thyroid derivatives
    Dextrothyroxine   Liothyronine
    Levothyroxine sodium   Thyroglobulin

E932.8 Antithyroid agents
    Iodides   Thiourea
    Thiouracil

E932.9 Other and unspecified hormones and synthetic substitutes

E933 Primarily systemic agents

E933.0 Antiallergic and antiemetic drugs
    Antihistamines   Diphenylpyraline
    Chlorpheniramine   Thonzylamine
    Diphenhydramine   Tripelennamine

> *Excludes:* *phenothiazine-based tranquilizers (E939.1)*

  ● Code new   ▲ Revision of   ④ ⑤ Fourth or fifth
     to this edition   existing code   digit required

E933.1 Antineoplastic and immunosuppressive drugs
 Azathioprine   Mechlorethamine hydrochloride
 Busulfan   Mercaptopurine
 Chlorambucil   Triethylenethiophosphoramide [thio-TEPA]
 Cyclophosphamide
 Cytarabine
 Fluorouracil

 Excludes: *antineoplastic antibiotics (E930.7)*

E933.2 Acidifying agents

E933.3 Alkalizing agents

E933.4 Enzymes, not elsewhere classified
 Penicillinase

E933.5 Vitamins, not elsewhere classified
 Vitamin A   Vitamin D

 Excludes: *nicotinic acid (E942.2)*
     vitamin K (E934.3)

E933.8 Other systemic agents, not elsewhere classified
 Heavy metal antagonists

E933.9 Unspecified systemic agent

E934 Agents primarily affecting blood constituents

E934.0 Iron and its compounds
 Ferric salts
 Ferrous sulphate and other ferrous salts

E934.1 Liver preparations and other antianemic agents
 Folic acid

E934.2 Anticoagulants
 Coumarin   Prothrombin synthesis inhibitor
 Heparin   Warfarin sodium
 Phenindione

E934.3 Vitamin K [phytonadione]

E934.4 Fibrinolysis-affecting drugs
 Aminocaproic acid   Streptokinase
 Streptodornase   Urokinase

E934.5 Anticoagulant antagonists and other coagulants
 Hexadimethrine bromide Protamine sulfate

E934.6 Gamma globulin

E934.7 Natural blood and blood products
 Blood plasma   Packed red cells
 Human fibrinogen   Whole blood

E934.8 Other agents affecting blood constituents
 Macromolecular blood substitutes

E934.9 Unspecified agent affecting blood constituents

E935 Analgesics, antipyretics, and antirheumatics

E935.0 Heroin
 Diacetylmorphine

E935.1 Methadone

E935.2 Other opiates and related narcotics
 Codeine [methylmorphine] Opium (alkaloids)
 Morphine   Meperidine [pethidine]

E935.3 Salicylates
 Acetylsalicylic acid [aspirin]
 Amino derivatives of salicylic acid
 Salicylic acid salts

E935.4 Aromatic analgesics, not elsewhere classified
 Acetanilid
 Paracetamol [acetaminophen]
 Phenacetin [acetophenetidin]

E935.5 Pyrazole derivatives
 Aminophenazone [aminopyrine]
 Phenylbutazone

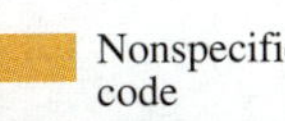

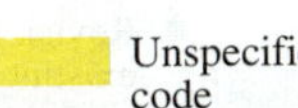

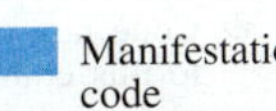

E935.6 **Antirheumatics [antiphlogistics]**
Gold salts   Indomethacin
Excludes: *salicylates (E935.3)*
steroids (E932.0)

E935.7 **Other non-narcotic analgesics**
Pyrabital

E935.8 **Other specified analgesics and antipyretics**
Pentazocine

E935.9 **Unspecified analgesic and antipyretic**

E936 **Anticonvulsants and anti-Parkinsonism drugs**

E936.0 **Oxazolidine derivatives**
Paramethadione   Trimethadione

E936.1 **Hydantoin derivatives**
Phenytoin

E936.2 **Succinimides**
Ethosuximide   Phensuximide

E936.3 **Other and unspecified anticonvulsants**
Beclamide   Primidone

E936.4 **Anti-Parkinsonism drugs**
Amantadine
Ethopropazine [profenamine]
Levodopa [L-dopa]

E937 **Sedatives and hypnotics**

E937.0 **Barbiturates**
Amobarbital [amylobarbitone]
Barbital [barbitone]
Butabarbital [butabarbitone]
Pentobarbital [pentobarbitone]
Phenobarbital [phenobarbitone]
Secobarbital [quinalbarbitone]

Excludes: *thiobarbiturates (E938.3)*

E937.1 **Chloral hydrate group**

E937.2 **Paraldehyde**

E937.3 **Bromine compounds**
Bromide   Carbromal (derivatives)

E937.4 **Methaqualone compounds**

E937.5 **Glutethimide group**

E937.6 **Mixed sedatives, not elsewhere classified**

E937.8 **Other sedatives and hypnotics**

E937.9 **Unspecified**
Sleeping:
  drug
  pill   } NOS
  tablet

E938 **Other central nervous system depressants and anesthetics**

E938.0 **Central nervous system muscle-tone depressants**
Chlorphenesin (carbamate)   Methocarbamol
Mephenesin

E938.1 **Halothane**

E938.2 **Other gaseous anesthetics**
Ether
Halogenated hydrocarbon derivatives, except halothane
Nitrous oxide

E938.3 **Intravenous anesthetics**
Ketamine   Thiobarbiturates, such as thiopental sodium
Methohexital
[methohexitone]

E938.4 **Other and unspecified general anesthetics**

● Code new   ▲ Revision of   ④ ⑤ Fourth or fifth
to this edition   existing code   digit required

E938.5 Surface and infiltration anesthetics
Cocaine   Procaine
Lidocaine [lignocaine]   Tetracaine

E938.6 Peripheral nerve- and plexus-blocking anesthetics

E938.7 Spinal anesthetics

E938.9 Other and unspecified local anesthetics

E939 Psychotropic agents

E939.0 Antidepressants
Amitriptyline   Monoamine oxidase [MAO] inhibitors
Imipramine

E939.1 Phenothiazine-based tranquilizers
Chlorpromazine   Prochlorperazine
Fluphenazine   Promazine
Phenothiazine

E939.2 Butyrophenone-based tranquilizers
Haloperidol   Trifluperidol
Spiperone

E939.3 Other antipsychotics, neuroleptics, and major tranquilizers

E939.4 Benzodiazepine-based tranquilizers
Chlordiazepoxide   Lorazepam
Diazepam   Medazepam
Flurazepam   Nitrazepam

E939.5 Other tranquilizers
Hydroxyzine   Meprobamate

E939.6 Psychodysleptics [hallucinogens]
Cannabis (derivatives)   Mescaline
Lysergide [LSD]   Psilocin
Marihuana (derivatives)   Psilocybin

E939.7 Psychostimulants
Amphetamine   Caffeine

> Excludes: *central appetite depressants (E947.0)*

E939.8 Other psychotropic agents

E939.9 Unspecified psychotropic agent

E940 Central nervous system stimulants

E940.0 Analeptics
Lobeline   Nikethamide

E940.1 Opiate antagonists
Levallorphan   Naloxone
Nalorphine

E940.8 Other specified central nervous system stimulants

E940.9 Unspecified central nervous system stimulant

E941 Drugs primarily affecting the autonomic nervous system

E941.0 Parasympathomimetics [cholinergics]
Acetylcholine   Pilocarpine
Anticholinesterase:
  organophosphorus
  reversible

E941.1 Parasympatholytics [anticholinergics and antimuscarinics] and spasmolytics
Atropine   Hyoscine [scopolamine]
Homatropine   Quaternary ammonium derivatives

> Excludes: *papaverine (E942.5)*

E941.2 Sympathomimetics [adrenergics]
Epinephrine [adrenalin]
Levarterenol [noradrenalin]

E941.3 Sympatholytics [antiadrenergics]
Phenoxybenzamine   Tolazoline hydrochloride

E941.9 Unspecified drug primarily affecting the autonomic nervous system

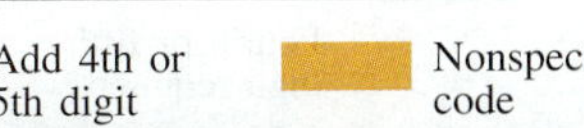

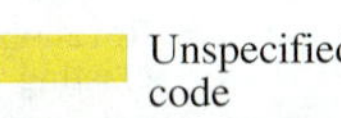

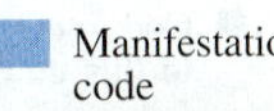

E942 Agents primarily affecting the cardiovascular system

E942.0 Cardiac rhythm regulators
Practolol
Procainamide
Propranolol
Quinidine

E942.1 Cardiotonic glycosides and drugs of similar action
Digitalis glycosides
Digoxin
Strophanthins

E942.2 Antilipemic and antiarteriosclerotic drugs
Cholestyramine
Clofibrate
Nicotinic acid derivatives
Sitosterols

> *Excludes:* *dextrothyroxine (E932.7)*

E942.3 Ganglion-blocking agents
Pentamethonium bromide

E942.4 Coronary vasodilators
Dipyridamole
Nitrates [nitroglycerin]
Nitrites
Prenylamine

E942.5 Other vasodilators
Cyclandelate
Diazoxide
Hydralazine
Papaverine

E942.6 Other antihypertensive agents
Clonidine
Guanethidine
Rauwolfia alkaloids
Reserpine

E942.7 Antivaricose drugs, including sclerosing agents
Monoethanolamine
Zinc salts

E942.8 Capillary-active drugs
Adrenochrome derivatives
Bioflavonoids
Metaraminol

E942.9 Other and unspecified agents primarily affecting the cardiovascular system

E943 Agents primarily affecting gastrointestinal system

E943.0 Antacids and antigastric secretion drugs
Aluminum hydroxide
Magnesium trisilicate

E943.1 Irritant cathartics
Bisacodyl
Castor oil
Phenolphthalein

E943.2 Emollient cathartics
Sodium dioctyl sulfosuccinate

E943.3 Other cathartics, including intestinal atonia drugs
Magnesium sulfate

E943.4 Digestants
Pancreatin
Papain
Pepsin

E943.5 Antidiarrheal drugs
Bismuth subcarbonate
Kaolin
Pectin

> *Excludes:* *anti-infectives (E930.0-E931.9)*

E943.6 Emetics

E943.8 Other specified agents primarily affecting the gastrointestinal system

E943.9 Unspecified agent primarily affecting the gastrointestinal system

E944 Water, mineral, and uric acid metabolism drugs

E944.0 Mercurial diuretics
Chlormerodrin
Mercaptomerin
Mercurophylline
Mersalyl

E944.1 Purine derivative diuretics
Theobromine
Theophylline

> *Excludes:* *aminophylline [theophylline ethylenediamine] (E945.7)*

E944.2 Carbonic acid anhydrase inhibitors
Acetazolamide

E944.3 Saluretics
Benzothiadiazides
Chlorothiazide group

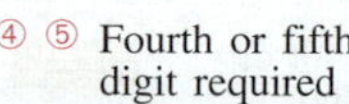

● Code new
to this edition

▲ Revision of
existing code

④ ⑤ Fourth or fifth
digit required

E944.4 **Other diuretics**
    Ethacrynic acid   Furosemide

E944.5 **Electrolytic, caloric, and water-balance agents**

E944.6 **Other mineral salts, not elsewhere classified**

E944.7 **Uric acid metabolism drugs**
    Cinchophen and congeners   Phenoquin
    Colchicine   Probenecid

E945 **Agents primarily acting on the smooth and skeletal muscles and respiratory system**

E945.0 **Oxytocic agents**
    Ergot alkaloids   Prostaglandins

E945.1 **Smooth muscle relaxants**
    Adiphenine
    Metaproterenol [orciprenaline]

    Excludes: papaverine (E942.5)

E945.2 **Skeletal muscle relaxants**
    Alcuronium chloride   Suxamethonium chloride

E945.3 **Other and unspecified drugs acting on muscles**

E945.4 **Antitussives**
    Dextromethorphan   Pipazethate hydrochloride

E945.5 **Expectorants**
    Acetylcysteine   Ipecacuanha
    Cocillana   Terpin hydrate
    Guaifenesin [glyceryl guaiacolate]

E945.6 **Anti-common cold drugs**

E945.7 **Antiasthmatics**
    Aminophylline [theophylline ethylenediamine]

E945.8 **Other and unspecified respiratory drugs**

E946 **Agents primarily affecting skin and mucous membrane, ophthalmological, otorhinolaryngological, and dental drugs**

E946.0 **Local anti-infectives and anti-inflammatory drugs**

E946.1 **Antipruritics**

E946.2 **Local astringents and local detergents**

E946.3 **Emollients, demulcents, and protectants**

E946.4 **Keratolytics, keratoplastics, other hair treatment drugs and preparations**

E946.5 **Eye anti-infectives and other eye drugs**
    Idoxuridine

E946.6 **Anti-infectives and other drugs and preparations for ear, nose, and throat**

E946.7 **Dental drugs topically applied**

E946.8 **Other agents primarily affecting skin and mucous membrane**
    Spermicides

E946.9 **Unspecified agent primarily affecting skin and mucous membrane**

E947 **Other and unspecified drugs and medicinal substances**

E947.0 **Dietetics**

E947.1 **Lipotropic drugs**

E947.2 **Antidotes and chelating agents, not elsewhere classified**

E947.3 **Alcohol deterrents**

E947.4 **Pharmaceutical excipients**

E947.8 **Other drugs and medicinal substances**
    Contrast media used for diagnostic x-ray procedures
    Diagnostic agents and kits

E947.9 **Unspecified drug or medicinal substance**

E948 **Bacterial vaccines**

E948.0 **BCG vaccine**

E948.1 **Typhoid and paratyphoid**

E948.2 **Cholera**

E948.3 **Plague**

E948.4 **Tetanus**

Add 4th or 5th digit   Nonspecific code   Unspecified code   Manifestation code

E948.5 Diphtheria

E948.6 Pertussis vaccine, including combinations with a pertussis component

E948.8 Other and unspecified bacterial vaccines

E948.9 Mixed bacterial vaccines, except combinations with a pertussis component

E949 Other vaccines and biological substances

> | *Excludes:* | *gamma globulin (E934.6)* |

E949.0 Smallpox vaccine

E949.1 Rabies vaccine

E949.2 Typhus vaccine

E949.3 Yellow fever vaccine

E949.4 Measles vaccine

E949.5 Poliomyelitis vaccine

E949.6 Other and unspecified viral and rickettsial vaccines
  Mumps vaccine

E949.7 Mixed viral-rickettsial and bacterial vaccines, except combinations with a pertussis component

> | *Excludes:* | *combinations with a pertussis component (E948.6)* |

E949.9 Other and unspecified vaccines and biological substances

SUICIDE AND SELF-INFLICTED INJURY (E950-E959)

Includes: injuries in suicide and attempted suicide
  self-inflicted injuries specified as intentional

E950 Suicide and self-inflicted poisoning by solid or liquid substances

E950.0 Analgesics, antipyretics, and antirheumatics

E950.1 Barbiturates

E950.2 Other sedatives and hypnotics

E950.3 Tranquilizers and other psychotropic agents

E950.4 Other specified drugs and medicinal substances

E950.5 Unspecified drug or medicinal substances

E950.6 Agricultural and horticultural chemical and pharmaceutical preparations other than plant foods and fertilizers

E950.7 Corrosive and caustic substances
  Suicide and self-inflicted poisoning by substances classifiable to E864

E950.8 Arsenic and its compounds

E950.9 Other and unspecified solid and liquid substances

E951 Suicide and self-inflicted poisoning by gases in domestic use

E951.0 Gas distributed by pipeline

E951.1 Liquefied petroleum gas distributed in mobile containers

E951.8 Other utility gas

E952 Suicide and self-inflicted poisoning by other gases and vapors

E952.0 Motor vehicle exhaust gas

E952.1 Other carbon monoxide

E952.8 Other specified gases and vapors

E952.9 Unspecified gases and vapors

E953 Suicide and self-inflicted injury by hanging, strangulation, and suffocation

E953.0 Hanging

E953.1 Suffocation by plastic bag

E953.8 Other specified means

E953.9 Unspecified means

E954 Suicide and self-inflicted injury by submersion [drowning]

E955 Suicide and self-inflicted injury by firearms, air guns and explosives

E955.0 Handgun

E955.1 Shotgun

● Code new
  to this edition   ▲ Revision of
  existing code   ④ ⑤ Fourth or fifth
  digit required

E955.2 **Hunting rifle**

E955.3 **Military firearms**

E955.4 **Other and unspecified firearm**
Gunshot NOS   Shot NOS

E955.5 **Explosives**

E955.6 **Air gun**
BB gun   Pellet gun

● E955.7 **Paintball gun**

E955.9 **Unspecified**

E956 **Suicide and self-inflicted injury by cutting and piercing instrument**

E957 **Suicide and self-inflicted injuries by jumping from high place**

E957.0 **Residential premises**

E957.1 **Other man-made structures**

E957.2 **Natural sites**

E957.9 **Unspecified**

E958 **Suicide and self-inflicted injury by other and unspecified means**

E958.0 **Jumping or lying before moving object**

E958.1 **Burns, fire**

E958.2 **Scald**

E958.3 **Extremes of cold**

E958.4 **Electrocution**

E958.5 **Crashing of motor vehicle**

E958.6 **Crashing of aircraft**

E958.7 **Caustic substances, except poisoning**

> *Excludes:* *poisoning by caustic substance (E950.7)*

E958.8 **Other specified means**

E958.9 **Unspecified means**

E959 **Late effects of self-inflicted injury**

> Note: This category is to be used to indicate circumstances classifiable to E950-E958 as the cause of death or disability from late effects, which are themselves classifiable elsewhere. The "late effects" include conditions reported as such or as sequelae which may occur at any time after the attempted suicide or self-inflicted injury.

HOMICIDE AND INJURY PURPOSELY INFLICTED BY OTHER PERSONS (E960-E969)

> Includes: injuries inflicted by another person with intent to injure or kill, by any means

> *Excludes:* *injuries due to:*
> *legal intervention (E970-E978)*
> *operations of war (E990-E999)*
> *terrorism (E979)*

E960 **Fight, brawl, rape**

E960.0 **Unarmed fight or brawl**
Beatings NOS
Brawl or fight with hands, fists, feet
Injured or killed in fight NOS

> *Excludes:* *homicidal:*
> *injury by weapons (E965.0-E966, E969)*
> *strangulation (E963)*
> *submersion (E964)*

E960.1 **Rape**

E961 **Assault by corrosive or caustic substance, except poisoning**
Injury or death purposely caused by corrosive or caustic substance, such as:
acid [any]
corrosive substance
vitriol

> *Excludes:* *burns from hot liquid (E968.3)*
> *chemical burns from swallowing a corrosive substance (E962.0-E962.9)*

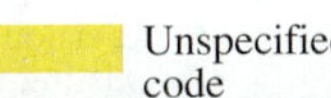

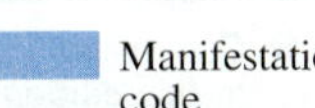

E962 Assault by poisoning

E962.0 Drugs and medicinal substances
Homicidal poisoning by any drug or medicinal substance

E962.1 Other solid and liquid substances

E962.2 Other gases and vapors

E962.9 Unspecified poisoning

E963 Assault by hanging and strangulation
Homicidal (attempt):
garrotting or ligature
hanging
strangulation
suffocation

E964 Assault by submersion [drowning]

E965 Assault by firearms and explosives

E965.0 Handgun
Pistol   Revolver

E965.1 Shotgun

E965.2 Hunting rifle

E965.3 Military firearms

E965.4 Other and unspecified firearm

E965.5 Antipersonnel bomb

E965.6 Gasoline bomb

E965.7 Letter bomb

E965.8 Other specified explosive
Bomb NOS (placed in) car
Bomb NOS (placed in)
house
Dynamite

E965.9 Unspecified explosive

E966 Assault by cutting and piercing instrument
Assassination (attempt), homicide (attempt) by any instrument classifiable under E920
Homicidal cut, any part of the body
Homicidal puncture, any part of the body
Homicidal stab, any part of the body
Stabbed, any part of the body

E967 Perpetrator of child and adult abuse
Note: selection of the correct perpetrator code is based on the relationship between the
perpetrator and the victim

E967.0 By father, stepfather or boyfriend
Male partner of child's parent or guardian

E967.1 By other specified person

E967.2 By mother, stepmother or girlfriend
Female partner of child's parent or guardian

E967.3 By spouse or partner
Abuse of spouse or partner by ex-spouse or ex-partner

E967.4 By child

E967.5 By sibling

E967.6 By grandparent

E967.7 By other relative

E967.8 By non-related caregiver

E967.9 By unspecified person

E968 Assault by other and unspecified means

E968.0 Fire
Arson   Homicidal burns NOS

> Excludes: *burns from hot liquid (E968.3)*

E968.1 Pushing from a high place

E968.2 Striking by blunt or thrown object

  ● Code new
to this edition   ▲ Revision of
existing code   ④ ⑤ Fourth or fifth
digit required

E968.3 Hot liquid
Homicidal burns by scalding

E968.4 Criminal neglect
Abandonment of child, infant, or other helpless person with intent to injure or kill

E968.5 Transport vehicle
Being struck by other vehicle or run down with intent to injure
Pushed in front of, thrown from, or dragged by moving vehicle with intent to injure

E968.6 Air gun
BB gun
Pellet gun

E968.7 Human bite

E968.8 Other specified means

E968.9 Unspecified means
Assassination (attempt) NOS   Manslaughter (nonaccidental)
Homicidal (attempt):   Murder (attempt) NOS
  injury NOS   Violence, non-accidental
  wound NOS

E969 Late effects of injury purposely inflicted by other person
Note: This category is to be used to indicate circumstances classifiable to E960-E968 as the cause of death or disability from late effects, which are themselves classifiable elsewhere. The "late effects" include conditions reported as such, or as sequelae which may occur at any time after the acute injury.

LEGAL INTERVENTION (E970-E978)

Includes: injuries inflicted by the police or other law-enforcing agents, including military on duty, in the course of arresting or attempting to arrest lawbreakers, suppressing disturbances, maintaining order, and other legal action
legal execution

Excludes: *injuries caused by civil insurrections (E990.0-E999)*

E970 Injury due to legal intervention by firearms
Gunshot wound   Injury by:
Injury by: rifle pellet or rubber bullet
  machine gun   shot NOS
  revolver

E971 Injury due to legal intervention by explosives
Injury by:
  dynamite
  explosive shell
  grenade
  mortar bomb

E972 Injury due to legal intervention by gas
Asphyxiation by gas
Injury by tear gas
Poisoning by gas

E973 Injury due to legal intervention by blunt object
Hit, struck by:
        baton (nightstick)
        blunt object
        stave

E974 Injury due to legal intervention by cutting and piercing instrument
Cut   Incised wound
Injured by bayonet   Stab wound

E975 Injury due to legal intervention by other specified means
Blow
Manhandling

E976 Injury due to legal intervention by unspecified means

E977 Late effects of injuries due to legal intervention
Note: This category is to be used to indicate circumstances classifiable to E970-E976 as the cause of death or disability from late effects, which are themselves classifiable elsewhere. The "late effects" include conditions reported as such, or as sequelae which may occur at any time after the acute injury due to legal intervention.

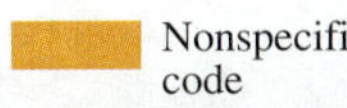

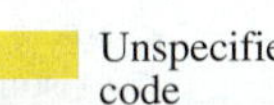

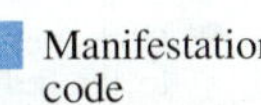

Manifestation
code

E978 Legal execution
All executions performed at the behest of the judiciary or ruling authority [whether permanent or temporary] as:

asphyxiation by gas	hanging
beheading, decapitation	poisoning
(by guillotine)	shooting
capital punishment	other specified means
electrocution	

TERRORISM (E979)

● **E979 Terrorism**
Injuries resulting from the unlawful use of force or violence against persons or property to intimidate or coerce a Government, the civilian population, or any segment thereof, in furtherance of political or social objective

● **E979.0 Terrorism involving explosion of marine weapons**
Depth-charge
Marine mine
Mine NOS at sea or in harbor
Sea-based artillery shell
Torpedo
Underwater blast

● **E979.1 Terrorism involving destruction of aircraft**
Aircraft used as a weapon
Aircraft:
    burned
    exploded
    shot down
Crushed by falling aircraft

● **E979.2 Terrorism involving other explosions and fragments**
Antipersonnel bomb (fragments)
Blast NOS
Explosion (of):
    artillery shell
    breech-block
    cannon block
    mortar bomb
    munitions being used in terrorism
    NOS
Fragments from:
    artillery shell
    bomb
    grenade
    guided missile
    land-mine
    rocket
    shell
    shrapnel
Mine NOS

● **E979.3 Terrorism involving fires, conflagration and hot substances**
Burning building or structure
    collapse of
    fall from
    hit by falling object in
    jump from
Conflagration NOS
Fire (causing):
    asphyxia
    burns
    NOS
    other injury
Melting of fittings and furniture in burning
Petrol bomb
Smouldering building or structure

● **E979.4 Terrorism involving firearms**

Bullet:	Pellets (shotgun)
carbine	
machine gun	
pistol	
rifle	
rubber (rifle)	

● Code new to this edition	▲ Revision of existing code	④ ⑤ Fourth or fifth digit required

● **E979.5 Terrorism involving nuclear weapons**
    Blast effects
    Exposure to ionizing radiation from nuclear weapon
    Fireball effects
    Heat from nuclear weapon
    Other direct and secondary effects of nuclear weapons

● **E979.6 Terrorism involving biological weapons**
    Anthrax
    Cholera
    Smallpox

● **E979.7 Terrorism involving chemical weapons**
    Gases, fumes, chemicals
    Hydrogen cyanide
    Phosgene
    Sarin

● **E979.8 Terrorism involving other means**
    Drowning and submersion
    Lasers
    Piercing or stabbing instruments
    Terrorism NOS

● **E979.9 Terrorism, secondary effects**
    Note: This code is for use to identify conditions occuring subsequent to a terrorist attack, not those that are due to the initial terrorist act.

        | Excludes: | *late effect of terrorist attack (E999.1)*

INJURY UNDETERMINED WHETHER ACCIDENTALLY OR PURPOSELY INFLICTED (E980-E989)

    Note: Categories E980-E989 are for use when it is unspecified or it cannot be determined whether the injuries are accidental (unintentional), suicide (attempted), or assault.

E980 Poisoning by solid or liquid substances, undetermined whether accidentally or purposely inflicted

    E980.0 Analgesics, antipyretics, and antirheumatics

    E980.1 Barbiturates

    E980.2 Other sedatives and hypnotics

    E980.3 Tranquilizers and other psychotropic agents

    E980.4 Other specified drugs and medicinal substances

    E980.5 Unspecified drug or medicinal substance

    E980.6 Corrosive and caustic substances
        Poisoning, undetermined whether accidental or purposeful, by substances classifiable to E864

    E980.7 Agricultural and horticultural chemical and pharmaceutical preparations other than plant foods and fertilizers

    E980.8 Arsenic and its compounds

    E980.9 Other and unspecified solid and liquid substances

E981 Poisoning by gases in domestic use, undetermined whether accidentally or purposely inflicted

    E981.0 Gas distributed by pipeline

    E981.1 Liquefied petroleum gas distributed in mobile containers

    E981.8 Other utility gas

E982 Poisoning by other gases, undetermined whether accidentally or purposely inflicted

    E982.0 Motor vehicle exhaust gas

    E982.1 Other carbon monoxide

    E982.8 Other specified gases and vapors

    E982.9 Unspecified gases and vapors

E983 Hanging, strangulation, or suffocation, undetermined whether accidentally or purposely inflicted

    E983.0 Hanging

    E983.1 Suffocation by plastic bag

    E983.8 Other specified means

    E983.9 Unspecified means

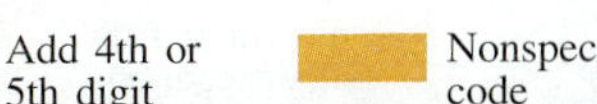

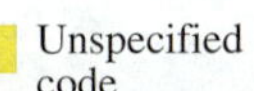

Unspecified code

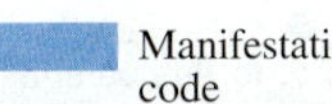

E984   Submersion [drowning], undetermined whether accidentally or purposely inflicted

E985   **Injury by firearms, air guns and explosives, undetermined whether accidentally or purposely inflicted**

   E985.0   Handgun

   E985.1   Shotgun

   E985.2   Hunting rifle

   E985.3   Military firearms

   E985.4   Other and unspecified firearm

   E985.5   Explosives

   E985.6   Air gun
         BB gun
         Pellet gun

   ● E985.7   Paintball gun

E986   **Injury by cutting and piercing instruments, undetermined whether accidentally or purposely inflicted**

E987   **Falling from high place, undetermined whether accidentally or purposely inflicted**

   E987.0   Residential premises

   E987.1   Other man-made structures

   E987.2   Natural sites

   E987.9   Unspecified site

E988   **Injury by other and unspecified means, undetermined whether accidentally or purposely inflicted**

   E988.0   Jumping or lying before moving object

   E988.1   Burns, fire

   E988.2   Scald

   E988.3   Extremes of cold

   E988.4   Electrocution

   E988.5   Crashing of motor vehicle

   E988.6   Crashing of aircraft

   E988.7   Caustic substances, except poisoning

   E988.8   Other specified means

   E988.9   Unspecified means

E989   **Late effects of injury, undetermined whether accidentally or purposely inflicted**

   Note: This category is to be used to indicate circumstances classifiable to E980-E988 as the cause of death or disability from late effects, which are themselves classifiable elsewhere. The "late effects" include conditions reported as such or as sequelae which may occur at any time after the acute injury, undetermined whether accidentally or purposely inflicted.

INJURY RESULTING FROM OPERATIONS OF WAR (E990-E999)

   Includes: injuries to military personnel and civilians caused by war and civil insurrections and occurring during the time of war and insurrection

   Excludes: *accidents during training of military personnel, manufacture of war material and transport, unless attributable to enemy action*

E990   **Injury due to war operations by fires and conflagrations**
   Includes: asphyxia, burns, or other injury originating from fire caused by a fire-producing device or indirectly by any conventional weapon

   E990.0   From gasoline bomb

   E990.9   From other and unspecified source

E991   **Injury due to war operations by bullets and fragments**

   E991.0   Rubber bullets (rifle)

   E991.1   Pellets (rifle)

● Code new
  to this edition

▲ Revision of
  existing code

④ ⑤ Fourth or fifth
  digit required

E991.2 Other bullets
Bullet [any, except rubber bullets and pellets]
carbine
machine gun
pistol
rifle
shotgun

E991.3 Antipersonnel bomb (fragments)

E991.9 Other and unspecified fragments
Fragments from:
artillery shell
bombs, except antipersonnel
grenade
guided missile

Fragments from:
land mine
rockets
shell
Shrapnel

E992 Injury due to war operations by explosion of marine weapons
Depth charge
Marine mines
Mine NOS, at sea or in harbor

Sea-based artillery shell
Torpedo
Underwater blast

E993 Injury due to war operations by other explosion
Accidental explosion of munitions
being used in war
Accidental explosion of own weapons
Air blast NOS
Blast NOS
Explosion NOS

Explosion of:
artillery shell
breech block
cannon block
mortar bomb
Injury by weapon burst

E994 Injury due to war operations by destruction of aircraft
Airplane:
burned
exploded
shot down

Crushed by falling airplane

E995 Injury due to war operations by other and unspecified forms of conventional warfare
Battle wounds
Bayonet injury

Drowned in war operations

E996 Injury due to war operations by nuclear weapons
Blast effects
Exposure to ionizing radiation from nuclear weapons
Fireball effects
Heat
Other direct and secondary effects of nuclear weapons

E997 Injury due to war operations by other forms of unconventional warfare

E997.0 Lasers

E997.1 Biological warfare

E997.2 Gases, fumes, and chemicals

E997.8 Other specified forms of unconventional warfare

E997.9 Unspecified form of unconventional warfare

E998 Injury due to war operations but occurring after cessation of hostilities
Injuries due to operations of war but occurring after cessation of hostilities by any means
classifiable under E990-E997
Injuries by explosion of bombs or mines placed in the course of operations of war, if the
explosion occurred after cessation of hostilities

▲ **E999 Late effect of injury due to war operations and terrorism**
Note: This category is to be used to indicate circumstances classifiable to E979, E990-E998 as the
cause of death or disability from late effects, which are themselves classifiable elsewhere.
The "late effects" include conditions reported as such or as sequelae which may occur at
any time after the acute injury, resulting from operations of war or terrorism.

● **E999.0 Late effect of injury due to war operations**

● **E999.1 Late effect of injury due to terrorism**

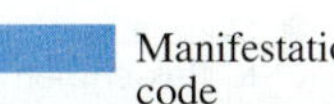

● Code new
to this edition

▲ Revision of
existing code

④ ⑤ Fourth or fifth
digit required

MORPHOLOGY OF NEOPLASMS

The World Health Organization has published an adaptation of the International Classification of Diseases for oncology (ICD-O). It contains a coded nomenclature for the morphology of neoplasms, which is reproduced here for those who wish to use it in conjunction with Chapter 2 of the *International Classification of Diseases, 9th Revision, Clinical Modification.*

The morphology code numbers consist of five digits; the first four identify the histological type of the neoplasm and the fifth indicates its behavior. The one-digit behavior code is as follows:

/0 Benign

/1 Uncertain whether benign or malignant
    Borderline malignancy

/2 Carcinoma in situ
    Intraepithelial
    Noninfiltrating
    Noninvasive

/3 Malignant, primary site

/6 Malignant, metastatic site
    Secondary site

/9 Malignant, uncertain whether primary or metastatic site

In the nomenclature below, the morphology code numbers include the behavior code appropriate to the histological type of neoplasm, but this behavior code should be changed if other reported information makes this necessary. For example, "chordoma (M9370/3)" is assumed to be malignant; the term "benign chordoma" should be coded M9370/0. Similarly, "superficial spreading adenocarcinoma (M8143/3)" described as "noninvasive" should be coded M8143/2 and "melanoma (M8720/3)" described as "secondary" should be coded M8720/6.

The following table shows the correspondence between the morphology code and the different sections of Chapter 2:

Morphology code Histology/Behavior			ICD-9-CM Chapter 2
Any	0	210-229	Benign neoplasms
M8000-M8004	1	239	Neoplasms of unspecified nature
M8010+	1	235-238	Neoplasms of uncertain behavior
Any	2	230-234	Carcinoma in situ
Any	3	140-195 200-208	Malignant neoplasms, stated or presumed to be primary
Any	6	196-198	Malignant neoplasms, stated or presumed to be secondary

The ICD-O behavior digit /9 is inapplicable in an ICD context, since all malignant neoplasms are presumed to be primary (/3) or secondary (/6) according to other information on the medical record.

Only the first-listed term of the full ICD-O morphology nomenclature appears against each code number in the list below. The ICD-9-CM Alphabetical Index (Volume 2), however, includes all the ICD-O synonyms as well as a number of other morphological names still likely to be encountered on medical records but omitted from ICD-O as outdated or otherwise undesirable.

A coding difficulty sometimes arises where a morphological diagnosis contains two qualifying adjectives that have different code numbers. An example is "transitional cell epidermoid carcinoma." "Transitional cell carcinoma NOS" is M8120/3 and "epidermoid carcinoma NOS" is M8070/3. In such circumstances, the higher number (M8120/3 in this example) should be used, as it is usually more specific.

CODED NOMENCLATURE FOR MORPHOLOGY OF NEOPLASMS

M800   **Neoplasms NOS**
M8000/0   *Neoplasm, benign*
M8000/1   *Neoplasm, uncertain whether benign or malignant*
M8000/3   *Neoplasm, malignant*
M8000/6   *Neoplasm, metastatic*
M8000/9   *Neoplasm, malignant, uncertain whether primary or metastatic*
M8001/0   *Tumor cells, benign*
M8001/1   *Tumor cells, uncertain whether benign or malignant*
M8001/3   *Tumor cells, malignant*
M8002/3   *Malignant tumor, small cell type*
M8003/3   *Malignant tumor, giant cell type*
M8004/3   *Malignant tumor, fusiform cell type*

M801-M804 Epithelial neoplasms NOS
M8010/0   *Epithelial tumor, benign*
M8010/2   *Carcinoma in situ NOS*
M8010/3   *Carcinoma NOS*
M8010/6   *Carcinoma, metastatic NOS*
M8010/9   *Carcinomatosis*
M8011/0   *Epithelioma, benign*
M8011/3   *Epithelioma, malignant*
M8012/3   *Large cell carcinoma NOS*
M8020/3   *Carcinoma, undifferentiated type NOS*
M8021/3   *Carcinoma, anaplastic type NOS*
M8022/3   *Pleomorphic carcinoma*
M8030/3   *Giant cell and spindle cell carcinoma*
M8031/3   *Giant cell carcinoma*
M8032/3   *Spindle cell carcinoma*
M8033/3   *Pseudosarcomatous carcinoma*
M8034/3   *Polygonal cell carcinoma*
M8035/3   *Spheroidal cell carcinoma*
M8040/1   *Tumorlet*
M8041/3   *Small cell carcinoma NOS*
M8042/3   *Oat cell carcinoma*
M8043/3   *Small cell carcinoma, fusiform cell type*

M805-M808 Papillary and squamous cell neoplasms
M8050/0   *Papilloma NOS (except Papilloma of urinary bladder M8120/1)*
M8050/2   *Papillary carcinoma in situ*
M8050/3   *Papillary carcinoma NOS*
M8051/0   *Verrucous papilloma*
M8051/3   *Verrucous carcinoma NOS*
M8052/0   *Squamous cell papilloma*
M8052/3   *Papillary squamous cell carcinoma*
M8053/0   *Inverted papilloma*
M8060/0   *Papillomatosis NOS*
M8070/2   *Squamous cell carcinoma in situ NOS*
M8070/3   *Squamous cell carcinoma NOS*
M8070/6   *Squamous cell carcinoma, metastatic NOS*
M8071/3   *Squamous cell carcinoma, keratinizing type NOS*
M8072/3   *Squamous cell carcinoma, large cell, nonkeratinizing type*
M8073/3   *Squamous cell carcinoma, small cell, nonkeratinizing type*
M8074/3   *Squamous cell carcinoma, spindle cell type*
M8075/3   *Adenoid squamous cell carcinoma*
M8076/2   *Squamous cell carcinoma in situ with questionable stromal invasion*
M8076/3   *Squamous cell carcinoma, microinvasive*
M8080/2   *Queyrat's erythroplasia*
M8081/2   *Bowen's disease*
M8082/3   *Lymphoepithelial carcinoma*

M809-M811 Basal cell neoplasms
M8090/1   *Basal cell tumor*
M8090/3   *Basal cell carcinoma NOS*
M8091/3   *Multicentric basal cell carcinoma*
M8092/3   *Basal cell carcinoma, morphea type*
M8093/3   *Basal cell carcinoma, fibroepithelial type*
M8094/3   *Basosquamous carcinoma*
M8095/3   *Metatypical carcinoma*
M8096/0   *Intraepidermal epithelioma of Jadassohn*
M8100/0   *Trichoepithelioma*
M8101/0   *Trichofolliculoma*

M8102/0	*Tricholemmoma*
M8110/0	*Pilomatrixoma*

M812-M813 Transitional cell papillomas and carcinomas

M8120/0	*Transitional cell papilloma NOS*
M8120/1	*Urothelial papilloma*
M8120/2	*Transitional cell carcinoma in situ*
M8120/3	*Transitional cell carcinoma NOS*
M8121/0	*Schneiderian papilloma*
M8121/1	*Transitional cell papilloma, inverted type*
M8121/3	*Schneiderian carcinoma*
M8122/3	*Transitional cell carcinoma, spindle cell type*
M8123/3	*Basaloid carcinoma*
M8124/3	*Cloacogenic carcinoma*
M8130/3	*Papillary transitional cell carcinoma*

M814-M838 Adenomas and adenocarcinomas

M8140/0	*Adenoma NOS*
M8140/1	*Bronchial adenoma NOS*
M8140/2	*Adenocarcinoma in situ*
M8140/3	*Adenocarcinoma NOS*
M8140/6	*Adenocarcinoma, metastatic NOS*
M8141/3	*Scirrhous adenocarcinoma*
M8142/3	*Linitis plastica*
M8143/3	*Superficial spreading adenocarcinoma*
M8144/3	*Adenocarcinoma, intestinal type*
M8145/3	*Carcinoma, diffuse type*
M8146/0	*Monomorphic adenoma*
M8147/0	*Basal cell adenoma*
M8150/0	*Islet cell adenoma*
M8150/3	*Islet cell carcinoma*
M8151/0	*Insulinoma NOS*
M8151/3	*Insulinoma, malignant*
M8152/0	*Glucagonoma NOS*
M8152/3	*Glucagonoma, malignant*
M8153/1	*Gastrinoma NOS*
M8153/3	*Gastrinoma, malignant*
M8154/3	*Mixed islet cell and exocrine adenocarcinoma*
M8160/0	*Bile duct adenoma*
M8160/3	*Cholangiocarcinoma*
M8161/0	*Bile duct cystadenoma*
M8161/3	*Bile duct cystadenocarcinoma*
M8170/0	*Liver cell adenoma*
M8170/3	*Hepatocellular carcinoma NOS*
M8180/0	*Hepatocholangioma, benign*
M8180/3	*Combined hepatocellular carcinoma and cholangiocarcinoma*
M8190/0	*Trabecular adenoma*
M8190/3	*Trabecular adenocarcinoma*
M8191/0	*Embryonal adenoma*
M8200/0	*Eccrine dermal cylindroma*
M8200/3	*Adenoid cystic carcinoma*
M8201/3	*Cribriform carcinoma*
M8210/0	*Adenomatous polyp NOS*
M8210/3	*Adenocarcinoma in adenomatous polyp*
M8211/0	*Tubular adenoma NOS*
M8211/3	*Tubular adenocarcinoma*
M8220/0	*Adenomatous polyposis coli*
M8220/3	*Adenocarcinoma in adenomatous polyposis coli*
M8221/0	*Multiple adenomatous polyps*
M8230/3	*Solid carcinoma NOS*
M8231/3	*Carcinoma simplex*
M8240/1	*Carcinoid tumor NOS*
M8240/3	*Carcinoid tumor, malignant*
M8241/1	*Carcinoid tumor, argentaffin NOS*
M8241/3	*Carcinoid tumor, argentaffin, malignant*
M8242/1	*Carcinoid tumor, nonargentaffin NOS*
M8242/3	*Carcinoid tumor, nonargentaffin, malignant*
M8243/3	*Mucocarcinoid tumor, malignant*
M8244/3	*Composite carcinoid*
M8250/1	*Pulmonary adenomatosis*
M8250/3	*Bronchiolo-alveolar adenocarcinoma*
M8251/0	*Alveolar adenoma*

M8251/3	*Alveolar adenocarcinoma*
M8260/0	*Papillary adenoma NOS*
M8260/3	*Papillary adenocarcinoma NOS*
M8261/1	*Villous adenoma NOS*
M8261/3	*Adenocarcinoma in villous adenoma*
M8262/3	*Villous adenocarcinoma*
M8263/0	*Tubulovillous adenoma*
M8270/0	*Chromophobe adenoma*
M8270/3	*Chromophobe carcinoma*
M8280/0	*Acidophil adenoma*
M8280/3	*Acidophil carcinoma*
M8281/0	*Mixed acidophil-basophil adenoma*
M8281/3	*Mixed acidophil-basophil carcinoma*
M8290/0	*Oxyphilic adenoma*
M8290/3	*Oxyphilic adenocarcinoma*
M8300/0	*Basophil adenoma*
M8300/3	*Basophil carcinoma*
M8310/0	*Clear cell adenoma*
M8310/3	*Clear cell adenocarcinoma NOS*
M8311/1	*Hypernephroid tumor*
M8312/3	*Renal cell carcinoma*
M8313/0	*Clear cell adenofibroma*
M8320/3	*Granular cell carcinoma*
M8321/0	*Chief cell adenoma*
M8322/0	*Water-clear cell adenoma*
M8322/3	*Water-clear cell adenocarcinoma*
M8323/0	*Mixed cell adenoma*
M8323/3	*Mixed cell adenocarcinoma*
M8324/0	*Lipoadenoma*
M8330/0	*Follicular adenoma*
M8330/3	*Follicular adenocarcinoma NOS*
M8331/3	*Follicular adenocarcinoma, well differentiated type*
M8332/3	*Follicular adenocarcinoma, trabecular type*
M8333/0	*Microfollicular adenoma*
M8334/0	*Macrofollicular adenoma*
M8340/3	*Papillary and follicular adenocarcinoma*
M8350/3	*Nonencapsulated sclerosing carcinoma*
M8360/1	*Multiple endocrine adenomas*
M8361/1	*Juxtaglomerular tumor*
M8370/0	*Adrenal cortical adenoma NOS*
M8370/3	*Adrenal cortical carcinoma*
M8371/0	*Adrenal cortical adenoma, compact cell type*
M8372/0	*Adrenal cortical adenoma, heavily pigmented variant*
M8373/0	*Adrenal cortical adenoma, clear cell type*
M8374/0	*Adrenal cortical adenoma, glomerulosa cell type*
M8375/0	*Adrenal cortical adenoma, mixed cell type*
M8380/0	*Endometrioid adenoma NOS*
M8380/1	*Endometrioid adenoma, borderline malignancy*
M8380/3	*Endometrioid carcinoma*
M8381/0	*Endometrioid adenofibroma NOS*
M8381/1	*Endometrioid adenofibroma, borderline malignancy*
M8381/3	*Endometrioid adenofibroma, malignant*

M839-M842 Adnexal and skin appendage neoplasms

M8390/0	*Skin appendage adenoma*
M8390/3	*Skin appendage carcinoma*
M8400/0	*Sweat gland adenoma*
M8400/1	*Sweat gland tumor NOS*
M8400/3	*Sweat gland adenocarcinoma*
M8401/0	*Apocrine adenoma*
M8401/3	*Apocrine adenocarcinoma*
M8402/0	*Eccrine acrospiroma*
M8403/0	*Eccrine spiradenoma*
M8404/0	*Hidrocystoma*
M8405/0	*Papillary hydradenoma*
M8406/0	*Papillary syringadenoma*
M8407/0	*Syringoma NOS*
M8410/0	*Sebaceous adenoma*
M8410/3	*Sebaceous adenocarcinoma*
M8420/0	*Ceruminous adenoma*
M8420/3	*Ceruminous adenocarcinoma*

M843   **Mucoepidermoid neoplasms**
M8430/1   *Mucoepidermoid tumor*
M8430/3   *Mucoepidermoid carcinoma*

M844-M849 Cystic, mucinous, and serous neoplasms
M8440/0   *Cystadenoma NOS*
M8440/3   *Cystadenocarcinoma NOS*
M8441/0   *Serous cystadenoma NOS*
M8441/1   *Serous cystadenoma, borderline malignancy*
M8441/3   *Serous cystadenocarcinoma NOS*
M8450/0   *Papillary cystadenoma NOS*
M8450/1   *Papillary cystadenoma, borderline malignancy*
M8450/3   *Papillary cystadenocarcinoma NOS*
M8460/0   *Papillary serous cystadenoma NOS*
M8460/1   *Papillary serous cystadenoma, borderline malignancy*
M8460/3   *Papillary serous cystadenocarcinoma*
M8461/0   *Serous surface papilloma NOS*
M8461/1   *Serous surface papilloma, borderline malignancy*
M8461/3   *Serous surface papillary carcinoma*
M8470/0   *Mucinous cystadenoma NOS*
M8470/1   *Mucinous cystadenoma, borderline malignancy*
M8470/3   *Mucinous cystadenocarcinoma NOS*
M8471/0   *Papillary mucinous cystadenoma NOS*
M8471/1   *Papillary mucinous cystadenoma, borderline malignancy*
M8471/3   *Papillary mucinous cystadenocarcinoma*
M8480/0   *Mucinous adenoma*
M8480/3   *Mucinous adenocarcinoma*
M8480/6   *Pseudomyxoma peritonei*
M8481/3   *Mucin-producing adenocarcinoma*
M8490/3   *Signet ring cell carcinoma*
M8490/6   *Metastatic signet ring cell carcinoma*

M850-M854 Ductal, lobular, and medullary neoplasms
M8500/2   *Intraductal carcinoma, noninfiltrating NOS*
M8500/3   *Infiltrating duct carcinoma*
M8501/2   *Comedocarcinoma, noninfiltrating*
M8501/3   *Comedocarcinoma NOS*
M8502/3   *Juvenile carcinoma of the breast*
M8503/0   *Intraductal papilloma*
M8503/2   *Noninfiltrating intraductal papillary adenocarcinoma*
M8504/0   *Intracystic papillary adenoma*
M8504/2   *Noninfiltrating intracystic carcinoma*
M8505/0   *Intraductal papillomatosis NOS*
M8506/0   *Subareolar duct papillomatosis*
M8510/3   *Medullary carcinoma NOS*
M8511/3   *Medullary carcinoma with amyloid stroma*
M8512/3   *Medullary carcinoma with lymphoid stroma*
M8520/2   *Lobular carcinoma in situ*
M8520/3   *Lobular carcinoma NOS*
M8521/3   *Infiltrating ductular carcinoma*
M8530/3   *Inflammatory carcinoma*
M8540/3   *Paget's disease, mammary*
M8541/3   *Paget's disease and infiltrating duct carcinoma of breast*
M8542/3   *Paget's disease, extramammary (except Paget's disease of bone)*

M855   **Acinar cell neoplasms**
M8550/0   *Acinar cell adenoma*
M8550/1   *Acinar cell tumor*
M8550/3   *Acinar cell carcinoma*

M856-M858 Complex epithelial neoplasms
M8560/3   *Adenosquamous carcinoma*
M8561/0   *Adenolymphoma*
M8570/3   *Adenocarcinoma with squamous metaplasia*
M8571/3   *Adenocarcinoma with cartilaginous and osseous metaplasia*
M8572/3   *Adenocarcinoma with spindle cell metaplasia*
M8573/3   *Adenocarcinoma with apocrine metaplasia*
M8580/0   *Thymoma, benign*
M8580/3   *Thymoma, malignant*

M859-M867 Specialized gonadal neoplasms
M8590/1   *Sex cord-stromal tumor*
M8600/0   *Thecoma NOS*
M8600/3   *Theca cell carcinoma*

M8610/0	*Luteoma NOS*
M8620/1	*Granulosa cell tumor NOS*
M8620/3	*Granulosa cell tumor, malignant*
M8621/1	*Granulosa cell-theca cell tumor*
M8630/0	*Androblastoma, benign*
M8630/1	*Androblastoma NOS*
M8630/3	*Androblastoma, malignant*
M8631/0	*Sertoli-Leydig cell tumor*
M8632/1	*Gynandroblastoma*
M8640/0	*Tubular androblastoma NOS*
M8640/3	*Sertoli cell carcinoma*
M8641/0	*Tubular androblastoma with lipid storage*
M8650/0	*Leydig cell tumor, benign*
M8650/1	*Leydig cell tumor NOS*
M8650/3	*Leydig cell tumor, malignant*
M8660/0	*Hilar cell tumor*
M8670/0	*Lipid cell tumor of ovary*
M8671/0	*Adrenal rest tumor*

M868-M871 Paragangliomas and glomus tumors

M8680/1	*Paraganglioma NOS*
M8680/3	*Paraganglioma, malignant*
M8681/1	*Sympathetic paraganglioma*
M8682/1	*Parasympathetic paraganglioma*
M8690/1	*Glomus jugulare tumor*
M8691/1	*Aortic body tumor*
M8692/1	*Carotid body tumor*
M8693/1	*Extra-adrenal paraganglioma NOS*
M8693/3	*Extra-adrenal paraganglioma, malignant*
M8700/0	*Pheochromocytoma NOS*
M8700/3	*Pheochromocytoma, malignant*
M8710/3	*Glomangiosarcoma*
M8711/0	*Glomus tumor*
M8712/0	*Glomangioma*

M872-M879 Nevi and melanomas

M8720/0	*Pigmented nevus NOS*
M8720/3	*Malignant melanoma NOS*
M8721/3	*Nodular melanoma*
M8722/0	*Balloon cell nevus*
M8722/3	*Balloon cell melanoma*
M8723/0	*Halo nevus*
M8724/0	*Fibrous papule of the nose*
M8725/0	*Neuronevus*
M8726/0	*Magnocellular nevus*
M8730/0	*Nonpigmented nevus*
M8730/3	*Amelanotic melanoma*
M8740/0	*Junctional nevus*
M8740/3	*Malignant melanoma in junctional nevus*
M8741/2	*Precancerous melanosis NOS*
M8741/3	*Malignant melanoma in precancerous melanosis*
M8742/2	*Hutchinson's melanotic freckle*
M8742/3	*Malignant melanoma in Hutchinson's melanotic freckle*
M8743/3	*Superficial spreading melanoma*
M8750/0	*Intradermal nevus*
M8760/0	*Compound nevus*
M8761/1	*Giant pigmented nevus*
M8761/3	*Malignant melanoma in giant pigmented nevus*
M8770/0	*Epithelioid and spindle cell nevus*
M8771/3	*Epithelioid cell melanoma*
M8772/3	*Spindle cell melanoma NOS*
M8773/3	*Spindle cell melanoma, type A*
M8774/3	*Spindle cell melanoma, type B*
M8775/3	*Mixed epithelioid and spindle cell melanoma*
M8780/0	*Blue nevus NOS*
M8780/3	*Blue nevus, malignant*
M8790/0	*Cellular blue nevus*

M880 Soft tissue tumors and sarcomas NOS

M8800/0	*Soft tissue tumor, benign*
M8800/3	*Sarcoma NOS*
M8800/9	*Sarcomatosis NOS*
M8801/3	*Spindle cell sarcoma*

M8802/3   *Giant cell sarcoma (except of bone M9250/3)*
M8803/3   *Small cell sarcoma*
M8804/3   *Epithelioid cell sarcoma*

M881-M883 Fibromatous neoplasms
M8810/0   *Fibroma NOS*
M8810/3   *Fibrosarcoma NOS*
M8811/0   *Fibromyxoma*
M8811/3   *Fibromyxosarcoma*
M8812/0   *Periosteal fibroma*
M8812/3   *Periosteal fibrosarcoma*
M8813/0   *Fascial fibroma*
M8813/3   *Fascial fibrosarcoma*
M8814/3   *Infantile fibrosarcoma*
M8820/0   *Elastofibroma*
M8821/1   *Aggressive fibromatosis*
M8822/1   *Abdominal fibromatosis*
M8823/1   *Desmoplastic fibroma*
M8830/0   *Fibrous histiocytoma NOS*
M8830/1   *Atypical fibrous histiocytoma*
M8830/3   *Fibrous histiocytoma, malignant*
M8831/0   *Fibroxanthoma NOS*
M8831/1   *Atypical fibroxanthoma*
M8831/3   *Fibroxanthoma, malignant*
M8832/0   *Dermatofibroma NOS*
M8832/1   *Dermatofibroma protuberans*
M8832/3   *Dermatofibrosarcoma NOS*

M884   Myxomatous neoplasms
M8840/0   *Myxoma NOS*
M8840/3   *Myxosarcoma*

M885-M888 Lipomatous neoplasms
M8850/0   *Lipoma NOS*
M8850/3   *Liposarcoma NOS*
M8851/0   *Fibrolipoma*
M8851/3   *Liposarcoma, well differentiated type*
M8852/0   *Fibromyxolipoma*
M8852/3   *Myxoid liposarcoma*
M8853/3   *Round cell liposarcoma*
M8854/3   *Pleomorphic liposarcoma*
M8855/3   *Mixed type liposarcoma*
M8856/0   *Intramuscular lipoma*
M8857/0   *Spindle cell lipoma*
M8860/0   *Angiomyolipoma*
M8860/3   *Angiomyoliposarcoma*
M8861/0   *Angiolipoma NOS*
M8861/1   *Angiolipoma, infiltrating*
M8870/0   *Myelolipoma*
M8880/0   *Hibernoma*
M8881/0   *Lipoblastomatosis*

M889-M892 Myomatous neoplasms
M8890/0   *Leiomyoma NOS*
M8890/1   *Intravascular leiomyomatosis*
M8890/3   *Leiomyosarcoma NOS*
M8891/1   *Epithelioid leiomyoma*
M8891/3   *Epithelioid leiomyosarcoma*
M8892/1   *Cellular leiomyoma*
M8893/0   *Bizarre leiomyoma*
M8894/0   *Angiomyoma*
M8894/3   *Angiomyosarcoma*
M8895/0   *Myoma*
M8895/3   *Myosarcoma*
M8900/0   *Rhabdomyoma NOS*
M8900/3   *Rhabdomyosarcoma NOS*
M8901/3   *Pleomorphic rhabdomyosarcoma*
M8902/3   *Mixed type rhabdomyosarcoma*
M8903/0   *Fetal rhabdomyoma*
M8904/0   *Adult rhabdomyoma*
M8910/3   *Embryonal rhabdomyosarcoma*
M8920/3   *Alveolar rhabdomyosarcoma*

M893-M899 Complex mixed and stromal neoplasms
M8930/3   *Endometrial stromal sarcoma*
M8931/1   *Endolymphatic stromal myosis*
M8932/0   *Adenomyoma*
M8940/0   *Pleomorphic adenoma*
M8940/3   *Mixed tumor, malignant NOS*
M8950/3   *Mullerian mixed tumor*
M8951/3   *Mesodermal mixed tumor*
M8960/1   *Mesoblastic nephroma*
M8960/3   *Nephroblastoma NOS*
M8961/3   *Epithelial nephroblastoma*
M8962/3   *Mesenchymal nephroblastoma*
M8970/3   *Hepatoblastoma*
M8980/3   *Carcinosarcoma NOS*
M8981/3   *Carcinosarcoma, embryonal type*
M8982/0   *Myoepithelioma*
M8990/0   *Mesenchymoma, benign*
M8990/1   *Mesenchymoma, NOS*
M8990/3   *Mesenchymoma, malignant*
M8991/3   *Embryonal sarcoma*

M900-M903 Fibroepithelial neoplasms
M9000/0   *Brenner tumor NOS*
M9000/1   *Brenner tumor, borderline malignancy*
M9000/3   *Brenner tumor, malignant*
M9010/0   *Fibroadenoma NOS*
M9011/0   *Intracanalicular fibroadenoma NOS*
M9012/0   *Pericanalicular fibroadenoma*
M9013/0   *Adenofibroma NOS*
M9014/0   *Serous adenofibroma*
M9015/0   *Mucinous adenofibroma*
M9020/0   *Cellular intracanalicular fibroadenoma*
M9020/1   *Cystosarcoma phyllodes NOS*
M9020/3   *Cystosarcoma phyllodes, malignant*
M9030/0   *Juvenile fibroadenoma*

M904   Synovial neoplasms
M9040/0   *Synovioma, benign*
M9040/3   *Synovial sarcoma NOS*
M9041/3   *Synovial sarcoma, spindle cell type*
M9042/3   *Synovial sarcoma, epithelioid cell type*
M9043/3   *Synovial sarcoma, biphasic type*
M9044/3   *Clear cell sarcoma of tendons and aponeuroses*

M905   Mesothelial neoplasms
M9050/0   *Mesothelioma, benign*
M9050/3   *Mesothelioma, malignant*
M9051/0   *Fibrous mesothelioma, benign*
M9051/3   *Fibrous mesothelioma, malignant*
M9052/0   *Epithelioid mesothelioma, benign*
M9052/3   *Epithelioid mesothelioma, malignant*
M9053/0   *Mesothelioma, biphasic type, benign*
M9053/3   *Mesothelioma, biphasic type, malignant*
M9054/0   *Adenomatoid tumor NOS*

M906-M909 Germ cell neoplasms
M9060/3   *Dysgerminoma*
M9061/3   *Seminoma NOS*
M9062/3   *Seminoma, anaplastic type*
M9063/3   *Spermatocytic seminoma*
M9064/3   *Germinoma*
M9070/3   *Embryonal carcinoma NOS*
M9071/3   *Endodermal sinus tumor*
M9072/3   *Polyembryoma*
M9073/1   *Gonadoblastoma*
M9080/0   *Teratoma, benign*
M9080/1   *Teratoma NOS*
M9080/3   *Teratoma, malignant NOS*
M9081/3   *Teratocarcinoma*
M9082/3   *Malignant teratoma, undifferentiated type*
M9083/3   *Malignant teratoma, intermediate type*
M9084/0   *Dermoid cyst*
M9084/3   *Dermoid cyst with malignant transformation*

M9090/0	*Struma ovarii NOS*
M9090/3	*Struma ovarii, malignant*
M9091/1	*Strumal carcinoid*

M910   **Trophoblastic neoplasms**
M9100/0	*Hydatidiform mole NOS*
M9100/1	*Invasive hydatidiform mole*
M9100/3	*Choriocarcinoma*
M9101/3	*Choriocarcinoma combined with teratoma*
M9102/3	*Malignant teratoma, trophoblastic*

M911   **Mesonephromas**
M9110/0	*Mesonephroma, benign*
M9110/1	*Mesonephric tumor*
M9110/3	*Mesonephroma, malignant*
M9111/1	*Endosalpingioma*

M912-M916   **Blood vessel tumors**
M9120/0	*Hemangioma NOS*
M9120/3	*Hemangiosarcoma*
M9121/0	*Cavernous hemangioma*
M9122/0	*Venous hemangioma*
M9123/0	*Racemose hemangioma*
M9124/3	*Kupffer cell sarcoma*
M9130/0	*Hemangioendothelioma, benign*
M9130/1	*Hemangioendothelioma NOS*
M9130/3	*Hemangioendothelioma, malignant*
M9131/0	*Capillary hemangioma*
M9132/0	*Intramuscular hemangioma*
M9140/3	*Kaposi's sarcoma*
M9141/0	*Angiokeratoma*
M9142/0	*Verrucous keratotic hemangioma*
M9150/0	*Hemangiopericytoma, benign*
M9150/1	*Hemangiopericytoma NOS*
M9150/3	*Hemangiopericytoma, malignant*
M9160/0	*Angiofibroma NOS*
M9161/1	*Hemangioblastoma*

M917   **Lymphatic vessel tumors**
M9170/0	*Lymphangioma NOS*
M9170/3	*Lymphangiosarcoma*
M9171/0	*Capillary lymphangioma*
M9172/0	*Cavernous lymphangioma*
M9173/0	*Cystic lymphangioma*
M9174/0	*Lymphangiomyoma*
M9174/1	*Lymphangiomyomatosis*
M9175/0	*Hemolymphangioma*

M918-M920   **Osteomas and osteosarcomas**
M9180/0	*Osteoma NOS*
M9180/3	*Osteosarcoma NOS*
M9181/3	*Chondroblastic osteosarcoma*
M9182/3	*Fibroblastic osteosarcoma*
M9183/3	*Telangiectatic osteosarcoma*
M9184/3	*Osteosarcoma in Paget's disease of bone*
M9190/3	*Juxtacortical osteosarcoma*
M9191/0	*Osteoid osteoma NOS*
M9200/0	*Osteoblastoma*

M921-M924   **Chondromatous neoplasms**
M9210/0	*Osteochondroma*
M9210/1	*Osteochondromatosis NOS*
M9220/0	*Chondroma NOS*
M9220/1	*Chondromatosis NOS*
M9220/3	*Chondrosarcoma NOS*
M9221/0	*Juxtacortical chondroma*
M9221/3	*Juxtacortical chondrosarcoma*
M9230/0	*Chondroblastoma NOS*
M9230/3	*Chondroblastoma, malignant*
M9240/3	*Mesenchymal chondrosarcoma*
M9241/0	*Chondromyxoid fibroma*

M925   **Giant cell tumors**
M9250/1	*Giant cell tumor of bone NOS*
M9250/3	*Giant cell tumor of bone, malignant*

M9251/1	*Giant cell tumor of soft parts NOS*
M9251/3	*Malignant giant cell tumor of soft parts*

M926 **Miscellaneous bone tumors**
M9260/3	*Ewing's sarcoma*
M9261/3	*Adamantinoma of long bones*
M9262/0	*Ossifying fibroma*

M927-M934 Odontogenic tumors
M9270/0	*Odontogenic tumor, benign*
M9270/1	*Odontogenic tumor NOS*
M9270/3	*Odontogenic tumor, malignant*
M9271/0	*Dentinoma*
M9272/0	*Cementoma NOS*
M9273/0	*Cementoblastoma, benign*
M9274/0	*Cementifying fibroma*
M9275/0	*Gigantiform cementoma*
M9280/0	*Odontoma NOS*
M9281/0	*Compound odontoma*
M9282/0	*Complex odontoma*
M9290/0	*Ameloblastic fibro-odontoma*
M9290/3	*Ameloblastic odontosarcoma*
M9300/0	*Adenomatoid odontogenic tumor*
M9301/0	*Calcifying odontogenic cyst*
M9310/0	*Ameloblastoma NOS*
M9310/3	*Ameloblastoma, malignant*
M9311/0	*Odontoameloblastoma*
M9312/0	*Squamous odontogenic tumor*
M9320/0	*Odontogenic myxoma*
M9321/0	*Odontogenic fibroma NOS*
M9330/0	*Ameloblastic fibroma*
M9330/3	*Ameloblastic fibrosarcoma*
M9340/0	*Calcifying epithelial odontogenic tumor*

M935-M937 Miscellaneous tumors
M9350/1	*Craniopharyngioma*
M9360/1	*Pinealoma*
M9361/1	*Pineocytoma*
M9362/3	*Pineoblastoma*
M9363/0	*Melanotic neuroectodermal tumor*
M9370/3	*Chordoma*

M938-M948 Gliomas
M9380/3	*Glioma, malignant*
M9381/3	*Gliomatosis cerebri*
M9382/3	*Mixed glioma*
M9383/1	*Subependymal glioma*
M9384/1	*Subependymal giant cell astrocytoma*
M9390/0	*Choroid plexus papilloma NOS*
M9390/3	*Choroid plexus papilloma, malignant*
M9391/3	*Ependymoma NOS*
M9392/3	*Ependymoma, anaplastic type*
M9393/1	*Papillary ependymoma*
M9394/1	*Myxopapillary ependymoma*
M9400/3	*Astrocytoma NOS*
M9401/3	*Astrocytoma, anaplastic type*
M9410/3	*Protoplasmic astrocytoma*
M9411/3	*Gemistocytic astrocytoma*
M9420/3	*Fibrillary astrocytoma*
M9421/3	*Pilocytic astrocytoma*
M9422/3	*Spongioblastoma NOS*
M9423/3	*Spongioblastoma polare*
M9430/3	*Astroblastoma*
M9440/3	*Glioblastoma NOS*
M9441/3	*Giant cell glioblastoma*
M9442/3	*Glioblastoma with sarcomatous component*
M9443/3	*Primitive polar spongioblastoma*
M9450/3	*Oligodendroglioma NOS*
M9451/3	*Oligodendroglioma, anaplastic type*
M9460/3	*Oligodendroblastoma*
M9470/3	*Medulloblastoma NOS*
M9471/3	*Desmoplastic medulloblastoma*
M9472/3	*Medullomyoblastoma*

M9480/3	*Cerebellar sarcoma NOS*
M9481/3	*Monstrocellular sarcoma*

M949-M952 Neuroepitheliomatous neoplasms

M9490/0	*Ganglioneuroma*
M9490/3	*Ganglioneuroblastoma*
M9491/0	*Ganglioneuromatosis*
M9500/3	*Neuroblastoma NOS*
M9501/3	*Medulloepithelioma NOS*
M9502/3	*Teratoid medulloepithelioma*
M9503/3	*Neuroepithelioma NOS*
M9504/3	*Spongioneuroblastoma*
M9505/1	*Ganglioglioma*
M9506/0	*Neurocytoma*
M9507/0	*Pacinian tumor*
M9510/3	*Retinoblastoma NOS*
M9511/3	*Retinoblastoma, differentiated type*
M9512/3	*Retinoblastoma, undifferentiated type*
M9520/3	*Olfactory neurogenic tumor*
M9521/3	*Esthesioneurocytoma*
M9522/3	*Esthesioneuroblastoma*
M9523/3	*Esthesioneuroepithelioma*

M953 Meningiomas

M9530/0	*Meningioma NOS*
M9530/1	*Meningiomatosis NOS*
M9530/3	*Meningioma, malignant*
M9531/0	*Meningotheliomatous meningioma*
M9532/0	*Fibrous meningioma*
M9533/0	*Psammomatous meningioma*
M9534/0	*Angiomatous meningioma*
M9535/0	*Hemangioblastic meningioma*
M9536/0	*Hemangiopericytic meningioma*
M9537/0	*Transitional meningioma*
M9538/1	*Papillary meningioma*
M9539/3	*Meningeal sarcomatosis*

M954-M957 Nerve sheath tumor

M9540/0	*Neurofibroma NOS*
M9540/1	*Neurofibromatosis NOS*
M9540/3	*Neurofibrosarcoma*
M9541/0	*Melanotic neurofibroma*
M9550/0	*Plexiform neurofibroma*
M9560/0	*Neurilemmoma NOS*
M9560/1	*Neurinomatosis*
M9560/3	*Neurilemmoma, malignant*
M9570/0	*Neuroma NOS*

M958 Granular cell tumors and alveolar soft part sarcoma

M9580/0	*Granular cell tumor NOS*
M9580/3	*Granular cell tumor, malignant*
M9581/3	*Alveolar soft part sarcoma*

M959-M963 Lymphomas, NOS or diffuse

M9590/0	*Lymphomatous tumor, benign*
M9590/3	*Malignant lymphoma NOS*
M9591/3	*Malignant lymphoma, non Hodgkin's type*
M9600/3	*Malignant lymphoma, undifferentiated cell type NOS*
M9601/3	*Malignant lymphoma, stem cell type*
M9602/3	*Malignant lymphoma, convoluted cell type NOS*
M9610/3	*Lymphosarcoma NOS*
M9611/3	*Malignant lymphoma, lymphoplasmacytoid type*
M9612/3	*Malignant lymphoma, immunoblastic type*
M9613/3	*Malignant lymphoma, mixed lymphocytic-histiocytic NOS*
M9614/3	*Malignant lymphoma, centroblastic-centrocytic, diffuse*
M9615/3	*Malignant lymphoma, follicular center cell NOS*
M9620/3	*Malignant lymphoma, lymphocytic, well differentiated NOS*
M9621/3	*Malignant lymphoma, lymphocytic, intermediate differentiation NOS*
M9622/3	*Malignant lymphoma, centrocytic*
M9623/3	*Malignant lymphoma, follicular center cell, cleaved NOS*
M9630/3	*Malignant lymphoma, lymphocytic, poorly differentiated NOS*
M9631/3	*Prolymphocytic lymphosarcoma*
M9632/3	*Malignant lymphoma, centroblastic type NOS*
M9633/3	*Malignant lymphoma, follicular center cell, noncleaved NOS*

M964   **Reticulosarcomas**
M9640/3   *Reticulosarcoma NOS*
M9641/3   *Reticulosarcoma, pleomorphic cell type*
M9642/3   *Reticulosarcoma, nodular*

M965-M966 Hodgkin's disease
M9650/3   *Hodgkin's disease NOS*
M9651/3   *Hodgkin's disease, lymphocytic predominance*
M9652/3   *Hodgkin's disease, mixed cellularity*
M9653/3   *Hodgkin's disease, lymphocytic depletion NOS*
M9654/3   *Hodgkin's disease, lymphocytic depletion, diffuse fibrosis*
M9655/3   *Hodgkin's disease, lymphocytic depletion, reticular type*
M9656/3   *Hodgkin's disease, nodular sclerosis NOS*
M9657/3   *Hodgkin's disease, nodular sclerosis, cellular phase*
M9660/3   *Hodgkin's paragranuloma*
M9661/3   *Hodgkin's granuloma*
M9662/3   *Hodgkin's sarcoma*

M969   **Lymphomas, nodular or follicular**
M9690/3   *Malignant lymphoma, nodular NOS*
M9691/3   *Malignant lymphoma, mixed lymphocytic-histiocytic, nodular*
M9692/3   *Malignant lymphoma, centroblastic-centrocytic, follicular*
M9693/3   *Malignant lymphoma, lymphocytic, well differentiated, nodular*
M9694/3   *Malignant lymphoma, lymphocytic, intermediate differentiation, nodular*
M9695/3   *Malignant lymphoma, follicular center cell, cleaved, follicular*
M9696/3   *Malignant lymphoma, lymphocytic, poorly differentiated, nodular*
M9697/3   *Malignant lymphoma, centroblastic type, follicular*
M9698/3   *Malignant lymphoma, follicular center cell, noncleaved, follicular*

M970   **Mycosis fungoides**
M9700/3   *Mycosis fungoides*
M9701/3   *Sezary's disease*

M971-M972 Miscellaneous reticuloendothelial neoplasms
M9710/3   *Microglioma*
M9720/3   *Malignant histiocytosis*
M9721/3   *Histiocytic medullary reticulosis*
M9722/3   *Letterer-Siwe's disease*

M973   **Plasma cell tumors**
M9730/3   *Plasma cell myeloma*
M9731/0   *Plasma cell tumor, benign*
M9731/1   *Plasmacytoma NOS*
M9731/3   *Plasma cell tumor, malignant*

M974   **Mast cell tumors**
M9740/1   *Mastocytoma NOS*
M9740/3   *Mast cell sarcoma*
M9741/3   *Malignant mastocytosis*

M975   **Burkitt's tumor**
M9750/3   *Burkitt's tumor*

M980-M994 Leukemias

M980   **Leukemias NOS**
M9800/3   *Leukemia NOS*
M9801/3   *Acute leukemia NOS*
M9802/3   *Subacute leukemia NOS*
M9803/3   *Chronic leukemia NOS*
M9804/3   *Aleukemic leukemia NOS*

M981   **Compound leukemias**
M9810/3   *Compound leukemia*

M982   **Lymphoid leukemias**
M9820/3   *Lymphoid leukemia NOS*
M9821/3   *Acute lymphoid leukemia*
M9822/3   *Subacute lymphoid leukemia*
M9823/3   *Chronic lymphoid leukemia*
M9824/3   *Aleukemic lymphoid leukemia*
M9825/3   *Prolymphocytic leukemia*

M983   **Plasma cell leukemias**
M9830/3   *Plasma cell leukemia*

M984   **Erythroleukemias**
M9840/3   *Erythroleukemia*
M9841/3   *Acute erythremia*

M9842/3	*Chronic erythremia*

M985   **Lymphosarcoma cell leukemias**
M9850/3   *Lymphosarcoma cell leukemia*

M986   **Myeloid leukemias**
M9860/3   *Myeloid leukemia NOS*
M9861/3   *Acute myeloid leukemia*
M9862/3   *Subacute myeloid leukemia*
M9863/3   *Chronic myeloid leukemia*
M9864/3   *Aleukemic myeloid leukemia*
M9865/3   *Neutrophilic leukemia*
M9866/3   *Acute promyelocytic leukemia*

M987   **Basophilic leukemias**
M9870/3   *Basophilic leukemia*

M988   **Eosinophilic leukemias**
M9880/3   *Eosinophilic leukemia*

M989   **Monocytic leukemias**
M9890/3   *Monocytic leukemia NOS*
M9891/3   *Acute monocytic leukemia*
M9892/3   *Subacute monocytic leukemia*
M9893/3   *Chronic monocytic leukemia*
M9894/3   *Aleukemic monocytic leukemia*

M990-M994   **Miscellaneous leukemias**
M9900/3   *Mast cell leukemia*
M9910/3   *Megakaryocytic leukemia*
M9920/3   *Megakaryocytic myelosis*
M9930/3   *Myeloid sarcoma*
M9940/3   *Hairy cell leukemia*

M995-M997   **Miscellaneous myeloproliferative and lymphoproliferative disorders**
M9950/1   *Polycythemia vera*
M9951/1   *Acute panmyelosis*
M9960/1   *Chronic myeloproliferative disease*
M9961/1   *Myelosclerosis with myeloid metaplasia*
M9962/1   *Idiopathic thrombocythemia*
M9970/1   *Chronic lymphoproliferative disease*

GLOSSARY OF MENTAL DISORDERS

The psychiatric terms which appear in Chapter 5, "Mental Disorders," are listed here in alphabetic sequence. Many of the glossary descriptions originally appeared in the section on Mental Disorders in the *International Classification of Diseases, 9th Revision*,[1] and others are included to define the psychiatric conditions added to *ICD-9-CM*. The additional definitions are based on material furnished by the American Psychiatric Association's Task Force on Nomenclature and Statistics[2] and from *A Psychiatric Glossary*.[3] In a few instances definitions were obtained from *Dorland's Illustrated Medical Dictionary*[4] and from *Stedman's Medical Dictionary, Illustrated*.[5]

1. Manual of the *International Classification of Diseases, Injuries, and Causes of Death*, 9th Revision. World Health Organization, Geneva, Switzerland, 1975.
2. American Psychiatric Association, Task Force on Nomenclature and Statistics, Robert L. Spitzer, Chairman.
3. A *Psychiatric Glossary*, Fourth Edition, American Psychiatric Association, Washington, D.C., 1975.
4. *Dorland's Illustrated Medical Dictionary*, Twenty-fifth Edition, W.B. Saunders Company, Philadelphia, 1974.
5. *Stedman's Medical Dictionary*, Illustrated, Twenty-third Edition, Williams and Wilkins, Baltimore, 1976.

Academic underachievement disorder: Failure to achieve in most school tasks despite adequate intellectual capacity, a supportive and encouraging social environment, and apparent effort. The failure occurs in the absence of a demonstrable specific learning disability and is caused by emotional conflict not clearly associated with any other mental disorder.[2]

Adaptation reaction—*see* Adjustment reaction

Adjustment reaction or disorder: Mild or transient disorders lasting longer than acute stress reactions which occur in individuals of any age without any apparent pre-existing mental disorder. Such disorders are often relatively circumscribed or situation-specific, are generally reversible, and usually last only a few months. They are usually closely related in time and content to stresses such as bereavement, migration, or other experiences. Reactions to major stress that last longer than a few days are also included. In children such disorders are associated with no significant distortion of development.[1]

    conduct disturbance: Mild or transient disorders in which the main disturbance predominantly involves a disturbance of conduct (e.g., an adolescent grief reaction resulting in aggressive or antisocial disorder).[1]

    depressive reaction: States of depression, not specifiable as manic-depressive, psychotic, or neurotic.[1]

        brief: Generally transient, in which the depressive symptoms are usually closely related in time and content to some stressful event.[1]

        prolonged: Generally long-lasting, usually developing in association with prolonged exposure to a stressful situation.[1]

    emotional disturbance: An adjustment disorder in which the main symptoms are emotional in type (e.g., anxiety, fear, worry) but not specifically depressive.[1]

    mixed conduct and emotional disturbance: An adjustment reaction in which both emotional disturbance and disturbance of conduct are prominent features.[1]

Affective psychoses: Mental disorders, usually recurrent, in which there is a severe disturbance of mood (mostly compounded of depression and anxiety but also manifested as elation, and excitement) which is accompanied by one or more of the following: delusions, perplexity, disturbed attitude to self, disorder of perception and behavior; these are all in keeping with the individual's prevailing mood (as are hallucinations when they occur). There is a strong tendency to suicide. For practical reasons, mild disorders of mood may also be included here if the symptoms match closely the descriptions given; this applies particularly to mild hypomania.[1]

    bipolar: A manic-depressive psychosis which has appeared in both the depressive and manic form, either alternating or separated by an interval of normality.[1]

        atypical: An episode of affective psychosis with some, but not all, of the features of the one form of the disorder in individuals who have had a previous episode of the other form of the disorder.[2]

        depressed: A manic-depressive psychosis, circular type, in which the depressive form is currently present.[1]

        manic: A manic-depressive psychosis, circular type, in which the manic form is currently present.[1]

        mixed: A manic-depressive psychosis, circular type, in which both manic and depressive symptoms are present at the same time.[1]

    depressed type: A manic-depressive psychosis in which there is a widespread depressed mood of gloom and wretchedness with some degree of anxiety. There is often reduced activity but there may be restlessness and agitation. There is marked tendency to recurrence; in a few cases this may be at regular intervals.[1]

atypical: An affective depressive disorder that cannot be classified as a manic-depressive psychosis, depressed type, or chronic depressive personality disorder, or as an adjustment disorder.[2]

manic type: A manic-depressive psychosis characterized by states of elation or excitement out of keeping with the individual's circumstances and varying from enhanced liveliness (hypomania) to violent, almost uncontrollable, excitement. Aggression and anger, flight of ideas, distractibility, impaired judgement, and grandiose ideas are common.[1]

mixed type: Manic-depressive psychosis syndromes corresponding to both the manic and depressed types, but which for other reasons cannot be classified more specifically.[1]

Aggressive personality—*see* Personality disorder, explosive type

Agoraphobia—*see* agoraphobia under Phobia

Alcohol dependence syndrome: A state, psychic and usually also physical, resulting from taking alcohol, characterized by behavioral and other responses that always include a compulsion to take alcohol on a continuous or periodic basis in order to experience its psychic effects, and sometimes to avoid the discomfort of its absence; tolerance may or may not be present. A person may be dependent on alcohol and other drugs; if so, also record the diagnosis of drug dependence to identify the agent. If alcohol dependence is associated with alcoholic psychosis or with physical complications, *both* diagnoses should be recorded.[1]

Alcohol intoxication

acute: A psychic and physical state resulting from alcohol ingestion characterized by slurred speech, unsteady gait, poor coordination, flushed facies, nystagmus, sluggish reflexes, fetor alcoholica, loud speech, emotional instability (e.g., jollity followed by lugubriousness), excessive conviviality, loquacity, and poorly inhibited sexual and aggressive behavior.[2]

idiosyncratic: Acute psychotic episodes induced by relatively small amounts of alcohol. These are regarded as individual idiosyncratic reactions to alcohol, not due to excessive consumption and without conspicuous neurological signs of intoxication.[1]

pathological—*see* Alcohol intoxication, idiosyncratic

Alcoholic psychoses: Organic psychotic states due mainly to excessive consumption of alcohol; defects of nutrition are thought to play an important role.[1]

alcohol abstinence syndrome—*see* alcohol withdrawal syndrome below

alcohol amnestic syndrome: A syndrome of prominent and lasting reduction of memory span, including striking loss of recent memory, disordered time appreciation and confabulation, occurring in alcoholics as the sequel to an acute alcoholic psychosis (especially delirium tremens) or, more rarely, in the course of chronic alcoholism. It is usually accompanied by peripheral neuritis and may be associated with Wernicke's encephalopathy.[1]

alcohol withdrawal delirium [delirium tremens]: Acute or subacute organic psychotic states in alcoholics, characterized by clouded consciousness, disorientation, fear, illusions, delusions, hallucinations of any kind, notably visual and tactile, and restlessness, tremor and sometimes fever.[1]

alcohol withdrawal hallucinosis: A psychosis usually of less than six months' duration, with slight or no clouding of consciousness and much anxious restlessness in which auditory hallucinations, mostly of voices uttering insults and threats, predominate.[1]

alcohol withdrawal syndrome: Tremor of hands, tongue, and eyelids following cessation of prolonged heavy drinking of alcohol. Nausea and vomiting, dry mouth, headache, heavy perspiration, fitful sleep, acute anxiety attacks, mood depression, feelings of guilt and remorse, and irritability are associated features.[2]

alcohol delirium—*see* alcohol withdrawal delirium above

alcoholic dementia: Nonhallucinatory dementias occurring in association with alcoholism, but not characterized by the features of either alcohol withdrawal delirium [delirium tremens] or alcohol amnestic syndrome [Korsakoff's alcoholic psychosis].[1]

alcoholic hallucinosis—*see* alcohol withdrawal hallucinosis above

alcoholic jealousy: Chronic paranoid psychosis characterized by delusional jealousy and associated with alcoholism.[1]

alcoholic paranoia—*see* Alcoholic jealousy

alcoholic polyneuritic psychosis—*see* alcohol amnestic syndrome above

Alcoholism

acute—*see* Alcohol intoxication, acute

chronic—*see* Alcohol dependence syndrome

Alexia: Loss of a previously possessed reading facility that cannot be explained by defective visual acuity.[3]

Amnesia, psychogenic: A form of dissociative hysteria in which there is a temporary disturbance in the ability to recall important personal information which has already been registered and stored in memory. The sudden onset of this disturbance in the absence of an underlying organic mental disorder, and the extent of the disturbance being too great to be explained by ordinary forgetfulness, are the essential features.[2]

Amnestic syndrome: A syndrome of prominent and lasting reduction of memory span, including striking loss of recent memory, disordered time appreciation, and confabulation. The commonest causes are chronic alcoholism [alcohol amnestic syndrome; Korsakoff's alcoholic psychosis], chronic barbiturate dependence, and malnutrition. An amnestic syndrome may be the predominating disturbance in the early states of presenile and senile dementia, arteriosclerotic dementia, and in encephalitis and other inflammatory and degenerative diseases in which there is particular bilateral involvement of the temporal lobes, and certain temporal lobe tumors.[2]

alcoholic—*see* alcohol amnestic syndrome under Alcoholic psychoses

Amoral personality—*see* Personality disorder, antisocial type

Anancastic [anankastic] neurosis—*see* Neurotic disorder, obsessive-compulsive

Anancastic [anankastic] personality—*see* Personality disorder, compulsive type

Anorexia nervosa: A disorder in which the main features are persistent active refusal to eat and marked loss of weight. The level of activity and alertness is characteristically high in relation to the degree of emaciation. Typically the disorder begins in teenage girls but it may sometimes begin before puberty and rarely it occurs in males. Amenorrhea is usual and there may be a variety of other physiological changes including slow pulse and respiration, low body temperature, and dependent edema. Unusual eating habits and attitudes toward food are typical and sometimes starvation follows or alternates with periods of overeating. The accompanying psychiatric symptoms are diverse.[1]

Anxiety hysteria—*see* phobia under Neurotic disorders

Anxiety state (neurotic): Apprehension, tension, or uneasiness that stems from the anticipation of danger, the source of which is largely unknown or unrecognized.[3]

atypical: An anxiety disorder that does not fulfill the criteria of generalized or panic attack anxiety. An example might be an individual with a single morbid fear.[2]

generalized: A disorder of at least six months' duration in which the predominant feature is limited to diffuse and persistent anxiety without the specific symptoms that characterize phobic disorders, panic disorder, or obsessive-compulsive disorder.[2]

panic attack: An episodic and often chronic, recurrent disorder in which the predominant features are anxiety attacks and nervousness. The anxiety attacks are manifested by discrete periods of sudden onset of intense apprehension, fearfulness, or terror often associated with feelings of impending doom.[2]

Aphasia, developmental: A delay in the production of spoken language. Rarely, there is also a developmental delay in the comprehension of speech sounds.[1]

Arteriosclerotic dementia: Dementia attributable, because of physical signs (on examination of the central nervous system), to degenerative arterial disease of the brain. Symptoms suggesting a focal lesion in the brain are common. There may be a fluctuating or patchy intellectual defect with insight, and an intermittent course is common. Clinical differentiation from senile or presenile dementia, which may coexist with it, may be very difficult or impossible. The diagnosis of cerebral atherosclerosis should also be recorded.[1]

Asocial personality—*see* Personality disorder, antisocial type

Astasia-abasia, hysterical: A form of conversion hysteria in which the individual is unable to stand or walk although the legs are otherwise under control.[4]

Asthenia, psychogenic—*see* neurasthenia under Neurotic disorders

Asthenic personality—*see* Personality disorder, dependent type

Attention deficit disorder—*see* attention deficit disorder under Hyperkinetic syndrome of childhood.

Autism, infantile: A syndrome present from birth or beginning almost invariably in the first 30 months. Responses to auditory and sometimes to visual stimuli are abnormal, and there are usually severe problems in the understanding of spoken language. Speech is delayed and, if it develops, is characterized by echolalia, the reversal of pronouns, immature grammatical structure, and inability to use abstract terms. There is generally an impairment in the social use of both verbal and gestural language. Problems in social relationships are most severe before the age of five years and include an impairment in the development of eye-to-eye gaze, social attachments, and cooperative play. Ritualistic behavior is usual and may include abnormal routines, resistance to change, attachment to odd objects and stereotyped patterns of play. The capacity for abstract or symbolic thought and for imaginative play is diminished. Intelligence ranges from severely subnormal to normal or above. Performance is usually better on tasks involving rote memory or visuospatial skills than on those requiring symbolic or linguistic skills.[1]

Avoidant personality—*see* Personality disorder, avoidant type

"Bad trips": Acute intoxication from hallucinogen abuse, manifested by hallucinatory states lasting only a few days or less.[1]

Barbiturate abuse: Cases where an individual has taken the drug to the detriment of his health or social functioning, in doses above or for periods beyond those normally regarded as therapeutic.[1]

Bestiality—*see* Zoophilia

Bipolar disorder—*see* Affective psychosis, bipolar

  atypical—*see* Affective psychosis, bipolar, atypical

Body-rocking—*see* Stereotyped repetitive movements

Borderline personality—*see* Personality disorder, borderline type

Borderline psychosis of childhood—*see* Psychosis, atypical childhood

Borderline schizophrenia—*see* Schizophrenia, latent

Bouffée délirante—*see* Paranoid reaction, acute

Briquet's disorder—*see* somatization disorder under Neurotic disorders

Bulimia: An episodic pattern of overeating [binge eating] accompanied by an awareness of the disordered eating pattern with a fear of not being able to stop eating voluntarily. Depressive moods and self-deprecating thoughts follow the episodes of binge eating.[2]

Catalepsy schizophrenia—*see* Schizophrenia, catatonic type

Catastrophic stress—*see* Gross stress reaction

Catatonia (schizophrenic)—*see* Schizophrenia, catatonic type

Character neurosis—*see* Personality disorders

Childhood autism—*see* Autism, infantile

Childhood type schizophrenia—*see* Psychosis, child

Chronic alcoholic brain syndrome—*see* alcoholic dementia under Alcoholic psychoses

Clay-eating—*see* Pica

Clumsiness syndrome—*see* coordination disorder under Developmental delay disorders, specific

Combat fatigue—*see* Posttraumatic disorder, acute

Compensation neurosis—*see* compensation neurosis under Neurotic disorders

Compulsive conduct disorder—*see* impulse control disorders under Conduct disorders

Compulsive neurosis—*see* Neurotic disorder, obsessive-compulsive

Compulsive personality—*see* Personality disorder, compulsive type

Concentration camp syndrome—*see* Posttraumatic stress disorder, prolonged

Conduct disorders: Disorders mainly involving aggressive and destructive behavior and disorders involving delinquency. It should be used for abnormal behavior, in individuals of any age, which gives rise to social disapproval but which is not part of any other psychiatric condition. Minor emotional disturbances may also be present. To be included, the behavior, as judged by its frequency, severity, and type of associations with other symptoms, must be abnormal in its context. Disturbances of conduct are distinguished from an adjustment reaction by a longer duration and by a lack of close relationship in time and content to some stress. They differ from a personality disorder by the absence of deeply ingrained maladaptive patterns of behavior present from adolescence or earlier.[1]

  impulse control disorders: A failure to resist an impulse, drive, or temptation to perform some action which is harmful to the individual or to others. The impulse may or may not be consciously resisted, and the act may or may not be premeditated or planned. Prior to committing the act, there is an increasing sense of tension, and at the time of committing the act, there is an experience of either pleasure, gratification, or release. Immediately following the act, there may or may not be genuine regret, self-reproach, or guilt.[2] *See also* Intermittent explosive disorder, Isolated explosive disorder, Kleptomania, Pathological gambling, and Pyromania.

  mixed disturbance of conduct and emotions: A disorder characterized by features of undersocialized and socialized disturbance of conduct, but in which there is also considerable emotional disturbance as shown, for example, by anxiety, misery, or obsessive manifestations.[1]

  socialized conduct disorder: Conduct disorders in individuals who have acquired the values or behavior of a delinquent peer group to whom they are loyal and with whom they characteristically steal, play truant, and stay out late at night. There may also be sexual promiscuity.[1]

  undersocialized conduct disturbance

    aggressive type: A disorder characterized by a persistent pattern of disrespect for the feelings and well-being of others (bullying, physical aggression, cruel behavior, hostility, verbal abusiveness, impudence, defiance, negativism), aggressive antisocial behavior (destructiveness, stealing, persistent lying, frequent truancy, and vandalism), and failure to develop close and stable relationships with others.[2]

unaggressive type: A disorder in which there is a lack of concern for the rights and feelings of others to a degree which indicates a failure to establish a normal degree of affection, empathy, or bond with others. There are two patterns of behavior found. In one, the child is fearful and timid, lacking self-assertiveness, resorts to self-protective and manipulative lying, indulges in whining demandingness and temper tantrums, feels rejected and unfairly treated, and is mistrustful of others. In the other pattern of the disorder, the child approaches others strictly for his own gains and acts exclusively because of exploitative and extractive goals. The child lies brazenly and steals, appearing to feel no guilt, and forms no social bonds to other individuals.[2]

Confusion, psychogenic—*see* Psychosis, reactive confusion

Confusion, reactive—*see* Psychosis, reactive confusion

Confusional state

    acute—*see* Delirium, acute

    epileptic—*see* Delirium, acute

    subacute—*see* Delirium, subacute

Conversion hysteria—*see* hysteria, conversion type under Neurotic disorders

Coordination disorder—*see* coordination disorder under Developmental delay disorders, specific

Culture shock: A form of stress reaction associated with an individual's assimilation into a new culture which is vastly different from that in which he was raised.[5]

Cyclic schizophrenia—*see* Schizophrenia, schizo-affective type

Cyclothymic personality or disorder—*see* Personality disorder, cyclothymic type

Delirium: Transient organic psychotic conditions with a short course in which there is a rapidly developing onset of disorganization of higher mental processes manifested by some degree of impairment of information processing, impaired or abnormal attention, perception, memory, and thinking. Clouded consciousness, confusion, disorientation, delusions, illusions, and often vivid hallucinations predominate in the clinical picture.[1,2]

    acute: short-lived states, lasting hours or days, of the above type.[1]

    subacute: states of the above type in which the symptoms, usually less florid, last for several weeks or longer, during which they may show marked fluctuations in intensity.[1]

Delirium tremens—*see* alcohol withdrawal delirium under Alcoholic psychoses

Delusions, systematized—*see* Paranoia

Dementia: A decrement in intellectual functioning of sufficient severity to interfere with occupational or social performance, or both. There is impairment of memory and abstract thinking, the ability to learn new skills, problem solving, and judgment. There is often also personality change or impairment in impulse control. Dementia in organic psychoses may be of a chronic or progressive nature, which if untreated are usually irreversible and terminal.[1,2]

    alcoholic—*see* alcoholic dementia under Alcoholic psychoses

    arteriosclerotic—*see* Arteriosclerotic dementia

    multi-infarct—*see* Arteriosclerotic dementia

    presenile—*see* Presenile dementia

    repeated infarct—*see* Arteriosclerotic dementia

    senile—*see* Senile dementia

Depersonalization syndrome—*see* depersonalization syndrome under Neurotic disorders

Depression: States of depression, usually of moderate but occasionally of marked intensity, which have no specifically manic-depressive or other psychotic depressive features, and which do not appear to be associated with stressful events or other features specified under neurotic depression.[1]

    anxiety—*see* depression under Neurotic disorders

    endogenous—*see* Affective psychosis, depressed type

    monopolar—*see* Affective psychosis, depressed type

    neurotic—*see* depression under Neurotic disorders

    psychotic—*see* Affective psychosis, depressed type

    psychotic reactive—*see* Psychosis, depressive

    reactive—*see* depression under Neurotic disorders

    reactive psychotic—*see* Psychosis, depressive

Depressive personality or character—*see* Personality disorder, chronic depressive type

Depressive reaction—*see* depressive reaction under Adjustment reaction

Depressive psychosis—*see* Affective psychosis, depressed type

Derealization (neurotic)—*see* depersonalization syndrome under Neurotic disorders

Developmental delay disorders, specific: A group of disorders in which a specific delay in development is the main feature. For many the delay is not explicable in terms of general intellectual retardation or of inadequate schooling. In each case development is related to biological maturation, but it is also influenced by nonbiological factors. A diagnosis of a specific developmental delay carries no etiological implications. A diagnosis of specific delay in development should not be made if it is due to a known neurological disorder.[1]

    arithmetical disorder: Disorders in which the main feature is a serious impairment in the development of arithmetical skills.[1]

    articulation disorder: A delay in the development of normal word-sound production resulting in defects of articulation. Omissions or substitutions of consonants are most frequent.[1]

    coordination disorder: Disorders in which the main feature is a serious impairment in the development of motor coordination which is not explicable in terms of general intellectual retardation. The clumsiness is commonly associated with perceptual difficulties.[1]

    mixed development disorder: A delay in the development of one specific skill (e.g., reading, arithmetic, speech, or coordination) is frequently associated with lesser delays in other skills. When this occurs the diagnosis should be made according to the skill most seriously impaired. The mixed category should be used only where the mixture of delayed skills is such that no one skill is preponderantly affected.[1]

    motor retardation—*see* coordination disorder above

    reading disorder or retardation: Disorders in which the main feature is a serious impairment in the development of reading or spelling skills which is not explicable in terms of general intellectual retardation or of inadequate schooling. Speech or language difficulties, impaired right-left differentiation, perceptuo-motor problems, and coding difficulties are frequently associated. Similar problems are often present in other members of the family. Adverse psychosocial factors may be present.[1]

    speech or language disorder: Disorders in which the main feature is a serious impairment in the development of speech or language (syntax or semantic) which is not explicable in terms of general intellectual retardation. Most commonly there is a delay in the development of normal word-sound production resulting in defects of articulation. Omissions or substitutions of consonants are most frequent. There may also be a delay in the production of spoken language. Rarely, there is also a developmental delay in the comprehension of sounds. Includes cases in which delay is largely due to environmental privation.[1]

Dipsomania—*see* Alcohol dependence syndrome

Disorganized schizophrenia—*see* Schizophrenia, disorganized type

Dissociative hysteria—*see* hysteria, dissociative type under Neurotic disorders

Drug abuse: Includes cases where an individual, for whom no other diagnosis is possible, has come under medical care because of the maladaptive effect of a drug on which he is not dependent (*see* Drug dependence) and that he has taken on his own initiative to the detriment of his health or social functioning. When drug abuse is secondary to a psychiatric disorder, record the disorder as an additional diagnosis.[1]

Drug dependence: A state, psychic and sometimes also physical, resulting from taking a drug, characterized by behavioral and other responses that always include a compulsion to take a drug on a continuous or periodic basis in order to experience its psychic effects, and sometimes to avoid the discomfort of its absence. Tolerance may or may not be present. A person may be dependent on more than one drug.[1]

Drug psychoses: Organic mental syndromes which are due to consumption of drugs (notably amphetamines, barbiturates, and opiate and LSD groups) and solvents. Some of the syndromes in this group are not as severe as most conditions labeled "psychotic," but they are included here for practical reasons. The drug should be identified, and also a diagnosis of drug dependence should be recorded, if present.[1]

    drug-induced hallucinosis: Hallucinatory states of more than a few days, but not more than a few months' duration, associated with large or prolonged intake of drugs, notably of the amphetamine and LSD groups. Auditory hallucinations usually predominate and there may be anxiety or restlessness. States following LSD or other hallucinogens lasting only a few days or less ["bad trips"] are not included.[1]

    drug-induced organic delusional syndrome: Paranoid states of more than a few days, but not more than a few months' duration, associated with large or prolonged intake of drugs, notably of the amphetamine and LSD groups.[1]

    drug withdrawal syndrome: States associated with drug withdrawal ranging from severe, as specified for alcohol withdrawal delirium [delirium tremens], to less severe states characterized by one or more symptoms such as convulsions, tremor, anxiety, restlessness, gastrointestinal and muscular complaints, and mild disorientation and memory disturbance.[1]

Drunkenness:

    acute—*see* Alcohol intoxication, acute

    pathologic—*see* Alcohol intoxication, idiosyncratic

    simple: A state of inebriation due to alcohol consumption without conspicuous neurological signs of intoxication.[2]

    sleep: An inability to fully arouse from the sleep state characterized by failure to attain full consciousness after arousal.[2]

Dyscalculia—*see* arithmetical disorder under Developmental delay disorders, specific

Dyslalia—*see* articulation disorder under Developmental delay disorders, specific

Dyslexia, developmental: A disorder in which the main feature is a serious impairment of reading skills which is not explicable in terms of general intellectual retardation or of inadequate schooling. Word-blindness and strephosymbolia (tendency to reverse letters and words in reading) are included.[1,3]

Dysmenorrhea, psychogenic: Painful menstruation due to disturbance of psychic control.[4]

Dyspareunia, functional—*see* functional dyspareunia under Psychosexual dysfunctions

Dyspraxia syndrome—*see* coordination disorder under Developmental delay disorders, specific

Dyssocial personality—*see* Personality disorder, antisocial type

Dysuria, psychogenic: Difficulty in passing urine due to psychic factors.[4]

Eating disorders: A group of disorders characterized by a conspicuous disturbance in eating behavior.[2] *See also* Bulimia, Pica, and Rumination, psychogenic.

Eccentric personality—*see* Personality disorder, eccentric type

Elective mutism: A pervasive and persistent refusal to speak in situations not attributable to a mental disorder. In some cases the behavior may manifest a form of withdrawal reaction to a specific stressful situation, or as a predominant feature in children exhibiting shyness or social withdrawal disorders.[2]

Emancipation disorder: An adjustment reaction in adolescents or young adults in which there is symptomatic expression (e.g., difficulty in making independent decisions, increased dependence on parental advice, adoption of values deliberately oppositional to parents) of a conflict over independence following the recent assumption of a status in which the individual is more independent of parental control or supervision.[2]

Emotional disturbances specific to childhood and adolescence: Less well-differentiated emotional disorders characteristic of the childhood period. When the emotional disorder takes the form of a neurosis, the appropriate diagnosis should be made. These disorders differ from adjustment reactions in terms of longer duration and by the lack of close relationship in time and content to some stress.[1] *See also* Academic underachievement disorder, Elective mutism, Identity disorder, Introverted disorder of childhood, Misery and unhappiness disorder, Oppositional disorder, Overanxious disorder, and Shyness disorder of childhood.

Encopresis: A disorder in which the main manifestation is the persistent voluntary or involuntary passage of formed stools of normal or near-normal consistency into places not intended for that purpose in the individual's own sociocultural setting. Sometimes the child has failed to gain bowel control, and sometimes he has gained control but then later again became encopretic. There may be a variety of associated psychiatric symptoms and there may be smearing of feces. The condition would not usually be diagnosed under the age of four years.[1]

Endogenous depression—*see* Affective psychosis, depressed type

Enuresis: A disorder in which the main manifestation is a persistent involuntary voiding of urine by day or night which is considered abnormal for the age of the individual. Sometimes the child will have failed to gain bladder control and in other cases he will have gained control and then lost it. Episodic or fluctuating enuresis should be included. The disorder would not usually be diagnosed under the age of four years.[1]

Epileptic confusional or twilight state—*see* Delirium, acute

Excitation

    catatonic—*see* Schizophrenia, catatonic type

    psychogenic—*see* Psychosis, excitative type

    reactive—*see* Psychosis, excitative type

Exhaustion delirium—*see* Stress reaction, acute

Exhibitionism: Sexual deviation in which the main sexual pleasure and gratification is derived from exposure of the genitals to a person of the opposite sex.[1]

Explosive personality disorder—*see* Personality disorder, explosive type

Factitious illness: A form of hysterical neurosis in which there are physical or psychological symptoms that are not real, genuine, or natural, which are produced by the individual and are under his voluntary control.[2]

physical symptom type: The presentation of physical symptoms that may be total fabrication, self-inflicted, an exaggeration or exacerbation of a pre-existing physical condition, or any combination or variation of these.[2]

psychological symptom type: The voluntary production of symptoms suggestive of a mental disorder. Behavior may mimic psychosis or, rather, the individual's idea of psychosis.[2]

Fanatic personality—*see* Personality disorder, paranoid type

Fatigue neurosis—*see* neurasthenia under Neurotic disorders

Feeble-minded—*see* Mental retardation, mild

Fetishism: A sexual deviation in which nonliving objects are utilized as a preferred or exclusive method of stimulating erotic arousal.[2]

Finger-flicking—*see* Stereotyped repetitive movements

Folie à deux—*see* Shared paranoid disorder

Frigidity: A psychosexual dysfunction in which there is partial or complete failure to attain or maintain the lubrication-swelling response of sexual excitement until completion of the sexual act.[2]

Frontal lobe syndrome: Changes in behavior following damage to the frontal areas of the brain or following interference with the connections of those areas. There is a general diminution of self-control, foresight, creativity, and spontaneity, which may be manifest as increased irritability, selfishness, restlessness and lack of concern for others. Conscientiousness and powers of concentration are often diminished, but measurable deterioration of intellect or memory is not necessarily present. The overall picture is often one of emotional dullness, lack of drive, and slowness; but, particularly in persons previously with energetic, restless, or aggressive characteristics, there may be a change towards impulsiveness, boastfulness, temper outbursts, silly fatuous humor, and the development of unrealistic ambitions; the direction of change usually depends upon the previous personality. A considerable degree of recovery is possible and may continue over the course of several years.[1]

Fugue, psychogenic: A form of dissociative hysteria characterized by an episode of wandering with inability to recall one's prior identity. Both onset and recovery are rapid. Following recovery there is no recollection of events which took place during the fugue state.[2]

Ganser's syndrome (hysterical): A form of factitious illness in which the patient voluntarily produces symptoms suggestive of a mental disorder.[2]

Gender identity disorder—*see* gender identity disorder under Psychosexual identity disorders

Gilles de la Tourette's disorder or syndrome—*see* Gilles de la Tourette's disorder under Tics

Grief reaction—*see* depressive reaction, brief under Adjustment reaction

Gross stress reaction—*see* Stress reaction, acute

Group delinquency—*see* socialized conduct disorder under Conduct disorders

Habit spasm—*see* chronic motor tic disorder under Tics

Hangover (alcohol)—*see* Drunkenness, simple

Head-banging—*see* Stereotyped repetitive movements

Hebephrenia—*see* Schizophrenia, disorganized type

Heller's syndrome—*see* Psychosis, disintegrative

High grade defect—*see* Mental retardation, mild

Homosexuality: Exclusive or predominant sexual attraction for persons of the same sex with or without physical relationship. Record homosexuality as a diagnosis whether or not it is considered as a mental disorder.[1]

Hospital addiction syndrome—*see* Munchausen syndrome

Hospital hoboes—*see* Munchausen syndrome

Hospitalism: A mild or transient adjustment reaction characterized by withdrawal seen in hospitalized patients. In young children this may be manifested by elective mutism.[1]

Hyperkinetic syndrome of childhood: Disorders in which the essential features are short attention-span and distractibility. In early childhood the most striking symptom is disinhibited, poorly organized and poorly regulated extreme overactivity but in adolescence this may be replaced by underactivity. Impulsiveness, marked mood fluctuations, and aggression are also common symptoms. Delays in the development of specific skills are often present and disturbed, poor relationships are common. If the hyperkinesis is symptomatic of an underlying disorder, the diagnosis of the underlying disorder is recorded instead.[1]

attention deficit disorder: Cases of hyperkinetic syndrome in which short attention span, distractibility, and overactivity are the main manifestations without significant disturbance of conduct or delay in specific skills.[1]

hyperkinesis with developmental delay: Cases in which the hyperkinetic syndrome is associated with speech delay, clumsiness, reading difficulties, or other delays of specific skills.[1]

hyperkinetic conduct disorder: Cases in which the hyperkinetic syndrome is associated with marked conduct disturbance but not developmental delay.[1]

Hypersomnia: A disorder of initiating arousal from sleep or maintaining wakefulness.

> **persistent:** Chronic difficulty in initiating arousal from sleep or maintaining wakefulness associated with major or minor depressive mental disorders.[2]

> **transient:** Episodes of difficulty in arousal from sleep or maintaining wakefulness associated with acute or intermittent emotional reactions or conflicts.[2]

Hypochondriasis—*see* hypochondriasis under Neurotic disorders

Hypomania—*see* Affective psychosis, manic type

Hypomanic personality—*see* Personality disorder, chronic hypomanic type

Hyposomnia—*see* Insomnia

Hysteria—*see* hysteria under Neurotic disorders

> **anxiety**—*see* phobia under Neurotic disorders

> **psychosis**—*see* Psychosis, reactive

>> **acute**—*see* Psychosis, excitative type

Hysterical personality—*see* Personality disorder, histrionic type

Identity disorder: An emotional disorder caused by distress over the inability to reconcile aspects of the self into a relatively coherent and acceptable sense of self, not secondary to another mental disorder. The disturbance is manifested by intense subjective distress regarding uncertainty about a variety of issues relating to identity, including long-term goals, career choice, friendship patterns, values, and loyalties.[2]

Idiocy—*see* Mental retardation, profound

Imbecile—*see* Mental retardation, moderate

Impotence: A psychosexual dysfunction in which there is partial or complete failure to attain or maintain erection until completion of the sexual act.[2]

Impulse control disorder—*see* impulse control disorders under Conduct disorders

Inadequate personality—*see* Personality disorder, dependent type

Induced paranoid disorder—*see* Shared paranoid disorder

Inebriety—*see* Drunkenness, simple

Infantile autism—*see* Autism, infantile

Insomnia: A disorder of initiating or maintaining sleep.[2]

> **persistent:** A chronic state of sleeplessness associated with chronic anxiety, major or minor depressive disorders, or psychoses.[2]

> **transient:** Episodes of sleeplessness associated with acute or intermittent emotional reactions or conflicts.[2]

Intermittent explosive disorder: Recurrent episodes of sudden and significant loss of control of aggressive impulses, not accounted for by any other mental disorder, which results in serious assault or destruction of property. The magnitude of the behavior during an episode is grossly out of proportion to any psychosocial stressors which may have played a role in eliciting the episode of lack of control. Following each episode there is genuine regret or self-reproach at the consequences of the action and the inability to control the aggressive impulse.[2]

Introverted disorder of childhood: An emotional disturbance in children chiefly manifested by a lack of interest in social relationships and indifference to social praise or criticism.[2]

Introverted personality—*see* Personality disorder, introverted type

Involutional melancholia—*see* Affective psychosis, depressed type

Involutional paranoid state—*see* Paraphrenia

Isolated explosive disorder: A disorder of impulse control in which there is a single discrete episode characterized by failure to resist an impulse which leads to a single, violent externally-directed act, which has a catastrophic impact on others, and for which the available information does not justify the diagnosis of another mental disorder.[2]

Isolated phobia—*see* simple phobia under Phobia

Jet lag syndrome: A phase-shift disruption of the 24-hour sleep-wake cycle due to rapid time-zone changes experienced in long-distance travel.[2]

Kanner's syndrome—*see* Autism, infantile

Kleptomania: A disorder of impulse control characterized by a recurrent failure to resist impulses to steal objects not for immediate use or their monetary value. An increasing sense of tension is experienced prior to committing the act, with an intense experience of gratification at the time of committing the theft.[2]

Korsakoff's psychosis:

    alcoholic—*see* alcohol amnestic syndrome under Alcoholic psychoses

    nonalcoholic—*see* Amnestic syndrome

Latent schizophrenia—*see* Schizophrenia, latent

Lesbianism—*see* Homosexuality

Lobotomy syndrome—*see* Frontal lobe syndrome

LSD reaction: Acute intoxication from hallucinogen abuse, manifested by hallucinatory states lasting only a few days or less.[1]

Major depressive disorder—*see* Affective psychosis, depressed type

Malingering: A clinical picture in which the predominant feature is the presentation of fake or grossly exaggerated physical or psychiatric illness apparently under voluntary control. In contrast to factitious illness, the symptoms produced in malingering are in pursuit of a goal which, when known, is recognizable and obviously understandable in light of knowledge of the individual's circumstances. Examples of understandable goals include, but are not limited to, becoming a "patient" in order to avoid conscription or military duty, avoid work, obtain financial compensation, evade criminal prosecution, and obtain drugs.[2]

Mania (monopolar)—*see* Affective psychosis, manic type

Manic-depressive psychosis

    circular type—*see* Affective psychosis, bipolar

    depressed type—*see* Affective psychosis, depressed type

    manic type—*see* Affective psychosis, manic type

    mixed type—*see* Affective psychosis, mixed type

Manic disorder—*see* Affective psychosis, manic type

    atypical—*see* Affective psychosis, manic type, atypical

Masochistic personality—*see* Personality disorder, masochistic type

Melancholia—*see* Affective psychoses

    involutional—*see* Affective psychosis, depressed type

Mental retardation: A condition of arrested or incomplete development of mind which is especially characterized by subnormality of intelligence. The coding should be made on the individual's *current* level of functioning *without regard to its nature* or causation, such as psychosis, cultural deprivation, Down's syndrome, etc. Where there is a specific cognitive handicap—such as in speech—the diagnosis of mental retardation should be based on assessments of cognition *outside the area of specific handicap.* The assessment of intellectual level should be based on whatever information is available, including clinical evidence, adaptive behavior, and psychometric findings. The IQ levels given are based on a test with a mean of 100 and a standard deviation of 15, such as the Wechsler scales. They are provided only as a guide and should not be applied rigidly. Mental retardation often involves psychiatric disturbances and may often develop as a result of some physical disease or injury. In these cases, an additional diagnosis should be recorded to identify any associated condition, psychiatric or physical.[1]

    mild mental retardation: IQ criteria 50-70. Individuals with this level of retardation are usually educable. During the pre-school period they can develop social and communication skills, have minimal retardation in sensorimotor areas, and often are not distinguished from normal children until a later age. During the school age period they can learn academic skills up to approximately the sixth-grade level. During the adult years, they can usually achieve social and vocational skills adequate for minimum self-support, but may need guidance and assistance when under social or economic stress.[2]

    moderate mental retardation: IQ criteria 35-49. Individuals with this level of retardation are usually trainable. During the pre-school period they can talk or learn to communicate. They have poor social awareness and fair motor development. During the school age period they can profit from training in social and occupational skills, but they are unlikely to progress beyond the second-grade level in academic subjects. During their adult years they may achieve self-maintenance in unskilled or semi-skilled work under sheltered conditions. They need supervision and guidance when under mild social or economic stress.[2]

    severe mental retardation: IQ criteria 20-34. Individuals with this level of retardation evidence poor motor development, minimal speech, and are generally unable to profit from training and self-help during the pre-school period. During the school age period they can talk or learn to communicate, can be trained in elementary health habits, and may profit from systematic habit training. During the adult years they may contribute partially to self-maintenance under complete supervision.[2]

profound mental retardation: IQ criteria under 20. Individuals with this level of retardation evidence minimal capacity for sensorimotor functioning and need nursing care during the pre-school period. During the school age period some further motor development may occur, and they may respond to minimal or limited training in self-help. During the adult years some motor and speech development may occur, and they may achieve very limited self-care and need nursing care.[2]

Merycism—*see* Rumination, psychogenic

Minimal brain dysfunction [MBD]—*see* Hyperkinetic syndrome of childhood

Misery and unhappiness disorder: An emotional disorder characteristic of childhood in which the main symptoms involve misery and unhappiness. There may also be eating and sleep disturbances.[1]

Mood swings (brief compensatory) (rebound): Mild disorders of mood (depression and anxiety or elation and excitement, occurring alternatingly or episodically) seen in affective psychosis.[1]

Motor tic disorders—*see* Tics

Motor-verbal tic disorder—*see* Gilles de la Tourette's disorder under Tics

Multi-infarct dementia or psychosis—*see* Arteriosclerotic dementia

Multiple operations syndrome—*see* Munchausen syndrome

Multiple personality: A form of dissociative hysteria in which there is the domination of the individual at any one time by one of two or more distinct personalities. Each personality is a full-integrated and complex unit with memories, behavior patterns, and social friendships which determine the nature of the individual's acts when uppermost in consciousness.[2]

Munchausen syndrome: A chronic form of factitious illness in which the individual demonstrates a plausible presentation of voluntarily produced physical symptomatology of such a degree that he is able to obtain and sustain multiple hospitalizations.[2]

Narcissistic personality—*see* Personality disorder, narcissistic type

Nervous debility—*see* neurasthenia under Neurotic disorders

Neurasthenia—*see* neurasthenia under Neurotic disorders

Neurotic delinquency—*see* mixed disturbance of conduct and emotions under Conduct disorders

Neurotic disorders: Neurotic disorders are mental disorders without any demonstrable organic basis in which the individual may have considerable insight and has unimpaired reality testing, in that he usually does not confuse his morbid subjective experiences and fantasies with external reality. Behavior may be greatly affected although usually remaining within socially acceptable limits, but personality is not disorganized. The principal manifestations include excessive anxiety, hysterical symptoms, phobias, obsessional and compulsive symptoms, and depression.[1]

    anxiety states: Various combinations of physical and mental manifestations of anxiety, not attributable to real danger and occurring either in attacks [*see* Anxiety state, panic attacks] or as a persisting state [*see* Anxiety state, generalized]. The anxiety is usually diffuse and may extend to panic. Other neurotic features such as obsessional or hysterical symptoms may be present but do not dominate the clinical picture.[1]

    compensation neurosis: Certain unconscious neurotic reactions in which features of secondary gain, such as a situational or financial advantage, are prominent.[3]

    depersonalization: A neurotic disorder with an unpleasant state of disturbed perception in which external objects or parts of one's own body are experienced as changed in their quality, unreal, remote, or automatized. The patient is aware of the subjective nature of the change he experiences. If depersonalization occurs as a feature of anxiety, schizophrenia, or other mental disorder, the condition is classified according to the major psychiatric disorder.[1]

    depression: A neurotic disorder characterized by disproportionate depression which has usually recognizably ensued on a distressing experience; it does not include among its features delusions or hallucinations, and there is often preoccupation with the psychic trauma which preceded the illness, e.g., loss of a cherished person or possession. Anxiety is also frequently present and mixed states of anxiety and depression should be included here. The distinction between depressive neurosis and psychosis should be made not only upon the degree of depression but also on the presence or absence of other neurotic and psychotic characteristics, and upon the degree of disturbance of the individual's behavior.[1]

    hypochondriasis: A neurotic disorder in which the conspicuous features are excessive concern with one's health in general or the integrity and functioning of some part of one's body, or less frequently, one's mind. It is usually associated with anxiety and depression. It may occur as a feature of some other severe mental disorder (e.g., manic-depressive psychosis, depressed type, schizophrenia, hysteria) and in that case should be classified according to the corresponding major disorder.[1]

    hysteria: A neurotic mental disorder in which motives, of which the patient seems unaware, produce either a restriction of the field of consciousness or disturbances of motor or sensory function which may seem to have psychological advantage or symbolic value.[1] There are three subtypes:

conversion type: The chief or only symptoms of the hysterical neurosis consist of psychogenic disturbance of function in some part of the body, e.g., paralysis, tremor, blindness, deafness, seizures.[1]

dissociative type: The most prominent feature of the hysterical neurosis is a narrowing of the field of consciousness which seems to serve an unconscious purpose and is commonly accompanied or followed by a selective amnesia. There may be dramatic but essentially superficial changes of personality [multiple personality], or sometimes the patient enters into a wandering state [fugue].[1]

factitious illness: Physical or psychological symptoms that are not real, genuine, or natural, which are produced by the individual and are under his voluntary control.[2]

neurasthenia: A neurotic disorder characterized by fatigue, irritability, headache, depression, insomnia, difficulty in concentration, and lack of capacity for enjoyment [anhedonia]. It may follow or accompany an infection or exhaustion, or arise from continued emotional stress. If neurasthenia is associated with a physical disorder, the latter should also be recorded as a diagnosis.[1]

obsessive-compulsive: States in which the outstanding symptom is a feeling of subjective compulsion, which must be resisted, to carry out some action, to dwell on an idea, to recall an experience, or to ruminate on an abstract topic. Unwanted thoughts which intrude, the insistency of words or ideas, ruminations or trains of thought are perceived by the individual to be inappropriate or nonsensical. The obsessional urge or idea is recognized as alien to the personality but as coming from within the self. Obsessional actions may be quasi-ritual performances designed to relieve anxiety, e.g., washing the hands to cope with contamination. Attempts to dispel the unwelcome thought or urges may lead to a severe inner struggle, with intense anxiety.[1]

occupational: A neurosis characterized by a functional disorder of a group of muscles used chiefly in one's occupation, marked by the occurrence of spasm, paresis, or incoordination on attempt to repeat the habitual movements (e.g., writers' cramp).[5]

phobic disorders: Neurotic states with abnormally intense dread of certain objects or specific situations which would not normally have that effect. If the anxiety tends to spread from a specified situation or object to a wider range of circumstances, it becomes akin to or identical with anxiety state and should be classified as such.[1] *See also* Phobia.

somatization disorder: A chronic, but fluctuating, neurotic disorder which begins early in life and is characterized by recurrent and multiple somatic complaints for which medical attention is sought but which are not apparently due to any physical illness. Complaints are presented in a dramatic, vague, or exaggerated way, or are part of a complicated medical history in which often many specific diagnoses have allegedly been made by other physicians. Complaints invariably refer to many organ systems (headache, fatigue, palpitations, fainting, nausea and vomiting, abdominal pains, bowel trouble, allergies, menstrual and sexual difficulties), and the individual frequently receives medical care from a number of physicians, sometimes simultaneously.[2]

Neurosis—*see* Neurotic disorders

Nightmares: Anxiety attacks occurring in dreams during REM sleep.[2]

Night terrors: A pathology of arousal from stage 4 sleep in which the individual experiences excessive terror and extreme panic (screaming, verbalizations), symptoms of autonomic activity, confusion, and poor recall for event.[2]

Nymphomania: Abnormal and excessive need or desire in the woman for sexual intercourse.[3]

Obsessional personality—*see* Personality disorder, compulsive type

Occupational neurosis—*see* Neurotic disorder, occupational

Oneirophrenia—*see* Schizophrenia, acute episode

Oppositional disorder of childhood or adolescence: A disorder characterized by pervasive opposition to all in authority regardless of self-interest, a continuous argumentativeness, and an unwillingness to respond to reasonable persuasion, not accounted for by a conduct disorder, adjustment disorder, or a psychosis of childhood. The oppositional behavior in this disorder is evoked by any demand, rule, suggestion, request, or admonishment placed on the individual.[2]

Organic affective syndrome: A clinical picture in which the predominating symptoms closely resemble those seen in either the depressive or manic affective disorders, occurring in the presence of evidence or history of a specific organic factor which is etiologically related to the disturbance, such as head trauma, endocranial tumors, and exocranial tumors secreting neurotoxic diatheses (e.g., pancreatic carcinoma). Excessive use of steroids, Cushing's syndrome, and other endocrine disorders may lead to an organic affective syndrome.[2]

Organic personality syndrome: Chronic, mild states of memory disturbance and intellectual deterioration, of nonpsychotic nature, often accompanied by increased irritability, querulousness, lassitude, and complaints of physical weakness. These states are often associated with old age, and may precede more severe states due to brain damage classifiable under senile or presenile dementia, dementia associated with other chronic organic psychotic brain syndromes, or delirium, delusions, hallucinosis, and depression in transient organic psychotic conditions.[1]

Organic psychosyndrome, focal (partial): A nonpsychotic organic mental disorder resembling the postconcussion syndrome associated with localized diseases of the brain or surrounding tissues.[1]

Organic psychotic conditions: Syndromes in which there is impairment of orientation, memory, comprehension, calculation, learning capacity, and judgment. These are the essential features but there may also be shallowness or lability of affect, or a more persistent disturbance of mood, lowering of ethical standards and exaggeration or emergence of personality traits, and diminished capacity for independent decision.[1] See also Alcohol psychoses, Arteriosclerotic dementia, Drug psychoses, Presenile dementia, and Senile dementia.

> **mixed paranoid and affective:** Organic psychosis in which depressive and paranoid symptoms are the main features.[1]

> **transient:** States characterized by clouded consciousness, confusion, disorientation, illusions, and often vivid hallucinations. They are usually due to some intra- or extracerebral toxic, infectious, metabolic or other systemic disturbance and are generally reversible. Depressive and paranoid symptoms may also be present but are not the main feature. The diagnosis of the associated physical or neurological condition should also be recorded.[1]

> > **acute delirium:** Short-lived states, lasting hours or days, of the above type.[1]

> > **subacute delirium:** States of the above type in which the symptoms, usually less florid, last for several weeks or longer during which they may show marked fluctuations in intensity.[1]

Organic reaction—*see* Organic psychotic conditions, transient

Overanxious disorder: An ill-defined emotional disorder characteristic of childhood in which the main symptoms involve anxiety and fearfulness.[1]

Panic disorder—*see* panic attack under Anxiety state

Paranoia: A rare chronic psychosis in which logically constructed systematized delusions have developed gradually without concomitant hallucinations or the schizophrenic type of disordered thinking. The delusions are mostly of grandeur (the paranoiac prophet or inventor), persecution, or somatic abnormality.[1]

> **alcoholic**—*see* alcoholic jealousy under Alcoholic psychoses

> **querulans:** A paranoid state which, though in many ways akin to schizophrenic or affective states, differs from other paranoid states and psychogenic paranoid psychosis.[1]

> **senile**—*see* Paraphrenia

Paranoid personality—*see* Personality disorder, paranoid type

Paranoid reaction, acute: Paranoid states apparently provoked by some emotional stress. The stress is often misconstrued as an attack or threat. Such states are particularly prone to occur in prisoners or as acute reactions to a strange and threatening environment, e.g., in immigrants.[1]

Paranoid schizophrenia—*see* Schizophrenia, paranoid type

Paranoid state

> **involutional**—*see* Paraphrenia

> **senile**—*see* Paraphrenia

> **simple:** A psychosis, acute or chronic, not classifiable as schizophrenia or affective psychosis, in which delusions, especially of being influenced, persecuted, or treated in some special way, are the main symptoms. The delusions are of a fairly fixed, elaborate, and systematized kind.[1]

Paranoid traits—*see* Personality disorder, paranoid type

Paraphilia—*see* Sexual deviations

Paraphrenia: Paranoid psychosis in which there are conspicuous hallucinations, often in several modalities. Affective symptoms and disordered thinking, if present, do not dominate the clinical picture, and the personality is well preserved.[1]

Paraphrenic schizophrenia—*see* Schizophrenia, paranoid type

Passive-aggressive personality — *see* Personality disorder, passive- aggressive type

Passive personality—*see* Personality disorder, dependent type

Pathological

> **alcohol intoxication**—*see* Alcohol intoxication, idiosyncratic

> **drug intoxication:** Individual idiosyncratic reactions to comparatively small quantities of a drug, which take the form of acute, brief psychotic states of any type.[1]

> **drunkenness**—*see* Alcohol intoxication, idiosyncratic

> **gambling:** A disorder of impulse control characterized by a chronic and progressive preoccupation with gambling and urge to gamble, with subsequent gambling behavior that compromises, disrupts, or damages personal, family, and vocational pursuits.[2]

> **personality**—*see* Personality disorder

Pedophilia: Sexual deviations in which an adult engages in sexual activity with a child of the same or opposite sex.[1]

Peregrinating patient—*see* Malingering

Personality disorders: Deeply ingrained maladaptive patterns of behavior generally recognizable by the time of adolescence or earlier and continuing throughout most of adult life, although often becoming less obvious in middle or old age. The personality is abnormal either in the balance of its components, their quality and expression, or in its total aspect. Because of this deviation or psychopathy the patient suffers or others have to suffer, and there is an adverse effect upon the individual or on society. It includes what is sometimes called psychopathic personality, but if this is determined primarily by malfunctioning of the brain, it should be classified as one of the nonpsychotic organic brain syndromes. When the patient exhibits an anomaly of personality directly related to his neurosis or psychosis, e.g., schizoid personality and schizophrenia or anancastic personality and obsessive compulsive neurosis, the relevant neurosis or psychosis which is in evidence should be diagnosed in addition.[1]

    affective type: A chronic personality disorder characterized by lifelong predominance of a pronounced mood. The illness does not have a clear onset, and there may be intermittent periods of disturbed mood separated by periods of normal mood.[1]

    anancastic [anankastic] type—*see* Personality disorder, compulsive type

    antisocial type: A personality disorder characterized by disregard for social obligations, lack of feeling for others, and impetuous violence or callous unconcern. There is a gross disparity between behavior and the prevailing social norms. Behavior is not readily modifiable by experience, including punishment. People with this personality are often affectively cold, and may be abnormally aggressive or irresponsible. Their tolerance to frustration is low; they blame others or offer plausible rationalizations for the behavior which brings them into conflict with society.[1]

    asthenic type—*see* Personality disorder, dependent type

    avoidant type: Individuals with this disorder exhibit excessive social inhibitions and shyness, a tendency to withdraw from opportunities for developing close relationships, and a fearful expectation that they will be belittled and humiliated. Desires for affection and acceptance are strong, but they are unwilling to enter relationships unless given unusually strong guarantees that they will be uncritically accepted. Therefore, they have few close relationships and suffer from feelings of loneliness and isolation.[2]

    borderline type: Individuals with this disorder are characterized by instability in a variety of areas, including interpersonal relationships, behavior, mood, and self image. Interpersonal relationships are often intense and unstable with marked shifts of attitude over time. Frequently there is impulsive and unpredictable behavior which is potentially physically self-damaging. There may be problems tolerating being alone, and chronic feelings of emptiness or boredom.[2]

    chronic depressive type: An affective personality disorder characterized by lifelong predominance of a chronic nonpsychotic disturbance involving either intermittent or sustained periods of depressed mood (marked by worry, pessimism, low output of energy, and a sense of futility).[2]

    chronic hypomanic type: An affective personality disorder characterized by lifelong predominance of a chronic nonpsychotic disturbance involving either intermittent or sustained periods of abnormally elevated mood (unshakable optimism and an enhanced zest for life and activity).[2]

    compulsive type: A personality disorder characterized by feelings of personal insecurity, doubt, and incompleteness leading to excessive conscientiousness, checking, stubbornness, and caution. There may be insistent and unwelcome thoughts or impulses which do not attain the severity of an obsessional neurosis. There is perfectionism and meticulous accuracy and a need to check repeatedly in an attempt to ensure this. Rigidity and excessive doubt may be conspicuous.[1]

    cyclothymic type: A chronic nonpsychotic disturbance involving depressed and elevated mood, lasting at least two years, separated by periods of normal mood.[2]

    dependent type: A personality disorder characterized by passive compliance with the wishes of elders and others and a weak inadequate response to the demands of daily life. Lack of vigor may show itself in the intellectual or emotional spheres; there is little capacity for enjoyment.[1]

    eccentric type: A personality disorder characterized by oddities of behavior which do not conform to the clinical syndromes of personality disorders described elsewhere.[2]

    explosive type: A personality disorder characterized by instability of mood with liability to intemperate outbursts of anger, hate, violence, or affection. Aggression may be expressed in words or in physical violence. The outbursts cannot readily be controlled by the affected persons, who are not otherwise prone to antisocial behavior.[1]

    histrionic type: A personality disorder characterized by shallow, labile affectivity, dependence on others, craving for appreciation and attention, suggestibility, and theatricality. There is often sexual immaturity, e.g., frigidity and over-responsiveness to stimuli. Under stress hysterical symptoms [neurosis] may develop.[1]

    hysterical type—*see* Personality disorder, histrionic type

    inadequate type—*see* Personality disorder, dependent type

introverted type: A form of schizoid personality in which the essential features are a profound defect in the ability to form social relationships and to respond to the usual forms of social reinforcements. Such patients are characteristically "loners" who do not appear distressed by their social distance and are not interested in greater social involvements.[2]

masochistic type: A personality disorder in which the individual appears to arrange life situations so as to be defeated and humiliated.[2]

narcissistic type: A personality disorder in which interpersonal difficulties are caused by an inflated sense of self-worth, and indifference to the welfare of others. Achievement deficits and social irresponsibilities are justified and sustained by a boastful arrogance, expansive fantasies, facile rationalization, and frank prevarication.[2]

paranoid type: A personality disorder in which there is excessive sensitiveness to setbacks or to what are taken to be humiliations and rebuffs, a tendency to distort experience by misconstruing the neutral or friendly actions of others as hostile or contemptuous, and a combative and tenacious sense of personal rights. There may be a proneness to jealousy or excessive self-importance. Such persons may feel helplessly humiliated and put upon; others, likewise excessively sensitive, are aggressive and insistent. In all cases there is excessive self-reference.[1]

passive-aggressive type: A personality disorder characterized by aggressive behavior manifested in passive ways, such as obstructionism, pouting, procrastination, intentional inefficiency, or stubbornness. The *aggression* often arises from resentment at failing to find gratification in a relationship with an individual or institution upon which the individual is overdependent.[3]

passive type—*see* Personality disorder, dependent type

schizoid type: A personality disorder in which there is withdrawal from affectional, social, and other contacts with autistic preference for fantasy and introspective reserve. Behavior may be slightly eccentric or indicate avoidance of competitive situations. Apparent coolness and detachment may mask an incapacity to express feeling.

schizotypal type: A form of schizoid personality in which individuals with this disorder manifest various oddities of thinking, perception, communication, and behavior. The disturbance in thinking may be expressed as magical thinking, ideas of reference, or paranoid ideation. Perceptual disturbances may include recurrent illusions and derealization [depersonalization]. Frequently, but not invariably, the behavioral manifestations include social isolation and constricted or inappropriate affect which interferes with rapport in face-to-face interaction without any of the frank psychotic features which characterize schizophrenia.[2]

Phobia: Neurotic states with abnormally intense dread of certain objects or specific situations which would not normally have that effect. If the anxiety tends to spread from a specified situation or object to a wider range of circumstances, it becomes akin to or identical with anxiety state, and should be classified as such.[1]

acrophobia: Fear of heights[3]

agoraphobia: fear of leaving the familiar setting of the home, and is almost always preceded by a phase during which there are recurrent panic attacks. Because of the anticipatory fear of helplessness when having a panic attack, the patient is reluctant or refuses to be alone, travel or walk alone, or to be in situations where there is no ready access to help, such as in crowds, closed or open spaces, or crowded stores.[2]

ailurophobia: Fear of cats[3]

algophobia: Fear of pain[3]

claustrophobia: Fear of closed spaces[3]

isolated phobia—*see* simple phobia below

mysophobia: Fear of dirt or germs[3]

obsessional—*see* Neurotic disorder, obsessive-compulsive

panphobia: Fear of everything[3]

simple phobia: Fear of a discrete object or situation which is neither fear of leaving the familiar setting of the home [agoraphobia], or of being observed by others in certain situations [social phobia]. Examples of simple phobia are fear of animals, acrophobia, and claustrophobia.

social phobia: Fear of situations in which the subject is exposed to possible scrutiny by others, and the possibility exists that he may act in a fashion that will be considered shameful. The most common social phobias are fears of public speaking, blushing, eating in public, writing in front of others, or using public lavatories.[2]

xenophobia: Fear of strangers[3]

Pica: Perverted appetite of nonorganic origin in which there is persistent eating of non-nutritional substances. Typically, infants ingest paint, plaster, string, hair, or cloth. Older children may have access to animal droppings, sand, bugs, leaves, or pebbles. In the adult, eating of starch or clay-earth has been observed.[2]

Postconcussion syndrome: States occurring after generalized contusion of the brain, in which the symptom picture may resemble that of the frontal lobe syndrome or that of any of the neurotic disorders, but in which in addition, headache, giddiness, fatigue, insomnia, and a subjective feeling of impaired intellectual ability are usually prominent. Mood may fluctuate, and quite ordinary stress may produce exaggerated fear and apprehension. There may be marked intolerance of mental and physical exertion, undue sensitivity to noise, and hypochondriacal preoccupation. The symptoms are more common in persons who have previously suffered from neurotic or personality disorders, or when there is a possibility of compensation. This syndrome is particularly associated with the closed type of head injury when signs of localized brain damage are slight or absent, but it may also occur in other conditions.[1]

Postcontusion syndrome or encephalopathy—*see* Postconcussion syndrome

Postencephalitic syndrome: A nonpsychotic organic mental disorder resembling the postconcussion syndrome associated with central nervous system infections.[1]

Postleucotomy syndrome—*see* Frontal lobe syndrome

Posttraumatic brain syndrome, nonpsychotic—*see* Postconcussion syndrome

Posttraumatic organic psychosis—*see* Organic psychotic conditions, transient

Posttraumatic stress disorder: The development of characteristic symptoms (re-experiencing the traumatic event, numbing of responsiveness to or involvement with the external world, and a variety of other autonomic, dysphoric, or cognitive symptoms) after experiencing a psychologically traumatic event or events outside the normal range of human experience (e.g., rape or assault, military combat, natural catastrophes such as flood or earthquake, or other disaster, such as airplane crash, fires, bombings).[2]

    acute: Brief, episodic, or recurrent disorders lasting less than six months' duration after the onset of trauma.[2]

    prolonged: Chronic disorders of the above type lasting six months or more following the trauma.[2]

Premature ejaculation—*see* premature ejaculation under Psychosexual dysfunction.

Prepsychotic schizophrenia—*see* Schizophrenia, latent

Presbyophrenia—*see* Organic personality syndrome

Presenile dementia: Dementia occuring usually before the age of 65 in patients with the relatively rare forms of diffuse or lobar cerebral atrophy. The associated neurological condition (e.g., Alzheimer's disease, Pick's disease, Jakob-Creutzfeldt disease) should also be recorded as a diagnosis.[1]

Prodromal schizophrenia—*see* Schizophrenia, latent

Pseudoneurotic schizophrenia—*see* Schizophrenia, latent

Psychalgia: Pains of mental origin, e.g., headache or backache, for which a more precise medical or psychiatric diagnosis cannot be made.[1]

Psychasthenia: A functional neurosis marked by stages of pathological fear or anxiety, obsessions, fixed ideas, tics, feelings of inadequacy, self-accusation, and peculiar feelings of strangeness, unreality, and depersonalization.[4]

Psychic shock: A sudden disturbance of mental equilibrium produced by strong emotion in response to physical or mental stress.[4]

Psychic factors associated with physical diseases: Mental disturbances or psychic factors of any type thought to have played a major part in the etiology of physical conditions, usually involving tissue damage, classified elsewhere. The mental disturbance is usually mild and nonspecific, and the psychic factors (worry, fear, conflict, etc.) may be present without any overt psychiatric disorder. Examples of these conditions are asthma, dermatitis, eczema, duodenal ulcer, ulcerative colitis, and urticaria, specified as due to psychogenic factors.
Use an additional diagnosis to identify the physical condition. In the rare instance that an overt psychiatric disorder is thought to have caused the physical condition, the psychiatric diagnosis should be recorded in addition.[1]

Psychoneurosis—*see* Neurotic disorders

Psycho-organic syndrome—*see* Organic psychotic conditions, transient

Psychopathic constitutional state—*see* Personality disorders

Psychopathic personality—*see* Personality disorders

Psychophysiological disorders: A variety of physical symptoms or types of physiological malfunctions of mental origin, not involving tissue damage, and usually mediated through the autonomic nervous system. The disorders are classified according to the body system involved. If the physical symptom is secondary to a psychiatric disorder classifiable elsewhere, the physical symptom is not classified as a psychophysiological disorder. If tissue damage is involved, then the diagnosis is classified as a *Psychic factor associated with diseases classified elsewhere.*[1]

Psychosexual dysfunctions: A group of disorders in which there is recurrent and persistent dysfunction encountered during sexual activity. The dysfunction may be lifelong or acquired, generalized or situational, and total or partial.[2]

functional dyspareunia: Recurrent and persistent genital pain associated with coitus.[2]

functional vaginismus: A history of recurrent and persistent involuntary spasm of the musculature of the outer one-third of the vagina that interferes with sexual activity.[2]

inhibited female orgasm: Recurrent and persistent inhibition of the female orgasm as manifested by a delay or absence of orgasm following a normal sexual excitement phase during sexual activity.[2]

inhibited male orgasm: Recurrent and persistent inhibition of the male orgasm as manifested by a delay or absence of either the emission or ejaculation phases, or more usually, both following an adequate phase of sexual excitement.[2]

inhibited sexual desire: Persistent inhibition of desire for engaging in a particular form of sexual activity.[2]

inhibited sexual excitement: Recurrent and persistent inhibition of sexual excitement during sexual activity, manifested either by partial or complete failure to attain or maintain erection until completion of the sexual act [impotence], or partial or complete failure to attain or maintain the lubrication-swelling response of sexual excitement until completion of the sexual act [frigidity].[2]

premature ejaculation: Ejaculation occurs before the individual wishes it, because of recurrent and persistent absence of reasonable voluntary control of ejaculation and orgasm during sexual activity.[2]

Psychosexual gender identity disorders: Behavior occurring in preadolescents of immature psychosexuality, or in adults, in which there is an incongruence between the individual's anatomic sex and gender identity.[2]

gender identity disorder: In children or in adults a condition in which the individual would prefer to be of the other sex, and strongly prefers the clothes, toys, activities, and companionship of the other sex. Cross-dressing is intermittent, although it may be frequent. In children the commonest form is feminism in boys.[2]

trans-sexualism: A psychosexual identity disorder centered around fixed beliefs that the overt bodily sex is wrong. The resulting behavior is directed towards either changing the sexual organs by operation, or completely concealing the bodily sex by adopting both the dress and behavior of the opposite sex.[1]

Psychosomatic disorders—*see* Psychophysiological disorders

Psychosis: Mental disorders in which impairment of mental function has developed to a degree that interferes grossly with insight, ability to meet some ordinary demands of life or to maintain adequate contact with reality. It is not an exact or well defined term. Mental retardation is excluded.[1]

affective—*see* Affective psychoses

alcoholic—*see* Alcoholic psychoses

atypical childhood: A variety of atypical infantile psychoses which may show some, but not all, of the features of infantile autism. Symptoms may include stereotyped repetitive movements, hyperkinesis, self-injury, retarded speech development, echolalia, and impaired social relationships. Such disorders may occur in children of any level of intelligence but are particularly common in those with mental retardation.[1]

borderline, of childhood—*see* Psychosis, atypical childhood

child: A group of disorders in children, characterized by distortions in the timing, rate, and sequence of many psychological functions involving language development and social relations in which the severe qualitative abnormalities are not normal for any stage of development.[2] See also Autism, infantile, Psychosis, disintegrative, Psychosis, atypical childhood.

depressive—*see* Affective psychosis, depressed type

depressive type: A depressive psychosis which can be similar in its symptoms to manic-depressive psychosis, depressed type but is apparently provoked by saddening stress such as a bereavement, or a severe disappointment or frustration. There may be less diurnal variation of symptoms than in manic-depressive psychosis, depressed type, and the delusions are more often understandable in the context of the life experiences. There is usually a serious disturbance of behavior, e.g., major suicidal attempt.[1]

disintegrative: A disorder in which normal or near-normal development for the first few years is followed by a loss of social skills and of speech, together with a severe disorder of emotions, behavior, and relationships. Usually this loss of speech and of social competence takes place over a period of a few months and is accompanied by the emergence of overactivity and of stereotypies. In most cases there is intellectual impairment, but this is not a necessary part of the disorder. The condition may follow overt brain disease, such as measles encephalitis, but it may also occur in the absence of any known organic brain disease or damage. Any associated neurological disorder should also be recorded.[1]

epileptic: An organic psychotic condition associated with epilepsy.[1]

excitative type: An affective psychosis similar in its symptoms to manic-depressive psychosis, manic type, but apparently provoked by emotional stress.[1]

hypomanic—*see* Affective psychosis, manic type

hysterical—*see* Psychosis, reactive

    acute—*see* Psychosis, excitative type

induced—*see* Shared paranoid disorder

infantile—*see* Autism, infantile

infective—*see* Organic psychotic conditions, transient

Korsakoff's:

    alcoholic—*see* alcohol amnestic syndrome under Alcoholic psychoses

    nonalcoholic—*see* Amnestic syndrome

manic-depressive—*see* Affective psychoses

multi-infarct—*see* Arteriosclerotic dementia

paranoid

    chronic—*see* Paranoia

    protracted reactive—*see* Psychosis, paranoid, psychogenic

    psychogenic: Psychogenic or reactive paranoid psychosis of any type which is more protracted than the reactions described under paranoid reaction, acute.[1]
        acute—*see* Paranoid reaction, acute

postpartum—*see* Psychosis, puerperal

psychogenic—*see* Psychosis, reactive

    depressive—*see* Psychosis, depressive type

puerperal: Any psychosis occurring within a fixed period (approximately 90 days) after childbirth.[3] The diagnosis should be classified according to the predominant symptoms or characteristics, such as schizophrenia, affective psychosis, paranoid states, or other specified psychosis.

reactive: A psychotic condition which is largely or entirely attributable to a recent life experience. This diagnosis is not used for the wider range of psychoses in which environmental factors play some, but not the *major,* part in etiology.[1]

    brief: A florid psychosis of at least a few hours' duration but lasting no more than two weeks, with sudden onset immediately following a severe environmental stress and eventually terminating in complete recovery to the pre-psychotic state.[2]

    confusion: Mental disorders with clouded consciousness, disorientation (though less marked than in organic confusion), and diminished accessibility often accompanied by excessive activity and apparently provoked by emotional stress.[1]

    depressive—*see* Psychosis, depressive type

schizo-affective—*see* Schizophrenia, schizo-affective type

schizophrenic—*see* Schizophrenia

schizophreniform—*see* Schizophrenia

    affective type—*See* Schizophrenia, schizo-affective type

    confusional type—*see* Schizophrenia, acute episode

senile—*see* Senile dementia, delusional type

Pyromania: A disorder of impulse control characterized by a recurrent failure to resist impulses to set fires without regard for the consequences, or with deliberate destructive intent. Invariably there is intense fascination with the setting of fires, seeing fires burn, and a satisfaction with the resultant destruction.[2]

Relationship problems of childhood: Emotional disorders characteristic of childhood in which the main symptoms involve relationship problems.[1]

Repeated infarct dementia—*see* Arteriosclerotic dementia

Residual schizophrenia—*.see* Schizophrenia, residual type

Restzustand (schizophrenia)—*see* Schizophrenia, residual type

Rumination:

    obsessional: The constant preoccupation with certain thoughts, with inability to dismiss them from the mind.[4] *see* Neurotic disorder, obsessive-compulsive.

    psychogenic: In children the regurgitation of food, with failure to thrive or weight loss developing after a period of normal functioning. Food is brought up without nausea, retching, or disgust. The food is then ejected from the mouth, or chewed and reswallowed.[2]

Sander's disease—*see* Paranoia

Satyriasis: Pathologic or exaggerated sexual desire or excitement in the man.[3]

Schizoid personality disorder—*see* Personality disorder, schizoid type

Schizophrenia: A group of psychoses in which there is a fundamental disturbance of personality, a characteristic distortion of thinking, often a sense of being controlled by alien forces, delusions which may be bizarre, disturbed perception, abnormal affect out of keeping with the real situation, and autism. Nevertheless, clear consciousness and intellectual capacity are usually maintained. The disturbance of personality involves its most basic functions which give the normal person his feeling of individuality, uniqueness, and self-direction. The most intimate thoughts, feelings, and acts are often felt to be known to or shared by others and explanatory delusions may develop, to the effect that natural or supernatural forces are at work to influence the schizophrenic person's thoughts and actions in ways that are often bizarre. He may see himself as the pivot of all that happens. Hallucinations, especially of hearing, are common and may comment on the patient or address him. Perception is frequently disturbed in other ways; there may be perplexity, irrelevant features may become all-important and accompanied by passivity feeling, may lead the patient to believe that everyday objects and situations possess a special, usually sinister, meaning intended for him. In the characteristic schizophrenic disturbance of thinking, peripheral and irrelevant features of a total concept, which are inhibited in normal directed mental activity, are brought to the forefront and utilized in place of the elements relevant and appropriate to the situation. Thus, thinking becomes vague, elliptical and obscure, and its expression in speech sometimes incomprehensible. Breaks and interpolations in the flow of consecutive thought are frequent, and the patient may be convinced that his thoughts are being withdrawn by some outside agency. Mood may be shallow, capricious, or incongruous. Ambivalence and disturbance of volition may appear as inertia, negativism, or stupor. Catatonia may be present. The diagnosis "schizophrenia" should not be made unless there is, or has been evident during the same illness, characteristic disturbance of thought, perception, mood, conduct, or personality—preferably in at least two of these areas. The diagnosis should not be restricted to conditions running a protracted, deteriorating, or chronic course. In addition to making the diagnosis on the criteria just given, effort should be made to specify one of the following subtypes of schizophrenia, according to the predominant symptoms.[1]

acute (undifferentiated): Schizophrenia of florid nature which cannot be classified as simple, catatonic, hebephrenic, paranoid, or any other types.[1]

acute episode: Schizophrenic disorders, other than simple, hebephrenic, catatonic, and paranoid, in which there is a dream-like state with slight clouding of consciousness and perplexity. External things, people, and events may become charged with personal significance for the patient. There may be ideas of reference and emotional turmoil. In many such cases remission occurs within a few weeks or months, even without treatment.[1]

atypical—*see* Schizophrenia, acute (undifferentiated)

borderline—*see* Schizophrenia, latent

catatonic type: Includes as an essential feature prominent psychomotor disturbances often alternating between extremes such as hyperkinesis and stupor, or automatic obedience and negativism. Constrained attitudes may be maintained for long periods: if the patient's limbs are put in some unnatural position they may be held there for some time after the external force has been removed. Severe excitement may be a striking feature of the condition. Depressive or hypomanic concomitants may be present.[1]

cenesthopathic—*see* Schizophrenia, acute (undifferentiated)

childhood type—*see* Psychosis, child

chronic undifferentiated—*see* Schizophrenia, residual

cyclic—*see* Schizophrenia, schizo-affective type

disorganized type: A form of schizophrenia in which affective changes are prominent, delusions and hallucinations fleeting and fragmentary, behavior irresponsible and unpredictable, and mannerisms common. The mood is shallow and inappropriate, accompanied by giggling or self-satisfied, self—absorbed smiling, or by a lofty manner, grimaces, mannerisms, pranks, hypochondriacal complaints, and reiterated phrases. Thought is disorganized. There is a tendency to remain solitary, and behavior seems empty of purpose and feeling. This form of schizophrenia usually starts between the ages of 15 and 25 years.[1]

hebephrenic type:—*see* Schizophrenia, disorganized type

latent: It has not been possible to produce a generally acceptable description for this condition. It is not recommended for general use, but a description is provided for those who believe it to be useful: a condition of eccentric or inconsequent behavior and anomalies of affect which give the impression of schizophrenia though no definite and characteristic schizophrenic anomalies, present or past, have been manifest.[1]

paranoid type: The form of schizophrenia in which relatively stable delusions, which may be accompanied by hallucinations, dominate the clinical picture. The delusions are frequently of persecution, but may take other forms (for example, of jealousy, exalted birth, Messianic mission, or bodily change). Hallucinations and erratic behavior may occur; in some cases conduct is seriously disturbed from the outset, thought disorder may be gross, and affective flattening with fragmentary delusions and hallucinations may develop.[1]

prepsychotic—*see* Schizophrenia, latent

prodromal—*see* Schizophrenia, latent

pseudoneurotic—*see* Schizophrenia, latent

residual: A chronic form of schizophrenia in which the symptoms that persist from the acute phase have mostly lost their sharpness. Emotional response is blunted and thought disorder, even when gross, does not prevent the accomplishment of routine work.[1]

schizo-affective type: A psychosis in which pronounced manic or depressive features are intermingled with schizophrenic features and which tends towards remission without permanent defect, but which is prone to recur. The diagnosis should be made only when both the affective and schizophrenic symptoms are pronounced.[1]

simple type: A psychosis in which there is insidious development of oddities of conduct, inability to meet the demands of society, and decline in total performance. Delusions and hallucinations are not in evidence and the condition is less obviously psychotic than are the hebephrenic, catatonic, and paranoid types of schizophrenia. With increasing social impoverishment vagrancy may ensue and the patient becomes self-absorbed, idle, and aimless. Because the schizophrenic symptoms are not clear-cut, diagnosis of this form should be made sparingly, if at all.[1]

simplex—*see* Schizophrenia, simple type

Schizophrenic syndrome of childhood—*see* Psychosis, child

Schizophreniform

attack—*see* Schizophrenia, acute episode

disorder—*see* Schizophrenia, acute episode

psychosis—*see* Schizophrenia

affective type—*see* Schizophrenia, schizo-affective type

confusional type—*see* Schizophrenia, acute episode

Schizotypal personality—Dementia occurring usually after the age of 65 in which any cerebral pathology other than that of senile atrophic change can be reasonably excluded.[1]

delirium: Senile dementia with a superimposed reversible episode of acute confusional state.[1]

delusional type: A type of senile dementia characterized by development in advanced old age, progressive in nature, in which delusions, varying from simple poorly formed paranoid delusions to highly formed paranoid delusional states, and hallucinations are also present.[1,2]

depressed type: A type of senile dementia characterized by development in advanced old age, progressive in nature, in which depressive features, ranging from mild to severe forms of manic-depressive affective psychosis, are also present. Disturbance of the sleep-waking cycle and preoccupation with dead people are often particularly prominent.[1,2]

paranoid type—*see* Senile dementia, delusional type

simple type—*see* Senile dementia

Sensitiver Beziehungswahn: A paranoid state which, though in many ways akin to schizophrenic or affective states, differs from paranoia, simple paranoid state, shared paranoid disorder, or psychogenic psychosis.[1]

Sensitivity reaction of childhood or adolescence—*see* Shyness disorder of childhood

Separation anxiety disorder: A clinical disorder in children in which the predominant disturbance is exaggerated distress at separation from parents, home, or other familial surroundings. When separation is instituted, the child may experience anxiety to the point of panic. In adults a similar disorder is seen in agoraphobic reactions.[2]

Sexual deviations: Abnormal sexual inclinations or behavior which are part of a referral problem. The limits and features of normal sexual behavior have not been stated absolutely in different societies and cultures, but are broadly such as serve approved social and biological purposes. The sexual activity of affected persons is directed primarily either towards people not of the opposite sex, or towards sexual acts not associated with coitus normally, or towards coitus performed under abnormal circumstances. If the anomalous behavior becomes manifest only during psychosis or other mental illness the condition should be classified under the major illness. It is common for more than one anomaly to occur together in the same individual; in that case the predominant deviation is classified. It is preferable not to diagnose sexual deviation in individuals who perform deviant sexual acts when normal sexual outlets are not available to them.[1] *see also* exhibitionism, Fetishism, Homosexuality, Nymphomania, Pedophilia, Satyriasis, Sexual masochism, Sexual sadism, Transvestism, Voyeurism, and Zoophilia.

Gender identity disorder and trans-sexualism are considered to be psychosexual gender identity disorders and are not included here.

Sexual masochism: A sexual deviation in which sexual arousal and pleasure is produced in an individual by his own physical or psychological suffering, and in which there are insistent and persistent fantasies wherein sexual excitement is produced as a result of suffering.[2]

Sexual sadism: A sexual deviation in which physical or psychological suffering inflicted on another person is utilized as a method of stimulating erotic excitement and orgasm, and in which there are insistent and persistent fantasies wherein sexual excitement is produced as a result of suffering inflicted on the partner.[2]

Shared paranoid disorder: Mainly delusional psychosis, usually chronic and often without florid features, which appears to have developed as a result of a close, if not dependent, relationship with another person who already has an established similar psychosis. The delusions are at least partly shared. The rare cases in which several persons are affected should also be included here.[1]

Shifting sleep-work schedule: A sleep disorder in which the phase- shift disruption of the 24-hour sleep-wake cycle occurs due to rapid changes in the individual's work schedule.[2]

Short sleeper: Individuals who typically need only 4-6 hours of sleep within the 24-hour cycle.[2]

Shyness disorder of childhood: A persistent and excessive shrinking from familiarity or contact with all strangers of sufficient severity as to interfere with peer functioning, yet there are warm and satisfying relationships with family members. A critical feature of this disorder is that the avoidant behavior with strangers persists even after prolonged exposure or contact.[2]

Sibling jealousy or rivalry: An emotional disorder related to competition between siblings for the love of a parent or for other recognition or gain.[3]

Simple phobia—*see* simple phobia under Phobia

Situational disturbance, acute—*see* Stress reaction, acute

Social phobia—*see* social phobia under Phobia

Social withdrawal of childhood—*see* Introverted disorder of childhood

Socialized conduct disorder—*see* socialized conduct disorder under Conduct disorders

Somatization disorder—*see* somatization disorder under Neurotic disorders

Somatoform disorder, atypical—*see* hypochondriasis under Neurotic disorders

Spasmus nutans—*see* Stereotyped repetitive movements

Specific academic or work inhibition: An adjustment reaction in which a specific academic or work inhibition occurs in an individual whose intellectual capacity, skills, and previous academic or work performance have been at least adequate, and in which the inhibition occurs despite apparent effort and is not due to any other mental disorder.[2]

Stammering—*see* Stuttering

Starch-eating—*see* Pica

Status postcommotio cerebri—*see* Postconcussion syndrome

Stereotyped repetitive movements: Disorders in which voluntary repetitive stereotyped movements, which are not due to any psychiatric or neurological condition, constitute the main feature. Includes head-banging, spasmus nutans, rocking, twirling, finger-flicking mannerisms, and eye poking. Such movements are particularly common in cases of mental retardation with sensory impairment or with environmental monotony.[1]

Stereotypies—*see* Stereotyped repetitive movements

Stress reaction

acute: Acute transient disorders of any severity and nature of emotions, consciousness, and psychomotor states (singly or in combination) which occur in individuals, without any apparent pre-existing mental disorder, in response to exceptional physical or mental stress, such as natural catastrophe or battle, and which usually subside within hours or days.[1]

chronic—*see* Adjustment reaction

Stupor

catatonic—*see* Schizophrenia, catatonic type

psychogenic—*see* Psychosis, reactive

Stuttering: Disorders in the rhythm of speech, in which the individual knows precisely what he wishes to say, but at the time is unable to say it because of an involuntary, repetitive prolongation or cessation of a sound.[1]

Subjective insomnia complaint: a complaint of insomnia made by the individual, which has not been investigated or proven.[2]

Systematized delusions—*see* Paranoia

Tension headache: Headache of mental origin for which a more precise medical or psychiatric diagnosis cannot be made.[1]

Tics: Disorders of no known organic origin in which the outstanding feature consists of quick, involuntary, apparently purposeless, and frequently repeated movements which are not due to any neurological condition. Any part of the body may be involved but the face is most frequently affected. Only one form of tic may be present, or there may be a combination of tics which are carried out simultaneously, alternatively, or consecutively.[1]

chronic motor tic disorder: A tic disorder starting in childhood and persisting into adult life. The tic is limited to no more than three motor areas, and rarely has a verbal component.[2]

Gilles de la Tourette's disorder [motor-verbal tic disorder]: a rare disorder occurring in individuals of any level of intelligence in which facial tics and tic-like throat noises become more marked and more generalized, and in which later whole words or short sentences (often with obscene content) are ejaculated spasmodically and involuntarily. There is some overlap with other varieties of tic.[1]

transient tic disorder of childhood: Facial or other tics beginning in childhood, but limited to one year in duration.[2]

Tobacco use disorder: Cases in which tobacco is used to the detriment of a person's health or social functioning or in which there is tobacco dependence. Dependence is included here rather than under drug dependence because tobacco differs from other drugs of dependence in its psychotoxic effects.[1]

Tranquilizer abuse: Cases where an individual has taken the drug to the detriment of his health or social functioning, in doses above or for periods beyond those normally regarded as therapeutic.[1]

Transient organic psychotic condition—*see* Organic psychotic conditions, transient

Trans-sexualism—*see* trans-sexualism under Psychosexual identity disorders

Transvestism: Sexual deviation in which there is recurrent and persistent dressing in clothes of the opposite sex, and initially in the early stage of the illness, for the purpose of sexual arousal.[2]

Twilight state

confusional—*see* Delirium, acute

psychogenic—*see* Psychosis, reactive confusion

Undersocialized conduct disorder—*see* undersocialized conduct disorder under Conduct disorders

Unsocialized aggressive disorder—*see* undersocialized conduct disorder, aggressive type under Conduct disorders

Vaginismus, functional—*see* functional vaginismus under Psychosexual dysfunctions

Vorbeireden: The symptom of the approximate answer or talking past the point, seen in the Ganser syndrome, a form of factitious illness.[2]

Voyeurism: A sexual deviation in which the individual repetitively seeks out situations in which he engages in looking at unsuspecting women who are either naked, in the act of disrobing, or engaging in sexual activity. The act of looking is accompanied by sexual excitement, frequently with orgasm. In its severe form, the act of peeping constitutes the preferred or exclusive sexual activity of the individual.[2]

Wernicke-Korsakoff syndrome—*see* alcohol amnestic syndrome under Alcoholic psychoses

Withdrawal reaction of childhood or adolescence—*see* Introverted disorder of childhood

Word-deafness: A developmental delay in the comprehension of speech sounds.[1]

Zoophilia: Sexual or anal intercourse with animals.[1]

1. Manual of the *International Classification of Diseases, Injuries, and Causes of Death.* 9th Revision. World Health Organization, Geneva, Switzerland, 1975.
2. American Psychiatric Association, Task Force on Nomenclature and Statistics, Robert L. Spitzer, Chairman.
3. *A Psychiatric Glossary*, Fourth Edition, American Psychiatric Association, Washington, D.C., 1975.
4. *Dorland's Illustrated Medical Dictionary.* Twenty-fifth Edition, W. B. Saunders Company, Philadelphia, 1974.
5. *Stedman's Medical Dictionary. Illustrated,* Twenty-third Edition, Williams and Wilkins, Baltimore, 1976.

CLASSIFICATION OF DRUGS BY AMERICAN HOSPITAL FORMULARY SERVICE LIST NUMBER AND THEIR ICD-9-CM EQUIVALENTS

The coding of adverse effects of drugs is keyed to the continually revised Hospital Formulary of the American Hospital Formulary Service (AHFS) published under the direction of the American Society of Hospital Pharmacists.

The following section gives the ICD-9-CM diagnosis code for each AHFS list.

	AHFS* LIST	ICD-9-CM Diagnosis Code
4:00	**ANTIHISTAMINE DRUGS**	963.0
8:00	**ANTI-INFECTIVE AGENTS**	
8:04	Amebacides	961.5
	hydroxyquinoline derivatives	961.3
	arsenical anti-infectives	961.1
8:08	Anthelmintics	961.6
	quinoline derivatives	961.3
8:12.04	Antifungal Antibiotics	960.1
	nonantibiotics	961.9
8:12.06	Cephalosporins	960.5
8:12.08	Chloramphenicol	960.2
8:12.12	The Erythromycins	960.3
8:12.16	The Penicillins	960.0
8:12.20	The Streptomycins	960.6
8:12.24	The Tetracyclines	960.4
8:12.28	Other Antibiotics	960.8
	antimycobacterial antibiotics	960.6
	macrolides	960.3
8:16	Antituberculars	961.8
	antibiotics	960.6
8:18	Antivirals	961.7
8:20	Plasmodicides (antimalarials)	961.4
8:24	Sulfonamides	961.0
8:26	The Sulfones	961.8
8:28	Treponemicides	961.2
8:32	Trichomonacides	961.5
	hydroxyquinoline derivatives	961.3
	nitrofuran derivatives	961.9
8:36	Urinary Germicides	961.9
	quinoline derivatives	961.3
8:40	Other Anti-Infectives	961.9
10:00	**ANTINEOPLASTIC AGENTS**	963.1
	antibiotics	960.7
	progestogens	962.2
12:00	**AUTONOMIC DRUGS**	
12:04	Parasympathomimetic (Cholinergic) Agents	971.0
12:08	Parasympatholytic (Cholinergic Blocking) Agents	971.1
12:12	Sympathomimetic (Adrenergic) Agents	971.2
12:16	Sympatholytic (Adrenergic Blocking) Agents	971.3
12:20	Skeletal Muscle Relaxants	975.2
	central nervous system muscle-tone depressants	968.0

AHFS* LIST		ICD-9-CM Diagnosis Code
16:00	**BLOOD DERIVATIVES**	964.7
20:00	**BLOOD FORMATION AND COAGULATION**	
20:04	Antianemia Drugs	964.1
20:04.04	Iron Preparations	964.0
20:04.08	Liver and Stomach Preparations	964.1
20:12.04	Anticoagulants	964.2
20:12.08	Antiheparin agents	964.5
20:12.12	Coagulants	964.5
20:12.16	Hemostatics	964.5
	capillary-active drugs	972.8
	fibrinolysis-affecting agents	964.4
	natural products	964.7
24:00	**CARDIOVASCULAR DRUGS**	
24:04	Cardiac Drugs	972.9
	cardiotonic agents	972.1
	rhythm regulators	972.0
24:06	Antilipemic Agents	972.2
	thyroid derivatives	962.7
24:08	Hypotensive Agents	972.6
	adrenergic blocking agents	971.3
	ganglion-blocking agents	972.3
	vasodilators	972.5
24:12	Vasodilating Agents	972.5
	coronary	972.4
	nicotinic acid derivatives	972.2
24:16	Sclerosing Agents	972.7
28:00	**CENTRAL NERVOUS SYSTEM DRUGS**	
28:04	General Anesthetics	968.4
	gaseous anesthetics	968.2
	halothane	968.1
	intravenous anesthetics	968.3
28:08	Analgesics and Antipyretics	965.9
	antirheumatics	965.6
	aromatic analgesics	965.4
	non-narcotics NEC	965.7
	opium alkaloids	965.00
	heroin	965.01
	methadone	965.02
	specified type NEC	965.09
	pyrazole derivatives	965.5
	salicylates	965.1
	specified type NEC	965.8
28:10	Narcotic Antagonists	970.1
28:12	Anticonvulsants	966.3
	barbiturates	967.0
	benzodiazepine-based tranquilizers	969.4
	bromides	967.3
	hydantoin derivatives	966.1
	oxazolidine derivative	966.0
	succinimides	966.2
28:16.04	Antidepressants	969.0
28:16.08	Tranquilizers	969.5
	benzodiazepine-based	969.4
	butyrophenone-based	969.2
	major NEC	969.3
	phenothiazine-based	969.1

* American Hospital Formulary Service

	AHFS* LIST	ICD-9-CM Diagnosis Code
28:16.12	Other Psychotherapeutic Agents	969.8
28:20	Respiratory and Cerebral Stimulants	970.9
	analeptics	970.0
	anorexigenic agents	977.0
	psychostimulants	969.7
	specified type NEC	970.8
28:24	Sedatives and Hypnotics	967.9
	barbiturates	967.0
	benzodiazepine-based tranquilizers	969.4
	chloral hydrate group	967.1
	glutethamide group	967.5
	intravenous anesthetics	968.3
	methaqualone	967.4
	paraldehyde	967.2
	phenothiazine-based tranquilizers	969.1
	specified type NEC	967.8
	thiobarbiturates	968.3
	tranquilizer NEC	969.5
36:00	**DIAGNOSTIC AGENTS**	977.8
40:00	**ELECTROLYTE, CALORIC, AND WATER BALANCE AGENTS NEC**	974.5
40:04	Acidifying Agents	963.2
40:08	Alkalinizing Agents	963.3
40:10	Ammonia Detoxicants	974.5
40:12	Replacement Solutions NEC	974.5
	plasma volume expanders	964.8
40:16	Sodium-Removing Resins	974.5
40:18	Potassium-Removing Resins	974.5
40:20	Caloric Agents	974.5
40:24	Salt and Sugar Substitutes	974.5
40:28	Diuretics NEC	974.4
	carbonic acid anhydrase inhibitors	974.2
	mercurials	974.0
	purine derivatives	974.1
	saluretics	974.3
40:36	Irrigating Solutions	974.5
40:40	Uricosuric Agents	974.7
44:00	**ENZYMES NEC**	963.4
	fibrinolysis-affecting agents	964.4
	gastric agents	973.4
48:00	**EXPECTORANTS AND COUGH PREPARATIONS**	
	antihistamine agents	963.0
	antitussives	975.4
	codeine derivatives	965.09
	expectorants	975.5
	narcotic agents NEC	965.09
52:00	**EYE, EAR, NOSE, AND THROAT PREPARATIONS**	
52:04	Anti-Infectives	
	ENT	976.6
	ophthalmic	976.5
52:04.04	Antibiotics	
	ENT	976.6
	ophthalmic	976.5

	AHFS* LIST	ICD-9-CM Diagnosis Code
52:04.06	Antivirals	
	ENT	976.6
	ophthalmic	976.5
52:04.08	Sulfonamides	
	ENT	976.6
	ophthalmic	976.5
52:04.12	Miscellaneous Anti-Infectives	
	ENT	976.6
	ophthalmic	976.5
52:08	Anti-Inflammatory Agents	
	ENT	976.6
	ophthalmic	976.5
52:10	Carbonic Anhydrase Inhibitors	974.2
52:12	Contact Lens Solutions	976.5
52:16	Local Anesthetics	968.5
52:20	Miotics	971.0
52:24	Mydriatics	
	adrenergics	971.2
	anticholinergics	971.1
	antimuscarinics	971.1
	parasympatholytics	971.1
	spasmolytics	971.1
	sympathomimetics	971.2
52:28	Mouth Washes and Gargles	976.6
52:32	Vasoconstrictors	971.2
52:36	Unclassified Agents	
	ENT	976.6
	ophthalmic	976.5
56:00	**GASTROINTESTINAL DRUGS**	
56:04	Antacids and Absorbants	973.0
56:08	Anti-Diarrhea Agents	973.5
56:10	Antiflatulents	973.8
56:12	Cathartics NEC	973.3
	emollients	973.2
	irritants	973.1
56:16	Digestants	973.4
56:20	Emetics and Antiemetics	
	antiemetics	963.0
	emetics	973.6
56:24	Lipotropic Agents	977.1
60:00	**GOLD COMPOUNDS**	965.6
64:00	**HEAVY METAL ANTAGONISTS**	963.8
68:00	**HORMONES AND SYNTHETIC SUBSTITUTES**	
68:04	Adrenals	962.0
68:08	Androgens	962.1
68:12	Contraceptives	962.2
68:16	Estrogens	962.2
68:18	Gonadotropins	962.4
68:20	Insulins and Antidiabetic Agents	962.3
68:20.08	Insulins	962.3
68:24	Parathyroid	962.6

	AHFS* LIST	ICD-9-CM Diagnosis Code
68:28	Pituitary	
	anterior	962.4
	posterior	962.5
68:32	Progestogens	962.2
68:34	Other Corpus Luteum Hormones	962.2
68:36	Thyroid and Antithyroid	
	antithyroid	962.8
	thyroid	962.7
72:00	**LOCAL ANESTHETICS NEC**	968.9
	topical (surface) agents	968.5
	infiltrating agents (intradermal) (subcutaneous) (submucosal)	968.5
	nerve blocking agents (peripheral) (plexus)(regional)	968.6
	spinal	968.7
76:00	**OXYTOCICS**	975.0
78:00	**RADIOACTIVE AGENTS**	990
80:00	**SERUMS, TOXOIDS, AND VACCINES**	
80:04	Serums	979.9
	immune globulin (gamma) (human)	964.6
80:08	Toxoids NEC	978.8
	diphtheria	978.5
	and tetanus	978.9
	with pertussis component	978.6
	tetanus	978.4
	and diphtheria	978.9
	with pertussis component	978.6
80:12	Vaccines NEC	979.9
	bacterial NEC	978.8
	with	
	other bacterial component	978.9
	pertussis component	978.6
	viral and rickettsial component	979.7
	rickettsial NEC	979.6
	with	
	bacterial component	979.7
	pertussis component	978.6
	viral component	979.7
	viral NEC	979.6
	with	
	bacterial component	979.7
	pertussis component	978.6
	rickettsial component	979.7
84:00	**SKIN AND MUCOUS MEMBRANE PREPARATIONS**	
84:04	Anti-Infectives	976.0
84:04.04	Antibiotics	976.0
84:04.08	Fungicides	976.0
84:04.12	Scabicides and Pediculicides	976.0
84:04.16	Miscellaneous Local Anti-Infectives	976.0
84:06	Anti-Inflammatory Agents	976.0
84:08	Antipruritics and Local Anesthetics	
	antipruritics	976.1
	local anesthetics	968.5
84:12	Astringents	976.2
84:16	Cell Stimulants and Proliferants	976.8
84:20	Detergents	976.2

	AHFS* LIST	ICD-9-CM Diagnosis Code
84:24	Emollients, Demulcents, and Protectants	976.3
84:28	Keratolytic Agents	976.4
84:32	Keratoplastic Agents	976.4
84:36	Miscellaneous Agents	976.8
86:00	**SPASMOLYTIC AGENTS**	975.1
	antiasthmatics	975.7
	papaverine	972.5
	theophyllin	974.1
88:00	**VITAMINS**	
88:04	Vitamin A	963.5
88:08	Vitamin B Complex	963.5
	hematopoietic vitamin	964.1
	nicotinic acid derivatives	972.2
88:12	Vitamin C	963.5
88:16	Vitamin D	963.5
88:20	Vitamin E	963.5
88:24	Vitamin K Activity	964.3
88:28	Multivitamin Preparations	963.5
92:00	**UNCLASSIFIED THERAPEUTIC AGENTS**	977.8

* American Hospital Formulary Service

CLASSIFICATION OF INDUSTRIAL ACCIDENTS
ACCORDING TO AGENCY

Annex B to the Resolution concerning Statistics of Employment Injuries adopted by the Tenth International Conference of Labor Statisticians on 12 October 1962

1 MACHINES

11 Prime-Movers, except Electrical Motors
111 Steam engines
112 Internal combustion engines
119 Others

12 Transmission Machinery
121 Transmission shafts
122 Transmission belts, cables, pulleys, pinions, chains, gears
129 Others

13 Metalworking Machines
131 Power presses
132 Lathes
133 Milling machines
134 Abrasive wheels
135 Mechanical shears
136 Forging machines
137 Rolling-mills
139 Others

14 Wood and Assimilated Machines
141 Circular saws
142 Other saws
143 Molding machines
144 Overhand planes
149 Others

15 Agricultural Machines
151 Reapers (including combine reapers)
152 Threshers
159 Others

16 Mining Machinery
161 Under-cutters
169 Others

19 Other Machines Not Elsewhere Classified
191 Earth-moving machines, excavating and scraping machines, except means of transport
192 Spinning, weaving and other textile machines
193 Machines for the manufacture of foodstuffs and beverages
194 Machines for the manufacture of paper
195 Printing machines
199 Others

2 MEANS OF TRANSPORT AND LIFTING EQUIPMENT

21 Lifting Machines and Appliances
211 Cranes
212 Lifts and elevators
213 Winches
214 Pulley blocks
219 Others

22 Means of Rail Transport
221 Inter-urban railways
222 Rail transport in mines, tunnels, quarries, industrial establishments, docks, etc.
229 Others

23 Other Wheeled Means of Transport, Excluding Rail Transport
231 Tractors
232 Lorries
233 Trucks
234 Motor vehicles, not elsewhere classified
235 Animal-drawn vehicles

2 MEANS OF TRANSPORT AND LIFTING EQUIPMENT *continued*

236 Hand-drawn vehicles
239 Others

24 Means of Air Transport

25 Means of Water Transport
251 Motorized means of water transport
252 Non-motorized means of water transport

26 Other Means of Transport
261 Cable-cars
262 Mechanical conveyors, except cable-cars
269 Others

3 OTHER EQUIPMENT

31 Pressure Vessels
311 Boilers
312 Pressurized containers
313 Pressurized piping and accessories
314 Gas cylinders
315 Caissons, diving equipment
319 Others

32 Furnaces, Ovens, Kilns
321 Blast furnaces
322 Refining furnaces
323 Other furnaces
324 Kilns
325 Ovens

33 Refrigerating Plants

34 Electrical Installations, Including Electric Motors, but Excluding Electric Hand Tools
341 Rotating machines
342 Conductors
343 Transformers
344 Control apparatus
349 Others

35 Electric Hand Tools

36 Tools, Implements, and Appliances, Except Electric Hand Tools
361 Power-driven hand tools, except electric hand tools
362 Hand tools, not power-driven
369 Others

37 Ladders, Mobile Ramps

38 Scaffolding

39 Other Equipment, Not Elsewhere Classified

4 MATERIALS, SUBSTANCES AND RADIATIONS

41 Explosives

42 Dusts, Gases, Liquids and Chemicals, Excluding Explosives
421 Dusts
422 Gases, vapors, fumes
423 Liquids, not elsewhere classified
424 Chemicals, not elsewhere classified

43 Flying Fragments

44 Radiations
441 Ionizing radiations
449 Others

49 Other Materials and Substances Not Elsewhere Classified

5 WORKING ENVIRONMENT

51 Outdoor
511 Weather

5 WORKING ENVIRONMENT *continued*

    512 Traffic and working surfaces
    513 Water
    519 Others

    52 Indoor
    521 Floors
    522 Confined quarters
    523 Stairs
    524 Other traffic and working surfaces
    525 Floor openings and wall openings
    526 Environmental factors (lighting, ventilation, temperature, noise, etc.)
    529 Others

    53 Underground
    531 Roofs and faces of mine roads and tunnels, etc.
    532 Floors of mine roads and tunnels, etc.
    533 Working-faces of mines, tunnels, etc.
    534 Mine shafts
    535 Fire
    536 Water
    539 Others

6 OTHER AGENCIES, NOT ELSEWHERE CLASSIFIED

    61 Animals
    611 Live animals
    612 Animals products

    69 Other Agencies, Not Elsewhere Classified

7 AGENCIES NOT CLASSIFIED FOR LACK OF SUFFICIENT DATA

LIST OF THREE-DIGIT CATEGORIES

1. INFECTIOUS AND PARASITIC DISEASES

Intestinal infectious diseases (001-009)

    001 Cholera
    002 Typhoid and paratyphoid fevers
    003 Other salmonella infections
    004 Shigellosis
    005 Other food poisoning (bacterial)
    006 Amebiasis
    007 Other protozoal intestinal diseases
    008 Intestinal infections due to other organisms
    009 Ill-defined intestinal infections

Tuberculosis (010-018)

    010 Primary tuberculous infection
    011 Pulmonary tuberculosis
    012 Other respiratory tuberculosis
    013 Tuberculosis of meninges and central nervous system
    014 Tuberculosis of intestines, peritoneum, and mesenteric glands
    015 Tuberculosis of bones and joints
    016 Tuberculosis of genitourinary system
    017 Tuberculosis of other organs
    018 Miliary tuberculosis

Zoonotic bacterial diseases (020-027)

    020 Plague
    021 Tularemia
    022 Anthrax
    023 Brucellosis
    024 Glanders
    025 Melioidosis
    026 Rat-bite fever
    027 Other zoonotic bacterial diseases

Other bacterial diseases (030-041)

    030 Leprosy
    031 Diseases due to other mycobacteria
    032 Diphtheria
    033 Whooping cough
    034 Streptococcal sore throat and scarlet fever
    035 Erysipelas
    036 Meningococcal infection
    037 Tetanus
    038 Septicemia
    039 Actinomycotic infections
    040 Other bacterial diseases
    041 Bacterial infection in conditions classified elsewhere and of unspecified site

Human immunodeficiency virus (042)

    042 Human immunodeficiency virus [HIV] disease

Poliomyelitis and other non-arthropod-borne viral diseases of central nervous system (045-049)

    045 Acute poliomyelitis
    046 Slow virus infection of central nervous system
    047 Meningitis due to enterovirus
    048 Other enterovirus diseases of central nervous system
    049 Other non-arthropod-borne viral diseases of central nervous system

Viral diseases accompanied by exanthem (050-057)

    050 Smallpox
    051 Cowpox and paravaccinia
    052 Chickenpox
    053 Herpes zoster
    054 Herpes simplex
    055 Measles
    056 Rubella
    057 Other viral exanthemata

1. INFECTIOUS AND PARASITIC DISEASES *continued*

Arthropod-borne viral diseases (060-066)

060	Yellow fever
061	Dengue
062	Mosquito-borne viral encephalitis
063	Tick-borne viral encephalitis
064	Viral encephalitis transmitted by other and unspecified arthropods
065	Arthropod-borne hemorrhagic fever
066	Other arthropod-borne viral diseases

Other diseases due to viruses and Chlamydiae (070-079)

070	Viral hepatitis
071	Rabies
072	Mumps
073	Ornithosis
074	Specific diseases due to Coxsackie virus
075	Infectious mononucleosis
076	Trachoma
077	Other diseases of conjunctiva due to viruses and Chlamydiae
078	Other diseases due to viruses and Chlamydiae
079	Viral and Chlamydial infection in conditions classified elsewhere and of unspecified site

Rickettsioses and other arthropod-borne diseases (080-088)

080	Louse-borne [epidemic] typhus
081	Other typhus
082	Tick-borne rickettsioses
083	Other rickettsioses
084	Malaria
085	Leishmaniasis
086	Trypanosomiasis
087	Relapsing fever
088	Other arthropod-borne diseases

Syphilis and other venereal diseases (090-099)

090	Congenital syphilis
091	Early syphilis, symptomatic
092	Early syphilis, latent
093	Cardiovascular syphilis
094	Neurosyphilis
095	Other forms of late syphilis, with symptoms
096	Late syphilis, latent
097	Other and unspecified syphilis
098	Gonococcal infections
099	Other venereal diseases

Other spirochetal diseases (100-104)

100	Leptospirosis
101	Vincent's angina
102	Yaws
103	Pinta
104	Other spirochetal infection

Mycoses (110-118)

110	Dermatophytosis
111	Dermatomycosis, other and unspecified
112	Candidiasis
114	Coccidioidomycosis
115	Histoplasmosis
116	Blastomycotic infection
117	Other mycoses
118	Opportunistic mycoses

Helminthiases (120-129)

120	Schistosomiasis [bilharziasis]
121	Other trematode infections
122	Echinococcosis
123	Other cestode infection
124	Trichinosis

1. INFECTIOUS AND PARASITIC DISEASES *continued*

125 Filarial infection and dracontiasis
126 Ancylostomiasis and necatoriasis
127 Other intestinal helminthiases
128 Other and unspecified helminthiases
129 Intestinal parasitism, unspecified

Other infectious and parasitic diseases (130-136)

130 Toxoplasmosis
131 Trichomoniasis
132 Pediculosis and phthirus infestation
133 Acariasis
134 Other infestation
135 Sarcoidosis
136 Other and unspecified infectious and parasitic diseases

Late effects of infectious and parasitic diseases (137-139)

137 Late effects of tuberculosis
138 Late effects of acute poliomyelitis
139 Late effects of other infectious and parasitic diseases

2. NEOPLASMS

Malignant neoplasm of lip, oral cavity, and pharynx (140-149)

140 Malignant neoplasm of lip
141 Malignant neoplasm of tongue
142 Malignant neoplasm of major salivary glands
143 Malignant neoplasm of gum
144 Malignant neoplasm of floor of mouth
145 Malignant neoplasm of other and unspecified parts of mouth
146 Malignant neoplasm of oropharynx
147 Malignant neoplasm of nasopharynx
148 Malignant neoplasm of hypopharynx
149 Malignant neoplasm of other and ill-defined sites within the lip, oral cavity, and pharynx

Malignant neoplasm of digestive organs and peritoneum (150-159)

150 Malignant neoplasm of esophagus
151 Malignant neoplasm of stomach
152 Malignant neoplasm of small intestine, including duodenum
153 Malignant neoplasm of colon
154 Malignant neoplasm of rectum, rectosigmoid junction, and anus
155 Malignant neoplasm of liver and intrahepatic bile ducts
156 Malignant neoplasm of gallbladder and extrahepatic bile ducts
157 Malignant neoplasm of pancreas
158 Malignant neoplasm of retroperitoneum and peritoneum
159 Malignant neoplasm of other and ill-defined sites within the digestive organs and peritoneum

Malignant neoplasm of respiratory and intrathoracic organs (160-165)

160 Malignant neoplasm of nasal cavities, middle ear, and accessory sinuses
161 Malignant neoplasm of larynx
162 Malignant neoplasm of trachea, bronchus, and lung
163 Malignant neoplasm of pleura
164 Malignant neoplasm of thymus, heart, and mediastinum
165 Malignant neoplasm of other and ill-defined sites within the respiratory system and intrathoracic organs

Malignant neoplasm of bone, connective tissue, skin, and breast (170-176)

170 Malignant neoplasm of bone and articular cartilage
171 Malignant neoplasm of connective and other soft tissue
172 Malignant melanoma of skin
173 Other malignant neoplasm of skin
174 Malignant neoplasm of female breast
175 Malignant neoplasm of male breast
176 Kaposi's sarcoma

Malignant neoplasm of genitourinary organs (179-189)

179 Malignant neoplasm of uterus, part unspecified
180 Malignant neoplasm of cervix uteri

2. NEOPLASMS *continued*

181   Malignant neoplasm of placenta
182   Malignant neoplasm of body of uterus
183   Malignant neoplasm of ovary and other uterine adnexa
184   Malignant neoplasm of other and unspecified female genital organs
185   Malignant neoplasm of prostate
186   Malignant neoplasm of testis
187   Malignant neoplasm of penis and other male genital organs
188   Malignant neoplasm of bladder
189   Malignant neoplasm of kidney and other and unspecified urinary organs

Malignant neoplasm of other and unspecified sites (190-199)

190   Malignant neoplasm of eye
191   Malignant neoplasm of brain
192   Malignant neoplasm of other and unspecified parts of nervous system
193   Malignant neoplasm of thyroid gland
194   Malignant neoplasm of other endocrine glands and related structures
195   Malignant neoplasm of other and ill-defined sites
196   Secondary and unspecified malignant neoplasm of lymph nodes
197   Secondary malignant neoplasm of respiratory and digestive systems
198   Secondary malignant neoplasm of other specified sites
199   Malignant neoplasm without specification of site

Malignant neoplasm of lymphatic and hematopoietic tissue (200-208)

200   Lymphosarcoma and reticulosarcoma
201   Hodgkin's disease
202   Other malignant neoplasm of lymphoid and histiocytic tissue
203   Multiple myeloma and immunoproliferative neoplasms
204   Lymphoid leukemia
205   Myeloid leukemia
206   Monocytic leukemia
207   Other specified leukemia
208   Leukemia of unspecified cell type

Benign neoplasms (210-229)

210   Benign neoplasm of lip, oral cavity, and pharynx
211   Benign neoplasm of other parts of digestive system
212   Benign neoplasm of respiratory and intrathoracic organs
213   Benign neoplasm of bone and articular cartilage
214   Lipoma
215   Other benign neoplasm of connective and other soft tissue
216   Benign neoplasm of skin
217   Benign neoplasm of breast
218   Uterine leiomyoma
219   Other benign neoplasm of uterus
220   Benign neoplasm of ovary
221   Benign neoplasm of other female genital organs
222   Benign neoplasm of male genital organs
223   Benign neoplasm of kidney and other urinary organs
224   Benign neoplasm of eye
225   Benign neoplasm of brain and other parts of nervous system
226   Benign neoplasm of thyroid gland
227   Benign neoplasm of other endocrine glands and related structures
228   Hemangioma and lymphangioma, any site
229   Benign neoplasm of other and unspecified sites

Carcinoma in situ (230-234)

230   Carcinoma in situ of digestive organs
231   Carcinoma in situ of respiratory system
232   Carcinoma in situ of skin
233   Carcinoma in situ of breast and genitourinary system
234   Carcinoma in situ of other and unspecified sites

Neoplasms of uncertain behavior (235-238)

235   Neoplasm of uncertain behavior of digestive and respiratory systems
236   Neoplasm of uncertain behavior of genitourinary organs
237   Neoplasm of uncertain behavior of endocrine glands and nervous system
238   Neoplasm of uncertain behavior of other and unspecified sites and tissues

2. NEOPLASMS *continued*

Neoplasm of unspecified nature (239)

239 Neoplasm of unspecified nature

3. ENDOCRINE, NUTRITIONAL AND METABOLIC DISEASES, AND IMMUNITY DISORDERS

Disorders of thyroid gland (240-246)

240 Simple and unspecified goiter
241 Nontoxic nodular goiter
242 Thyrotoxicosis with or without goiter
243 Congenital hypothyroidism
244 Acquired hypothyroidism
245 Thyroiditis
246 Other disorders of thyroid

Diseases of other endocrine glands (250-259)

250 Diabetes mellitus
251 Other disorders of pancreatic internal secretion
252 Disorders of parathyroid gland
253 Disorders of the pituitary gland and its hypothalamic control
254 Diseases of thymus gland
255 Disorders of adrenal glands
256 Ovarian dysfunction
257 Testicular dysfunction
258 Polyglandular dysfunction and related disorders
259 Other endocrine disorders

Nutritional deficiencies (260-269)

260 Kwashiorkor
261 Nutritional marasmus
262 Other severe protein-calorie malnutrition
263 Other and unspecified protein-calorie malnutrition
264 Vitamin A deficiency
265 Thiamine and niacin deficiency states
266 Deficiency of B-complex components
267 Ascorbic acid deficiency
268 Vitamin D deficiency
269 Other nutritional deficiencies

Other metabolic disorders and immunity disorders (270-279)

270 Disorders of amino-acid transport and metabolism
271 Disorders of carbohydrate transport and metabolism
272 Disorders of lipoid metabolism
273 Disorders of plasma protein metabolism
274 Gout
275 Disorders of mineral metabolism
276 Disorders of fluid, electrolyte, and acid-base balance
277 Other and unspecified disorders of metabolism
278 Obesity and other hyperalimentation
279 Disorders involving the immune mechanism

4. DISEASES OF THE BLOOD AND BLOOD-FORMING ORGANS

Diseases of blood and blood-forming organs (280-289)

280 Iron deficiency anemias
281 Other deficiency anemias
282 Hereditary hemolytic anemias
283 Acquired hemolytic anemias
284 Aplastic anemia
285 Other and unspecified anemias
286 Coagulation defects
287 Purpura and other hemorrhagic conditions
288 Diseases of white blood cells
289 Other diseases of blood and blood-forming organs

5. MENTAL DISORDERS

Organic psychotic conditions (290-294)
- 290 Senile and presenile organic psychotic conditions
- 291 Alcoholic psychoses
- 292 Drug psychoses
- 293 Transient organic psychotic conditions
- 294 Other organic psychotic conditions (chronic)

Other psychoses (295-299)
- 295 Schizophrenic psychoses
- 296 Affective psychoses
- 297 Paranoid states (Delusional disorders)
- 298 Other nonorganic psychoses
- 299 Psychoses with origin specific to childhood

Neurotic disorders, personality disorders, and other nonpsychotic mental disorders (300-316)
- 300 Neurotic disorders
- 301 Personality disorders
- 302 Sexual deviations and disorders
- 303 Alcohol dependence syndrome
- 304 Drug dependence
- 305 Nondependent abuse of drugs
- 306 Physiological malfunction arising from mental factors
- 307 Special symptoms or syndromes, not elsewhere classified
- 308 Acute reaction to stress
- 309 Adjustment reaction
- 310 Specific nonpsychotic mental disorders due to organic brain damage
- 311 Depressive disorder, not elsewhere classified
- 312 Disturbance of conduct, not elsewhere classified
- 313 Disturbance of emotions specific to childhood and adolescence
- 314 Hyperkinetic syndrome of childhood
- 315 Specific delays in development
- 316 Psychic factors associated with diseases classified elsewhere

Mental retardation (317-319)
- 317 Mild mental retardation
- 318 Other specified mental retardation
- 319 Unspecified mental retardation

6. DISEASES OF THE NERVOUS SYSTEM AND SENSE ORGANS

Inflammatory diseases of the central nervous system (320-326)
- 320 Bacterial meningitis
- 321 Meningitis due to other organisms
- 322 Meningitis of unspecified cause
- 323 Encephalitis, myelitis, and encephalomyelitis
- 324 Intracranial and intraspinal abscess
- 325 Phlebitis and thrombophlebitis of intracranial venous sinuses
- 326 Late effects of intracranial abscess or pyogenic infection

Hereditary and degenerative diseases of the central nervous system (330-337)
- 330 Cerebral degenerations usually manifest in childhood
- 331 Other cerebral degenerations
- 332 Parkinson's disease
- 333 Other extrapyramidal disease and abnormal movement disorders
- 334 Spinocerebellar disease
- 335 Anterior horn cell disease
- 336 Other diseases of spinal cord
- 337 Disorders of the autonomic nervous system

Other disorders of the central nervous system (340-349)
- 340 Multiple sclerosis
- 341 Other demyelinating diseases of central nervous system
- 342 Hemiplegia and hemiparesis
- 343 Infantile cerebral palsy
- 344 Other paralytic syndromes
- 345 Epilepsy
- 346 Migraine
- 347 Cataplexy and narcolepsy

6. DISEASES OF THE NERVOUS SYSTEM AND SENSE ORGANS *continued*

348 Other conditions of brain
349 Other and unspecified disorders of the nervous system

Disorders of the peripheral nervous system (350-359)

350 Trigeminal nerve disorders
351 Facial nerve disorders
352 Disorders of other cranial nerves
353 Nerve root and plexus disorders
354 Mononeuritis of upper limb and mononeuritis multiplex
355 Mononeuritis of lower limb and unspecified site
356 Hereditary and idiopathic peripheral neuropathy
357 Inflammatory and toxic neuropathy
358 Myoneural disorders
359 Muscular dystrophies and other myopathies

Disorders of the eye and adnexa (360-379)

360 Disorders of the globe
361 Retinal detachments and defects
362 Other retinal disorders
363 Chorioretinal inflammations and scars and other disorders of choroid
364 Disorders of iris and ciliary body
365 Glaucoma
366 Cataract
367 Disorders of refraction and accommodation
368 Visual disturbances
369 Blindness and low vision
370 Keratitis
371 Corneal opacity and other disorders of cornea
372 Disorders of conjunctiva
373 Inflammation of eyelids
374 Other disorders of eyelids
375 Disorders of lacrimal system
376 Disorders of the orbit
377 Disorders of optic nerve and visual pathways
378 Strabismus and other disorders of binocular eye movements
379 Other disorders of eye

Diseases of the ear and mastoid process (380-389)

380 Disorders of external ear
381 Nonsuppurative otitis media and Eustachian tube disorders
382 Suppurative and unspecified otitis media
383 Mastoiditis and related conditions
384 Other disorders of tympanic membrane
385 Other disorders of middle ear and mastoid
386 Vertiginous syndromes and other disorders of vestibular system
387 Otosclerosis
388 Other disorders of ear
389 Hearing loss

7. DISEASES OF THE CIRCULATORY SYSTEM

Acute rheumatic fever (390-392)

390 Rheumatic fever without mention of heart involvement
391 Rheumatic fever with heart involvement
392 Rheumatic chorea

Chronic rheumatic heart disease (393-398)

393 Chronic rheumatic pericarditis
394 Diseases of mitral valve
395 Diseases of aortic valve
396 Diseases of mitral and aortic valves
397 Diseases of other endocardial structures
398 Other rheumatic heart disease

Hypertensive disease (401-405)

401 Essential hypertension
402 Hypertensive heart disease
403 Hypertensive renal disease

7. DISEASES OF THE CIRCULATORY SYSTEM *continued*

 404 Hypertensive heart and renal disease
 405 Secondary hypertension

Ischemic heart disease (410-414)
 410 Acute myocardial infarction
 411 Other acute and subacute form of ischemic heart disease
 412 Old myocardial infarction
 413 Angina pectoris
 414 Other forms of chronic ischemic heart disease

Diseases of pulmonary circulation (415-417)
 415 Acute pulmonary heart disease
 416 Chronic pulmonary heart disease
 417 Other diseases of pulmonary circulation

Other forms of heart disease (420-429)
 420 Acute pericarditis
 421 Acute and subacute endocarditis
 422 Acute myocarditis
 423 Other diseases of pericardium
 424 Other diseases of endocardium
 425 Cardiomyopathy
 426 Conduction disorders
 427 Cardiac dysrhythmias
 428 Heart failure
 429 Ill-defined descriptions and complications of heart disease

Cerebrovascular disease (430-438)
 430 Subarachnoid hemorrhage
 431 Intracerebral hemorrhage
 432 Other and unspecified intracranial hemorrhage
 433 Occlusion and stenosis of precerebral arteries
 434 Occlusion of cerebral arteries
 435 Transient cerebral ischemia
 436 Acute but ill-defined cerebrovascular disease
 437 Other and ill-defined cerebrovascular disease
 438 Late effects of cerebrovascular disease

Diseases of arteries, arterioles, and capillaries (440-448)
 440 Atherosclerosis
 441 Aortic aneurysm and dissection
 442 Other aneurysm
 443 Other peripheral vascular disease
 444 Arterial embolism and thrombosis
 445 Atheroembolism
 446 Polyarteritis nodosa and allied conditions
 447 Other disorders of arteries and arterioles
 448 Diseases of capillaries

Diseases of veins and lymphatics, and other diseases of circulatory system (451-459)
 451 Phlebitis and thrombophlebitis
 452 Portal vein thrombosis
 453 Other venous embolism and thrombosis
 454 Varicose veins of lower extremities
 455 Hemorrhoids
 456 Varicose veins of other sites
 457 Noninfective disorders of lymphatic channels
 458 Hypotension
 459 Other disorders of circulatory system

8. DISEASES OF THE RESPIRATORY SYSTEM

Acute respiratory infections (460-466)
 460 Acute nasopharyngitis [common cold]
 461 Acute sinusitis
 462 Acute pharyngitis
 463 Acute tonsillitis
 464 Acute laryngitis and tracheitis

8. DISEASES OF THE RESPIRATORY SYSTEM *continued*

465 Acute upper respiratory infections of multiple or unspecified sites
466 Acute bronchitis and bronchiolitis

Other diseases of upper respiratory tract (470-478)
470 Deviated nasal septum
471 Nasal polyps
472 Chronic pharyngitis and nasopharyngitis
473 Chronic sinusitis
474 Chronic disease of tonsils and adenoids
475 Peritonsillar abscess
476 Chronic laryngitis and laryngotracheitis
477 Allergic rhinitis
478 Other diseases of upper respiratory tract

Pneumonia and influenza (480-487)
480 Viral pneumonia
481 Pneumococcal pneumonia [Streptococcus pneumoniae pneumonia]
482 Other bacterial pneumonia
483 Pneumonia due to other specified organism
484 Pneumonia in infectious diseases classified elsewhere
485 Bronchopneumonia, organism unspecified
486 Pneumonia, organism unspecified
487 Influenza

Chronic obstructive pulmonary disease and allied conditions (490-496)
490 Bronchitis, not specified as acute or chronic
491 Chronic bronchitis
492 Emphysema
493 Asthma
494 Bronchiectasis
495 Extrinsic allergic alveolitis
496 Chronic airway obstruction, not elsewhere classified

Pneumoconioses and other lung diseases due to external agents (500-508)
500 Coalworkers' pneumoconiosis
501 Asbestosis
502 Pneumoconiosis due to other silica or silicates
503 Pneumoconiosis due to other inorganic dust
504 Pneumopathy due to inhalation of other dust
505 Pneumoconiosis, unspecified
506 Respiratory conditions due to chemical fumes and vapors
507 Pneumonitis due to solids and liquids
508 Respiratory conditions due to other and unspecified external agents

Other diseases of respiratory system (510-519)
510 Empyema
511 Pleurisy
512 Pneumothorax
513 Abscess of lung and mediastinum
514 Pulmonary congestion and hypostasis
515 Postinflammatory pulmonary fibrosis
516 Other alveolar and parietoalveolar pneumopathy
517 Lung involvement in conditions classified elsewhere
518 Other diseases of lung
519 Other diseases of respiratory system

9. DISEASES OF THE DIGESTIVE SYSTEM

Diseases of oral cavity, salivary glands, and jaws (520-529)
520 Disorders of tooth development and eruption
521 Diseases of hard tissues of teeth
522 Diseases of pulp and periapical tissues
523 Gingival and periodontal diseases
524 Dentofacial anomalies, including malocclusion
525 Other diseases and conditions of the teeth and supporting structures
526 Diseases of the jaws
527 Diseases of the salivary glands
528 Diseases of the oral soft tissues, excluding lesions specific for gingiva and tongue
529 Diseases and other conditions of the tongue

9. DISEASES OF THE DIGESTIVE SYSTEM *continued*

Diseases of esophagus, stomach, and duodenum (530-537)

530 Diseases of esophagus
531 Gastric ulcer
532 Duodenal ulcer
533 Peptic ulcer, site unspecified
534 Gastrojejunal ulcer
535 Gastritis and duodenitis
536 Disorders of function of stomach
537 Other disorders of stomach and duodenum

Appendicitis (540-543)

540 Acute appendicitis
541 Appendicitis, unqualified
542 Other appendicitis
543 Other diseases of appendix

Hernia of abdominal cavity (550-553)

550 Inguinal hernia
551 Other hernia of abdominal cavity, with gangrene
552 Other hernia of abdominal cavity, with obstruction, but without mention of gangrene
553 Other hernia of abdominal cavity without mention of obstruction or gangrene

Noninfectious enteritis and colitis (555-558)

555 Regional enteritis
556 Ulcerative colitis
557 Vascular insufficiency of intestine
558 Other and unspecified noninfectious gastroenteritis and colitis

Other diseases of intestines and peritoneum (560-569)

560 Intestinal obstruction without mention of hernia
562 Diverticula of intestine
564 Functional digestive disorders, not elsewhere classified
565 Anal fissure and fistula
566 Abscess of anal and rectal regions
567 Peritonitis
568 Other disorders of peritoneum
569 Other disorders of intestine

Other diseases of digestive system (570-579)

570 Acute and subacute necrosis of liver
571 Chronic liver disease and cirrhosis
572 Liver abscess and sequelae of chronic liver disease
573 Other disorders of liver
574 Cholelithiasis
575 Other disorders of gallbladder
576 Other disorders of biliary tract
577 Diseases of pancreas
578 Gastrointestinal hemorrhage
579 Intestinal malabsorption

10. DISEASES OF THE GENITOURINARY SYSTEM

Nephritis, nephrotic syndrome, and nephrosis (580-589)

580 Acute glomerulonephritis
581 Nephrotic syndrome
582 Chronic glomerulonephritis
583 Nephritis and nephropathy, not specified as acute or chronic
584 Acute renal failure
585 Chronic renal failure
586 Renal failure, unspecified
587 Renal sclerosis, unspecified
588 Disorders resulting from impaired renal function
589 Small kidney of unknown cause

Other diseases of urinary system (590-599)

590 Infections of kidney
591 Hydronephrosis
592 Calculus of kidney and ureter
593 Other disorders of kidney and ureter

10. DISEASES OF THE GENITOURINARY SYSTEM *continued*

594 Calculus of lower urinary tract
595 Cystitis
596 Other disorders of bladder
597 Urethritis, not sexually transmitted, and urethral syndrome
598 Urethral stricture
599 Other disorders of urethra and urinary tract

Diseases of male genital organs (600-608)

600 Hyperplasia of prostate
601 Inflammatory diseases of prostate
602 Other disorders of prostate
603 Hydrocele
604 Orchitis and epididymitis
605 Redundant prepuce and phimosis
606 Infertility, male
607 Disorders of penis
608 Other disorders of male genital organs

Disorders of breast (610-611)

610 Benign mammary dysplasias
611 Other disorders of breast

Inflammatory disease of female pelvic organs (614-616)

614 Inflammatory disease of ovary, fallopian tube, pelvic cellular tissue, and peritoneum
615 Inflammatory diseases of uterus, except cervix
616 Inflammatory disease of cervix, vagina, and vulva

Other disorders of female genital tract (617-629)

617 Endometriosis
618 Genital prolapse
619 Fistula involving female genital tract
620 Noninflammatory disorders of ovary, fallopian tube, and broad ligament
621 Disorders of uterus, not elsewhere classified
622 Noninflammatory disorders of cervix
623 Noninflammatory disorders of vagina
624 Noninflammatory disorders of vulva and perineum
625 Pain and other symptoms associated with female genital organs
626 Disorders of menstruation and other abnormal bleeding from female genital tract
627 Menopausal and postmenopausal disorders
628 Infertility, female
629 Other disorders of female genital organs

11. COMPLICATIONS OF PREGNANCY, CHILDBIRTH AND THE PUERPERIUM

Ectopic and molar pregnancy (630-633)

630 Hydatidiform mole
631 Other abnormal product of conception
632 Missed abortion
633 Ectopic pregnancy

Other pregnancy with abortive outcome (634-639)

634 Abortion
635 Legally induced abortion
636 Illegally induced abortion
637 Unspecified abortion
638 Failed attempted abortion
639 Complications following abortion and ectopic and molar pregnancies

Complications mainly related to pregnancy (640-648)

640 Hemorrhage in early pregnancy
641 Antepartum hemorrhage, abruptio placentae, and placenta previa
642 Hypertension complicating pregnancy, childbirth, and the puerperium
643 Excessive vomiting in pregnancy
644 Early or threatened labor
645 Late pregnancy
646 Other complications of pregnancy, not elsewhere classified
647 Infective and parasitic conditions in the mother classifiable elsewhere but complicating pregnancy, childbirth, and the puerperium
648 Other current conditions in the mother classifiable elsewhere but complicating pregnancy, childbirth, and the puerperium

11. COMPLICATIONS OF PREGNANCY, CHILDBIRTH AND THE PUERPERIUM *continued*

Normal delivery, and other indications for care in pregnancy, labor, and delivery (650-659)

650 Normal delivery
651 Multiple gestation
652 Malposition and malpresentation of fetus
653 Disproportion
654 Abnormality of organs and soft tissues of pelvis
655 Known or suspected fetal abnormality affecting management of mother
656 Other fetal and placental problems affecting management of mother
657 Polyhydramnios
658 Other problems associated with amniotic cavity and membranes
659 Other indications for care or intervention related to labor and delivery and not elsewhere classified

Complications occurring mainly in the course of labor and delivery (660-669)

660 Obstructed labor
661 Abnormality of forces of labor
662 Long labor
663 Umbilical cord complications
664 Trauma to perineum and vulva during delivery
665 Other obstetrical trauma
666 Postpartum hemorrhage
667 Retained placenta or membranes, without hemorrhage
668 Complications of the administration of anesthetic or other sedation in labor and delivery
669 Other complications of labor and delivery, not elsewhere classified

Complications of the puerperium (670-677)

670 Major puerperal infection
671 Venous complications in pregnancy and the puerperium
672 Pyrexia of unknown origin during the puerperium
673 Obstetrical pulmonary embolism
674 Other and unspecified complications of the puerperium, not elsewhere classified
675 Infections of the breast and nipple associated with childbirth
676 Other disorders of the breast associated with childbirth, and disorders of lactation
677 Late effect of complication of pregnancy, childbirth, and the puerperium

12. DISEASES OF THE SKIN AND SUBCUTANEOUS TISSUE

Infections of skin and subcutaneous tissue (680-686)

680 Carbuncle and furuncle
681 Cellulitis and abscess of finger and toe
682 Other cellulitis and abscess
683 Acute lymphadenitis
684 Impetigo
685 Pilonidal cyst
686 Other local infections of skin and subcutaneous tissue

Other inflammatory conditions of skin and subcutaneous tissue (690-698)

690 Erythematosquamous dermatosis
691 Atopic dermatitis and related conditions
692 Contact dermatitis and other eczema
693 Dermatitis due to substances taken internally
694 Bullous dermatoses
695 Erythematous conditions
696 Psoriasis and similar disorders
697 Lichen
698 Pruritus and related conditions

Other diseases of skin and subcutaneous tissue (700-709)

700 Corns and callosities
701 Other hypertrophic and atrophic conditions of skin
702 Other dermatoses
703 Diseases of nail
704 Diseases of hair and hair follicles
705 Disorders of sweat glands
706 Diseases of sebaceous glands
707 Chronic ulcer of skin

12. DISEASES OF THE SKIN AND SUBCUTANEOUS TISSUE *continued*

708 Urticaria
709 Other disorders of skin and subcutaneous tissue

13. DISEASES OF THE MUSCULOSKELETAL SYSTEM AND CONNECTIVE TISSUE

Arthropathies and related disorders (710-719)

710 Diffuse diseases of connective tissue
711 Arthropathy associated with infections
712 Crystal arthropathies
713 Arthropathy associated with other disorders classified elsewhere
714 Rheumatoid arthritis and other inflammatory polyarthropathies
715 Osteoarthrosis and allied disorders
716 Other and unspecified arthropathies
717 Internal derangement of knee
718 Other derangement of joint
719 Other and unspecified disorder of joint

Dorsopathies (720-724)

720 Ankylosing spondylitis and other inflammatory spondylopathies
721 Spondylosis and allied disorders
722 Intervertebral disc disorders
723 Other disorders of cervical region
724 Other and unspecified disorders of back

Rheumatism, excluding the back (725-729)

725 Polymyalgia rheumatica
726 Peripheral enthesopathies and allied syndromes
727 Other disorders of synovium, tendon, and bursa
728 Disorders of muscle, ligament, and fascia
729 Other disorders of soft tissues

Osteopathies, chondropathies, and acquired musculoskeletal deformities (730-739)

730 Osteomyelitis, periostitis, and other infections involving bone
731 Osteitis deformans and osteopathies associated with other disorders classified
    elsewhere
732 Osteochondropathies
733 Other disorders of bone and cartilage
734 Flat foot
735 Acquired deformities of toe
736 Other acquired deformities of limbs
737 Curvature of spine
738 Other acquired deformity
739 Nonallopathic lesions, not elsewhere classified

14. CONGENITAL ANOMALIES

740 Anencephalus and similar anomalies
741 Spina bifida
742 Other congenital anomalies of nervous system
743 Congenital anomalies of eye
744 Congenital anomalies of ear, face, and neck
745 Bulbus cordis anomalies and anomalies of cardiac septal closure
746 Other congenital anomalies of heart
747 Other congenital anomalies of circulatory system
748 Congenital anomalies of respiratory system
749 Cleft palate and cleft lip
750 Other congenital anomalies of upper alimentary tract
751 Other congenital anomalies of digestive system
752 Congenital anomalies of genital organs
753 Congenital anomalies of urinary system
754 Certain congenital musculoskeletal deformities
755 Other congenital anomalies of limbs
756 Other congenital musculoskeletal anomalies
757 Congenital anomalies of the integument
758 Chromosomal anomalies
759 Other and unspecified congenital anomalies

15. CERTAIN CONDITIONS ORIGINATING IN THE PERINATAL PERIOD

Maternal causes of perinatal morbidity and mortality (760-763)

760 Fetus or newborn affected by maternal conditions which may be unrelated to present pregnancy
761 Fetus or newborn affected by maternal complications of pregnancy
762 Fetus or newborn affected by complications of placenta, cord, and membranes
763 Fetus or newborn affected by other complications of labor and delivery

Other conditions originating in the perinatal period (764-779)

764 Slow fetal growth and fetal malnutrition
765 Disorders relating to short gestation and low birthweight
766 Disorders relating to long gestation and high birthweight
767 Birth trauma
768 Intrauterine hypoxia and birth asphyxia
769 Respiratory distress syndrome
770 Other respiratory conditions of fetus and newborn
771 Infections specific to the perinatal period
772 Fetal and neonatal hemorrhage
773 Hemolytic disease of fetus or newborn, due to isoimmunization
774 Other perinatal jaundice
775 Endocrine and metabolic disturbances specific to the fetus and newborn
776 Hematological disorders of fetus and newborn
777 Perinatal disorders of digestive system
778 Conditions involving the integument and temperature regulation of fetus and newborn
779 Other and ill-defined conditions originating in the perinatal period

16. SYMPTOMS, SIGNS, AND ILL-DEFINED CONDITIONS

Symptoms (780-789)

780 General symptoms
781 Symptoms involving nervous and musculoskeletal systems
782 Symptoms involving skin and other integumentary tissue
783 Symptoms concerning nutrition, metabolism, and development
784 Symptoms involving head and neck
785 Symptoms involving cardiovascular system
786 Symptoms involving respiratory system and other chest symptoms
787 Symptoms involving digestive system
788 Symptoms involving urinary system
789 Other symptoms involving abdomen and pelvis

Nonspecific abnormal findings (790-796)

790 Nonspecific findings on examination of blood
791 Nonspecific findings on examination of urine
792 Nonspecific abnormal findings in other body substances
793 Nonspecific abnormal findings on radiological and other examination of body structure
794 Nonspecific abnormal results of function studies
795 Nonspecific abnormal histological and immunological findings
796 Other nonspecific abnormal findings

Ill-defined and unknown causes of morbidity and mortality (797-799)

797 Senility without mention of psychosis
798 Sudden death, cause unknown
799 Other ill-defined and unknown causes of morbidity and mortality

17. INJURY AND POISONING

Fracture of skull (800-804)

800 Fracture of vault of skull
801 Fracture of base of skull
802 Fracture of face bones
803 Other and unqualified skull fractures
804 Multiple fractures involving skull or face with other bones

Fracture of neck and trunk (805-809)

805 Fracture of vertebral column without mention of spinal cord injury
806 Fracture of vertebral column with spinal cord injury
807 Fracture of rib(s), sternum, larynx, and trachea
808 Fracture of pelvis
809 Ill-defined fractures of bones of trunk

17. INJURY AND POISONING *continued*

Fracture of upper limb (810-819)

- 810 Fracture of clavicle
- 811 Fracture of scapula
- 812 Fracture of humerus
- 813 Fracture of radius and ulna
- 814 Fracture of carpal bone(s)
- 815 Fracture of metacarpal bone(s)
- 816 Fracture of one or more phalanges of hand
- 817 Multiple fractures of hand bones
- 818 Ill-defined fractures of upper limb
- 819 Multiple fractures involving both upper limbs, and upper limb with rib(s) and sternum

Fracture of lower limb (820-829)

- 820 Fracture of neck of femur
- 821 Fracture of other and unspecified parts of femur
- 822 Fracture of patella
- 823 Fracture of tibia and fibula
- 824 Fracture of ankle
- 825 Fracture of one or more tarsal and metatarsal bones
- 826 Fracture of one or more phalanges of foot
- 827 Other, multiple, and ill-defined fractures of lower limb
- 828 Multiple fractures involving both lower limbs, lower with upper limb, and lower limb(s) with rib(s) and sternum
- 829 Fracture of unspecified bones

Dislocation (830-839)

- 830 Dislocation of jaw
- 831 Dislocation of shoulder
- 832 Dislocation of elbow
- 833 Dislocation of wrist
- 834 Dislocation of finger
- 835 Dislocation of hip
- 836 Dislocation of knee
- 837 Dislocation of ankle
- 838 Dislocation of foot
- 839 Other, multiple, and ill-defined dislocations

Sprains and strains of joints and adjacent muscles (840-848)

- 840 Sprains and strains of shoulder and upper arm
- 841 Sprains and strains of elbow and forearm
- 842 Sprains and strains of wrist and hand
- 843 Sprains and strains of hip and thigh
- 844 Sprains and strains of knee and leg
- 845 Sprains and strains of ankle and foot
- 846 Sprains and strains of sacroiliac region
- 847 Sprains and strains of other and unspecified parts of back
- 848 Other and ill-defined sprains and strains

Intracranial injury, excluding those with skull fracture (850-854)

- 850 Concussion
- 851 Cerebral laceration and contusion
- 852 Subarachnoid, subdural, and extradural hemorrhage, following injury
- 853 Other and unspecified intracranial hemorrhage following injury
- 854 Intracranial injury of other and unspecified nature

Internal injury of thorax, abdomen, and pelvis (860-869)

- 860 Traumatic pneumothorax and hemothorax
- 861 Injury to heart and lung
- 862 Injury to other and unspecified intrathoracic organs
- 863 Injury to gastrointestinal tract
- 864 Injury to liver
- 865 Injury to spleen
- 866 Injury to kidney
- 867 Injury to pelvic organs
- 868 Injury to other intra-abdominal organs
- 869 Internal injury to unspecified or ill-defined organs

17. INJURY AND POISONING *continued*

Open wound of head, neck, and trunk (870-879)

870 Open wound of ocular adnexa
871 Open wound of eyeball
872 Open wound of ear
873 Other open wound of head
874 Open wound of neck
875 Open wound of chest (wall)
876 Open wound of back
877 Open wound of buttock
878 Open wound of genital organs (external), including traumatic amputation
879 Open wound of other and unspecified sites, except limbs

Open wound of upper limb (880-887)

880 Open wound of shoulder and upper arm
881 Open wound of elbow, forearm, and wrist
882 Open wound of hand except finger(s) alone
883 Open wound of finger(s)
884 Multiple and unspecified open wound of upper limb
885 Traumatic amputation of thumb (complete) (partial)
886 Traumatic amputation of other finger(s) (complete) (partial)
887 Traumatic amputation of arm and hand (complete) (partial)

Open wound of lower limb (890-897)

890 Open wound of hip and thigh
891 Open wound of knee, leg [except thigh], and ankle
892 Open wound of foot except toe(s) alone
893 Open wound of toe(s)
894 Multiple and unspecified open wound of lower limb
895 Traumatic amputation of toe(s) (complete) (partial)
896 Traumatic amputation of foot (complete) (partial)
897 Traumatic amputation of leg(s) (complete) (partial)

Injury to blood vessels (900-904)

900 Injury to blood vessels of head and neck
901 Injury to blood vessels of thorax
902 Injury to blood vessels of abdomen and pelvis
903 Injury to blood vessels of upper extremity
904 Injury to blood vessels of lower extremity and unspecified sites

Late effects of injuries, poisonings, toxic effects, and other external causes (905-909)

905 Late effects of musculoskeletal and connective tissue injuries
906 Late effects of injuries to skin and subcutaneous tissues
907 Late effects of injuries to the nervous system
908 Late effects of other and unspecified injuries
909 Late effects of other and unspecified external causes

Superficial injury (910-919)

910 Superficial injury of face, neck, and scalp except eye
911 Superficial injury of trunk
912 Superficial injury of shoulder and upper arm
913 Superficial injury of elbow, forearm, and wrist
914 Superficial injury of hand(s) except finger(s) alone
915 Superficial injury of finger(s)
916 Superficial injury of hip, thigh, leg, and ankle
917 Superficial injury of foot and toe(s)
918 Superficial injury of eye and adnexa
919 Superficial injury of other, multiple, and unspecified sites

Contusion with intact skin surface (920-924)

920 Contusion of face, scalp, and neck except eye(s)
921 Contusion of eye and adnexa
922 Contusion of trunk
923 Contusion of upper limb
924 Contusion of lower limb and of other and unspecified sites

Crushing injury (925-929)

925 Crushing injury of face, scalp, and neck
926 Crushing injury of trunk
927 Crushing injury of upper limb

17. INJURY AND POISONING *continued*

- 928 Crushing injury of lower limb
- 929 Crushing injury of multiple and unspecified sites

Effects of foreign body entering through orifice (930-939)

- 930 Foreign body on external eye
- 931 Foreign body in ear
- 932 Foreign body in nose
- 933 Foreign body in pharynx and larynx
- 934 Foreign body in trachea, bronchus, and lung
- 935 Foreign body in mouth, esophagus, and stomach
- 936 Foreign body in intestine and colon
- 937 Foreign body in anus and rectum
- 938 Foreign body in digestive system, unspecified
- 939 Foreign body in genitourinary tract

Burns (940-949)

- 940 Burn confined to eye and adnexa
- 941 Burn of face, head, and neck
- 942 Burn of trunk
- 943 Burn of upper limb, except wrist and hand
- 944 Burn of wrist(s) and hand(s)
- 945 Burn of lower limb(s)
- 946 Burns of multiple specified sites
- 947 Burn of internal organs
- 948 Burns classified according to extent of body surface involved
- 949 Burn, unspecified

Injury to nerves and spinal cord (950-957)

- 950 Injury to optic nerve and pathways
- 951 Injury to other cranial nerve(s)
- 952 Spinal cord injury without evidence of spinal bone injury
- 953 Injury to nerve roots and spinal plexus
- 954 Injury to other nerve(s) of trunk excluding shoulder and pelvic girdles
- 955 Injury to peripheral nerve(s) of shoulder girdle and upper limb
- 956 Injury to peripheral nerve(s) of pelvic girdle and lower limb
- 957 Injury to other and unspecified nerves

Certain traumatic complications and unspecified injuries (958-959)

- 958 Certain early complications of trauma
- 959 Injury, other and unspecified

Poisoning by drugs, medicinal and biological substances (960-979)

- 960 Poisoning by antibiotics
- 961 Poisoning by other anti-infectives
- 962 Poisoning by hormones and synthetic substitutes
- 963 Poisoning by primarily systemic agents
- 964 Poisoning by agents primarily affecting blood constituents
- 965 Poisoning by analgesics, antipyretics, and antirheumatics
- 966 Poisoning by anticonvulsants and anti-Parkinsonism drugs
- 967 Poisoning by sedatives and hypnotics
- 968 Poisoning by other central nervous system depressants and anesthetics
- 969 Poisoning by psychotropic agents
- 970 Poisoning by central nervous system stimulants
- 971 Poisoning by drugs primarily affecting the autonomic nervous system
- 972 Poisoning by agents primarily affecting the cardiovascular system
- 973 Poisoning by agents primarily affecting the gastrointestinal system
- 974 Poisoning by water, mineral, and uric acid metabolism drugs
- 975 Poisoning by agents primarily acting on the smooth and skeletal muscles and respiratory system
- 976 Poisoning by agents primarily affecting skin and mucous membrane, ophthalmological, otorhinolaryngological, and dental drugs
- 977 Poisoning by other and unspecified drugs and medicinals
- 978 Poisoning by bacterial vaccines
- 979 Poisoning by other vaccines and biological substances

Toxic effects of substances chiefly nonmedicinal as to source (980-989)

- 980 Toxic effect of alcohol
- 981 Toxic effect of petroleum products
- 982 Toxic effect of solvents other than petroleum-based

17. INJURY AND POISONING *continued*

    983   Toxic effect of corrosive aromatics, acids, and caustic alkalis
    984   Toxic effect of lead and its compounds (including fumes)
    985   Toxic effect of other metals
    986   Toxic effect of carbon monoxide
    987   Toxic effect of other gases, fumes, or vapors
    988   Toxic effect of noxious substances eaten as food
    989   Toxic effect of other substances, chiefly nonmedicinal as to source

Other and unspecified effects of external causes (990-995)

    990   Effects of radiation, unspecified
    991   Effects of reduced temperature
    992   Effects of heat and light
    993   Effects of air pressure
    994   Effects of other external causes
    995   Certain adverse effects, not elsewhere classified

Complications of surgical and medical care, not elsewhere classified (996-999)

    996   Complications peculiar to certain specified procedures
    997   Complications affecting specified body systems, not elsewhere classified
    998   Other complications of procedures, not elsewhere classified
    999   Complications of medical care, not elsewhere classified

SUPPLEMENTARY CLASSIFICATION OF FACTORS INFLUENCING HEALTH STATUS AND CONTACT WITH HEALTH SERVICES

Persons with potential health hazards related to communicable diseases (V01-V06)

    V01   Contact with or exposure to communicable diseases
    V02   Carrier or suspected carrier of infectious diseases
    V03   Need for prophylactic vaccination and inoculation against bacterial diseases
    V04   Need for prophylactic vaccination and inoculation against certain viral diseases
    V05   Need for other prophylactic vaccination and inoculation against single diseases
    V06   Need for prophylactic vaccination and inoculation against combinations of diseases

Persons with need for isolation, other potential health hazards and prophylactic measures (V07-V09)

    V07   Need for isolation and other prophylactic measures
    V08   Asymptomatic human immunodeficiency virus (HIV) infection status
    V09   Infection with drug-resistant microorganisms

Persons with potential health hazards related to personal and family history (V10-V19)

    V10   Personal history of malignant neoplasm
    V11   Personal history of mental disorder
    V12   Personal history of certain other diseases
    V13   Personal history of other diseases
    V14   Personal history of allergy to medicinal agents
    V15   Other personal history presenting hazards to health
    V16   Family history of malignant neoplasm
    V17   Family history of certain chronic disabling diseases
    V18   Family history of certain other specific conditions
    V19   Family history of other conditions

Persons encountering health services in circumstances related to reproduction and development (V20-V29)

    V20   Health supervision of infant or child
    V21   Constitutional states in development
    V22   Normal pregnancy
    V23   Supervision of high-risk pregnancy
    V24   Postpartum care and examination
    V25   Encounter for contraceptive management
    V26   Procreative management
    V27   Outcome of delivery
    V28   Antenatal screening
    V29   Observation and evaluation of newborns and infants for suspected condition not found

Liveborn infants according to type of birth (V30-V39)

    V30   Single liveborn
    V31   Twin, mate liveborn
    V32   Twin, mate stillborn
    V33   Twin, unspecified
    V34   Other multiple, mates all liveborn

SUPPLEMENTARY CLASSIFICATION...HEALTH STATUS/HEALTH SERVICES *continued*

V35 Other multiple, mates all stillborn
V36 Other multiple, mates live- and stillborn
V37 Other multiple, unspecified
V39 Unspecified

Persons with a condition influencing their health status (V40-V49)

V40 Mental and behavioral problems
V41 Problems with special senses and other special functions
V42 Organ or tissue replaced by transplant
V43 Organ or tissue replaced by other means
V44 Artificial opening status
V45 Other postsurgical states
V46 Other dependence on machines
V47 Other problems with internal organs
V48 Problems with head, neck, and trunk
V49 Other conditions influencing health status

Persons encountering health services for specific procedures and aftercare (V50-V59)

V50 Elective surgery for purposes other than remedying health states
V51 Aftercare involving the use of plastic surgery
V52 Fitting and adjustment of prosthetic device and implant
V53 Fitting and adjustment of other device
V54 Other orthopedic aftercare
V55 Attention to artificial openings
V56 Encounter for dialysis and dialysis catheter care
V57 Care involving use of rehabilitation procedures
V58 Encounter for other and unspecified procedures and aftercare
V59 Donors

Persons encountering health services in other circumstances (V60-V69)

V60 Housing, household, and economic circumstances
V61 Other family circumstances
V62 Other psychosocial circumstances
V63 Unavailability of other medical facilities for care
V64 Persons encountering health services for specific procedures, not carried out
V65 Other persons seeking consultation without complaint or sickness
V66 Convalescence and palliative care
V67 Follow-up examination
V68 Encounters for administrative purposes
V69 Problems related to lifestyle

Persons without reported diagnosis encountered during examination and investigation of individuals and populations (V70-V82)

V70 General medical examination
V71 Observation and evaluation for suspected conditions not found
V72 Special investigations and examinations
V73 Special screening examination for viral and chlamydial diseases
V74 Special screening examination for bacterial and spirochetal diseases
V75 Special screening examination for other infectious diseases
V76 Special screening for malignant neoplasms
V77 Special screening for endocrine, nutritional, metabolic, and immunity disorders
V78 Special screening for disorders of blood and blood-forming organs
V79 Special screening for mental disorders and developmental handicaps
V80 Special screening for neurological, eye, and ear diseases
V81 Special screening for cardiovascular, respiratory, and genitourinary diseases
V82 Special screening for other conditions
V83 Genetic carrier status

SUPPLEMENTARY CLASSIFICATION OF EXTERNAL CAUSES OF INJURY AND POISONING

Railway accidents (E800-E807)

E800 Railway accident involving collision with rolling stock
E801 Railway accident involving collision with other object
E802 Railway accident involving derailment without antecedent collision
E803 Railway accident involving explosion, fire, or burning
E804 Fall in, on, or from railway train
E805 Hit by rolling stock

SUPPLEMENTARY CLASSIFICATION...INJURY AND POISONING *continued*

    E806 Other specified railway accident
    E807 Railway accident of unspecified nature

Motor vehicle traffic accidents (E810-E819)

    E810 Motor vehicle traffic accident involving collision with train
    E811 Motor vehicle traffic accident involving re-entrant collision with another motor vehicle
    E812 Other motor vehicle traffic accident involving collision with another motor vehicle
    E813 Motor vehicle traffic accident involving collision with other vehicle
    E814 Motor vehicle traffic accident involving collision with pedestrian
    E815 Other motor vehicle traffic accident involving collision on the highway
    E816 Motor vehicle traffic accident due to loss of control, without collision on the highway
    E817 Noncollision motor vehicle traffic accident while boarding or alighting
    E818 Other noncollision motor vehicle traffic accident
    E819 Motor vehicle traffic accident of unspecified nature

Motor vehicle nontraffic accidents (E820-E825)

    E820 Nontraffic accident involving motor-driven snow vehicle
    E821 Nontraffic accident involving other off-road motor vehicle
    E822 Other motor vehicle nontraffic accident involving collision with moving object
    E823 Other motor vehicle nontraffic accident involving collision with stationary object
    E824 Other motor vehicle nontraffic accident while boarding and alighting
    E825 Other motor vehicle nontraffic accident of other and unspecified nature

Other road vehicle accidents (E826-E829)

    E826 Pedal cycle accident
    E827 Animal-drawn vehicle accident
    E828 Accident involving animal being ridden
    E829 Other road vehicle accidents

Water transport accidents (E830-E838)

    E830 Accident to watercraft causing submersion
    E831 Accident to watercraft causing other injury
    E832 Other accidental submersion or drowning in water transport accident
    E833 Fall on stairs or ladders in water transport
    E834 Other fall from one level to another in water transport
    E835 Other and unspecified fall in water transport
    E836 Machinery accident in water transport
    E837 Explosion, fire, or burning in watercraft
    E838 Other and unspecified water transport accident

Air and space transport accidents (E840-E845)

    E840 Accident to powered aircraft at takeoff or landing
    E841 Accident to powered aircraft, other and unspecified
    E842 Accident to unpowered aircraft
    E843 Fall in, on, or from aircraft
    E844 Other specified air transport accidents
    E845 Accident involving spacecraft

Vehicle accidents, not elsewhere classifiable (E846-E849)

    E846 Accidents involving powered vehicles used solely within the buildings and premises
            of an industrial or commercial establishment
    E847 Accidents involving cable cars not running on rails
    E848 Accidents involving other vehicles, not elsewhere classifiable
    E849 Place of occurrence

Accidental poisoning by drugs, medicinal substances, and biologicals (E850-E858)

    E850 Accidental poisoning by analgesics, antipyretics, and antirheumatics
    E851 Accidental poisoning by barbiturates
    E852 Accidental poisoning by other sedatives and hypnotics
    E853 Accidental poisoning by tranquilizers
    E854 Accidental poisoning by other psychotropic agents
    E855 Accidental poisoning by other drugs acting on central and autonomic nervous systems
    E856 Accidental poisoning by antibiotics
    E857 Accidental poisoning by other anti-infectives
    E858 Accidental poisoning by other drugs

Accidental poisoning by other solid and liquid substances, gases, and vapors (E860-E869)

    E860 Accidental poisoning by alcohol, not elsewhere classified
    E861 Accidental poisoning by cleansing and polishing agents, disinfectants, paints, and
            varnishes

SUPPLEMENTARY CLASSIFICATION...INJURY AND POISONING *continued*

E862 Accidental poisoning by petroleum products, other solvents and their vapors, not elsewhere classified

E863 Accidental poisoning by agricultural and horticultural chemical and pharmaceutical preparations other than plant foods and fertilizers

E864 Accidental poisoning by corrosives and caustics, not elsewhere classified

E865 Accidental poisoning from poisonous foodstuffs and poisonous plants

E866 Accidental poisoning by other and unspecified solid and liquid substances

E867 Accidental poisoning by gas distributed by pipeline

E868 Accidental poisoning by other utility gas and other carbon monoxide

E869 Accidental poisoning by other gases and vapors

Misadventures to patients during surgical and medical care (E870-E876)

E870 Accidental cut, puncture, perforation, or hemorrhage during medical care

E871 Foreign object left in body during procedure

E872 Failure of sterile precautions during procedure

E873 Failure in dosage

E874 Mechanical failure of instrument or apparatus during procedure

E875 Contaminated or infected blood, other fluid, drug, or biological substance

E876 Other and unspecified misadventures during medical care

Surgical and medical procedures as the cause of abnormal reaction of patient or later complication, without mention of misadventure at the time of procedure (E878-E879)

E878 Surgical operation and other surgical procedures as the cause of abnormal reaction of patient, or of later complication, without mention of misadventure at the time of operation

E879 Other procedures, without mention of misadventure at the time of procedure, as the cause of abnormal reaction of patient, or of later complication

Accidental falls (E880-E888)

E880 Fall on or from stairs or steps

E881 Fall on or from ladders or scaffolding

E882 Fall from or out of building or other structure

E883 Fall into hole or other opening in surface

E884 Other fall from one level to another

E885 Fall on same level from slipping, tripping, or stumbling

E886 Fall on same level from collision, pushing or shoving, by or with other person

E887 Fracture, cause unspecified

E888 Other and unspecified fall

Accidents caused by fire and flames (E890-E899)

E890 Conflagration in private dwelling

E891 Conflagration in other and unspecified building or structure

E892 Conflagration not in building or structure

E893 Accident caused by ignition of clothing

E894 Ignition of highly inflammable material

E895 Accident caused by controlled fire in private dwelling

E896 Accident caused by controlled fire in other and unspecified building or structure

E897 Accident caused by controlled fire not in building or structure

E898 Accident caused by other specified fire and flames

E899 Accident caused by unspecified fire

Accidents due to natural and environmental factors (E900-E909)

E900 Excessive heat

E901 Excessive cold

E902 High and low air pressure and changes in air pressure

E903 Travel and motion

E904 Hunger, thirst, exposure, and neglect

E905 Venomous animals and plants as the cause of poisoning and toxic reactions

E906 Other injury caused by animals

E907 Lightning

E908 Cataclysmic storms, and floods resulting from storms

E909 Cataclysmic earth surface movements and eruptions

Accidents caused by submersion, suffocation, and foreign bodies (E910-E915)

E910 Accidental drowning and submersion

E911 Inhalation and ingestion of food causing obstruction of respiratory tract or suffocation

E912 Inhalation and ingestion of other object causing obstruction of respiratory tract or suffocation

E913 Accidental mechanical suffocation

SUPPLEMENTARY CLASSIFICATION...INJURY AND POISONING *continued*

E914 Foreign body accidentally entering eye and adnexa
E915 Foreign body accidentally entering other orifice

Other accidents (E916-E928)
E916 Struck accidentally by falling object
E917 Striking against or struck accidentally by objects or persons
E918 Caught accidentally in or between objects
E919 Accidents caused by machinery
E920 Accidents caused by cutting and piercing instruments or objects
E921 Accident caused by explosion of pressure vessel
E922 Accident caused by firearm and air gun missile
E923 Accident caused by explosive material
E924 Accident caused by hot substance or object, caustic or corrosive material, and steam
E925 Accident caused by electric current
E926 Exposure to radiation
E927 Overexertion and strenuous movements
E928 Other and unspecified environmental and accidental causes

Late effects of accidental injury (E929)
E929 Late effects of accidental injury

Drugs, medicinal and biological substances causing adverse effects in therapeutic use (E930-E949)
E930 Antibiotics
E931 Other anti-infectives
E932 Hormones and synthetic substitutes
E933 Primarily systemic agents
E934 Agents primarily affecting blood constituents
E935 Analgesics, antipyretics, and antirheumatics
E936 Anticonvulsants and anti-Parkinsonism drugs
E937 Sedatives and hypnotics
E938 Other central nervous system depressants and anesthetics
E939 Psychotropic agents
E940 Central nervous system stimulants
E941 Drugs primarily affecting the autonomic nervous system
E942 Agents primarily affecting the cardiovascular system
E943 Agents primarily affecting gastrointestinal system
E944 Water, mineral, and uric acid metabolism drugs
E945 Agents primarily acting on the smooth and skeletal muscles and respiratory system
E946 Agents primarily affecting skin and mucous membrane, ophthalmological,
    otorhinolaryngological, and dental drugs
E947 Other and unspecified drugs and medicinal substances
E948 Bacterial vaccines
E949 Other vaccines and biological substances

Suicide and self-inflicted injury (E950-E959)
E950 Suicide and self-inflicted poisoning by solid or liquid substances
E951 Suicide and self-inflicted poisoning by gases in domestic use
E952 Suicide and self-inflicted poisoning by other gases and vapors
E953 Suicide and self inflicted injury by hanging, strangulation, and suffocation
E954 Suicide and self-inflicted injury by submersion [drowning]
E955 Suicide and self-inflicted injury by firearms, air guns and explosives
E956 Suicide and self-inflicted injury by cutting and piercing instruments
E957 Suicide and self-inflicted injuries by jumping from high place
E958 Suicide and self-inflicted injury by other and unspecified means
E959 Late effects of self-inflicted injury

Homicide and injury purposely inflicted by other persons (E960-E969)
E960 Fight, brawl, and rape
E961 Assault by corrosive or caustic substance, except poisoning
E962 Assault by poisoning
E963 Assault by hanging and strangulation
E964 Assault by submersion [drowning]
E965 Assault by firearms and explosives
E966 Assault by cutting and piercing instrument
E967 Perpetrator of child and adult abuse
E968 Assault by other and unspecified means
E969 Late effects of injury purposely inflicted by other person

SUPPLEMENTARY CLASSIFICATION...INJURY AND POISONING *continued*

Legal intervention (E970-E978)

E970 Injury due to legal intervention by firearms
E971 Injury due to legal intervention by explosives
E972 Injury due to legal intervention by gas
E973 Injury due to legal intervention by blunt object
E974 Injury due to legal intervention by cutting and piercing instruments
E975 Injury due to legal intervention by other specified means
E976 Injury due to legal intervention by unspecified means
E977 Late effects of injuries due to legal intervention
E978 Legal execution
E979 Terrorism

Injury undetermined whether accidentally or purposely inflicted (E980-E989)

E980 Poisoning by solid or liquid substances, undetermined whether accidentally or
purposely inflicted
E981 Poisoning by gases in domestic use, undetermined whether accidentally or purposely
inflicted
E982 Poisoning by other gases, undetermined whether accidentally or purposely inflicted
E983 Hanging, strangulation, or suffocation, undetermined whether accidentally or
purposely inflicted
E984 Submersion [drowning], undetermined whether accidentally or purposely inflicted
E985 Injury by firearms, air guns and explosives, undetermined whether accidentally or
purposely inflicted
E986 Injury by cutting and piercing instruments, undetermined whether accidentally or
purposely inflicted
E987 Falling from high place, undetermined whether accidentally or purposely inflicted
E988 Injury by other and unspecified means, undetermined whether accidentally or
purposely inflicted
E989 Late effects of injury, undetermined whether accidentally or purposely inflicted

Injury resulting from operations of war (E990-E999)

E990 Injury due to war operations by fires and conflagrations
E991 Injury due to war operations by bullets and fragments
E992 Injury due to war operations by explosion of marine weapons
E993 Injury due to war operations by other explosion
E994 Injury due to war operations by destruction of aircraft
E995 Injury due to war operations by other and unspecified forms of conventional warfare
E996 Injury due to war operations by nuclear weapons
E997 Injury due to war operations by other forms of unconventional warfare
E998 Injury due to war operations but occurring after cessation of hostilities
E999 Late effects of injury due to war operations and terrorism

DISEASES: ALPHABETIC INDEX
VOLUME 2

A

AAV (disease) (illness) (infection)—*see* Human immunodeficiency virus (disease) (illness) (infection)

Abactio —*see* Abortion, induced

Abactus venter —*see* Abortion, induced

Abarognosis 781.99

Abasia (-astasia) 307.9
  atactica 781.3
  choreic 781.3
  hysterical 300.11
  paroxysmal trepidant 781.3
  spastic 781.3
  trembling 781.3
  trepidans 781.3

Abderhalden-Kaufmann-Lignac syndrome (cystinosis) 270.0

Abdomen, abdominal —*see also* condition
  accordion 306.4
  acute 789.0
  angina 557.1
  burst 868.00
  convulsive equivalent (*see also* Epilepsy) 345.5
  heart 746.87
  muscle deficiency syndrome 756.79
  obstipum 756.79

Abdominalgia 789.0
  periodic 277.3

Abduction contracture, hip or other joint —*see* Contraction, joint

Abercrombie's syndrome (amyloid degeneration) 277.3

Aberrant (congenital)—*see also* Malposition, congenital
  adrenal gland 759.1
  blood vessel NEC 747.60
    arteriovenous NEC 747.60
    cerebrovascular 747.81
    gastrointestinal 747.61
    lower limb 747.64
    renal 747.62
    spinal 747.82
    upper limb 747.63
  breast 757.6
  endocrine gland NEC 759.2
  gastrointestinal vessel (peripheral) 747.61
  hepatic duct 751.69
  lower limb vessel (peripheral) 747.64
  pancreas 751.7
  parathyroid gland 759.2
  peripheral vascular vessel NEC 747.60
  pituitary gland (pharyngeal) 759.2
  renal blood vessel 747.62
  sebaceous glands, mucous membrane, mouth 750.26
  spinal vessel 747.82
  spleen 759.0
  testis (descent) 752.51
  thymus gland 759.2
  thyroid gland 759.2
  upper limb vessel (peripheral) 747.63

Aberratio
  lactis 757.6
  testis 752.51

Aberration —*see also* Anomaly
  chromosome—*see* Anomaly, chromosome(s)
  distantial 368.9
  mental (*see also* Disorder, mental, nonpsychotic) 300.9

Abetalipoproteinemia 272.5

Abionarce 780.79

Abiotrophy 799.8

Ablatio
  placentae—*see* Placenta, ablatio
  retinae (*see also* Detachment, retina) 361.9

Ablation
  pituitary (gland) (with hypofunction) 253.7
  placenta—*see* Placenta, ablatio
  uterus 621.8

Ablepharia, ablepharon, ablephary 743.62

Ablepsia —*see* Blindness

Ablepsy —*see* Blindness

Ablutomania 300.3

Abnormal, abnormality, abnormalities —*see also* Anomaly
  acid-base balance 276.4
    fetus or newborn—*see* Distress, fetal
  adaptation curve, dark 368.63
  alveolar ridge 525.9
  amnion 658.9
    affecting fetus or newborn 762.9
  anatomical relationship NEC 759.9
  apertures, congenital, diaphragm 756.6
  auditory perception NEC 388.40
  autosomes NEC 758.5
    13 758.1
    18 758.2
    21 or 22 758.0
    D$_1$ 758.1
    E$_3$ 758.2
    G 758.0
  ballistocardiogram 794.39
  basal metabolic rate (BMR) 794.7
  biosynthesis, testicular androgen 257.2
  blood level (of)
    cobalt 790.6
    copper 790.6
    iron 790.6
    lithium 790.6
    magnesium 790.6
    mineral 790.6
    zinc 790.6
  blood pressure
    elevated (without diagnosis of hypertension) 796.2
    low (*see also* Hypotension) 458.9
      reading (incidental) (isolated) (nonspecific) 796.3
  bowel sounds 787.5
  breathing behavior—*see* Respiration
  caloric test 794.19
  cervix (acquired) NEC 622.9
    congenital 752.40
    in pregnancy or childbirth 654.6
      causing obstructed labor 660.2
        affecting fetus or newborn 763.1
  chemistry, blood NEC 790.6
  chest sounds 786.7
  chorion 658.9
    affecting fetus or newborn 762.9
  chromosomal NEC 758.89
    analysis, nonspecific result 795.2
    autosomes (*see also* Abnormal, autosomes NEC) 758.5
    fetal, (suspected) affecting management of pregnancy 655.1
    sex 758.81

Abnormal, abnormality . . .—*continued*
narrowness, eyelid 743.62
optokinetic response 379.57
organs or tissues of pelvis NEC
in pregnancy or childbirth 654.9
affecting fetus or newborn 763.89
causing obstructed labor 660.2
affecting fetus or newborn 763.1
origin—*see* Malposition, congenital
palmar creases 757.2
Papanicolaou (smear)
cervix 795.00
atypical squamous cell changes of
undetermined significance
favor benign (ASCUS favor benign)
795.01
favor dysplasia (ASCUS favor dysplasia)
795.02
nonspecific finding NEC 795.09
other site 795.1
parturition
affecting fetus or newborn 763.9
mother—*see* Delivery, complicated
pelvis (bony)—*see* Deformity, pelvis
percussion, chest 786.7
periods (grossly) (see also Menstruation) 626.9
phonocardiogram 794.39
placenta—*see* Placenta, abnormal
plantar reflex 796.1
plasma protein—*see* Deficiency, plasma, protein
pleural folds 748.8
position—*see also* Malposition
gravid uterus 654.4
causing obstructed labor 660.2
affecting fetus or newborn 763.1
posture NEC 781.92
presentation (fetus)—*see* Presentation, fetus,
abnormal
product of conception NEC 631
puberty—*see* Puberty
pulmonary
artery 747.3
function, newborn 770.89
test results 794.2
ventilation, newborn 770.89
hyperventilation 786.01
pulsations in neck 785.1
pupil reflexes 379.40
quality of milk 676.8
radiological examination 793.9
abdomen NEC 793.6
biliary tract 793.3
breast 793.89
mammogram NOS 793.80
mammographic microcalcification 793.81
gastrointestinal tract 793.4
genitourinary organs 793.5
head 793.0
intrathoracic organ NEC 793.2
lung (field) 793.1
musculoskeletal system 793.7
retroperitoneum 793.6
skin and subcutaneous tissue 793.9
skull 793.0
red blood cells 790.09
morphology 790.09
volume 790.09
reflex NEC 796.1
renal function test 794.4
respiration signs—*see* Respiration
response to nerve stimulation 794.10

Abnormal, abnormality . . .—*continued*
retinal correspondence 368.34
rhythm, heart—*see also* Arrhythmia fetus—*see*
Distress, fetal
saliva 792.4
scan
brain 794.09
kidney 794.4
liver 794.8
lung 794.2
thyroid 794.5
secretion
gastrin 251.5
glucagon 251.4
semen 792.2
serum level (of)
acid phosphatase 790.5
alkaline phosphatase 790.5
amylase 790.5
enzymes NEC 790.5
lipase 790.5
shape
cornea 743.41
gallbladder 751.69
gravid uterus 654.4
affecting fetus or newborn 763.89
causing obstructed labor 660.2
affecting fetus or newborn 763.1
head (see also Anomaly, skull) 756.0
organ or site, congenital NEC—*see* Distortion
sinus venosus 747.40
size
fetus, complicating delivery 653.5
causing obstructed labor 660.1
gallbladder 751.69
head (*see also* Anomaly, skull) 756.0
organ or site, congenital NEC—*see* Distortion
teeth 520.2
skin and appendages, congenital NEC 757.9
soft parts of pelvis—*see* Abnormal, organs or
tissues of pelvis
spermatozoa 792.2
sputum (amount) (color) (excessive) (odor)
(purulent) 786.4
stool NEC 787.7
bloody 578.1
occult 792.1
bulky 787.7
color (dark) (light) 792.1
content (fat) (mucus) (pus) 792.1
occult blood 792.1
synchondrosis 756.9
test results without manifest disease—*see*
Findings, abnormal
thebesian valve 746.9
thermography—*see* Findings, abnormal,
structure
threshold, cones or rods (eye) 368.63
thyroid-binding globulin 246.8
thyroid product 246.8
toxicology (findings) NEC 796.0
tracheal cartilage (congenital) 748.3
transport protein 273.8
ultrasound results—*see* Findings, abnormal,
structure
umbilical cord
affecting fetus or newborn 762.6
complicating delivery 663.9
specified NEC 663.8
union
cricoid cartilage and thyroid cartilage 748.3

Abnormal, abnormality . . .—*continued*
　　larynx and trachea 748.3
　　thyroid cartilage and hyoid bone 748.3
　urination NEC 788.69
　　psychogenic 306.53
　　stream
　　　intermittent 788.61
　　　slowing 788.62
　　　splitting 788.61
　　　weak 788.62
　urine (constituents) NEC 791.9
　uterine hemorrhage (*see also* Hemorrhage,
　　　uterus) 626.9
　　climacteric 627.0
　　postmenopausal 627.1
　vagina (acquired) (congenital)
　　in pregnancy or childbirth 654.7
　　　affecting fetus or newborn 763.89
　　　causing obstructed labor 660.2
　　　　affecting fetus or newborn 763.1
　vascular sounds 785.9
　vectorcardiogram 794.39
　visually evoked potential (VEP) 794.13
　vulva (acquired) (congenital)
　　in pregnancy or childbirth 654.8
　　　affecting fetus or newborn 763.89
　　　causing obstructed labor 660.2
　　　　affecting fetus or newborn 763.1
　weight
　　gain 783.1
　　　of pregnancy 646.1
　　　　with hypertension—see Toxemia, of
　　　　　pregnancy
　　loss 783.21
　x-ray examination—*see* Abnormal, radiological
　　examination
Abnormally formed uterus —*see* Anomaly,
　uterus
Abnormity (any organ or part)—*see* Anomaly
ABO
　hemolytic disease 773.1
　incompatibility reaction 999.6
Abocclusion 524.2
Abolition, language 784.69
Aborter, habitual or recurrent NEC
　without current pregnancy 629.9
　current abortion (*see also* Abortion,
　　spontaneous) 634.9
　　affecting fetus or newborn 761.8
　observation in current pregnancy 646.3
Abortion (complete) (incomplete) (inevitable)
　　(with retained products of conception) 637.9

> *Note—Use the following fifth-digit*
> *subclassification with categories 634-637:*
>
> *0　unspecified*
> *1　incomplete*
> *2　complete*

　with
　　complication(s) (any) following previous
　　　abortion—*see* category 639
　　damage to pelvic organ (laceration) (rupture)
　　　(tear) 637.2
　　embolism (air) (amniotic fluid) (blood clot)
　　　(pulmonary) (pyemic) (septic) (soap) 637.6
　　genital tract and pelvic infection 637.0
　　hemorrhage, delayed or excessive 637.1
　　metabolic disorder 637.4
　　renal failure (acute) 637.3
　　sepsis (genital tract) (pelvic organ) 637.0

Abortion—*continued*
　　urinary tract 637.7
　　shock (postoperative) (septic) 637.5
　　specified complication NEC 637.7
　　toxemia 637.3
　　unspecified complication(s) 637.8
　　urinary tract infection 637.7
　accidental—*see* Abortion, spontaneous
　artificial—*see* Abortion, induced
　attempted (failed)—*see* Abortion, failed
　criminal—*see* Abortion, illegal
　early—*see* Abortion, spontaneous
　elective—*see* Abortion, legal
　failed (legal) 638.9
　　with
　　　damage to pelvic organ (laceration)
　　　　(rupture) (tear) 638.2
　　　embolism (air) (amniotic fluid) (blood clot)
　　　　(pulmonary) (pyemic) (septic) (soap)
　　　　638.6
　　　genital tract and pelvic infection 638.0
　　　hemorrhage, delayed or excessive 638.1
　　　metabolic disorder 638.4
　　　renal failure (acute) 638.3
　　　sepsis (genital tract) (pelvic organ) 638.0
　　　　urinary tract 638.7
　　　shock (postoperative) (septic) 638.5
　　　specified complication NEC 638.7
　　　toxemia 638.3
　　　unspecified complication(s) 638.8
　　　urinary tract infection 638.7
　fetal indication—*see* Abortion, legal
　fetus 779.6
　following threatened abortion—*see* Abortion,
　　by type
　habitual or recurrent (care during pregnancy)
　　646.3
　　with current abortion (*see also* Abortion,
　　　spontaneous) 634.9
　　affecting fetus or newborn 761.8
　　without current pregnancy 629.9
　homicidal—*see* Abortion, illegal
　illegal 636.9
　　with
　　　damage to pelvic organ (laceration)
　　　　(rupture) (tear) 636.2
　　　embolism (air) (amniotic fluid) (blood clot)
　　　　(pulmonary) (pyemic) (septic) (soap)
　　　　636.6
　　　genital tract and pelvic infection 636.0
　　　hemorrhage, delayed or excessive 636.1
　　　metabolic disorder 636.4
　　　renal failure 636.3
　　　sepsis (genital tract) (pelvic organ) 636.0
　　　　urinary tract 636.7
　　　shock (postoperative) (septic) 636.5
　　　specified complication NEC 636.7
　　　toxemia 636.3
　　　unspecified complication(s) 636.8
　　　urinary tract infection 636.7
　　fetus 779.6
　induced 637.9
　　illegal—*see* Abortion, illegal
　　legal indications—*see* Abortion, legal
　　medical indications—*see* Abortion, legal
　　therapeutic—*see* Abortion, legal
　late—*see* Abortion, spontaneous
　legal (legal indication) (medical indication)
　　　(under medical supervision) 635.9

Abortion—*continued*
  with
    damage to pelvic organ (laceration)
        (rupture) (tear) 635.2
    embolism (air) (amniotic fluid) (blood clot)
        (pulmonary) (pyemic) (septic) (soap)
        635.6
    genital tract and pelvic infection 635.0
    hemorrhage, delayed or excessive 635.1
    metabolic disorder 635.4
    renal failure (acute) 635.3
    sepsis (genital tract) (pelvic organ) 635.0
        urinary tract 635.7
    shock (postoperative) (septic) 635.5
    specified complication NEC 635.7
    toxemia 635.3
    unspecified complication(s) 635.8
    urinary tract infection 635.7
  fetus 779.6
  medical indication—*see* Abortion, legal
  mental hygiene problem—*see* Abortion, legal
  missed 632
  operative—*see* Abortion, legal
  psychiatric indication—*see* Abortion, legal
  recurrent—*see* Abortion, spontaneous
  self-induced—*see* Abortion, illegal
  septic—*see* Abortion, by type, with sepsis
  spontaneous 634.9
    with
      damage to pelvic organ (laceration)
          (rupture) (tear) 634.2
      embolism (air) (amniotic fluid) (blood clot)
          (pulmonary) (pyemic) (septic) (soap)
          634.6
      genital tract and pelvic infection 634.0
      hemorrhage, delayed or excessive 634.1
      metabolic disorder 634.4
      renal failure 634.3
      sepsis (genital tract) (pelvic organ) 634.0
          urinary tract 634.7
      shock (postoperative) (septic) 634.5
      specified complication NEC 634.7
      toxemia 634.3
      unspecified complication(s) 634.8
      urinary tract infection 634.7
    fetus 761.8
    threatened 640.0
      affecting fetus or newborn 762.1
  surgical—*see* Abortion, legal
  therapeutic—*see* Abortion, legal
  threatened 640.0
    affecting fetus or newborn 762.1
  tubal—*see* Pregnancy, tubal
  voluntary—*see* Abortion, legal
Abortus fever 023.9
Aboulomania 301.6
Abrachia 755.20
Abrachiatism 755.20
Abrachiocephalia 759.89
Abrachiocephalus 759.89
Abrami's disease (acquired hemolytic jaundice)
    283.9
Abramov-Fiedler myocarditis (acute isolated
    myocarditis) 422.91
Abrasion —*see also* Injury, superficial, by site
  cornea 918.1
  dental 521.2
  teeth, tooth (dentifrice) (habitual) (hard tissues)
      (occupational) (ritual) (traditional) (wedge
      defect) 521.2

Abrikossov's tumor (M9580/0)—*see also*
    Neoplasm, connective tissue, benign
  malignant (M9580/3)—*see* Neoplasm,
      connective tissue, malignant
Abrism 988.8
Abruption, placenta —*see* Placenta, abruptio
Abruptio placentae —*see* Placenta, abruptio
Abscess (acute) (chronic) (infectional)
    (lymphangitic) (metastatic) (multiple)
    (pyogenic) (septic) (with lymphangitis) (*see*
    also Cellulitis) 682.9
  abdomen, abdominal
    cavity—*see* Abscess, peritoneum
    wall 682.2
  abdominopelvic—*see* Abscess, peritoneum
  accessory sinus (chronic) (*see also* Sinusitis)
      473.9
  adrenal (capsule) (gland) 255.8
  alveolar 522.5
    with sinus 522.7
  amebic 006.3
    bladder 006.8
    brain (with liver or lung abscess) 006.5
    liver (without mention of brain or lung
        abscess) 006.3
      with
        brain abscess (and lung abscess) 006.5
        lung abscess 006.4
    lung (with liver abscess) 006.4
      with brain abscess 006.5
    seminal vesicle 006.8
    specified site NEC 006.8
    spleen 006.8
  anaerobic 040.0
  ankle 682.6
  anorectal 566
  antecubital space 682.3
  antrum (chronic) (Highmore) (*see also*
      Sinusitis, maxillary) 473.0
  anus 566
  apical (tooth) 522.5
    with sinus (alveolar) 522.7
  appendix 540.1
  areola (acute) (chronic) (nonpuerperal) 611.0
    puerperal, postpartum 675.1
  arm (any part, above wrist) 682.3
  artery (wall) 447.2
  atheromatous 447.2
  auditory canal (external) 380.10
  auricle (ear) (staphylococcal) (streptococcal)
      380.10
  axilla, axillary (region) 682.3
    lymph gland or node 683
  back (any part) 682.2
  Bartholin's gland 616.3
    with
      abortion—*see* Abortion, by type, with sepsis
      ectopic pregnancy (*see also* categories
          633.0-633.9) 639.0
      molar pregnancy (*see also* categories
          630-632) 639.0
    complicating pregnancy or puerperium 646.6
    following
      abortion 639.0
      ectopic or molar pregnancy 639.0
  bartholinian 616.3
  Bezold's 383.01
  bile, biliary, duct or tract (*see also*
      Cholecystitis) 576.8
  bilharziasis 120.1

Abscess—*continued*
  bladder (wall) 595.89
    amebic 006.8
  bone (subperiosteal) (*see also* Osteomyelitis)
    730.0
    accessory sinus (chronic) (*see also* Sinusitis)
      473.9
    acute 730.0
    chronic or old 730.1
    jaw (lower) (upper) 526.4
    mastoid—*see* Mastoiditis, acute
    petrous (*see also* Petrositis) 383.20
    spinal (tuberculous) (*see also* Tuberculosis)
      015.0 *[730.88]*
      nontuberculous 730.08
  bowel 569.5
  brain (any part) 324.0
    amebic (with liver or lung abscess) 006.5
    cystic 324.0
    late effect—*see* category 326
    otogenic 324.0
    tuberculous (*see also* Tuberculosis) 013.3
  breast (acute) (chronic) (nonpuerperal) 611.0
    newborn 771.5
    puerperal, postpartum 675.1
    tuberculous (*see also* Tuberculosis) 017.9
  broad ligament (chronic) (*see also* Disease,
    pelvis, inflammatory) 614.4
    acute 614.3
  Brodie's (chronic) (localized) (*see also*
    Osteomyelitis) 730.1
  bronchus 519.1
  buccal cavity 528.3
  bulbourethral gland 597.0
  bursa 727.89
    pharyngeal 478.29
  buttock 682.5
  canaliculus, breast 611.0
  canthus 372.20
  cartilage 733.99
  cecum 569.5
    with appendicitis 540.1
  cerebellum, cerebellar 324.0
    late effect—*see* category 326
  cerebral (embolic) 324.0
    late effect—*see* category 326
  cervical (neck region) 682.1
    lymph gland or node 683
    stump (*see also* Cervicitis) 616.0
  cervix (stump) (uteri) (*see also* Cervicitis) 616.0
  cheek, external 682.0
    inner 528.3
  chest 510.9
    with fistula 510.0
    wall 682.2
  chin 682.0
  choroid 363.00
  ciliary body 364.3
  circumtonsillar 475
  cold (tuberculous)—*see also* Tuberculosis,
    abscess
    articular—*see* Tuberculosis, joint
  colon (wall) 569.5
  colostomy or enterostomy 569.6
  conjunctiva 372.00
  connective tissue NEC 682.9
  cornea 370.55
    with ulcer 370.00
  corpus
    cavernosum 607.2
    luteum (*see also* Salpingo-oophoritis) 614.2

Abscess—*continued*
  Cowper's gland 597.0
  cranium 324.0
  cul-de-sac (Douglas') (posterior) (*see also*
    Disease, pelvis, inflammatory) 614.4
    acute 614.3
  dental 522.5
    with sinus (alveolar) 522.7
  dentoalveolar 522.5
    with sinus (alveolar) 522.7
  diaphragm, diaphragmatic—*see* Abscess,
    peritoneum
  digit NEC 681.9
  Douglas' cul-de-sac or pouch (*see also* Disease,
    pelvis, inflammatory) 614.4
    acute 614.3
  Dubois' 090.5
  ductless gland 259.8
  ear
    acute 382.00
    external 380.10
    inner 386.30
    middle—*see* Otitis media
  elbow 682.3
  endamebic—*see* Abscess, amebic
  entamebic—*see* Abscess, amebic
  enterostomy 569.6
  epididymis 604.0
  epidural 324.9
    brain 324.0
    late effect—*see* category 326
    spinal cord 324.1
  epiglottis 478.79
  epiploon, epiploic—*see* Abscess, peritoneum
  erysipelatous (*see also* Erysipelas) 035
  esophagus 530.19
  ethmoid (bone) (chronic) (sinus) (*see also*
    Sinusitis, ethmoidal) 473.2
  external auditory canal 380.10
  extradural 324.9
    brain 324.0
    late effect—*see* category 326
    spinal cord 324.1
  extraperitoneal—*see* Abscess, peritoneum
  eye 360.00
  eyelid 373.13
  face (any part, except eye) 682.0
  fallopian tube (*see also* Salpingo-oophoritis)
    614.2
  fascia 728.89
  fauces 478.29
  fecal 569.5
  femoral (region) 682.6
  filaria, filarial (*see also* Infestation, filarial)
    125.9
  finger (any) (intrathecal) (periosteal)
    (subcutaneous) (subcuticular) 681.00
  fistulous NEC 682.9
  flank 682.2
  foot (except toe) 682.7
  forearm 682.3
  forehead 682.0
  frontal (sinus) (chronic) (*see also* Sinusitis,
    frontal) 473.1
  gallbladder (*see also* Cholecystitis, acute) 575.0
  gastric 535.0
  genital organ or tract NEC
    female 616.9
      with
        abortion—*see* Abortion, by type, with
          sepsis

Abscess—*continued*
    ectopic pregnancy (*see also* categories 633.0-633.9) 639.0
    molar pregnancy (*see also* categories 630-632) 639.0
  following
    abortion 639.0
    ectopic or molar pregnancy 639.0
  puerperal, postpartum, childbirth 670
  male 608.4
genitourinary system, tuberculous (*see also* Tuberculosis) 016.9
gingival 523.3
gland, glandular (lymph) (acute) NEC 683
glottis 478.79
gluteal (region) 682.5
gonorrheal NEC (*see also* Gonococcus) 098.0
groin 682.2
gum 523.3
hand (except finger or thumb) 682.4
head (except face) 682.8
heart 429.89
heel 682.7
helminthic (*see also* Infestation, by specific parasite) 128.9
hepatic 572.0
  amebic (*see also* Abscess, liver, amebic) 006.3
  duct 576.8
hip 682.6
  tuberculous (active) (*see also* Tuberculosis) 015.1
ileocecal 540.1
ileostomy (bud) 569.6
iliac (region) 682.2
  fossa 540.1
iliopsoas (tuberculous) (*see also* Tuberculosis) 015.0 *[730.88]*
  nontuberculous 728.89
infraclavicular (fossa) 682.3
inguinal (region) 682.2
  lymph gland or node 683
intersphincteric (anus) 566
intestine, intestinal 569.5
  rectal 566
intra-abdominal (*see also* Abscess, peritoneum) 567.2
  postoperative 998.59
intracranial 324.0
  late effect—*see* category 326
intramammary—*see* Abscess, breast
intramastoid (*see also* Mastoiditis, acute) 383.00
intraorbital 376.01
intraperitoneal—*see* Abscess, peritoneum
intraspinal 324.1
  late effect—*see* category 326
intratonsillar 475
iris 364.3
ischiorectal 566
jaw (bone) (lower) (upper) 526.4
  skin 682.0
joint (*see also* Arthritis, pyogenic) 711.0
  vertebral (tuberculous) (*see also* Tuberculosis) 015.0 *[730.88]*
    nontuberculous 724.8
kidney 590.2
  with
    abortion—*see* Abortion, by type, with urinary tract infection
    calculus 592.0
    ectopic pregnancy (*see also* categories 633.0-633.9) 639.8

Abscess—*continued*
  molar pregnancy (*see also* categories 630-632) 639.8
complicating pregnancy or puerperium 646.6
  affecting fetus or newborn 760.1
following
  abortion 639.8
  ectopic or molar pregnancy 639.8
knee 682.6
  joint 711.06
  tuberculous (active) (*see also* Tuberculosis) 015.2
labium (majus) (minus) 616.4
  complicating pregnancy, childbirth, or puerperium 646.6
lacrimal (passages) (sac) (*see also* Dacryocystitis) 375.30
  caruncle 375.30
  gland (*see also* Dacryoadenitis) 375.00
lacunar 597.0
larynx 478.79
lateral (alveolar) 522.5
  with sinus 522.7
leg, except foot 682.6
lens 360.00
lid 373.13
lingual 529.0
  tonsil 475
lip 528.5
Littre's gland 597.0
liver 572.0
  amebic 006.3
    with
      brain abscess (and lung abscess) 006.5
      lung abscess 006.4
  due to Entamoeba histolytica 006.3
  dysenteric (*see also* Abscess, liver, amebic) 006.3
  pyogenic 572.0
  tropical (*see also* Abscess, liver, amebic) 006.3
loin (region) 682.2
lumbar (tuberculous) (*see also* Tuberculosis) 015.0 *[730.88]*
  nontuberculous 682.2
lung (miliary) (putrid) 513.0
  amebic (with liver abscess) 006.4
    with brain abscess 006.5
lymph, lymphatic, gland or node (acute) 683
  any site, except mesenteric 683
  mesentery 289.2
lymphangitic, acute—*see* Cellulitis
malar 526.4
mammary gland—*see* Abscess, breast
marginal (anus) 566
mastoid (process) (*see also* Mastoiditis, acute) 383.00
  subperiosteal 383.01
maxilla, maxillary 526.4
  molar (tooth) 522.5
    with sinus 522.7
  premolar 522.5
  sinus (chronic) (*see also* Sinusitis, maxillary) 473.0
mediastinum 513.1
meibomian gland 373.12
meninges (*see also* Meningitis) 320.9
mesentery, mesenteric—*see* Abscess, peritoneum
mesosalpinx (*see also* Salpingo-oophoritis) 614.2
milk 675.1

Abscess—*continued*
  suprapelvic (*see also* Disease, pelvis,
      inflammatory) 614.4
    acute 614.3
  suprapubic 682.2
  suprarenal (capsule) (gland) 255.8
  sweat gland 705.89
  syphilitic 095.8
  teeth, tooth (root) 522.5
    with sinus (alveolar) 522.7
    supporting structures NEC 523.3
  temple 682.0
  temporal region 682.0
  temporosphenoidal 324.0
    late effect—*see* category 326
  tendon (sheath) 727.89
  testicle—*see* Orchitis
  thecal 728.89
  thigh (acquired) 682.6
  thorax 510.9
    with fistula 510.0
  throat 478.29
  thumb (intrathecal) (periosteal) (subcutaneous)
      (subcuticular) 681.00
  thymus (gland) 254.1
  thyroid (gland) 245.0
  toe (any) (intrathecal) (periosteal)
      (subcutaneous) (subcuticular) 681.10
  tongue (staphylococcal) 529.0
  tonsil(s) (lingual) 475
  tonsillopharyngeal 475
  tooth, teeth (root) 522.5
    with sinus (alveolar) 522.7
    supporting structure NEC 523.3
  trachea 478.9
  trunk 682.2
  tubal (*see also* Salpingo-oophoritis) 614.2
  tuberculous—*see* Tuberculosis, abscess
  tubo-ovarian (*see also* Salpingo-oophoritis)
      614.2
  tunica vaginalis 608.4
  umbilicus NEC 682.2
    newborn 771.4
  upper arm 682.3
  upper respiratory 478.9
  urachus 682.2
  urethra (gland) 597.0
  urinary 597.0
  uterus, uterine (wall) (*see also* Endometritis)
      615.9
    ligament (*see also* Disease, pelvis,
        inflammatory) 614.4
      acute 614.3
    neck (*see also* Cervicitis) 616.0
  uvula 528.3
  vagina (wall) (*see also* Vaginitis) 616.10
  vaginorectal (*see also* Vaginitis) 616.10
  vas deferens 608.4
  vermiform appendix 540.1
  vertebra (column) (tuberculous) (*see also*
      Tuberculosis) 015.0 *[730.88]*
    nontuberculous 730.0
  vesical 595.89
  vesicouterine pouch (*see also* Disease, pelvis,
      inflammatory) 614.4
  vitreous (humor) (pneumococcal) 360.04
  vocal cord 478.5
  von Bezold's 383.01
  vulva 616.4
    complicating pregnancy, childbirth, or
        puerperium 646.6

Abscess—*continued*
  vulvovaginal gland (*see also* Vaginitis) 616.3
  web-space 682.4
  wrist 682.4
Absence (organ or part) (complete or partial)
  acoustic nerve 742.8
  adrenal (gland) (congenital) 759.1
    acquired V45.79
  albumin (blood) 273.8
  alimentary tract (complete) (congenital) (partial)
      751.8
    lower 751.5
    upper 750.8
  alpha-fucosidase 271.8
  alveolar process (acquired) 525.8
    congenital 750.26
  anus, anal (canal) (congenital) 751.2
  aorta (congenital) 747.22
  aortic valve (congenital) 746.89
  appendix, congenital 751.2
  arm (acquired) V49.60
    above elbow V49.66
    below elbow V49.65
    congenital (*see also* Deformity, reduction,
        upper limb) 755.20
      lower—*see* Absence, forearm, congenital
      upper (complete) (partial) (with absence of
          distal elements, incomplete) 755.24
        with
          complete absence of distal elements
              755.21
          forearm (incomplete) 755.23
  artery (congenital) (peripheral) NEC (*see also*
      Anomaly, peripheral vascular system)
      747.60
    brain 747.81
    cerebral 747.81
    coronary 746.85
    pulmonary 747.3
    umbilical 747.5
  atrial septum 745.69
  auditory canal (congenital) (external) 744.01
  auricle (ear) (with stenosis or atresia of auditory
      canal), congenital 744.01
  bile, biliary duct (common) or passage
      (congenital) 751.61
  bladder (acquired) V45.74
    congenital 753.8
  bone (congenital) NEC 756.9
    marrow 284.9
      acquired (secondary) 284.8
      congenital 284.0
      hereditary 284.0
      idiopathic 284.9
    skull 756.0
  bowel sounds 787.5
  brain 740.0
    specified part 742.2
  breast(s) (acquired) V45.71
    congenital 757.6
  broad ligament (congenital) 752.19
  bronchus (congenital) 748.3
  calvarium, calvaria (skull) 756.0
  canaliculus lacrimalis, congenital 743.65
  carpal(s) (congenital) (complete) (partial) (with
      absence of distal elements, incomplete) (*see
      also* Deformity, reduction, upper limb)
      755.28
    with complete absence of distal elements
        755.21
  cartilage 756.9

Absence—*continued*
  humerus, congenital (complete) (partial) (with
    absence of distal elements, incomplete) (*see
    also* Deformity, reduction, upper limb)
    755.24
    with
      complete absence of distal elements 755.21
      radius and ulna (incomplete) 755.23
  hymen (congenital) 752.49
  ileum (acquired) (postoperative) (posttraumatic)
    V45.72
    congenital 751.1
  immunoglobulin, isolated NEC 279.03
    IgA 279.01
    IgG 279.03
    IgM 279.02
  incus (acquired) 385.24
    congenital 744.04
  internal ear (congenital) 744.05
  intestine (acquired) (small) V45.72
    congenital 751.1
      large 751.2
    large V45.72
      congenital 751.2
  iris (congenital) 743.45
  jaw—*see* Absence, mandible
  jejunum (acquired) V45.72
    congenital 751.1
  joint, congenital NEC 755.8
  kidney(s) (acquired) V45.73
    congenital 753.0
  labium (congenital) (majus) (minus) 752.49
  labyrinth, membranous 744.05
  lacrimal apparatus (congenital) 743.65
  larynx (congenital) 748.3
  leg (acquired) V49.70
    above knee V49.76
    below knee V49.75
    congenital (partial) (unilateral) (*see also*
      Deformity, reduction, lower limb) 755.31
      lower (complete) (partial) (with absence of
        distal elements, incomplete) 755.35
        with
          complete absence of distal elements
            (foot and toes) 755.31
          thigh (incomplete) 755.33
            with complete absence of distal
              elements 755.31
      upper—*see* Absence, femur
  lens (congenital) 743.35
    acquired 379.31
  ligament, broad (congenital) 752.19
  limb (acquired)
    congenital (complete) (partial) (*see also*
      Deformity, reduction) 755.4
      lower 755.30
        complete 755.31
        incomplete 755.32
        longitudinal—*see* Deficiency, lower limb,
          longitudinal
        transverse 755.31
      upper 755.20
        complete 755.21
        incomplete 755.22
        longitudinal—*see* Deficiency, upper limb,
          longitudinal
        transverse 755.21
    lower NEC V49.70
    upper NEC V49.60
  lip 750.26
  liver (congenital) (lobe) 751.69

Absence—*continued*
  lumbar (congenital) (vertebra) 756.13
    isthmus 756.11
    pars articularis 756.11
  lumen—*see* Atresia
  lung (bilateral) (congenital) (fissure) (lobe)
    (unilateral) 748.5
    acquired (any part) V45.76
  mandible (congenital) 524.09
  maxilla (congenital) 524.09
  menstruation 626.0
  metacarpal(s), congenital (complete) (partial)
    (with absence of distal elements,
      incomplete) (*see also* Deformity, reduction,
      upper limb) 755.28
    with all fingers, complete 755.21
  metatarsal(s), congenital (complete) (partial)
    (with absence of distal elements,
      incomplete) (*see also* Deformity, reduction,
      lower limb) 755.38
    with complete absence of distal elements
      755.31
  muscle (congenital) (pectoral) 756.81
    ocular 743.69
  musculoskeletal system (congenital) NEC 756.9
  nail(s) (congenital) 757.5
  neck, part 744.89
  nerve 742.8
  nervous system, part NEC 742.8
  neutrophil 288.0
  nipple (congenital) 757.6
  nose (congenital) 748.1
    acquired 738.0
  nuclear 742.8
  ocular muscle (congenital) 743.69
  organ
    of Corti (congenital) 744.05
    or site
      acquired V45.79
      congenital NEC 759.89
  osseous meatus (ear) 744.03
  ovary (acquired) V45.77
    congenital 752.0
  oviduct (acquired) V45.77
    congenital 752.19
  pancreas (congenital) 751.7
    acquired (postoperative) (posttraumatic)
      V45.79
  parathyroid gland (congenital) 759.2
  parotid gland(s) (congenital) 750.21
  patella, congenital 755.64
  pelvic girdle (congenital) 755.69
  penis (congenital) 752.69
    acquired V45.77
  pericardium (congenital) 746.89
  perineal body (congenital) 756.81
  phalange(s), congenital 755.4
    lower limb (complete) (intercalary) (partial)
      (terminal) (*see also* Deformity, reduction,
      lower limb) 755.39
      meaning all toes (complete) (partial) 755.31
      transverse 755.31
    upper limb (complete) (intercalary) (partial)
      (terminal) (*see also* Deformity, reduction,
      upper limb) 755.29
      meaning all digits (complete) (partial)
        755.21
      transverse 755.21
  pituitary gland (congenital) 759.2
  postoperative—*see* Absence, by site, acquired
  prostate (congenital) 752.8

Absence—*continued*
     complete absence of distal elements 755.21
     humerus (incomplete) 755.23
 umbilical artery (congenital) 747.5
 ureter (congenital) 753.4
  acquired V45.74
 urethra, congenital 753.8
  acquired V45.74
 urinary system, part NEC, congenital 753.8
  acquired V45.74
 uterus (acquired)V45.77
  congenital 752.3
 uvula (congenital) 750.26
 vagina, congenital 752.49
  acquired V45.77
 vas deferens (congenital) 752.8
  acquired V45.77
 vein (congenital) (peripheral) NEC (*see also* Anomaly, peripheral vascular system) 747.60
  brain 747.81
  great 747.49
  portal 747.49
  pulmonary 747.49
 vena cava (congenital) (inferior) (superior) 747.49
 ventral horn cell 742.59
 ventricular septum 745.3
 vermis of cerebellum 742.2
 vertebra, congenital 756.13
 vulva, congenital 752.49
Absentia epileptica (*see also* Epilepsy) 345.0
Absinthemia (*see also* Dependence) 304.6
Absinthism (*see also* Dependence) 304.6
Absorbent system disease 459.89
Absorption
 alcohol, through placenta or breast milk 760.71
 antibiotics, through placenta or breast milk 760.74
 anti-infective, through placenta or breast milk 760.74
 chemical NEC 989.9
  specified chemical or substance—*see* Table of drugs and chemicals
  through placenta or breast milk (fetus or newborn) 760.70
   alcohol 760.71
   anti-infective agents 760.74
   cocaine 760.75
   "crack" 760.75
   diethylstilbestrol [DES] 760.76
   hallucinogenic agents 760.73
   medicinal agents NEC 760.79
   narcotics 760.72
   obstetric anesthetic or analgesic drug 763.5
   specified agent NEC 760.79
   suspected, affecting management of pregnancy 655.5
 cocaine, through placenta or breast milk 760.75
 drug NEC (*see also* Reaction, drug)
  through placenta or breast milk (fetus or newborn) 760.70
   alcohol 760.71
   anti-infective agents 760.74
   cocaine 760.75
   "crack" 760.75
   diethylstilbestrol (DES) 760.76
   hallucinogenic agents 760.73
   medicinal agents NEC 760.79
   narcotics 760.72

Absorption—*continued*
   obstetric anesthetic or analgesic drug 763.5
   specified agent NEC 760.79
   suspected, affecting management of pregnancy 655.5
 fat, disturbance 579.8
 hallucinogenic agents, through placenta or breast milk 760.73
 immune sera, through placenta or breast milk 760.79
 lactose defect 271.3
 medicinal agents NEC, through placenta or breast milk 760.79
 narcotics, through placenta or breast milk 760.72
 noxious substance,—*see* Absorption, chemical
 protein, disturbance 579.8
 pus or septic, general—*see* Septicemia
 quinine, through placenta or breast milk 760.74
 toxic substance—*see* Absorption, chemical
 uremic—*see* Uremia
Abstinence symptoms or syndrome
 alcohol 291.81
 drug 292.0
Abt-Letterer-Siwe syndrome (acute histiocytosis X) (M9722/3) 202.5
Abulia 799.8
Abulomania 301.6
Abuse
 adult 995.80
  emotional 995.82
  multiple forms 995.85
  neglect (nutritional) 995.84
  physical 995.81
  psychological 995.82
  sexual 995.83
 alcohol (*see also* Alcoholism) 305.0
  dependent 303.9
  non-dependent 305.0
 child 995.50
  counseling
   perpetrator
    non-parent V62.83
    parent V61.22
   victim V61.21
  emotional 995.51
  multiple forms 995.59
  neglect (nutritional) 995.52
  physical 995.54
   shaken infant syndrome 995.55
  psychological 995.51
  sexual 995.53
 drugs, nondependent 305.9

> *Note—Use the following fifth-digit subclassification with the following codes: 305.0, 305.2-305.9:*
>
> *0 unspecified*
> *1 continuous*
> *2 episodic*
> *3 in remission*

  amphetamine type 305.7
  antidepressants 305.8
  barbiturates 305.4
  caffeine 305.9
  cannabis 305.2
  cocaine type 305.6
  hallucinogens 305.3
  hashish 305.2
  LSD 305.3
  marijuana 305.2

Abuse—*continued*
  mixed 305.9
    morphine type 305.5
    opioid type 305.5
    phencyclidine (PCP) 305.9
    specified NEC 305.9
    tranquilizers 305.4
  spouse 995.80
  tobacco 305.1
Acalcerosis 275.40
Acalcicosis 275.40
Acalculia 784.69
  developmental 315.1
Acanthocheilonemiasis 125.4
Acanthocytosis 272.5
Acanthokeratodermia 701.1
Acantholysis 701.8
  bullosa 757.39
Acanthoma (benign) (M8070/0)—*see also*
  Neoplasm, by site, benign
  malignant (M8070/3)—*see* Neoplasm, by site,
    malignant
Acanthosis (acquired) (nigricans) 701.2
  adult 701.2
  benign (congenital) 757.39
  congenital 757.39
  glycogenic
    esophagus 530.8
  juvenile 701.2
  tongue 529.8
Acanthrocytosis 272.5
Acapnia 276.3
Acarbia 276.2
Acardia 759.89
Acardiacus amorphus 759.89
Acardiotrophia 429.1
Acardius 759.89
Acariasis 133.9
  sarcoptic 133.0
Acaridiasis 133.9
Acarinosis 133.9
Acariosis 133.9
Acarodermatitis 133.9
  urticarioides 133.9
Acarophobia 300.29
Acatalasemia 277.8
Acatalasia 277.8
Acatamathesia 784.69
Acataphasia 784.5
Acathisia 781.0
  due to drugs 333.99
Acceleration, accelerated
  atrioventricular conduction 426.7
  idioventricular rhythm 427.89
Accessory (congenital)
  adrenal gland 759.1
  anus 751.5
  appendix 751.5
  atrioventricular conduction 426.7
  auditory ossicles 744.04
  auricle (ear) 744.1
  autosome(s) NEC 758.5
    21 or 22 758.0
  biliary duct or passage 751.69
  bladder 753.8
  blood vessels (peripheral) (congenital) NEC
    (*see also* Anomaly, peripheral vascular
    system) 747.60
    cerebral 747.81
    coronary 746.85
  bone NEC 756.9

Accessory—*continued*
  foot 755.67
  breast tissue, axilla 757.6
  carpal bones 755.56
  cecum 751.5
  cervix 752.49
  chromosome(s) NEC 758.5
    13-15 758.1
    16-18 758.2
    21 or 22 758.0
    autosome(s) NEC 758.5
    D_1 758.1
    E_3 758.2
    G 758.0
    sex 758.81
  coronary artery 746.85
  cusp(s), heart valve NEC 746.89
    pulmonary 746.09
  cystic duct 751.69
  digits 755.00
  ear (auricle) (lobe) 744.1
  endocrine gland NEC 759.2
  external os 752.49
  eyelid 743.62
  eye muscle 743.69
  face bone(s) 756.0
  fallopian tube (fimbria) (ostium) 752.19
  fingers 755.01
  foreskin 605
  frontonasal process 756.0
  gallbladder 751.69
  genital organ(s)
    female 752.8
      external 752.49
      internal NEC 752.8
    male NEC 752.8
      penis 752.69
  genitourinary organs NEC 752.8
  heart 746.89
    valve NEC 746.89
      pulmonary 746.09
  hepatic ducts 751.69
  hymen 752.49
  intestine (large) (small) 751.5
  kidney 753.3
  lacrimal canal 743.65
  leaflet, heart valve NEC 746.89
    pulmonary 746.09
  ligament, broad 752.19
  liver (duct) 751.69
  lobule (ear) 744.1
  lung (lobe) 748.69
  muscle 756.82
  navicular of carpus 755.56
  nervous system, part NEC 742.8
  nipple 757.6
  nose 748.1
  organ or site NEC—*see* Anomaly, specified
    type NEC
  ovary 752.0
  oviduct 752.19
  pancreas 751.7
  parathyroid gland 759.2
  parotid gland (and duct) 750.22
  pituitary gland 759.2
  placental lobe—*see* Placenta, abnormal
  preauricular appendage 744.1
  prepuce 605
  renal arteries (multiple) 747.62
  rib 756.3
    cervical 756.2

Acidemia 276.2
  arginosuccinic 270.6
  fetal
    affecting management of pregnancy 656.3
    before onset of labor, in liveborn infant 768.2
    during labor, in liveborn infant 768.3
    intrauterine—*see* Distress, fetal 656.3
    unspecified as to time of onset, in liveborn
      infant 768.4
  pipecolic 270.7
Acidity, gastric (high) (low) 536.8
  psychogenic 306.4
Acidocytopenia 288.0
Acidocytosis 288.3
Acidopenia 288.0
Acidosis 276.2
  diabetic 250.1
  fetal, affecting newborn 768.9
  fetal, affecting management of pregnancy 656.8
  kidney tubular 588.8
  lactic 276.2
  metabolic NEC 276.2
    with respiratory acidosis 276.4
    late, of newborn 775.7
  renal
    hyperchloremic 588.8
    tubular (distal) (proximal) 588.8
  respiratory 276.2
    complicated by
      metabolic acidosis 276.4
      metabolic alkalosis 276.4
Aciduria 791.9
  arginosuccinic 270.6
  beta-aminoisobutyric (BAIB) 277.2
  glycolic 271.8
  methylmalonic 270.3
    with glycinemia 270.7
  organic 270.9
  orotic (congenital) (hereditary) (pyrimidine
    deficiency) 281.4
Acladiosis 111.8
  skin 111.8
Aclasis
  diaphyseal 756.4
  tarsoepiphyseal 756.59
Acleistocardia 745.5
Aclusion 524.4
Acmesthesia 782.0
Acne (pustular) (vulgaris) 706.1
  agminata (*see also* Tuberculosis) 017.0
  artificialis 706.1
  atrophica 706.0
  cachecticorum (Hebra) 706.1
  conglobata 706.1
  conjunctiva 706.1
  cystic 706.1
  decalvans 704.09
  erythematosa 695.3
  eyelid 706.1
  frontalis 706.0
  indurata 706.1
  keloid 706.1
  lupoid 706.0
  necrotic, necrotica 706.0
    miliaris 704.8
  nodular 706.1
  occupational 706.1
  papulosa 706.1
  rodens 706.0
  rosacea 695.3
  scorbutica 267

Acne—*continued*
  scrofulosorum (Bazin) (*see also* Tuberculosis)
    017.0
  summer 692.72
  tropical 706.1
  varioliformis 706.0
Acneiform drug eruptions 692.3
Acnitis (primary) (*see also* Tuberculosis) 017.0
Acomia 704.00
Acontractile bladder 344.61
Aconuresis (*see also* Incontinence) 788.30
Acosta's disease 993.2
Acousma 780.1
Acoustic —*see* condition
Acousticophobia 300.29
Acquired —*see* condition
Acquired immunodeficiency syndrome —*see*
  Human immunodeficiency virus (disease)
  (illness) (infection)
Acragnosis 781.99
Acrania (monster) 740.0
Acroagnosis 781.99
Acroasphyxia, chronic 443.89
Acrobrachycephaly 756.0
Acrobystiolith 608.89
Acrobystitis 607.2
Acrocephalopolysyndactyly 755.55
Acrocephalosyndactyly 755.55
Acrocephaly 756.0
Acrochondrohyperplasia 759.82
Acrocyanosis 443.89
  newborn 770.83
Acrodermatitis 686.8
  atrophicans (chronica) 701.8
  continua (Hallopeau) 696.1
  enteropathica 686.8
  Hallopeau's 696.1
  perstans 696.1
  pustulosa continua 696.1
  recalcitrant pustular 696.1
Acrodynia 985.0
Acrodysplasia 755.55
Acrohyperhidrosis 780.8
Acrokeratosis verruciformis 757.39
Acromastitis 611.0
Acromegaly, acromegalia (skin) 253.0
Acromelalgia 443.89
Acromicria, acromikria 756.59
Acronyx 703.0
Acropachy, thyroid (*see also* Thyrotoxicosis)
  242.9
Acropachyderma 757.39
Acroparesthesia 443.89
  simple (Schultz's type) 443.89
  vasomotor (Nothnagel's type) 443.89
Acropathy thyroid (*see also* Thyrotoxicosis)
  242.9
Acrophobia 300.29
Acroposthitis 607.2
Acroscleriasis (*see also* Scleroderma) 710.1
Acroscleroderma (*see also* Scleroderma) 710.1
Acrosclerosis (*see also* Scleroderma) 710.1
Acrosphacelus 785.4
Acrosphenosyndactylia 755.55
Acrospiroma, eccrine (M8402/0)—*see*
  Neoplasm, skin, benign
Acrostealgia 732.9
Acrosyndactyly (*see also* Syndactylism) 755.10
Acrotrophodynia 991.4

Note—The list of adjectival modifiers below is not exhaustive. A description of adenocarcinoma that does not appear in this list should be coded in the same manner as carcinoma with that description. Thus, "mixed acidophil-basophil adenocarcinoma," should be coded in the same manner as "mixed acidophil-basophil carcinoma," which appears in the list under "Carcinoma."

Except where otherwise indicated, the morphological varieties of adenocarcinoma in the list below should be coded by site as for "Neoplasm, malignant."

Adenocarcinoma—*continued*
  in situ (M8140/2)—*see* Neoplasm, by site, in
      situ
  intestinal type (M8144/3)
    specified site—*see* Neoplasm, by site,
        malignant
    unspecified site 151.9
  intraductal (noninfiltrating) (M8500/2)
    papillary (M8503/2)
      specified site—*see* Neoplasm, by site, in situ
      unspecified site 233.0
    specified site—*see* Neoplasm, by site, in situ
    unspecified site 233.0
  islet cell (M8150/3)
    and exocrine, mixed (M8154/3)
      specified site—*see* Neoplasm, by site,
          malignant
      unspecified site 157.9
    pancreas 157.4
    specified site NEC—*see* Neoplasm, by site,
        malignant
    unspecified site 157.4
  lobular (M8520/3)
    specified site—*see* Neoplasm, by site,
        malignant
    unspecified site 174.9
  medullary (M8510/3)
  mesonephric (M9110/3)
  mixed cell (M8323/3)
  mucinous (M8480/3)
  mucin-producing (M8481/3)
  mucoid (M8480/3)—*see also* Neoplasm, by
      site, malignant
    cell (M8300/3)
      specified site—*see* Neoplasm, by site,
          malignant
      unspecified site 194.3
  nonencapsulated sclerosing (M8350/3) 193
  oncocytic (M8290/3)
  oxyphilic (M8290/3)
  papillary (M8260/3)
    and follicular (M8340/3) 193
    intraductal (noninfiltrating) (M8503/2)
      specified site—*see* Neoplasm, by site, in situ
      unspecified site 233.0
    serous (M8460/3)
      specified site—*see* Neoplasm, by site,
          malignant
      unspecified site 183.0
  papillocystic (M8450/3)
    specified site—*see* Neoplasm, by site,
        malignant
    unspecified site 183.0
  pseudomucinous (M8470/3)
    specified site—*see* Neoplasm, by site,
        malignant
    unspecified site 183.0
  renal cell (M8312/3) 189.0
  sebaceous (M8410/3)
  serous (M8441/3)—*see also* Neoplasm, by site,
      malignant
    papillary
      specified site—*see* Neoplasm, by site,
          malignant
      unspecified site 183.0
  signet ring cell (M8490/3)
  superficial spreading (M8143/3)
  sweat gland (M8400/3)—*see* Neoplasm, skin,
      malignant
  trabecular (M8190/3)
  tubular (M8211/3)

Adenocarcinoma—*continued*
  villous (M8262/3)
  water-clear cell (M8322/3) 194.1
Adenofibroma (M9013/0)
  clear cell (M8313/0)—*see* Neoplasm, by site,
      benign
  endometrioid (M8381/0) 220
    borderline malignancy (M8381/1) 236.2
    malignant (M8381/3) 183.0
  mucinous (M9015/0)
    specified site—*see* Neoplasm, by site, benign
    unspecified site 220
  prostate 600.2
  serous (M9014/0)
    specified site—*see* Neoplasm, by site, benign
    unspecified site 220
  specified site—*see* Neoplasm, by site, benign
  unspecified site 220
Adenofibrosis
  breast 610.2
  endometrioid 617.0
Adenoiditis 474.01
  acute 463
  chronic 474.01
    with chronic tonsillitis 474.02
Adenoids (congenital) (of nasal fossa) 474.9
  hypertrophy 474.12
  vegetations 474.2
Adenolipomatosis (symmetrical) 272.8
Adenolymphoma (M8561/0)
  specified site—*see* Neoplasm, by site, benign
  unspecified 210.2
Adenoma (sessile) (M8140/0)—*see also*
    Neoplasm, by site, benign

> *Note—Except where otherwise indicated, the*
> *morphological varieties of adenoma in the list*
> *below should be coded by site as for*
> *"Neoplasm, benign."*

  acidophil (M8280/0)
    specified site—*see* Neoplasm, by site, benign
    unspecified site 227.3
  acinar (cell) (M8550/0)
  acinic cell (M8550/0)
  adrenal (cortex) (cortical) (functioning)
      (M8370/0) 227.0
    clear cell type (M8373/0) 227.0
    compact cell type (M8371/0) 227.0
    glomerulosa cell type (M8374/0) 227.0
    heavily pigmented variant (M8372/0) 227.0
    mixed cell type (M8375/0) 227.0
  alpha cell (M8152/0)
    pancreas 211.7
    specified site NEC—*see* Neoplasm, by site,
        benign
    unspecified site 211.7
  alveolar (M8251/0)
  apocrine (M8401/0)
    breast 217
    specified site NEC—*see* Neoplasm, skin,
        benign
    unspecified site 216.9
  basal cell (M8147/0)
  basophil (M8300/0)
    specified site—*see* Neoplasm, by site, benign
    unspecified site 227.3
  beta cell (M8151/0)
    pancreas 211.7
    specified site NEC—*see* Neoplasm, by site,
        benign
    unspecified site 211.7

Adenoma—*continued*
  bile duct (M8160/0) 211.5
  black (M8372/0) 227.0
  bronchial (M8140/1) 235.7
    carcinoid type (M8240/3)—*see* Neoplasm,
      lung, malignant
    cylindroid type (M8200/3)—*see* Neoplasm,
      lung, malignant
  ceruminous (M8420/0) 216.2
  chief cell (M8321/0) 227.1
  chromophobe (M8270/0)
    (specified site—*see* Neoplasm, by site, benign
    unspecified site 227.3
  clear cell (M8310/0)
  colloid (M8334/0)
    specified site—*see* Neoplasm, by site, benign
    unspecified site 226
  cylindroid type, bronchus (M8200/3)—*see*
      Neoplasm, lung, malignant
  duct (M8503/0)
  embryonal (M8191/0)
  endocrine, multiple (M8360/1)
    single specified site—*see* Neoplasm, by site,
      uncertain behavior
    two or more specified sites 237.4
    unspecified site 237.4
  endometrioid (M8380/0)—*see also* Neoplasm,
      by site, benign
    borderline malignancy (M8380/1)—*see*
      Neoplasm, by site, uncertain behavior
  eosinophil (M8280/0)
    specified site—*see* Neoplasm, by site, benign
    unspecified site 227.3
  fetal (M8333/0)
    specified site—*see* Neoplasm, by site, benign
    unspecified site 226
  follicular (M8330/0)
    specified site—*see* Neoplasm, by site, benign
    unspecified site 226
  hepatocellular (M8170/0) 211.5
  Hürthle cell (M8290/0) 226
  intracystic papillary (M8504/0)
  islet cell (functioning) (M8150/0)
    pancreas 211.7
    specified site NEC—*see* Neoplasm, by site,
      benign
    unspecified site 211.7
  liver cell (M8170/0) 211.5
  macrofollicular (M8334/0)
    specified site NEC—*see* Neoplasm, by site,
      benign
    unspecified site 226
  malignant, malignum (M8140/3)—*see*
      Neoplasm, by site, malignant
  mesonephric (M9110/0)
  microfollicular (M8333/0)
    specified site—*see* Neoplasm, by site, benign
    unspecified site 226
  mixed cell (M8323/0)
  monomorphic (M8146/0)
  mucinous (M8480/0)
  mucoid cell (M8300/0)
    specified site—*see* Neoplasm, by site, benign
    unspecified site 227.3
  multiple endocrine (M8360/1)
    single specified site—*see* Neoplasm, by site,
      uncertain behavior
    two or more specified sites 237.4
    unspecified site 237.4
  nipple (M8506/0) 217
  oncocytic (M8290/0)

Adenoma—*continued*
  oxyphilic (M8290/0)
  papillary (M8260/0)—*see also* Neoplasm, by
      site, benign
    intracystic (M8504/0)
  papillotubular (M8263/0)
  Pick's tubular (M8640/0)
    specified site—*see* Neoplasm, by site, benign
    unspecified site
      female 220
      male 222.0
  pleomorphic (M8940/0)
  polypoid (M8210/0)
  prostate (benign) 600.2
  rete cell 222.0
  sebaceous, sebaceum (gland) (senile)
      (M8410/0)—*see also* Neoplasm, skin,
      benign
    disseminata 759.5
  Sertoli cell (M8640/0)
    specified site—*see* Neoplasm, by site, benign
    unspecified site
      female 220
      male 222.0
  skin appendage (M8390/0)—*see* Neoplasm,
      skin, benign
  sudoriferous gland (M8400/0)—*see* Neoplasm,
      skin, benign
  sweat gland or duct (M8400/0)—*see* Neoplasm,
      skin, benign
  testicular (M8640/0)
    specified site—*see* Neoplasm, by site, benign
    unspecified site
      female 220
      male 222.0
  thyroid 226
  trabecular (M8190/0)
  tubular (M8211/0)—*see also* Neoplasm, by site,
      benign
    papillary (M8460/3)
    Pick's (M8640/0)
      specified site—*see* Neoplasm, by site,
        benign
      unspecified site
        female 220
        male 222.0
  tubulovillous (M8263/0)
  villoglandular (M8263/0)
  villous (M8261/1)—*see* Neoplasm, by site,
      uncertain behavior
  water-clear cell (M8322/0) 227.1
  wolffian duct (M9110/0)
Adenomatosis (M8220/0)
  endocrine (multiple) (M8360/1)
    single specified site—*see* Neoplasm, by site,
      uncertain behavior
    two or more specified sites 237.4
    unspecified site 237.4
  erosive of nipple (M8506/0) 217
  pluriendocrine   *see* Adenomatosis, endocrine
  pulmonary (M8250/1) 235.7
    malignant (M8250/3)—*see* Neoplasm, lung,
      malignant
  specified site—*see* Neoplasm, by site, benign
  unspecified site 211.3
Adenomatous
    cyst, thyroid (gland)—*see* Goiter, nodular
    goiter (nontoxic) (*see also* Goiter, nodular)
      241.9
    toxic or with hyperthyroidism 242.3

Adhesion—*continued*
  omentum (*see also* Adhesions, peritoneum)
    568.0
  organ or site, congenital NEC—*see* Anomaly,
    specified type NEC
  ovary 614.6
    congenital (to cecum, kidney, or omentum)
      752.0
  parauterine 614.6
  parovarian 614.6
  pelvic (peritoneal)
    female 614.6
    male (*see also* Adhesions, peritoneum) 568.0
    postpartal (old) 614.6
    tuberculous (*see also* Tuberculosis) 016.9
  penis to scrotum (congenital) 752.69
  periappendiceal (*see also* Adhesions,
    peritoneum) 568.0
  pericardium (nonrheumatic) 423.1
    rheumatic 393
    tuberculous (*see also* Tuberculosis) 017.9
      [420.0]
  pericholecystic 575.8
  perigastric (*see also* Adhesions, peritoneum)
    568.0
  periovarian 614.6
  periprostatic 602.8
  perirectal (*see also* Adhesions, peritoneum)
    568.0
  perirenal 593.89
  peritoneum, peritoneal (fibrous) (postoperative)
    568.0
    with obstruction (intestinal) 560.81
      with hernia—*see also* Hernia, by site, with
        obstruction
        gangrenous—*see* Hernia, by site, with
          gangrene
      duodenum 537.3
    congenital 751.4
    female, (postoperative) (postinfective) 614.6
    pelvic, female 614.6
    pelvic, male 568.0
    postpartal, pelvic 614.6
    to uterus 614.6
  peritubal 614.6
  periureteral 593.89
  periuterine 621.5
  perivesical 596.8
  perivesicular (seminal vesicle) 608.89
  pleura, pleuritic 511.0
    tuberculous (*see also* Tuberculosis, pleura)
      012.0
  pleuropericardial 511.0
  postoperative (gastrointestinal tract) *(See also*
    Adhesions, peritoneum) 568.0
    eyelid 997.99
      surgically created V45.69
    urethra 598.2
  postpartal, old 624.4
  preputial, prepuce 605
  pulmonary 511.0
  pylorus (*see also* Adhesions, peritoneum) 568.0
  Rosenmüller's fossa 478.29
  sciatic nerve 355.0
  seminal vesicle 608.89
  shoulder (joint) 726.0
  sigmoid flexure (*see also* Adhesions,
    peritoneum) 568.0
  spermatic cord (acquired) 608.89
    congenital 752.8
  spinal canal 349.2

Adhesion—*continued*
  nerve 355.9
    root 724.9
      cervical NEC 723.4
      lumbar NEC 724.4
      lumbosacral 724.4
      thoracic 724.4
  stomach (*see also* Adhesions, peritoneum) 568.0
  subscapular 726.2
  tendonitis 726.90
    shoulder 726.0
  testicle 608.89
  tongue (congenital) (to gum or roof of mouth)
    750.12
    acquired 529.8
  trachea 519.1
  tubo-ovarian 614.6
  tunica vaginalis 608.89
  ureter 593.89
  uterus 621.5
    to abdominal wall 614.6
      in pregnancy or childbirth 654.4
        affecting fetus or newborn 763.89
  vagina (chronic) (postoperative) (postradiation)
    623.2
  vaginitis (congenital) 752.49
  vesical 596.8
  vitreous 379.29
Adie (-Holmes) syndrome (tonic pupillary
  reaction) 379.46
Adiponecrosis neonatorum 778.1
Adiposa dolorosa 272.8
Adiposalgia 272.8
Adiposis 278.0
  cerebralis 253.8
  dolorosa 272.8
  tuberosa simplex 272.8
Adiposity 278.0
  heart (*see also* Degeneration, myocardial) 429.1
  localized 278.1
Adiposogenital dystrophy 253.8
Adjustment
  prosthesis or other device—*see* Fitting of
  reaction—*see* Reaction, adjustment
Administration, prophylactic
  antibiotics V07.39
  antitoxin, any V07.2
  antivenin V07.2
  chemotherapeutic agent NEC V07.39
  chemotherapy NEC V07.39
  diphtheria antitoxin V07.2
  fluoride V07.31
  gamma globulin V07.2
  immune sera (gamma globulin) V07.2
  passive immunization agent V07.2
  RhoGAM V07.2
Admission (encounter)
  as organ donor—*see* Donor
  by mistake V68.9
  for
    adequacy testing (for)
      hemodialysis V56.31
      peritoneal dialysis V56.32
    adjustment (of)
      artificial
        arm (complete) (partial) V52.0
        eye V52.2
        leg (complete) (partial) V52.1
      brain neuropacemaker V53.02
      breast
        implant V50.1

Admission—*continued*
    prosthesis V52.4
    cardiac device V53.39
      defibrillator, automatic implantable V53.32
      pacemaker V53.31
        carotid sinus V53.39
    catheter
      non-vascular V58.82
      vascular V58.81
    cerebral ventricle (communicating) shunt V53.01
    colostomy belt V53.5
    contact lenses V53.1
    cystostomy device V53.6
    dental prosthesis V52.3
    device NEC V53.9
      abdominal V53.5
      cardiac V53.39
        defibrillator, automatic implantable V53.32
        pacemaker V53.31
          carotid sinus V53.39
      cerebral ventricle (communicating) shunt V53.01
      intrauterine contraceptive V25.1
      nervous system V53.09
      orthodontic V53.4
      prosthetic V52.9
        breast V52.4
        dental V52.3
        eye V52.2
        specified type NEC V52.8
      special senses V53.09
      substitution
        auditory V53.09
        nervous system V53.09
        visual V53.09
      urinary V53.6
    dialysis catheter
      extracorporeal V56.1
      peritoneal V56.2
    diaphragm (contraceptive) V25.02
    hearing aid V53.2
    ileostomy device V53.5
    intestinal appliance or device NEC V53.5
    intrauterine contraceptive device V25.1
    neuropacemaker (brain) (peripheral nerve) (spinal cord) V53.02
    orthodontic device V53.4
    orthopedic (device) V53.7
      brace V53.7
      cast V53.7
      shoes V53.7
    pacemaker
      brain V53.02
      cardiac V53.31
      carotid sinus V53.39
      peripheral nerve V53.02
      spinal cord V53.02
    prosthesis V52.9
      arm (complete) (partial) V52.0
      breast V52.4
      dental V52.3
      eye V52.2
      leg (complete) (partial) V52.1
      specified type NEC V52.8
    spectacles V53.1
    wheelchair V53.8
  adoption referral or proceedings V68.89
  aftercare (*see also* Aftercare) V58.9
    cardiac pacemaker V53.31

Admission—*continued*
  chemotherapy V58.1
  dialysis
    extracorporeal (renal) V56.0
    peritoneal V56.8
    renal V56.0
  fracture (*see also* Aftercare, fracture) V54.9
  medical NEC V58.89
  orthopedic V54.9
    specified care NEC V54.89
    specified type NEC V54.8
  pacemaker device
    brain V53.02
    cardiac V53.31
    carotid sinus V53.39
    nervous system V53.02
    spinal cord V53.02
  postoperative NEC V58.49
    wound closure, planned V58.41
  postpartum
    immediately after delivery V24.0
    routine follow-up V24.2
  postradiation V58.0
  radiation therapy V58.0
  removal of
    non-vascular catheter V58.82
    vascular catheter V58.81
    specified NEC V58.89
      removal of vascular catheter V58.81
    surgical NEC V58.49
      wound closure, planned V58.41
  artificial insemination V26.1
  attention to artificial opening (of) V55.9
    artificial vagina V55.7
    colostomy V55.3
    cystostomy V55.5
    enterostomy V55.4
    gastrostomy V55.1
    ileostomy V55.2
    jejunostomy V55.4
    nephrostomy V55.6
    specified site NEC V55.8
      intestinal tract V55.4
      urinary tract V55.6
    tracheostomy V55.0
    ureterostomy V55.6
    urethrostomy V55.6
  battery replacement
    cardiac pacemaker V53.31
  boarding V65.0
  breast
    augmentation or reduction V50.1
    removal, prophylactic V50.41
  change of
    cardiac pacemaker (battery) V53.31
    carotid sinus pacemaker V53.39
    catheter in artificial opening—*see* Attention to, artificial, opening
    dressing V58.3
    fixation device
      external V54.89
      internal V54.0
    Kirschner wire V54.89
    neuropacemaker device (brain) (peripheral nerve) (spinal cord) V53.02
    pacemaker device
      brain V53.02
      cardiac V53.31
      carotid sinus V53.39
      nervous system V53.02
    plaster cast V54.89

Admission—*continued*
    splint, external V54.89
    Steinmann pin V54.89
    surgical dressing V58.3
    traction device V54.89
  checkup only V70.0
  chemotherapy V58.1
  circumcision, ritual or routine (in absence of
    medical indication) V50.2
  clinical research investigation (control)
    (normal comparison) (participant) V70.7
  closure of artificial opening—*see* Attention to,
    artificial, opening
  contraceptive
    counseling V25.09
    management V25.9
      specified type NEC V25.8
  convalescence following V66.9
    chemotherapy V66.2
    psychotherapy V66.3
    radiotherapy V66.1
    surgery V66.0
    treatment (for) V66.5
      combined V66.6
      fracture V66.4
      mental disorder NEC V66.3
      specified condition NEC V66.5
  cosmetic surgery NEC V50.1
    following healed injury or operation V51
  counseling (*see also* Counseling) V65.40
    without complaint or sickness V65.49
    contraceptive management V25.09
    dietary V65.3
    exercise V65.41
    for
      nonattending third party V65.1
      victim of abuse
        child V61.21
        partner or spouse V61.11
    genetic V26.3
    gonorrhea V65.45
    HIV V65.44
    human immunodeficiency virus V65.44
    injury prevention V65.43
    procreative management V26.4
    sexually transmitted disease NEC V65.45
      HIV V65.44
    specified reason NEC V65.49
    substance use and abuse V65.42
    syphilis V65.45
    victim of abuse
      child V61.21
      partner or spouse V61.11
  desensitization to allergens V07.1
  dialysis V56.0
    catheter
      fitting and adjustment
        extracorporeal V56.1
        peritoneal V56.2
      removal or replacement
        extracorporeal V56.1
        peritoneal V56.2
    extracorporeal (renal) V56.0
    peritoneal V56.8
    renal V56.0
  dietary surveillance and counseling V65.3
  drug monitoring, therapeutic V58.83
  ear piercing V50.3
  elective surgery V50.9
    breast
      augmentation or reduction V50.1

Admission—*continued*
    removal, prophylactic V50.41
  circumcision, ritual or routine (in absence of
    medical indication) V50.2
  cosmetic NEC V50.1
    following healed injury or operation V51
  ear piercing V50.3
  face-lift V50.1
  hair transplant V50.0
  plastic
    cosmetic NEC V50.1
    following healed injury or operation V51
  prophylactic organ removal V50.49
    breast V50.41
    ovary V50.42
  repair of scarred tissue (following healed
    injury or operation) V51
  specified type NEC V50.8
  end-of-life care V66.7
  examination (*see also* Examination) V70.9
    administrative purpose NEC V70.3
    adoption V70.3
    allergy V72.7
    at health care facility V70.0
    athletic team V70.3
    camp V70.3
    cardiovascular, preoperative V72.81
    clinical research investigation (control)
      (participant) V70.7
    dental V72.2
    developmental testing (child) (infant) V20.2
    donor (potential) V70.8
    driver's license V70.3
    ear V72.1
    employment V70.5
    eye V72.0
    follow-up (routine)—*see* Examination,
      follow-up
    for admission to
      old age home V70.3
      school V70.3
    general V70.9
      specified reason NEC V70.8
    gynecological V72.3
    health supervision (child) (infant) V20.2
    hearing V72.1
    immigration V70.3
    insurance certification V70.3
    laboratory V72.6
    marriage license V70.3
    medical (general) (*see also* Examination,
      medical) V70.9
    medicolegal reasons V70.4
    naturalization V70.3
    pelvic (annual) (periodic) V72.3
    postpartum checkup V24.2
    pregnancy (possible) (unconfirmed) V72.4
    preoperative V72.84
      cardiovascular V72.81
      respiratory V72.82
      specified NEC V72.83
    prison V70.3
    psychiatric (general) V70.2
      requested by authority V70.1
    radiological NEC V72.5
    respiratory, preoperative V72.82
    school V70.3
    screening—*see* Screening
    skin hypersensitivity V72.7
    specified type NEC V72.85
    sport competition V70.3

Admission—*continued*

vision V72.0
well baby and child care V20.2
exercise therapy V57.1
face-lift, cosmetic reason V50.1
fitting (of)
artificial
arm (complete) (partial) V52.0
eye V52.2
leg (complete) (partial) V52.1
biliary drainage tube V58.82
brain neuropacemaker V53.02
breast V52.4
implant V50.1
prosthesis V52.4
cardiac pacemaker V53.31
catheter
non-vascular V58.82
vascular V58.81
cerebral ventricle (communicating) shunt
V53.01
chest tube V58.82
colostomy belt V53.5
contact lenses V53.1
cystostomy device V53.6
dental prosthesis V52.3
device NEC V53.9
abdominal V53.5
cerebral ventricle (communicating) shunt
V53.01
intrauterine contraceptive V25.1
nervous system V53.09
orthodontic V53.4
prosthetic V52.9
breast V52.4
dental V52.3
eye V52.2
special senses V53.09
substitution
auditory V53.09
nervous system V53.09
visual V53.09
diaphragm (contraceptive) V25.02
fistula (sinus tract) drainage tube V58.82
hearing aid V53.2
ileostomy device V53.5
intestinal appliance or device NEC V53.5
intrauterine contraceptive device V25.1
neuropacemaker (brain) (peripheral nerve)
(spinal cord) V53.02
orthodontic device V53.4
orthopedic (device) V53.7
brace V53.7
cast V53.7
shoes V53.7
pacemaker
brain V53.02
cardiac V53.31
carotid sinus V53.39
spinal cord V53.02
pleural drainage tube V58.82
prosthesis V52.9
arm (complete) (partial) V52.0
breast V52.4
dental V52.3
eye V52.2
leg (complete) (partial) V52.1
specified type NEC V52.8
spectacles V53.1
wheelchair V53.8

Admission—*continued*

follow-up examination (routine) (following)
V67.9
cancer chemotherapy V67.2
chemotherapy V67.2
high-risk medication NEC V67.51
injury NEC V67.59
psychiatric V67.3
psychotherapy V67.3
radiotherapy V67.1
specified surgery NEC V67.09
surgery V67.00
vaginal pap smear V67.01
treatment (for) V67.9
combined V67.6
fracture V67.4
involving high-risk medication NEC
V67.51
mental disorder V67.3
specified NEC V67.59
hair transplant, for cosmetic reason V50.0
health advice, education, or instruction V65.4
hospice care V66.7
insertion (of)
subdermal implantable contraceptive V25.5
intrauterine device
insertion V25.1
management V25.42
investigation to determine further disposition
V63.8
isolation V07.0
issue of
medical certificate NEC V68.0
repeat prescription NEC V68.1
contraceptive device NEC V25.49
kidney dialysis V56.0
mental health evaluation V70.2
requested by authority V70.1
nonmedical reason NEC V68.89
nursing care evaluation V63.8
observation (without need for further medical
care) (*see also* Observation) V71.9
accident V71.4
alleged rape or seduction V71.5
criminal assault V71.6
following accident V71.4
at work V71.3
foreign body ingestion V71.89
growth and development variations,
childhood V21.0
inflicted injury NEC V71.6
ingestion of deleterious agent or foreign
body V71.89
injury V71.6
malignant neoplasm V71.1
mental disorder V71.09
newborn—*see* Observation, suspected
condition, newborn
rape V71.5
specified NEC V71.89
suspected disorder V71.9
abuse V71.81
accident V71.4
at work V71.3
benign neoplasm V71.89
cardiovascular V71.7
exposure
anthrax V71.82
biological agent NEC V71.83
heart V71.7
inflicted injury NEC V71.6

Aerodontalgia 993.2
Aeroembolism 993.3
Aerogenes capsulatus infection (*see also*
  Gangrene, gas) 040.0
Aero-otitis media 993.0
Aerophagy, aerophagia 306.4
  psychogenic 306.4
Aerosinusitis 993.1
Aerotitis 993.0
Affection, affections —*see also* Disease
  sacroiliac (joint), old 724.6
  shoulder region NEC 726.2
Afibrinogenemia 286.3
  acquired 286.6
  congenital 286.3
  postpartum 666.3
African
  sleeping sickness 086.5
  tick fever 087.1
  trypanosomiasis 086.5
    Gambian 086.3
    Rhodesian 086.4
Aftercare V58.9
  artificial openings—*see* Attention to, artificial,
    opening
  blood transfusion without reported diagnosis
    V58.2
  breathing exercise V57.0
  cardiac device V53.39
    defibrillator, automatic implantable V53.32
    pacemaker V53.31
      carotid sinus V53.39
  carotid sinus pacemaker V53.39
  cerebral ventricle (communicating) shunt
    V53.01
  chemotherapy session (adjunctive)
    (maintenance) V58.1
  defibrillator, automatic implantable cardiac
    V53.32
  exercise (remedial) (therapeutic) V57.1
    breathing V57.0
  extracorporeal dialysis (intermittent) (treatment)
    V56.0
  following surgery NEC V58.49
    for
      injury V58.43
      neoplasm V58.42
      trauma V58.43
    joint replacement V54.81
    of
      circulatory system V58.73
      digestive system V58.75
      genital organs V58.76
      genitourinary system V58.76
      musculoskeletal system V58.78
      nervous system V58.72
      oral cavity V58.75
      respiratory system V58.74
      sense organs V58.71
      skin V58.77
      subcutaneous tissue V58.77
      teeth V58.75
      urinary system V58.76
    wound closure, planned V58.41
  fracture V54.9
    healing V54.89
      pathologic
        arm V54.20
          lower V54.22
          upper V54.21
        hip V54.23

Aftercare—*continued*
    leg V54.24
      lower V54.26
      upper V54.25
      specified site NEC V54.29
      vertebrae V54.27
    traumatic
      arm V54.10
        lower V54.12
        upper V54.11
      hip V54.13
      leg V54.14
        lower V54.16
        upper V54.15
      specified site NEC V54.19
      vertebrae V54.17
    removal of
      external fixation device V54.89
      internal fixation device V54.0
    specified care NEC V54.89
  gait training V57.1
    for use of artificial limb(s) V57.81
  involving
    dialysis (intermittent) (treatment)
      extracorporeal V56.0
      peritoneal V56.8
      renal V56.0
    gait training V57.1
      for use of artificial limb(s) V57.81
    orthoptic training V57.4
    orthotic training V57.81
    radiotherapy session V58.0
    removal of
      dressings V58.3
      fixation device
        external V54.89
        internal V54.0
      fracture plate V54.0
      pins V54.0
      plaster cast V54.89
      rods V54.0
      screws V54.0
      surgical dressings V58.3
      sutures V58.3
      traction device, external V54.89
  neuropacemaker (brain) (peripheral nerve)
    (spinal cord) V53.02
  occupational therapy V57.21
  orthodontic V58.5
  orthopedic V54.9
    change of external fixation or traction device
      V54.89
    following joint replacement V54.81
    removal of fixation device
      external V54.89
      internal V54.0
    specified care NEC V54.89
  orthoptic training V57.4
  orthotic training V57.81
  pacemaker
    brain V53.02
    cardiac V53.31
    carotid sinus V53.39
    peripheral nerve V53.02
    spinal cord V53.02
  peritoneal dialysis (intermittent) (treatment)
    V56.8
  physical therapy NEC V57.1
    breathing exercises V57.0
  radiotherapy session V58.0
  rehabilitation procedure V57.9

Agenesis—*continued*
  larynx 748.3
  leg NEC (*see also* Deformity, reduction, lower
    limb) 755.30
  lens 743.35
  limb (complete) (partial) (*see also* Deformity,
    reduction) 755.4
    lower NEC 755.30
    upper 755.20
  lip 750.26
  liver 751.69
  lung (bilateral) (fissures) (lobe) (unilateral)
    748.5
  mandible 524.09
  maxilla 524.09
  metacarpus NEC 755.28
  metatarsus NEC 755.38
  muscle (any) 756.81
  musculoskeletal system NEC 756.9
  nail(s) 757.5
  neck, part 744.89
  nerve 742.8
  nervous system, part NEC 742.8
  nipple 757.6
  nose 748.1
  nuclear 742.8
  organ
    of Corti 744.05
    or site not listed—*see* Anomaly, specified
      type NEC
  osseous meatus (ear) 744.03
  ovary 752.0
  oviduct 752.19
  pancreas 751.7
  parathyroid (gland) 759.2
  patella 755.64
  pelvic girdle (complete) (partial) 755.69
  penis 752.69
  pericardium 746.89
  perineal body 756.81
  pituitary (gland) 759.2
  prostate 752.8
  pulmonary
    artery 747.3
    trunk 747.3
    vein 747.49
  punctum lacrimale 743.65
  radioulnar NEC (*see also* Absence, forearm,
    congenital) 755.25
  radius NEC (*see also* Absence, radius,
    congenital) 755.26
  rectum 751.2
  renal 753.0
  respiratory organ NEC 748.9
  rib 756.3
  roof of orbit 742.0
  round ligament 752.8
  sacrum 756.13
  salivary gland 750.21
  scapula 755.59
  scrotum 752.8
  seminal duct or tract 752.8
  septum
    atrial 745.69
    between aorta and pulmonary artery 745.0
    ventricular 745.3
  shoulder girdle (complete) (partial) 755.59
  skull (bone) 756.0
    with
      anencephalus 740.0
      encephalocele 742.0

Agenesis—*continued*
  hydrocephalus 742.3
    with spina bifida (*see also* Spina bifida)
      741.0
    microcephalus 742.1
  spermatic cord 752.8
  spinal cord 742.59
  spine 756.13
    lumbar 756.13
      isthmus 756.11
      pars articularis 756.11
  spleen 759.0
  sternum 756.3
  stomach 750.7
  tarsus NEC 755.38
  tendon 756.81
  testicular 752.8
  testis 752.8
  thymus (gland) 759.2
  thyroid (gland) 243
    cartilage 748.3
  tibia NEC (*see also* Absence, tibia, congenital)
    755.36
  tibiofibular NEC 755.35
  toe (complete) (partial) (*see also* Absence, toe,
    congenital) 755.39
  tongue 750.11
  trachea (cartilage) 748.3
  ulna NEC (*see also* Absence, ulna, congenital)
    755.27
  ureter 753.4
  urethra 753.8
  urinary tract NEC 753.8
  uterus 752.3
  uvula 750.26
  vagina 752.49
  vas deferens 752.8
  vein(s) (peripheral) NEC (*see also* Anomaly,
    peripheral vascular system) 747.60
    brain 747.81
    great 747.49
    portal 747.49
    pulmonary 747.49
  vena cava (inferior) (superior) 747.49
  vermis of cerebellum 742.2
  vertebra 756.13
    lumbar 756.13
      isthmus 756.11
      pars articularis 756.11
  vulva 752.49
Ageusia (*see also* Disturbance, sensation) 781.1
Aggressiveness 301.3
Aggressive outburst (*see also* Disturbance,
  conduct) 312.0
  in children and adolescents 313.9
Aging skin 701.8
Agitated —*see* condition
Agitation 307.9
  catatonic (*see also* Schizophrenia) 295.2
Aglossia (congenital) 750.11
Aglycogenosis 271.0
Agnail (finger) (with lymphangitis) 681.02
Agnosia (body image) (tactile) 784.69
  verbal 784.69
    auditory 784.69
      secondary to organic lesion 784.69
    developmental 315.8
    secondary to organic lesion 784.69
    visual 784.69
      developmental 315.8
      secondary to organic lesion 784.69

Agnosia—*continued*
  visual 368.16
    developmental 315.31
Agoraphobia 300.22
  with panic attacks 300.21
Agrammatism 784.69
Agranulocytopenia 288.0
Agranulocytosis (angina) (chronic) (cyclical)
    (genetic) (infantile) (periodic) (pernicious)
    288.0
Agraphia (absolute) 784.69
  with alexia 784.61
  developmental 315.39
Agrypnia (*see also* Insomnia) 780.52
Ague (*see also* Malaria) 084.6
  brass-founders' 985.8
  dumb 084.6
  tertian 084.1
Agyria 742.2
Ahumada-del Castillo syndrome (nonpuerperal
    galactorrhea and amenorrhea) 253.1
AIDS 042
AIDS-associated retrovirus (disease) (illness)
    042
  infection—*see* Human immunodeficiency virus,
    infection
AIDS-associated virus (disease) (illness) 042
  infection—*see* Human immunodeficiency virus,
    infection
AIDS-like disease (illness) (syndrome) 042
AIDS-related complex 042
AIDS-related conditions 042
AIDS-related virus (disease) (illness) 042
  infection—*see* Human immunodeficiency virus,
    infection
AIDS virus (disease) (illness) 042
  infection—*see* Human immunodeficiency virus,
    infection
Ailment, heart —*see* Disease, heart
Ailurophobia 300.29
Ainhum (disease) 136.0
Air
  anterior mediastinum 518.1
  compressed, disease 993.3
  embolism (any site) (artery) (cerebral) 958.0
    with
      abortion—*see* Abortion, by type, with
        embolism
      ectopic pregnancy (*see also* categories
        633.0-633.9) 639.6
      molar pregnancy (*see also* categories
        630-632) 639.6
      due to implanted device—*see* Complications,
        due to (presence of) any device, implant,
        or graft classified to 996.0-996.5 NEC
      following
        abortion 639.6
        ectopic or molar pregnancy 639.6
      infusion, perfusion, or transfusion 999.1
    in pregnancy, childbirth, or puerperium 673.0
    traumatic 958.0
  hunger 786.09
    psychogenic 306.1
  leak (lung) (pulmonary) (thorax) 512.8
    iatrogenic 512.1
    postoperative 512.1
  rarefied, effects of—*see* Effect, adverse, high
    altitude
  sickness 994.6
Airplane sickness 994.6
Akathisia, acathisia 781.0
  due to drugs 333.99

Akinesia algeria 352.6
Akiyami 100.89
Akureyri disease (epidemic neuromyasthenia)
    049.8
Alacrima (congenital) 743.65
Alactasia (hereditary) 271.3
Alalia 784.3
  developmental 315.31
    receptive-expressive 315.32
  secondary to organic lesion 784.3
Alaninemia 270.8
Alastrim 050.1
Albarrán's disease (colibacilluria) 791.9
Albers-Schönberg's disease (marble bones)
    756.52
Albert's disease 726.71
Albinism, albino (choroid) (cutaneous) (eye)
    (generalized) (isolated) (ocular)
    (oculocutaneous) (partial) 270.2
Albinismus 270.2
Albright (-Martin) (-Bantam) disease
    (pseudohypoparathyroidism) 275.49
Albright (-McCune) (-Sternberg) syndrome
    (osteitis fibrosa disseminata) 756.59
Albuminous —*see* condition
Albuminuria, albuminuric (acute) (chronic)
    (subacute) 791.0
  Bence-Jones 791.0
  cardiac 785.9
  complicating pregnancy, childbirth, or
    puerperium 646.2
    with hypertension—*see* Toxemia, of
      pregnancy
    affecting fetus or newborn 760.1
  cyclic 593.6
  gestational 646.2
  gravidarum 646.2
    with hypertension—*see* Toxemia, of
      pregnancy
    affecting fetus or newborn 760.1
  heart 785.9
  idiopathic 593.6
  orthostatic 593.6
  postural 593.6
  pre-eclamptic (mild) 642.4
    affecting fetus or newborn 760.0
    severe 642.5
      affecting fetus or newborn 760.0
  recurrent physiologic 593.6
  scarlatinal 034.1
Albumosuria 791.0
  Bence-Jones 791.0
  myelopathic (M9730/3) 203.0
Alcaptonuria 270.2
Alcohol, alcoholic
  abstinance 291.81
  acute intoxication 305.0
    with dependence 303.0
  addiction (*see also* Alcoholism) 303.9
    maternal
      with suspected fetal damage affecting
        management of pregnancy 655.4
      affecting fetus or newborn 760.71
  amnestic disorder, persisting 291.1
  anxiety 291.89
  brain syndrome, chronic 291.2
  cardiopathy 425.5
  chronic (*see also* Alcoholism) 303.9
  cirrhosis (liver) 571.2
  delirium 291.0
    acute 291.0

Alcohol, alcoholic—*continued*
   chronic 291.1
      tremens 291.0
      withdrawal 291.0
   dementia NEC 291.2
   deterioration 291.2
   drunkenness (simple) 305.0
   hallucinosis (acute) 291.3
   insanity 291.9
   intoxication (acute) 305.0
      with dependence 303.0
      pathological 291.4
   jealousy 291.5
   Korsakoff's, Korsakov's, Korsakow's 291.1
   liver NEC 571.3
      acute 571.1
      chronic 571.2
   mania (acute) (chronic) 291.9
   mood 291.89
   paranoia 291.5
   paranoid (type) psychosis 291.5
   pellagra 265.2
   poisoning, accidental (acute) NEC 980.9
      specified type of alcohol—*see* Table of drugs
         and chemicals
   psychosis (*see also* Psychosis, alcoholic) 291.9
      Korsakoff's, Korsakov's, Korsakow's 291.1
      polyneuritic 291.1
         with
            delusions 291.5
            hallucinations 291.3
   withdrawal symptoms, syndrome NEC 291.81
      delirium 291.0
      hallucinosis 291.3
Alcoholism 303.9

> *Note—Use the following fifth-digit*
> *subclassification with category 303:*
>
> *0 unspecified*
> *1 continuous*
> *2 episodic*
> *3 in remission*

   with psychosis (*see also* Psychosis, alcoholic)
      291.9
   acute 303.0
   chronic 303.9
      with psychosis 291.9
   complicating pregnancy, childbirth, or
      puerperium 648.4
      affecting fetus or newborn 760.71
   history V11.3
   Korsakoff's, Korsakov's, Korsakow's 291.1
   suspected damage to fetus affecting
      management of pregnancy 655.4
Alder's anomaly or syndrome (leukocyte
   granulation anomaly) 288.2
Alder-Reilly anomaly (leukocyte granulation)
   288.2
Aldosteronism (primary) (secondary) 255.1
   congenital 255.1
Aldosteronoma (M8370/1) 237.2
Aldrich (-Wiskott) syndrome
   (eczema-thrombocytopenia) 279.12
Aleppo boil 085.1
Aleukemic —*see* condition

Aleukia
   congenital 288.0
   hemorrhagica 284.9
      acquired (secondary) 284.8
      congenital 284.0
      idiopathic 284.9
   splenica 289.4
Alexia (congenital) (developmental) 315.01
   secondary to organic lesion 784.61
Algoneurodystrophy 733.7
Algophobia 300.29
Alibert's disease (mycosis fungoides) (M9700/3)
   202.1
Alibert-Bazin disease (M9700/3) 202.1
Alice in Wonderland syndrome 293.89
Alienation, mental (*see also* Psychosis) 298.9
Alkalemia 276.3
Alkalosis 276.3
   metabolic 276.3
      with respiratory acidosis 276.4
   respiratory 276.3
Alkaptonuria 270.2
Allen-Masters syndrome 620.6
Allergic bronchopulmonary aspergillosis 518.6
Allergy, allergic (reaction) 995.3
   air-borne substance (*see also* Fever, hay) 477.9
      specified allergen NEC 477.8
   alveolitis (extrinsic) 495.9
      due to
         Aspergillus clavatus 495.4
         cryptostroma corticale 495.6
         organisms (fungal, thermophilic
            actinomycete, other) growing in
            ventilation (air conditioning systems)
            495.7
      specified type NEC 495.8
   anaphylactic shock 999.4
      due to
         food—*see* Anaphylactic shock, due to, food
   angioneurotic edema 995.1
   animal (dander) (epidermal) (hair) 477.8
   arthritis (*see also* Arthritis, allergic) 716.2
   asthma—*see* Asthma
   bee sting (anaphylactic shock) 989.5
   biological—*see* Allergy, drug
   bronchial asthma—*see* Asthma
   conjunctivitis (eczematous) 372.14
   dander (animal) 477.8
   dandruff 477.8
   dermatitis (venenata)—*see* Dermatitis
   diathesis V15.09
   drug, medicinal substance, and biological (any)
      (correct medicinal substance properly
      administered) (external) (internal) 995.2
      wrong substance given or taken NEC 977.9
         specified drug or substance—*see* Table of
            drugs and chemicals
   dust (house) (stock) 477.8
   eczema—*see* Eczema
   endophthalmitis 360.19
   epidermal (animal) 477.8
   feathers 477.8
   food (any) (ingested) 693.1
      atopic 691.8
      in contact with skin 692.5
   gastritis 535.4
   gastroenteritis 558.3
   gastrointestinal 558.3
   grain 477.0
   grass (pollen) 477.0
      asthma (*see also* Asthma) 493.0

Allergy, allergic—*continued*
  hay fever 477.0
  hair (animal) 477.8
  hay fever (grass) (pollen) (ragweed) (tree) (*see*
    also Fever, hay) 477.9
  history (of) V15.09
    to
      eggs V15.03
      food additives V15.05
      insect bite V15.06
      latex V15.07
      milk products V15.02
      nuts V15.05
        peanuts V15.01
      radiographic dye V15.08
      seafood V15.04
      specified food NEC V15.05
      spider bite V15.06
  horse serum—*see* Allergy, serum
  inhalant 477.9
    dust 477.8
    pollen 477.0
    specified allergen other than pollen 477.8
  kapok 477.8
  medicine—*see* Allergy, drug
  migraine 346.2
  pannus 370.62
  pneumonia 518.3
  pollen (any) (hay fever) 477.0
    asthma (*see also* Asthma) 493.0
  primrose 477.0
  primula 477.0
  purpura 287.0
  ragweed (pollen) (Senecio jacobae) 477.0
    asthma (*see also* Asthma) 493.0
    hay fever 477.0
  respiratory (*see also* Allergy, inhalant) 477.9
    due to
      drug—*see* Allergy, drug
      food—*see* Allergy, food
  rhinitis (*see also* Fever, hay) 477.9
    due to food 477.1
  rose 477.0
  Senecio jacobae 477.0
  serum (prophylactic) (therapeutic) 999.5
    anaphylactic shock 999.4
  shock (anaphylactic)
    due to
      adverse effect of correct medicinal
        substance properly administered 995.0
      food—*see* Anaphylactic shock, due to, food
    from serum or immunization 999.5
      anaphylactic 999.4
  sinusitis (*see also* Fever, hay) 477.9
  skin reaction 692.9
    specified substance—*see* Dermatitis, due to
  tree (any) (hay fever) (pollen) 477.0
    asthma (*see also* Asthma) 493.0
  upper respiratory (*see also* Fever, hay) 477.9
  urethritis 597.89
  urticaria 708.0
  vaccine—*see* Allergy, serum
Allescheriosis 117.6
Alligator skin disease (ichthyosis congenita)
  757.1
  acquired 701.1
Allocheiria, allochiria (*see also* Disturbance,
  sensation) 782.0
Almeida's disease (Brazilian blastomycosis)
  116.1

Alopecia (atrophicans) (pregnancy) (premature)
  (senile) 704.00
  adnata 757.4
  areata 704.01
  (celsi 704.01
  cicatrisata 704.09
  circumscripta 704.01
  congenital, congenitalis 757.4
  disseminata 704.01
  effluvium (telogen) 704.02
  febrile 704.09
  generalisata 704.09
  hereditaria 704.09
  marginalis 704.01
  mucinosa 704.09
  postinfectional 704.09
  seborrheica 704.09
  specific 091.82
  syphilitic (secondary) 091.82
  telogen effluvium 704.02
  totalis 704.09
  toxica 704.09
  universalis 704.09
  x-ray 704.09
Alper's disease 330.8
Alpha-lipoproteinemia 272.4
Alpha thalassemia 282.4
Alphos 696.1
Alpine sickness 993.2
Alport's syndrome (hereditary
  hematuria-nephropathy-deafness) 759.89
Alteration (of), altered
  awareness 780.09
    transient 780.02
  consciousness 780.09
    persistent vegetative state 780.03
    transient 780.02
  mental status 780.99
Alternaria (infection) 118
Alternating —*see* condition
Altitude, high (effects)—*see* Effect, adverse,
  high altitude
Aluminosis (of lung) 503
Alvarez syndrome (transient cerebral ischemia)
  435.9
Alveolar capillary block syndrome 516.3
Alveolitis
  allergic (extrinsic) 495.9
    due to organisms (fungal, thermophilic
      actinomycete, other) growing in
      ventilation (air conditioning systems)
      495.7
    specified type NEC 495.8
  due to
    Aspergillus clavatus 495.4
    Cryptostroma corticale 495.6
  fibrosing (chronic) (cryptogenic) (lung) 516.3
    idiopathic 516.3
    rheumatoid 714.81
  jaw 526.5
  sicca dolorosa 526.5
Alveolus, alveolar —*see* condition
Alymphocytosis (pure) 279.2
Alymphoplasia, thymic 279.2
Alzheimer's
  dementia (senile)
    with behavioral disturbance 331.0 *[294.11]*
    without behavioral disturbance 331.0 *[294.10]*
  disease or sclerosis 331.0
    with dementia—*see* Alzheimer's, dementia
Amastia (*see also* Absence, breast) 611.8

Amaurosis (acquired) (congenital) (*see also*
　　Blindness) 369.00
　fugax 362.34
　hysterical 300.11
　Leber's (congenital) 362.76
　tobacco 377.34
　uremic—*see* Uremia
Amaurotic familial idiocy (infantile) (juvenile)
　　(late) 330.1
Ambisexual 752.7
Amblyopia (acquired) (congenital) (partial)
　　368.00
　color 368.59
　　acquired 368.55
　deprivation 368.02
　ex anopsia 368.00
　hysterical 300.11
　nocturnal 368.60
　　vitamin A deficiency 264.5
　refractive 368.03
　strabismic 368.01
　suppression 368.01
　tobacco 377.34
　toxic NEC 377.34
　uremic—*see* Uremia
Ameba, amebic (histolytica)–*see also* Amebiasis
　abscess 006.3
　　bladder 006.8
　　brain (with liver and lung abscess) 006.5
　　liver 006.3
　　　with
　　　　brain abscess (and lung abscess) 006.5
　　　　lung abscess 006.4
　　　lung (with liver abscess) 006.4
　　　　with brain abscess 006.5
　　　seminal vesicle 006.8
　　　spleen 006.8
　carrier (suspected of) V02.2
　meningoencephalitis
　　due to Naegleria (gruberi) 136.2
　　primary 136.2
Amebiasis NEC 006.9
　with
　　brain abscess (with liver or lung abscess)
　　　006.5
　　liver abscess (without mention of brain or
　　　lung abscess) 006.3
　　lung abscess (with liver abscess) 006.4
　　　with brain abscess 006.5
　acute 006.0
　bladder 006.8
　chronic 006.1
　cutaneous 006.6
　cutis 006.6
　due to organism other than Entamoeba
　　histolytica 007.8
　hepatic (*see also* Abscess, liver, amebic) 006.3
　nondysenteric 006.2
　seminal vesicle 006.8
　specified
　　organism NEC 007.8
　　site NEC 006.8
Ameboma 006.8
Amelia 755.4
　lower limb 755.31
　upper limb 755.21
Ameloblastoma (M9310/0) 213.1
　jaw (bone) (lower) 213.1
　　upper 213.0
　long bones (M9261/3)—*see* Neoplasm, bone,
　　malignant

Ameloblastoma—*continued*
　malignant (M9310/3) 170.1
　　jaw (bone) (lower) 170.1
　　　upper 170.0
　mandible 213.1
　tibial (M9261/3) 170.7
Amelogenesis imperfecta 520.5
　nonhereditaria (segmentalis) 520.4
Amenorrhea (primary) (secondary) 626.0
　due to ovarian dysfunction 256.8
　hyperhormonal 256.8
Amentia (*see also* Retardation, mental) 319
　Meynert's (nonalcoholic) 294.0
　　alcoholic 291.1
　nevoid 759.6
American
　leishmaniasis 085.5
　mountain tick fever 066.1
　trypanosomiasis—*see* Trypanosomiasis,
　　American
Ametropia (*see also* Disorder, accommodation)
　　367.9
Amianthosis 501
Amimia 784.69
Amino acid
　deficiency 270.9
　　anemia 281.4
　metabolic disorder (*see also* Disorder, amino
　　acid) 270.9
Aminoaciduria 270.9
　imidazole 270.5
Amnesia (retrograde) 780.99
　auditory 784.69
　　developmental 315.31
　　secondary to organic lesion 784.69
　hysterical or dissociative type 300.12
　psychogenic 300.12
　transient global 437.7
Amnestic (confabulatory) syndrome 294.0
　alcohol-induced 291.1
　drug-induced 292.83
　posttraumatic 294.0
Amniocentesis screening (for) V28.2
　alphafetoprotein level, raised V28.1
　chromosomal anomalies V28.0
Amnion, amniotic —*see also* condition
　nodosum 658.8
Amnionitis (complicating pregnancy) 658.4
　affecting fetus or newborn 762.7
Amoral trends 301.7
Amotio retinae (*see also* Detachment, retina)
　　361.9
Ampulla
　lower esophagus 530.89
　phrenic 530.89
Amputation
　any part of fetus, to facilitate delivery 763.89
　cervix (supravaginal) (uteri) 622.8
　　in pregnancy or childbirth 654.6
　　　affecting fetus or newborn 763.89
　clitoris—*see* Wound, open, clitoris
　congenital
　　lower limb 755.31
　　upper limb 755.21
　neuroma (traumatic)—*see also* Injury, nerve, by
　　site
　　surgical complications (late) 997.61
　penis—*see* Amputation, traumatic, penis
　status (without complication)—*see* Absence, by
　　site, acquired
　stump (surgical)(posttraumatic)

Amputation—*continued*
  abnormal, painful, or with complication (late) 997.60
  healed or old NEC —*see also* Absence, by site, acquired
    lower V49.70
    upper V49.60
  traumatic (complete) (partial)

> *Note—"Complicated" includes traumatic amputation with delayed healing, delayed treatment, foreign body, or infection.*

    arm 887.4
      at or above elbow 887.2
        complicated 887.3
      below elbow 887.0
        complicated 887.1
      both (bilateral) (any level(s)) 887.6
        complicated 887.7
      complicated 887.5
      finger(s) (one or both hands) 886.0
        with thumb(s) 885.0
          complicated 885.1
        complicated 886.1
      foot (except toe(s) only) 896.0
        and other leg 897.6
          complicated 897.7
        both (bilateral) 896.2
          complicated 896.3
        complicated 896.1
      toe(s) only (one or both feet) 895.0
        complicated 895.1
    genital organ(s) (external) NEC 878.8
      complicated 878.9
    hand (except finger(s) only) 887.0
      and other arm 887.6
        complicated 887.7
      both (bilateral) 887.6
        complicated 887.7
      complicated 887.1
      finger(s) (one or both hands) 886.0
        with thumb(s) 885.0
          complicated 885.1
        complicated 886.1
      thumb(s) (with fingers of either hand) 885.0
        complicated 885.1
    head 874.9
    late effect—*see* Late, effects (of), amputation
    leg 897.4
      and other foot 897.6
        complicated 897.7
      at or above knee 897.2
        complicated 897.3
      below knee 897.0
        complicated 897.1
      both (bilateral) 897.6
        complicated 897.7
      complicated 897.5
    lower limb(s) except toe(s)—*see* Amputation, traumatic, leg
    nose—*see* Wound, open, nose
    penis 878.0
      complicated 878.1
    sites other than limbs—*see* Wound, open, by site
    thumb(s) (with finger(s) of either hand) 885.0
      complicated 885.1
    toe(s) (one or both feet) 895.0
      complicated 895.1
    upper limb(s)—*see* Amputation, traumatic, arm

Amputee (bilateral) (old) —*see also* Absence, by site, acquired V49.70
Amusia 784.69
  developmental 315.39
  secondary to organic lesion 784.69
Amyelencephalus 740.0
Amyelia 742.59
Amygdalitis— *see* Tonsillitis
Amygdalolith 474.8
Amyloid disease or degeneration 277.3
  heart 277.3 *[425.7]*
Amyloidosis (familial) (general) (generalized) (genetic) (primary) (secondary) 277.3
  with lung involvement 277.3 *[517.8]*
  heart 277.3 *[425.7]*
  nephropathic 277.3 *[583.81]*
  neuropathic (Portuguese) (Swiss) 277.3 *[357.4]*
  pulmonary 277.3 *[517.8]*
  systemic, inherited 277.3
Amylopectinosis (brancher enzyme deficiency) 271.0
Amylophagia 307.52
Amyoplasia, congenita 756.89
Amyotonia 728.2
  congenita 358.8
Amyotrophia, amyotrophy, amyotrophic 728.2
  congenita 756.89
  diabetic 250.6 *[358.1]*
  lateral sclerosis (syndrome) 335.20
  neuralgic 353.5
  sclerosis (lateral) 335.20
  spinal progressive 335.21
Anacidity
  gastric 536.0
  psychogenic 306.4
Anaerosis of newborn 768.9
Analbuminemia 273.8
Analgesia (*see also* Anesthesia) 782.0
Analphalipoproteinemia 272.5
Anaphylactic shock or reaction (correct substance properly administered) 995.0
  due to
    food 995.60
      additives 995.66
      crustaceans 995.62
      eggs 995.68
      fish 995.65
      fruits 995.63
      milk products 995.67
      nuts (tree) 995.64
      peanuts 995.61
      seeds 995.64
      specified NEC 995.69
      tree nuts 995.64
      vegetables 995.63
    immunization 999.4
    overdose or wrong substance given or taken 977.9
    specified drug—*see* Table of drugs and chemicals
  following sting(s) 989.5
  purpura 287.0
  serum 999.4
Anaphylactoid shock or reaction —*see* Anaphylactic shock
Anaphylaxis —*see* Anaphylactic shock
Anaplasia, cervix 622.1
Anarthria 784.5
Anarthritic rheumatoid disease 446.5

Anasarca 782.3
  cardiac (*see also* Failure, heart) 428.0
  fetus or newborn 778.0
  lung 514
  nutritional 262
  pulmonary 514
  renal (*see also* Nephrosis) 581.9
Anaspadias 752.62
Anastomosis
  aneurysmal—*see* Aneurysm
  arteriovenous, congenital NEC (*see also*
     Anomaly, arteriovenous) 747.60
    ruptured, of brain (*see also* Hemorrhage,
      subarachnoid) 430
  intestinal 569.89
    complicated NEC 997.4
     involving urinary tract 997.5
  retinal and choroidal vessels 743.58
    acquired 362.17
Anatomical narrow angle (glaucoma) 365.02
Ancylostoma (infection) (infestation) 126.9
  americanus 126.1
  braziliense 126.2
  caninum 126.8
  ceylanicum 126.3
  duodenale 126.0
  Necator americanus 126.1
Ancylostomiasis (intestinal) 126.9
  Ancylostoma
    americanus 126.1
    caninum 126.8
    ceylanicum 126.3
    duodenale 126.0
  braziliense 126.2
  Necator americanus 126.1
Anders' disease or syndrome (adiposis tuberosa
  simplex) 272.8
Andersen's glycogen storage disease 271.0
Anderson's disease 272.7
Andes disease 993.2
Andrews' disease (bacterid) 686.8
Androblastoma (M8630/1)
  benign (M8630/0)
    specified site—*see* Neoplasm, by site, benign
    unspecified site
      female 220
      male 222.0
  malignant (M8630/3)
    specified site—*see* Neoplasm, by site,
     malignant
    unspecified site
      female 183.0
      male 186.9
  specified site—*see* Neoplasm, by site, uncertain
    behavior
  tubular (M8640/0)
    with lipid storage (M8641/0)
      specified site—*see* Neoplasm, by site,
       benign
      unspecified site
        female 220
        male 222.0
    specified site—*see* Neoplasm, by site, benign
    unspecified site
      female 220
      male 222.0
  unspecified site
    female 236.2
    male 236.4

Android pelvis 755.69
  with disproportion (fetopelvic) 653.3
    affecting fetus or newborn 763.1
    causing obstructed labor 660.1
     affecting fetus or newborn 763.1
Anectasis, pulmonary (newborn or fetus) 770.5
Anemia 285.9
  in
    chronic illness NEC 285.29
    end-stage renal disease 285.21
    neoplastic disease 285.22
  of chronic illness NEC 285.29
  with
    disorder of
      anaerobic glycolysis 282.3
      pentose phosphate pathway 282.2
    koilonychia 280.9
  6-phosphogluconic dehydrogenase deficiency
    282.2
  achlorhydric 280.9
  achrestic 281.8
  Addison's (pernicious) 281.0
  Addison-Biermer (pernicious) 281.0
  agranulocytic 288.0
  amino acid deficiency 281.4
  aplastic 284.9
    acquired (secondary) 284.8
    congenital 284.0
    constitutional 284.0
    due to
      chronic systemic disease 284.8
      drugs 284.8
      infection 284.8
      radiation 284.8
    idiopathic 284.9
    myxedema 244.9
    of or complicating pregnancy 648.2
    red cell (acquired) (pure) (with thymoma)
     284.8
      congenital 284.0
    specified type NEC 284.8
    toxic (paralytic) 284.8
  aregenerative 284.9
    congenital 284.0
  asiderotic 280.9
  atypical (primary) 285.9
  autohemolysis of Selwyn and Dacie (type I)
    282.2
  autoimmune hemolytic 283.0
  Baghdad Spring 282.2
  Balantidium coli 007.0
  Biermer's (pernicious) 281.0
  blood loss (chronic) 280.0
    acute 285.1
  bothriocephalus 123.4
  brickmakers' (*see also* Ancylostomiasis) 126.9
  cerebral 437.8
  childhood 285.9
  chlorotic 280.9
  chronica congenita aregenerativa 284.0
  chronic simple 281.9
  combined system disease NEC 281.0 *[336.2]*
    due to dietary deficiency 281.1 *[336.2]*
  complicating pregnancy or childbirth 648.2
  congenital (following fetal blood loss) 776.5
    aplastic 284.0
    due to isoimmunization NEC 773.2
    Heinz-body 282.7
    hereditary hemolytic NEC 282.9
    nonspherocytic
      Type I 282.2

Anemia—*continued*
  acquired 283.9
    with hemoglobinuria NEC 283.2
    autoimmune (cold type) (idiopathic)
      (primary) (secondary) (symptomatic)
      (warm type) 283.0
    due to
      cold reactive antibodies 283.0
      drug exposure 283.0
      warm reactive antibodies 283.0
    fragmentation 283.19
    idiopathic (chronic) 283.9
    infectious 283.19
      autoimmune 283.0
    non-autoimmune NEC 283.10
    toxic 283.19
    traumatic cardiac 283.19
  acute 283.9
    due to enzyme deficiency NEC 282.3
    fetus or newborn (*see also* Disease,
      hemolytic) 773.2
      late 773.5
    Lederer's (acquired infectious hemolytic
      anemia) 283.19
  autoimmune (acquired) 283.0
  chronic 282.9
    idiopathic 283.9
  cold type (secondary) (symptomatic) 283.0
  congenital (spherocytic) (*see also*
    Spherocytosis) 282.0
    nonspherocytic—*see* Anemia, hemolytic,
      nonspherocytic, congenital
  drug-induced 283.0
    enzyme deficiency 282.2
  due to
    cardiac conditions 283.19
    drugs 283.0
    enzyme deficiency NEC 282.3
      drug-induced 282.2
    presence of shunt or other internal prosthetic
      device 283.19
    thrombotic thrombocytopenic purpura 446.6
  elliptocytotic (*see also* Elliptocytosis) 282.1
  familial 282.9
  hereditary 282.9
    due to enzyme deficiency NEC 282.3
    specified NEC 282.8
  idiopathic (chronic) 283.9
  infectious (acquired) 283.19
  mechanical 283.19
  microangiopathic 283.19
  non-autoimmune NEC 283.10
  nonspherocytic
    congenital or hereditary NEC 282.3
      glucose-6-phosphate dehydrogenase
        deficiency 282.2
      pyruvate kinase (PK) deficiency 282.3
      type I 282.2
      type II 282.3
    type I 282.2
    type II 282.3
  of or complicating pregnancy 648.2
  resulting from presence of shunt or other
    internal prosthetic device 283.19
  secondary 283.19
    autoimmune 283.0
  sickle-cell—*see* Disease, sickle-cell
  Stransky-Regala type (Hb-E) (*see also*
    Disease, hemoglobin) 282.7
  symptomatic 283.19
    autoimmune 283.0

Anemia—*continued*
  toxic (acquired) 283.19
  uremic (adult) (child) 283.11
  warm type (secondary) (symptomatic) 283.0
  hemorrhagic (chronic) 280.0
    acute 285.1
  HEMPAS 285.8
  hereditary erythroblast multinuclearity- positive
    acidified serum test 285.8
  Herrick's (hemoglobin S disease) 282.61
  hexokinase deficiency 282.3
  high A$_2$ 282.4
  hookworm (*see also* Ancylostomiasis) 126.9
  hypochromic (idiopathic) (microcytic)
    (normoblastic) 280.9
    with iron loading 285.0
    due to blood loss (chronic) 280.0
      acute 285.1
    familial sex linked 285.0
    pyridoxine-responsive 285.0
  hypoplasia, red blood cells 284.8
    congenital or familial 284.0
  hypoplastic (idiopathic) 284.9
    congenital 284.0
    familial 284.0
    of childhood 284.0
  idiopathic 285.9
    hemolytic, chronic 283.9
  infantile 285.9
  infective, infectional 285.9
  intertropical (*see also* Ancylostomiasis) 126.9
  iron (Fe) deficiency 280.9
    due to blood loss (chronic) 280.0
      acute 285.1
    of or complicating pregnancy 648.2
    specified NEC 280.8
  Jaksch's (pseudoleukemia infantum) 285.8
  Joseph-Diamond-Blackfan (congenital
    hypoplastic) 284.0
  labyrinth 386.50
  Lederer's (acquired infectious hemolytic
    anemia) 283.19
  leptocytosis (hereditary) 282.4
  leukoerythroblastic 285.8
  macrocytic 281.9
    nutritional 281.2
    of or complicating pregnancy 648.2
    tropical 281.2
  malabsorption (familial), selective B$_{12}$ with
    proteinuria 281.1
  malarial (*see also* Malaria) 084.6
  malignant (progressive) 281.0
  malnutrition 281.9
  marsh (*see also* Malaria) 084.6
  Mediterranean (with hemoglobinopathy) 282.4
  megaloblastic 281.9
    combined B$_{12}$ and folate deficiency 281.3
    nutritional (of infancy) 281.2
    of infancy 281.2
    of or complicating pregnancy 648.2
    refractory 281.3
    specified NEC 281.3
  megalocytic 281.9
  microangiopathic hemolytic 283.19
  microcytic (hypochromic) 280.9
    due to blood loss (chronic) 280.0
      acute 285.1
    familial 282.4
    hypochromic 280.9
  microdrepanocytosis 282.4
  miners' (*see also* Ancylostomiasis) 126.9

Anemia—*continued*
  myelopathic 285.8
  myelophthisic (normocytic) 285.8
  newborn (*see also* Disease, hemolytic) 773.2
    due to isoimmunization (*see also* Disease,
      hemolytic) 773.2
    late, due to isoimmunization 773.5
    posthemorrhagic 776.5
  nonregenerative 284.9
  nonspherocytic hemolytic—*see* Anemia,
    hemolytic, nonspherocytic
  normocytic (infectional) (not due to blood loss)
    285.9
    due to blood loss (chronic) 280.0
      acute 285.1
    myelophthisic 284.8
  nutritional (deficiency) 281.9
    with
      poor iron absorption 280.9
      specified deficiency NEC 281.8
    due to inadequate dietary iron intake 280.1
    megaloblastic (of infancy) 281.2
  of childhood (*see also* Thalassemia) 282.4
  of or complicating pregnancy 648.2
    affecting fetus or newborn 760.8
  of prematurity 776.6
  orotic aciduric (congenital) (hereditary) 281.4
  osteosclerotic 289.8
  ovalocytosis (hereditary) (*see also*
    Elliptocytosis) 282.1
  paludal (*see also* Malaria) 084.6
  pentose phosphate pathway deficiency 282.2
  pernicious (combined system disease)
    (congenital) (dorsolateral spinal
    degeneration) (juvenile) (myelopathy)
    (neuropathy) (posterior sclerosis) (primary)
    (progressive) (spleen) 281.0
    of or complicating pregnancy 648.2
  pleochromic 285.9
    of sprue 281.8
  portal 285.8
  posthemorrhagic (chronic) 280.0
    acute 285.1
    newborn 776.5
  pressure 285.9
  primary 285.9
  profound 285.9
  progressive 285.9
    malignant 281.0
    pernicious 281.0
  protein-deficiency 281.4
  pseudoleukemica infantum 285.8
  puerperal 648.2
  pure red cell 284.8
    congenital 284.0
  pyridoxine-responsive (hypochromic) 285.0
  pyruvate kinase (PK) deficiency 282.3
  refractoria sideroblastica 285.0
  refractory (primary) 284.9
    with hemochromatosis 285.0
    megaloblastic 281.3
    sideroblastic 285.0
    sideropenic 280.9
  Rietti-Greppi-Micheli (thalassemia minor) 282.4
  scorbutic 281.8
  secondary (to) 285.9
    blood loss (chronic) 280.0
      acute 285.1
    hemorrhage 280.0
      acute 285.1
    inadequate dietary iron intake 280.1

Anemia—*continued*
  semiplastic 284.9
  septic 285.9
  sickle-cell (*see also* Disease, sickle-cell) 282.60
  sideroachrestic 285.0
  sideroblastic (acquired) (any type) (congenital)
    (drug-induced) (due to disease) (hereditary)
    (primary) (refractory) (secondary)
    (sex-linked hypochromic) (vitamin B_6
    responsive) 285.0
  sideropenic (refractory) 280.9
    due to blood loss (chronic) 280.0
      acute 285.1
  simple chronic 281.9
  specified type NEC 285.8
  spherocytic (hereditary) (*see also*
    Spherocytosis) 282.0
  splenic 285.8
    familial (Gaucher's) 272.7
  splenomegalic 285.8
  stomatocytosis 282.8
  syphilitic 095.8
  target cell (oval) 282.4
  thalassemia 282.4
  thrombocytopenic (*see also* Thrombocytopenia)
    287.5
  toxic 284.8
  triosephosphate isomerase deficiency 282.3
  tropical, macrocytic 281.2
  tuberculous (*see also* Tuberculosis) 017.9
  vegan's 281.1
  vitamin
    B_6-responsive 285.0
    B_{12} deficiency (dietary) 281.1
      pernicious 281.0
  von Jaksch's (pseudoleukemia infantum) 285.8
  Witts' (achlorhydric anemia) 280.9
  Zuelzer (-Ogden) (nutritional megaloblastic
    anemia) 281.2
Anencephalus, anencephaly 740.0
  fetal, affecting management of pregnancy 655.0
Anergasia (*see also* Psychosis, organic) 294.9
  senile 290.0
Anesthesia, anesthetic 782.0
  complication or reaction NEC 995.2
    due to
      correct substance properly administered
        995.2
      overdose or wrong substance given 968.4
        specified anesthetic—*see* Table of drugs
        and chemicals
  cornea 371.81
  death from
    correct substance properly administered 995.4
    during delivery 668.9
    overdose or wrong substance given 968.4
      specified anesthetic—*see* Table of drugs
      and chemicals
  eye 371.81
  functional 300.11
  hyperesthetic, thalamic 348.8
  hysterical 300.11
  local skin lesion 782.0
  olfactory 781.1
  sexual (psychogenic) 302.72
  shock
    due to
      correct substance properly administered
        995.4
      overdose or wrong substance given 968.4

Anesthesia, anesthetic—*continued*
    specified anesthetic—*see* Table of drugs
        and chemicals
  skin 782.0
  tactile 782.0
  testicular 608.9
  thermal 782.0
Anetoderma (maculosum) 701.3
Aneuploidy NEC 758.5
Aneurin deficiency 265.1
Aneurysm (anastomotic) (artery) (cirsoid)
  (diffuse) (false) (fusiform) (multiple)
  (ruptured) (saccular) (varicose) 442.9
  abdominal (aorta) 441.4
    ruptured 441.3
    syphilitic 093.0
  aorta, aortic (nonsyphilitic) 441.9
    abdominal 441.4
      dissecting 441.02
      ruptured 441.3
      syphilitic 093.0
    arch 441.2
      ruptured 441.1
    arteriosclerotic NEC 441.9
      ruptured 441.5
    ascending 441.2
      ruptured 441.1
    congenital 747.29
    descending 441.9
      abdominal 441.4
        ruptured 441.3
      ruptured 441.5
      thoracic 441.2
        ruptured 441.1
    dissecting 441.00
      abdominal 441.02
      thoracic 441.01
      thoracoabdominal 441.03
    due to coarctation (aorta) 747.10
    ruptured 441.5
    sinus, right 747.29
    syphilitic 093.0
    thoracoabdominal 441.7
      ruptured 441.6
    thorax, thoracic (arch) (nonsyphilitic) 441.2
      dissecting 441.01
      ruptured 441.1
      syphilitic 093.0
    transverse 441.2
      ruptured 441.1
    valve (heart) (*see also* Endocarditis, aortic)
      424.1
  arteriosclerotic NEC 442.9
    cerebral 437.3
      ruptured (*see also* Hemorrhage,
        subarachnoid) 430
  arteriovenous (congenital) (peripheral) NEC
    (*see also* Anomaly, arteriovenous) 747.60
    acquired NEC 447.0
    brain 437.3
      ruptured (*see also* Hemorrhage,
        subarachnoid) 430
    coronary 414.11
    pulmonary 417.0
  brain (cerebral) 747.81
    ruptured (*see also* Hemorrhage,
      subarachnoid) 430
  coronary 746.85
  pulmonary 747.3
  retina 743.58
  specified site NEC 747.89

Aneurysm—*continued*
  acquired 447.0
  traumatic (*see also* Injury, blood vessel, by
    site) 904.9
  basal—*see* Aneurysm, brain
  berry (congenital) (ruptured) (*see also*
    Hemorrhage, subarachnoid) 430
  brain 437.3
    arteriosclerotic 437.3
      ruptured (*see also* Hemorrhage,
        subarachnoid) 430
    arteriovenous 747.81
      acquired 437.3
        ruptured (*see also* Hemorrhage,
          subarachnoid) 430
      ruptured (*see also* Hemorrhage,
        subarachnoid) 430
    berry (congenital) (ruptured) (*see also*
      Hemorrhage, subarachnoid) 430
    congenital 747.81
      ruptured (*see also* Hemorrhage,
        subarachnoid) 430
    meninges 437.3
      ruptured (*see also* Hemorrhage,
        subarachnoid) 430
    miliary (congenital) (ruptured) (*see also*
      Hemorrhage, subarachnoid) 430
    mycotic 421.0
      ruptured (*see also* Hemorrhage,
        subarachnoid) 430
    nonruptured 437.3
    ruptured (*see also* Hemorrhage, subarachnoid)
      430
    syphilitic 094.87
    syphilitic (hemorrhage) 094.87
    traumatic—*see* Injury, intracranial
  cardiac (false) (*see also* Aneurysm, heart)
    414.10
  carotid artery (common) (external) 442.81
    internal (intracranial portion) 437.3
      extracranial portion 442.81
      ruptured into brain (*see also* Hemorrhage,
        subarachnoid) 430
      syphilitic 093.89
      intracranial 094.87
  cavernous sinus (*see also* Aneurysm, brain)
    437.3
    arteriovenous 747.81
      ruptured (*see also* Hemorrhage,
        subarachnoid) 430
    congenital 747.81
      ruptured (*see also* Hemorrhage,
        subarachnoid) 430
  celiac 442.84
  central nervous system, syphilitic 094.89
  cerebral—*see* Aneurysm, brain
  chest—*see* Aneurysm, thorax
  circle of Willis (*see also* Aneurysm, brain) 437.3
    congenital 747.81
      ruptured (*see also* Hemorrhage,
        subarachnoid) 430
    ruptured (*see also* Hemorrhage, subarachnoid)
      430
  common iliac artery 442.2
  congenital (peripheral) NEC 747.60
    brain 747.81
      ruptured (*see also* Hemorrhage,
        subarachnoid) 430
    cerebral—*see* Aneurysm, brain, congenital
    coronary 746.85
    gastrointestinal 747.61

Aneurysm—*continued*
  lower limb 747.64
  pulmonary 747.3
  renal 747.62
  retina 743.58
  specified site NEC 747.89
  spinal 747.82
  upper limb 747.63
 conjunctiva 372.74
 conus arteriosus (*see also* Aneurysm, heart)
   414.10
 coronary (arteriosclerotic) (artery) (vein) (*see*
   also Aneurysm, heart) 414.11
  arteriovenous 746.85
  congenital 746.85
  syphilitic 093.89
 cylindrical 441.9
  ruptured 441.5
  syphilitic 093.9
 dissecting 442.9
  aorta 441.00
   abdominal 441.02
   thoracic 441.01
   thoracoabdominal 441.03
  syphilitic 093.9
 ductus arteriosus 747.0
 embolic—*see* Embolism, artery
 endocardial, infective (any valve) 421.0
 femoral 442.3
 gastroduodenal 442.84
 gastroepiploic 442.84
 heart (chronic or with a stated duration of over 8
   weeks) (infectional) (wall) 414.10
  acute or with a stated duration of 8 weeks or
    less (*see also* Infarct, myocardium) 410.9
  congenital 746.89
  valve—*see* Endocarditis
 hepatic 442.84
 iliac (common) 442.2
 infective (any valve) 421.0
 innominate (nonsyphilitic) 442.89
  syphilitic 093.89
 interauricular septum (*see also* Aneurysm,
   heart) 414.10
 interventricular septum (*see also* Aneurysm,
   heart) 414.10
 intracranial—*see* Aneurysm, brain
 intrathoracic (nonsyphilitic) 441.2
  ruptured 441.1
  syphilitic 093.0
 jugular vein 453.8
 lower extremity 442.3
 lung (pulmonary artery) 417.1
 malignant 093.9
 mediastinal (nonsyphilitic) 442.89
  syphilitic 093.89
 miliary (congenital) (ruptured) (*see also*
   Hemorrhage, subarachnoid) 430
 mitral (heart) (valve) 424.0
 mural (arteriovenous) (heart) (*see also*
   Aneurysm, heart) 414.10
 mycotic, any site 421.0
  ruptured, brain (*see also* Hemorrhage,
    subarachnoid) 430
 myocardium (*see also* Aneurysm, heart) 414.10
 neck 442.81
 pancreaticoduodenal 442.84
 patent ductus arteriosus 747.0
 peripheral NEC 442.89
  congenital NEC (*see also* Aneurysm,
   congenital) 747.60

Aneurysm—*continued*
 popliteal 442.3
 pulmonary 417.1
  arteriovenous 747.3
   acquired 417.0
  syphilitic 093.89
  valve (heart) (*see also* Endocarditis,
   pulmonary) 424.3
 racemose 442.9
  congenital (peripheral) NEC 747.60
 radial 442.0
 Rasmussen's (*see also* Tuberculosis) 011.2
 renal 442.1
 retinal (acquired) 362.17
  congenital 743.58
  diabetic 250.5 *[362.01]*
 sinus, aortic (of Valsalva) 747.29
 specified site NEC 442.89
 spinal (cord) 442.89
  congenital 747.82
  syphilitic (hemorrhage) 094.89
 spleen, splenic 442.83
 subclavian 442.82
  syphilitic 093.89
 superior mesenteric 442.84
 syphilitic 093.9
  aorta 093.0
  central nervous system 094.89
  congenital 090.5
  spine, spinal 094.89
 thoracoabdominal 441.7
  ruptured 441.6
 thorax, thoracic (arch) (nonsyphilitic) 441.2
  dissecting 441.01
  ruptured 441.1
  syphilitic 093.0
 traumatic (complication) (early)—*see* Injury,
   blood vessel, by site
 tricuspid (heart) (valve)—*see* Endocarditis,
   tricuspid
 ulnar 442.0
 upper extremity 442.0
 valve, valvular—*see* Endocarditis
 venous 456.8
  congenital NEC (*see also* Aneurysm,
   congenital) 747.60
 ventricle (arteriovenous) (*see also* Aneurysm,
   heart) 414.10
 visceral artery NEC 442.84
Angiectasis 459.89
Angiectopia 459.9
Angiitis 447.6
 allergic granulomatous 446.4
 hypersensitivity 446.20
  Goodpasture's syndrome 446.21
  specified NEC 446.29
 necrotizing 446.0
 Wegener's (necrotizing respiratory
   granulomatosis) 446.4
Angina (attack) (cardiac) (chest) (effort) (heart)
   (pectoris) (syndrome) (vasomotor) 413.9
 abdominal 557.1
 agranulocytic 288.0
 aphthous 074.0
 catarrhal 462
 crescendo 411.1
 croupous 464.4
 cruris 443.9
  due to atherosclerosis NEC (*see also*
   Arteriosclerosis, extremities) 440.20
 decubitus 413.0

Angina—*continued*
 diphtheritic (membranous) 032.0
 erysipelatous 034.0
 erythematous 462
 exudative, chronic 476.0
 faucium 478.29
 gangrenous 462
  diphtheritic 032.0
 infectious 462
 initial 411.1
 intestinal 557.1
 ludovici 528.3
 Ludwig's 528.3
 malignant 462
  diphtheritic 032.0
 membranous 464.4
  diphtheritic 032.0
 mesenteric 557.1
 monocytic 075
 nocturnal 413.0
 phlegmonous 475
  diphtheritic 032.0
 preinfarctional 411.1
 Prinzmetal's 413.1
 progressive 411.1
 pseudomembranous 101
 psychogenic 306.2
 pultaceous, diphtheritic 032.0
 scarlatinal 034.1
 septic 034.0
 simple 462
 stable NEC 413.9
 staphylococcal 462
 streptococcal 034.0
 stridulous, diphtheritic 032.3
 syphilitic 093.9
  congenital 090.5
 tonsil 475
 trachealis 464.4
 unstable 411.1
 variant 413.1
 Vincent's 101
Angioblastoma (M9161/1)—*see* Neoplasm,
 connective tissue, uncertain behavior
Angiocholecystitis (*see also* Cholecystitis, acute)
 575.0
Angiocholitis (*see also* Cholecystitis, acute) 576.1
Angiodysgensis spinalis 336.1
Angiodysplasia (intestinalis) (intestine) 569.84
 with hemorrhage 569.85
 duodenum 537.82
  with hemorrhage 537.83
 stomach 537.82
  with hemorrhage 537.83
Angioedema (allergic) (any site) (with urticaria)
 995.1
 hereditary 277.6
Angioendothelioma (M9130/1)—*see also*
 Neoplasm, by site, uncertain behavior
 benign (M9130/0) (*see also* Hemangioma, by
  site) 228.00
 bone (M9260/3)—*see* Neoplasm, bone,
  malignant
 Ewing's (M9260/3)—*see* Neoplasm, bone,
  malignant
 nervous system (M9130/0) 228.09
Angiofibroma (M9160/0)—*see also* Neoplasm,
 by site, benign
 juvenile (M9160/0) 210.7
  specified site—*see* Neoplasm, by site, benign
  unspecified site 210.7
Angiohemophilia (A) (B) 286.4

Angioid streaks (choroid) (retina) 363.43
Angiokeratoma (M9141/0)—*see also* Neoplasm,
 skin, benign
 corporis diffusum 272.7
Angiokeratosis
 diffuse 272.7
Angioleiomyoma (M8894/0)—*see* Neoplasm,
 connective tissue, benign
Angioleucitis 683
Angiolipoma (M8861/0) (*see also* Lipoma, by
 site) 214.9
 infiltrating (M8861/1)—*see* Neoplasm,
  connective tissue, uncertain behavior
Angioma (M9120/0) (*see also* Hemangioma, by
 site) 228.00
 capillary 448.1
 hemorrhagicum hereditaria 448.0
 malignant (M9120/3)—*see* Neoplasm,
  connective tissue, malignant
 pigmentosum et atrophicum 757.33
 placenta—*see* Placenta, abnormal
 plexiform (M9131/0)—*see* Hemangioma, by site
 senile 448.1
 serpiginosum 709.1
 spider 448.1
 stellate 448.1
Angiomatosis 757.32
 bacillary 083.8
 corporis diffusum universale 272.7
 cutaneocerebral 759.6
 encephalocutaneous 759.6
 encephalofacial 759.6
 encephalotrigeminal 759.6
 hemorrhagic familial 448.0
 hereditary familial 448.0
 heredofamilial 448.0
 meningo-oculofacial 759.6
 multiple sites 228.09
 neuro-oculocutaneous 759.6
 retina (Hippel's disease) 759.6
 retinocerebellosa 759.6
 retinocerebral 759.6
 systemic 228.09
Angiomyolipoma (M8860/0)
 specified site—*see* Neoplasm, connective
  tissue, benign
 unspecified site 223.0
Angiomyoliposarcoma (M8860/3)—*see*
 Neoplasm, connective tissue, malignant
Angiomyoma (M8894/0)—*see* Neoplasm,
 connective tissue, benign
Angiomyosarcoma (M8894/3)—*see* Neoplasm,
 connective tissue, malignant
Angioneurosis 306.2
Angioneurotic edema (allergic) (any site) (with
 urticaria) 995.1
 hereditary 277.6
Angiopathia, angiopathy 459.9
 diabetic (peripheral) 250.7 *[443.81]*
 peripheral 443.9
  diabetic 250.7 *[443.81]*
  specified type NEC 443.89
 retinae syphilitica 093.89
 retinalis (juvenilis) 362.18
  background 362.10
  diabetic 250.5 *[362.01]*
  proliferative 362.29
  tuberculous (*see also* Tuberculosis) 017.3
   [362.18]
Angiosarcoma (M9120/3)—*see* Neoplasm,
 connective tissue, malignant
Angiosclerosis —*see* Arteriosclerosis

Angioscotoma, enlarged 368.42
Angiospasm 443.9
  brachial plexus 353.0
  cerebral 435.9
  cervical plexus 353.2
  nerve
    arm 354.9
      axillary 353.0
      median 354.1
      ulnar 354.2
    autonomic (*see also* Neuropathy, peripheral,
      autonomic) 337.9
    axillary 353.0
    leg 355.8
      plantar 355.6
    lower extremity—*see* Angiospasm, nerve, leg
    median 354.1
    peripheral NEC 355.9
    spinal NEC 355.9
    sympathetic (*see also* Neuropathy, peripheral,
      autonomic) 337.9
    ulnar 354.2
    upper extremity—*see* Angiospasm, nerve, arm
  peripheral NEC 443.9
  traumatic 443.9
    foot 443.9
    leg 443.9
    vessel 443.9
Angiospastic disease or edema 443.9
Anguillulosis 127.2
Angulation
  cecum (*see also* Obstruction, intestine) 560.9
  coccyx (acquired) 738.6
    congenital 756.19
  femur (acquired) 736.39
    congenital 755.69
  intestine (large) (small) (*see also* Obstruction,
    intestine) 560.9
  sacrum (acquired) 738.5
    congenital 756.19
  sigmoid (flexure) (*see also* Obstruction,
    intestine) 560.9
  spine (*see also* Curvature, spine) 737.9
  tibia (acquired) 736.89
    congenital 755.69
  ureter 593.3
  wrist (acquired) 736.09
    congenital 755.59
Angulus infectiosus 686.8
Anhedonia 302.72
Anhidrosis (lid) (neurogenic) (thermogenic)
  705.0
Anhydration 276.5
  with
    hypernatremia 276.0
    hyponatremia 276.1
Anhydremia 276.5
  with
    hypernatremia 276.0
    hyponatremia 276.1
Anidrosis 705.0
Aniridia (congenital) 743.45
Anisakiasis (infection) (infestation) 127.1
Anisakis larva infestation 127.1
Aniseikonia 367.32
Anisocoria (pupil) 379.41
  congenital 743.46
Anisocytosis 790.09
Anisometropia (congenital) 367.31
Ankle —*see* condition

Ankyloblepharon (acquired) (eyelid) 374.46
  filiforme (adnatum) (congenital) 743.62
  total 743.62
Ankylodactly (*see also* Syndactylism) 755.10
Ankyloglossia 750.0
Ankylosis (fibrous) (osseous) 718.50
  ankle 718.57
  any joint, produced by surgical fusion V45.4
  cricoarytenoid (cartilage) (joint) (larynx) 478.79
  dental 521.6
  ear ossicle NEC 385.22
    malleus 385.21
  elbow 718.52
  finger 718.54
  hip 718.55
  incostapedial joint (infectional) 385.22
  joint, produced by surgical fusion NEC V45.4
  knee 718.56
  lumbosacral (joint) 724.6
  malleus 385.21
  multiple sites 718.59
  postoperative (status) V45.4
  sacroiliac (joint) 724.6
  shoulder 718.51
  specified site NEC 718.58
  spine NEC 724.9
  surgical V45.4
  teeth, tooth (hard tissues) 521.6
  temporomandibular joint 524.61
  wrist 718.53
Ankylostoma— *see* Ancylostoma
Ankylostomiasis (intestinal)—*see*
  Ancylostomiasis
Ankylurethria (*see also* Stricture, urethra) 598.9
Annular —*see also* condition
  detachment, cervix 622.8
  organ or site, congenital NEC—*see* Distortion
  pancreas (congenital) 751.7
Anodontia (complete) (partial) (vera) 520.0
  with abnormal spacing 524.3
  acquired 525.10
    causing malocclusion 524.3
    due to
      caries 525.13
      extraction 525.10
      periodontal disease 525.12
      trauma 525.11
Anomaly, anomalous (congenital) (unspecified
  type) 759.9
  abdomen 759.9
  abdominal wall 756.70
  acoustic nerve 742.9
  adrenal (gland) 759.1
  Alder (-Reilly) (leukocyte granulation) 288.2
  alimentary tract 751.9
    lower 751.5
    specified type NEC 751.8
    upper (any part, except tongue) 750.9
      tongue 750.10
        specified type NEC 750.19
  alveolar ridge (process) 525.8
  ankle (joint) 755.69
  anus, anal (canal) 751.5
  aorta, aortic 747.20
    arch 747.21
    coarctation (postductal) (preductal) 747.10
    cusp or valve NEC 746.9
    septum 745.0
    specified type NEC 747.29
  aorticopulmonary septum 745.0
  apertures, diaphragm 756.6

Anomaly, anomalous—*continued*
  Chédiak-Higashi (-Steinbrinck) (congenital
     gigantism of peroxidase granules) 288.2
  cheek 744.9
  chest (wall) 756.3
  chin 744.9
    specified type NEC 744.89
  chordae tendineae 746.9
  choroid 743.9
    plexus 742.9
  chromosomes, chromosomal 758.9
    13 (13-15) 758.1
    18 (16-18) 758.2
    21 or 22 758.0
    autosomes NEC (*see also* Abnormality,
     autosomes) 758.5
     deletion 758.3
    Christchurch 758.3
    D_1 758.1
    E_3 758.2
    G 758.0
    mitochondrial 758.9
    mosaics 758.89
    sex 758.81
     complement, XO 758.6
     complement, XXX 758.81
     complement, XYY 758.81
     gonadal dysgenesis 758.6
     Klinefelter's 758.7
     Turner's 758.6
    trisomy 21 758.0
  cilia 743.9
  circulatory system 747.9
    specified type NEC 747.89
  clavicle 755.51
  clitoris 752.40
  coccyx 756.10
  colon 751.5
  common duct 751.60
  communication
    coronary artery 746.85
    left ventricle with right atrium 745.4
  concha (ear) 744.3
  connection
    renal vessels with kidney 747.62
    total pulmonary venous 747.41
  connective tissue 756.9
    specified type NEC 756.89
  cornea 743.9
    shape 743.41
    size 743.41
    specified type NEC 743.49
  coronary
    artery 746.85
    vein 746.89
  cranium—*see* Anomaly, skull
  cricoid cartilage 748.3
  cushion, endocardial 745.60
    specified type NEC 745.69
  cystic duct 751.60
  dental arch relationship 524.2
  dentition 520.6
  dentofacial NEC 524.9
    functional 524.5
    specified type NEC 524.8
  dermatoglyphic 757.2
  Descemet's membrane 743.9
    specified type NEC 743.49
  development
    cervix 752.40
    vagina 752.40

Anomaly, anomalous—*continued*
  vulva 752.40
  diaphragm, diaphragmatic (apertures) NEC
    756.6
  digestive organ(s) or system 751.9
    lower 751.5
    specified type NEC 751.8
    upper 750.9
  distribution, coronary artery 746.85
  ductus
    arteriosus 747.0
    Botalli 747.0
  duodenum 751.5
  dura 742.9
    brain 742.4
    spinal cord 742.59
  ear 744.3
    causing impairment of hearing 744.00
     specified type NEC 744.09
    external 744.3
     causing impairment of hearing 744.02
     specified type NEC 744.29
    inner (causing impairment of hearing) 744.05
    middle, except ossicles (causing impairment
     of hearing) 744.03
     ossicles 744.04
    ossicles 744.04
    prominent auricle 744.29
    specified type NEC 744.29
     with hearing impairment 744.09
  Ebstein's (heart) 746.2
    tricuspid valve 746.2
  ectodermal 757.9
  Eisenmenger's (ventricular septal defect) 745.4
  ejaculatory duct 752.9
    specified type NEC 752.8
  elbow (joint) 755.50
  endocardial cushion 745.60
    specified type NEC 745.69
  endocrine gland NEC 759.2
  epididymis 752.9
  epiglottis 748.3
  esophagus 750.9
    specified type NEC 750.4
  Eustachian tube 744.3
    specified type NEC 744.24
  eye (any part) 743.9
    adnexa 743.9
     specified type NEC 743.69
    anophthalmos 743.00
    anterior
     chamber and related structures 743.9
      angle 743.9
       specified type NEC 743.44
      specified type NEC 743.44
     segment 743.9
      combined 743.48
      multiple 743.48
      specified type NEC 743.49
    cataract (*see also* Cataract) 743.30
    glaucoma (*see also* Buphthalmia) 743.20
    lid 743.9
     specified type NEC 743.63
    microphthalmos (*see also* Microphthalmos)
     743.10
    posterior segment 743.9
     specified type NEC 743.59
     vascular 743.58
     vitreous 743.9
      specified type NEC 743.51
    ptosis (eyelid) 743.61

Anomaly, anomalous—*continued*
  retina 743.9
    specified type NEC 743.59
  sclera 743.9
    specified type NEC 743.47
  specified type NEC 743.8
  eyebrow 744.89
  eyelid 743.9
    specified type NEC 743.63
  face (any part) 744.9
    bone(s) 756.0
    specified type NEC 744.89
  fallopian tube 752.10
    specified type NEC 752.19
  fascia 756.9
    specified type NEC 756.89
  femur 755.60
  fibula 755.60
  finger 755.50
    supernumerary 755.01
    webbed (*see also* Syndactylism, fingers) 755.11
  fixation, intestine 751.4
  flexion (joint) 755.9
    hip or thigh (*see also* Dislocation, hip, congenital) 754.30
  folds, heart 746.9
  foot 755.67
  foramen
    Botalli 745.5
    ovale 745.5
  forearm 755.50
  forehead (*see also* Anomaly, skull) 756.0
  form, teeth 520.2
  fovea centralis 743.9
  frontal bone (*see also* Anomaly, skull) 756.0
  gallbladder 751.60
  Gartner's duct 752.11
  gastrointestinal tract 751.9
    specified type NEC 751.8
    vessel 747.61
  genitalia, genital organ(s) or system
    female 752.9
      external 752.40
        specified type NEC 752.49
      internal NEC 752.9
    male (external and internal) 752.9
      epispadias 752.62
      hidden penis 752.65
      hydrocele, congenital 778.6
      hypospadias 752.61
      micropenis 752.64
      testis, undescended 752.51
        retractile 752.52
    specified type NEC 752.8
  genitourinary NEC 752.9
  Gerbode 745.4
  globe (eye) 743.9
  glottis 748.3
  granulation or granulocyte, genetic 288.2
    constitutional 288.2
    leukocyte 288.2
  gum 750.9
  gyri 742.9
  hair 757.9
    specified type NEC 757.4
  hand 755.50
  hard tissue formation in pulp 522.3
  head (*see also* Anomaly, skull) 756.0
  heart 746.9
    auricle 746.9

Anomaly, anomalous—*continued*
    bands 746.9
    fibroelastosis cordis 425.3
    folds 746.9
    malposition 746.87
    maternal, affecting fetus or newborn 760.3
    obstructive NEC 746.84
    patent ductus arteriosus (Botalli) 747.0
    septum 745.9
      acquired 429.71
      aortic 745.0
      aorticopulmonary 745.0
      atrial 745.5
      auricular 745.5
      between aorta and pulmonary artery 745.0
      endocardial cushion type 745.60
        specified type NEC 745.69
      interatrial 745.5
      interventricular 745.4
        with pulmonary stenosis or atresia, dextraposition of aorta, and hypertrophy of right ventricle 745.2
        acquired 429.71
      specified type NEC 745.8
      ventricular 745.4
        with pulmonary stenosis or atresia, dextraposition of aorta, and hypertrophy of right ventricle 745.2
        acquired 429.71
    specified type NEC 746.89
    tetralogy of Fallot 745.2
    valve NEC 746.9
      aortic 746.9
        atresia 746.89
        bicuspid valve 746.4
        insufficiency 746.4
        specified type NEC 746.89
        stenosis 746.3
          subaortic 746.81
          supravalvular 747.22
      mitral 746.9
        atresia 746.89
        insufficiency 746.6
        specified type NEC 746.89
        stenosis 746.5
      pulmonary 746.00
        atresia 746.01
        insufficiency 746.09
        stenosis 746.02
          infundibular 746.83
          subvalvular 746.83
      tricuspid 746.9
        atresia 746.1
        stenosis 746.1
    ventricle 746.9
  heel 755.67
  Hegglin's 288.2
  hemianencephaly 740.0
  hemicephaly 740.0
  hemicrania 740.0
  hepatic duct 751.60
  hip (joint) 755.63
  hourglass
    bladder 753.8
    gallbladder 751.69
    stomach 750.7
  humerus 755.50
  hymen 752.40
  hypersegmentation of neutrophils, hereditary 288.2
  hypophyseal 759.2

Anomaly, anomalous—*continued*
  musculoskeletal system, except limbs 756.9
  nail 757.5
  neck 744.89
  nerve 742.8
    acoustic 742.8
    optic 742.8
  nervous system 742.8
  nipple 757.6
  nose 748.1
  organ NEC 759.89
    of Corti 744.05
  osseous meatus (ear) 744.03
  ovary 752.0
  oviduct 752.19
  pancreas 751.7
  parathyroid 759.2
  patella 755.64
  pelvic girdle 755.69
  penis 752.69
  pericardium 746.89
  peripheral vascular system NEC (*see also*
    Anomaly, peripheral vascular system)
    747.60
  pharynx 750.29
  pituitary 759.2
  prostate 752.8
  radius 755.59
  rectum 751.5
  respiratory system 748.8
  rib 756.3
  round ligament 752.8
  sacrum 756.19
  salivary duct or gland 750.26
  scapula 755.59
  sclera 743.47
  scrotum 752.8
  seminal duct or tract 752.8
  shoulder girdle 755.59
  site NEC 759.89
  skin 757.39
  skull (bone(s)) 756.0
    with
      anencephalus 740.0
      encephalocele 742.0
      hydrocephalus 742.3
        with spina bifida (*see also* Spina bifida)
        741.0
      microcephalus 742.1
  specified organ or site NEC 759.89
  spermatic cord 752.8
  spinal cord 742.59
  spine 756.19
  spleen 759.0
  sternum 756.3
  stomach 750.7
  tarsus 755.67
  tendon 756.89
  testis 752.8
  thorax (wall) 756.3
  thymus 759.2
  thyroid (gland) 759.2
    cartilage 748.3
  tibia 755.69
  toe 755.66
  tongue 750.19
  trachea (cartilage) 748.3
  ulna 755.59
  urachus 753.7
  ureter 753.4
    obstructive 753.29

Anomaly, anomalous—*continued*
  urethra 753.8
    obstructive 753.6
  urinary tract 753.8
  uterus 752.3
  uvula 750.26
  vagina 752.49
  vascular NEC (*see also* Anomaly, peripheral
    vascular system) 747.60
    brain 747.81
  vas deferens 752.8
  vein(s) (peripheral) NEC (*see also* Anomaly,
    peripheral vascular system) 747.60
    brain 747.81
    great 747.49
    portal 747.49
    pulmonary 747.49
  vena cava (inferior) (superior) 747.49
  vertebra 756.19
  vulva 752.49
spermatic cord 752.9
spine, spinal 756.10
  column 756.10
  cord 742.9
    meningocele (*see also* Spina bifida) 741.9
    specified type NEC 742.59
    spina bifida (*see also* Spina bifida) 741.9
    vessel 747.82
  meninges 742.59
  nerve root 742.9
spleen 759.0
Sprengel's 755.52
sternum 756.3
stomach 750.9
  specified type NEC 750.7
submaxillary gland 750.9
superior vena cava 747.40
talipes—*see* Talipes
tarsus 755.67
  with complete absence of distal elements
    755.31
teeth, tooth NEC 520.9
  position 524.3
  spacing 524.3
tendon 756.9
  specified type NEC 756.89
termination
  coronary artery 746.85
testis 752.9
thebesian valve 746.9
thigh 755.60
  flexion (*see also* Subluxation, congenital, hip)
    754.32
thorax (wall) 756.3
throat 750.9
thumb 755.50
  supernumerary 755.01
thymus gland 759.2
thyroid (gland) 759.2
  cartilage 748.3
tibia 755.60
  saber 090.5
toe 755.66
  supernumerary 755.02
  webbed (*see also* Syndactylism, toes) 755.13
tongue 750.10
  specified type NEC 750.19
trachea, tracheal 748.3
  cartilage 748.3
  rings 748.3
tragus 744.3

Anomaly, anomalous—*continued*
  transverse aortic arch 747.21
  trichromata 368.59
  trichromatopsia 368.59
  tricuspid (leaflet) (valve) 746.9
    atresia 746.1
    Ebstein's 746.2
    specified type NEC 746.89
    stenosis 746.1
  trunk 759.9
  Uhl's (hypoplasia of myocardium, right
     ventricle) 746.84
  ulna 755.50
  umbilicus 759.9
    artery 747.5
  union, trachea with larynx 748.3
  unspecified site 759.9
  upper extremity 755.50
    vessel 747.63
  urachus 753.7
    specified type NEC 753.7
  ureter 753.9
    obstructive 753.20
    specified type NEC 753.4
     obstructive 753.29
  urethra (valve) 753.9
    obstructive 753.6
    specified type NEC 753.8
  urinary tract or system (any part, except
     urachus) 753.9
    specified type NEC 753.8
    urachus 753.7
  uterus 752.3
    with only one functioning horn 752.3
    in pregnancy or childbirth 654.0
     affecting fetus or newborn 763.89
     causing obstructed labor 660.2
      affecting fetus or newborn 763.1
  uvula 750.9
  vagina 752.40
  valleculae 748.3
  valve (heart) NEC 746.9
    formation, ureter 753.29
    pulmonary 746.00
    specified type NEC 746.89
  vascular NEC (*see also* Anomaly, peripheral
     vascular system) 747.60
    ring 747.21
  vas deferens 752.9
  vein(s) (peripheral) NEC (*see also* Anomaly,
     peripheral vascular system) 747.60
    brain 747.81
    cerebral 747.81
    coronary 746.89
    great 747.40
     specified type NEC 747.49
    portal 747.40
    pulmonary 747.40
    retina 743.9
  vena cava (inferior) (superior) 747.40
  venous return (pulmonary) 747.49
    partial 747.42
    total 747.41
  ventricle, ventricular (heart) 746.9
    bands 746.9
    folds 746.9
    septa 745.4
  vertebra 756.10
  vesicourethral orifice 753.9
  vessels NEC (*see also* Anomaly, peripheral
     vascular system) 747.60

Anomaly, anomalous—*continued*
  optic papilla 743.9
  vitelline duct 751.0
  vitreous humor 743.9
    specified type NEC 743.51
  vulva 752.40
  wrist (joint) 755.50
Anomia 784.69
Anonychia 757.5
  acquired 703.8
Anophthalmos, anophthalmus (clinical)
    (congenital) (globe) 743.00
  acquired V45.78
Anopsia (altitudinal) (quadrant) 368.46
Anorchia 752.8
Anorchism, anorchidism 752.8
Anorexia 783.0
  hysterical 300.11
  nervosa 307.1
Anosmia (*see also* Disturbance, sensation) 781.1
  hysterical 300.11
  postinfectional 478.9
  psychogenic 306.7
  traumatic 951.8
Anosognosia 780.99
Anosphrasia 781.1
Anosteoplasia 756.50
Anotia 744.09
Anovulatory cycle 628.0
Anoxemia 799.0
  newborn 768.9
Anoxia 799.0
  altitude 993.2
  cerebral 348.1
    with
     abortion—*see* Abortion, by type,
      with specified complication NEC
     ectopic pregnancy (*see also* categories
      633.0-633.9) 639.8
     molar pregnancy (*see also* categories
      630-632) 639.8
    complicating
     delivery (cesarean) (instrumental) 669.4
     ectopic or molar pregnancy 639.8
     obstetric anesthesia or sedation 668.2
    during or resulting from a procedure 997.01
    following
     abortion 639.8
     ectopic or molar pregnancy 639.8
    newborn (*see also* Distress, fetal, liveborn
     infant) 768.9
  due to drowning 994.1
  fetal, affecting newborn 768.9
  heart—*see* Insufficiency, coronary
  high altitude 993.2
  intrauterine
    fetal death (before onset of labor) 768.0
     during labor 768.1
    liveborn infant—*see* Distress, fetal, liveborn
     infant
  myocardial—*see* Insufficiency, coronary
  newborn 768.9
    mild or moderate 768.6
    severe 768.5
  pathological 799.0
Anteflexion —*see* Anteversion
Antenatal
  care, normal pregnancy V22.1
    first V22.0
  screening (for) V28.9
    based on amniocentesis NEC V28.2

Antenatal—*continued*
    chromosomal anomalies V28.0
      raised alphafetoprotein levels V28.1
    chromosomal anomalies V28.0
    fetal growth retardation using ultrasonics V28.4
    isoimmunization V28.5
    malformations using ultrasonics V28.3
    raised alphafetoprotein levels in amniotic fluid V28.1
    specified condition NEC V28.8
    Streptococcus B V28.6
Antepartum —*see* condition
Anterior —*see also* condition
    spinal artery compression syndrome 721.1
Antero-occlusion 524.2
Anteversion
    cervix (*see also* Anteversion, uterus) 621.6
    femur (neck), congenital 755.63
    uterus, uterine (cervix) (postinfectional) (postpartal, old) 621.6
      congenital 752.3
      in pregnancy or childbirth 654.4
        affecting fetus or newborn 763.89
        causing obstructed labor 660.2
          affecting fetus or newborn 763.1
Anthracosilicosis (occupational) 500
Anthracosis (lung) (occupational) 500
    lingua 529.3
Anthrax 022.9
    with pneumonia 022.1 *[484.5]*
    colitis 022.2
    cutaneous 022.0
    gastrointestinal 022.2
    intestinal 022.2
    pulmonary 022.1
    respiratory 022.1
    septicemia 022.3—
    specified manifestation NEC 022.8
Anthropoid pelvis 755.69
    with disproportion (fetopelvic) 653.2
      affecting fetus or newborn 763.1
      causing obstructed labor 660.1
        affecting fetus or newborn 763.1
Anthropophobia 300.29
Antibioma, breast 611.0
Antibodies
    maternal (blood group) (*see also* Incompatibility) 656.2
    anti-D, cord blood 656.1
      fetus or newborn 773.0
Antibody deficiency syndrome
    agammaglobulinemic 279.00
    congenital 279.04
    hypogammaglobulinemic 279.00
Anticoagulant, circulating (*see also* Circulating anticoagulants) 286.5
Antimongolism syndrome 758.3
Antimonial cholera 985.4
Antisocial personality 301.7
Antithrombinemia (*see also* Circulating anticoagulants) 286.5
Antithromboplastinemia (*see also* Circulating anticoagulants) 286.5
Antithromboplastinogenemia (*see also* Circulating anticoagulants) 286.5
Antitoxin complication or reaction —*see* Complications, vaccination
Anton (-Babinski) syndrome (hemiasomatognosia) 307.9
Antritis (chronic) 473.0
  acute 461.0

Antrum, antral —*see* condition
Anuria 788.5
    with
      abortion—*see* Abortion, by type, with renal failure
      ectopic pregnancy (*see also* categories 633.0-633.9) 639.3
      molar pregnancy (*see also* categories 630-632) 639.3
    calculus (impacted) (recurrent) 592.9
      kidney 592.0
      ureter 592.1
    congenital 753.3
    due to a procedure 997.5
    following
      abortion 639.3
      ectopic or molar pregnancy 639.3
    newborn 753.3
    postrenal 593.4
    puerperal, postpartum, childbirth 669.3
    specified as due to a procedure 997.5
    sulfonamide
      correct substance properly administered 788.5
      overdose or wrong substance given or taken 961.0
    traumatic (following crushing) 958.5
Anus, anal —*see* condition
Anusitis 569.49
Anxiety (neurosis) (reaction) (state) 300.00
    alcohol-induced 291.89
    depression 300.4
    drug-induced 292.89
    due to or associated with physical condition 293.84
    generalized 300.02
    hysteria 300.20
    in
      acute stress reaction 308.0
      transient adjustment reaction 309.24
    panic type 300.01
    separation, abnormal 309.21
    syndrome (organic) (transient) 293.84
Aorta, aortic —*see* condition
Aortectasia 441.9
Aortitis (nonsyphilitic) 447.6
    arteriosclerotic 440.0
    calcific 447.6
    Döhle-Heller 093.1
    luetic 093.1
    rheumatic (*see also* Endocarditis, acute, rheumatic) 391.1
    rheumatoid—*see* Arthritis, rheumatoid
    specific 093.1
    syphilitic 093.1
      congenital 090.5
Apathetic thyroid storm (*see also* Thyrotoxicosis) 242.9
Apepsia 536.8
    achlorhydric 536.0
    psychogenic 306.4
Aperistalsis, esophagus 530.0
Apert's syndrome (acrocephalosyndactyly) 755.55
Apert-Gallais syndrome (adrenogenital) 255.2
Apertognathia 524.2
Aphagia 787.2
    psychogenic 307.1
Aphakia (acquired) (bilateral) (postoperative) (unilateral) 379.31
    congenital 743.35

Aphalangia (congenital) 755.4
 lower limb (complete) (intercalary) (partial)
   (terminal) 755.39
   meaning all digits (complete) (partial) 755.31
   transverse 755.31
 upper limb (complete) (intercalary) (partial)
   (terminal) 755.29
   meaning all digits (complete) (partial) 755.21
   transverse 755.21
Aphasia (amnestic) (ataxic) (auditory) (Broca's)
   (choreatic) (classic) (expressive) (global)
   (ideational) (ideokinetic) (ideomotor) (jargon)
   (motor) (nominal) (receptive) (semantic)
   (sensory) (syntactic) (verbal) (visual)
   (Wernicke's) 784.3
 developmental 315.31
 syphilis, tertiary 094.89
 uremic—*see* Uremia
Aphemia 784.3
 uremic—*see* Uremia
Aphonia 784.41
 clericorum 784.49
 hysterical 300.11
 organic 784.41
 psychogenic 306.1
Aphthae, aphthous —*see also* condition
 Bednar's 528.2
 cachectic 529.0
 epizootic 078.4
 fever 078.4
 oral 528.2
 stomatitis 528.2
 thrush 112.0
 ulcer (oral) (recurrent) 528.2
   genital organ(s) NEC
     female 629.8
     male 608.89
   larynx 478.79
Apical —*see* condition
Aplasia —*see also* Agenesis
 alveolar process (acquired) 525.8
   congenital 750.26
 aorta (congenital) 747.22
 aortic valve (congenital) 746.89
 axialis extracorticalis (congenital) 330.0
 bone marrow (myeloid) 284.9
   acquired (secondary) 284.8
   congenital 284.0
   idiopathic 284.9
 brain 740.0
   specified part 742.2
 breast 757.6
 bronchus 748.3
 cementum 520.4
 cerebellar 742.2
 congenital pure red cell 284.0
 corpus callosum 742.2
 erythrocyte 284.8
   congenital 284.0
 extracortical axial 330.0
 eye (congenital) 743.00
 fovea centralis (congenital) 743.55
 germinal (cell) 606.0
 iris 743.45
 labyrinth, membranous 744.05
 limb (congenital) 755.4
   lower NEC 755.30
   upper NEC 755.20
 lung (bilateral) (congenital) (unilateral) 748.5
 nervous system NEC 742.8
 nuclear 742.8

Aplasia—*continued*
 ovary 752.0
 Pelizaeus-Merzbacher 330.0
 prostate (congenital) 752.8
 red cell (pure) (with thymoma) 284.8
   acquired (secondary) 284.8
   congenital 284.0
   hereditary 284.0
   of infants 284.0
   primary 284.0
 round ligament (congenital) 752.8
 salivary gland 750.21
 skin (congenital) 757.39
 spinal cord 742.59
 spleen 759.0
 testis (congenital) 752.8
 thymic, with immunodeficiency 279.2
 thyroid 243
 uterus 752.3
 ventral horn cell 742.59
Apleuria 756.3
Apnea, apneic (spells) 786.03
 newborn, neonatorum 770.81
   essential 770.81
   obstructive 770.82
   primary 770.81
   sleep 770.81
   specified NEC 770.82
 psychogenic 306.1
 sleep NEC 780.57
   with
     hypersomnia 780.53
     hyposomnia 780.51
     insomnia 780.51
     sleep disturbance NEC 780.57
Apneumatosis newborn 770.4
Apodia 755.31
Apophysitis (bone) (*see also* Osteochondrosis)
   732.9
 calcaneus 732.5
 juvenile 732.6
Apoplectiform convulsions (*see also* Disease,
   cerebrovascular, acute) 436
Apoplexia, apoplexy, apoplectic (*see also*
   Disease, cerebrovascular, acute) 436
 abdominal 569.89
 adrenal 036.3
 attack 436
 basilar (*see also* Disease, cerebrovascular,
   acute) 436
 brain (*see also* Disease, cerebrovascular, acute)
   436
 bulbar (*see also* Disease, cerebrovascular,
   acute) 436
 capillary (*see also* Disease, cerebrovascular,
   acute) 436
 cardiac (*see also* Infarct, myocardium) 410.9
 cerebral (*see also* Disease, cerebrovascular,
   acute) 436
 chorea (*see also* Disease, cerebrovascular,
   acute) 436
 congestive (*see also* Disease, cerebrovascular,
   acute) 436
   newborn 767.4
 embolic (*see also* Embolism, brain) 434.1
 fetus 767.0
 fit (*see also* Disease, cerebrovascular, acute) 436
 healed or old V12.59
 heart (auricle) (ventricle) (*see also* Infarct,
   myocardium) 410.9
 heat 992.0

Apoplexia, apoplexy, apoplectic—*continued*
  hemiplegia (*see also* Disease, cerebrovascular,
    acute) 436
  hemorrhagic (stroke) (*see also* Hemorrhage,
    brain) 432.9
  ingravescent (*see also* Disease, cerebrovascular,
    acute) 436
  late effect—*see* Late effect(s) (of)
    cerebrovascular disease
  lung—*see* Embolism, pulmonary
  meninges, hemorrhagic (*see also* Hemorrhage,
    subarachnoid) 430
  neonatorum 767.0
  newborn 767.0
  pancreatitis 577.0
  placenta 641.2
  progressive (*see also* Disease, cerebrovascular,
    acute) 436
  pulmonary (artery) (vein)—*see* Embolism,
    pulmonary
  sanguineous (*see also* Disease, cerebrovascular,
    acute) 436
  seizure (*see also* Disease, cerebrovascular,
    acute) 436
  serous (*see also* Disease, cerebrovascular,
    acute) 436
  spleen 289.59
  stroke (*see also* Disease, cerebrovascular, acute)
    436
  thrombotic (*see also* Thrombosis, brain) 434.0
  uremic—*see* Uremia
  uteroplacental 641.2
Appendage
  fallopian tube (cyst of Morgagni) 752.11
  intestine (epiploic) 751.5
  preauricular 744.1
  testicular (organ of Morgagni) 752.8
Appendicitis 541
  with
    perforation, peritonitis (generalized), or
      rupture 540.0
      with peritoneal abscess 540.1
    peritoneal abscess 540.1
  acute (catarrhal) (fulminating) (gangrenous)
    (inflammatory) (obstructive) (retrocecal)
    (suppurative) 540.9
    with
      perforation, peritonitis, or rupture 540.0
        with peritoneal abscess 540.1
      peritoneal abscess 540.1
  amebic 006.8
  chronic (recurrent) 542
  exacerbation—*see* Appendicitis, acute
  fulminating—*see* Appendicitis, acute
  gangrenous—*see* Appendicitis, acute
  healed (obliterative) 542
  interval 542
  neurogenic 542
  obstructive 542
  pneumococcal 541
  recurrent 542
  relapsing 542
  retrocecal 541
  subacute (adhesive) 542
  subsiding 542
  suppurative—*see* Appendicitis, acute
  tuberculous (*see also* Tuberculosis) 014.8
Appendiclausis 543.9
Appendicolithiasis 543.9
Appendicopathia oxyurica 127.4

Appendix, appendicular —*see also* condition
  Morgagni (male) 752.8
  fallopian tube 752.11
Appetite
  depraved 307.52
  excessive 783.6
    psychogenic 307.51
  lack or loss (*see also* Anorexia) 783.0
    nonorganic origin 307.59
  perverted 307.52
    hysterical 300.11
Apprehension, apprehensiveness (abnormal)
  (state) 300.00
  specified type NEC 300.09
Approximal wear 521.1
Apraxia (classic) (ideational) (ideokinetic)
  (ideomotor) (motor) 784.69
  oculomotor, congenital 379.51
  verbal 784.69
Aptyalism 527.7
Aqueous misdirection 365.83
Arabicum elephantiasis (*see also* Infestation,
  filarial) 125.9
Arachnidism 989.5
Arachnitis —*see* Meningitis
Arachnodactyly 759.82
Arachnoidism 989.5
Arachnoiditis (acute) (adhesive) (basic) (brain)
  (cerebrospinal) (chiasmal) (chronic) (spinal)
  (*see also* Meningitis) 322.9
  meningococcal (chronic) 036.0
  syphilitic 094.2
  tuberculous (*see also* Tuberculosis, meninges)
    013.0
Araneism 989.5
Arboencephalitis, Australian 062.4
Arborization block (heart) 426.6
Arbor virus, arbovirus (infection) NEC 066.9
ARC 042
Arches —*see* condition
Arcuatus uterus 752.3
Arcus (cornea)
  juvenilis 743.43
    interfering with vision 743.42
  senilis 371.41
Arc-welders' lung 503
Arc-welders' syndrome (photokeratitis) 370.24
Areflexia 796.1
Areola —*see* condition
Argentaffinoma (M8241/1)—*see also*
  Neoplasm, by site, uncertain behavior
  benign (M8241/0)—*see* Neoplasm, by site,
    benign
  malignant (M8241/3)—*see* Neoplasm, by site,
    malignant
  syndrome 259.2
Argentinian hemorrhagic fever 078.7
Arginosuccinicaciduria 270.6
Argonz-Del Castillo syndrome (nonpuerperal
  galactorrhea and amenorrhea) 253.1
Argyll-Robertson phenomenon pupil, or
  syndrome (syphilitic) 094.89
  atypical 379.45
  nonluetic 379.45
  nonsyphilitic 379.45
  reversed 379.45
Argyria, argyriasis NEC 985.8
  conjunctiva 372.55
  cornea 371.16
  from drug or medicinal agent

Argyria, argyriasis—*continued*
correct substance properly administered
709.09
overdose or wrong substance given or taken
961.2
Arhinencephaly 742.2
Arias-Stella phenomenon 621.3
Ariboflavinosis 266.0
Arizona enteritis 008.1
Arm —*see* condition
Armenian disease 277.3
Arnold-Chiari obstruction or syndrome (*see also* Spina bifida) 741.0
type I 348.4
type II (*see also* Spina bifida) 741.0
type III 742.0
type IV 742.2
Arrest, arrested
active phase of labor 661.1
affecting fetus or newborn 763.7
any plane in pelvis
complicating delivery 660.1
affecting fetus or newborn 763.1
bone marrow (*see also* Anemia, aplastic) 284.9
cardiac 427.5
with
abortion—*see* Abortion, by type, with
specified complication NEC
ectopic pregnancy (*see also* categories
633.0-633.9) 639.8
molar pregnancy (*see also* categories
630-632) 639.8
complicating
anesthesia
correct substance properly administered
427.5
obstetric 668.1
overdose or wrong substance given 968.4
specified anesthetic—*see* Table of drugs
and chemicals
delivery (cesarean) (instrumental) 669.4
ectopic or molar pregnancy 639.8
surgery (nontherapeutic) (therapeutic) 997.1
fetus or newborn 779.89
following
abortion 639.8
ectopic or molar pregnancy 639.8
postoperative (immediate) 997.1
long-term effect of cardiac surgery 429.4
cardiorespiratory (*see also* Arrest, cardiac) 427.5
deep transverse 660.3
affecting fetus or newborn 763.1
development or growth
bone 733.91
child 783.40
fetus 764.9
affecting management of pregnancy 656.5
tracheal rings 748.3
epiphyseal 733.91
granulopoiesis 288.0
heart—*see* Arrest, cardiac
respiratory 799.1
newborn 770.89
sinus 426.6
transverse (deep) 660.3
affecting fetus or newborn 763.1
Arrhenoblastoma (M8630.1)
benign (M8630/0)
specified site—*see* Neoplasm, by site, benign
unspecified site
female 220

Arrhenoblastoma—*continued*
male 222.0
malignant (M8630/3)
specified site— *see* Neoplasm, by site,
malignant
unspecified site
female 183.0
male 186.9
specified site—*see* Neoplasm, by site, uncertain
behavior
unspecified site
female 236.2
male 236.4
Arrhinencephaly 742.2
due to
trisomy 13 (13-15) 758.1
trisomy 18 (16-l8) 758.2
Arrhythmia (auricle) (cardiac) (cordis) (gallop
rhythm) (juvenile) (nodal) (reflex) (sinus)
(supraventricular) (transitory) (ventricle) 427.9
bigeminal rhythm 427.89
block 426.9
bradycardia 427.89
contractions, premature 427.60
coronary sinus 427.89
ectopic 427.89
extrasystolic 427.60
postoperative 997.1
psychogenic 306.2
vagal 780.2
Arrillaga-Ayerza syndrome (pulmonary artery
sclerosis with pulmonary hypertension) 416.0
Arsenical
dermatitis 692.4
keratosis 692.4
pigmentation 985.1
from drug or medicinal agent
correct substance properly administered
709.09
overdose or wrong substance given or taken
961.1
Arsenism 985.1
from drug or medicinal agent
correct substance properly administered 692.4
overdose or wrong substance given or taken
961.1
Arterial —*see* condition
Arteriectasis 447.8
Arteriofibrosis —*see* Arteriosclerosis
Arteriolar sclerosis —*see* Arteriosclerosis
Arteriolith —*see* Arteriosclerosis
Arteriolitis 447.6
necrotizing, kidney 447.5
renal—*see* Hypertension, kidney
Arteriolosclerosis —*see* Arteriosclerosis
Arterionephrosclerosis (*see also* Hypertension,
kidney) 403.90
Arteriopathy 447.9
Arteriosclerosis, arteriosclerotic (artery)
(deformans) (diffuse) (disease) (endarteritis)
(general) (obliterans) (obliterative) (occlusive)
(senile) (with calcification) 440.9
with
gangrene 440.24
psychosis (*see also* Psychosis,
arteriosclerotic) 290.40
ulceration 440.23
aorta 440.0
arteries of extremities NEC — *see*
Arteriosclerosis, extremities

Arthritis, arthritic (acute) (chronic) (subacute)
716.9

> *Note—Use the following fifth-digit subclassification with categories 711-712, 715-716:*
>
> 0 *site unspecified*
> 1 *shoulder region*
> 2 *upper arm*
> 3 *forearm*
> 4 *hand*
> 5 *pelvic region and thigh*
> 6 *lower leg*
> 7 *ankle and foot*
> 8 *other specified sites*
> 9 *multiple sites*

allergic 716.2
ankylosing (crippling) (spine) 720.0
  sites other than spine 716.9
atrophic 714.0
  spine 720.9
back (*see also* Arthritis, spine) 721.90
Bechterew's (ankylosing spondylitis) 720.0
blennorrhagic 098.50
cervical, cervicodorsal (*see also* Spondylosis,
  cervical) 721.0
Charcot's 094.0 *[713.5]*
  diabetic 250.6 *[713.5]*
  syringomyelic 336.0 *[713.5]*
  tabetic 094.0 *[713.5]*
chylous (*see also* Filariasis) 125.9 *[711.7]*
climacteric NEC 716.3
coccyx 721.8
cricoarytenoid 478.79
crystal (-induced)—*see* Arthritis, due to crystals
deformans (*see also* Osteoarthrosis) 715.9
  spine 721.90
    with myelopathy 721.91
degenerative (*see also* Osteoarthrosis) 715.9
  idiopathic 715.09
  polyarticular 715.09
  spine 721.90
    with myelopathy 721.91
dermatoarthritis, lipoid 272.8 *[713.0]*
due to or associated with
  acromegaly 253.0 *[713.0]*
  actinomycosis 039.8 *[711.4]*
  amyloidosis 277.3 *[713.7]*
  bacterial disease NEC 040.89 *[711.4]*
  Behçet's syndrome 136.1 *[711.2]*
  blastomycosis 116.0 *[711.6]*
  brucellosis (*see also* Brucellosis) 023.9
    [711.4]
  caisson disease 993.3
  coccidioidomycosis 114.3 *[711.6]*
  coliform (Escherichia coli) 711.0
  colitis, ulcerative (*see also* Colitis, ulcerative)
    556.9 *[713.1]*
  cowpox 051.0 *[711.5]*
  crystals (*see also* Gout)
    dicalcium phosphate 275.49 *[712.1]*
    pyrophosphate 275.49 *[712.2]*
    specified NEC 275.49 *[712.8]*
  dermatoarthritis, lipoid 272.8 *[713.0]*
  dermatological disorder NEC 709.9 *[713.3]*
  diabetes 250.6 *[713.5]*
  diphtheria 032.89 *[711.4]*
  dracontiasis 125.7 *[711.7]*
  dysentery 009.0 *[711.3]*

Arthritis, arthritic—*continued*
endocrine disorder NEC 259.9 *[713.0]*
enteritis NEC 009.1 *[711.3]*
  infectious (*see also* Enteritis, infectious)
    009.0 *[711.3]*
    specified organism NEC 008.8 *[711.3]*
  regional (*see also* Enteritis, regional) 555.9
    [713.1]
  specified organism NEC 008.8 *[711.3]*
epiphyseal slip, nontraumatic (old) 716.8
erysipelas 035 *[711.4]*
erythema
  epidemic 026.1
  multiforme 695.1 *[713.3]*
  nodosum 695.2 *[713.3]*
Escherichia coli 711.0
filariasis NEC 125.9 *[711.7]*
gastrointestinal condition NEC 569.9 *[713.1]*
glanders 024 *[711.4]*
Gonococcus 098.50
gout 274.0
H. influenzae 711.0
helminthiasis NEC 128.9 *[711.7]*
hematological disorder NEC 289.9 *[713.2]*
hemochromatosis 275.0 *[713.0]*
hemoglobinopathy NEC (*see also* Disease,
  hemoglobin) 282.7 *[713.2]*
hemophilia (*see also* Hemophilia) 286.0
  [713.2]
Hemophilus influenzae (H. influenzae) 711.0
Henoch (-Schönlein) purpura 287.0 *[713.6]*
histoplasmosis NEC (*see also* Histoplasmosis)
  115.99 *[711.6]*
hyperparathyroidism 252.0 *[713.0]*
hypersensitivity reaction NEC 995.3 *[713.6]*
hypogammaglobulinemia (*see also*
  Hypogammaglobulinemia) 279.00 *[713.0]*
hypothyroidism NEC 244.9 *[713.0]*
infection (*see also* Arthritis, infectious) 711.9
infectious disease NEC 136.9 *[711.8]*
leprosy (*see also* Leprosy) 030.9 *[711.4]*
leukemia NEC (M9800/3) 208.9 *[713.2]*
lipoid dermatoarthritis 272.8 *[713.0]*
Lyme disease 088.81 *[711.8]*
meaning Osteoarthritis—*see* Osteoarthrosis
Mediterranean fever, familial 277.3 *[713.7]*
meningococcal infection 036.82
metabolic disorder NEC 277.9 *[713.0]*
multiple myelomatosis (M9730/3) 203.0
  [713.2]
mumps 072.79 *[711.5]*
mycobacteria 031.8 *[711.4]*
mycosis NEC 117.9 *[711.6]*
neurological disorder NEC 349.9 *[713.5]*
ochronosis 270.2 *[713.0]*
O'Nyong Nyong 066.3 *[711.5]*
parasitic disease NEC 136.9 *[711.8]*
paratyphoid fever (*see also* Fever,
  paratyphoid) 002.9 *[711.3]*
Pneumococcus 711.0
poliomyelitis (*see also* Poliomyelitis) 045.9
  [711.5]
Pseudomonas 711.0
psoriasis 696.0
pyogenic organism (E. coli) (H. influenzae)
  (Pseudomonas) (Streptococcus) 711.0
rat-bite fever 026.1 *[711.4]*
regional enteritis (*see also* Enteritis, regional)
  555.9 *[713.1]*
Reiter's disease 099.3 *[711.1]*
respiratory disorder NEC 519.9 *[713.4]*

Arthritis, arthritic—*continued*
  reticulosis, malignant (M9720/3) 202.3
    [713.2]
  rubella 056.71
  salmonellosis 003.23
  sarcoidosis 135 *[713.7]*
  serum sickness 999.5 *[713.6]*
  Staphylococcus 711.0
  Streptococcus 711.0
  syphilis (*see also* Syphilis) 094.0 *[711.4]*
  syringomyelia 336.0 *[713.5]*
  thalassemia 282.4 *[713.2]*
  tuberculosis (*see also* Tuberculosis, arthritis)
    015.9 *[711.4]*
  typhoid fever 002.0 *[711.3]*
  ulcerative colitis (*see also* Colitis, ulcerative)
    556.9 *[713.1]*
  urethritis
    nongonococcal (*see also* Urethritis,
      nongonococcal) 099.40 *[711.1]*
    nonspecific (*see also* Urethritis,
      nongonococcal) 099.40 *[711.1]*
    Reiter's 099.3 *[711.1]*
  viral disease NEC 079.99 *[711.5]*
 erythema epidemic 026.1
 gonococcal 098.50
 gouty (acute) 274.0
 hypertrophic (*see also* Osteoarthrosis) 715.9
  spine 721.90
    with myelopathy 721.91
 idiopathic, blennorrheal 099.3
 in caisson disease 993.3 *[713.8]*
 infectious or infective (acute) (chronic)
  (subacute) NEC 711.9
  nonpyogenic 711.9
  spine 720.9
 inflammatory NEC 714.9
 juvenile rheumatoid (chronic) (polyarticular)
  714.30
  acute 714.31
  monoarticular 714.33
  pauciarticular 714.32
 lumbar (*see also* Spondylosis, lumbar) 721.3
 meningococcal 036.82
 menopausal NEC 716.3
 migratory—*see* Fever, rheumatic
 neuropathic (Charcot's) 094.0 *[713.5]*
  diabetic 250.6 *[713.5]*
  nonsyphilitic NEC 349.9 *[713.5]*
  syringomyelic 336.0 *[713.5]*
  tabetic 094.0 *[713.5]*
 nodosa (*see also* Osteoarthrosis) 715.9
  spine 721.90
    with myelopathy 721.91
 nonpyogenic NEC 716.9
  spine 721.90
    with myelopathy 721.91
 ochronotic 270.2 *[713.0]*
 palindromic (*see also* Rheumatism,
  palindromic) 719.3
 pneumococcal 711.0
 postdysenteric 009.0 *[711.3]*
 postrheumatic, chronic (Jaccoud's) 714.4
 primary progressive 714.0
  spine 720.9
 proliferative 714.0
  spine 720.0
 psoriatic 696.0
 purulent 711.0
 pyogenic or pyemic 711.0

Arthritis, arthritic—*continued*
 rheumatic 714.0
  acute or subacute—*see* Fever, rheumatic
  chronic 714.0
  spine 720.9
 rheumatoid (nodular) 714.0
  with
    splenoadenomegaly and leukopenia 714.1
    visceral or systemic involvement 714.2
  aortitis 714.89
  carditis 714.2
  heart disease 714.2
  juvenile (chronic) (polyarticular) 714.30
    acute 714.31
    monoarticular 714.33
    pauciarticular 714.32
  spine 720.0
 rubella 056.71
 sacral, sacroiliac, sacrococcygeal (*see also*
  Spondylosis, sacral) 721.3
 scorbutic 267
 senile or senescent (*see also* Osteoarthrosis)
  715.9
  spine 721.90
    with myelopathy 721.91
 septic 711.0
 serum (nontherapeutic) (therapeutic) 999.5
  [713.6]
 specified form NEC 716.8
 spine 721.90
  with myelopathy 721.91
  atrophic 720.9
  degenerative 721.90
    with myelopathy 721.91
  hypertrophic (with deformity) 721.90
    with myelopathy 721.91
  infectious or infective NEC 720.9
  Marie-Strümpell 720.0
  nonpyogenic 721.90
    with myelopathy 721.91
  pyogenic 720.9
  rheumatoid 720.0
  traumatic (old) 721.7
  tuberculous (*see also* Tuberculosis) 015.0
    [720.81]
 staphylococcal 711.0
 streptococcal 711.0
 suppurative 711.0
 syphilitic 094.0 *[713.5]*
  congenital 090.49 *[713.5]*
 syphilitica deformans (Charcot) 094.0 *[713.5]*
 temporomandibular joint 524.69
 thoracic (*see also* Spondylosis, thoracic) 721.2
 toxic of menopause 716.3
 transient 716.4
 traumatic (chronic) (old) (post) 716.1
  current injury—*see* nature of injury
 tuberculous (*see also* Tuberculosis, arthritis)
  015.9 *[711.4]*
 urethritica 099.3 *[711.1]*
 urica, uratic 274.0
 venereal 099.3 *[711.1]*
 vertebral (*see also* Arthritis, spine) 721.90
 villous 716.8
 von Bechterew's 720.0
Arthrocele (*see also* Effusion, joint) 719.0
Arthrochondritis —*see* Arthritis
Arthrodesis status V45.4
Arthrodynia (*see also* Pain, joint) 719.4
 psychogenic 307.89
Arthrodysplasia 755.9
Arthrofibrosis, joint (*see also* Ankylosis) 718.5

Arthrogryposis 728.3
  multiplex, congenita 754.89
Arthrokatadysis 715.35
Arthrolithiasis 274.0
Arthro-onychodysplasia 756.89
Arthro-osteo-onychodysplasia 756.89
Arthropathy (*see also* Arthritis) 716.9

Note—Use the following fifth-digit subclassification with categories 711-712, 716:

0 *site unspecified*
1 *shoulder region*
2 *upper arm*
3 *forearm*
4 *hand*
5 *pelvic region and thigh*
6 *lower leg*
7 *ankle and foot*
8 *other specified sites*
9 *multiple sites*

  Behçet's 136.1 *[711.2]*
  Charcot's 094.0 *[713.5]*
    diabetic 250.6 *[713.5]*
    syringomyelic 336.0 *[713.5]*
    tabetic 094.0 *[713.5]*
  crystal (-induced)—*see* Arthritis, due to crystals
  gouty 274.0
  neurogenic, neuropathic (Charcot's) (tabetic)
      094.0 *[713.5]*
    diabetic 250.6 *[713.5]*
    nonsyphilitic NEC 349.9 *[713.5]*
    syringomyelic 336.0 *[713.5]*
  postdysenteric NEC 009.0 *[711.3]*
  postrheumatic, chronic (Jaccoud's) 714.4
  psoriatic 696.0
  pulmonary 731.2
  specified NEC 716.8
  syringomyelia 336.0 *[713.5]*
  tabes dorsalis 094.0 *[713.5]*
  tabetic 094.0 *[713.5]*
  transient 716.4
  traumatic 716.1
  uric acid 274.0
Arthrophyte (*see also* Loose, body, joint) 718.1
Arthrophytis 719.80
  ankle 719.87
  elbow 719.82
  foot 719.87
  hand 719.84
  hip 719.85
  knee 719.86
  multiple sites 719.89
  pelvic region 719.85
  shoulder (region) 719.81
  specified site NEC 719.88
  wrist 719.83
Arthropyosis (*see also* Arthritis, pyogenic) 711.0
Arthrosis (deformans) (degenerative) (*see also*
    Osteoarthrosis) 715.9
  Charcot's 094.0 *[713.5]*
  polyarticular 715.09
  spine (*see also* Spondylosis) 721.90
Arthus' phenomenon 995.2
  due to
    correct substance properly administered 995.2
    overdose or wrong substance given or taken
        977.9
      specified drug—*see* Table of drugs and
          chemicals
    serum 999.5

Articular —*see also* condition
  disc disorder (reducing or non-reducing) 524.63
  spondylolisthesis 756.12
Artificial
  device (prosthetic)—*see* Fitting, device
  insemination V26.1
  menopause (states) (symptoms) (syndrome)
      627.4
  opening status (functioning) (without
      complication) V44.9
    anus (colostomy) V44.3
    colostomy V44.3
    cystostomy V44.50
      appendico-vesicostomy V44.52
      cutaneous-vesicostomy V44.51
      specified type NEC V44.59
    enterostomy V44.4
    gastrostomy V44.1
    ileostomy V44.2
    intestinal tract NEC V44.4
    jejunostomy V44.4
    nephrostomy V44.6
    specified site NEC V44.8
    tracheostomy V44.0
    ureterostomy V44.6
    urethrostomy V44.6
    urinary tract NEC V44.6
    vagina V44.7
  vagina status V44.7
ARV (disease) (illness) (infection)—*see* Human
    immunodeficiency virus (disease) (illness)
    (infection)
Arytenoid —*see* condition
Asbestosis (occupational) 501
Asboe-Hansen's disease (incontinentia
    pigmenti) 757.33
Ascariasis (intestinal) (lung) 127.0
Ascaridiasis 127.0
Ascaridosis 127.0
Ascaris 127.0
  lumbricoides (infestation) 127.0
  pneumonia 127.0
Ascending —*see* condition
Aschoff's bodies (*see also* Myocarditis,
    rheumatic) 398.0
Ascites 789.5
  abdominal NEC 789.5
  cancerous (M8000/6) 197.6
  cardiac 428.0
  chylous (nonfilarial) 457.8
    filarial (*see also* Infestation, filarial) 125.9
  congenital 778.0
  due to S. japonicum 120.2
  fetal, causing fetopelvic disproportion 653.7
  heart 428.0
  joint (*see also* Effusion, joint) 719.0
  malignant (M8000/6) 197.6
  pseudochylous 789.5
  syphilitic 095.2
  tuberculous (*see also* Tuberculosis) 014.0
Ascorbic acid (vitamin C) deficiency (scurvy)
    267
ASCUS (atypical squamous cell changes of
    undetermined significance)
  favor benign 795.01
  favor dysplasia 795.02
ASCVD (arteriosclerotic cardiovascular disease)
    429.2
Aseptic —*see* condition
Asherman's syndrome 621.5
Asialia 527.7
Asiatic cholera (*see also* Cholera) 001.9

Asocial personality or trends 301.7
Asomatognosia 781.8
Aspergillosis 117.3
  with pneumonia 117.3 *[484.6]*
  allergic bronchopulmonary 518.6
  nonsyphilitic NEC 117.3
Aspergillus (flavus) (fumigatus) (infection) (terreus) 117.3
Aspermatogenesis 606.0
Aspermia (testis) 606.0
Asphyxia, asphyxiation (by) 799.0
  antenatal—*see* Distress, fetal
  bedclothes 994.7
  birth (*see also* Asphyxia, newborn) 768.9
  bunny bag 994.7
  carbon monoxide 986
  caul (*see also* Asphyxia, newborn) 768.9
  cave-in 994.7
    crushing—*see* Injury, internal, intrathoracic organs
  constriction 994.7
  crushing—*see* Injury, internal, intrathoracic organs
  drowning 994.1
  fetal, affecting newborn 768.9
  food or foreign body (in larynx) 933.1
    bronchioles 934.8
    bronchus (main) 934.1
    lung 934.8
    nasopharynx 933.0
    nose, nasal passages 932
    pharynx 933.0
    respiratory tract 934.9
      specified part NEC 934.8
    throat 933.0
    trachea 934.0
  gas, fumes, or vapor NEC 987.9
    specified—*see* Table of drugs and chemicals
  gravitational changes 994.7
  hanging 994.7
  inhalation—*see* Inhalation
  intrauterine
    fetal death (before onset of labor) 768.0
      during labor 768.1
    liveborn infant—*see* Distress, fetal, liveborn infant
  local 443.0
  mechanical 994.7
    during birth (*see also* Distress, fetal) 768.9
  mucus 933.1
    bronchus (main) 934.1
    larynx 933.1
    lung 934.8
    nasal passages 932
    newborn 770.1
    pharynx 933.0
    respiratory tract 934.9
      specified part NEC 934.8
    throat 933.0
    trachea 934.0
    vaginal (fetus or newborn) 770.1
  newborn 768.9
    blue 768.6
    livida 768.6
    mild or moderate 768.6
    pallida 768.5
    severe 768.5
    white 768.5
    with neurologic involvement 768.5
  pathological 799.0
  plastic bag 994.7

Asphyxia, Asphyxiation—*continued*
  postnatal (*see also* Asphyxia, newborn) 768.9
    mechanical 994.7
  pressure 994.7
  reticularis 782.61
  strangulation 994.7
  submersion 994.1
  traumatic NEC—*see* Injury, internal, intrathoracic organs
  vomiting, vomitus—*see* Asphyxia, food or foreign body
Aspiration
  acid pulmonary (syndrome) 997.3
    obstetric 668.0
  amniotic fluid 770.1
  bronchitis 507.0
  contents of birth canal 770.1
  fetal pneumonitis 770.1
  food, foreign body, or gasoline (with asphyxiation)—*see* Asphyxia, food or foreign body
  meconium 770.1
  mucus 933.1
    into
      bronchus (main) 934.1
      lung 934.8
      respiratory tract 934.9
        specified part NEC 934.8
      trachea 934.0
    newborn 770.1
    vaginal (fetus or newborn) 770.1
  newborn 770.1
  pneumonia 507.0
  pneumonitis 507.0
    fetus or newborn 770.1
    obstetric 668.0
  syndrome of newborn (massive) (meconium) 770.1
  vernix caseosa 770.1
Asplenia 759.0
  with mesocardia 746.87
Assam fever 085.0
Assimilation, pelvis
  with disproportion 653.2
    affecting fetus or newborn 763.1
    causing obstructed labor 660.1
      affecting fetus or newborn 763.1
Assmann's focus (*see also* Tuberculosis) 011.0
Astasia (-abasia) 307.9
  hysterical 300.11
Asteatosis 706.8
  cutis 706.8
Astereognosis 780.99
Asterixis 781.3
  in liver disease 572.8
Asteroid hyalitis 379.22
Asthenia, asthenic 780.79
  cardiac (*see also* Failure, heart) 428.9
    psychogenic 306.2
  cardiovascular (*see also* Failure, heart) 428.9
    psychogenic 306.2
  heart (*see also* Failure, heart) 428.9
    psychogenic 306.2
  hysterical 300.11
  myocardial (*see also* Failure, heart) 428.9
    psychogenic 306.2
  nervous 300.5
  neurocirculatory 306.2
  neurotic 300.5
  psychogenic 300.5
  psychoneurotic 300.5

Asthenia, asthenic—*continued*
  psychophysiologic 300.5
  reaction, psychoneurotic 300.5
  senile 797
  Stiller's 780.79
  tropical anhidrotic 705.1
Asthenopia 368.13
  accommodative 367.4
  hysterical (muscular) 300.11
  psychogenic 306.7
Asthenospermia 792.2
Asthma, asthmatic (bronchial) (catarrh)
    (spasmodic) 493.9

Note—Use the following fifth-digit
subclassification with category 493:

0 without mention of status asthmaticus or acute
exacerbation or unspecified
1 with status asthmaticus
2 with acute exacerbation

  with
    chronic obstructive pulmonary disease
      (COPD) 493.2
    hay fever 493.0
    rhinitis, allergic 493.0
  allergic 493.9
    stated cause (external allergen) 493.0
  atopic 493.0
  cardiac (*see also* Failure, ventricular, left) 428.1
  cardiobronchial (*see also* Failure, ventricular,
    left) 428.1
  cardiorenal (*see also* Hypertension, cardiorenal)
    404.90
  childhood 493.0
  colliers' 500
  croup 493.9
  detergent 507.8
  due to
    detergent 507.8
    inhalation of fumes 506.3
    internal immunological process 493.0
  endogenous (intrinsic) 493.1
  eosinophilic 518.3
  exogenous (cosmetics) (dander or dust) (drugs)
    (dust) (feathers) (food) (hay) (platinum)
    (pollen) 493.0
  extrinsic 493.0
  grinders' 502
  hay 493.0
  heart (*see also* Failure, ventricular, left) 428.1
  IgE 493.0
  infective 493.1
  intrinsic 493.1
  Kopp's 254.8
  late-onset 493.1
  meat-wrappers' 506.9
  Millar's (laryngismus stridulus) 478.75
  millstone makers' 502
  miners' 500
  Monday morning 504
  New Orleans (epidemic) 493.0
  platinum 493.0
  pneumoconiotic (occupational) NEC 505
  potters' 502
  psychogenic 316 *[493.9]*
  pulmonary eosinophilic 518.3
  red cedar 495.8
  Rostan's (*see also* Failure, ventricular, left)
    428.1
  sandblasters' 502

Asthma, asthmatic—*continued*
  sequoiosis 495.8
  stonemasons' 502
  thymic 254.8
  tuberculous (*see also* Tuberculosis, pulmonary)
    011.9
  Wichmann's (laryngismus stridulus) 478.75
  wood 495.8
Astigmatism (compound) (congenital) 367.20
  irregular 367.22
  regular 367.21
Astroblastoma (M9430/3)
  nose 748.1
  specified site—*see* Neoplasm, by site,
    malignant
  unspecified site 191.9
Astrocytoma (cystic) (M9400/3)
  anaplastic type (M9401/3)
    specified site—*see* Neoplasm, by site,
      malignant
    unspecified site 191.9
  fibrillary (M9420/3)
    specified site—*see* Neoplasm, by site,
      malignant
    unspecified site 191.9
  fibrous (M9420/3)
    specified site—*see* Neoplasm, by site,
      malignant
    unspecified site 191.9
  gemistocytic (M9411/3)
    specified site—*see* Neoplasm, by site,
      malignant
    unspecified site 191.9
  juvenile (M9421/3)
    specified site—*see* Neoplasm, by site,
      malignant
    unspecified site 191.9
  nose 748.1
  pilocytic (M9421/3)
    specified site—*see* Neoplasm, by site,
      malignant
    unspecified site 191.9
  piloid (M9421/3)
    specified site—*see* Neoplasm, by site,
      malignant
    unspecified site 191.9
  protoplasmic (M9410/3)
    specified site—*see* Neoplasm, by site,
      malignant
    unspecified site 191.9
  specified site—*see* Neoplasm, by site, malignant
  subependymal (M9383/1) 237.5
    giant cell (M9384/1) 237.5
  unspecified site 191.9
Astroglioma (M9400/3)
  nose 748.1
  specified site—*see* Neoplasm, by site, malignant
  unspecified site 191.9
Asymbolia 784.60
Asymmetrical breathing 786.09
Asymmetry —*see also* Distortion
  chest 786.9
  face 754.0
  jaw NEC 524.12
    maxillary 524.11
  pelvis with disproportion 653.0
    affecting fetus or newborn 763.1
    causing obstructed labor 660.1
      affecting fetus or newborn 763.1
Asynergia 781.3
Asynergy 781.3
  ventricular 429.89

Atresia, atretic—*continued*
  aorta 747.22
    with hypoplasia of ascending aorta and
      defective development of left ventricle
      (with mitral valve atresia) 746.7
    arch 747.11
    ring 747.21
  aortic (orifice) (valve) 746.89
    arch 747.11
  aqueduct of Sylvius 742.3
    with spina bifida (*see also* Spina bifida) 741.0
  artery NEC (*see also* Atresia, blood vessel)
    747.60
    cerebral 747.81
    coronary 746.85
    eye 743.58
    pulmonary 747.3
    umbilical 747.5
  auditory canal (external) 744.02
  bile, biliary duct (common) or passage 751.61
    acquired (*see also* Obstruction, biliary) 576.2
  bladder (neck) 753.6
  blood vessel (peripheral) NEC 747.60
    cerebral 747.81
    gastrointestinal 747.61
    lower limb 747.64
    pulmonary artery 747.3
    renal 747.62
    spinal 747.82
    upper limb 747.63
  bronchus 748.3
  canal, ear 744.02
  cardiac
    valve 746.89
      aortic 746.89
      mitral 746.89
      pulmonary 746.01
      tricuspid 746.1
  cecum 751.2
  cervix (acquired) 622.4
    congenital 752.49
    in pregnancy or childbirth 654.6
      affecting fetus or newborn 763.89
      causing obstructed labor 660.2
        affecting fetus or newborn 763.1
  choana 748.0
  colon 751.2
  cystic duct 751.61
    acquired 575.8
      with obstruction (*see also* Obstruction,
        gallbladder) 575.2
  digestive organs NEC 751.8
  duodenum 751.1
  ear canal 744.02
  ejaculatory duct 752.8
  epiglottis 748.3
  esophagus 750.3
  Eustachian tube 744.24
  fallopian tube (acquired) 628.2
    congenital 752.19
  follicular cyst 620.0
  foramen of
    Luschka 742.3
      with spina bifida (*see also* Spina bifida)
        741.0
    Magendie 742.3
      with spina bifida (*see also* Spina bifida)
        741.0
  gallbladder 751.69
  genital organ
    external

Atresia, atretic—*continued*
    female 752.49
    male NEC 752.8
      penis 752.69
    internal
      female 752.8
      male 752.8
  glottis 748.3
  gullet 750.3
  heart
    valve NEC 746.89
      aortic 746.89
      mitral 746.89
      pulmonary 746.01
      tricuspid 746.1
  hymen 752.42
    acquired 623.3
    postinfective 623.3
  ileum 751.1
  intestine (small) 751.1
    large 751.2
  iris, filtration angle (*see also* Buphthalmia)
    743.20
  jejunum 751.1
  kidney 753.3
  lacrimal, apparatus 743.65
    acquired—*see* Stenosis, lacrimal
  larynx 748.3
  ligament, broad 752.19
  lung 748.5
  meatus urinarius 753.6
  mitral valve 746.89
    with atresia or hypoplasia of aortic orifice or
      valve, with hypoplasia of ascending aorta
      and defective development of left
      ventricle 746.7
  nares (anterior) (posterior) 748.0
  nasolacrimal duct 743.65
  nasopharynx 748.8
  nose, nostril 748.0
    acquired 738.0
  organ or site NEC—*see* Anomaly, specified
    type NEC
  osseous meatus (ear) 744.03
  oviduct (acquired) 628.2
    congenital 752.19
  parotid duct 750.23
    acquired 527.8
  pulmonary (artery) 747.3
    valve 746.01
    vein 747.49
  pulmonic 746.01
  pupil 743.46
  rectum 751.2
  salivary duct or gland 750.23
    acquired 527.8
  sublingual duct 750.23
    acquired 527.8
  submaxillary duct or gland 750.23
    acquired 527.8
  trachea 748.3
  tricuspid valve 746.1
  ureter 753.29
  ureteropelvic junction 753.21
  ureterovesical orifice 753.22
  urethra (valvular) 753.6
  urinary tract NEC 753.29
  uterus 752.3
    acquired 621.8
  vagina (acquired) 623.2
    congenital 752.49

Atresia, atretic—*continued*
  postgonococcal (old) 098.2
  postinfectional 623.2
  senile 623.2
  vascular NEC (*see also* Atresia, blood vessel) 747.60
    cerebral 747.81
  vas deferens 752.8
  vein NEC (*see also* Atresia, blood vessel) 747.60
    cardiac 746.89
    great 747.49
    portal 747.49
    pulmonary 747.49
  vena cava (inferior) (superior) 747.49
  vesicourethral orifice 753.6
  vulva 752.49
    acquired 624.8
Atrichia, atrichosis 704.00
  congenital (universal) 757.4
Atrioventricularis commune 745.69
Atrophia —*see also* Atrophy
  alba 709.09
  cutis 701.8
    idiopathica progressiva 701.8
    senilis 701.8
  dermatological, diffuse (idiopathic) 701.8
  flava hepatis (acuta) (subacuta) (*see also* Necrosis, liver) 570
  gyrata of choroid and retina (central) 363.54
    generalized 363.57
  senilis 797
    dermatological 701.8
  unguium 703.8
    congenita 757.5
Atrophoderma, atrophodermia 701.9
  diffusum (idiopathic) 701.8
  maculatum 701.3
    et striatum 701.3
      due to syphilis 095.8
    syphilitic 091.3
  neuriticum 701.8
  pigmentosum 757.33
  reticulatum symmetricum faciei 701.8
  senile 701.8
  symmetrical 701.8
  vermiculata 701.8
Atrophy, atrophic
  adrenal (autoimmune) (capsule) (cortex) (gland) 255.4
    with hypofunction 255.4
  alveolar process or ridge (edentulous) 525.2
  appendix 543.9
  Aran-Duchenne muscular 335.21
  arm 728.2
  arteriosclerotic—*see* Arteriosclerosis
  arthritis 714.0
    spine 720.9
  bile duct (any) 576.8
  bladder 596.8
  blanche (of Milian) 701.3
  bone (senile) 733.99
    due to
      disuse 733.7
      infection 733.99
      tabes dorsalis (neurogenic) 094.0
    posttraumatic 733.99
  brain (cortex) (progressive) 331.9
    with dementia 290.10
    Alzheimer's 331.0
      with dementia—*see* Alzheimer's dementia

Atrophy, atrophic—*continued*
  circumscribed (Pick's) 331.1
    with dementia
      with behavioral disturbance 331.1 *[294.11]*
      without behavioral disturbance 331.1 *[294.10]*
  congenital 742.4
  hereditary 331.9
  senile 331.2
  breast 611.4
    puerperal, postpartum 676.3
  buccal cavity 528.9
  cardiac (brown) (senile) (*see also* Degeneration, myocardial) 429.1
  cartilage (infectional) (joint) 733.99
  cast, plaster of Paris 728.2
  cerebellar—*see* Atrophy, brain
  cerebral—*see* Atrophy, brain
  cervix (endometrium) (mucosa) (myometrium) (senile) (uteri) 622.8
    menopausal 627.8
  Charcot-Marie-Tooth 356.1
  choroid 363.40
    diffuse secondary 363.42
    hereditary (*see also* Dystrophy, choroid) 363.50
      gyrate
        central 363.54
        diffuse 363.57
        generalized 363.57
    senile 363.41
  ciliary body 364.57
  colloid, degenerative 701.3
  conjunctiva (senile) 372.89
  corpus cavernosum 607.89
  cortical (*see also* Atrophy, brain) 331.9
  Cruveilhier's 335.21
  cystic duct 576.8
  dacryosialadenopathy 710.2
  degenerative
    colloid 701.3
    senile 701.3
  Déjérine-Thomas 333.0
  diffuse idiopathic, dermatological 701.8
  disuse
    bone 733.7
    muscle 728.2
  Duchenne-Aran 335.21
  ear 388.9
  edentulous alveolar ridge 525.2
  emphysema, lung 492.8
  endometrium (senile) 621.8
    cervix 622.8
  enteric 569.89
  epididymis 608.3
  eyeball, cause unknown 360.41
  eyelid (senile) 374.50
  facial (skin) 701.9
  facioscapulohumeral (Landouzy-Déjérine) 359.1
  fallopian tube (senile), acquired 620.3
  fatty, thymus (gland) 254.8
  gallbladder 575.8
  gastric 537.89
  gastritis (chronic) 535.1
  gastrointestinal 569.89
  genital organ, male 608.89
  glandular 289.3
  globe (phthisis bulbi) 360.41
  gum 523.2
  hair 704.2

Atrophy, atrophic—*continued*
   associated with retinal dystrophy 377.13
      dominant hereditary 377.16
      glaucomatous 377.14
      hereditary (dominant) (Leber's) 377.16
      Leber's (hereditary) 377.16
      partial 377.15
      postinflammatory 377.12
      primary 377.11
      syphilitic 094.84
         congenital 090.49
         tabes dorsalis 094.0
   orbit 376.45
   ovary (senile), acquired 620.3
   oviduct (senile), acquired 620.3
   palsy, diffuse 335.20
   pancreas (duct) (senile) 577.8
   papillary muscle 429.81
   paralysis 355.9
   parotid gland 527.0
   patches skin 701.3
      senile 701.8
   penis 607.89
   pharyngitis 472.1
   pharynx 478.29
   pluriglandular 258.8
   polyarthritis 714.0
   prostate 602.2
   pseudohypertrophic 359.1
   renal (*see also* Sclerosis, renal) 587
   reticulata 701.8
   retina (*see also* Degeneration, retina) 362.60
      hereditary (*see also* Dystrophy, retina) 362.70
   rhinitis 472.0
   salivary duct or gland 527.0
   scar NEC 709.2
   sclerosis, lobar (of brain) 331.0
      with dementia
         with behavioral disturbance 331.1 *[294.11]*
         without behavioral disturbance 331.1
            [294.10]
   scrotum 608.89
   seminal vesicle 608.89
   senile 797
      degenerative, of skin 701.3
   skin (patches) (senile) 701.8
   spermatic cord 608.89
   spinal (cord) 336.8
      acute 336.8
      muscular (chronic) 335.10
         adult 335.19
         familial 335.11
         juvenile 335.10
      paralysis 335.10
         acute (*see also* Poliomyelitis, with paralysis)
            045.1
   spine (column) 733.99
   spleen (senile) 289.59
   spots (skin) 701.3
      senile 701.8
   stomach 537.89
   striate and macular 701.3
      syphilitic 095.8
   subcutaneous 701.9
      due to injection 999.9
   sublingual gland 527.0
   submaxillary gland 527.0
   Sudeck's 733.7
   suprarenal (autoimmune) (capsule) (gland) 255.4
      with hypofunction 255.4
   tarso-orbital fascia, congenital 743.66

Atrophy, atrophic—*continued*
   testis 608.3
   thenar, partial 354.0
   throat 478.29
   thymus (fat) 254.8
   thyroid (gland) 246.8
      with
         cretinism 243
         myxedema 244.9
      congenital 243
   tongue (senile) 529.8
      papillae 529.4
      smooth 529.4
   trachea 519.1
   tunica vaginalis 608.89
   turbinate 733.99
   tympanic membrane (nonflaccid) 384.82
      flaccid 384.81
   ulcer (*see also* Ulcer, skin) 707.9
   upper respiratory tract 478.9
   uterus, uterine (acquired) (senile) 621.8
      cervix 622.8
      due to radiation (intended effect) 621.8
   vagina (senile) 627.3
   vascular 459.89
   vas deferens 608.89
   vertebra (senile) 733.99
   vulva (primary) (senile) 624.1
   Werdnig-Hoffmann 335.0
   yellow (acute) (congenital) (liver) (subacute)
      (*see also* Necrosis, liver) 570
      chronic 571.8
      resulting from administration of blood,
         plasma, serum, or other biological
         substance (within 8 months of
         administration)—*see* Hepatitis, viral

Attack
   akinetic (*see also* Epilepsy) 345.0
   angina—*see* Angina
   apoplectic (*see also* Disease, cerebrovascular,
      acute) 436
   benign shuddering 333.93
   bilious—*see* Vomiting
   cataleptic 300.11
   cerebral (*see also* Disease, cerebrovascular,
      acute) 436
   coronary (*see also* Infarct, myocardium) 410.9
   cyanotic, newborn 770.83
   epileptic (*see also* Epilepsy) 345.9
   epileptiform 780.39
   heart (*see also* Infarct, myocardium) 410.9
   hemiplegia (*see also* Disease, cerebrovascular,
      acute) 436
   hysterical 300.11
   jacksonian (*see also* Epilepsy) 345.5
   myocardium, myocardial (*see also* Infarct,
      myocardium) 410.9
   myoclonic (*see also* Epilepsy) 345.1
   panic 300.01
   paralysis (*see also* Disease, cerebrovascular,
      acute) 436
   paroxysmal 780.39
   psychomotor (*see also* Epilepsy) 345.4
   salaam (*see also* Epilepsy) 345.6
   schizophreniform (*see also* Schizophrenia) 295.4
   sensory and motor 780.39
   syncope 780.2
   toxic, cerebral 780.39
   transient ischemic (TIA) 435.9
   unconsciousness 780.2
      hysterical 300.11

Attack—*continued*
  vasomotor 780.2
  vasovagal (idiopathic) (paroxysmal) 780.2
Attention to
  artificial
    opening (of) V55.9
      digestive tract NEC V55.4
      specified site NEC V55.8
      urinary tract NEC V55.6
      vagina V55.7
  colostomy V55.3
  cystostomy V55.5
  gastrostomy V55.1
  ileostomy V55.2
  jejunostomy V55.4
  nephrostomy V55.6
  surgical dressings V58.3
  sutures V58.3
  tracheostomy V55.0
  ureterostomy V55.6
  urethrostomy V55.6
Attrition
  gum 523.2
  teeth (excessive) (hard tissues) 521.1
Atypical —*see also* condition
  distribution, vessel (congenital) (peripheral)
    NEC 747.60
  endometrium 621.9
  glandular cell changes of undetermined
    significance
    favor benign (AGCUS favor benign) 795.01
    favor dysplasia (AGCUS favor dysplasia)
      795.02
  kidney 593.89
  squamous cell changes of undetermined
    significance
    favor benign (ASCUS favor benign) 795.01
    favor dysplasia (ASCUS favor dysplasia)
      795.02
Atypism, cervix 622.1
Audible tinnitus (*see also* Tinnitus) 388.30
Auditory —*see* condition
Audry's syndrome (acropachyderma) 757.39
Aujeszky's disease 078.89
Aura, jacksonian (*see also* Epilepsy) 345.5
Aurantiasis, cutis 278.3
Auricle, auricular —*see* condition
Auriculotemporal syndrome 350.8
Australian
  Q fever 083.0
  X disease 062.4
Autism, autistic (child) (infantile) 299.0
Autodigestion 799.8
Autoerythrocyte sensitization 287.2
Autographism 708.3
Autoimmune
  cold sensitivity 283.0
  disease NEC 279.4
  hemolytic anemia 283.0
  thyroiditis 245.2
Autoinfection, septic —*see* Septicemia
Autointoxication 799.8
Automatism 348.8
  epileptic (*see also* Epilepsy) 345.4
  paroxysmal, idiopathic (*see also* Epilepsy) 345.4
Autonomic, autonomous
  bladder 596.54
    neurogenic 596.54
      with cauda equine 344.61
  dysreflexia 337.3

Autonomic, autonomous— *continued*
  faciocephalalgia (*see also* Neuropathy,
    peripheral, autonomic) 337.9
  hysterical seizure 300.11
  imbalance (*see also* Neuropathy, peripheral,
    autonomic) 337.9
Autophony 388.40
Autosensitivity, erythrocyte 287.2
Autotopagnosia 780.99
Autotoxemia 799.8
Autumn —*see* condition
Avellis' syndrome 344.89
Aviators
  disease or sickness (*see* also Effect, adverse,
    high altitude) 993.2
  ear 993.0
  effort syndrome 306.2
Avitaminosis (multiple NEC) (*see also*
  Deficiency, vitamin) 269.2
  A 264.9
  B 266.9
    with
      beriberi 265.0
      pellagra 265.2
  B_1 265.1
  B_2 266.0
  B_6 266.1
  B_{12} 266.2
  C (with scurvy) 267
  D 268.9
    with
      osteomalacia 268.2
      rickets 268.0
  E 269.1
  G 266.0
  H 269.1
  K 269.0
  multiple 269.2
  nicotinic acid 265.2
  P 269.1
Avulsion (traumatic) 879.8
  blood vessel—*see* Injury, blood vessel, by site
  cartilage—*see also* Dislocation, by site
    knee, current (*see also* Tear, meniscus) 836.2
    symphyseal (inner), complicating delivery
      665.6
  complicated 879.9
  diaphragm—*see* Injury, internal, diaphragm
  ear—*see* Wound, open, ear
  epiphysis of bone—*see* Fracture, by site
  external site other than limb—*see* Wound, open,
    by site
  eye 871.3
  fingernail—*see* Wound, open, finger
  fracture—*see* Fracture, by site
  genital organs, external—*see* Wound, open,
    genital organs
  head (intracranial) NEC—*see also* Injury,
    intracranial, with open intracranial wound
    complete 874.9
    external site NEC 873.8
      complicated 873.9
  internal organ or site—*see* Injury, internal, by
    site
  joint—*see also* Dislocation, by site
    capsule—*see* Sprain, by site
  ligament—*see* Sprain, by site
  limb—*see also* Amputation, traumatic, by site
    skin and subcutaneous tissue—*see* Wound,
      open, by site
  muscle—*see* Sprain, by site

Avulsion—*continued*
  nerve (root)—*see* Injury, nerve, by site
  scalp—*see* Wound, open, scalp
  skin and subcutaneous tissue—*see* Wound,
    open, by site
  symphyseal cartilage (inner), complicating
    delivery 665.6
  tendon—*see also* Sprain, by site
    with open wound—*see* Wound, open, by site
  toenail—*see* Wound, open, toe(s)
  tooth 873.63
    complicated 873.73
Awareness of heart beat 785.1
Axe grinders' disease 502
Axenfeld's anomaly or syndrome 743.44
Axilla, axillary —*see also* condition
  breast 757.6
Axonotmesis —*see* Injury, nerve, by site
Ayala's disease 756.89
Ayerza's disease or syndrome (pulmonary
  artery sclerosis with pulmonary hypertension)
  416.0
Azoospermia 606.0
Azorean disease (of the nervous system) 334.8
Azotemia 790.6
  meaning uremia (*see also* Uremia) 586
Aztec ear 744.29
Azygos lobe, lung (fissure) 748.69

B

Baader's syndrome (erythema multiforme exudativum) 695.1
Baastrup's syndrome 721.5
Babesiasis 088.82
Babesiosis 088.82
Babington's disease (familial hemorrhagic telangiectasia) 448.0
Babinski's syndrome (cardiovascular syphilis) 093.89
Babinski-Fröhlich syndrome (adiposogenital dystrophy) 253.8
Babinski-Nageotte syndrome 344.89
Bacillary —*see* condition
Bacilluria 791.9
  asymptomatic, in pregnancy or puerperium 646.5
  tuberculous (*see also* Tuberculosis) 016.9
Bacillus—*see also* **Infection, bacillus**
  abortus infection 023.1
  anthracis infection 022.9
  coli
    infection 041.4
      generalized 038.42
      intestinal 008.00
    pyemia 038.42
    septicemia 038.42
  Flexner's 004.1
  fusiformis infestation 101
  mallei infection 024
  Shiga's 004.0
  suipestifer infection (*see also* Infection, Salmonella) 003.9
Back —*see* condition
Backache (postural) 724.5
  psychogenic 307.89
  sacroiliac 724.6
Backflow (pyelovenous) (*see also* Disease, renal) 593.9
Backknee (*see also* Genu, recurvatum) 736.5
Bacteremia (*see also* Infection, bacillus) 790.7
  with
    sepsis—*see* Septicemia
  during
    labor 659.3
    pregnancy 647.8
  newborn 771.83
Bacteria
  in blood (*see also* Bacteremia) 790.7
  in urine (*see also* Bacteriuria) 599.0
Bacterial —*see* condition
Bactericholia (*see also* Cholecystitis, acute) 575.0
Bacterid, bacteride (Andrews' pustular) 686.8
Bacteriuria, bacteruria 791.9
  with
    urinary tract infection 599.0
  asymptomatic 791.9
    in pregnancy or puerperium 646.5
      affecting fetus or newborn 760.1
Bad
  breath 784.9
  heart—*see* Disease, heart
  trip (*see also* Abuse, drugs, nondependent) 305.3
Baehr-Schiffrin disease (thrombotic thrombocytopenic purpura) 446.6
Baelz's disease (cheilitis glandularis apostematosa) 528.5
Baerensprung's disease (eczema marginatum) 110.3

Bagassosis (occupational) 495.1
Baghdad boil 085.1
Bagratuni's syndrome (temporal arteritis) 446.5
Baker's
  cyst (knee) 727.51
    tuberculous (*see also* Tuberculosis) 015.2
  itch 692.89
Bakwin-Krida syndrome (craniometaphyseal dysplasia) 756.89
Balanitis (circinata) (gangraenosa) (infectious) (vulgaris) 607.1
  amebic 006.8
  candidal 112.2
  chlamydial 099.53
  due to Ducrey's bacillus 099.0
  erosiva circinata et gangraenosa 607.1
  gangrenous 607.1
  gonococcal (acute) 098.0
    chronic or duration of 2 months or over 098.2
  nongonococcal 607.1
  phagedenic 607.1
  venereal NEC 099.8
  xerotica obliterans 607.81
Balanoposthitis 607.1
  chlamydial 099.53
  gonococcal (acute) 098.0
    chronic or duration of 2 months or over 098.2
  ulcerative NEC 099.8
Balanorrhagia —*see* Balanitis
Balantidiasis 007.0
Balantidiosis 007.0
Balbuties, balbutio 307.0
Bald
  patches on scalp 704.00
  tongue 529.4
Baldness (*see also* Alopecia) 704.00
Balfour's disease (chloroma) 205.3
Balint's syndrome (psychic paralysis of visual fixation) 368.16
Balkan grippe 083.0
Ball
  food 938
  hair 938
Ballantyne (-Runge) syndrome (postmaturity) 766.2
Balloon disease (*see also* Effect, adverse, high altitude) 993.2
Ballooning posterior leaflet syndrome 424.0
Baló's disease or concentric sclerosis 341.1
Bamberger's disease (hypertrophic pulmonary osteoarthropathy) 731.2
Bamberger-Marie disease (hypertrophic pulmonary osteoarthropathy) 731.2
Bamboo spine 720.0
Bancroft's filariasis 125.0
Band(s)
  adhesive (*see also* Adhesions, peritoneum) 568.0
  amniotic 658.8
    affecting fetus or newborn 762.8
  anomalous or congenital—*see also* Anomaly, specified type NEC
    atrial 746.9
    heart 746.9
    intestine 751.4
    omentum 751.4
    ventricular 746.9
  cervix 622.3
  gallbladder (congenital) 751.69

Band(s)—*continued*
  intestinal (adhesive) (*see also* Adhesions,
    peritoneum) 568.0
    congenital 751.4
  obstructive (*see also* Obstruction, intestine)
    560.81
  periappendiceal (congenital) 751.4
  peritoneal (adhesive) (*see also* Adhesions,
    peritoneum) 568.0
    with intestinal obstruction 560.81
    congenital 751.4
  uterus 621.5
  vagina 623.2
Bandl's ring (contraction)
  complicating delivery 661.4
    affecting fetus or newborn 763.7
Bang's disease (Brucella abortus) 023.1
Bangkok hemorrhagic fever 065.4
Bannister's disease 995.1
Bantam-Albright-Martin disease
  (pseudohypoparathyroidism) 275.49
Banti's disease or syndrome (with cirrhosis)
  (with portal hypertension)—*see* Cirrhosis,
  liver
Bar
  calcaneocuboid 755.67
  calcaneonavicular 755.67
  cubonavicular 755.67
  prostate 600.9
  talocalcaneal 755.67
Baragnosis 780.99
Barasheh, barashek 266.2
Barcoo disease or rot (*see also* Ulcer, skin) 707.9
Bard-Pic syndrome (carcinoma, head of
  pancreas) 157.0
Bärensprung's disease (eczema marginatum)
  110.3
Baritosis 503
Barium lung disease 503
Barlow's syndrome (meaning mitral valve
  prolapse) 424.0
Barlow (-Möller) disease or syndrome (meaning
  infantile scurvy) 267
Barodontalgia 993.2
Baron Münchausen syndrome 301.51
Barosinusitis 993.1
Barotitis 993.0
Barotrauma 993.2
  odontalgia 993.2
  otitic 993.0
  sinus 993.1
Barraquer's disease or syndrome (progressive
  lipodystrophy) 272.6
Barré-Guillain syndrome 357.0
Barré-Liéou syndrome (posterior cervical
  sympathetic) 723.2
Barrel chest 738.3
Barrett's syndrome or ulcer (chronic peptic
  ulcer of esophagus) 530.2
Bársony-Polgár syndrome (corkscrew
  esophagus) 530.5
Bársony-Teschendorf syndrome (corkscrew
  esophagus) 530.5
Bartholin's
  adenitis (*see also* Bartholinitis) 616.8
  gland—*see* condition
Bartholinitis (suppurating) 616.8
  gonococcal (acute) 098.0
    chronic or duration of 2 months or over 098.2
Bartonellosis 088.0

Bartter's syndrome (secondary
  hyperaldosteronism with juxtaglomerular
  hyperplasia) 255.1
Basal—*see* **condition**
Basan's (hidrotic) ectodermal dysplasia 757.31
Baseball finger 842.13
Basedow's disease or syndrome (exophthalmic
  goiter) 242.0
Basic —*see* condition
Basilar —*see* condition
Bason's (hidrotic) ectodermal dysplasia 757.31
Basopenia 288.0
Basophilia 288.8
Basophilism (corticoadrenal) (Cushing's)
  (pituitary) (thymic) 255.0
Bassen-Kornzweig syndrome
  (abetalipoproteinemia) 272.5
Bat ear 744.29
Bateman's
  disease 078.0
  purpura (senile) 287.2
Bathing cramp 994.1
Bathophobia 300.23
Batten's disease, retina 330.1 *[362.71]*
Batten-Mayou disease 330.1 *[362.71]*
Batten-Steinert syndrome 359.2
Battered
  adult (syndrome) 995.81
  baby or child (syndrome) 995.54
  spouse (syndrome) 995.81
Battey mycobacterium infection 031.0
Battledore placenta —*see* Placenta, abnormal
Battle exhaustion (*see also* Reaction, stress,
  acute) 308.9
Baumgarten-Cruveilhier (cirrhosis) disease, or
  syndrome 571.5
Bauxite
  fibrosis (of lung) 503
  workers' disease 503
Bayle's disease (dementia paralytica) 094.1
Bazin's disease (primary) (*see also* Tuberculosis)
  017.1
Beach ear 380.12
Beaded hair (congenital) 757.4
Beard's disease (neurasthenia) 300.5
Bearn-Kunkel (-Slater) syndrome (lupoid
  hepatitis) 571.49
Beat
  elbow 727.2
  hand 727.2
  knee 727.2
Beats
  ectopic 427.60
  escaped, heart 427.60
    postoperative 997.1
  premature (nodal) 427.60
    atrial 427.61
    auricular 427.61
    postoperative 997.1
    specified type NEC 427.69
    supraventricular 427.61
    ventricular 427.69
Beau's
  disease or syndrome (*see also* Degeneration,
    myocardial) 429.1
  lines (transverse furrows on fingernails) 703.8
Bechterew's disease (ankylosing spondylitis)
  720.0
Bechterew-Strümpell-Marie syndrome
  (ankylosing spondylitis) 720.0

Bifid—*continued*
uvula 749.02
with cleft lip (*see also* Cleft, palate, with cleft lip) 749.20
Biforis uterus (suprasimplex) 752.3
Bifurcation (congenital)—*see also* Imperfect, closure
gallbladder 751.69
kidney pelvis 753.3
renal pelvis 753.3
rib 756.3
tongue 750.13
trachea 748.3
ureter 753.4
urethra 753.8
uvula 749.02
with cleft lip (*see also* Cleft, palate, with cleft lip) 749.20
vertebra 756.19
Bigeminal pulse 427.89
Bigeminy 427.89
Big spleen syndrome 289.4
Bilateral —*see* condition
Bile duct —*see* condition
Bile pigments in urine 791.4
Bilharziasis (*see also* Schistosomiasis) 120.9
chyluria 120.0
cutaneous 120.3
galacturia 120.0
hematochyluria 120.0
intestinal 120.1
lipemia 120.9
lipuria 120.0
Oriental 120.2
piarhemia 120.9
pulmonary 120.2
tropical hematuria 120.0
vesical 120.0
Biliary —*see* condition
Bilious (attack)—*see also* Vomiting
fever, hemoglobinuric 084.8
Bilirubinuria 791.4
Biliuria 791.4
Billroth's disease
meningocele (*see also* Spina bifida) 741.9
Bilobate placenta —*see* Placenta, abnormal
Bilocular
heart 745.7
stomach 536.8
Bing-Horton syndrome (histamine cephalgia) 346.2
Binswanger's disease or dementia 290.12
Biörck (-Thorson) syndrome (malignant carcinoid) 259.2
Biparta, bipartite —*see also* Imperfect, closure
carpal scaphoid 755.59
patella 755.64
placenta—*see* Placenta, abnormal
vagina 752.49
Bird
face 756.0
fanciers' lung or disease 495.2
Bird's disease (oxaluria) 271.8
Birth
abnormal fetus or newborn 763.9
accident, fetus or newborn—*see* Birth, injury
complications in mother—*see* Delivery, complicated
compression during NEC 767.9
defect—*see* Anomaly
delayed, fetus 763.9

Birth—*continued*
difficult NEC, affecting fetus or newborn 763.9
dry, affecting fetus or newborn 761.1
forced, NEC, affecting fetus or newborn 763.89
forceps, affecting fetus or newborn 763.2
hematoma of sternomastoid 767.8
immature 765.1
extremely 765.0
inattention, after or at 995.52
induced, affecting fetus or newborn 763.89
infant—*see* Newborn
injury NEC 767.9
adrenal gland 767.8
basal ganglia 767.0
brachial plexus (paralysis) 767.6
brain (compression) (pressure) 767.0
cerebellum 767.0
cerebral hemorrhage 767.0
conjunctiva 767.8
eye 767.8
fracture
bone, any except clavicle or spine 767.3
clavicle 767.2
femur 767.3
humerus 767.3
long bone 767.3
radius and ulna 767.3
skeleton NEC 767.3
skull 767.3
spine 767.4
tibia and fibula 767.3
hematoma 767.8
liver (subcapsular) 767.8
mastoid 767.8
skull 767.1
sternomastoid 767.8
testes 767.8
vulva 767.8
intracranial (edema) 767.0
laceration
brain 767.0
by scalpel 767.8
peripheral nerve 767.7
liver 767.8
meninges
brain 767.0
spinal cord 767.4
nerves (cranial, peripheral) 767.7
brachial plexus 767.6
facial 767.5
paralysis 767.7
brachial plexus 767.6
Erb (-Duchenne) 767.6
facial nerve 767.5
Klumpke (-Déjérine) 767.6
radial nerve 767.6
spinal (cord) (hemorrhage) (laceration) (rupture) 767.4
rupture
intracranial 767.0
liver 767.8
spinal cord 767.4
spleen 767.8
viscera 767.8
scalp 767.1
scalpel wound 767.8
shock, newborn 779.89
skeleton NEC 767.3
specified NEC 767.8
spinal cord 767.4
spleen 767.8

Bleeding—*continued*
  rectum, rectal 569.3
  tendencies (*see also* Defect, coagulation) 286.9
  throat 784.8
  umbilical stump 772.3
  umbilicus 789.9
  unrelated to menstrual cycle 626.6
  uterus, uterine 626.9
    climacteric 627.0
    dysfunctional 626.8
    functional 626.8
    unrelated to menstrual cycle 626.6
  vagina, vaginal 623.8
    functional 626.8
  vicarious 625.8
Blennorrhagia, blennorrhagic —*see*
    Blennorrhea
Blennorrhea (acute) 098.0
  adultorum 098.40
  alveolaris 523.4
  chronic or duration of 2 months or over 098.2
  gonococcal (neonatorum) 098.40
  inclusion (neonatal) (newborn) 771.6
  neonatorum 098.40
Blepharelosis (*see also* Entropion) 374.00
Blepharitis (eyelid) 373.00
  angularis 373.01
  ciliaris 373.00
    with ulcer 373.01
  marginal 373.00
    with ulcer 373.01
  scrofulous (*see also* Tuberculosis) 017.3
    [373.00]
  squamous 373.02
  ulcerative 373.01
Blepharochalasis 374.34
  congenital 743.62
Blepharoclonus 333.81
Blepharoconjunctivitis (*see also* Conjunctivitis)
    372.20
  angular 372.21
  contact 372.22
Blepharophimosis (eyelid) 374.46
  congenital 743.62
Blepharoplegia 374.89
Blepharoptosis 374.30
  congenital 743.61
Blepharopyorrhea 098.49
Blepharospasm 333.81
Blessig's cyst 362.62
Blighted ovum 631
Blind
  bronchus (congenital) 748.3
  eye—*see also* Blindness
    hypertensive 360.42
    hypotensive 360.41
  loop syndrome (postoperative) 579.2
  sac, fallopian tube (congenital) 752.19
  spot, enlarged 368.42
  tract or tube (congenital) NEC—*see* Atresia
Blindness (acquired) (congenital) (both eyes)
    369.00
  blast 921.3
    with nerve injury—*see* Injury, nerve, optic
  Bright's—*see* Uremia
  color (congenital) 368.59
    acquired 368.55
    blue 368.53
    green 368.52
    red 368.51
    total 368.54

Blindness—*continued*
  concussion 950.9
  cortical 377.75
  day 368.10
    acquired 368.10
    congenital 368.10
    hereditary 368.10
    specified type NEC 368.10
  due to
    injury NEC 950.9
    refractive error—*see* Error, refractive
  eclipse (total) 363.31
  emotional 300.11
  hysterical 300.11
  legal (both eyes) (USA definition) 369.4
    with impairment of better (less impaired) eye
      near-total 369.02
        with
          lesser eye impairment 369.02
            near-total 369.04
            total 369.03
      profound 369.05
        with
          lesser eye impairment 369.05
            near-total 369.07
            profound 369.08
            total 369.06
      severe 369.21
        with
          lesser eye impairment 369.21
            blind 369.11
            near-total 369.13
            profound 369.14
            severe 369.22
            total 369.12
    total
      with lesser eye impairment total 369.01
  mind 784.69
  moderate
    both eyes 369.25
      with impairment of lesser eye (specified as)
        blind, not further specified 369.15
        low vision, not further specified 369.23
        near-total 369.17
        profound 369.18
        severe 369.24
        total 369.16
    one eye 369.74
      with vision of other eye (specified as)
        near-normal 369.75
        normal 369.76
  near-total
    both eyes 369.04
      with impairment of lesser eye (specified as)
        blind, not further specified 369.02
        total 369.03
    one eye 369.64
      with vision of other eye (specified as)
        near-normal 369.65
        normal 369.66
  night 368.60
    acquired 368.62
    congenital (Japanese) 368.61
    hereditary 368.61
    specified type NEC 368.69
    vitamin A deficiency 264.5
  nocturnal—*see* Blindness, night
  one eye 369.60
    with low vision of other eye 369.10
  profound
    both eyes 369.08

Blindness—*continued*
    with impairment of lesser eye (specified as)
      blind, not further specified 369.05
      near-total 369.07
      total 369.06
    one eye 369.67
      with vision of other eye (specified as)
        near-normal 369.68
        normal 369.69
  psychic 784.69
  severe
    both eyes 369.22
      with impairment of lesser eye (specified as)
        blind, not further specified 369.11
        low vision, not further specified 369.21
        near-total 369.13
        profound 369.14
        total 369.12
    one eye 369.71
      with vision of other eye (specified as)
        near-normal 369.72
        normal 369.73
  snow 370.24
  sun 363.31
  temporary 368.12
  total
    both eyes 369.01
    one eye 369.61
      with vision of other eye (specified as)
        near-normal 369.62
        normal 369.63
  transient 368.12
  traumatic NEC 950.9
  word (developmental) 315.01
    acquired 784.61
    secondary to organic lesion 784.61
Blister —*see also* Injury, superficial, by site
  beetle dermatitis 692.89
  due to burn—*see* Burn, by site, second degree
  fever 054.9
  multiple, skin, nontraumatic 709.8
Bloating 787.3
Bloch-Siemens syndrome (incontinentia
    pigmenti) 757.33
Bloch-Stauffer dyshormonal dermatosis 757.33
Bloch-Sulzberger disease or syndrome
    (incontinentia pigmenti) (melanoblastosis)
    757.33
Block
  alveolar capillary 516.3
  arborization (heart) 426.6
  arrhythmic 426.9
  atrioventricular (AV) (incomplete) (partial)
    426.10
    with
      2:1 atrioventricular response block 426.13
      atrioventricular dissociation 426.0
    first degree (incomplete) 426.11
    second degree (Mobitz type I) 426.13
      Mobitz (type) II 426.12
    third degree 426.0
    complete 426.0
      congenital 746.86
    congenital 746.86
    Mobitz (incomplete)
      type I (Wenckebach's) 426.13
      type II 426.12
    partial 426.13
  auriculoventricular (*see also* Block,
    atrioventricular) 426.10
    complete 426.0

Block—*continued*
  congenital 746.86
  congenital 746.86
  bifascicular (cardiac) 426.53
  bundle branch (complete) (false) (incomplete)
    426.50
    bilateral 426.53
    left (complete) (main stem) 426.3
      with right bundle branch block 426.53
      anterior fascicular 426.2
        with
          posterior fascicular block 426.3
          right bundle branch block 426.52
      hemiblock 426.2
      incomplete 426.2
        with right bundle branch block 426.53
      posterior fascicular 426.2
        with
          anterior fascicular block 426.3
          right bundle branch block 426.51
    right 426.4
      with
        left bundle branch block (incomplete)
          (main stem) 426.53
        left fascicular block 426.53
          anterior 426.52
          posterior 426.51
    Wilson's type 426.4
  cardiac 426.9
  conduction 426.9
    complete 426.0
  Eustachian tube (*see also* Obstruction,
    Eustachian tube) 381.60
  fascicular (left anterior) (left posterior) 426.2
  foramen Magendie (acquired) 331.3
    congenital 742.3
      with spina bifida (*see also* Spina bifida)
        741.0
  heart 426.9
    first degree (atrioventricular) 426.11
    second degree (atrioventricular) 426.13
    third degree (atrioventricular) 426.0
    bundle branch (complete) (false) (incomplete)
      426.50
      bilateral 426.53
      left (*see also* Block, bundle branch, left)
        426.3
      right (*see also* Block, bundle branch, right)
        426.4
    complete (atrioventricular) 426.0
    congenital 746.86
    incomplete 426.13
    intra-atrial 426.6
    intraventricular NEC 426.6
    sinoatrial 426.6
    specified type NEC 426.6
  hepatic vein 453.0
  intraventricular (diffuse) (myofibrillar) 426.6
    bundle branch (complete) (false) (incomplete)
      426.50
      bilateral 426.53
      left (*see also* Block, bundle branch, left)
        426.3
      right (*see also* Block, bundle branch, right)
        426.4
  kidney (*see also* Disease, renal) 593.9
    postcystoscopic 997.5
  myocardial (*see also* Block, heart) 426.9
  nodal 426.10
  optic nerve 377.49
  organ or site (congenital) NEC—*see* Atresia

Boil —*continued*
  finger (any) 680.4
  flank 680.2
  foot (any part) 680.7
  forearm 680.3
  Gafsa 085.1
  genital organ, male 608.4
  gluteal (region) 680.5
  groin 680.2
  hand (any part) 680.4
  head (any part, except face) 680.8
  heel 680.7
  hip 680.6
  knee 680.6
  labia 616.4
  lacrimal (*see also* Dacryocystitis) 375.30
    gland (*see also* Dacryoadenitis) 375.00
    passages (duct) (sac) (*see also* Dacryocystitis) 375.30
  leg, any part except foot 680.6
  multiple sites 680.9
  Natal 085.1
  neck 680.1
  nose (external) (septum) 680.0
  orbit, orbital 376.01
  partes posteriores 680.5
  pectoral region 680.2
  penis 607.2
  perineum 680.2
  pinna 680.0
  scalp (any part) 680.8
  scrotum 608.4
  seminal vesicle 608.0
  shoulder 680.3
  skin NEC 680.9
  specified site NEC 680.8
  spermatic cord 608.4
  temple (region) 680.0
  testis 608.4
  thigh 680.6
  thumb 680.4
  toe (any) 680.7
  tropical 085.1
  trunk 680.2
  tunica vaginalis 608.4
  umbilicus 680.2
  upper arm 680.3
  vas deferens 608.4
  vulva 616.4
  wrist 680.4
Bold hives (*see also* Urticaria) 708.9
Bolivian hemorrhagic fever 078.7
Bombé, iris 364.74
Bomford-Rhoads anemia (refractory) 284.9
Bone —*see* condition
Bonnevie-Ullrich syndrome 758.6
Bonnier's syndrome 386.19
Bonvale Dam fever 780.79
Bony block of joint 718.80
  ankle 718.87
  elbow 718.82
  foot 718.87
  hand 718.84
  hip 718.85
  knee 718.86
  multiple sites 718.89
  pelvic region 718.85
  shoulder (region) 718.81
  specified site NEC 718.88
  wrist 718.83

Borderline
  intellectual functioning V62.89
  pelvis 653.1
    with obstruction during labor 660.1
      affecting fetus or newborn 763.1
  psychosis (*see also* Schizophrenia) 295.5
    of childhood (*see also* Psychosis, childhood) 299.8
  schizophrenia (*see also* Schizophrenia) 295.5
Borna disease 062.9
Bornholm disease (epidemic pleurodynia) 074.1
Borrelia vincentii (mouth) (pharynx) (tonsils) 101
Bostock's catarrh (*see also* Fever, hay) 477.9
Boston exanthem 048
Botalli, ductus (patent) (persistent) 747.0
Bothriocephalus latus infestation 123.4
Botulism 005.1
Bouba (*see also* Yaws) 102.9
Bouffée délirante 298.3
Bouillaud's disease or syndrome (rheumatic heart disease) 391.9
Bourneville's disease (tuberous sclerosis) 759.5
Boutonneuse fever 082.1
Boutonniere
  deformity (finger) 736.21
  hand (intrinsic) 736.21
Bouveret (-Hoffmann) disease or syndrome (paroxysmal tachycardia) 427.2
Bovine heart —*see* Hypertrophy, cardiac
Bowel —*see* condition
Bowen's
  dermatosis (precancerous) (M8081/2)—*see* Neoplasm, skin, in situ
  disease (M8081/2)—*see* Neoplasm, skin, in situ
  epithelioma (M8081/2)—*see* Neoplasm, skin, in situ
  type
    epidermoid carcinoma in situ (M8081/2)—*see* Neoplasm, skin, in situ
    intraepidermal squamous cell carcinoma (M8081/2)–*see* Neoplasm, skin, in situ
Bowing
  femur 736.89
    congenital 754.42
  fibula 736.89
    congenital 754.43
  forearm 736.09
    away from midline (cubitus valgus) 736.01
    toward midline (cubitus varus) 736.02
  leg(s), long bones, congenital 754.44
  radius 736.09
    away from midline (cubitus valgus) 736.01
    toward midline (cubitus varus) 736.02
  tibia 736.89
    congenital 754.43
Bowleg (s) 736.42
  congenital 754.44
  rachitic 268.1
Boyd's dysentery 004.2
Brachial —*see* condition
Brachman-de Lange syndrome (Amsterdam dwarf, mental retardation, and brachycephaly) 759.89
Brachycardia 427.89
Brachycephaly 756.0
Brachymorphism and ectopia lentis 759.89
Bradley's disease (epidemic vomiting) 078.82
Bradycardia 427.89
  chronic (sinus) 427.81
  newborn 779.81

Broken—*continued*
  implant or internal device—*see* listing under
    Complications, mechanical
  neck—*see* Fracture, vertebra, cervical
  nose 802.0
    open 802.1
  tooth, teeth 873.63
    complicated 873.73
Bromhidrosis 705.89
Bromidism, bromism
  acute 967.3
    correct substance properly administered
      349.82
    overdose or wrong substance given or taken
      967.3
  chronic (*see also* Dependence) 304.1
Bromidrosiphobia 300.23
Bromidrosis 705.89
Bronchi, bronchial —*see* condition
Bronchiectasis (cylindrical) (diffuse) (fusiform)
    (localized) (moniliform) (postinfectious)
    (recurrent) (saccular) 494.0
  with acute exacerbation 494.1
  congenital 748.61
  tuberculosis (*see also* Tuberculosis) 011.5
Bronchiolectasis —*see* Bronchiectasis
Bronchiolitis (acute) (infectious) (subacute)
    466.19
  with
    bronchospasm or obstruction 466.19
    influenza, flu, or grippe 487.1
  catarrhal (acute) (subacute) 466.19
  chemical 506.0
    chronic 506.4
  chronic (obliterative) 491.8
  due to external agent—*see* Bronchitis, acute,
    due to
  fibrosa obliterans 491.8
  influenzal 487.1
  obliterans 491.8
    status post lung transplant 996.84
    with organizing pneumonia (B.O.O.P.) 516.8
  obliterative (chronic) (diffuse) (subacute) 491.8
    due to fumes or vapors 506.4
  respiratory syncytial virus 466.11
  vesicular—*see* Pneumonia, broncho-
Bronchitis (diffuse) (hypostatic) (infectious)
    (inflammatory) (simple) 490
  with
    emphysema—*see* Emphysema
    influenza, flu, or grippe 487.1
    obstruction airway, chronic 491.20
      with acute exacerbation 491.21
    tracheitis 490
      acute or subacute 466.0
        with bronchospasm or obstruction 466.0
      chronic 491.8
  acute or subacute 466.0
    with
      bronchospasm 466.0
      chronic
        bronchitis (obstructive) 491.21
        obstructive pulmonary disease (COPD)
          491.21
      obstruction 466.0
      tracheitis 466.0
    chemical (due to fumes or vapors) 506.0
    due to
      fumes or vapors 506.0
      radiation 508.8
  allergic (acute) (*see also* Asthma) 493.9

Bronchitis—*continued*
  arachidic 934.1
  aspiration 507.0
    due to fumes or vapors 506.0
  asthmatic (acute) 493.90
    with
      acute exacerbation 493.92
      status asthmaticus 493.91
    chronic 493.2
  capillary 466.19
    with bronchospasm or obstruction 466.19
    chronic 491.8
  caseous (*see also* Tuberculosis) 011.3
  Castellani's 104.8
  catarrhal 490
    acute—*see* Bronchitis, acute
    chronic 491.0
  chemical (acute) (subacute) 506.0
    chronic 506.4
    due to fumes or vapors (acute) (subacute)
      506.0
      chronic 506.4
  chronic 491.9
    with
      tracheitis (chronic) 491.8
    asthmatic 493.2
    catarrhal 491.0
    chemical (due to fumes and vapors) 506.4
    due to
      fumes or vapors (chemical) (inhalation)
        506.4
      radiation 508.8
      tobacco smoking 491.0
    mucopurulent 491.1
    obstructive 491.20
      with acute bronchitis or acute exacerbation
        491.21
    purulent 491.1
    simple 491.0
    specified type NEC 491.8
  croupous 466.0
    with bronchospasm or obstruction 466.0
    due to fumes or vapors 506.0
  emphysematous 491.20
    with acute bronchitis or acute exacerbation
      491.21
  exudative 466.0
  fetid (chronic) (recurrent) 491.1
  fibrinous, acute or subacute 466.0
    with bronchospasm or obstruction 466.0
  grippal 487.1
  influenzal 487.1
  membranous, acute or subacute 466.0
    with bronchospasm or obstruction 466.0
  moulders' 502
  mucopurulent (chronic) (recurrent) 491.1
    acute or subacute 466.0
  non-obstructive 491.0
  obliterans 491.8
  obstructive (chronic) 491.20
    with acute bronchitis or acute exacerbation
      491.21
  pituitous 491.1
  plastic (inflammatory) 466.0
  pneumococcal, acute or subacute 466.0
    with bronchospasm or obstruction 466.0
  pseudomembranous 466.0

Burn—*continued*
  second degree 942.21
  third degree 942.31
    deep 942.41
      with loss of body part 942.51
  brow—*see* Burn, forehead
  buttock(s)—*see* Burn, back
  canthus (eye) 940.1
    chemical 940.0
  cervix (uteri) 947.4
  cheek (cutaneous) 941.07
    with
      face or head—*see* Burn, head, multiple sites
    first degree 941.17
    second degree 941.27
    third degree 941.37
      deep 941.47
        with loss of body part 941.57
  chest wall (anterior) 942.02
    with
      trunk—*see* Burn, trunk, multiple sites
    first degree 942.12
    second degree 942.22
    third degree 942.32
      deep 942.42
        with loss of body part 942.52
  chin 941.04
    with
      face or head—*see* Burn, head, multiple sites
    first degree 941.14
    second degree 941.24
    third degree 941.34
      deep 941.44
        with loss of body part 941.54
  clitoris—*see* Burn, genitourinary organs,
    external
  colon 947.3
  conjunctiva (and cornea) 940.4
    chemical
      acid 940.3
      alkaline 940.2
  cornea (and conjunctiva) 940.4
    chemical
      acid 940.3
      alkaline 940.2
  costal region—*see* Burn, chest wall
  due to ingested chemical agent—*see* Burn,
    internal organs
  ear (auricle) (canal) (drum) (external) 941.01
    with
      face or head—*see* Burn, head, multiple sites
    first degree 941.11
    second degree 941.21
    third degree 941.31
      deep 941.41
        with loss of a body part 941.51
  elbow 943.02
    with
      hand(s) and wrist(s)—*see* Burn, multiple
        specified sites
      upper limb(s) except hand(s) or
        wrist(s)—*see also* Burn, arm(s),
        multiple sites
    first degree 943.12
    second degree 943.22
    third degree 943.32
      deep 943.42
        with loss of body part 943.52
  electricity, electric current—*see* Burn, by site
  entire body—*see* Burn, multiple, specified sites

Burn—*continued*
  epididymis—*see* Burn, genitourinary organs,
    external
  epigastric region—*see* Burn, abdomen
  epiglottis 947.1
  esophagus 947.2
  extent (percent of body surface)
    less than 10 percent 948.0
    10-19 percent 948.1
    20-29 percent 948.2
    30-39 percent 948.3
    40-49 percent 948.4
    50-59 percent 948.5
    60-69 percent 948.6
    70-79 percent 948.7
    80-89 percent 948.8
    90 percent or more 948.9
  extremity
    lower—*see* Burn, leg
    upper—*see* Burn, arm(s)
  eye(s) (and adnexa) (only) 940.9
    with
      face, head, or neck 941.02
        first degree 941.12
        second degree 941.22
        third degree 941.32
          deep 941.42
            with loss of body part 941.52
      other sites (classifiable to more than one
        category in 940-945)—*see* Burn,
        multiple, specified sites
      resulting rupture and destruction of eyeball
        940.5
    specified part—*see* Burn, by site
  eyeball—*see also* Burn, eye
    with resulting rupture and destruction of
      eyeball 940.5
  eyelid(s) 940.1
    chemical 940.0
  face—*see* Burn, head
  finger (nail) (subungual) 944.01
    with
      hand(s)—*see* Burn, hand(s), multiple sites
      other sites—*see* Burn, multiple, specified
        sites
      thumb 944.04
        first degree 944.14
        second degree 944.24
        third degree 944.34
          deep 944.44
            with loss of body part 944.54
    first degree 944.11
    second degree 944.21
    third degree 944.31
      deep 944.41
        with loss of body part 944.51
    multiple (digits) 944.03
      with thumb—*see* Burn, finger, with thumb
      first degree 944.13
      second degree 944.23
      third degree 944.33
        deep 944.43
          with loss of body part 944.53
  flank—*see* Burn, abdomen
  foot 945.02
    with
      lower limb(s)—*see* Burn, leg, multiple sites
    first degree 945.12
    second degree 945.22
    third degree 945.32
      deep 945.42

Burn—*continued*
trachea 947.1
trunk 942.00
first degree 942.10
second degree 942.20
third degree 942.30
deep 942.40
with loss of body part 942.50
multiple sites 942.09
first degree 942.19
second degree 942.29
third degree 942.39
deep 942.49
with loss of body part 942.59
specified site NEC 942.09
first degree 942.19
second degree 942.29
third degree 942.39
deep 942.49
with loss of body part 942.59
tunica vaginalis—*see* Burn, genitourinary
organs, external
tympanic membrane—*see* Burn, ear
tympanum—*see* Burn, ear
ultraviolet 692.82
unspecified site (multiple) 949.0
with extent of body surface involved specified
less than 10 percent 948.0
10-19 percent 948.1
20-29 percent 948.2
30-39 percent 948.3
40-49 percent 948.4
50-59 percent 948.5
60-69 percent 948.6
70-79 percent 948.7
80-89 percent 948.8
90 percent or more 948.9
first degree 949.1
second degree 949.2
third degree 949.3
deep 949.4
with loss of body part 949.5
uterus 947.4
uvula 947.0
vagina 947.4
vulva—*see* Burn, genitourinary organs, external
wrist(s) 944.07
with
hand(s)—*see* Burn, hand(s), multiple sites
first degree 944.17
second degree 944.27
third degree 944.37
deep 944.47
with loss of body part 944.57
Burnett's syndrome (milk-alkali) 999.9
Burnier's syndrome (hypophyseal dwarfism)
253.3
Burning
feet syndrome 266.2
sensation (*see also* Disturbance, sensation) 782.0
tongue 529.6
Burns' disease (osteochondrosis, lower ulna)
732.3
Bursa —*see also* condition
pharynx 478.29
Bursitis NEC 727.3
Achilles tendon 726.71
adhesive 726.90
shoulder 726.0
ankle 726.79
buttock 726.5

Bursitis—*continued*
calcaneal 726.79
collateral ligament
fibular 726.63
tibial 726.62
Duplay's 726.2
elbow 726.33
finger 726.8
foot 726.79
gonococcal 098.52
hand 726.4
hip 726.5
infrapatellar 726.69
ischiogluteal 726.5
knee 726.60
occupational NEC 727.2
olecranon 726.33
pes anserinus 726.61
pharyngeal 478.29
popliteal 727.51
prepatellar 726.65
radiohumeral 727.3
scapulohumeral 726.19
adhesive 726.0
shoulder 726.10
adhesive 726.0
subacromial 726.19
adhesive 726.0
subcoracoid 726.19
subdeltoid 726.19
adhesive 726.0
subpatellar 726.69
syphilitic 095.7
Thornwaldt's, Tornwaldt's (pharyngeal) 478.29
toe 726.79
trochanteric area 726.5
wrist 726.4
Burst stitches or sutures (complication of
surgery) (external) 998.32
internal 998.31
Buruli ulcer 031.1
Bury's disease (erythema elevatum diutinum)
695.89
Buschke's disease or scleredema (adultorum)
710.1
Busquet's disease (osteoperiostitis) (*see also*
Osteomyelitis) 730.1
Busse-Buschke disease (cryptococcosis) 117.5
Buttock —*see* condition
Button
Biskra 085.1
Delhi 085.1
oriental 085.1
Buttonhole hand (intrinsic) 736.21
Bwamba fever (encephalitis) 066.3
Byssinosis (occupational) 504
Bywaters' syndrome 958.5

C

Cacergasia 300.9
Cachexia 799.4
  cancerous (M8000/3) 199.1
  cardiac—*see* Disease, heart
  dehydration 276.5
    with
      hypernatremia 276.0
      hyponatremia 276.1
  due to malnutrition 261
  exophthalmic 242.0
  heart—*see* Disease, heart
  hypophyseal 253.2
  hypopituitary 253.2
  lead 984.9
    specified type of lead—*see* Table of drugs and
      chemicals
  malaria 084.9
  malignant (M8000/3) 199.1
  marsh 084.9
  nervous 300.5
  old age 797
  pachydermic—*see* Hypothyroidism
  paludal 084.9
  pituitary (postpartum) 253.2
  renal (*see also* Disease, renal) 593.9
  saturnine 984.9
    specified type of lead—*see* Table of drugs and
      chemicals
  senile 797
  Simmonds' (pituitary cachexia) 253.2
  splenica 289.59
  strumipriva (*see also* Hypothyroidism) 244.9
  tuberculous NEC (*see also* Tuberculosis) 011.9
café au lait spots 709.09
Caffey's disease or syndrome (infantile cortical
    hyperostosis) 756.59
Caisson disease 993.3
Caked breast (puerperal, postpartum) 676.2
Cake kidney 753.3
Calabar swelling 125.2
Calcaneal spur 726.73
Calcaneoapophysitis 732.5
Calcaneonavicular bar 755.67
Calcareous —*see* condition
Calcicosis (occupational) 502
Calciferol (vitamin D) deficiency 268.9
  with
    osteomalacia 268.2
    rickets (*see also* Rickets) 268.0
Calcification
  adrenal (capsule) (gland) 255.4
    tuberculous (*see also* Tuberculosis) 017.6
  aorta 440.0
  artery (annular)—*see* Arteriosclerosis
  auricle (ear) 380.89
  bladder 596.8
    due to S. hematobium 120.0
  brain (cortex)—*see* Calcification, cerebral
  bronchus 519.1
  bursa 727.82
  cardiac (*see also* Degeneration, myocardial)
    429.1
  cartilage (postinfectional) 733.99
  cerebral (cortex) 348.8
    artery 437.0
  cervix (uteri) 622.8
  choroid plexus 349.2
  conjunctiva 372.54

Calcification—*continued*
  corpora cavernosa (penis) 607.89
  cortex (brain)—*see* Calcification, cerebral
  dental pulp (nodular) 522.2
  dentinal papilla 520.4
  disc, intervertebral 722.90
    cervical, cervicothoracic 722.91
    lumbar, lumbosacral 722.93
    thoracic, thoracolumbar 722.92
  fallopian tube 620.8
  falx cerebri—*see* Calcification, cerebral
  fascia 728.89
  gallbladder 575.8
  general 275.40
  heart (*see also* Degeneration, myocardial) 429.1
    valve—*see* Endocarditis
  intervertebral cartilage or disc (postinfectional)
    722.90
    cervical, cervicothoracic 722.91
    lumbar, lumbosacral 722.93
    thoracic, thoracolumbar 722.92
  intracranial—*see* Calcification, cerebral
  intraspinal ligament 728.89
  joint 719.80
    ankle 719.87
    elbow 719.82
    foot 719.87
    hand 719.84
    hip 719.85
    knee 719.86
    multiple sites 719.89
    pelvic region 719.85
    shoulder (region) 719.81
    specified site NEC 719.88
    wrist 719.83
  kidney 593.89
    tuberculous (*see also* Tuberculosis) 016.0
  larynx (senile) 478.79
  lens 366.8
  ligament 728.89
    intraspinal 728.89
    knee (medial collateral) 717.89
  lung 518.89
    active 518.89
    postinfectional 518.89
    tuberculous (*see also* Tuberculosis,
      pulmonary) 011.9
  lymph gland or node (postinfectional) 289.3
    tuberculous (*see also* Tuberculosis, lymph
      gland) 017.2
  massive (paraplegic) 728.10
  medial NEC (*see also* Arteriosclerosis,
    extremities) 440.20
  meninges (cerebral) 349.2
  metastatic 275.40
  Mönckeberg's—*see* Arteriosclerosis
  muscle 728.10
    heterotopic, postoperative 728.13
  myocardium, myocardial (*see also*
    Degeneration, myocardial) 429.1
  ovary 620.8
  pancreas 577.8
  penis 607.99
  periarticular 728.89
  pericardium (*see also* Pericarditis) 423.8
  pineal gland 259.8
  pleura 511.0
    postinfectional 518.89

Calcification—*continued*
   tuberculous (*see also* Tuberculosis, pleura)
      012.0
  pulp (dental) (nodular) 522.2
  renal 593.89
  rider's bone 733.99
  sclera 379.16
  semilunar cartilage 717.89
  spleen 289.59
  subcutaneous 709.3
  suprarenal (capsule) (gland) 255.4
  tendon (sheath) 727.82
    with bursitis, synovitis or tenosynovitis 727.82
  trachea 519.1
  ureter 593.89
  uterus 621.8
  vitreous 379.29
Calcified —*see also* Calcification
  hematoma NEC 959.9
Calcinosis (generalized) (interstitial) (tumoral)
    (universalis) 275.49
  circumscripta 709.3
  cutis 709.3
  intervertebralis 275.49 *[722.90]*
  Raynaud's
     phenomenonsclerodactylytelangiectasis
     (CRST) 710.1
Calcium
  blood
    high (*see also* Hypercalcemia) 275.42
    low (*see also* Hypocalcemia) 275.41
  deposits—*see also* Calcification, by site
    in bursa 727.82
    in tendon (sheath) 727.82
      with bursitis, synovitis or tenosynovitis
       727.82
  salts or soaps in vitreous 379.22
Calciuria 791.9
Calculi —*see* Calculus
Calculosis, intrahepatic —*see*
  Choledocholithiasis
Calculus, calculi, calculous 592.9
  ampulla of Vater—*see* Choledocholithiasis
  anuria (impacted) (recurrent) 592.0
  appendix 543.9
  bile duct (any)—*see* Choledocholithiasis
  biliary—*see* Cholelithiasis
  bilirubin, multiple—*see* Cholelithiasis
  bladder (encysted) (impacted) (urinary) 594.1
    diverticulum 594.0
  bronchus 518.89
  calyx (kidney) (renal) 592.0
    congenital 753.3
  cholesterol (pure) (solitary)—*see* Cholelithiasis
  common duct (bile)—*see* Choledocholithiasis
  conjunctiva 372.54
  cystic 594.1
    duct—*see* Cholelithiasis
  dental 523.6
    subgingival 523.6
    supragingival 523.6
  epididymis 608.89
  gallbladder—*see also* Cholelithiasis
    congenital 751.69
  hepatic (duct)—*see* Choledocholithiasis
  intestine (impaction) (obstruction) 560.39
  kidney (impacted) (multiple) (pelvis) (recurrent)
    (staghorn) 592.0
    congenital 753.3
  lacrimal (passages) 375.57
  liver (impacted)—*see* Choledocholithiasis

Calculus, calculi, calculous—*continued*
  lung 518.89
  nephritic (impacted) (recurrent) 592.0
  nose 478.1
  pancreas (duct) 577.8
  parotid gland 527.5
  pelvis, encysted 592.0
  prostate 602.0
  pulmonary 518.89
  renal (impacted) (recurrent) 592.0
    congenital 753.3
  salivary (duct) (gland) 527.5
  seminal vesicle 608.89
  staghorn 592.0
  Stensen's duct 527.5
  sublingual duct or gland 527.5
    congenital 750.26
  submaxillary duct, gland, or region 527.5
  suburethral 594.8
  tonsil 474.8
  tooth, teeth 523.6
  tunica vaginalis 608.89
  ureter (impacted) (recurrent) 592.1
  urethra (impacted) 594.2
  urinary (duct) (impacted) (passage) (tract) 592.9
    lower tract NEC 594.9
      specified site 594.8
  vagina 623.8
  vesical (impacted) 594.1
  Wharton's duct 527.5
Caliectasis 593.89
California
  disease 114.0
  encephalitis 062.5
Caligo cornea 371.03
Callositas, callosity (infected) 700
Callus (infected) 700
  bone 726.91
  excessive, following fracture—*see also* Late,
    effect (of), fracture
Calvé (-Perthes) disease (osteochondrosis,
    femoral capital) 732.1
Calvities (*see also* Alopecia) 704.00
Cameroon fever (*see also* Malaria) 084.6
Camptocormia 300.11
Camptodactyly (congenital) 755.59
Camurati-Engelmann disease (diaphyseal
    sclerosis) 756.59
Canal— *see* condition
Canaliculitis (lacrimal) (acute) 375.31
  Actinomyces 039.8
  chronic 375.41
Canavan's disease 330.0
Cancer (M8000/3)—*see also* Neoplasm, by site,
  malignant

> *Note—The term "cancer" when modified by an adjective or adjectival phrase indicating a morphological type should be coded in the same manner as "carcinoma" with that adjective or phrase. Thus, "squamous-cell cancer" should be coded in the same manner as "squamous-cell carcinoma," which appears in the list under "Carcinoma."*

  bile duct type (M8160/3), liver 155.1
  hepatocellular (M8170/3) 155.0
Cancerous (M8000/3)—*see* Neoplasm, by site,
  malignant
Cancerphobia 300.29
Cancrum oris 528.1

Candidiasis, candidal 112.9
  with pneumonia 112.4
  balanitis 112.2
  congenital 771.7
  disseminated 112.5
  endocarditis 112.81
  esophagus 112.84
  intertrigo 112.3
  intestine 112.85
  lung 112.4
  meningitis 112.83
  mouth 112.0
  nails 112.3
  neonatal 771.7
  onychia 112.3
  otitis externa 112.82
  otomycosis 112.82
  paronychia 112.3
  perionyxis 112.3
  pneumonia 112.4
  pneumonitis 112.4
  skin 112.3
  specified site NEC 112.89
  systemic 112.5
  urogenital site NEC 112.2
  vagina 112.1
  vulva 112.1
  vulvovaginitis 112.1
Candidiosis —*see* Candidiasis
Candiru infection or infestation 136.8
Canities (premature) 704.3
  congenital 757.4
Canker (mouth) (sore) 528.2
  rash 034.1
Cannabinosis 504
Canton fever 081.9
Cap
  cradle 690.11
Capillariasis 127.5
Capillary —*see* condition
Caplan's syndrome 714.81
Caplan-Colinet syndrome 714.81
Capsule —*see* condition
Capsulitis (joint) 726.90
  adhesive (shoulder) 726.0
  hip 726.5
  knee 726.60
  labyrinthine 387.8
  thyroid 245.9
  wrist 726.4
Caput
  crepitus 756.0
  medusae 456.8
  succedaneum 767.1
Carapata disease 087.1
Carate —*see* Pinta
Carboxyhemoglobinemia 986
Carbuncle 680.9
  abdominal wall 680.2
  ankle 680.6
  anus 680.5
  arm (any part, above wrist) 680.3
  auditory canal, external 680.0
  axilla 680.3
  back (any part) 680.2
  breast 680.2
  buttock 680.5
  chest wall 680.2
  corpus cavernosum 607.2
  ear (any part) (external) 680.0
  eyelid 373.13

Carbuncle—*continued*
  face (any part, except eye) 680.0
  finger (any) 680.4
  flank 680.2
  foot (any part) 680.7
  forearm 680.3
  genital organ (male) 608.4
  gluteal (region) 680.5
  groin 680.2
  hand (any part) 680.4
  head (any part, except face) 680.8
  heel 680.7
  hip 680.6
  kidney (*see also* Abscess, kidney) 590.2
  knee 680.6
  labia 616.4
  lacrimal
    gland (*see also* Dacryoadenitis) 375.00
    passages (duct) (sac) (*see also* Dacryocystitis) 375.30
  leg, any part except foot 680.6
  lower extremity, any part except foot 680.6
  malignant 022.0
  multiple sites 680.9
  neck 680.1
  nose (external) (septum) 680.0
  orbit, orbital 376.01
  partes posteriores 680.5
  pectoral region 680.2
  penis 607.2
  perineum 680.2
  pinna 680.0
  scalp (any part) 680.8
  scrotum 608.4
  seminal vesicle 608.0
  shoulder 680.3
  skin NEC 680.9
  specified site NEC 680.8
  spermatic cord 608.4
  temple (region) 680.0
  testis 608.4
  thigh 680.6
  thumb 680.4
  toe (any) 680.7
  trunk 680.2
  tunica vaginalis 608.4
  umbilicus 680.2
  upper arm 680.3
  urethra 597.0
  vas deferens 608.4
  vulva 616.4
  wrist 680.4
Carbunculus (*see also* Carbuncle) 680.9
Carcinoid (tumor) (M8240/1)—*see also*
    Neoplasm, by site, uncertain behavior
  and struma ovarii (M9091/1) 236.2
  argentaffin (M8241/1)—*see* Neoplasm, by site,
      uncertain behavior
    malignant (M8241/3)—*see* Neoplasm, by site,
        malignant
  benign (M9091/0) 220
  composite (M8244/3)—*see* Neoplasm, by site,
      malignant
  goblet cell (M8243/3)—*see* Neoplasm, by site,
      malignant
  malignant (M8240/3)—*see* Neoplasm, by site,
      malignant
  nonargentaffin (M8242/1)—*see also* Neoplasm,
      by site, uncertain behavior
    malignant (M8242/3)—*see* Neoplasm, by site,
        malignant

Carcinoma—*continued*
  fibroepithelial type basal cell (M8093/3)—*see*
    Neoplasm, skin, malignant
  follicular (M8330/3)
    and papillary (mixed) (M8340/3) 193
    moderately differentiated type (M8332/3) 193
    pure follicle type (M8331/3) 193
    specified site—*see* Neoplasm, by site,
      malignant
    trabecular type (M8332/3) 193
    unspecified site 193
    well differentiated type (M8331/3) 193
  gelatinous (M8480/3)
  giant cell (M8031/3)
    and spindle cell (M8030/3)
  granular cell (M8320/3)
  granulosa cell (M8620/3) 183.0
  hepatic cell (M8170/3) 155.0
  hepatocellular (M8170/3) 155.0
    and bile duct, mixed (M8180/3)
      155.0
  hepatocholangiolitic (M8180/3) 155.0
  Hurthle cell (thyroid) 193
  hypernephroid (M8311/3)
  in
    adenomatous
      polyp (M8210/3)
      polyposis coli (M8220/3) 153.9
    pleomorphic adenoma (M8940/3)
    polypoid adenoma (M8210/3)
    situ (M8010/3)—*see* Carcinoma,
      in situ
    tubular adenoma (M8210/3)
    villous adenoma (M8261/3)
  infiltrating duct (M8500/3)
    with Paget's disease (M8541/3)—*see*
      Neoplasm, breast, malignant
    specified site—*see* Neoplasm, by site,
      malignant
    unspecified site 174.9
  inflammatory (M8530/3)
    specified site—*see* Neoplasm, by site,
      malignant
    unspecified site 174.9
  in situ (M8010/2)—*see also* Neoplasm, by site,
    in situ
    epidermoid (M8070/2)—*see also* Neoplasm,
      by site, in situ
      with questionable stromal invasion
        (M8076/2)
        specified site—*see* Neoplasm, by site, in
          situ
        unspecified site 233.1
      Bowen's type (M8081/2)—*see* Neoplasm,
        skin, in situ
    intraductal (M8500/2)
      specified site—*see* Neoplasm, by site, in situ
      unspecified site 233.0
    lobular (M8520/2)
      specified site—*see* Neoplasm, by site, in situ
      unspecified site 233.0
    papillary (M8050/2)—*see* Neoplasm, by site,
      in situ
    squamous cell (M8070/2)—*see also*
      Neoplasm, by site, in situ
    with questionable stromal invasion (M8076/2)
      specified site—*see* Neoplasm, by site, in
        situ
      unspecified site 233.1
    transitional cell (M8120/2)—*see* Neoplasm,
      by site, in situ

Carcinoma—*continued*
  intestinal type (M8144/3)
    specified site—*see* Neoplasm, by site,
      malignant
    unspecified site 151.9
  intraductal (noninfiltrating) (M8500/2)
    papillary (M8503/2)
      specified site—*see* Neoplasm, by site, in situ
      unspecified site 233.0
    specified site—*see* Neoplasm, by site, in situ
    unspecified site 233.0
  intraepidermal (M8070/2)—*see also* Neoplasm,
    skin, in situ
    squamous cell, Bowen's type (M8081/2)—*see*
      Neoplasm, skin, in situ
  intraepithelial (M8010/2)—*see also* Neoplasm,
    by site, in situ
    squamous cell (M8072/2)—*see* Neoplasm, by
      site, in situ
  intraosseous (M9270/3) 170.1
    upper jaw (bone) 170.0
  islet cell (M8150/3)
    and exocrine, mixed (M8154/3)
      specified site—*see* Neoplasm, by site,
        malignant
      unspecified site 157.9
    pancreas 157.4
    specified site NEC—*see* Neoplasm, by site,
      malignant
    unspecified site 157.4
  juvenile, breast (M8502/3)—*see* Neoplasm,
    breast, malignant
  Kulchitsky's cell (carcinoid tumor of intestine)
    259.2
  large cell (M8012/3)
    squamous cell, nonkeratinizing type
      (M8072/3)
  Leydig cell (testis) (M8650/3)
    specified site—*see* Neoplasm, by site,
      malignant
    unspecified site 186.9
      female 183.0
      male 186.9
  liver cell (M8170/3) 155.0
  lobular (infiltrating) (M8520/3)
    non-infiltrating (M8520/3)
      specified site—*see* Neoplasm, by site, in situ
      unspecified site 233.0
    specified site—*see* Neoplasm, by site,
      malignant
    unspecified site 174.9
  lymphoepithelial (M8082/3)
  medullary (M8510/3)
    with
      amyloid stroma (M8511/3)
        specified site—*see* Neoplasm, by site,
          malignant
        unspecified site 193
      lymphoid stroma (M8512/3)
        specified site—*see* Neoplasm, by site,
          malignant
        unspecified site 174.9
  mesometanephric (M9110/3)
  mesonephric (M9110/3)
  metastatic (M8010/6)—*see* Metastasis, cancer
  metatypical (M8095/3)—*see* Neoplasm, skin,
    malignant
  morphea type basal cell (M8092/3)—*see*
    Neoplasm, skin, malignant
  mucinous (M8480/3)
  mucin-producing (M8481/3)

Carcinoma—*continued*
  tubular (M8211/3)
  undifferentiated type (M8020/3)
  urothelial (M8120/3)
  ventriculi 151.9
  verrucous (epidermoid) (squamous cell)
    (M8051/3)
  villous (M8262/3)
  water-clear cell (M8322/3) 194.1
  wolffian duct (M9110/3)
Carcinomaphobia 300.29
Carcinomatosis
  peritonei (M8010/6) 197.6
  specified site NEC (M8010/3)—*see* Neoplasm,
    by site, malignant
  unspecified site (M8010/6) 199.0
Carcinosarcoma (M8980/3)—*see also*
  Neoplasm, by site, malignant
  embryonal type (M8981/3)—*see* Neoplasm, by
    site, malignant
Cardia, cardial —*see* condition
Cardiac —*see also* condition
  death—*see* Disease, heart
  device
    defibrillator, automatic implantable V45.02
    in situ NEC V45.00
    pacemaker
      cardiac
        fitting or adjustment V53.3
        in situ V45.01
      carotid sinus
        fitting or adjustment V53.3
        in situ V45.09
  pacemaker—*see* Cardiac, device, pacemaker
  tamponade 423.9
Cardialgia (*see also* Pain, precordial) 786.51
Cardiectasis —*see* Hypertrophy, cardiac
Cardiochalasia 530.81
Cardiomalacia (*see also* Degeneration,
  myocardial) 429.1
Cardiomegalia glycogenica diffusa 271.0
Cardiomegaly (*see also* Hypertrophy, cardiac)
  429.3
  congenital 746.89
  glycogen 271.0
  hypertensive (*see also* Hypertension, heart)
    402.90
  idiopathic 429.3
Cardiomyoliposis (*see also* Degeneration,
  myocardial) 429.1
Cardiomyopathy (congestive) (constrictive)
  (familial) (infiltrative) (obstructive)
  (restrictive) (sporadic) 425.4
  alcoholic 425.5
  amyloid 277.3 *[425.7]*
  beriberi 265.0 *[425.7]*
  cobalt-beer 425.5
  congenital 425.3
  due to
    amyloidosis 277.3 *[425.7]*
    beriberi 265.0 *[425.7]*
    cardiac glycogenesis 271.0 *[425.7]*
    Chagas' disease 086.0
    Friedreich's ataxia 334.0 *[425.8]*
    mucopolysaccharidosis 277.5 *[425.7]*
    myotonia atrophica 359.2 *[425.8]*
    progressive muscular dystrophy 359.1 *[425.8]*
    sarcoidosis 135 *[425.8]*

Cardiomyopathy—*continued*
  glycogen storage 271.0 *[425.7]*
  hypertensive—*see* Hypertension, with, heart
    involvement
  hypertrophic
    nonobstructive 425.4
    obstructive 425.1
      congenital 746.84
  idiopathic (concentric) 425.4
  in
    Chagas' disease 086.0
    sarcoidosis 135 *[425.8]*
  ischemic 414.8
  metabolic NEC 277.9 *[425.7]*
    amyloid 277.3 *[425.7]*
    thyrotoxic (*see also* Thyrotoxicosis) 242.9
      [425.7]
    thyrotoxicosis (*see also* Thyrotoxicosis) 242.9
      [425.7]
  nutritional 269.9 *[425.7]*
    beriberi 265.0 *[425.7]*
  obscure of Africa 425.2
  postpartum 674.8
  primary 425.4
  secondary 425.9
  thyrotoxic (*see also* Thyrotoxicosis) 242.9
    [425.7]
  toxic NEC 425.9
  tuberculous (*see also* Tuberculosis) 017.9
    [425.8]
Cardionephritis —*see* Hypertension, cardiorenal
Cardionephropathy —*see* Hypertension,
  cardiorenal
Cardionephrosis —*see* Hypertension,
  cardiorenal
Cardioneurosis 306.2
Cardiopathia nigra 416.0
Cardiopathy (*see also* Disease, heart) 429.9
  hypertensive (*see also* Hypertension, heart)
    402.90
  idiopathic 425.4
  mucopolysaccharidosis 277.5 *[425.7]*
Cardiopericarditis (*see also* Pericarditis) 423.9
Cardiophobia 300.29
Cardioptosis 746.87
Cardiorenal —*see* condition
Cardiorrhexis (*see also* Infarct, myocardium)
  410.9
Cardiosclerosis —*see* Arteriosclerosis, coronary
Cardiosis —*see* Disease, heart
Cardiospasm (esophagus) (reflex) (stomach)
  530.0
  congenital 750.7
Cardiostenosis —*see* Disease, heart
Cardiosymphysis 423.1
Cardiothyrotoxicosis —*see* Hyperthyroidism
Cardiovascular —*see* condition
Carditis (acute) (bacterial) (chronic) (subacute)
  429.89
  Coxsackie 074.20
  hypertensive (*see also* Hypertension, heart)
    402.90
  meningococcal 036.40
  rheumatic—*see* Disease, heart, rheumatic
  rheumatoid 714.2
Care (of)
  child (routine) V20.1
  convalescent following V66.9
    chemotherapy V66.2
    medical NEC V66.5
    psychotherapy V66.3

Care—*continued*
  radiotherapy V66.1
  surgery V66.0
  surgical NEC V66.0
  treatment (for) V66.5
    combined V66.6
    fracture V66.4
    mental disorder NEC V66.3
    specified type NEC V66.5
  end-of-life care V66.7
  family member (handicapped) (sick)
    creating problem for family V61.49
    provided away from home for holiday relief
      V60.5
    unavailable, due to
      absence (person rendering care) (sufferer)
        V60.4
      inability (any reason) of person rendering
        care V60.4
  holiday relief V60.5
  hospice V66.7
  lack of (at or after birth) (infant) (child) 995.52
    adult 995.84
  lactation of mother V24.1
  palliative V66.7
  postpartum
    immediately after delivery V24.0
    routine follow-up V24.2
  prenatal V22.1
    first pregnancy V22.0
    high risk pregnancy V23.9
      specified problem NEC V23.8
  terminal V66.7
  unavailable, due to
    absence of person rendering care V60.4
    inability (any reason) of person rendering care
      V60.4
  well baby V20.1
Caries (bone) (*see also* Tuberculosis, bone)
    015.9 *[730.8]*
  arrested 521.04
  cementum 521.03
  cerebrospinal (tuberculous) 015.0 *[730.88]*
  dental (acute) (chronic) (incipient) (infected)
    521.09
    with pulp exposure 521.03
    extending to
      dentine 521.02
      pulp 521.03
    other specified NEC 521.09
  dentin (acute) (chronic) 521.02
  enamel (acute) (chronic) (incipient) 521.01
  external meatus 380.89
  hip (*see also* Tuberculosis) 015.1 *[730.85]*
  knee 015.2 *[730.86]*
  labyrinth 386.8
  limb NEC 015.7 *[730.88]*
  mastoid (chronic) (process) 383.1
  middle ear 385.89
  nose 015.7 *[730.88]*
  orbit 015.7 *[730.88]*
  ossicle 385.24
  petrous bone 383.20
  sacrum (tuberculous) 015.0 *[730.88]*
  spine, spinal (column) (tuberculous) 015.0
    [730.88]
  syphilitic 095.5
    congenital 090.0 *[730.8]*
  teeth (internal) 521.00
    initial 521.01
  vertebra (column) (tuberculous) 015.0 *[730.88]*
Carini's syndrome (ichthyosis congenita) 757.1

Carious teeth 521.00
Carneous mole 631
Carnosinemia 270.5
Carotid body or sinus syndrome 337.0
Carotidynia 337.0
Carotinemia (dietary) 278.3
Carotinosis (cutis) (skin) 278.3
Carpal tunnel syndrome 354.0
Carpenter's syndrome 759.89
Carpopedal spasm (*see also* Tetany) 781.7
Carpoptosis 736.05
Carrier (suspected) of
  amebiasis V02.2
  bacterial disease (meningococcal,
    staphylococcal, streptococcal) NEC V02.59
  cholera V02.0
  cystic fibrosis gene V83.81
  defective gene V83.89
  diphtheria V02.4
  dysentery (bacillary) V02.3
    amebic V02.2
  Endamoeba histolytica V02.2
  gastrointestinal pathogens NEC V02.3
  genetic defect V83.89
  gonorrhea V02.7
  group B streptococcus V02.51
  HAA (hepatitis Australian-antigen) V02.61
  hemophilia A (asymptomatic) V83.01
    symptomatic V83.02
  hepatitis V02.60
    Australian-antigen (HAA) V02.61
    B V02.61
    C V02.62
    serum V02.61
    specified type NEC V02.69
    viral V02.60
  infective organism NEC V02.9
  malaria V02.9
  paratyphoid V02.3
  Salmonella V02.3
    typhosa V02.1
  serum hepatitis V02.61
  Shigella V02.3
  Staphylococcus NEC V02.59
  Streptococcus NEC V02.52
    group B V02.51
  typhoid V02.1
  venereal disease NEC V02.8
Carrión's disease (Bartonellosis) 088.0
Car sickness 994.6
Carter's
  relapsing fever (Asiatic) 087.0
Cartilage —*see* condition
Caruncle (inflamed)
  abscess, lacrimal (*see also* Dacryocystitis)
    375.30
  conjunctiva 372.00
    acute 372.00
  eyelid 373.00
  labium (majus) (minus) 616.8
  lacrimal 375.30
  urethra (benign) 599.3
  vagina (wall) 616.8
Cascade stomach 537.6
Caseation lymphatic gland (*see also*
  Tuberculosis) 017.2
Caseous
  bronchitis—*see* Tuberculosis, pulmonary
  meningitis 013.0
  pneumonia—*see* Tuberculosis, pulmonary
Cassidy (-Scholte) syndrome (malignant
  carcinoid) 259.2

Catarrh, catarrhal—*continued*
  cervix, cervical (canal) (uteri)—*see* Cervicitis
  chest (*see also* Bronchitis) 490
  chronic 472.0
  congestion 472.0
  conjunctivitis 372.03
  due to syphilis 095.9
    congenital 090.0
  enteric—*see* Enteritis
  epidemic 487.1
  Eustachian 381.50
  eye (acute) (vernal) 372.03
  fauces (*see also* Pharyngitis) 462
  febrile 460
  fibrinous acute 466.0
  gastroenteric—*see* Enteritis
  gastrointestinal—*see* Enteritis
  gingivitis 523.0
  hay (*see also* Fever, hay) 477.9
  infectious 460
  intestinal—*see* Enteritis
  larynx (*see also* Laryngitis, chronic) 476.0
  liver 070.1
    with hepatic coma 070.0
  lung (*see also* Bronchitis) 490
    acute 466.0
    chronic 491.0
  middle ear (chronic)—*see* Otitis media, chronic
  mouth 528.0
  nasal (chronic) (*see also* Rhinitis) 472.0
    acute 460
  nasobronchial 472.2
  nasopharyngeal (chronic) 472.2
    acute 460
  nose—*see* Catarrh, nasal
  ophthalmia 372.03
  pneumococcal, acute 466.0
  pulmonary (*see also* Bronchitis) 490
    acute 466.0
    chronic 491.0
  spring (eye) 372.13
  suffocating (*see also* Asthma) 493.9
  summer (hay) (*see also* Fever, hay) 477.9
  throat 472.1
  tracheitis 464.10
    with obstruction 464.11
  tubotympanal 381.4
    acute (*see also* Otitis media, acute,
        nonsuppurative) 381.00
    chronic 381.10
  vasomotor (*see also* Fever, hay) 477.9
  vesical (bladder)—*see* Cystitis
Catarrhus aestivus (*see also* Fever, hay) 477.9
Catastrophe, cerebral (*see also* Disease,
    cerebrovascular, acute) 436
Catatonia, catatonic (acute) 781.99
  agitation 295.2
  dementia (praecox) 295.2
  due to or associated with physical condition
      293.89
  excitation 295.2
  excited type 295.2
  schizophrenia 295.2
  stupor 295.2
  with
    affective psychosis —*see* Psychosis, affective)
Cat-scratch —*see also* Injury, superficial
  disease or fever 078.3
Cauda equina —*see also* condition syndrome
    344.60
Cauliflower ear 738.7
Caul over face 768.9

Causalgia 355.9
  lower limb 355.71
  upper limb 354.4
Cause
  external, general effects NEC 994.9
  not stated 799.9
  unknown 799.9
Caustic burn —*see also* Burn, by site
  from swallowing caustic or corrosive
      substance—*see* Burn, internal organs
Cavare's disease (familial periodic paralysis)
    359.3
Cave-in, injury
  crushing (severe) (*see also* Crush, by site) 869.1
  suffocation 994.7
Cavernitis (penis) 607.2
  lymph vessel—*see* Lymphangioma
Cavernositis 607.2
Cavernous —*see* condition
Cavitation of lung (*see also* Tuberculosis) 011.2
  nontuberculous 518.89
  primary, progressive 010.8
Cavity
  lung—*see* Cavitation of lung
  optic papilla 743.57
  pulmonary—*see* Cavitation of lung
  teeth 521.00
  vitreous (humor) 379.21
Cavovarus foot, congenital 754.59
Cavus foot (congenital) 754.71
  acquired 736.73
Cazenave's
  disease (pemphigus) NEC 694.4
  lupus (erythematosus) 695.4
Cecitis —*see* Appendicitis
Cecocele —*see* Hernia
Cecum —*see* condition
Celiac
  artery compression syndrome 447.4
  disease 579.0
  infantilism 579.0
Cell, cellular —*see also* condition
  anterior chamber (eye) (positive aqueous ray)
      364.04
Cellulitis (diffuse) (with lymphangitis) (*see also*
    Abscess) 682.9
  abdominal wall 682.2
  anaerobic (*see also* Gas gangrene) 040.0
  ankle 682.6
  anus 566
  areola 611.0
  arm (any part, above wrist) 682.3
  auditory canal (external) 380.10
  axilla 682.3
  back (any part) 682.2
  breast 611.0
    postpartum 675.1
  broad ligament (*see also* Disease, pelvis,
      inflammatory) 614.4
    acute 614.3
  buttock 682.5
  cervical (neck region) 682.1
  cervix (uteri) (*see also* Cervicitis) 616.0
  cheek, external 682.0
    internal 528.3
  chest wall 682.2
  chronic NEC 682.9
  colostomy 569.61
  corpus cavernosum 607.2
  digit 681.9

Cellulitis—*continued*
  Douglas' cul-de-sac or pouch (chronic) (*see also* Disease, pelvis, inflammatory) 614.4
    acute 614.3
  drainage site (following operation) 998.59
  ear, external 380.10
  enterostomy 569.61
  erysipelar (*see also* Erysipelas) 035
  eyelid 373.13
  face (any part, except eye) 682.0
  finger (intrathecal) (periosteal) (subcutaneous) (subcuticular) 681.00
  flank 682.2
  foot (except toe) 682.7
  forearm 682.3
  gangrenous (*see also* Gangrene) 785.4
  genital organ NEC
    female—*see* Abscess, genital organ, female
    male 608.4
  glottis 478.71
  gluteal (region) 682.5
  gonococcal NEC 098.0
  groin 682.2
  hand (except finger or thumb) 682.4
  head (except face) NEC 682.8
  heel 682.7
  hip 682.6
  jaw (region) 682.0
  knee 682.6
  labium (majus) (minus) (*see also* Vulvitis) 616.10
  larynx 478.71
  leg, except foot 682.6
  lip 528.5
  mammary gland 611.0
  mouth (floor) 528.3
  multiple sites NEC 682.9
  nasopharynx 478.21
  navel 682.2
    newborn NEC 771.4
  neck (region) 682.1
  nipple 611.0
  nose 478.1
    external 682.0
  orbit, orbital 376.01
  palate (soft) 528.3
  pectoral (region) 682.2
  pelvis, pelvic
    with
      abortion—*see* Abortion, by type, with sepsis
      ectopic pregnancy (*see also* categories 633.0-633.9) 639.0
      molar pregnancy (*see also* categories 630-632) 639.0
    female (*see also* Disease, pelvis, inflammatory) 614.4
      acute 614.3
    following
      abortion 639.0
      ectopic or molar pregnancy 639.0
    male (*see also* Abscess, peritoneum) 567.2
    puerperal, postpartum, childbirth 670
  penis 607.2
  perineal, perineum 682.2
  perirectal 566
  peritonsillar 475
  periurethral 597.0
  periuterine (*see also* Disease, pelvis, inflammatory) 614.4
    acute 614.3
  pharynx 478.21

Cellulitis—*continued*
  phlegmonous NEC 682.9
  rectum 566
  retromammary 611.0
  retroperitoneal (*see also* Peritonitis) 567.2
  round ligament (*see also* Disease, pelvis, inflammatory) 614.4
    acute 614.3
  scalp (any part) 682.8
    dissecting 704.8
  scrotum 608.4
  seminal vesicle 608.0
  septic NEC 682.9
  shoulder 682.3
  specified sites NEC 682.8
  spermatic cord 608.4
  submandibular (region) (space) (triangle) 682.0
    gland 527.3
  submaxillary 528.3
    gland 527.3
  submental (pyogenic) 682.0
    gland 527.3
  suppurative NEC 682.9
  testis 608.4
  thigh 682.6
  thumb (intrathecal) (periosteal) (subcutaneous) (subcuticular) 681.00
  toe (intrathecal) (periosteal) (subcutaneous) (subcuticular) 681.10
  tonsil 475
  trunk 682.2
  tuberculous (primary) (*see also* Tuberculosis) 017.0
  tunica vaginalis 608.4
  umbilical 682.2
    newborn NEC 771.4
  vaccinal 999.3
  vagina—*see* Vaginitis
  vas deferens 608.4
  vocal cords 478.5
  vulva (*see also* Vulvitis) 616.10
  wrist 682.4
Cementoblastoma, benign (M9273/0) 213.1
  upper jaw (bone) 213.0
Cementoma (M9273/0) 213.1
  gigantiform (M9276/0) 213.1
    upper jaw (bone) 213.0
  upper jaw (bone) 213.0
Cementoperiostitis 523.4
Cephalgia, cephalalgia (*see also* Headache) 784.0
  histamine 346.2
  nonorganic origin 307.81
  psychogenic 307.81
  tension 307.81
Cephalhematocele, cephalematocele
  due to birth injury 767.1
  fetus or newborn 767.1
  traumatic (*see also* Contusion, head) 920
Cephalhematoma, cephalematoma (calcified)
  due to birth injury 767.1
  fetus or newborn 767.1
  traumatic (*see also* Contusion, head) 920
Cephalic —*see* condition
Cephalitis —*see* Encephalitis
Cephalocele 742.0
Cephaloma —*see* Neoplasm, by site, malignant
Cephalomenia 625.8
Cephalopelvic —*see* condition
Cercomoniasis 007.3
Cerebellitis —*see* Encephalitis

Cerebellum (cerebellar)—*see* condition
Cerebral —*see* condition
Cerebritis —*see* Encephalitis
Cerebrohepatorenal syndrome 759.89
Cerebromacular degeneration 330.1
Cerebromalacia (*see also* Softening, brain) 434.9
Cerebrosidosis 272.7
Cerebrospasticity —*see* Palsy, cerebral
Cerebrospinal —*see* condition
Cerebrum —*see* condition
Ceroid storage disease 272.7
Cerumen (accumulation) (impacted) 380.4
Cervical —*see also* condition
  auricle 744.43
  rib 756.2
Cervicalgia 723.1
Cervicitis (acute) (chronic) (nonvenereal)
    (subacute) (with erosion or ectropion) 616.0
  with
    abortion—*see* Abortion, by type, with sepsis
    ectopic pregnancy (*see also* categories
        633.0-633.9) 639.0
    molar pregnancy (*see also* categories
        630-632) 639.0
    ulceration 616.0
  chlamydial 099.53
  complicating pregnancy or puerperium 646.6
    affecting fetus or newborn 760.8
  following
    abortion 639.0
    ectopic or molar pregnancy 639.0
  gonococcal (acute) 098.15
    chronic or duration of 2 months or more
        098.35
  senile (atrophic) 616.0
  syphilitic 095.8
  trichomonal 131.09
  tuberculous (*see also* Tuberculosis) 016.7
Cervicoaural fistula 744.49
Cervicocolpitis (emphysematosa) (*see also*
    Cervicitis) 616.0
Cervix —*see* condition
Cesarean delivery, operation or section NEC
    669.7
  affecting fetus or newborn 763.4
  post mortem, affecting fetus or newborn 761.6
  previous, affecting management of pregnancy
    654.2
Céstan's syndrome 344.89
Céstan-Chenais paralysis 344.89
Céstan-Raymond syndrome 433.8
Cestode infestation NEC 123.9
  specified type NEC 123.8
Cestodiasis 123.9
Chaberts' disease 022.9
Chacaleh 266.2
Chafing 709.8
Chagas' disease (*see also* Trypanosomiasis,
    American) 086.2
  with heart involvement 086.0
Chagres fever 084.0
Chalasia (cardiac sphincter) 530.81
Chalazion 373.2
Chalazoderma 757.39
Chalcosis 360.24
  cornea 371.15
  crystalline lens 360.24 *[366.34]*
  retina 360.24.
Chalicosis (occupational) (pulmonum) 502

Chancre (any genital site) (hard) (indurated)
    (infecting) (primary) (recurrent) 091.0
  congenital 090.0
  conjunctiva 091.2
  Ducrey's 099.0
  extragenital 091.2
  eyelid 091.2
  Hunterian 091.0
  lip (syphilis) 091.2
  mixed 099.8
  nipple 091.2
  Nisbet's 099.0
  of
    carate 103.0
    pinta 103.0
    yaws 102.0
  palate, soft 091.2
  phagedenic 099.0
  Ricord's 091.0
  Rollet's (syphilitic) 091.0
  seronegative 091.0
  seropositive 091.0
  simple 099.0
  soft 099.0
    bubo 099.0
  urethra 091.0
  yaws 102.0
Chancriform syndrome 114.1
Chancroid 099.0
  anus 099.0
  penis (Ducrey's bacillus) 099.0
  perineum 099.0
  rectum 099.0
  scrotum 099.0
  urethra 099.0
  vulva 099.0
Chandipura fever 066.8
Chandler's disease (osteochondritis dissecans,
    hip) 732.7
Change (s) (of)—*see also* Removal of
  arteriosclerotic—*see* Arteriosclerosis
  battery
    cardiac pacemaker V53.31
  bone 733.90
    diabetic 250.8 *[731.8]*
    in disease, unknown cause 733.90
  bowel habits 787.99
  cardiorenal (vascular) (*see also* Hypertension,
      cardiorenal) 404.90
  cardiovascular—*see* Disease, cardiovascular
  circulatory 459.9
  cognitive or personality change of other type,
      nonpsychotic 310.1
  color, teeth, tooth
    during formation 520.8
    posteruptive 521.7
  contraceptive device V25.42
  cornea, corneal
    degenerative NEC 371.40
    membrane NEC 371.30
    senile 371.41
  coronary (*see also* Ischemia, heart) 414.9
  degenerative
    chamber angle (anterior) (iris) 364.56
    ciliary body 364.57
    spine or vertebra (*see also* Spondylosis)
        721.90
  dental pulp, regressive 522.2
  dressing V58.3
  fixation device V54.89
    external V54.89

Change(s) (of)—*continued*
 internal V54.0
 heart—*see also* Disease, heart
 hip joint 718.95
 hyperplastic larynx 478.79
 hypertrophic
  nasal sinus (*see also* Sinusitis) 473.9
  turbinate, nasal 478.0
  upper respiratory tract 478.9
 inflammatory—*see* Inflammation
 joint (*see also* Derangement, joint) 718.90
  sacroiliac 724.6
 Kirschner wire V54.89
 knee 717.9
 macular, congenital 743.55
 malignant (M——/3)—*see also* Neoplasm, by
  site, malignant

---

*Note—for malignant change occurring in a
neoplasm, use the appropriate M code with
behavior digit /3 e.g., malignant change in
uterine fibroid—M8890/3. For malignant
change occurring in a nonneoplastic condition
(e.g., gastric ulcer) use the M code M8000/3.*

---

 mental (status) NEC 780.99
  due to or associated with physical
    condition—*see* Syndrome, brain
 myocardium, myocardial—*see* Degeneration,
   myocardial
 of life (*see also* Menopause) 627.2
 pacemaker battery (cardiac) V53.31
 peripheral nerve 355.9
 personality (nonpsychotic) NEC 310.1
 plaster cast V54.89
 refractive, transient 367.81
 regressive, dental pulp 522.2
 retina 362.9
  myopic (degenerative) (malignant) 360.21
  vascular appearance 362.13
 sacroiliac joint 724.6
 scleral 379.19
  degenerative 379.16
 senile (*see also* Senility) 797
 sensory (*see also* Disturbance, sensation) 782.0
 skin texture 782.8
 spinal cord 336.9
 splint, external V54.89
 subdermal implantable contraceptive V25.5
 suture V58.3
 traction device V54.89
 trophic 355.9
  arm NEC 354.9
  leg NEC 355.8
  lower extremity NEC 355.8
  upper extremity NEC 354.9
 vascular 459.9
 vasomotor 443.9
 voice 784.49
  psychogenic 306.1
Changing sleep-work schedule, affecting sleep
 307.45
Changuinola fever 066.0
Chapping skin 709.8
Character
 depressive 301.12
Charcot's
 arthropathy 094.0 *[713.5]*
 cirrhosis—*see* Cirrhosis, biliary
 disease 094.0
  spinal cord 094.0

Charcot's—*continued*
 fever (biliary) (hepatic) (intermittent)—*see*
   Choledocholithiasis
 joint (disease) 094.0 *[713.5]*
  diabetic 250.6 *[713.5]*
  syringomyelic 336.0 *[713.5]*
 syndrome (intermittent claudication) 443.9
  due to atherosclerosis 440.21
**Charcot-Marie-Tooth disease, paralysis, or syn-
  drome** 356.1
Charleyhorse (quadriceps) 843.8
 muscle, except quadriceps—*see* Sprain, by site
Charlouis' disease (*see also* Yaws) 102.9
Chauffeur's fracture —*see* Fracture, ulna,
  lower end
Cheadle (-Möller) (-Barlow) disease or
  syndrome (infantile scurvy) 267
Checking (of)
 contraceptive device (intrauterine) V25.42
 device
  fixation V54.89
   external V54.89
   internal V54.0
  traction V54.89
 Kirschner wire V54.89
 plaster cast V54.89
 splint, external V54.89
Checkup
 following treatment—*see* Examination
 health V70.0
 infant (not sick) V20.2
 pregnancy (normal) V22.1
  first V22.0
  high risk pregnancy V23.9
   specified problem NEC V23.8
Chédiak-Higashi (-Steinbrinck) anomaly,
  disease, or syndrome (congenital gigantism of
  peroxidase granules) 288.2
Cheek —*see also* condition
 biting 528.9
Cheese itch 133.8
Cheese washers' lung 495.8
Cheilitis 528.5
 actinic (due to sun) 692.72
  chronic NEC 692.74
   due to radiation, except from sun 692.82
  due to radiation, except from sun 692.82
 acute 528.5
 angular 528.5
 catarrhal 528.5
 chronic 528.5
 exfoliative 528.5
 gangrenous 528.5
 glandularis apostematosa 528.5
 granulomatosa 351.8
 infectional 528.5
 membranous 528.5
 Miescher's 351.8
 suppurative 528.5
 ulcerative 528.5
 vesicular 528.5
Cheilodynia 528.5
Cheilopalatoschisis (*see also* Cleft, palate, with
  cleft lip) 749.20
Cheilophagia 528.9
Cheiloschisis (*see also* Cleft, lip) 749.10
Cheilosis 528.5
 with pellagra 265.2
 angular 528.5
 due to
  dietary deficiency 266.0
  vitamin deficiency 266.0

Cheiromegaly 729.89
Cheiropompholyx 705.81
Cheloid (*see also* Keloid) 701.4
Chemical burn —*see also* Burn, by site
  from swallowing chemical—*see* Burn, internal
    organs
Chemodectoma (M8693/1)—*see*
  Paraganglioma, nonchromaffin
Chemoprophylaxis NEC V07.39
Chemosis, conjunctiva 372.73
Chemotherapy
  convalescence V66.2
  encounter (for) V58.1
  maintenance V58.1
  prophylactic NEC V07.39
    fluoride V07.31
Cherubism 526.89
Chest —*see* condition
Cheyne-Stokes respiration (periodic) 786.04
Chiari's
  disease or syndrome (hepatic vein thrombosis)
    453.0
  malformation
    type I 348.4
    type II (*see also* Spina bifida) 741.0
    type III 742.0
    type IV 742.2
  network 746.89
Chiari-Frommel syndrome 676.6
Chicago disease (North American
  blastomycosis) 116.0
Chickenpox (*see also* Varicella) 052.9
  vaccination and inoculation (prophylactic) V05.4
Chiclero ulcer 085.4
Chiggers 133.8
Chignon 111.2
  fetus or newborn (from vacuum extraction)
    767.1
Chigoe disease 134.1
Chikungunya fever 066.3
Chilaiditi's syndrome (subphrenic displacement,
  colon) 751.4
Chilblains 991.5
  lupus 991.5
Child
  behavior causing concern V61.20
Childbed fever 670
Childbirth —*see also* Delivery
  puerperal complications—*see* Puerperal
Childhood, period of rapid growth V21.0
Chill (s) 780.99
  with fever 780.6
  congestive 780.99
    in malarial regions 084.6
  septic—*see* Septicemia
  urethral 599.84
Chilomastigiasis 007.8
Chin —*see* condition
Chinese dysentery 004.9
Chiropractic dislocation (*see also* Lesion,
  nonallopathic, by site) 739.9
Chitral fever 066.0
Chlamydia, chlamydial -*see* **condition**
Chloasma 709.09
  cachecticorum 709.09
  eyelid 374.52
    congenital 757.33
    hyperthyroid 242.0
  gravidarum 646.8
  idiopathic 709.09
  skin 709.09
  symptomatic 709.09

Chloroma (M9930/3) 205.3
Chlorosis 280.9
  Egyptian (*see also* Ancylostomiasis) 126.9
  miners' (*see also* Ancylostomiasis) 126.9
Chlorotic anemia 280.9
Chocolate cyst (ovary) 617.1
Choked
  disk or disc—*see* Papilledema
  on food, phlegm, or vomitus NEC (*see also*
    Asphyxia, food) 933.1
  phlegm 933.1
  while vomiting NEC (*see also* Asphyxia, food)
    933.1
Chokes (resulting from bends) 993.3
Choking sensation 784.9
Cholangiectasis (*see also* Disease, gallbladder)
  575.8
Cholangiocarcinoma (M8160/3)
  and hepatocellular carcinoma, combined
    (M8180/3) 155.0
  liver 155.1
  specified site NEC—*see* Neoplasm, by site,
    malignant
  unspecified site 155.1
Cholangiohepatitis 575.8
  due to fluke infestation 121.1
Cholangiohepatoma (M8180/3) 155.0
Cholangiolitis (acute) (chronic) (extrahepatic)
  (gangrenous) 576.1
  intrahepatic 575.8
  paratyphoidal (*see also* Fever, paratyphoid)
    002.9
  typhoidal 002.0
Cholangioma (M8160/0) 211.5
  malignant—*see* Cholangiocarcinoma
Cholangitis (acute) (ascending) (catarrhal)
  (chronic) (infective) (malignant) (primary)
  (recurrent) (sclerosing) (secondary)
  (stenosing) (suppurative) 576.1
  chronic nonsuppurative destructive 571.6
  nonsuppurative destructive (chronic) 571.6
Cholecystdocholithiasis —*see*
  Choledocholithiasis
Cholecystitis 575.10
  with
    calculus, stones in
      bile duct (common) (hepatic)—*see*
        Choledocholithiasis
      gallbladder—*see* Cholelithiasis
  acute and chronic 575.12
  chronic 575.11
  emphysematous (acute) (*see also* Cholecystitis,
    acute) 575.0
  gangrenous (*see also* Cholecystitis, acute) 575.0
  paratyphoidal, current (*see also* Fever,
    paratyphoid) 002.9
  suppurative (*see also* Cholecystitis, acute) 575.0
  typhoidal 002.0
Choledochitis (suppurative) 576.1
Choledocholith —*see* Choledocholithiasis
Choledocholithiasis 574.5

> *Note—Use the following fifth-digit*
> *subclassification with category 574:*
>
> *0 without mention of obstruction*
> *1 with obstruction*

  with
    cholecystitis 574.4
      acute 574.3
      chronic 574.4

Choledocholithiasis—*continued*
  cholelithiasis 574.9
    with
      cholecystitis 574.7
        acute 574.6
          and chronic 574.8
        chronic 574.7
Cholelithiasis (impacted) (multiple) 574.2

> *Note—Use the following fifth-digit*
> *subclassification with category 574:*
>
> *0 without mention of obstruction*
> *1 with obstruction*

  with
    cholecystitis 574.1
      acute 574.0
      chronic 574.1
    choledocholithiasis 574.9
      with
        cholecystitis 574.7
          acute 574.6
            and chronic 574.8
          chronic cholecystitis 574.7
Cholemia (*see also* Jaundice) 782.4
  familial 277.4
  Gilbert's (familial nonhemolytic) 277.4
Cholemic gallstone —*see* Cholelithiasis
Choleperitoneum, choleperitonitis (*see also*
    Disease, gallbladder) 567.8
Cholera (algid) (Asiatic) (asphyctic) (epidemic)
    (gravis) (Indian) (malignant) (morbus)
    (pestilential) (spasmodic) 001.9
  antimonial 985.4
  carrier (suspected) of V02.0
  classical 001.0
  contact V01.0
  due to
    Vibrio
      cholerae (Inaba, Ogawa, Hikojima
        serotypes) 001.0
        El Tor 001.1
  El Tor 001.1
  exposure to V01.0
  vaccination, prophylactic (against) V03.0
Cholerine (*see also* Cholera) 001.9
Cholestasis 576.8
Cholesteatoma (ear) 385.30
  attic (primary) 385.31
  diffuse 385.35
  external ear (canal) 380.21
  marginal (middle ear) 385.32
    with involvement of mastoid cavity 385.33
    secondary (with middle ear involvement)
      385.33
  mastoid cavity 385.30
  middle ear (secondary) 385.32
    with involvement of mastoid cavity 385.33
  postmastoidectomy cavity (recurrent) 383.32
  primary 385.31
  recurrent, postmastoidectomy cavity 383.32
  secondary (middle ear) 385.32
    with involvement of mastoid cavity 385.33
Cholesteatosis (middle ear) (*see also*
    Cholesteatoma) 385.30
  diffuse 385.35
Cholesteremia 272.0
Cholesterin
  granuloma, middle ear 385.82
  in vitreous 379.22

Cholesterol
  deposit
    retina 362.82
    vitreous 379.22
  imbibition of gallbladder (*see also* Disease,
    gallbladder) 575.6
Cholesterolemia 272.0
  essential 272.0
  familial 272.0
  hereditary 272.0
Cholesterosis, cholesterolosis (gallbladder) 575.6
  middle ear (*see also* Cholesteatoma) 385.30
  with
    cholecystitis—*see* Cholecystitis
    cholelithiasis—*see* Cholelithiasis
Cholocolic fistula (*see also* Fistula, gallbladder)
    575.5
Choluria 791.4
Chondritis (purulent) 733.99
  costal 733.6
    Tietze's 733.6
  patella, posttraumatic 717.7
  posttraumatica patellae 717.7
  tuberculous (active) (*see also* Tuberculosis)
    015.9
    intervertebral 015.0 *[730.88]*
Chondroangiopathia calcarea seu punctate
    756.59
Chondroblastoma (M9230/0)—*see also*
    Neoplasm, bone, benign
  malignant (M9230/3)—*see* Neoplasm, bone,
    malignant
Chondrocalcinosis (articular) (crystal
    deposition) (dihydrate) (*see also* Arthritis, due
    to, crystals) 275.49 *[712.3]*
  due to
    calcium pyrophosphate 275.49 *[712.2]*
    dicalcium phosphate crystals 275.49 *[712.1]*
    pyrophosphate crystals 275.4 *[712.2]*
Chondrodermatitis nodularis helicis 380.00
Chondrodysplasia 756.4
  angiomatose 756.4
  calcificans congenita 756.59
  epiphysialis punctata 756.59
  hereditary deforming 756.4
Chondrodystrophia (fetalis) 756.4
  calcarea 756.4
  calcificans congenita 756.59
  fetalis hypoplastica 756.59
  hypoplastica calcinosa 756.59
  punctata 756.59
  tarda 277.5
Chondrodystrophy (familial) (hypoplastic) 756.4
Chondroectodermal dysplasia 756.55
Chondrolysis 733.99
Chondroma (M9220/0)—*see also* Neoplasm
    cartilage, benign
  juxtacortical (M9221/0)—*see* Neoplasm, bone,
    benign
  periosteal (M9221/0)—*see* Neoplasm, bone,
    benign
Chondromalacia 733.92
  epiglottis (congenital) 748.3
  generalized 733.92
  knee 717.7
  larynx (congenital) 748.3
  localized, except patella 733.92
  patella, patellae 717.7
  systemic 733.92
  tibial plateau 733.92
  trachea (congenital) 748.3

Chondromatosis (M9220/1)—*see* Neoplasm,
  cartilage, uncertain behavior
Chondromyxosarcoma (M9220/3)—*see*
  Neoplasm, cartilage, malignant
Chondro-osteodysplasia (Morquio-Brailsford
  type) 277.5

Chondro-osteodystrophy 277.5
Chondro-osteodystrophy 277.5
Chondro-osteoma (M9210/0)—*see* Neoplasm,
  bone, benign
Chondropathia tuberosa 733.6
Chondrosarcoma (M9220/3)—*see also*
  Neoplasm, cartilage, malignant
  juxtacortical (M9221/3)—*see* Neoplasm, bone,
    malignant
  mesenchymal (M9240/3)—*see* Neoplasm,
    connective tissue, malignant
Chordae tendineae rupture (chronic) 429.5
Chordee (nonvenereal) 607.89
  congenital 752.63
  gonococcal 098.2
Chorditis (fibrinous) (nodosa) (tuberosa) 478.5
Chordoma (M9370/3)—*see* Neoplasm, by site,
  malignant
Chorea (gravis) (minor) (spasmodic) 333.5
  with
    heart involvement—*see* Chorea with
      rheumatic heart disease
    rheumatic heart disease (chronic, inactive, or
      quiescent) (conditions classifiable to
      393-398)—*see also* Rheumatic heart
      condition involved
      active or acute (conditions classifiable to
        391) 392.0
  acute—*see* Chorea, Sydenham's
  apoplectic (*see also* Disease, cerebrovascular,
    acute) 436
  chronic 333.4
  electric 049.8
  gravidarum—*see* Eclampsia, pregnancy
  habit 307.22
  hereditary 333.4
  Huntington's 333.4
  posthemiplegic 344.89
  pregnancy—*see* Eclampsia, pregnancy
  progressive 333.4
    chronic 333.4
    hereditary 333.4
  rheumatic (chronic) 392.9
    with heart disease or involvement—*see*
      Chorea, with rheumatic heart disease
  senile 333.5
  Sydenham's 392.9
    with heart involvement—*see* Chorea, with
      rheumatic heart disease
    nonrheumatic 333.5
  variabilis 307.23
Choreoathetosis (paroxysmal) 333.5
Chorioadenoma (destruens) (M9100/1) 236.1
Chorioamnionitis 658.4
  affecting fetus or newborn 762.7
Chorioangioma (M9120/0) 219.8
Choriocarcinoma (M9100/3)
  combined with
    embryonal carcinoma (M9101/3)—*see*
      Neoplasm, by site, malignant
    teratoma (M9101/3)—*see* Neoplasm, by site,
      malignant
  specified site—*see* Neoplasm, by site, malignant

Choriocarcinoma—*continued*
  unspecified site
    female 181
    male 186.9
Chorioencephalitis, lymphocytic (acute)
  (serous) 049.0
Chorioepithelioma (M9100/3)—*see*
  Choriocarcinoma
Choriomeningitis (acute) (benign) (lymphocytic)
  (serous) 049.0
Chorionepithelioma (M9100/3)—*see*
  Choriocarcinoma
Chorionitis (*see also* Scleroderma) 710.1
Chorioretinitis 363.20
  disseminated 363.10
    generalized 363.13
    in
      neurosyphilis 094.83
      secondary syphilis 091.51
    peripheral 363.12
    posterior pole 363.11
    tuberculous (*see also* Tuberculosis) 017.3
      [363.13]
  due to
    histoplasmosis (*see also* Histoplasmosis)
      115.92
    toxoplasmosis (acquired) 130.2
      congenital (active) 771.2
  focal 363.00
    juxtapapillary 363.01
    peripheral 363.04
    posterior pole NEC 363.03
  juxtapapillaris, juxtapapillary 363.01
  progressive myopia (degeneration) 360.21
  syphilitic (secondary) 091.51
    congenital (early) 090.0 *[363.13]*
      late 090.5 *[363.13]*
    late 095.8 *[363.13]*
  tuberculous (*see also* Tuberculosis) 017.3
    [363.13]
Choristoma —*see* Neoplasm, by site, benign
Choroid —*see* condition
Choroideremia, choroidermia (initial stage)
  (late stage) (partial or total atrophy) 363.55
Choroiditis (*see also* Chorioretinitis) 363.20
  leprous 030.9 *[363.13]*
  senile guttate 363.41
  sympathetic 360.11
  syphilitic (secondary) 091.51
    congenital (early) 090.0 *[363.13]*
      late 090.5 *[363.13]*
    late 095.8 *[363.13]*
  Tay's 363.41
  tuberculous (*see also* Tuberculosis) 017.3
    [363.13]
Choroidopathy NEC 363.9
  degenerative (*see also* Degeneration, choroid)
    363.40
  hereditary (*see also* Dystrophy, choroid) 363.50
  specified type NEC 363.8
Choroidoretinitis —*see* Chorioretinitis
Choroidosis, central serous 362.41
Choroidretinopathy, serous 362.41
Christian's syndrome (chronic histiocytosis X)
  277.8
Christian-Weber disease (nodular
  nonsuppurative panniculitis) 729.30
Christmas disease 286.1
Chromaffinoma (M8700/0)—*see also*
  Neoplasm, by site, benign
  malignant (M8700/3)—*see* Neoplasm, by site,
    malignant

Closure—*continued*
congenital 743.65
neonatal 375.55
nose (congenital) 748.0
acquired 738.0
vagina 623.2
valve—*see* Endocarditis
vulva 624.8
Clot (blood)
artery (obstruction) (occlusion) (*see also* Embolism) 444.9
bladder 596.7
brain (extradural or intradural) (*see also* Thrombosis, brain) 434.0
late effect—*see* Late effect(s) (of) cerebrovascular disease
circulation 444.9
heart (*see also* Infarct, myocardium) 410.9
vein (*see also* Thrombosis) 453.9
Clotting defect NEC (*see also* Defect, coagulation) 286.9
Clouded state 780.09
epileptic (*see also* Epilepsy) 345.9
paroxysmal (idiopathic) (*see also* Epilepsy) 345.9
Clouding
corneal graft 996.51
Cloudy
antrum, antra 473.0
dialysis effluent 792.5
Clouston's (hidrotic) ectodermal dysplasia 757.31
Clubbing of fingers 781.5
Clubfinger 736.29
acquired 736.29
congenital 754.89
Clubfoot (congenital) 754.70
acquired 736.71
equinovarus 754.51
paralytic 736.71
Club hand (congenital) 754.89
acquired 736.07
Clubnail (acquired) 703.8
congenital 757.5
Clump kidney 753.3
Clumsiness 781.3
syndrome 315.4
Cluttering 307.0
Clutton's joints 090.5
Coagulation, intravascular (diffuse) (disseminated) (*see also* Fibrinolysis) 286.6
newborn 776.2
Coagulopathy (*see also* Defect, coagulation) 286.9
consumption 286.6
intravascular (disseminated) NEC 286.6
newborn 776.2
Coalition
calcaneoscaphoid 755.67
calcaneus 755.67
tarsal 755.67
Coal miners'
elbow 727.2
lung 500
Coal workers' lung or pneumoconiosis 500
Coarctation
aorta (postductal) (preductal) 747.10
pulmonary artery 747.3
Coated tongue 529.3
Coats' disease 362.12
Cocainism (*see also* Dependence) 304.2
Coccidioidal granuloma 114.3

Coccidioidomycosis 114.9
with pneumonia 114.0
cutaneous (primary) 114.1
disseminated 114.3
extrapulmonary (primary) 114.1
lung 114.5
acute 114.0
chronic 114.4
primary 114.0
meninges 114.2
primary (pulmonary) 114.0
acute 114.0
prostate 114.3
pulmonary 114.5
acute 114.0
chronic 114.4
primary 114.0
specified site NEC 114.3
Coccidioidosis 114.9
lung 114.5
acute 114.0
chronic 114.4
primary 114.0
meninges 114.2
Coccidiosis (colitis) (diarrhea) (dysentery) 007.2
Cocciuria 791.9
Coccus in urine 791.9
Coccydynia 724.79
Coccygodynia 724.79
Coccyx —*see* condition
Cochin-China
diarrhea 579.1
anguilluliasis 127.2
ulcer 085.1
Cock's peculiar tumor 706.2
Cockayne's disease or syndrome (microcephaly and dwarfism) 759.89
Cockayne-Weber syndrome (epidermolysis bullosa) 757.39
Cocked-up toe 735.2
Codman's tumor (benign chondroblastoma) (M9230/0)—*see* Neoplasm, bone, benign
Coenurosis 123.8
Coffee workers' lung 495.8
Cogan's syndrome 370.52
congenital oculomotor apraxia 379.51
nonsyphilitic interstitial keratitis 370.52
Coiling, umbilical cord —*see* Complications, umbilical cord
Coitus, painful (female) 625.0
male 608.89
psychogenic 302.76
Cold 460
with influenza, flu, or grippe 487.1
abscess—*see also* Tuberculosis, abscess
articular—*see* Tuberculosis, joint
agglutinin
disease (chronic) or syndrome 283.0
hemoglobinuria 283.0
paroxysmal (cold) (nocturnal) 283.2
allergic (*see also* Fever, hay) 477.9
bronchus or chest—*see* Bronchitis
with grippe or influenza 487.1
common (head) 460
vaccination, prophylactic (against) V04.7
deep 464.10
effects of 991.9
specified effect NEC 991.8
excessive 991.9
specified effect NEC 991.8
exhaustion from 991.8

Cold —*continued*
  exposure to 991.9
    specified effect NEC 991.8
  grippy 487.1
  head 460
  injury syndrome (newborn) 778.2
  intolerance 780.99
  on lung—*see* Bronchitis
  rose 477.0
  sensitivity, autoimmune 283.0
  virus 460
Coldsore (*see also* Herpes, simplex) 054.9
Colibacillosis 041.4
  generalized 038.42
Colibacilluria 791.9
Colic (recurrent) 789.0
  abdomen 789.0
    (recurrent)psychogenic 307.89
  appendicular 543.9
  appendix 543.9
  bile duct—*see* Choledocholithiasis
  biliary—*see* Cholelithiasis
  bilious—*see* Cholelithiasis
  common duct—*see* Choledocholithiasis
  Devonshire NEC 984.9
    specified type of lead—*see* Table of drugs and
      chemicals
  flatulent 787.3
  gallbladder or gallstone—*see* Cholelithiasis
  gastric 536.8
  hepatic (duct)—*see* Choledocholithiasis
  hysterical 300.11
  infantile 789.0
  intestinal 789.0
  kidney 788.0
  lead NEC 984.9
    specified type of lead—*see* Table of drugs and
      chemicals
  liver (duct)—*see* Choledocholithiasis
  mucous 564.9
    psychogenic 316 *[564.9]*
  nephritic 788.0
  painter's NEC 984.9
  pancreas 577.8
  psychogenic 306.4
  renal 788.0
  saturnine NEC 984.9
    specified type of lead—*see* Table of drugs and
      chemicals
  spasmodic 789.0
  ureter 788.0
  urethral 599.84
    due to calculus 594.2
  uterus 625.8
    menstrual 625.3
  vermicular 543.9
  virus 460
  worm NEC 128.9
Colicystitis (*see also* Cystitis) 595.9
Colitis (acute) (catarrhal) (croupous) (cystica
  superficialis) (exudative) (hemorrhagic)
  (noninfectious) (phlegmonous) (presumed
  noninfectious) 558.9
  adaptive 564.9
  allergic 558.3
  amebic (*see also* Amebiasis) 006.9
    nondysenteric 006.2
  anthrax 022.2
  bacillary (*see also* Infection, Shigella) 004.9
  balantidial 007.0
  chronic 558.9

Colitis—*continued*
  ulcerative (*see also* Colitis, ulcerative) 556.9
  coccidial 007.2
  dietetic 558.9
  due to radiation 558.1
  functional 558.9
  gangrenous 009.0
  giardial 007.1
  granulomatous 555.1
  gravis (*see also* Colitis, ulcerative) 556.9
  infectious (*see also* Enteritis, due to, specific
    organism) 009.0
    presumed 009.1
  ischemic 557.9
    acute 557.0
    chronic 557.1
    due to mesenteric artery insufficiency 557.1
  membranous 564.9
    psychogenic 316 *[564.9]*
  mucous 564.9
    psychogenic 316 *[564.9]*
  necrotic 009.0
  polyposa (*see also* Colitis, ulcerative) 556.9
  protozoal NEC 007.9
  pseudomembranous 008.45
  pseudomucinous 564.9
  regional 555.1
  segmental 555.1
  septic (*see also* Enteritis, due to, specific
    organism) 009.0
  spastic 564.9
    psychogenic 316 *[564.9]*
  staphylococcus 008.41
    food 005.0
  thromboulcerative 557.0
  toxic 558.2
  transmural 555.1
  trichomonal 007.3
  tuberculous (ulcerative) 014.8
  ulcerative (chronic) (idiopathic) (nonspecific)
    556.9
    entero- 556.0
    fulminant 557.0
    ileo- 556.1
    left-sided 556.5
    procto- 556.2
    proctosigmoid 556.3
    psychogenic 316 *[556]*
    specified NEC 556.8
    universal 556.6
Collagen disease NEC 710.9
  nonvascular 710.9
  vascular (allergic) (*see also* Angiitis,
    hypersensitivity) 446.20
Collagenosis (*see also* Collagen disease) 710.9
  cardiovascular 425.4
  mediastinal 519.3
Collapse 780.2
  adrenal 255.8
  cardiorenal (*see also* Hypertension, cardiorenal)
    404.90
  cardiorespiratory 785.51
    fetus or newborn 779.89
  cardiovascular (*see also* Disease, heart) 785.51
    fetus or newborn 779.89
  circulatory (peripheral) 785.59
    with
      abortion—*see* Abortion, by type, with shock
      ectopic pregnancy (*see also* categories
        633.0-633.9) 639.5

Collapse—*continued*
>> molar pregnancy (*see also* categories
>>> 630-632) 639.5
>> during or after labor and delivery 669.1
>> fetus or newborn 779.89
>> following
>>> abortion 639.5
>>> ectopic or molar pregnancy 639.5
> during or after labor and delivery 669.1
>> fetus or newborn 779.89
> external ear canal 380.50
>> secondary to
>>> inflammation 380.53
>>> surgery 380.52
>>> trauma 380.51
> general 780.2
> heart—*see* Disease, heart
> heat 992.1
> hysterical 300.11
> labyrinth, membranous (congenital) 744.05
> lung (massive) (*see also* Atelectasis) 518.0
>> pressure, during labor 668.0
> myocardial—*see* Disease, heart
> nervous (*see also* Disorder, mental,
>> nonpsychotic) 300.9
> neurocirculatory 306.2
> nose 738.0
> postoperative (cardiovascular) 998.0
> pulmonary (*see also* Atelectasis) 518.0
>> fetus or newborn 770.5
>>> partial 770.5
>>> primary 770.4
> thorax 512.8
>> iatrogenic 512.1
>> postoperative 512.1
> trachea 519.1
> valvular—*see* Endocarditis
> vascular (peripheral) 785.59
>> with
>>> abortion—*see* Abortion, by type, with shock
>>> ectopic pregnancy (*see also* categories
>>>> 633.0-633.9) 639.5
>>> molar pregnancy (*see also* categories
>>>> 630-632) 639.5
>> cerebral (*see also* Disease, cerebrovascular,
>>> acute) 436
>> during or after labor and delivery 669.1
>> fetus or newborn 779.89
>> following
>>> abortion 639.5
>>> ectopic or molar pregnancy 639.5
> vasomotor 785.59
> vertebra 733.13
Collateral —*see also* condition
> circulation (venous) 459.89
> dilation, veins 459.89
Colles' fracture (closed) (reversed) (separation)
> 813.41
> open 813.51
Collet's syndrome 352.6
Collet-Sicard syndrome 352.6
Colliculitis urethralis (*see also* Urethritis) 597.89
Colliers'
> asthma 500
> lung 500
> phthisis (*see also* Tuberculosis) 011.4
Collodion baby (ichthyosis congenita) 757.1
Colloid milium 709.3

Coloboma NEC 743.49
> choroid 743.59
> fundus 743.52
> iris 743.46
> lens 743.36
> lids 743.62
> optic disc (congenital) 743.57
>> acquired 377.23
> retina 743.56
> sclera 743.47
Coloenteritis —*see* Enteritis
Colon —*see* condition
Coloptosis 569.89
Color
> amblyopia NEC 368.59
>> acquired 368.55
> blindness NEC (congenital) 368.59
>> acquired 368.55
Colostomy
> attention to V55.3
> fitting or adjustment V53.5
> malfunctioning 569.62
> status V44.3
Colpitis (*see also* Vaginitis) 616.10
Colpocele 618.6
Colpocystitis (*see also* Vaginitis) 616.10
Colporrhexis 665.4
Colpospasm 625.1
Column, spinal, vertebral —*see* condition
Coma 780.01
> apoplectic (*see also* Disease, cerebrovascular,
>> acute) 436
> diabetic (with ketoacidosis) 250.3
>> hyperosmolar 250.2
> eclamptic (*see also* Eclampsia) 780.39
> epileptic 345.3
> hepatic 572.2
> hyperglycemic 250.2
> hyperosmolar (diabetic) (nonketotic) 250.2
> hypoglycemic 251.0
>> diabetic 250.3
> insulin 250.3
>> hyperosmolar 250.2
>> non-diabetic 251.0
>> organic hyperinsulinism 251.0
> Kussmaul's (diabetic) 250.3
> liver 572.2
> newborn 779.2
> prediabetic 250.2
> uremic—*see* Uremia
Combat fatigue (*see also* Reaction, stress, acute)
> 308.9
Combined —*see* condition
Comedo 706.1
Comedocarcinoma (M8501/3)—*see also*
> Neoplasm, breast, malignant
> noninfiltrating (M8501/2)
>> specified site—*see* Neoplasm, by site, in situ
>> unspecified site 233.0
Comedomastitis 610.4
Comedones 706.1
> lanugo 757.4
Comma bacillus, carrier (suspected) of V02.3
Comminuted fracture —*see* Fracture, by site
Common
> aortopulmonary trunk 745.0
> atrioventricular canal (defect) 745.69
> atrium 745.69
> cold (head) 460
>> vaccination, prophylactic (against) V04.7
> truncus (arteriosus) 745.0
> ventricle 745.3

Commotio (current)
   cerebri (*see also* Concussion, brain) 850.9
      with skull fracture—*see* Fracture, skull, by site
   retinae 921.3
   spinalis—*see* Injury, spinal, by site
Commotion (current)
   brain (without skull fracture) (*see also*
      Concussion, brain) 850.9
      with skull fracture—*see* Fracture, skull, by site
   spinal cord—*see* Injury, spinal, by site
Communication
   abnormal—*see also* Fistula
     between
       base of aorta and pulmonary artery 745.0
       left ventricle and right atrium 745.4
       pericardial sac and pleural sac 748.8
       pulmonary artery and pulmonary vein 747.3
     congenital, between uterus and anterior
       abdominal wall 752.3
      bladder 752.3
      intestine 752.3
      rectum 752.3
   left ventricular-right atrial 745.4
   pulmonary artery-pulmonary vein 747.3
Compensation
   broken—*see* Failure, heart
   failure—*see* Failure, heart
   neurosis, psychoneurosis 300.11
Complaint —*see also* Disease
   bowel, functional 564.9
     psychogenic 306.4
   intestine, functional 564.9
     psychogenic 306.4
   kidney (*see also* Disease, renal) 593.9
   liver 573.9
   miners' 500
Complete —*see* condition
Complex
   cardiorenal (*see also* Hypertension, cardiorenal)
     404.90
   castration 300.9
   Costen's 524.60
   ego-dystonic homosexuality 302.0
   Eisenmenger's (ventricular septal defect) 745.4
   homosexual, ego-dystonic 302.0
   hypersexual 302.89
   inferiority 301.9
   jumped process
     spine—*see* Dislocation, vertebra
   primary, tuberculosis (*see also* Tuberculosis)
     010.0
   Taussig-Bing (transposition, aorta and
     overriding pulmonary artery) 745.11
Complications
   abortion NEC—*see* categories 634-639
   accidental puncture or laceration during a
     procedure 998.2
   amputation stump (late) (surgical) 997.60
     traumatic—*see* Amputation, traumatic
   anastomosis (and bypass)—*see also*
     Complications, due to (presence of) any
     device, implant, or graft classified to
     996.0-996.5 NEC
     hemorrhage NEC 998.11
     intestinal (internal) NEC 997.4
      involving urinary tract 997.5
     mechanical—*see* Complications, mechanical,
      graft
     urinary tract (involving intestinal tract) 997.5
   anesthesia, anesthetic NEC (*see also*
     Anesthesia, complication) 995.2

Complications—*continued*
   in labor and delivery 668.9
     affecting fetus or newborn 763.5
     cardiac 668.1
     central nervous system 668.2
     pulmonary 668.0
     specified type NEC 668.8
   aortocoronary (bypass) graft 996.03
     atherosclerosis —*see* Arteriosclerosis,
      coronary
     embolism 996.72
     occlusion NEC 996.72
     thrombus 996.72
   arthroplasty 996.4
   artificial opening
     cecostomy 569.60
     colostomy 569.6
     cystostomy 997.5
     enterostomy 569.60
     gastrostomy 536.40
     ileostomy 569.60
     jejunostomy 569.60
     nephrostomy 997.5
     tracheostomy 519.00
     ureterostomy 997.5
     urethrostomy 997.5
   bile duct implant (prosthetic) NEC 996.79
     infection or inflammation 996.69
     mechanical 996.59
   bleeding (intraoperative) (postoperative) 998.11
   blood vessel graft 996.1
     aortocoronary 996.03
      atherosclerosis —*see* Arteriosclerosis,
       coronary
      embolism 996.72
      occlusion NEC 996.72
      thrombus 996.72
     atherosclerosis —*see* Arteriosclerosis,
      extremities
     embolism 996.74
     occlusion NEC 996.74
     thrombus 996.74
   bone growth stimulator NEC 996.78
     infection or inflammation 996.67
   bone marrow transplant 996.85
   breast implant (prosthetic) NEC 996.79
     infection or inflammation 996.69
     mechanical 996.54
   bypass—*see also* Complications, anastomosis
     aortocoronary 996.03
      atherosclerosis —*see* Arteriosclerosis,
       coronary
      embolism 996.72
      occlusion NEC 996.72
      thrombus 996.72
     carotid artery 996.1
      atherosclerosis —*see* Arteriosclerosis,
       extremities
      embolism 996.74
      occlusion NEC 996.74
      thrombus 996.74
   cardiac (*see also* Disease, heart) 429.9
     device, implant, or graft NEC 996.72
      infection or inflammation 996.61
      long-term effect 429.4
       mechanical (*see also* Complications,
        mechanical, by type) 996.00
       valve prosthesis 996.71
        infection or inflammation 996.61
     postoperative NEC 997.1
      long-term effect 429.4

Complications—*continued*
  bone marrow 996.85
  corneal NEC 996.79
    infection or inflammation 996.69
    rejection or reaction 996.51
  mechanical—*see* Complications, mechanical,
      graft
  organ (immune or nonimmune cause) (partial)
      (total) 996.80
    bone marrow 996.85
    heart 996.83
    intestines 996.87
    kidney 996.81
    liver 996.82
    lung 996.84
    pancreas 996.86
    specified NEC 996.89
  skin NEC 996.79
    infection or inflammation 996.69
    rejection 996.52
      artificial 996.55
      decellularized allodermis 996.55
  heart—*see also* Disease, heart
    transplant (immune or nonimmune cause)
        996.83
  hematoma (intraoperative) (postoperative)
      998.12
  hemorrhage (intraoperative) (postoperative)
      998.11
  hyperalimentation therapy NEC 999.9
  immunization (procedure)—*see* Complications,
      vaccination
  implant—*see also* Complications, due to
      (presence of) any device, implant, or graft
      classified to 996.0-996.5 NEC
    mechanical—*see* Complications, mechanical,
        implant
  infection and inflammation
    due to (presence of) any device, implant, or
        graft classified to 996.0-996.5 NEC 996.60
      arterial NEC 996.62
        coronary 996.61
        renal dialysis 996.62
      arteriovenous fistula or shunt 996.62
      bone growth stimulator 996.67
      breast 996.69
      cardiac 996.61
      catheter NEC 996.69
        peritoneal 996.68
        spinal 996.63
        urinary, indwelling 996.64
        vascular NEC 996.62
        ventricular shunt 996.63
      coronary artery bypass 996.61
      electrodes
        brain 996.63
        heart 996.61
      gastrointestinal NEC 996.69
      genitourinary NEC 996.65
        indwelling urinary catheter 996.64
      heart valve 996.61
      infusion pump 996.62
      intrauterine contraceptive device 996.65
      joint prosthesis, internal 996.66
      ocular lens 996.69
      orbital (implant) 996.69
      orthopedic NEC 996.67
        joint, internal 996.66
      specified type NEC 996.69
      urinary catheter, indwelling 996.64
      ventricular shunt 996.63

Complications—*continued*
  infusion (procedure) 999.9
    blood—*see* Complications, transfusion
    infection NEC 999.3
    sepsis NEC 999.3
  inhalation therapy NEC 999.9
  injection (procedure) 999.9
    drug reaction (*see also* Reaction, drug) 995.2
    infection NEC 999.3
    sepsis NEC 999.3
    serum (prophylactic) (therapeutic)—*see*
        Complications, vaccination
    vaccine (any)—*see* Complications, vaccination
  inoculation (any)—*see* Complications,
      vaccination
  internal device (catheter) (electronic) (fixation)
      (prosthetic) NEC—*see also* Complications,
      due to (presence of) any device, implant, or
      graft classified to 996.0-996.5 NEC
    mechanical—*see* Complications, mechanical
  intestinal transplant (immune or nonimmune
      cause) 996.87
  intraoperative bleeding or hemorrhage 998.11
  intrauterine contraceptive device (*see also*
      Complications, contraceptive device) 996.76
    infection or inflammation 996.65
    with fetal damage affecting management of
        pregnancy 655.8
  jejunostomy 569.60
  kidney transplant (immune or nonimmune
      cause) 996.81
  labor 669.9
    specified condition NEC 669.8
  liver transplant (immune or nonimmune cause)
      996.82
  lumbar puncture 349.0
  mechanical
    anastomosis—*see* Complications, mechanical,
        graft
    bypass—*see* Complications, mechanical, graft
    catheter NEC 996.59
      cardiac 996.09
      cystostomy 996.39
      dialysis (hemodialysis) 996.1
        peritoneal 996.56
      during a procedure 998.2
      urethral, indwelling 996.31
    colostomy 569.62
    device NEC 996.59
      balloon (counterpulsation), intra-aortic 996.1
      cardiac 996.00
        automatic implantable defibrillator 996.04
        long-term effect 429.4
        specified NEC 996.09
      contraceptive, intrauterine 996.32
      counterpulsation, intra-aortic 996.1
      fixation, external, with internal components
          996.4
      fixation, internal (nail, rod, plate) 996.4
      genitourinary 996.30
        specified NEC 996.39
      nervous system 996.2
      orthopedic, internal 996.4
      prosthetic NEC 996.59
      umbrella, vena cava 996.1
      vascular 996.1
    dorsal column stimulator 996.2
    electrode NEC 996.59
      brain 996.2
      cardiac 996.01
      spinal column 996.2

Complications—*continued*
  mechanical NEC (*see also* Complications, mechanical) 996.59
  puerperium NEC (*see also* Puerperal) 674.9
  puncture, spinal 349.0
  pyelogram 997.5
  radiation 990
  radiotherapy 990
  reattached
    body part, except extremity 996.99
    extremity (infection) (rejection) 996.90
      arm(s) 996.94
      digit(s) (hand) 996.93
        foot 996.95
      finger(s) 996.93
      foot 996.95
      forearm 996.91
      hand 996.92
      leg 996.96
      lower NEC 996.96
      toe(s) 996.95
      upper NEC 996.94
  reimplant—*see also* Complications, due to (presence of) any device, implant, or graft classified to 996.0-996.5 NEC
    bone marrow 996.85
    extremity (*see also* Complications, reattached, extremity) 996.90
    due to infection 996.90
    mechanical—*see* Complications, mechanical, reimplant
    organ (immune or nonimmune cause) (partial) (total) (*see also* Complications, transplant, organ, by site) 996.80
  renal allograft 996.81
  renal dialysis—*see* Complications, dialysis
  respiratory 519.9
    device, implant or graft NEC 996.79
      infection or inflammation 996.69
      mechanical 996.59
    distress syndrome, adult, following trauma or surgery 518.5
    insufficiency, acute, postoperative 518.5
    postoperative NEC 997.3
    therapy NEC 999.9
  sedation during labor and delivery 668.9
    affecting fetus or newborn 763.5
    cardiac 668.1
    central nervous system 668.2
    pulmonary 668.0
    specified type NEC 668.8
  seroma (intraoperative) (postoperative) (noninfected) 998.13
    infected 998.51
  shunt—*see also* Complications, due to (presence of) any device, implant, or graft classified to 996.0-996.5 NEC
    mechanical—*see* Complications, mechanical, shunt
  specified body system NEC
    device, implant, or graft—*see* Complications, due to (presence of) any device, implant, or graft classified to 996.0-996.5 NEC
    postoperative NEC 997.99
  spinal puncture or tap 349.0
  stoma, external
    gastrointestinal tract
      colostomy 569.60
      enterostomy 569.60
      gastrostomy 536.40
    urinary tract 997.5

Complications—*continued*
  surgical procedures 998.9
    accidental puncture or laceration 998.2
    amputation stump (late) 997.60
    anastomosis—*see* Complications, anastomosis
    burst stitches or sutures (external) 998.32
      internal 998.31
    cardiac 997.1
      long-term effect following cardiac surgery 429.4
    cataract fragments in eye 998.82
    catheter device—*see* Complications, catheter device
    cecostomy malfunction 569.62
    colostomy malfunction 569.62
    cystostomy malfunction 997.5
    dehiscence (of incision) (external) 998.32
      internal 998.31
    dialysis NEC (*see also* Complications, dialysis) 999.9
    disruption
      anastomosis (internal)—*see* Complications, mechanical, graft
      internal suture (line) 998.31
      wound (external) 998.32
        internal 998.31
    dumping syndrome (postgastrectomy) 564.2
    elephantiasis or lymphedema 997.99
      postmastectomy 457.0
    emphysema (surgical) 998.81
    enterostomy malfunction 569.62
    evisceration 998.32
    fistula (persistent postoperative) 998.6
    foreign body inadvertently left in wound (sponge) (suture) (swab) 998.4
    from nonabsorbable surgical material (Dacron) (mesh) (permanent suture) (reinforcing) (Teflon)—*see* Complications, due to (presence of) any device, implant, or graft classified to 996.0-996.5 NEC
    gastrointestinal NEC 997.4
    gastrostomy malfunction 536.42
    hematoma 998.12
    hemorrhage 998.11
    ileostomy malfunction 569.62
    internal prosthetic device NEC (*see also* Complications, internal device) 996.70
      hemolytic anemia 283.19
      infection or inflammation 996.60
      malfunction—*see* Complications, mechanical
      mechanical complication—*see* Complications, mechanical
      thrombus 996.70
    jejunostomy malfunction 569.62
    nervous system NEC 997.00
    obstruction, internal anastomosis—*see* Complications, mechanical, graft
    other body system NEC 997.99
    peripheral vascular NEC 997.2
    postcardiotomy syndrome 429.4
    postcholecystectomy syndrome 576.0
    postcommissurotomy syndrome 429.4
    postgastrectomy dumping syndrome 564.2
    postmastectomy lymphedema syndrome 457.0
    postmastoidectomy 383.30
      cholesteatoma, recurrent 383.32
      cyst, mucosal 383.31
      granulation 383.33
      inflammation, chronic 383.33

Concretion—*continued*
  intestine (impaction) (obstruction) 560.39
  lacrimal (passages) 375.57
  prepuce (male) 605
    female (clitoris) 624.8
  salivary gland (any) 527.5
  seminal vesicle 608.89
  stomach 537.89
  tonsil 474.8
Concussion (current) 850.9
  with
    loss of consciousness 850.5
      brief (less than one hour) 850.1
      moderate (1-24 hours) 850.2
      prolonged (more than 24 hours) (with
          complete recovery) (with return to
          pre-existing conscious level) 850.3
        without return to pre-existing conscious
          level 850.4
    mental confusion or disorientation (without
        loss of consciousness) 850.0
      with loss of consciousness—*see*
          Concussion, with, loss of consciousness
  without loss of consciousness 850.0
  blast (air) (hydraulic) (immersion) (underwater)
      869.0
    with open wound into cavity 869.1
    abdomen or thorax—*see* Injury, internal, by
      site
    brain—*see* Concussion, brain
    ear (acoustic nerve trauma) 951.5
      with perforation, tympanic membrane—*see*
          Wound, open, ear drum
    thorax—*see* Injury, internal, intrathoracic
      organs NEC
  brain or cerebral (without skull fracture) 850.9
    with
      loss of consciousness 850.5
        brief (less than one hour) 850.1
        moderate (1-24 hours) 850.2
        prolonged (more than 24 hours) (with
            complete recovery) (with return to
            pre-existing conscious level) 850.3
          without return to pre-existing conscious
            level 850.4
      mental confusion or disorientation (without
          loss of consciousness) 850.0
        with loss of consciousness—*see*
            Concussion, brain, with, loss of
            consciousness
      skull fracture—*see* Fracture, skull, by site
    without loss of consciousness 850.0
  cauda equina 952.4
  cerebral—*see* Concussion, brain
  conus medullaris (spine) 952.4
  hydraulic—*see* Concussion, blast
  internal organs—*see* Injury, internal, by site
  labyrinth—*see* Injury, intracranial
  ocular 921.3
  osseous labyrinth—*see* Injury, intracranial
  spinal (cord)—*see also* Injury, spinal, by site
    due to
      broken
        back—*see* Fracture, vertebra, by site, with
          spinal cord injury
        neck—*see* Fracture, vertebra, cervical,
          with spinal cord injury
      fracture, fracture dislocation, or
          compression fracture of spine or
          vertebra—*see* Fracture, vertebra, by site,
          with spinal cord injury

Concussion—*continued*
  syndrome 310.2
  underwater blast—*see* Concussion, blast
Condition —*see also* Disease
  psychiatric 298.9
  respiratory NEC 519.9
    acute or subacute NEC 519.9
      due to
        external agent 508.9
          specified type NEC 508.8
        fumes or vapors (chemical) (inhalation)
          506.3
        radiation 508.0
    chronic NEC 519.9
      due to
        external agent 508.9
          specified type NEC 508.8
        fumes or vapors (chemical) (inhalation)
          506.4
        radiation 508.1
    due to
      external agent 508.9
        specified type NEC 508.8
      fumes or vapors (chemical) (inhalation)
        506.9
Conduct disturbance (*see also* Disturbance,
    conduct) 312.9
  adjustment reaction 309.3
  hyperkinetic 314.2
Condyloma NEC 078.10
  acuminatum 078.11
  gonorrheal 098.0
  latum 091.3
  syphilitic 091.3
    congenital 090.0
  venereal, syphilitic 091.3
Confinement —*see* Delivery
Conflagration —*see also* Burn, by site
  asphyxia (by inhalation of smoke, gases, fumes,
      or vapors) 987.9
    specified agent—*see* Table of drugs and
      chemicals
Conflict
  family V61.9
    specified circumstance NEC V61.8
  interpersonal NEC V62.81
  marital V61.10
    involving divorce or estrangement V61.0
  parent-child V61.20
  partner V61.10
Confluent —*see* condition
Confusion, confused (mental) (state) (*see also*
    State, confusional) 298.9
  acute 293.0
  epileptic 293.0
  postoperative 293.9
  psychogenic 298.2
  reactive (from emotional stress, psychological
      trauma) 298.2
  subacute 293.1
Congelation 991.9
Congenital —*see also* condition
  aortic septum 747.29
  intrinsic factor deficiency 281.0
  malformation—*see* Anomaly
Congestion, congestive (chronic) (passive)
  asphyxia, newborn 768.9
  bladder 596.8
  bowel 569.89
  brain (*see also* Disease, cerebrovascular NEC)
    437.8

Conjunctivitis—*continued*
  of Beal 077.3
  parasitic 372.15
    filariasis (*see also* Filariasis) 125.9 *[372.15]*
    mucocutaneous leishmaniasis 085.5 *[372.15]*
  Parinaud's 372.02
  petrificans 372.39
  phlyctenular 370.31
  pseudomembranous 372.04
    diphtheritic 032.81
  purulent 372.03
  Reiter's 099.3 *[372.33]*
  rosacea 695.3 *[372.31]*
  serous 372.01
    viral 077.99
  simple chronic 372.11
  specified NEC 372.39
  sunlamp 372.04
  swimming pool 077.0
  trachomatous (follicular) 076.1
    acute 076.0
    late effect 139.1
  traumatic NEC 372.39
  tuberculous (*see also* Tuberculosis) 017.3
    [370.31]
  tularemic 021.3
  tularensis 021.3
  vernal 372.13
    limbar 372.13 *[370.32]*
  viral 077.99
    acute hemorrhagic 077.4
    specified NEC 077.8
Conjunctivochalasis 372.81
Conjunctoblepharitis —*see* Conjunctivitis
Conn (-Louis) syndrome (primary aldosteronism)
    255.1
Connective tissue —*see* condition
Conradi (-Hünermann) syndrome or disease
    (chondrodysplasia calcificans congenita)
    756.59
Consanguinity V19.7
Consecutive —*see* condition
Consolidated lung (base)—*see* Pneumonia, lobar
Constipation 564.00
  atonic 564.09
  drug induced
    correct substance properly administered
      564.09
    overdose or wrong substance given or taken
      977.9
      specified drug—*see* Table of drugs and
        chemicals
  neurogenic 564.09
  other specified NEC 564.09
  outlet dysfunction 564.02
  psychogenic 306.4
  simple 564.00
  slow transit 564.01
  spastic 564.09
Constitutional —*see also* condition
  arterial hypotension (*see also* Hypotension)
    458.9
  obesity 278.00
    morbid 278.01
  psychopathic state 301.9
  short stature in childhood 783.43
  state, developmental V21.9
    specified development NEC V21.8
  substandard 301.6
Constitutionally substandard 301.6

Constriction
  anomalous, meningeal bands or folds 742.8
  aortic arch (congenital) 747.10
  asphyxiation or suffocation by 994.7
  bronchus 519.1
  canal, ear (*see also* Stricture, ear canal,
    acquired) 380.50
  duodenum 537.3
  gallbladder (*see also* Obstruction, gallbladder)
    575.2
    congenital 751.69
  intestine (*see also* Obstruction, intestine) 560.9
  larynx 478.74
    congenital 748.3
  meningeal bands or folds, anomalous 742.8
  organ or site, congenital NEC—*see* Atresia
  prepuce (congenital) 605
  pylorus 537.0
    adult hypertrophic 537.0
    congenital or infantile 750.5
    newborn 750.5
  ring (uterus) 661.4
    affecting fetus or newborn 763.7
  spastic—*see also* Spasm
    ureter 593.3
    urethra—*see* Stricture, urethra
  stomach 537.89
  ureter 593.3
  urethra—*see* Stricture, urethra
  visual field (functional) (peripheral) 368.45
Constrictive —*see* condition
Consultation V65.9
  medical—*see also* Counseling, medical
  specified reason NEC V65.8
  without complaint or sickness V65.9
    feared complaint unfounded V65.5
    specified reason NEC V65.8
Consumption —*see* Tuberculosis
Contact
  with
    AIDS virus V01.7
    anthrax V01.81
    cholera V01.0
    communicable disease V01.9
      specified type NEC V01.89
      viral NEC V01.7
    German measles V01.4
    gonorrhea V01.6
    HIV V01.7
    human immunodeficiency virus V01.7
    parasitic disease NEC V01.89
    poliomyelitis V01.2
    rabies V01.5
    rubella V01.4
    smallpox V01.3
    syphilis V01.6
    tuberculosis V01.1
    venereal disease V01.6
    viral disease NEC V01.7
  dermatitis—*see* Dermatitis
Contamination, food (*see also* Poisoning, food)
    005.9
Contraception, contraceptive
  advice NEC V25.09
    family planning V25.09
    fitting of diaphragm V25.02
    prescribing or use of
      oral contraceptive agent V25.01
      specified agent NEC V25.02
  counseling NEC V25.09
    family planning V25.09

Contraception, contraceptive—*continued*
   fitting of diaphragm V25.02
     prescribing or use of
       oral contraceptive agent V25.01
       specified agent NEC V25.02
   device (in situ) V45.59
     causing menorrhagia 996.76
     checking V25.42
     complications 996.32
     insertion V25.1
     intrauterine V45.51
     reinsertion V25.42
     removal V25.42
     subdermal V45.52
   fitting of diaphragm V25.02
   insertion
     intrauterine contraceptive device V25.1
     subdermal implantable V25.5
   maintenance V25.40
     examination V25.40
       intrauterine device V25.42
       oral contraceptive V25.41
        specified method NEC V25.49
        subdermal implantable V25.43
     intrauterine device V25.42
     oral contraceptive V25.41
     specified method NEC V25.49
     subdermal implantable V25.43
   management NEC V25.49
   prescription
     oral contraceptive agent V25.01
       repeat V25.41
     specified agent NEC V25.02
       repeat V25.49
   sterilization V25.2
   surveillance V25.40
     intrauterine device V25.42
     oral contraceptive agent V25.41
     specified method NEC V25.49
     subdermal implantable V25.43

Contraction, contracture, contracted
   Achilles tendon (*see also* Short, tendon,
     Achilles) 727.81
   anus 564.89
   axilla 729.9
   bile duct (*see also* Disease, biliary) 576.8
   bladder 596.8
     neck or sphincter 596.0
   bowel (*see also* Obstruction, intestine) 560.9
   Braxton Hicks 644.1
   bronchus 519.1
   burn (old)—*see* Cicatrix
   cecum (*see also* Obstruction, intestine) 560.9
   cervix (*see also* Stricture, cervix) 622.4
     congenital 752.49
   cicatricial—*see* Cicatrix
   colon (*see also* Obstruction, intestine) 560.9
   conjunctiva trachomatous, active 076.1
     late effect 139.1
   Dupuytren's 728.6
   eyelid 374.41
   eye socket (after enucleation) 372.64
   face 729.9
   fascia (lata) (postural) 728.89
     Dupuytren's 728.6
     palmar 728.6
     plantar 728.71
   finger NEC 736.29
     congenital 755.59
     joint (*see also* Contraction, joint) 718.44
   flaccid, paralytic

Contraction—*continued*
    joint (*see also* Contraction, joint) 718.4
    muscle 728.85
     ocular 378.50
   gallbladder (*see also* Obstruction, gallbladder)
     575.2
   hamstring 728.89
    tendon 727.81
   heart valve—*see* Endocarditis
   Hicks' 644.1
   hip (*see also* Contraction, joint) 718.4
   hourglass
    bladder 596.8
     congenital 753.8
    gallbladder (*see also* Obstruction, gallbladder)
     575.2
     congenital 751.69
    stomach 536.8
     congenital 750.7
     psychogenic 306.4
    uterus 661.4
     affecting fetus or newborn 763.7
   hysterical 300.11
   infantile (*see also* Epilepsy) 345.6
   internal os (*see also* Stricture, cervix) 622.4
   intestine (*see also* Obstruction, intestine) 560.9
   joint (abduction) (acquired) (adduction)
     (flexion) (rotation) 718.40
    ankle 718.47
    congenital NEC 755.8
     generalized or multiple 754.89
      lower limb joints 754.89
     hip (*see also* Subluxation, congenital, hip)
      754.32
     lower limb (including pelvic girdle) not
      involving hip 754.89
     upper limb (including shoulder girdle) 755.59
    elbow 718.42
    foot 718.47
    hand 718.44
    hip 718.45
    hysterical 300.11
    knee 718.46
    multiple sites 718.49
    pelvic region 718.45
    shoulder (region) 718.41
    specified site NEC 718.48
    wrist 718.43
   kidney (granular) (secondary) (*see also*
     Sclerosis, renal) 587
    congenital 753.3
    hydronephritic 591
    pyelonephritic (*see also* Pyelitis, chronic)
     590.00
    tuberculous (*see also* Tuberculosis) 016.0
   ligament 728.89
    congenital 756.89
   liver—*see* Cirrhosis, liver
   muscle (postinfectional) (postural) NEC 728.85
    congenital 756.89
     sternocleidomastoid 754.1
    extraocular 378.60
    eye (extrinsic) (*see also* Strabismus) 378.9
     paralytic (*see also* Strabismus, paralytic)
      378.50
    flaccid 728.85
    hysterical 300.11
    ischemic (Volkmann's) 958.6
    paralytic 728.85
    posttraumatic 958.6
    psychogenic 306.0

Note—Use the following fifth-digit subclassification with categories 851-854:

0 unspecified state of consciousness
1 with no loss of consciousness
2 with brief [less than one hour] loss of consciousness
3 with moderate [1-24 hours] loss of consciousness
4 with prolonged [more than 24 hours] loss of consciousness and return to pre-existing conscious level
5 with prolonged [more than 24 hours] loss of consciousness, without return to pre-existing conscious level
Use fifth-digit 5 to designate when a patient is unconscious and dies before regaining conciousness, regardless of the duration of the loss of conciousness
6 with loss of consciousness of unspecified duration
9 with concussion, unspecified

Contusion—*continued*
>with
>>open intracranial wound 851.9
>>skull fracture—*see* Fracture, skull, by site
>cerebellum 851.4
>>with open intracranial wound 851.5
>cortex 851.0
>>with open intracranial wound 851.1
>occipital lobe 851.4
>>with open intracranial wound 851.5
>stem 851.4
>>with open intracranial wound 851.5
>breast 922.0
>brow (and other part(s) of neck, scalp, or face, except eye) 920
>buttock 922.32
>canthus 921.1
>cardiac 861.01
>>with open wound into thorax 861.11
>cauda equina (spine) 952.4
>cerebellum—*see* Contusion, brain, cerebellum
>cerebral—*see* Contusion, brain
>cheek(s) (and other part(s) of neck, scalp, or face, except eye) 920
>chest (wall) 922.1
>chin (and other part(s) of neck, scalp, or face, except eye) 920
>clitoris 922.4
>conjunctiva 921.1
>conus medullaris (spine) 952.4
>cornea 921.3
>corpus cavernosum 922.4
>cortex (brain) (cerebral)—*see* Contusion, brain, cortex
>costal region 922.1
>ear (and other part(s) of neck, scalp, or face except eye) 920
>elbow 923.11
>>with forearm 923.10
>epididymis 922.4
>epigastric region 922.2
>eye NEC 921.9
>eyeball 921.3
>eyelid(s) (and periocular area) 921.1
>face (and neck, or scalp any part, except eye) 920
>femoral triangle 922.2
>fetus or newborn 772.6
>finger(s) (nail) (subungual) 923.3
>flank 922.2
>foot (with ankle) (excluding toe(s)) 924.20
>forearm (and elbow) 923.10
>forehead (and other part(s) of neck, scalp, or face, except eye) 920
>genital organs, external 922.4
>globe (eye) 921.3
>groin 922.2
>gum(s) (and other part(s) of neck, scalp, or face, except eye) 920
>hand(s) (except fingers alone) 923.20
>head (any part, except eye) (and face) (and neck) 920
>heart—*see* Contusion, cardiac
>heel 924.20
>hip 924.01
>>with thigh 924.00
>iliac region 922.2
>inguinal region 922.2
>internal organs (abdomen, chest, or pelvis) NEC—*see* Injury, internal, by site
>interscapular region 922.33

Contusion—*continued*
>iris (eye) 921.3
>kidney 866.01
>>with open wound into cavity 866.11
>knee 924.11
>>with lower leg 924.10
>labium (majus) (minus) 922.4
>lacrimal apparatus, gland, or sac 921.1
>larynx (and other part(s) of neck, scalp, or face, except eye) 920
>late effect—*see* Late, effects (of), contusion
>leg 924.5
>>lower (with knee) 924.10
>lens 921.3
>lingual (and other part(s) of neck, scalp, or face, except eye) 920
>lip(s) (and other part(s) of neck, scalp, or face, except eye) 920
>liver 864.01
>>with
>>>laceration—*see* Laceration, liver
>>>open wound into cavity 864.11
>lower extremity 924.5
>>multiple sites 924.4
>lumbar region 922.31
>lung 861.21
>>with open wound into thorax 861.31
>malar region (and other part(s) of neck, scalp, or face, except eye) 920
>mandibular joint (and other part(s) of neck, scalp, or face, except eye) 920
>mastoid region (and other part(s) of neck, scalp, or face, except eye) 920
>membrane, brain—*see* Contusion, brain
>midthoracic region 922.1
>mouth (and other part(s) of neck, scalp, or face, except eye) 920
>multiple sites (not classifiable to same three-digit category) 924.8
>>lower limb 924.4
>>trunk 922.8
>>upper limb 923.8
>muscle NEC 924.9
>myocardium—*see* Contusion, cardiac
>nasal (septum) (and other part(s) of neck, scalp, or face, except eye) 920
>neck (and scalp, or face any part, except eye) 920
>nerve—*see* Injury, nerve, by site
>continuednose (and other part(s) of neck, scalp, or face, except eye) 920
>occipital region (scalp) (and neck or face, except eye) 920
>>lobe—*see* Contusion, brain, occipital lobe
>orbit (region) (tissues) 921.2
>palate (soft) (and other part(s) of neck, scalp, or face, except eye) 920
>parietal region (scalp) (and neck, or face, except eye) 920
>>lobe—*see* Contusion, brain
>penis 922.4
>pericardium—*see* Contusion, cardiac
>perineum 922.4
>periocular area 921.1
>pharynx (and other part(s) of neck, scalp, or face, except eye) 920
>popliteal space (*see also* Contusion, knee) 924.11
>prepuce 922.4
>pubic region 922.4
>pudenda 922.4

Contusion—*continued*
  pulmonary—*see* Contusion, lung
  quadriceps femoralis 924.00
  rib cage 922.1
  sacral region 922.32
  salivary ducts or glands (and other part(s) of
      neck, scalp, or face, except eye) 920
  scalp (and neck, or face any part, except eye)
      920
  scapular region 923.01
    with shoulder or upper arm 923.09
  sclera (eye) 921.3
  scrotum 922.4
  shoulder 923.00
    with upper arm or axillar regions 923.09
  skin NEC 924.9
  skull 920
  spermatic cord 922.4
  spinal cord—*see also* Injury, spinal, by site
    cauda equina 952.4
    conus medullaris 952.4
  spleen 865.01
    with open wound into cavity 865.11
  sternal region 922.1
  stomach—*see* Injury, internal, stomach
  subconjunctival 921.1
  subcutaneous NEC 924.9
  submaxillary region (and other part(s) of neck,
      scalp, or face, except eye) 920
  submental region (and other part(s) of neck,
      scalp, or face, except eye) 920
  subperiosteal NEC 924.9
  supraclavicular fossa (and other part(s) of neck,
      scalp, or face, except eye) 920
  supraorbital (and other part(s) of neck, scalp, or
      face, except eye) 920
  temple (region) (and other part(s) of neck, scalp,
      or face, except eye) 920
  testis 922.4
  thigh (and hip) 924.00
  thorax 922.1
    organ—*see* Injury, internal, intrathoracic
  throat (and other part(s) of neck, scalp, or face,
      except eye) 920
  thumb(s) (nail) (subungual) 923.3
  toe(s) (nail) (subungual) 924.3
  tongue (and other part(s) of neck, scalp, or face,
      except eye) 920
  trunk 922.9
    multiple sites 922.8
    specified site—*see* Contusion, by site
  tunica vaginalis 922.4
  tympanum (membrane) (and other part(s) of
      neck, scalp, or face, except eye) 920
  upper extremity 923.9
    multiple sites 923.8
  uvula (and other part(s) of neck, scalp, or face,
      except eye) 920
  vagina 922.4
  vocal cord(s) (and other part(s) of neck, scalp,
      or face, except eye) 920
  vulva 922.4
  wrist 923.21
    with hand(s), except finger(s) alone 923.20
Conus (any type) (congenital) 743.57
  acquired 371.60
  medullaris syndrome 336.8
Convalescence (following) V66.9
  chemotherapy V66.2
  medical NEC V66.5
  psychotherapy V66.3

Convalescence—*continued*
  radiotherapy V66.1
  surgery NEC V66.0
  treatment (for) NEC V66.5
    combined V66.6
    fracture V66.4
    mental disorder NEC V66.3
    specified disorder NEC V66.5
Conversion
  hysteria, hysterical, any type 300.11
  laparoscopic surgical procedure to open
      procedure V64.4
  neurosis, any 300.11
  reaction, any 300.11
Converter, tuberculosis (test reaction) 795.5
Convulsions (idiopathic) 780.39
  apoplectiform (*see also* Disease,
      cerebrovascular, acute) 436
  brain 780.39
  cerebral 780.39
  cerebrospinal 780.39
  due to trauma NEC—*see* Injury, intracranial
  eclamptic (*see also* Eclampsia) 780.39
  epileptic (*see also* Epilepsy) 345.9
  epileptiform (*see also* Seizure, epileptiform)
      780.39
  epileptoid (*see also* Seizure, epileptiform)
      780.39
  ether
    anesthetic
      correct substance properly administered
          780.39
      overdose or wrong substance given 968.2
    other specified type—*see* Table of drugs and
        chemicals
  febrile 780.31
  generalized 780.39
  hysterical 300.11
  infantile 780.39
    epilepsy—*see* Epilepsy
  internal 780.39
  jacksonian (*see also* Epilepsy) 345.5
  myoclonic 333.2
  newborn 779.0
  paretic 094.1
  pregnancy (nephritic) (uremic)—*see* Eclampsia,
      pregnancy
  psychomotor (*see also* Epilepsy) 345.4
  puerperal, postpartum—*see* Eclampsia,
      pregnancy
  recurrent 780.39
    epileptic—*see* Epilepsy
  reflex 781.0
  repetitive 780.39
    epileptic—*see* Epilepsy
  salaam (*see also* Epilepsy) 345.6
  scarlatinal 034.1
  spasmodic 780.39
  tetanus, tetanic (*see also* Tetanus) 037
  thymic 254.8
  uncinate 780.39
  uremic 586
Convulsive —*see also* Convulsions
  disorder or state 780.39
    epileptic—*see* Epilepsy
  equivalent, abdominal (*see also* Epilepsy) 345.5
Cooke-Apert-Gallais syndrome (adrenogenital)
    255.2
Cooley's anemia (erythroblastic) 282.4
Coolie itch 126.9

Cooper's
 disease 610.1
 hernia—*see* Hernia, Cooper's
Coordination disturbance 781.3
Copper wire arteries, retina 362.13
Copra itch 133.8
Coprolith 560.39
Coprophilia 302.89
Coproporphyria, hereditary 277.1
Coprostasis 560.39
 with hernia—*see also* Hernia, by site, with
  obstruction
   gangrenous—*see* Hernia, by site, with
    gangrene
Cor
 biloculare 745.7
 bovinum—*see* Hypertrophy, cardiac
 bovis—*see also* Hypertrophy, cardiac
 pulmonale (chronic) 416.9
  acute 415.0
 triatriatum, triatrium 746.82
 triloculare 745.8
  biatriatum 745.3
  biventriculare 745.69
Corbus' disease 607.1
Cord —*see also* condition
 around neck (tightly) (with compression)
  affecting fetus or newborn 762.5
  complicating delivery 663.1
   without compression 663.3
    affecting fetus or newborn 762.6
 bladder NEC 344.61
  tabetic 094.0
 prolapse
  affecting fetus or newborn 762.4
  complicating delivery 663.0
Cord's angiopathy (*see also* Tuberculosis) 017.3
 [362.18]
Cordis ectopia 746.87
Corditis (spermatic) 608.4
Corectopia 743.46
Cori type glycogen storage disease —*see*
 Disease, glycogen storage
Cork-handlers' disease or lung 495.3
Corkscrew esophagus 530.5
Corlett's pyosis (impetigo) 684
Corn (infected) 700
Cornea—*see also* condition
 donor V59.5
 guttata (dystrophy) 371.57
 plana 743.41
Cornelia de Lange's syndrome (Amsterdam
 dwarf, mental retardation, and brachycephaly)
 759.89
Cornual gestation or pregnancy —*see*
 Pregnancy, cornual
Cornu cutaneum 702.8
Coronary (artery)—*see also* condition
 arising from aorta or pulmonary trunk 746.85
Corpora —*see also* condition
 amylacea (prostate) 602.8
 cavernosa—*see* condition
Corpulence (*see also* Obesity) 278.0
Corpus —*see* condition
Corrigan's disease —*see* Insufficiency, aortic
Corrosive burn —*see* Burn, by site
Corsican fever (*see also* Malaria) 084.6
Cortical —*see also* condition
 blindness 377.75
 necrosis, kidney (bilateral) 583.6
Corticoadrenal —*see* condition
Corticosexual syndrome 255.2

Coryza (acute) 460
 with grippe or influenza 487.1
 syphilitic 095.8
  congenital (chronic) 090.0
Costen's syndrome or complex 524.60
Costiveness (*see also* Constipation) 564.00
Costochondritis 733.6
Cotard's syndrome (paranoia) 297.1
Cot death 798.0
Cotungo's disease 724.3
Cough 786.2
 with hemorrhage (*see also* Hemoptysis) 786.3
 affected 786.2
 bronchial 786.2
  with grippe or influenza 487.1
 chronic 786.2
 epidemic 786.2
 functional 306.1
 hemorrhagic 786.3
 hysterical 300.11
 laryngeal, spasmodic 786.2
 nervous 786.2
 psychogenic 306.1
 smokers' 491.0
 tea tasters' 112.89
Counseling NEC V65.40
 without complaint or sickness V65.49
 abuse victim NEC V62.89
  child V61.21
  partner V61.11
  spouse V61.11
 child abuse, maltreatment, or neglect V61.21
 contraceptive NEC V25.09
  device (intrauterine) V25.02
  maintenance V25.40
   intrauterine contraceptive device V25.42
   oral contraceptive (pill) V25.41
   specified type NEC V25.49
   subdermal implantable V25.43
  management NEC V25.9
  oral contraceptive (pill) V25.01
  prescription NEC V25.02
   oral contraceptive (pill) V25.01
    repeat prescription V25.41
   repeat prescription V25.40
  subdermal implantable V25.43
  surveillance V25.40
 dietary V65.3
 exercise V65.41
 explanation of
  investigation finding NEC V65.49
  medication NEC V65.49
 family planning V25.09
 for nonattending third party V65.1
 genetic V26.3
 gonorrhea V65.45
 health (advice) (education) (instruction) NEC
  V65.49
 HIV V65.44
 human immunodeficiency virus V65.44
 injury prevention V65.43
 marital V61.10
 medical (for) V65.9
  boarding school resident V60.6
  condition not demonstrated V65.5
  feared complaint and no disease found V65.5
  institutional resident V60.6
  on behalf of another V65.1
  person living alone V60.3
 parent-child conflict V61.20
  specified problem NEC V61.29

Crepitus—*continued*
　foot 719.67
　hand 719.64
　hip 719.65
　knee 719.66
　multiple sites 719.69
　pelvic region 719.65
　shoulder (region) 719.61
　specified site NEC 719.68
　wrist 719.63
Crescent or conus choroid, congenital 743.57
Cretin, cretinism (athyrotic) (congenital)
　　(endemic) (metabolic) (nongoitrous)
　　(sporadic) 243
　goitrous (sporadic) 246.1
　pelvis (dwarf type) (male type) 243
　　with disproportion (fetopelvic) 653.1
　　　affecting fetus or newborn 763.1
　　　causing obstructed labor 660.1
　　　　affecting fetus or newborn 763.1
　pituitary 253.3
Cretinoid degeneration 243
Creutzfeldt-Jakob disease (syndrome) 046.1
　with dementia
　　with behavioral disturbance 046.1 *[294.11]*
　　without behavioral disturbance 046.1 *[294.10]*
Crib death 798.0
Cribriform hymen 752.49
Cri-du-chat syndrome 758.3
Crigler-Najjar disease or syndrome (congenital
　　hyperbilirubinemia) 277.4
Crimean hemorrhagic fever 065.0
Criminalism 301.7
Crisis
　abdomen 789.0
　addisonian (acute adrenocortical insufficiency)
　　255.4
　adrenal (cortical) 255.4
　asthmatic—*see* Asthma
　brain, cerebral (*see also* Disease,
　　cerebrovascular, acute) 436
　celiac 579.0
　Dietl's 593.4
　emotional NEC 309.29
　　acute reaction to stress 308.0
　　adjustment reaction 309.9
　　specific to childhood and adolescence 313.9
　gastric (tabetic) 094.0
　glaucomatocyclitic 364.22
　heart (*see also* Failure, heart) 428.9
　hypertensive—*see* Hypertension
　nitritoid
　　correct substance properly administered 458.2
　　overdose or wrong substance given or taken
　　　961.1
　oculogyric 378.87
　　psychogenic 306.7
　Pel's 094.0
　psychosexual identity 302.6
　rectum 094.0
　renal 593.81
　sickle cell 282.62
　stomach (tabetic) 094.0
　tabetic 094.0
　thyroid (*see also* Thyrotoxicosis) 242.9
　thyrotoxic (*see also* Thyrotoxicosis) 242.9
　vascular—*see* Disease, cerebrovascular, acute
Crocq's disease (acrocyanosis) 443.89
Crohn's disease (*see also* Enteritis, regional)
　555.9
Cronkhite-Canada syndrome 211.3
Crooked septum, nasal 470

Cross
　birth (of fetus) complicating delivery 652.3
　　with successful version 652.1
　　causing obstructed labor 660.0
　bite, anterior or posterior 524.2
　eye (*see also* Esotropia) 378.00
Crossed ectopia of kidney 753.3
Crossfoot 754.50
Croup, croupus (acute) (angina) (catarrhal)
　　(infective) (inflammatory) (laryngeal)
　　(membranous) (nondiphtheritic)
　　(pseudomembranous) 464.4
　asthmatic (*see also* Asthma) 493.9
　bronchial 466.0
　diphtheritic (membranous) 032.3
　false 478.75
　spasmodic 478.75
　　diphtheritic 032.3
　stridulous 478.75
　　diphtheritic 032.3
Crouzon's disease (craniofacial dysostosis) 756.0
Crowding, teeth 524.3
CRST syndrome (cutaneous systemic sclerosis)
　710.1
Cruchet's disease (encephalitis lethargica) 049.8
Cruelty in children (*see also* Disturbance,
　　conduct) 312.9
Crural ulcer (*see also* Ulcer, lower extremity)
　707.10
Crush, crushed, crushing (injury) 929.9
　with
　　fracture—*see* Fracture, by site
　abdomen 926.19
　　internal—*see* Injury, internal, abdomen
　ankle 928.21
　　with other parts of foot 928.20
　arm 927.9
　　lower (and elbow) 927.10
　　upper 927.03
　　　with shoulder or axillary region 927.09
　axilla 927.02
　　with shoulder or upper arm 927.09
　back 926.11
　breast 926.19
　buttock 926.12
　cheek 925.1
　chest—*see* Injury, internal, chest
　ear 925.1
　elbow 927.11
　　with forearm 927.10
　face 925.1
　finger(s) 927.3
　　with hand(s) 927.20
　　　and wrist(s) 927.21
　flank 926.19
　foot, excluding toe(s) alone (with ankle) 928.20
　forearm (and elbow) 927.10
　genitalia, external (female) (male) 926.0
　　internal—*see* Injury, internal, genital organ
　　　NEC
　hand, except finger(s) alone (and wrist) 927.20
　head—*see* Fracture, skull, by site
　heel 928.20
　hip 928.01
　　with thigh 928.00
　internal organ (abdomen, chest, or pelvis)—*see*
　　Injury, internal, by site
　knee 928.11
　　with leg, lower 928.10
　labium (majus) (minus) 926.0
　larynx 925.2

Cutis—*continued*
laxa 756.83
senilis 701.8
marmorata 782.61
osteosis 709.3
pendula 756.83
acquired 701.8
rhomboidalis nuchae 701.8
verticis gyrata 757.39
acquired 701.8
Cyanopathy, newborn 770.83
Cyanosis 782.5
autotoxic 289.7
common atrioventricular canal 745.69
congenital 770.83
conjunctiva 372.71
due to
endocardial cushion defect 745.60
nonclosure, foramen botalli 745.5
patent foramen botalli 745.5
persistent foramen ovale 745.5
enterogenous 289.7
fetus or newborn 770.83
ostium primum defect 745.61
paroxysmal digital 443.0
retina, retinal 362.10
Cycle
anovulatory 628.0
menstrual, irregular 626.4
Cyclencephaly 759.89
Cyclical vomiting 536.2
psychogenic 306.4
Cyclitic membrane 364.74
Cyclitis (*see also* Iridocyclitis) 364.3
acute 364.00
primary 364.01
recurrent 364.02
chronic 364.10
in
sarcoidosis 135 *[364.11]*
tuberculosis (*see also* Tuberculosis) 017.3
[364.11]
Fuchs' heterochromic 364.21
granulomatous 364.10
lens induced 364.23
nongranulomatous 364.00
posterior 363.21
primary 364.01
recurrent 364.02
secondary (noninfectious) 364.04
infectious 364.03
subacute 364.00
primary 364.01
recurrent 364.02
Cyclokeratitis —*see* Keratitis
Cyclophoria 378.44
Cyclopia, cyclops 759.89
Cycloplegia 367.51
Cyclospasm 367.53
Cyclosporiasis 007.5
Cyclothymia 301.13
Cyclothymic personality 301.13
Cyclotropia 378.33
Cyesis —*see* Pregnancy
Cylindroma (M8200/3)—*see also* Neoplasm, by
site, malignant
eccrine dermal (M8200/0)—*see* Neoplasm,
skin, benign
skin (M8200/0)—*see* Neoplasm, skin, benign
Cylindruria 791.7
Cyllosoma 759.89

Cynanche
diphtheritic 032.3
tonsillaris 475
Cynorexia 783.6
Cyphosis —*see* Kyphosis
Cyprus fever (*see also* Brucellosis) 023.9
Cyriax's syndrome (slipping rib) 733.99
Cyst (mucus) (retention) (serous) (simple)

> *Note—In general, cysts are not neoplastic and are classified to the appropriate category for disease of the specified anatomical site. This generalization does not apply to certain types of cysts which are neoplastic in nature, for example, dermoid, nor does it apply to cysts of certain structures, for example, branchial cleft, which are classified as developmental anomalies. The following listing includes some of the most frequently reported sites of cysts as well as qualifiers which indicate the type of cyst. The latter qualifiers usually are not repeated under the anatomical sites. Since the code assignment for a given site may vary depending upon the type of cyst, the coder should refer to the listings under the specified type of cyst before consideration is given to the site.*

accessory, fallopian tube 752.11
adenoid (infected) 474.8
adrenal gland 255.8
congenital 759.1
air, lung 518.89
allantoic 753.7
alveolar process (jaw bone) 526.2
amnion, amniotic 658.8
anterior chamber (eye) 364.60
exudative 364.62
implantation (surgical) (traumatic) 364.61
parasitic 360.13
anterior nasopalatine 526.1
antrum 478.1
anus 569.49
apical (periodontal) (tooth) 522.8
appendix 543.9
arachnoid, brain 348.0
arytenoid 478.79
auricle 706.2
Baker's (knee) 727.51
tuberculous (*see also* Tuberculosis) 015.2
Bartholin's gland or duct 616.2
bile duct (*see also* Disease, biliary) 576.8
bladder (multiple) (trigone) 596.8
Blessig's 362.62
blood, endocardial (*see also* Endocarditis)
424.90
blue dome 610.0
bone (local) 733.20
aneurysmal 733.22
jaw 526.2
developmental (odontogenic) 526.0
fissural 526.1
latent 526.89
solitary 733.21
unicameral 733.21
brain 348.0
congenital 742.4
hydatid (*see also* Echinococcus) 122.9
third ventricle (colloid) 742.4
branchial (cleft) 744.42
branchiogenic 744.42

Cyst —*continued*
  breast (benign) (blue dome) (pedunculated)
    (solitary) (traumatic) 610.0
    involution 610.4
    sebaceous 610.8
  broad ligament (benign) 620.8
    embryonic 752.11
  bronchogenic (mediastinal) (sequestration)
    518.89
    congenital 748.4
  buccal 528.4
  bulbourethral gland (Cowper's) 599.89
  bursa, bursal 727.49
    pharyngeal 478.26
  calcifying odontogenic (M9301/0) 213.1
    upper jaw (bone) 213.0
  canal of Nuck (acquired) (serous) 629.1
    congenital 752.41
  canthus 372.75
  carcinomatous (M8010/3)—*see* Neoplasm, by
    site, malignant
  cartilage (joint)—*see* Derangement, joint
  cauda equina 336.8
  cavum septi pellucidi NEC 348.0
  celomic (pericardium) 746.89
  cerebellopontine (angle)—*see* Cyst, brain
  cerebellum—*see* Cyst, brain
  cerebral—*see* Cyst, brain
  cervical lateral 744.42
  cervix 622.8
    embryonal 752.41
    nabothian (gland) 616.0
  chamber, anterior (eye) 364.60
    exudative 364.62
    implantation (surgical) (traumatic) 364.61
    parasitic 360.13
  chiasmal, optic NEC (*see also* Lesion,
    chiasmal) 377.54
  chocolate (ovary) 617.1
  choledochal (congenital) 751.69
    acquired 576.8
  choledochus 751.69
  chorion 658.8
  choroid plexus 348.0
  chyle, mesentery 457.8
  ciliary body 364.60
    exudative 364.64
    implantation 364.61
    primary 364.63
  clitoris 624.8
  coccyx (*see also* Cyst, bone) 733.20
  colloid
    third ventricle (brain) 742.4
    thyroid gland—*see* Goiter
  colon 569.89
  common (bile) duct (*see also* Disease, biliary)
    576.8
  congenital NEC 759.89
    adrenal glands 759.1
    epiglottis 748.3
    esophagus 750.4
    fallopian tube 752.11
    kidney 753.10
      multiple 753.19
      single 753.11
    larynx 748.3
    liver 751.62
    lung 748.4
    mediastinum 748.8
    ovary 752.0
    oviduct 752.11

Cyst —*continued*
  pancreas 751.7
  periurethral (tissue) 753.8
  prepuce NEC 752.69
    penis 752.69
  sublingual 750.26
  submaxillary gland 750.26
  thymus (gland) 759.2
  tongue 750.19
  ureterovesical orifice 753.4
  vulva 752.41
  conjunctiva 372.75
  cornea 371.23
  corpora quadrigemina 348.0
  corpus
    albicans (ovary) 620.2
    luteum (ruptured) 620.1
  Cowper's gland (benign) (infected) 599.89
  cranial meninges 348.0
  craniobuccal pouch 253.8
  craniopharyngeal pouch 253.8
  cystic duct (*see also* Disease, gallbladder) 575.8
  Cysticercus (any site) 123.1
  Dandy-Walker 742.3
    with spina bifida (*see also* Spina bifida) 741.0
  dental 522.8
    developmental 526.0
    eruption 526.0
    lateral periodontal 526.0
    primordial (keratocyst) 526.0
    root 522.8
  dentigerous 526.0
    mandible 526.0
    maxilla 526.0
  dermoid (M9084/0)—*see also* Neoplasm, by
    site, benign
    with malignant transformation (M9084/3)
      183.0
    implantation
      external area or site (skin) NEC 709.8
      iris 364.61
      skin 709.8
      vagina 623.8
      vulva 624.8
    mouth 528.4
    oral soft tissue 528.4
    sacrococcygeal 685.1
      with abscess 685.0
  developmental of ovary, ovarian 752.0
  dura (cerebral) 348.0
    spinal 349.2
  ear (external) 706.2
  echinococcal (*see also* Echinococcus) 122.9
  embryonal
    cervix uteri 752.41
    genitalia, female external 752.41
    uterus 752.3
    vagina 752.41
  endometrial 621.8
    ectopic 617.9
  endometrium (uterus) 621.8
    ectopic—*see* Endometriosis
  enteric 751.5
  enterogenous 751.5
  epidermal (inclusion) (*see also* Cyst, skin) 706.2
  epidermoid (inclusion) (*see also* Cyst, skin)
    706.2
    mouth 528.4
    not of skin—*see* Cyst, by site
    oral soft tissue 528.4
  epididymis 608.89

Cyst —*continued*
  epiglottis 478.79
  epiphysis cerebri 259.8
  epithelial (inclusion) (*see also* Cyst, skin) 706.2
  epoophoron 752.11
  eruption 526.0
  esophagus 530.89
  ethmoid sinus 478.1
  eye (retention) 379.8
    congenital 743.03
    posterior segment, congenital 743.54
  eyebrow 706.2
  eyelid (sebaceous) 374.84
    infected 373.13
    sweat glands or ducts 374.84
  falciform ligament (inflammatory) 573.8
  fallopian tube 620.8
  female genital organs NEC 629.8
  fimbrial (congenital) 752.11
  fissural (oral region) 526.1
  follicle (atretic) (graafian) (ovarian) 620.0
    nabothian (gland) 616.0
  follicular (atretic) (ovarian) 620.0
    dentigerous 526.0
  frontal sinus 478.1
  gallbladder or duct 575.8
  ganglion 727.43
  Gartner's duct 752.11
  gas, of mesentery 568.89
  gingiva 523.8
  gland of moll 374.84
  globulomaxillary 526.1
  graafian follicle 620.0
  granulosal lutein 620.2
  hemangiomatous (M9121/0) (*see also*
    Hemangioma) 228.00
  hydatid (*see also* Echinococcus) 122.9
    fallopian tube (Morgagni) 752.11
    liver NEC 122.8
    lung NEC 122.9
    Morgagni 752.8
      fallopian tube 752.11
    specified site NEC 122.9
  hymen 623.8
    embryonal 752.41
  hypopharynx 478.26
  hypophysis, hypophyseal (duct) (recurrent)
    253.8
    cerebri 253.8
  implantation (dermoid)
    anterior chamber (eye) 364.61
    external area or site (skin) NEC 709.8
    iris 364.61
    vagina 623.8
    vulva 624.8
  incisor, incisive canal 526.1
  inclusion (epidermal) (epithelial) (epidermoid)
    (mucous) (squamous) (*see also* Cyst, skin)
    706.2
    not of skin—*see* Neoplasm, by site, benign
  intestine (large) (small) 569.89
  intracranial—*see* Cyst, brain
  intraligamentous 728.89
    knee 717.89
  intrasellar 253.8
  iris (idiopathic) 364.60
    exudative 364.62
    implantation (surgical) (traumatic) 364.61
    miotic pupillary 364.55
    parasitic 360.13
  Iwanoff's 362.62

Cyst —*continued*
  jaw (bone) (aneurysmal) (extravasation)
    (hemorrhagic) (traumatic) 526.2
    developmental (odontogenic) 526.0
    fissural 526.1
  keratin 706.2
  kidney (congenital) 753.10
    acquired 593.2
    calyceal (*see also* Hydronephrosis) 591
    multiple 753.19
    pyelogenic (*see also* Hydronephrosis) 591
    simple 593.2
    single 753.11
    solitary (not congenital) 593.2
  labium (majus) (minus) 624.8
    sebaceous 624.8
  lacrimal
    apparatus 375.43
    gland or sac 375.12
  larynx 478.79
  lens 379.39
    congenital 743.39
  lip (gland) 528.5
  liver 573.8
    congenital 751.62
    hydatid (*see also* Echinococcus) 122.8
      granulosis 122.0
      multilocularis 122.5
  lung 518.89
    congenital 748.4
    giant bullous 492.0
  lutein 620.1
  lymphangiomatous (M9173/0) 228.1
  lymphoepithelial
    mouth 528.4
    oral soft tissue 528.4
  macula 362.54
  malignant (M8000/3)—*see* Neoplasm, by site,
    malignant
  mammary gland (sweat gland) (*see also* Cyst,
    breast) 610.0
  mandible 526.2
    dentigerous 526.0
    radicular 522.8
  maxilla 526.2
    dentigerous 526.0
    radicular 522.8
  median
    anterior maxillary 526.1
    palatal 526.1
  mediastinum (congenital) 748.8
  meibomian (gland) (retention) 373.2
    infected 373.12
  membrane, brain 348.0
  meninges (cerebral) 348.0
    spinal 349.2
  meniscus knee 717.5
  mesentery, mesenteric (gas) 568.89
    chyle 457.8
    gas 568.89
  mesonephric duct 752.8
  mesothelial
    peritoneum 568.89
    pleura (peritoneal) 568.89
  milk 611.5
  miotic pupillary (iris) 364.55
  Morgagni (hydatid) 752.8
    fallopian tube 752.11
  mouth 528.4
  mullerian duct 752.8
  multilocular (ovary) (M8000/1) 239.5

Cyst —*continued*
  eyelid 374.84
    genital organ NEC
      female 629.8
      male 608.89
    scrotum 706.2
  semilunar cartilage (knee) (multiple) 717.5
  seminal vesicle 608.89
  serous (ovary) 620.2
  sinus (antral) (ethmoidal) (frontal) (maxillary)
    (nasal) (sphenoidal) 478.1
  Skene's gland 599.89
  skin (epidermal) (epidermoid, inclusion)
    (epithelial) (inclusion) (retention)
    (sebaceous) 706.2
    breast 610.8
    eyelid 374.84
    genital organ NEC
      female 629.8
      male 608.89
    neoplastic 216.3
    scrotum 706.2
    sweat gland or duct 705.89
  solitary
    bone 733.21
    kidney 593.2
  spermatic cord 608.89
  sphenoid sinus 478.1
  spinal meninges 349.2
  spine (*see also* Cyst, bone) 733.20
  spleen NEC 289.59
    congenital 759.0
    hydatid (*see also* Echinococcus) 122.9
  spring water (pericardium) 746.89
  subarachnoid 348.0
    intrasellar 793.0
  subdural (cerebral) 348.0
    spinal cord 349.2
  sublingual gland 527.6
    mucous extravasation or retention 527.6
  submaxillary gland 527.6
    mucous extravasation or retention 527.6
  suburethral 599.89
  suprarenal gland 255.8
  suprasellar—*see* Cyst, brain
  sweat gland or duct 705.89
  sympathetic nervous system 337.9
  synovial 727.40
    popliteal space 727.51
  Tarlov's 355.9
  tarsal 373.2
  tendon (sheath) 727.42
  testis 608.89
  theca-lutein (ovary) 620.2
  Thornwaldt's, Tornwaldt's 478.26
  thymus (gland) 254.8
  thyroglossal (duct) (infected) (persistent) 759.2
  thyroid (gland) 246.2
    adenomatous—*see* Goiter, nodular
    colloid (*see also* Goiter) 240.9
  thyrolingual duct (infected) (persistent) 759.2
  tongue (mucous) 529.8
  tonsil 474.8
  tooth (dental root) 522.8
  tubo-ovarian 620.8
    inflammatory 614.1
  tunica vaginalis 608.89
  turbinate (nose) (*see also* Cyst, bone) 733.20
  Tyson's gland (benign) (infected) 607.89
  umbilicus 759.89
  urachus 753.7

Cyst —*continued*
  ureter 593.89
  ureterovesical orifice 593.89
    congenital 753.4
  urethra 599.84
  urethral gland (Cowper's) 599.89
  uterine
    ligament 620.8
      embryonic 752.11
    tube 620.8
  uterus (body) (corpus) (recurrent) 621.8
    embryonal 752.3
  utricle (ear) 386.8
    prostatic 599.89
  utriculus masculinus 599.89
  vagina, vaginal (squamous cell) (wall) 623.8
    embryonal 752.41
    implantation 623.8
    inclusion 623.8
  vallecula, vallecular 478.79
  ventricle, neuroepithelial 348.0
  verumontanum 599.89
  vesical (orifice) 596.8
  vitreous humor 379.29
  vulva (sweat glands) 624.8
    congenital 752.41
    implantation 624.8
    inclusion 624.8
    sebaceous gland 624.8
  vulvovaginal gland 624.8
  wolffian 752.8

Cystadenocarcinoma (M8440/3)—*see also*
  Neoplasm, by site, malignant
  bile duct type (M8161/3) 155.1
  endometrioid (M8380/3)—*see* Neoplasm, by
    site, malignant
  mucinous (M8470/3)
    papillary (M8471/3)
      specified site—*see* Neoplasm, by site,
        malignant
      unspecified site 183.0
    specified site—*see* Neoplasm, by site,
      malignant
    unspecified site 183.0
  papillary (M8450/3)
    mucinous (M8471/3)
      specified site—*see* Neoplasm, by site,
        malignant
      unspecified site 183.0
    pseudomucinous (M8471/3)
      specified site—*see* Neoplasm, by site,
        malignant
      unspecified site 183.0
    serous (M8460/3)
      specified site—*see* Neoplasm, by site,
        malignant
      unspecified site 183.0
    specified site—*see* Neoplasm, by site,
      malignant
    unspecified 183.0
  pseudomucinous (M8470/3)
    papillary (M8471/3)
      specified site—*see* Neoplasm, by site,
        malignant
      unspecified site 183.0
    specified site—*see* Neoplasm, by site,
      malignant
    unspecified site 183.0
  serous (M8441/3)
    papillary (M8460/3)

Cystadenocarcinoma—*continued*
    specified site—*see* Neoplasm, by site,
      malignant
    unspecified site 183.0
  specified site—*see* Neoplasm, by site,
    malignant
  unspecified site 183.0
Cystadenofibroma (M9013/0)
  clear cell (M8313/0)—*see* Neoplasm, by site,
    benign
  endometrioid (M8381/0) 220
    borderline malignancy (M8381/1) 236.2
    malignant (M8381/3) 183.0
  mucinous (M9015/0)
    specified site—*see* Neoplasm, by site, benign
    unspecified site 220
  serous (M9014/0)
    specified site—*see* Neoplasm, by site, benign
    unspecified site 220
  specified site—*see* Neoplasm, by site, benign
  unspecified site 220
Cystadenoma (M8440/0)—*see also* Neoplasm,
  by site, benign
  bile duct (M8161/0) 211.5
  endometrioid (M8380/0)—*see also* Neoplasm,
    by site, benign
    borderline malignancy (M8380/1)—*see*
      Neoplasm, by site, uncertain behavior
  malignant (M8440/3)—*see* Neoplasm, by site,
    malignant
  mucinous (M8470/0)
    borderline malignancy (M8470/1)
      specified site—*see* Neoplasm, uncertain
        behavior
      unspecified site 236.2
    papillary (M8471/0)
      borderline malignancy (M8471/1)
        specified site—*see* Neoplasm, by site,
          uncertain behavior
        unspecified site 236.2
      specified site—*see* Neoplasm, by site,
        benign
      unspecified site 220
    specified site—*see* Neoplasm, by site, benign
    unspecified site 220
  papillary (M8450/0)
    borderline malignancy (M8450/1)
      specified site—*see* Neoplasm, by site,
        uncertain behavior
      unspecified site 236.2
    lymphomatosum (M8561/0) 210.2
    mucinous (M8471/0)
      borderline malignancy (M8471/1)
        specified site—*see* Neoplasm, by site,
          uncertain behavior
        unspecified site 236.2
      specified site—*see* Neoplasm, by site,
        benign
      unspecified site 220
    pseudomucinous (M8471/0)
      borderline malignancy (M8471/1)
        specified site—*see* Neoplasm, by site,
          uncertain behavior
        unspecified site 236.2
      specified site—*see* Neoplasm, by site,
        benign
      unspecified site 220
    serous (M8460/0)
      borderline malignancy (M8460/1)
        specified site—*see* Neoplasm, by site,
          uncertain behavior

Cystadenoma—*continued*
    unspecified site 236.2
      specified site—*see* Neoplasm, by site,
        benign
      unspecified site 220
    specified site—*see* Neoplasm, by site, benign
    unspecified site 220
  pseudomucinous (M8470/0)
    borderline malignancy (M8470/1)
      specified site—*see* Neoplasm, by site,
        uncertain behavior
      unspecified site 236.2
    papillary (M8471/0)
      borderline malignancy (M8471/1)
        specified site—*see* Neoplasm, by site,
          uncertain behavior
        unspecified site 236.2
      specified site—*see* Neoplasm, by site,
        benign
      unspecified site 220
    specified site—*see* Neoplasm, by site, benign
    unspecified site 220
  serous (M8441/0)
    borderline malignancy (M8441/1)
      specified site—*see* Neoplasm, by site,
        uncertain behavior
      unspecified site 236.2
    papillary (M8460/0)
      borderline malignancy (M8460/1)
        specified site—*see* Neoplasm, by site,
          uncertain behavior
        unspecified site 236.2
      specified site—*see* Neoplasm, by site,
        benign
      unspecified site 220
    specified site—*see* Neoplasm, by site, benign
    unspecified site 220
  thyroid 226
Cystathioninemia 270.4
Cystathioninuria 270.4
Cystic —*see also* condition
  breast, chronic 610.1
  corpora lutea 620.1
  degeneration, congenital
    brain 742.4
    kidney (*see also* Cystic, disease, kidney)
      753.10
  disease
    breast, chronic 610.1
    kidney, congenital 753.10
      medullary 753.16
      multiple 753.19
      polycystic—*see* Polycystic, kidney
      single 753.11
      specified NEC 753.19
    liver, congenital 751.62
    lung 518.89
      congenital 748.4
    pancreas, congenital 751.7
    semilunar cartilage 717.5
  duct—*see* condition
  eyeball, congenital 743.03
  fibrosis (pancreas) 277.00
    with
      manifestations
        gastrointestinal 277.03
        pulmonary 277.02
        specified NEC 277.09
      meconium ileus 277.01
      pulmonary exacerbation 277.02
  hygroma (M9173/0) 228.1

Cystic—*continued*
  kidney, congenital 753.10
    medullary 753.16
    multiple 753.19
    polycystic—*see* Polycystic, kidney
    single 753.11
    specified NEC 753.19
  liver, congenital 751.62
  lung 518.89
    congenital 748.4
  mass—*see* Cyst
  mastitis, chronic 610.1
  ovary 620.2
  pancreas, congenital 751.7
Cysticerciasis 123.1
Cysticercosis (mammary) (subretinal) 123.1
Cysticercus 123.1
  cellulosae infestation 123.1
Cystinosis (malignant) 270.0
Cystinuria 270.0
Cystitis (bacillary) (colli) (diffuse) (exudative)
    (hemorrhagic) (purulent) (recurrent) (septic)
    (suppurative) (ulcerative) 595.9
  with
    abortion—*see* Abortion, by type, with urinary
      tract infection
    ectopic pregnancy (*see also* categories
      633.0-633.9) 639.8
    fibrosis 595.1
    leukoplakia 595.1
    malakoplakia 595.1
    metaplasia 595.1
    molar pregnancy (*see also* categories
      630-632) 639.8
  actinomycotic 039.8 *[595.4]*
  acute 595.0
    of trigone 595.3
  allergic 595.89
  amebic 006.8 *[595.4]*
  bilharzial 120.9 *[595.4]*
  blennorrhagic (acute) 098.11
    chronic or duration of 2 months or more
      098.31
  bullous 595.89
  calculous 594.1
  chlamydial 099.53
  chronic 595.2
    interstitial 595.1
    of trigone 595.3
  complicating pregnancy, childbirth, or
      puerperium 646.6
    affecting fetus or newborn 760.1
  cystic(a) 595.81
  diphtheritic 032.84
  echinococcal
    granulosus 122.3 *[595.4]*
    multilocularis 122.6 *[595.4]*
  emphysematous 595.89
  encysted 595.81
  follicular 595.3
  following
    abortion 639.8
    ectopic or molar pregnancy 639.8
  gangrenous 595.89
  glandularis 595.89
  gonococcal (acute) 098.11
    chronic or duration of 2 months or more
      098.31
  incrusted 595.89
  interstitial 595.1
  irradiation 595.82

Cystitis—*continued*
  irritation 595.89
  malignant 595.89
  monilial 112.2
  of trigone 595.3
  panmural 595.1
  polyposa 595.89
  prostatic 601.3
  radiation 595.82
  Reiter's (abacterial) 099.3
  specified NEC 595.89
  subacute 595.2
  submucous 595.1
  syphilitic 095.8
  trichomoniasis 131.09
  tuberculous (*see also* Tuberculosis) 016.1
  ulcerative 595.1
Cystocele (-rectocele)
  female (without uterine prolapse) 618.0
    with uterine prolapse 618.4
      complete 618.3
      incomplete 618.2
  in pregnancy or childbirth 654.4
    affecting fetus or newborn 763.89
    causing obstructed labor 660.2
      affecting fetus or newborn 763.1
  male 596.8
Cystoid
  cicatrix limbus 372.64
  degeneration macula 362.53
Cystolithiasis 594.1
Cystoma (M8440/0)—*see also* Neoplasm, by
    site, benign
  endometrial, ovary 617.1
  mucinous (M8470/0)
    specified site—*see* Neoplasm, by site, benign
    unspecified site 220
  serous (M8441/0)
    specified site—*see* Neoplasm, by site, benign
    unspecified site 220
  simple (ovary) 620.2
Cystoplegia 596.53
Cystoptosis 596.8
Cystopyelitis (*see also* Pyelitis) 590.80
Cystorrhagia 596.8
Cystosarcoma phyllodes (M9020/1) 238.3
  benign (M9020/0) 217
  malignant (M9020/3)—*see* Neoplasm, breast,
    malignant
Cystostomy status V44.50
  appendico-vesicostomy V44.52
  cutaneous-vesicostomy V44.51
  specified type NEC V44.59
  with complication 997.5
Cystourethritis (*see also* Urethritis) 597.89
Cystourethrocele (*see also* Cystocele)
  female (without uterine prolapse) 618.0
    with uterine prolapse 618.4
      complete 618.3
      incomplete 618.2
  male 596.8
Cytomegalic inclusion disease 078.5
  congenital 771.1
Cytomycosis, reticuloendothelial (*see also*
    Histoplasmosis, American) 115.00

D

Daae (-Finsen) disease (epidemic pleurodynia) 074.1
Dabney's grip 074.1
Da Costa's syndrome (neurocirculatory asthenia) 306.2
Dacryoadenitis, dacryadenitis 375.00
  acute 375.01
  chronic 375.02
Dacryocystitis 375.30
  acute 375.32
  chronic 375.42
  neonatal 771.6
  phlegmonous 375.33
  syphilitic 095.8
    congenital 090.0
  trachomatous, active 076.1
    late effect 139.1
  tuberculous (*see also* Tuberculosis) 017.3
Dacryocystoblennorrhea 375.42
Dacryocystocele 375.43
Dacryolith, dacryolithiasis 375.57
Dacryoma 375.43
Dacryopericystitis (acute) (subacute) 375.32
  chronic 375.42
Dacryops 375.11
Dacryosialadenopathy, atrophic 710.2
Dacryostenosis 375.56
  congenital 743.65
Dactylitis 686.9
  bone (*see also* Osteomyelitis) 730.2
  sickle-cell 282.61
  syphilitic 095.5
  tuberculous (*see also* Tuberculosis) 015.5
Dactylolysis spontanea 136.0
Dactylosymphysis (*see also* Syndactylism) 755.10
Damage
  arteriosclerotic—*see* Arteriosclerosis
  brain 348.9
    anoxic, hypoxic 348.1
      during or resulting from a procedure 997.01
    child NEC 343.9
    due to birth injury 767.0
    minimal (child) (*see also* Hyperkinesia) 314.9
    newborn 767.0
  cardiac—*see also* Disease, heart
  cardiorenal (vascular) (*see also* Hypertension, cardiorenal) 404.90
  central nervous system—*see* Damage, brain
  cerebral NEC—*see* Damage, brain
  coccyx, complicating delivery 665.6
  coronary (*see also* Ischemia, heart) 414.9
  eye, birth injury 767.8
  heart—*see also* Disease, heart
    valve—*see* Endocarditis
  hypothalamus NEC 348.9
  liver 571.9
    alcoholic 571.3
  myocardium (*see also* Degeneration, myocardial) 429.1
  pelvic
    joint or ligament, during delivery 665.6
    organ NEC
      with
        abortion—*see* Abortion, by type, with damage to pelvic organs
        ectopic pregnancy (*see also* categories 633.0-633.9) 639.2

Damage—*continued*
      molar pregnancy (*see also* categories 630-632) 639.2
    during delivery 665.5
    following
      abortion 639.2
      ectopic or molar pregnancy 639.2
  renal (*see also* Disease, renal) 593.9
  skin, solar 692.79
    acute 692.72
    chronic 692.74
  subendocardium, subendocardial (*see also* Degeneration, myocardial) 429.1
  vascular 459.9
Dameshek's syndrome (erythroblastic anemia) 282.4
Dana-Putnam syndrome (subacute combined sclerosis with pernicious anemia) 281.0 *[336.2]*
Danbolt (-Closs) syndrome (acrodermatitis enteropathica) 686.8
Dandruff 690.18
Dandy fever 061
Dandy-Walker deformity or syndrome (atresia, foramen of Magendie) 742.3
  with spina bifida (*see also* Spina bifida) 741.0
Dangle foot 736.79
Danielssen's disease (anesthetic leprosy) 030.1
Danlos' syndrome 756.83
Darier's disease (congenital) (keratosis follicularis) 757.39
  due to vitamin A deficiency 264.8
  meaning erythema annulare centrifugum 695.0
Darier-Roussy sarcoid 135
Darling's
  disease (*see also* Histoplasmosis, American) 115.00
  histoplasmosis (*see also* Histoplasmosis, American) 115.00
Dartre 054.9
Darwin's tubercle 744.29
Davidson's anemia (refractory) 284.9
Davies' disease 425.0
Davies-Colley syndrome (slipping rib) 733.99
Dawson's encephalitis 046.2
Day blindness (*see also* Blindness, day) 368.60
Dead
  fetus
    retained (in utero) 656.4
      early pregnancy (death before 22 completed weeks gestation) 632
      late (death after 22 completed weeks gestation) 656.4
    syndrome 641.3
  labyrinth 386.50
  ovum, retained 631
Deaf and dumb NEC 389.7
Deaf mutism (acquired) (congenital) NEC 389.7
  endemic 243
  hysterical 300.11
  syphilitic, congenital 090.0

Deafness (acquired) (bilateral) (both ears)
(complete) (congenital) (hereditary) (middle
ear) (partial) (unilateral) 389.9
  with blue sclera and fragility of bone 756.51
  auditory fatigue 389.9
  aviation 993.0
    nerve injury 951.5
  boilermakers' 951.5
  central 389.14
    with conductive hearing loss 389.2
  conductive (air) 389.00
    with sensorineural hearing loss 389.2
    combined types 389.08
    external ear 389.01
    inner ear 389.04
    middle ear 389.03
    multiple types 389.08
    tympanic membrane 389.02
  emotional (complete) 300.11
  functional (complete) 300.11
  high frequency 389.8
  hysterical (complete) 300.11
  injury 951.5
  low frequency 389.8
  mental 784.69
  mixed conductive and sensorineural 389.2
  nerve 389.12
    with conductive hearing loss 389.2
  neural 389.12
    with conductive hearing loss 389.2
  noise-induced 388.12
    nerve injury 951.5
  nonspeaking 389.7
  perceptive 389.10
    with conductive hearing loss 389.2
    central 389.14
    combined types 389.18
    multiple types 389.18
    neural 389.12
    sensory 389.11
  psychogenic (complete) 306.7
  sensorineural (*see also* Deafness, perceptive)
    389.10
  sensory 389.11
    with conductive hearing loss 389.2
  specified type NEC 389.8
  sudden NEC 388.2
  syphilitic 094.89
  transient ischemic 388.02
  transmission—*see* Deafness, conductive
  traumatic 951.5
  word (secondary to organic lesion) 784.69
    developmental 315.31
Death
  after delivery (cause not stated) (sudden) 674.9
  anesthetic
    due to
      correct substance properly administered
        995.4
      overdose or wrong substance given 968.4
        specified anesthetic—*see* Table of drugs
          and chemicals
    during delivery 668.9
  brain 348.8
  cardiac—*see* Disease, heart
  cause unknown 798.2
  cot (infant) 798.0
  crib (infant) 798.0

Death—*continued*
  fetus, fetal (cause not stated) (intrauterine) 779.9
    early, with retention (before 22 completed
      weeks gestation) 632
    from asphyxia or anoxia (before labor) 768.0
      during labor 768.1
    late, affecting management of pregnancy
      (after 22 completed weeks gestation) 656.4
  from pregnancy NEC 646.9
  instantaneous 798.1
  intrauterine (*see also* Death, fetus) 779.9
    complicating pregnancy 656.4
  maternal, affecting fetus or newborn 761.6
  neonatal NEC 779.9
  sudden (cause unknown) 798.1
    during delivery 669.9
      under anesthesia NEC 668.9
    infant, syndrome (SIDS) 798.0
    puerperal, during puerperium 674.9
  unattended (cause unknown) 798.9
  under anesthesia NEC
    due to
      correct substance properly administered
        995.4
      overdose or wrong substance given 968.4
        specified anesthetic—*see* Table of drugs
          and chemicals
    during delivery 668.9
  violent 798.1
de Beurmann-Gougerot disease (sporotrichosis)
  117.1
Debility (general) (infantile) (postinfectional)
  799.3
  with nutritional difficulty 269.9
  congenital or neonatal NEC 779.9
  nervous 300.5
  old age 797
  senile 797
Débove's disease (splenomegaly) 789.2
Decalcification
  bone (*see also* Osteoporosis) 733.00
  teeth 521.8
Decapitation 874.9
  fetal (to facilitate delivery) 763.89
Decapsulation, kidney 593.89
Decay
  dental 521.00
  senile 797
  tooth, teeth 521.00
Decensus, uterus —*see* Prolapse, uterus
Deciduitis (acute)
  with
    abortion—*see* Abortion, by type, with sepsis
    ectopic pregnancy (*see also* categories
      633.0-633.9) 639.0
    molar pregnancy (*see also* categories
      630-632) 639.0
  affecting fetus or newborn 760.8
  following
    abortion 639.0
    ectopic or molar pregnancy 639.0
  in pregnancy 646.6
  puerperal, postpartum 670
Deciduoma malignum (M9100/3) 181
Deciduous tooth (retained) 520.6
Decline (general) (*see also* Debility) 799.3

Decompensation
  cardiac (acute) (chronic) (*see also* Disease,
      heart) 429.9
    failure—*see* Failure, heart
  cardiorenal (*see also* Hypertension, cardiorenal)
      404.90
  cardiovascular (*see also* Disease,
      cardiovascular) 429.2
  heart (*see also* Disease, heart) 429.9
    failure—*see* Failure, heart
  hepatic 572.2
  myocardial (acute) (chronic) (*see also* Disease,
      heart) 429.9
    failure—*see* Failure, heart
  respiratory 519.9
Decompression sickness 993.3
Decrease, decreased
  blood
    platelets (*see also* Thrombocytopenia) 287.5
    pressure 796.3
      due to shock following
        injury 958.4
        operation 998.0
  cardiac reserve—*see* Disease, heart
  estrogen 256.39
    postablative 256.2
  fetal movements 655.7
  fragility of erythrocytes 289.8
  function
    adrenal (cortex) 255.4
      medulla 255.5
    ovary in hypopituitarism 253.4
    parenchyma of pancreas 577.8
    pituitary (gland) (lobe) (anterior) 253.2
      posterior (lobe) 253.8
  functional activity 780.99
  glucose 790.2
  haptoglobin (serum) NEC 273.8
  platelets (*see also* Thrombocytopenia) 287.5
  pulse pressure 785.9
  respiration due to shock following injury 958.4
  tear secretion NEC 375.15
  tolerance
    fat 579.8
    glucose 790.2
    salt and water 276.9
  vision NEC 369.9
Decubital gangrene 707.0 *[785.4]*
Decubiti (*see also* Decubitus) 707.0
Decubitus (ulcer) 707.0
  with gangrene 707.0 *[785.4]*
Deepening acetabulum 718.85
Defect, defective 759.9
  3-beta-hydroxysteroid dehydrogenase 255.2
  11-hydroxylase 255.2
  21-hydroxylase 255.2
  abdominal wall, congenital 756.70
  aorticopulmonary septum 745.0
  aortic septal 745.0
  atrial septal (ostium secundum type) 745.5
    acquired 429.71
    ostium primum type 745.61
    sinus venosus 745.8
  atrioventricular
    canal 745.69
    septum 745.4
      acquired 429.71
  atrium secundum 745.5
    acquired 429.71
  auricular septal 745.5
    acquired 429.71

Defect, defective—*continued*
  bilirubin excretion 277.4
  biosynthesis, testicular androgen 257.2
  bulbar septum 745.0
  butanol-insoluble iodide 246.1
  chromosome—*see* Anomaly, chromosome
  circulation (acquired) 459.9
    congenital 747.9
    newborn 747.9
  clotting NEC (*see also* Defect, coagulation)
      286.9
  coagulation (factor) (*see also* Deficiency,
      coagulation factor) 286.9
    with
      abortion—*see* Abortion, by type, with
        hemorrhage
      ectopic pregnancy (*see also* categories
        634-638) 639.1
      molar pregnancy (*see also* categories
        630-632) 639.1
    acquired (any) 286.7
    antepartum or intrapartum 641.3
      affecting fetus or newborn 762.1
    causing hemorrhage of pregnancy or delivery
        641.3
    due to
      liver disease 286.7
      vitamin K deficiency 286.7
    newborn, transient 776.3
    postpartum 666.3
    specified type NEC 286.3
  conduction (heart) 426.9
    bone (*see also* Deafness, conductive) 389.00
  congenital, organ or site NEC—*see also*
      Anomaly
  circulation 747.9
  Descemet's membrane 743.9
    specified type NEC 743.49
  diaphragm 756.6
  ectodermal 757.9
  esophagus 750.9
  pulmonic cusps—*see* Anomaly, heart valve
  respiratory system 748.9
    specified type NEC 748.8
  cushion endocardial 745.60
  dentin (hereditary) 520.5
  Descemet's membrane (congenital) 743.9
    acquired 371.30
    specific type NEC 743.49
  deutan 368.52
  developmental—*see also* Anomaly, by site
    cauda equina 742.59
    left ventricle 746.9
      with atresia or hypoplasia of aortic orifice or
        valve, with hypoplasia of ascending
        aorta 746.7
      in hypoplastic left heart syndrome 746.7
    testis 752.9
    vessel 747.9
  diaphragm
    with elevation, eventration, or hernia—*see*
      Hernia, diaphragm
    congenital 756.6
      with elevation, eventration, or hernia 756.6
      gross (with elevation, eventration, or hernia)
        756.6
  ectodermal, congenital 757.9
  Eisenmenger's (ventricular septal defect) 745.4
  endocardial cushion 745.60
    specified type NEC 745.69

Defect, defective—*continued*
  esophagus, congenital 750.9
  extensor retinaculum 728.9
  fibrin polymerization (*see also* Defect,
    coagulation) 286.3
  filling
    biliary tract 793.3
    bladder 793.5
    gallbladder 793.3
    kidney 793.5
    stomach 793.4
    ureter 793.5
  fossa ovalis 745.5
  gene, carrier (suspected) of V83.89
  Gerbode 745.4
  glaucomatous, without elevated tension 365.89
  Hageman (factor) (*see also* Defect, coagulation)
    286.3
  hearing (*see also* Deafness) 389.9
  high grade 317
  homogentisic acid 270.2
  interatrial septal 745.5
    acquired 429.71
  interauricular septal 745.5
    acquired 429.71
  interventricular septal 745.4
    with pulmonary stenosis or atresia,
      dextroposition of aorta, and hypertrophy
      of right ventricle 745.2
    acquired 429.71
    in tetralogy of Fallot 745.2
  iodide trapping 246.1
  iodotyrosine dehalogenase 246.1
  kynureninase 270.2
  learning, specific 315.2
  mental (*see also* Retardation, mental) 319
  osteochondral NEC 738.8
  ostium
    primum 745.61
    secundum 745.5
  pericardium 746.89
  peroxidase-binding 246.1
  placental blood supply—*see* Placenta,
    insufficiency
  platelet (qualitative) 287.1
    constitutional 286.4
  postural, spine 737.9
  protan 368.51
  pulmonic cusps, congenital 746.00
  renal pelvis 753.9
    obstructive 753.29
    specified type NEC 753.3
  respiratory system, congenital 748.9
    specified type NEC 748.8
  retina, retinal 361.30
    with detachment (*see also* Detachment, retina,
      with retinal defect) 361.00
    multiple 361.33
      with detachment 361.02
    nerve fiber bundle 362.85
    single 361.30
      with detachment 361.01
  septal (closure) (heart) NEC 745.9
    acquired 429.71
    atrial 745.5
    specified type NEC 745.8
  speech NEC 784.5
    developmental 315.39
    secondary to organic lesion 784.5
  Taussig-Bing (transposition, aorta and
    overriding pulmonary artery) 745.11

Defect, defective—*continued*
  teeth, wedge 521.2
  thyroid hormone synthesis 246.1
  tritan 368.53
  ureter 753.9
    obstructive 753.29
  vascular (acquired) (local) 459.9
    congenital (peripheral) NEC 747.60
      gastrointestinal 747.61
      lower limb 747.64
      renal 747.62
      specified NEC 747.69
      spinal 747.82
      upper limb 747.63
  ventricular septal 745.4
    with pulmonary stenosis or atresia,
      dextraposition of aorta, and hypertrophy
      of right ventricle 745.2
    acquired 429.71
    atrioventricular canal type 745.69
    between infundibulum and anterior portion
      745.4
    in tetralogy of Fallot 745.2
    isolated anterior 745.4
  vision NEC 369.9
  visual field 368.40
    arcuate 368.43
    heteronymous, bilateral 368.47
    homonymous, bilateral 368.46
    localized NEC 368.44
    nasal step 368.44
    peripheral 368.44
    sector 368.43
  voice 784.40
  wedge, teeth (abrasion) 521.2
Defeminization syndrome 255.2
Deferentitis 608.4
  gonorrheal (acute) 098.14
    chronic or duration of 2 months or over 098.34
Defibrination syndrome (*see also* Fibrinolysis)
  286.6
Deficiency, deficient
  3-beta-hydroxysteroid dehydrogenase 255.2
  6-phosphogluconic dehydrogenase (anemia)
    282.2
  11-beta-hydroxylase 255.2
  17-alpha-hydroxylase 255.2
  18-hydroxysteroid dehydrogenase 255.2
  20-alpha-hydroxylase 255.2
  21-hydroxylase 255.2
  abdominal muscle syndrome 756.79
  accelerator globulin (Ac G) (blood) (*see also*
    Defect, coagulation) 286.3
  AC globulin (congenital) (*see also* Defect,
    coagulation) 286.3
    acquired 286.7
  activating factor (blood) (*see also* Defect,
    coagulation) 286.3
  adenohypophyseal 253.2
  adenosine deaminase 277.2
  aldolase (hereditary) 271.2
  alpha-1-antitrypsin 277.6
  alpha-1-trypsin inhibitor 277.6
  alpha-fucosidase 271.8
  alpha-lipoprotein 272.5
  alpha-mannosidase 271.8
  amino acid 270.9
  anemia—*see* Anemia, deficiency
  aneurin 265.1
    with beriberi 265.0

Deficiency, deficient—*continued*
  antibody NEC 279.00
  antidiuretic hormone 253.5
  antihemophilic
    factor (A) 286.0
      B 286.1
      C 286.2
    globulin (AHG) NEC 286.0
  antitrypsin 277.6
  argininosuccinate synthetase or lyase 270.6
  ascorbic acid (with scurvy) 267
  autoprothrombin
    I (*see also* Defect, coagulation) 286.3
    II 286.1
    C (*see also* Defect, coagulation) 286.3
  bile salt 579.8
  biotin 266.2
  biotinidase 277.6
  bradykinase-1 277.6
  brancher enzyme (amylopectinosis) 271.0
  calciferol 268.9
    with
      osteomalacia 268.2
      rickets (*see also* Rickets) 268.0
  calcium 275.40
    dietary 269.3
  calorie, severe 261
  carbamyl phosphate synthetase 270.6
  cardiac (*see also* Insufficiency, myocardial)
      428.0
  carnitine palmityl transferase 791.3
  carotene 264.9
  Carr factor (*see also* Defect, coagulation) 286.9
  central nervous system 349.9
  ceruloplasmin 275.1
  cevitamic acid (with scurvy) 267
  choline 266.2
  Christmas factor 286.1
  chromium 269.3
  citrin 269.1
  clotting (blood) (*see also* Defect, coagulation)
      286.9
  coagulation factor NEC 286.9
    with
      abortion—*see* Abortion, by type, with
          hemorrhage
      ectopic pregnancy (*see also* categories
          634-638) 639.1
      molar pregnancy (*see also* categories
          630-632) 639.1
    acquired (any) 286.7
    antepartum or intrapartum 641.3
      affecting fetus or newborn 762.1
    due to
      liver disease 286.7
      vitamin K deficiency 286.7
    newborn, transient 776.3
    postpartum 666.3
    specified type NEC 286.3
  color vision (congenital) 368.59
    acquired 368.55
  combined, two or more coagulation factors (*see
      also* Defect, coagulation) 286.9
  complement factor NEC 279.8
  contact factor (*see also* Defect, coagulation)
      286.3
  copper NEC 275.1
  corticoadrenal 255.4
  craniofacial axis 756.0
  cyanocobalamin (vitamin B₁₂) 266.2

Deficiency, deficient—*continued*
  debrancher enzyme (limit dextrinosis) 271.0
  desmolase 255.2
  diet 269.9
  dihydrofolate reductase 281.2
  dihydropteridine reductase 270.1
  disaccharidase (intestinal) 271.3
  disease NEC 269.9
  ear(s) V48.8
  edema 262
  endocrine 259.9
  enzymes, circulating NEC (*see also* Deficiency,
      by specific enzyme) 277.6
  ergosterol 268.9
    with
      osteomalacia 268.2
      rickets (*see also* Rickets) 268.0
  erythrocytic glutathione (anemia) 282.2
  eyelid(s) V48.8
  factor (*see also* Defect, coagulation) 286.9
    I (congenital) (fibrinogen) 286.3
      antepartum or intrapartum 641.3
        affecting fetus or newborn 762.1
      newborn, transient 776.3
      postpartum 666.3
    II (congenital) (prothrombin) 286.3
    V (congenital) (labile) 286.3
    VII (congenital) (stable) 286.3
    VIII (congenital) (functional) 286.0
      with
        functional defect 286.0
        vascular defect 286.4
    IX (Christmas) (congenital) (functional) 286.1
    X (congenital) (Stuart-Prower) 286.3
    XI (congenital) (plasma thromboplastin
        antecedent) 286.2
    XII (congenital) (Hageman) 286.3
    XIII (congenital) (fibrin stabilizing) 286.3
    Hageman 286.3
    multiple (congenital) 286.9
      acquired 286.7
  fibrinase (*see also* Defect, coagulation) 286.3
  fibrinogen (congenital) (*see also* Defect,
      coagulation) 286.3
    acquired 286.6
  fibrin stabilizing factor (congenital) (*see also*
      Defect, coagulation) 286.3
    acquired 286.7
  finger—*see* Absence, finger
  Fletcher factor (*see also* Defect, coagulation)
      286.9
  fluorine 269.3
  folate, anemia 281.2
  folic acid (vitamin Bc) 266.2
    anemia 281.2
  follicle-stimulating hormone (FSH) 253.4
  fructokinase 271.2
  fructose-1, 6-diphosphate 271.2
  fructose-1-phosphate aldolase 271.2
  FSH (follicle stimulating hormone) 253.4
  fucosidase 271.8
  galactokinase 271.1
  galactose-1-phosphate uridyl transferase 271.1
  gamma globulin in blood 279.00
  glass factor (*see also* Defect, coagulation) 286.3
  glucocorticoid 255.4
  glucose-6-phosphatase 271.0
  glucose-6-phosphate dehydrogenase anemia
      282.2
  glucuronyl transferase 277.4
  glutathione-reductase (anemia) 282.2

Deficiency, deficient—*continued*
  glycogen synthetase 271.0
  growth hormone 253.3
  Hageman factor (congenital) (*see also* Defect,
     coagulation) 286.3
  head V48.0
  hemoglobin (*see also* Anemia) 285.9
  hepatophosphorylase 271.0
  hexose monophosphate (HMP) shunt 282.2
  HGH (human growth hormone) 253.3
  HG-PRT 277.2
  homogentisic acid oxidase 270.2
  hormone—*see also* Deficiency, by specific
     hormone
    anterior pituitary (isolated) (partial) NEC
      253.4
      growth (human) 253.3
    follicle-stimulating 253.4
    growth (human) (isolated) 253.3
    human growth 253.3
    interstitial cell-stimulating 253.4
    luteinizing 253.4
    melanocyte-stimulating 253.4
    testicular 257.2
  human growth hormone 253.3
  humoral 279.00
    with
      hyper-IgM 279.05
        autosomal recessive 279.05
        X-linked 279.05
      increased IgM 279.05
    congenital hypogammaglobulinemia 279.04
    non-sex-linked 279.06
    selective immunoglobulin NEC 279.03
      IgA 279.01
      IgG 279.03
      IgM 279.02
        increased 279.05
    specified NEC 279.09
  hydroxylase 255.2
  hypoxanthine-guanine
     phosphoribosyltransferase (HG-PRT) 277.2
  ICSH (interstitial cell-stimulating hormone)
     253.4
  immunity NEC 279.3
    cell-mediated 279.10
      with
        hyperimmunoglobulinemia 279.2
        thrombocytopenia and eczema 279.12
      specified NEC 279.19
    combined (severe) 279.2
      syndrome 279.2
    common variable 279.06
    humoral NEC 279.00
    IgA (secretory) 279.01
    IgG 279.03
    IgM 279.02
  immunoglobulin, selective NEC 279.03
    IgA 279.01
    IgG 279.03
    IgM 279.02
  inositol (B complex) 266.2
  interferon 279.4
  internal organ V47.0
  interstitial cell-stimulating hormone (ICSH)
     253.4
  intrinsic (urethral) sphincter (ISD) 599.82
  intrinsic factor (Castle's) (congenital) 281.0
  invertase 271.3
  iodine 269.3
  iron, anemia 280.9

Deficiency, deficient—*continued*
  labile factor (congenital) (*see also* Defect,
     coagulation) 286.3
    acquired 286.7
  lacrimal fluid (acquired) 375.15
    congenital 743.64
  lactase 271.3
  Laki-Lorand factor (*see also* Defect,
     coagulation) 286.3
  lecithin-cholesterol acyltranferase 272.5
  LH (luteinizing hormone) 253.4
  limb V49.0
    lower V49.0
      congenital (*see also* Deficiency, lower limb,
        congenital) 755.30
    upper V49.0
      congenital (*see also* Deficiency, upper limb,
        congenital) 755.20
  lipocaic 577.8
  lipoid (high-density) 272.5
  lipoprotein (familial) (high density) 272.5
  liver phosphorylase 271.0
  lower limb V49.0
    congenital 755.30
      with complete absence of distal elements
        755.31
      longitudinal (complete) (partial) (with distal
        deficiencies, incomplete) 755.32
        with complete absence of distal elements
         755.31
        combined femoral, tibial, fibular
         (incomplete) 755.33
        femoral 755.34
        fibular 755.37
        metatarsal(s) 755.38
        phalange(s) 755.39
         meaning all digits 755.31
        tarsal(s) 755.38
        tibia 755.36
        tibiofibular 755.35
      transverse 755.31
  luteinizing hormone (LH) 253.4
  lysosomal alpha-1, 4 glucosidase 271.0
  magnesium 275.2
  mannosidase 271.8
  melanocyte-stimulating hormone (MSH) 253.4
  menadione (vitamin K) 269.0
    newborn 776.0
  mental (familial) (hereditary) (*see also*
     Retardation, mental) 319
  mineral NEC 269.3
  molybdenum 269.3
  moral 301.7
  multiple, syndrome 260
  myocardial (*see also* Insufficiency myocardial)
     428.0
  myophosphorylase 271.0
  NADH (DPNH) -methemoglobin-reductase
     (congenital) 289.7
  NADH diaphorase or reductase (congenital)
     289.7
  neck V48.1
  niacin (amide) (-tryptophan) 265.2
  nicotinamide 265.2
  nicotinic acid (amide) 265.2
  nose V48.8
  number of teeth (*see also* Anodontia) 520.0
  nutrition, nutritional 269.9
    specified NEC 269.8

Deformity—*continued*
  caruncle, lacrimal (congenital) 743.9
    acquired 375.69
  cascade, stomach 537.6
  cecum (congenital) 751.5
    acquired 569.89
  cerebral (congenital) 742.9
    acquired 348.8
  cervix (acquired) (uterus) 622.8
    congenital 752.40
  cheek (acquired) 738.19
    congenital 744.9
  chest (wall) (acquired) 738.3
    congenital 754.89
    late effect of rickets 268.1
  chin (acquired) 738.19
    congenital 744.9
  choroid (congenital) 743.9
    acquired 363.8
    plexus (congenital) 742.9
      acquired 349.2
  cicatricial—*see* Cicatrix
  cilia (congenital) 743.9
    acquired 374.89
  circulatory system (congenital) 747.9
  clavicle (acquired) 738.8
    congenital 755.51
  clitoris (congenital) 752.40
    acquired 624.8
  clubfoot—*see* Clubfoot
  coccyx (acquired) 738.6
    congenital 756.10
  colon (congenital) 751.5
    acquired 569.89
  concha (ear) (congenital) (*see also* Deformity,
     ear) 744.3
    acquired 380.32
  congenital, organ or site not listed (*see also*
     Anomaly) 759.9
  cornea (congenital) 743.9
    acquired 371.70
  coronary artery (congenital) 746.85
    acquired (*see also* Ischemia, heart) 414.9
  cranium (acquired) 738.19
    congenital (*see also* Deformity, skull,
      congenital) 756.0
  cricoid cartilage (congenital) 748.3
    acquired 478.79
  cystic duct (congenital) 751.60
    acquired 575.8
  Dandy-Walker 742.3
    with spina bifida (*see also* Spina bifida) 741.0
  diaphragm (congenital) 756.6
    acquired 738.8
  digestive organ(s) or system (congenital) NEC
     751.9
    specified type NEC 751.8
  ductus arteriosus 747.0
  duodenal bulb 537.89
  duodenum (congenital) 751.5
    acquired 537.89
  dura (congenital) 742.9
    brain 742.4
      acquired 349.2
    spinal 742.59
      acquired 349.2

Deformity—*continued*
  ear (congenital) 744.3
    acquired 380.32
    auricle 744.3
      causing impairment of hearing 744.02
    causing impairment of hearing 744.00
    external 744.3
      causing impairment of hearing 744.02
    internal 744.05
    lobule 744.3
    middle 744.03
      ossicles 744.04
    ossicles 744.04
  ectodermal (congenital) NEC 757.9
    specified type NEC 757.8
  ejaculatory duct (congenital) 752.9
    acquired 608.89
  elbow (joint) (acquired) 736.00
    congenital 755.50
    contraction 718.42
  endocrine gland NEC 759.2
  epididymis (congenital) 752.9
    acquired 608.89
    torsion 608.2
  epiglottis (congenital) 748.3
    acquired 478.79
  esophagus (congenital) 750.9
    acquired 530.89
  Eustachian tube (congenital) NEC 744.3
    specified type NEC 744.24
  extremity (acquired) 736.9
    congenital, except reduction deformity 755.9
      lower 755.60
      upper 755.50
    reduction—*see* Deformity, reduction
  eye (congenital) 743.9
    acquired 379.8
    muscle 743.9
  eyebrow (congenital) 744.89
  eyelid (congenital) 743.9
    acquired 374.89
    specified type NEC 743.62
  face (acquired) 738.19
    congenital (any part) 744.9
      due to intrauterine malposition and pressure
        754.0
  fallopian tube (congenital) 752.10
    acquired 620.8
  femur (acquired) 736.89
    congenital 755.60
  fetal
    with fetopelvic disproportion 653.7
      affecting fetus or newborn 763.1
    causing obstructed labor 660.1
      affecting fetus or newborn 763.1
    known or suspected, affecting management of
      pregnancy 655.9
  finger (acquired) 736.20
    boutonniere type 736.21
    congenital 755.50
    flexion contracture 718.44
    swan neck 736.22
  flexion (joint) (acquired) 736.9
    congenital NEC 755.9
    hip or thigh (acquired) 736.39
      congenital (*see also* Subluxation,
        congenital, hip) 754.32

Deformity—*continued*
　foot (acquired) 736.70
　　cavovarus 736.75
　　　congenital 754.59
　　congenital NEC 754.70
　　　specified type NEC 754.79
　　valgus (acquired) 736.79
　　　congenital 754.60
　　　　specified type NEC 754.69
　　varus (acquired) 736.79
　　　congenital 754.50
　　　　specified type NEC 754.59
　forearm (acquired) 736.00
　　congenital 755.50
　forehead (acquired) 738.19
　　congenital (*see also* Deformity, skull,
　　　congenital) 756.0
　frontal bone (acquired) 738.19
　　congenital (*see also* Deformity, skull,
　　　congenital) 756.0
　gallbladder (congenital) 751.60
　　acquired 575.8
　gastrointestinal tract (congenital) NEC 751.9
　　acquired 569.89
　　specified type NEC 751.8
　genitalia, genital organ(s) or system NEC
　　congenital 752.9
　　female (congenital) 752.9
　　　acquired 629.8
　　　external 752.40
　　　internal 752.9
　　male (congenital) 752.9
　　　acquired 608.89
　globe (eye) (congenital) 743.9
　　acquired 360.89
　gum (congenital) 750.9
　　acquired 523.9
　gunstock 736.02
　hand (acquired) 736.00
　　claw 736.06
　　congenital 755.50
　　minus (and plus) (intrinsic) 736.09
　　pill roller (intrinsic) 736.09
　　plus (and minus) (intrinsic) 736.09
　　swan neck (intrinsic) 736.09
　head (acquired) 738.10
　　congenital (*see also* Deformity, skull,
　　　congenital) 756.0
　　specified NEC 738.19
　heart (congenital) 746.9
　　auricle (congenital) 746.9
　　septum 745.9
　　　auricular 745.5
　　　specified type NEC 745.8
　　　ventricular 745.4
　　valve (congenital) NEC 746.9
　　　acquired—*see* Endocarditis
　　　pulmonary (congenital) 746.00
　　　specified type NEC 746.89
　　ventricle (congenital) 746.9
　heel (acquired) 736.76
　　congenital 755.67
　hepatic duct (congenital) 751.60
　　acquired 576.8
　　　with calculus, choledocholithiasis, or
　　　　stones—*see* Choledocholithiasis
　hip (joint) (acquired) 736.30
　　congenital NEC 755.63
　　flexion 718.45
　　　congenital (*see also* Subluxation,
　　　　congenital, hip) 754.32

Deformity—*continued*
　hourglass—*see* Contraction, hourglass
　humerus (acquired) 736.89
　　congenital 755.50
　hymen (congenital) 752.40
　hypophyseal (congenital) 759.2
　ileocecal (coil) (valve) (congenital) 751.5
　　acquired 569.89
　ileum (intestine) (congenital) 751.5
　　acquired 569.89
　ilium (acquired) 738.6
　　congenital 755.60
　integument (congenital) 757.9
　intervertebral cartilage or disc (acquired)—*see
　　also* Displacement, intervertebral disc
　　congenital 756.10
　intestine (large) (small) (congenital) 751.5
　　acquired 569.89
　iris (acquired) 364.75
　　congenital 743.9
　　prolapse 364.8
　ischium (acquired) 738.6
　　congenital 755.60
　jaw (acquired) (congenital) NEC 524.9
　　due to intrauterine malposition and pressure
　　　754.0
　joint (acquired) NEC 738.8
　　congenital 755.9
　　contraction (abduction) (adduction)
　　　(extension) (flexion)—*see* Contraction,
　　　joint
　kidney(s) (calyx) (pelvis) (congenital) 753.9
　　acquired 593.89
　　vessel 747.62
　　　acquired 459.9
　Klippel-Feil (brevicollis) 756.16
　knee (acquired) NEC 736.6
　　congenital 755.64
　labium (majus) (minus) (congenital) 752.40
　　acquired 624.8
　lacrimal apparatus or duct (congenital) 743.9
　　acquired 375.69
　larynx (muscle) (congenital) 748.3
　　acquired 478.79
　　web (glottic) (subglottic) 748.2
　leg (lower) (upper) (acquired) NEC 736.89
　　congenital 755.60
　　reduction—*see* Deformity, reduction, lower
　　　limb
　lens (congenital) 743.9
　　acquired 379.39
　lid (fold) (congenital) 743.9
　　acquired 374.89
　ligament (acquired) 728.9
　　congenital 756.9
　limb (acquired) 736.9
　　congenital, except reduction deformity 755.9
　　　lower 755.60
　　　　reduction (*see also* Deformity, reduction,
　　　　　lower limb) 755.30
　　　upper 755.50
　　　　reduction (*see also* Deformity, reduction,
　　　　　lower limb) 755.20
　　specified NEC 736.89
　lip (congenital) NEC 750.9
　　acquired 528.5
　　specified type NEC 750.26

Deformity—*continued*
reduction (extremity) (limb) 755.4
  brain 742.2
  lower limb 755.30
    with complete absence of distal elements
      755.31
    longitudinal (complete) (partial) (with distal
        deficiencies, incomplete) 755.32
      with complete absence of distal elements
        755.31
    combined femoral, tibial, fibular
        (incomplete) 755.33
    femoral 755.34
    fibular 755.37
    metatarsal(s) 755.38
    phalange(s) 755.39
      meaning all digits 755.31
    tarsal(s) 755.38
    tibia 755.36
    tibiofibular 755.35
    transverse 755.31
  upper limb 755.20
    with complete absence of distal elements
      755.21
    longitudinal (complete) (partial) (with distal
        deficiencies, incomplete) 755.22
      with complete absence of distal elements
        755.21
    carpal(s) 755.28
    combined humeral, radial, ulnar
        (incomplete) 755.23
    humeral 755.24
    metacarpal(s) 755.28
    phalange(s) 755.29
      meaning all digits 755.21
    radial 755.26
    radioulnar 755.25
    ulnar 755.27
  transverse (complete) (partial) 755.21
renal—*see* Deformity, kidney
respiratory system (congenital) 748.9
  specified type NEC 748.8
rib (acquired) 738.3
  congenital 756.3
    cervical 756.2
rotation (joint) (acquired) 736.9
  congenital 755.9
  hip or thigh 736.39
    congenital (*see also* Subluxation,
        congenital, hip) 754.32
sacroiliac joint (congenital) 755.69
  acquired 738.5
sacrum (acquired) 738.5
  congenital 756.10
saddle
  back 737.8
  nose 738.0
    syphilitic 090.5
salivary gland or duct (congenital) 750.9
  acquired 527.8
scapula (acquired) 736.89
  congenital 755.50
scrotum (congenital) 752.9
  acquired 608.89
sebaceous gland, acquired 706.8
seminal tract or duct (congenital) 752.9
  acquired 608.89
septum (nasal) (acquired) 470
  congenital 748.1

Deformity—*continued*
shoulder (joint) (acquired) 736.89
  congenital 755.50
    specified type NEC 755.59
  contraction 718.41
sigmoid (flexure) (congenital) 751.5
  acquired 569.89
sinus of Valsalva 747.29
skin (congenital) 757.9
  acquired NEC 709.8
skull (acquired) 738.19
  congenital 756.0
    with
      anencephalus 740.0
      encephalocele 742.0
      hydrocephalus 742.3
        with spina bifida (*see also* Spina bifida)
          741.0
      microcephalus 742.1
    due to intrauterine malposition and pressure
      754.0
soft parts, organs or tissues (of pelvis)
  in pregnancy or childbirth NEC 654.9
    affecting fetus or newborn 763.89
    causing obstructed labor 660.2
      affecting fetus or newborn 763.1
spermatic cord (congenital) 752.9
  acquired 608.89
    torsion 608.2
spinal
  column—*see* Deformity, spine
  cord (congenital) 742.9
    acquired 336.8
    vessel (congenital) 747.82
  nerve root (congenital) 742.9
    acquired 724.9
  vessel 747.82
spine (acquired) NEC 738.5
  congenital 756.10
    due to intrauterine malposition and pressure
      754.2
  kyphoscoliotic (*see also* Kyphoscoliosis)
      737.30
  kyphotic (*see also* Kyphosis) 737.10
  lordotic (*see also* Lordosis) 737.20
  rachitic 268.1
  scoliotic (*see also* Scoliosis) 737.30
spleen
  acquired 289.59
  congenital 759.0
Sprengel's (congenital) 755.52
sternum (acquired) 738.3
  congenital 756.3
stomach (congenital) 750.9
  acquired 537.89
submaxillary gland (congenital) 750.9
  acquired 527.8
swan neck (acquired)
  finger 736.22
  hand 736.09
talipes—*see* Talipes
teeth, tooth NEC 520.9
testis (congenital) 752.9
  acquired 608.89
    torsion 608.2
thigh (acquired) 736.89
  congenital 755.60
thorax (acquired) (wall) 738.3
  congenital 754.89
  late effect of rickets 268.1

Deformity—*continued*
  thumb (acquired) 736.20
    congenital 755.50
  thymus (tissue) (congenital) 759.2
  thyroid (gland) (congenital) 759.2
    cartilage 748.3
      acquired 478.79
  tibia (acquired) 736.89
    congenital 755.60
    saber 090.5
  toe (acquired) 735.9
    congenital 755.66
    specified NEC 735.8
  tongue (congenital) 750.10
    acquired 529.8
  tooth, teeth NEC 520.9
  trachea (rings) (congenital) 748.3
    acquired 519.1
  transverse aortic arch (congenital) 747.21
  tricuspid (leaflets) (valve) (congenital) 746.9
    acquired—*see* Endocarditis, tricuspid
    atresia or stenosis 746.1
    specified type NEC 746.89
  trunk (acquired) 738.3
    congenital 759.9
  ulna (acquired) 736.00
    congenital 755.50
  upper extremity—*see* Deformity, arm
  urachus (congenital) 753.7
  ureter (opening) (congenital) 753.9
    acquired 593.89
  urethra (valve) (congenital) 753.9
    acquired 599.84
  urinary tract or system (congenital) 753.9
    urachus 753.7
  uterus (congenital) 752.3
    acquired 621.8
  uvula (congenital) 750.9
    acquired 528.9
  vagina (congenital) 752.40
    acquired 623.8
  valve, valvular (heart) (congenital) 746.9
    acquired—*see* Endocarditis
    pulmonary 746.00
    specified type NEC 746.89
  vascular (congenital) (peripheral) NEC 747.60
    acquired 459.9
    gastrointestinal 747.61
    lower limb 747.64
    renal 747.62
    specified site NEC 747.69
    spinal 747.82
    upper limb 747.63
  vas deferens (congenital) 752.9
    acquired 608.89
  vein (congenital) NEC (*see also* Deformity,
      vascular) 747.60
    brain 747.81
    coronary 746.9
    great 747.40
  vena cava (inferior) (superior) (congenital)
      747.40
  vertebra—*see* Deformity, spine
  vesicourethral orifice (acquired) 596.8
    congenital NEC 753.9
      specified type NEC 753.8
  vessels of optic papilla (congenital) 743.9
  visual field (contraction) 368.45
  vitreous humor (congenital) 743.9
    acquired 379.29

Deformity—*continued*
  vulva (congenital) 752.40
    acquired 624.8
  wrist (joint) (acquired) 736.00
    congenital 755.50
    contraction 718.43
    valgus 736.03
      congenital 755.59
    varus 736.04
      congenital 755.59
Degeneration, degenerative
  adrenal (capsule) (gland) 255.8
    with hypofunction 255.4
    fatty 255.8
    hyaline 255.8
    infectional 255.8
    lardaceous 277.3
  amyloid (any site) (general) 277.3
  anterior cornua, spinal cord 336.8
  aorta, aortic 440.0
    fatty 447.8
    valve (heart) (*see also* Endocarditis, aortic)
        424.1
  arteriovascular—*see* Arteriosclerosis
  artery, arterial (atheromatous) (calcareous)—*see
      also* Arteriosclerosis
    amyloid 277.3
    lardaceous 277.3
    medial NEC (*see also* Arteriosclerosis,
        extremities) 440.20
  articular cartilage NEC (*see also* Disorder,
      cartilage, articular) 718.0
    elbow 718.02
    knee 717.5
    patella 717.7
    shoulder 718.01
    spine (*see also* Spondylosis) 721.90
  atheromatous—*see* Arteriosclerosis
  bacony (any site) 277.3
  basal nuclei or ganglia NEC 333.0
  bone 733.90
  brachial plexus 353.0
  brain (cortical) (progressive) 331.9
    arteriosclerotic 437.0
    childhood 330.9
      specified type NEC 330.8
    congenital 742.4
    cystic 348.0
      congenital 742.4
    familial NEC 331.89
    grey matter 330.8
    heredofamilial NEC 331.89
    in
      alcoholism 303.9 *[331.7]*
      beriberi 265.0 *[331.7]*
      cerebrovascular disease 437.9 *[331.7]*
      congenital hydrocephalus 742.3 *[331.7]*
        with spina bifida (*see also* Spina bifida)
            741.0 *[331.7]*
      Fabry's disease 272.7 *[330.2]*
      Gaucher's disease 272.7 *[330.2]*
      Hunter's disease or syndrome 277.5 *[330.3]*
      lipidosis
        cerebral 330.1
        generalized 272.7 *[330.2]*
      mucopolysaccharidosis 277.5 *[330.3]*
      myxedema (*see also* Myxedema) 244.9
          [331.7]
      neoplastic disease NEC (M8000/1) 239.9
          [331.7]
      Niemann-Pick disease 272.7 *[330.2]*

Degeneration, degenerative—*continued*
    sphingolipidosis 272.7 *[330.2]*
    vitamin B₁₂ deficiency 266.2 *[331.7]*
  motor centers 331.89
  senile 331.2
  specified type NEC 331.89
 breast—*see* Disease, breast
 Bruch's membrane 363.40
 bundle of His 426.50
  left 426.3
  right 426.4
 calcareous NEC 275.49
 capillaries 448.9
  amyloid 277.3
  fatty 448.9
  lardaceous 277.3
 cardiac (brown) (calcareous) (fatty) (fibrous)
    (hyaline) (mural) (muscular) (pigmentary)
    (senile) (with arteriosclerosis) (*see also*
    Degeneration, myocardial) 429.1
  valve, valvular—*see* Endocarditis
 cardiorenal (*see also* Hypertension, cardiorenal)
    404.90
 cardiovascular (*see also* Disease,
    cardiovascular) 429.2
  renal (*see also* Hypertension, cardiorenal)
    404.90
 cartilage (joint)—*see* Derangement, joint
 cerebellar NEC 334.9
  primary (hereditary) (sporadic) 334.2
 cerebral—*see* Degeneration, brain
 cerebromacular 330.1
 cerebrovascular 437.1
  due to hypertension 437.2
  late effect—*see* Late effect(s) (of)
    cerebrovascular disease
 cervical plexus 353.2
 cervix 622.8
  due to radiation (intended effect) 622.8
    adverse effect or misadventure 622.8
 changes, spine or vertebra (*see also*
    Spondylosis) 721.90
 chitinous 277.3
 chorioretinal 363.40
  congenital 743.53
  hereditary 363.50
 choroid (colloid) (drusen) 363.40
  hereditary 363.50
  senile 363.41
    diffuse secondary 363.42
 cochlear 386.8
 collateral ligament (knee) (medial) 717.82
  lateral 717.81
 combined (spinal cord) (subacute) 266.2 *[336.2]*
  with anemia (pernicious) 281.0 *[336.2]*
    due to dietary deficiency 281.1 *[336.2]*
  due to vitamin B₁₂ deficiency anemia (dietary)
    281.1 *[336.2]*
 conjunctiva 372.50
  amyloid 277.3 *[372.50]*
 cornea 371.40
  calcerous 371.44
  familial (hereditary) (*see also* Dystrophy,
    cornea) 371.50
    macular 371.55
    reticular 371.54
  hyaline (of old scars) 371.41
  marginal (Terrien's) 371.48
  mosaic (shagreen) 371.41
  nodular 371.46
  peripheral 371.48

Degeneration, degenerative—*continued*
 senile 371.41
 cortical (cerebellar) (parenchymatous) 334.2
  alcoholic 303.9 *[334.4]*
  diffuse, due to arteriopathy 437.0
 corticostriatal-spinal 334.8
 cretinoid 243
 cruciate ligament (knee) (posterior) 717.84
  anterior 717.83
 cutis 709.3
  amyloid 277.3
 dental pulp 522.2
 disc disease—*see* Degeneration, intervertebral
  disc
 dorsolateral (spinal cord)—*see* Degeneration,
  combined
 endocardial 424.90
 extrapyramidal NEC 333.90
 eye NEC 360.40
  macular (*see also* Degeneration, macula)
    362.50
    congenital 362.75
    hereditary 362.76
 fatty (diffuse) (general) 272.8
  liver 571.8
    alcoholic 571.0
  localized site—*see* Degeneration, by site, fatty
  placenta—*see* Placenta, abnormal
 globe (eye) NEC 360.40
  macular—*see* Degeneration, macula
 grey matter 330.8
 heart (brown) (calcareous) (fatty) (fibrous)
    (hyaline) (mural) (muscular) (pigmentary)
    (senile) (with arteriosclerosis) (*see also*
    Degeneration, myocardial) 429.1
  amyloid 277.3 *[425.7]*
  atheromatous —*see* Arteriosclerosis, coronary
  gouty 274.82
  hypertensive (*see also* Hypertension, heart)
    402.90
  ischemic 414.9
  valve, valvular—*see* Endocarditis
 hepatolenticular (Wilson's) 275.1
 hepatorenal 572.4
 heredofamilial
  brain NEC 331.89
  spinal cord NEC 336.8
 hyaline (diffuse) (generalized) 728.9
  localized—*see also* Degeneration, by site
    cornea 371.41
    keratitis 371.41
 hypertensive vascular—*see* Hypertension
 infrapatellar fat pad 729.31
 internal semilunar cartilage 717.3
 intervertebral disc 722.6
  with myelopathy 722.70
  cervical, cervicothoracic 722.4
    with myelopathy 722.71
  lumbar, lumbosacral 722.52
    with myelopathy 722.73
  thoracic, thoracolumbar 722.51
    with myelopathy 722.72
 intestine 569.89
  amyloid 277.3
  lardaceous 277.3
 iris (generalized) (*see also* Atrophy, iris) 364.59
  pigmentary 364.53
  pupillary margin 364.54
 ischemic—*see* Ischemia
 joint disease (*see also* Osteoarthrosis) 715.9
  multiple sites 715.09

Dehydration (cachexia) 276.5
  with
    hypernatremia 276.0
    hyponatremia 276.1
  newborn 775.5
Deiters' nucleus syndrome 386.19
Déjérine's disease 356.0
Déjérine-Klumpke paralysis 767.6
Déjérine-Roussy syndrome 348.8
Déjérine-Sottas disease or neuropathy
  (hypertrophic) 356.0
Déjérine-Thomas atrophy or syndrome 333.0
de Lange's syndrome (Amsterdam dwarf,
  mental retardation, and brachycephaly) 759.89
Delay, delayed
  adaptation, cones or rods 368.63
  any plane in pelvis
    affecting fetus or newborn 763.1
    complicating delivery 660.1
  birth or delivery NEC 662.1
    affecting fetus or newborn 763.9
    second twin, triplet, or multiple mate 662.3
  closure—*see also* Fistula
    cranial suture 756.0
    fontanel 756.0
  coagulation NEC 790.92
  conduction (cardiac) (ventricular) 426.9
  delivery NEC 662.1
    second twin, triplet, etc. 662.3
      affecting fetus or newborn 763.89
  development
    in childhood 783.40
      physiological 783.40
    intellectual NEC 315.9
    learning NEC 315.2
    reading 315.00
    sexual 259.0
    speech 315.39
      associated with hyperkinesis 314.1
    spelling 315.09
  gastric emptying 536.8
  menarche 256.39
    due to pituitary hypofunction 253.4
  menstruation (cause unknown) 626.8
  milestone in childhood 783.42
  motility—*see* Hypomotility
  passage of meconium (newborn) 777.1
  primary respiration 768.9
  puberty 259.0
  sexual maturation, female 259.0
Del Castillo's syndrome (germinal aplasia) 606.0
Deleage's disease 359.89
Delhi (boil) (button) (sore) 085.1
Delinquency (juvenile) 312.9
  group (*see also* Disturbance, conduct) 312.2
  neurotic 312.4
Delirium, delirious 780.09
  acute (psychotic) 293.0
  alcoholic 291.0
    acute 291.0
    chronic 291.1
  alcoholicum 291.0
  chronic (*see also* Psychosis) 293.89
    due to or associated with physical
      condition—*see* Psychosis, organic
  drug-induced 292.81
  eclamptic (*see also* Eclampsia) 780.39
  exhaustion (*see also* Reaction, stress, acute)
    308.9
  hysterical 300.11

Delirium, delirious—*continued*
  in
    presenile dementia 290.11
    senile dementia 290.3
  induced by drug 292.81
  manic, maniacal (acute) (*see also* Psychosis,
    affective) 296.0
    recurrent episode 296.1
    single episode 296.0
  puerperal 293.9
  senile 290.3
  subacute (psychotic) 293.1
  thyroid (*see also* Thyrotoxicosis) 242.9
  traumatic—*see also* Injury, intracranial
    with
      lesion, spinal cord—*see* Injury, spinal, by
        site
      shock, spinal—*see* Injury, spinal, by site
  tremens (impending) 291.0
  uremic—*see* Uremia
  withdrawal
    alcoholic (acute) 291.0
      chronic 291.1
    drug 292.0
Delivery

> Note—Use the following fifth-digit
> subclassification with categories 640-648,
> 651-676:
>
> *0 unspecified as to episode of care*
> *1 delivered, with or without mention of*
> *antepartum condition*
> *2 delivered, with mention of*
> *postpartum complication*
> *3 antepartum condition or complication*
> *4 postpartum condition or*
> *complication*

  breech (assisted) (spontaneous) 652.2
    affecting fetus or newborn 763.0
    extraction NEC 669.6
  cesarean (for) 669.7
    abnormal
      cervix 654.6
      pelvic organs or tissues 654.9
      pelvis (bony) (major) NEC 653.0
      presentation or position 652.9
        in multiple gestation 652.6
      size, fetus 653.5
      soft parts (of pelvis) 654.9
      uterus, congenital 654.0
      vagina 654.7
      . vulva 654.8
    abruptio placentae 641.2
    acromion presentation 652.8
    affecting fetus or newborn 763.4
    anteversion, cervix or uterus 654.4
    atony, uterus 666.1
    bicornis or bicornuate uterus 654.0
    breech presentation 652.2
    brow presentation 652.4
    cephalopelvic disproportion (normally formed
      fetus) 653.4
    chin presentation 652.4
    cicatrix of cervix 654.6
    contracted pelvis (general) 653.1
      inlet 653.2
      outlet 653.3
    cord presentation or prolapse 663.0
    cystocele 654.4

Delivery—*continued*
- deformity (acquired) (congenital)
  - pelvic organs or tissues NEC 654.9
  - pelvis (bony) NEC 653.0
- displacement, uterus NEC 654.4
- disproportion NEC 653.9
- distress
  - fetal 656.8
  - maternal 669.0
- eclampsia 642.6
- face presentation 652.4
- failed
  - forceps 660.7
  - trial of labor NEC 660.6
  - vacuum extraction 660.7
  - ventouse 660.7
- fetal deformity 653.7
- fetal-maternal hemorrhage 656.0
- fetus, fetal
  - distress 656.8
  - prematurity 656.8
- fibroid (tumor) (uterus) 654.1
- footling 652.8
  - with successful version 652.1
- hemorrhage (antepartum) (intrapartum) NEC 641.9
- hydrocephalic fetus 653.6
- incarceration of uterus 654.3
- incoordinate uterine action 661.4
- inertia, uterus 661.2
  - primary 661.0
  - secondary 661.1
- lateroversion, uterus or cervix 654.4
- mal lie 652.9
- malposition
  - fetus 652.9
    - in multiple gestation 652.6
  - pelvic organs or tissues NEC 654.9
  - uterus NEC or cervix 654.4
- malpresentation NEC 652.9
  - in multiple gestation 652.6
- maternal
  - diabetes mellitus 648.0
  - heart disease NEC 648.6
- meconium in liquor 656.8
  - staining only 792.3
- oblique presentation 652.3
- oversize fetus 653.5
- pelvic tumor NEC 654.9
- placental insufficiency 656.5
- placenta previa 641.0
  - with hemorrhage 641.1
- poor dilation, cervix 661.0
- pre-eclampsia 642.4
  - severe 642.5
- previous
  - cesarean delivery 654.2
  - surgery (to)
    - cervix 654.6
    - gynecological NEC 654.9
    - uterus NEC 654.9
      - from previous cesarean delivery 654.2
    - vagina 654.7
- prolapse
  - arm or hand 652.7
  - uterus 654.4
- prolonged labor 662.1
- rectocele 654.4
- retroversion, uterus or cervix 654.3

Delivery—*continued*
- rigid
  - cervix 654.6
  - pelvic floor 654.4
  - perineum 654.8
  - vagina 654.7
  - vulva 654.8
- sacculation, pregnant uterus 654.4
- scar(s)
  - cervix 654.6
  - cesarean delivery 654.2
  - uterus NEC 654.9
    - due to previous cesarean delivery 654.2
- Shirodkar suture in situ 654.5
- shoulder presentation 652.8
- stenosis or stricture, cervix 654.6
- transverse presentation or lie 652.3
- tumor, pelvic organs or tissues NEC 654.4
- umbilical cord presentation or prolapse 663.0
- completely normal case—*see category* 650
- complicated (by) NEC 669.9
  - abdominal tumor, fetal 653.7
    - causing obstructed labor 660.1
  - abnormal, abnormality of
    - cervix 654.6
      - causing obstructed labor 660.2
    - forces of labor 661.9
    - formation of uterus 654.0
    - pelvic organs or tissues 654.9
      - causing obstructed labor 660.2
    - pelvis (bony) (major) NEC 653.0
      - causing obstructed labor 660.1
    - presentation or position NEC 652.9
      - causing obstructed labor 660.0
    - size, fetus 653.5
      - causing obstructed labor 660.1
    - soft parts (of pelvis) 654.9
      - causing obstructed labor 660.2
    - uterine contractions NEC 661.9
    - uterus (formation) 654.0
      - causing obstructed labor 660.2
    - vagina 654.7
      - causing obstructed labor 660.2
  - abnormally formed uterus (any type) (congenital) 654.0
    - causing obstructed labor 660.2
  - acromion presentation 652.8
    - causing obstructed labor 660.0
  - adherent placenta 667.0
    - with hemorrhage 666.0
  - adhesions, uterus (to abdominal wall) 654.4
  - advanced maternal age NEC 659.6
    - multigravida 659.6
    - primigravida 659.5
  - air embolism 673.0
  - amnionitis 658.4
  - amniotic fluid embolism 673.1
  - anesthetic death 668.9
  - annular detachment, cervix 665.3
  - antepartum hemorrhage—*see* Delivery, complicated, hemorrhage
  - anteversion, cervix or uterus 654.4
    - causing obstructed labor 660.2
  - apoplexy 674.0
    - placenta 641.2
  - arrested active phase 661.1
  - asymmetrical pelvis bone 653.0
    - causing obstructed labor 660.1
  - atony, uterus (hypotonic) (inertia) 666.1
    - hypertonic 661.4
  - Bandl's ring 661.4

Delivery—*continued*
  battledore placenta—*see* Placenta, abnormal
  bicornis or bicornuate uterus 654.0
    causing obstructed labor 660.2
  birth injury to mother NEC 665.9
  bleeding (*see also* Delivery, complicated,
    hemorrhage) 641.9
  breech presentation (assisted) (buttocks)
    (complete) (frank) (spontaneous) 652.2
    with successful version 652.1
  brow presentation 652.4
  cephalopelvic disproportion (normally formed
    fetus) 653.4
    causing obstructed labor 660.1
  cerebral hemorrhage 674.0
  cervical dystocia 661.0
  chin presentation 652.4
    causing obstructed labor 660.0
  cicatrix
    cervix 654.6
      causing obstructed labor 660.2
    vagina 654.7
      causing obstructed labor 660.2
  colporrhexis 665.4
    with perineal laceration 664.0
  compound presentation 652.8
    causing obstructed labor 660.0
  compression of cord (umbilical) 663.2
    around neck 663.1
    cord prolapsed 663.0
  contraction, contracted pelvis 653.1
    causing obstructed labor 660.1
    general 653.1
      causing obstructed labor 660.1
    inlet 653.2
      causing obstructed labor 660.1
    midpelvic 653.8
      causing obstructed labor 660.1
    midplane 653.8
      causing obstructed labor 660.1
    outlet 653.3
      causing obstructed labor 660.1
  contraction ring 661.4
  cord (umbilical) 663.9
    around neck, tightly or with compression
      663.1
      without compression 663.3
    bruising 663.6
    complication NEC 663.9
      specified type NEC 663.8
    compression NEC 663.2
    entanglement NEC 663.3
      with compression 663.2
    forelying 663.0
    hematoma 663.6
    marginal attachment 663.8
    presentation 663.0
    prolapse (complete) (occult) (partial) 663.0
    short 663.4
    specified complication NEC 663.8
    thrombosis (vessels) 663.6
    vascular lesion 663.6
    velamentous insertion 663.8
  Couvelaire uterus 641.2
  cretin pelvis (dwarf type) (male type) 653.1
    causing obstructed labor 660.1
  crossbirth 652.3
    with successful version 652.1
    causing obstructed labor 660.0
  cyst (Gartner's duct) 654.7

Delivery—*continued*
  cystocele 654.4
    causing obstructed labor 660.2
  death of fetus (near term) 656.4
    early (before 22 completed weeks'
      gestation) 632
  deformity (acquired) (congenital)
    fetus 653.7
      causing obstructed labor 660.1
    pelvic organs or tissues NEC 654.9
      causing obstructed labor 660.2
    pelvis (bony) NEC 653.0
      causing obstructed labor 660.1
  delay, delayed
    delivery in multiple pregnancy 662.3
      due to locked mates 660.5
    following rupture of membranes
      (spontaneous) 658.2
      artificial 658.3
  depressed fetal heart tones 659.7
  diastasis recti 665.8
  dilatation
    bladder 654.4
      causing obstructed labor 660.2
    cervix, incomplete, poor or slow 661.0
  diseased placenta 656.7
  displacement uterus NEC 654.4
    causing obstructed labor 660.2
  disproportion NEC 653.9
    causing obstructed labor 660.1
  disruptio uteri—*see* Delivery, complicated,
    rupture, uterus
  distress
    fetal 656.8
    maternal 669.0
  double uterus (congenital) 654.0
    causing obstructed labor 660.2
  dropsy amnion 657
  dysfunction, uterus 661.9
    hypertonic 661.4
    hypotonic 661.2
      primary 661.0
      secondary 661.1
    incoordinate 661.4
  dystocia
    cervical 661.0
    fetal—*see* Delivery, complicated, abnormal,
      presentation
    maternal—*see* Delivery, complicated,
      prolonged labor
    pelvic—*see* Delivery, complicated,
      contraction pelvis
    positional 652.8
    shoulder girdle 660.4
  eclampsia 642.6
  ectopic kidney 654.4
    causing obstructed labor 660.2
  edema, cervix 654.6
    causing obstructed labor 660.2
  effusion, amniotic fluid 658.1
  elderly multigravida 659.6
  elderly primigravida 659.5
  embolism (pulmonary) 673.2
    air 673.0
    amniotic fluid 673.1
    blood-clot 673.2
    cerebral 674.0
    fat 673.8
    pyemic 673.3
    septic 673.3

Delivery—*continued*
    prolapse (complete) (occult) (partial) 663.0
    unstable lie 652.0
      causing obstructed labor 660.0
    uterine
      inertia (*see also* Delivery, complicated,
        inertia, uterus) 661.2
        spasm 661.4
    vasa previa 663.5
    velamentous insertion of cord 663.8
    young maternal age 659.8
  delayed NEC 662.1
    following rupture of membranes
      (spontaneous) 658.2
      artificial 658.3
    second twin, triplet, etc. 662.3
  difficult NEC 669.9
    previous, affecting management of pregnancy
      or childbirth V23.49
    specified type NEC 669.8
  early onset (spontaneous) 644.2
  forceps NEC 669.5
    affecting fetus or newborn 763.2
  footling 652.8
    with successful version 652.1
  missed (at or near term) 656.4
  multiple gestation NEC 651.9
    with fetal loss and retention of one or more
      fetus(es) 651.6
    specified type NEC 651.8
      with fetal loss and retention of one or more
        fetus(es) 651.6
  nonviable infant 656.4
  normal—*see* category 650
  precipitate 661.3
    affecting fetus or newborn 763.6
  premature NEC (before 37 completed weeks
    gestation) 644.2
    previous, affecting management of pregnancy
      V23.41
  quadruplet NEC 651.2
    with fetal loss and retention of one or more
      fetus(es) 651.5
  quintuplet NEC 651.8
    with fetal loss and retention of one or more
      fetus(es) 651.6
  sextuplet NEC 651.8
    with fetal loss and retention of one or more
      fetus(es) 651.6
  specified complication NEC 669.8
  stillbirth (near term) NEC 656.4
    early (before 22 completed weeks' gestation)
      632
  term pregnancy (live birth) NEC—*see* category
    650
    stillbirth NEC 656.4
  threatened premature 644.2
  triplets NEC 651.1
    with fetal loss and retention of one or more
      fetus(es) 651.4
    delayed delivery (one or more mates) 662.3
    locked mates 660.5
  twins NEC 651.0
    with fetal loss and retention of one or more
      fetus(es) 651.3
    delayed delivery (one or more mates) 662.3
    locked mates 660.5
  uncomplicated—*see* category 650
  vacuum extractor NEC 669.5
    affecting fetus or newborn 763.3
  ventouse NEC 669.5
    affecting fetus or newborn 763.3

Dellen, cornea 371.41
Delusions (paranoid) 297.9
  grandiose 297.1
  parasitosis 300.29
  systematized 297.1
Dementia 294.8
  alcoholic (*see also* Psychosis, alcoholic) 291.2
  Alzheimer's—*see* Alzheimer's dementia
  arteriosclerotic (simple type) (uncomplicated)
    290.40
    with
      acute confusional state 290.41
      delirium 290.41
      delusional features 290.42
      depressive features 290.43
    depressed type 290.43
    paranoid type 290.42
  Binswanger's 290.12
  catatonic (acute) (*see also* Schizophrenia) 295.2
  congenital (*see also* Retardation, mental) 319
  degenerative 290.9
    presenile-onset—*see* Dementia, presenile
    senile-onset—*see* Dementia, senile
  developmental (*see also* Schizophrenia) 295.9
  dialysis 294.8
    transient 293.9
  due to or associated with condition(s) classified
    elsewhere
    Alzheimer's
      with behavioral disturbance 331.0 *[294.11]*
      without behavioral disturbance 331.0
        [294.10]
    cerebral lipidoses
      with behavioral disturbance 330.1 *[294.11]*
      without behavioral disturbance 330.1
        [294.10]
    epilepsy
      with behavioral disturbance 345.9 *[294.11]*
      without behavioral disturbance 345.9
        [294.10]
    hepatolenticular degeneration
      with behavioral disturbance 275.1 *[294.11]*
      without behavioral disturbance 275.1
        [294.10]
    HIV
      with behavioral disturbance 042 *[294.11]*
      without behavioral disturbance 042 *[294.10]*
    Huntington's chorea
      with behavioral disturbance 333.4 *[294.11]*
      without behavioral disturbance 333.4
        [294.10]
    Jakob-Creutzfeldt disease
      with behavioral disturbance 046.1 *[294.11]*
      without behavioral disturbance 046.1
        [294.10]
    multiple sclerosis
      with behavioral disturbance 340 *[294.11]*
      without behavioral disturbance 340 *[294.10]*
    neurosyphilis
      with behavioral disturbance 094.9 *[294.11]*
      without behavioral disturbance 094.9
        [294.10]
    Pelizaeus-Merzbacher disease
      with behavioral disturbance 333.0 *[294.11]*
      without behavioral disturbance 333.0
        [294.10]
    Pick's disease
      with behavioral disturbance 331.1 *[294.11]*
      without behavioral disturbance 331.1
        [294.10]

Dementia—*continued*
  polyarteritis nodosa
    with behavioral disturbance 446.0 *[294.11]*
    without behavioral disturbance 446.0
      [294.10]
  syphilis
    with behavioral disturbance 094.1 *[294.11]*
    without behavioral disturbance 094.1
      [294.10]
  Wilson's disease
    with behavioral disturbance 275.1 *[294.11]*
    without behavioral disturbance 275.1
      [294.10]
  hebephrenic (acute) 295.1
  Heller's (infantile psychosis) (*see also*
    Psychosis, childhood) 299.1
  idiopathic 290.9
    presenile-onset—*see* Dementia, presenile
    senile-onset—*see* Dementia, senile
  in
    arteriosclerotic brain disease 290.40
    senility 290.0
  induced by drug 292.82
  infantile, infantilia (*see also* Psychosis,
    childhood) 299.0
  multi-infarct (cerebrovascular) (*see also*
    Dementia, arteriosclerotic) 290.40
  old age 290.0
  paralytica, paralytic 094.1
    juvenilis 090.40
    syphilitic 094.1
      congenital 090.40
    tabetic form 094.1
  paranoid (*see also* Schizophrenia) 295.3
  paraphrenic (*see also* Schizophrenia) 295.3
  paretic 094.1
  praecox (*see also* Schizophrenia) 295.9
  presenile 290.10
    with
      acute confusional state 290.11
      delirium 290.11
      delusional features 290.12
      depressive features 290.13
    depressed type 290.13
    paranoid type 290.12
    simple type 290.10
    uncomplicated 290.10
  primary (acute) (*see also* Schizophrenia) 295.0
  progressive, syphilitic 094.1
  puerperal—*see* Psychosis, puerperal
  schizophrenic (*see also* Schizophrenia) 295.9
  senile 290.0
    with
      acute confusional state 290.3
      delirium 290.3
      delusional features 290.20
      depressive features 290.21
    depressed type 290.21
    exhaustion 290.0
    paranoid type 290.20
  simple type (acute) (*see also* Schizophrenia)
    295.0
  simplex (acute) (*see also* Schizophrenia) 295.0
  syphilitic 094.1
  uremic—*see* Uremia
  vascular 290.40
Demerol dependence (*see also* Dependence)
  304.0
Demineralization, ankle (*see also* Osteoporosis)
  733.00
Demodex folliculorum (infestation) 133.8
de Morgan's spots (senile angiomas) 448.1

Demyelinating
  polyneuritis, chronic inflammatory 357.81
Demyelination, demyelinization
  central nervous system 341.9
    specified NEC 341.8
  corpus callosum (central) 341.8
  global 340
Dengue (fever) 061
  sandfly 061
  vaccination, prophylactic (against) V05.1
  virus hemorrhagic fever 065.4
Dens
  evaginatus 520.2
  in dente 520.2
  invaginatus 520.2
Density
  increased, bone (disseminated) (generalized)
    (spotted) 733.99
  lung (nodular) 518.89
Dental —*see also* condition
  examination only V72.2
Dentia praecox 520.6
Denticles (in pulp) 522.2
Dentigerous cyst 526.0
Dentin
  irregular (in pulp) 522.3
  opalescent 520.5
  secondary (in pulp) 522.3
  sensitive 521.8
Dentinogenesis imperfecta 520.5
Dentinoma (M9271/0) 213.1
  upper jaw (bone) 213.0
Dentition 520.7
  abnormal 520.6
  anomaly 520.6
  delayed 520.6
  difficult 520.7
  disorder of 520.6
  precocious 520.6
  retarded 520.6
Denture sore (mouth) 528.9
Dependence

> *Note—Use the following fifth-digit*
> *subclassification with category 304:*
>
> *0 unspecified*
> *1 continuous*
> *2 episodic*
> *3 in remission*

  with
    withdrawal symptoms
      alcohol 291.81
      drug 292.0
  14-hydroxy-dihydromorphinone 304.0
  absinthe 304.6
  acemorphan 304.0
  acetanilid(e) 304.6
  acetophenetidin 304.6
  acetorphine 304.0
  acetyldihydrocodeine 304.0
  acetyldihydrocodeinone 304.0
  Adalin 304.1
  Afghanistan black 304.3
  agrypnal 304.1
  alcohol, alcoholic (ethyl) (methyl) (wood) 303.9
    maternal, with suspected fetal damage
      affecting management of pregnancy 655.4
  allobarbitone 304.1
  allonal 304.1
  allylisopropylacetylurea 304.1

Dependence—*continued*
  alphaprodine (hydrochloride) 304.0
  Alurate 304.1
  Alvodine 304.0
  amethocaine 304.6
  amidone 304.0
  amidopyrine 304.6
  aminopyrine 304.6
  amobarbital 304.1
  amphetamine(s) (type) (drugs classifiable to 969.7) 304.4
  amylene hydrate 304.6
  amylobarbitone 304.1
  amylocaine 304.6
  Amytal (sodium) 304.1
  analgesic (drug) NEC 304.6
    synthetic with morphine-like effect 304.0
  anesthetic (agent) (drug) (gas) (general) (local) NEC 304.6
  Angel dust 304.6
  anileridine 304.0
  antipyrine 304.6
  aprobarbital 304.1
  aprobarbitone 304.1
  atropine 304.6
  Avertin (bromide) 304.6
  barbenyl 304.1
  barbital(s) 304.1
  barbitone 304.1
  barbiturate(s) (compounds) (drugs classifiable to 967.0) 304.1
  barbituric acid (and compounds) 304.1
  benzedrine 304.4
  benzylmorphine 304.0
  Beta-chlor 304.1
  bhang 304.3
  blue velvet 304.0
  Brevital 304.1
  bromal (hydrate) 304.1
  bromide(s) NEC 304.1
  bromine compounds NEC 304.1
  bromisovalum 304.1
  bromoform 304.1
  Bromo-seltzer 304.1
  bromural 304.1
  butabarbital (sodium) 304.1
  butabarpal 304.1
  butallylonal 304.1
  butethal 304.1
  buthalitone (sodium) 304.1
  Butisol 304.1
  butobarbitone 304.1
  butyl chloral (hydrate) 304.1
  caffeine 304.4
  cannabis (indica) (sativa) (resin) (derivatives) (type) 304.3
  carbamazepine 304.6
  Carbrital 304.1
  carbromal 304.1
  carisoprodol 304.6
  Catha (edulis) 304.4
  chloral (betaine) (hydrate) 304.1
  chloralamide 304.1
  chloralformamide 304.1
  chloralose 304.1
  chlordiazepoxide 304.1
  Chloretone 304.1
  chlorobutanol 304.1
  chlorodyne 304.1
  chloroform 304.6
  Cliradon 304.0

Dependence—*continued*
  coca (leaf) and derivatives 304.2
  cocaine 304.2
    hydrochloride 304.2
    salt (any) 304.2
  codeine 304.0
  combination of drugs (excluding morphine or opioid type drug) NEC 304.8
    morphine or opioid type drug with any other drug 304.7
  croton-chloral 304.1
  cyclobarbital 304.1
  cyclobarbitone 304.1
  dagga 304.3
  Delvinal 304.1
  Demerol 304.0
  desocodeine 304.0
  desomorphine 304.0
  desoxyephedrine 304.4
  DET 304.5
  dexamphetamine 304.4
  dexedrine 304.4
  dextromethorphan 304.0
  dextromoramide 304.0
  dextronorpseudophedrine 304.4
  dextrorphan 304.0
  diacetylmorphine 304.0
  Dial 304.1
  diallylbarbituric acid 304.1
  diamorphine 304.0
  diazepam 304.1
  dibucaine 304.6
  dichloroethane 304.6
  diethyl barbituric acid 304.1
  diethylsulfone-diethylmethane 304.1
  difencloxazine 304.0
  dihydrocodeine 304.0
  dihydrocodeinone 304.0
  dihydrohydroxycodeinone 304.0
  dihydroisocodeine 304.0
  dihydromorphine 304.0
  dihydromorphinone 304.0
  dihydroxcodeinone 304.0
  Dilaudid 304.0
  dimenhydrinate 304.6
  dimethylmeperidine 304.0
  dimethyltriptamine 304.5
  Dionin 304.0
  diphenoxylate 304.6
  dipipanone 304.0
  d-lysergic acid diethylamide 304.5
  DMT 304.5
  Dolophine 304.0
  DOM 304.2
  Doriden 304.1
  dormiral 304.1
  Dormison 304.1
  Dromoran 304.0
  drug NEC 304.9
    analgesic NEC 304.6
    combination (excluding morphine or opioid type drug) NEC 304.8
      morphine or opioid type drug with any other drug 304.7
    complicating pregnancy, childbirth, or puerperium 648.3
      affecting fetus or newborn 779.5
    hallucinogenic 304.5
    hypnotic NEC 304.1
    narcotic NEC 304.9
    psychostimulant NEC 304.4

Dependence—*continued*
Neravan 304.1
neurobarb 304.1
nicotine 305.1
Nisentil 304.0
nitrous oxide 304.6
Noctec 304.1
Noludar 304.1
nonbarbiturate sedatives and tranquilizers with
 similar effect 304.1
noptil 304.1
normorphine 304.0
noscapine 304.0
Novocaine 304.6
Numorphan 304.0
nunol 304.1
Nupercaine 304.6
Oblivon 304.1
on
 aspirator V46.0
 hyperbaric chamber V46.8
 iron lung V46.1
 machine (enabling) V46.9
  specified type NEC V46.8
 Possum (Patient-Operated-Selector-
  Mechanism) V46.8
 renal dialysis machine V45.1
 respirator V46.1
 supplemental oxygen V46.2
opiate 304.0
opioids 304.0
opioid type drug 304.0
 with any other drug 304.7
opium (alkaloids) (derivatives) (tincture) 304.0
ortal 304.1
Oxazepam 304.1
oxycodone 304.0
oxymorphone 304.0
Palfium 304.0
Panadol 304.6
pantopium 304.0
pantopon 304.0
papaverine 304.0
paracetamol 304.6
paracodin 304.0
paraldehyde 304.1
paregoric 304.0
Parzone 304.0
PCP (phencyclidine) 304.6
Pearly Gates 304.5
pentazocine 304.0
pentobarbital 304.1
pentobarbitone (sodium) 304.1
Pentothal 304.1
Percaine 304.6
Percodan 304.0
Perichlor 304.1
Pernocton 304.1
Pernoston 304.1
peronine 304.0
pethidine (hydrochloride) 304.0
petrichloral 304.1
peyote 304.5
Phanodorn 304.1
phenacetin 304.6
phenadoxone 304.0
phenaglycodol 304.1
phenazocine 304.0
phencyclidine 304.6
phenmetrazine 304.4
phenobal 304.1

Dependence—*continued*
phenobarbital 304.1
phenobarbitone 304.1
phenomorphan 304.0
phenonyl 304.1
phenoperidine 304.0
pholcodine 304.0
piminodine 304.0
Pipadone 304.0
Pitkin's solution 304.6
Placidyl 304.1
polysubstance 304.8
Pontocaine 304.6
pot 304.3
potassium bromide 304.1
Preludin 304.4
Prinadol 304.0
probarbital 304.1
procaine 304.6
propanal 304.1
propoxyphene 304.6
psilocibin 304.5
psilocin 304.5
psilocybin 304.5
psilocyline 304.5
psilocyn 304.5
psychedelic agents 304.5
psychostimulant NEC 304.4
psychotomimetic agents 304.5
pyrahexyl 304.3
Pyramidon 304.6
quinalbarbitone 304.1
racemoramide 304.0
racemorphan 304.0
Rela 304.6
scopolamine 304.6
secobarbital 304.1
Seconal 304.1
sedative NEC 304.1
 nonbarbiturate with barbiturate effect 304.1
Sedormid 304.1
sernyl 304.1
sodium bromide 304.1
Soma 304.6
Somnal 304.1
Somnos 304.1
Soneryl 304.1
soporific (drug) NEC 304.1
specified drug NEC 304.6
speed 304.4
spinocaine 304.6
Stovaine 304.6
STP 304.5
stramonium 304.6
Sulfonal 304.1
sulfonethylmethane 304.1
sulfonmethane 304.1
Surital 304.1
synthetic drug with morphine-like effect 304.0
talbutal 304.1
tetracaine 304.6
tetrahydrocannabinol 304.3
tetronal 304.1
THC 304.3
thebacon 304.0
thebaine 304.0
thiamil 304.1
thiamylal 304.1
thiopental 304.1
tobacco 305.1
toluene, toluol 304.6

Dependence—*continued*
　tranquilizer NEC 304.1
　　nonbarbiturate with barbiturate effect 304.1
　tribromacetaldehyde 304.6
　tribromethanol 304.6
　tribromomethane 304.6
　trichloroethanol 304.6
　trichoroethyl phosphate 304.1
　triclofos 304.1
　Trional 304.1
　Tuinal 304.1
　Turkish Green 304.3
　urethan(e) 304.6
　Valium 304.1
　Valmid 304.1
　veganin 304.0
　veramon 304.1
　Veronal 304.1
　versidyne 304.6
　vinbarbital 304.1
　vinbarbitone 304.1
　vinyl bitone 304.1
　vitamin B$_6$ 266.1
　wine 303.9
　Zactane 304.6
Dependency
　passive 301.6
　reactions 301.6
Depersonalization (episode, in neurotic state)
　　(neurotic) (syndrome) 300.6
Depletion
　carbohydrates 271.9
　complement factor 279.8
　extracellular fluid 276.5
　plasma 276.5
　potassium 276.8
　　nephropathy 588.8
　salt or sodium 276.1
　　causing heat exhaustion or prostration 992.4
　　nephropathy 593.9
　volume 276.5
　　extracellular fluid 276.5
　　plasma 276.5
Deposit
　argentous, cornea 371.16
　bone, in Boeck's sarcoid 135
　calcareous, calcium—*see* Calcification
　cholesterol
　　retina 362.82
　　skin 709.3
　　vitreous (humor) 379.22
　conjunctival 372.56
　cornea, corneal NEC 371.10
　　argentous 371.16
　　in
　　　cystinosis 270.0 *[371.15]*
　　　mucopolysaccharidosis 277.5 *[371.15]*
　crystalline, vitreous (humor) 379.22
　hemosiderin, in old scars of cornea 371.11
　metallic, in lens 366.45
　skin 709.3
　teeth, tooth (betel) (black) (green) (materia alba)
　　(orange) (soft) (tobacco) 523.6
　urate, in kidney (*see also* Disease, renal) 593.9
Depraved appetite 307.52

Depression 311
　acute (*see also* Psychosis, affective) 296.2
　　recurrent episode 296.3
　　single episode 296.2
　agitated (*see also* Psychosis, affective) 296.2
　　recurrent episode 296.3
　　single episode 296.2
　anaclitic 309.21
　anxiety 300.4
　arches 734
　　congenital 754.61
　autogenous (*see also* Psychosis, affective) 296.2
　　recurrent episode 296.3
　　single episode 296.2
　basal metabolic rate (BMR) 794.7
　bone marrow 289.9
　central nervous system 799.1
　　newborn 779.2
　cerebral 331.9
　　newborn 779.2
　cerebrovascular 437.8
　　newborn 779.2
　chest wall 738.3
　endogenous (*see also* Psychosis, affective) 296.2
　　recurrent episode 296.3
　　single episode 296.2
　functional activity 780.99
　hysterical 300.11
　involutional, climacteric, or menopausal (*see
　　also* Psychosis, affective) 296.2
　　recurrent episode 296.3
　　single episode 296.2
　manic (*see also* Psychosis, affective) 296.80
　medullary 348.8
　　newborn 779.2
　mental 300.4
　metatarsal heads—*see* Depression, arches
　metatarsus—*see* Depression, arches
　monopolar (*see also* Psychosis, affective) 296.2
　　recurrent episode 296.3
　　single episode 296.2
　nervous 300.4
　neurotic 300.4
　nose 738.0
　postpartum 648.4
　psychogenic 300.4
　　reactive 298.0
　psychoneurotic 300.4
　psychotic (*see also* Psychosis, affective) 296.2
　　reactive 298.0
　　recurrent episode 296.3
　　single episode 296.2
　reactive 300.4
　　neurotic 300.4
　　psychogenic 298.0
　　psychoneurotic 300.4
　　psychotic 298.0
　recurrent 296.3
　respiratory center 348.8
　　newborn 770.89
　scapula 736.89
　senile 290.21
　situational (acute) (brief) 309.0
　　prolonged 309.1
　skull 754.0
　sternum 738.3
　visual field 368.40

Depressive reaction —*see also* Reaction,
   depressive
  acute (transient) 309.0
    with anxiety 309.28
  prolonged 309.1
  situational (acute) 309.0
    prolonged 309.1
Deprivation
  cultural V62.4
  emotional V62.89
    affecting
      adult 995.82
      infant or child 995.51
  food 994.2
    specific substance NEC 269.8
  protein (familial) (kwashiorkor) 260
  social V62.4
    affecting
      adult 995.82
      infant or child 995.51
  symptoms, syndrome
    alcohol 291.81
    drug 292.0
  vitamins (*see also* Deficiency, vitamin) 269.2
  water 994.3
de Quervain's
  disease (tendon sheath) 727.04
  thyroiditis (subacute granulomatous thyroiditis)
    245.1
Derangement
  ankle (internal) 718.97
    current injury (*see also* Dislocation, ankle)
      837.0
    recurrent 718.37
  cartilage (articular) NEC (*see also* Disorder,
    cartilage, articular) 718.0
    knee 717.9
      recurrent 718.36
    recurrent 718.3
  collateral ligament (knee) (medial) (tibial)
    717.82
    current injury 844.1
      lateral (fibular) 844.0
    lateral (fibular) 717.81
      current injury 844.0
  cruciate ligament (knee) (posterior) 717.84
    anterior 717.83
      current injury 844.2
    current injury 844.2
  elbow (internal) 718.92
    current injury (*see also* Dislocation, elbow)
      832.00
    recurrent 718.32
  gastrointestinal 536.9
  heart—*see* Disease, heart
  hip (joint) (internal) (old) 718.95
    current injury (*see also* Dislocation, hip)
      835.00
    recurrent 718.35
  intervertebral disc—*see* Displacement,
    intervertebral disc
  joint (internal) 718.90
    ankle 718.97
    current injury—*see also* Dislocation, by site
      knee, meniscus or cartilage (*see also* Tear,
        meniscus) 836.2
    elbow 718.92
    foot 718.97
    hand 718.94
    hip 718.95
    knee 717.9

Derangement—*continued*
    multiple sites 718.99
    pelvic region 718.95
    recurrent 718.30
      ankle 718.37
      elbow 718.32
      foot 718.37
      hand 718.34
      hip 718.35
      knee 718.36
      multiple sites 718.39
      pelvic region 718.35
      shoulder (region) 718.31
      specified site NEC 718.38
      temporomandibular (old) 524.69
      wrist 718.33
    shoulder (region) 718.91
    specified site NEC 718.98
    spine NEC 724.9
    temporomandibular 524.69
    wrist 718.93
  knee (cartilage) (internal) 717.9
    current injury (*see also* Tear, meniscus) 836.2
    ligament 717.89
      capsular 717.85
      collateral—*see* Derangement, collateral
        ligament
      cruciate—*see* Derangement, cruciate
        ligament
      specified NEC 717.85
    recurrent 718.36
  low back NEC 724.9
  meniscus NEC (knee) 717.5
    current injury (*see also* Tear, meniscus) 836.2
    lateral 717.40
      anterior horn 717.42
      posterior horn 717.43
      specified NEC 717.49
    medial 717.3
      anterior horn 717.1
      posterior horn 717.2
    recurrent 718.3
    site other than knee—*see* Disorder, cartilage,
      articular
  mental (*see also* Psychosis) 298.9
  rotator cuff (recurrent) (tear) 726.10
    current 840.4
  sacroiliac (old) 724.6
    current—*see* Dislocation, sacroiliac
  semilunar cartilage (knee) 717.5
    current injury 836.2
      lateral 836.1
      medial 836.0
    recurrent 718.3
  shoulder (internal) 718.91
    current injury (*see also* Dislocation, shoulder)
      831.00
    recurrent 718.31
  spine (recurrent) NEC 724.9
    current—*see* Dislocation, spine
  temporomandibular (internal) (joint) (old)
    524.69
    current—*see* Dislocation, jaw
Dercum's disease or syndrome (adiposis
  dolorosa) 272.8
Derealization (neurotic) 300.6
Dermal —*see* condition
Dermaphytid —*see* Dermatophytosis
Dermatergosis —*see* Dermatitis

Dermatitis (allergic) (contact) (occupational)
  (venenata) 692.9
 ab igne 692.82
 acneiform 692.9
 actinic (due to sun) 692.70
  acute 692.72
  chronic NEC 692.74
  other than from sun NEC 692.82
 ambustionis
  due to
    burn or scald—*see* Burn, by site
    sunburn (*see also* Sunburn) 692.71
 amebic 006.6
 ammonia 691.0
 anaphylactoid NEC 692.9
 arsenical 692.4
 artefacta 698.4
  psychogenic 316 *[698.4]*
 asthmatic 691.8
 atopic (allergic) (intrinsic) 691.8
  psychogenic 316 *[691.8]*
 atrophicans 701.8
  diffusa 701.8
  maculosa 701.3
 berlock, berloque 692.72
 blastomycetic 116.0
 blister beetle 692.89
 Brucella NEC 023.9
 bullosa 694.9
  striata pratensis 692.6
 bullous 694.9
  mucosynechial, atrophic 694.60
    with ocular involvement 694.61
  seasonal 694.8
 calorica
  due to
    burn or scald—*see* Burn, by site
    cold 692.89
    sunburn (*see also* Sunburn) 692.71
 caterpillar 692.89
 cercarial 120.3
 combustionis
  due to
    burn or scald—*see* Burn, by site
    sunburn (*see also* Sunburn) 692.71
 congelationis 991.5
 contusiformis 695.2
 diabetic 250.8
 diaper 691.0
 diphtheritica 032.85
 due to
  acetone 692.2
  acids 692.4
  adhesive plaster 692.4
  alcohol (skin contact) (substances classifiable
    to 980.0-980.9) 692.4
    taken internally 693.8
  alkalis 692.4
  allergy NEC 692.9
  ammonia (household) (liquid) 692.4
  arnica 692.3
  arsenic 692.4
    taken internally 693.8
  blister beetle 692.89
  cantharides 692.3
  carbon disulphide 692.2
  caterpillar 692.89
  caustics 692.4
  cereal (ingested) 693.1
    contact with skin 692.5

Dermatitis—*continued*
 chemical(s) NEC 692.4
  internal 693.8
  irritant NEC 692.4
  taken internally 693.8
 chlorocompounds 692.2
 coffee (ingested) 693.1
  contact with skin 692.5
 cold weather 692.89
 cosmetics 692.81
 cyclohexanes 692.2
 deodorant 692.81
 detergents 692.0
 dichromate 692.4
 drugs and medicinals (correct substance
    properly administered) (internal use) 693.0
  external (in contact with skin) 692.3
    wrong substance given or taken 976.9
      specified substance—*see* Table of drugs
        and chemicals
    wrong substance given or taken 977.9
      specified substance—*see* Table of drugs
        and chemicals
 dyes 692.89
  hair 692.89
 epidermophytosis—*see* Dermatophytosis
 esters 692.2
 external irritant NEC 692.9
  specified agent NEC 692.89
 eye shadow 692.81
 fish (ingested) 693.1
  contact with skin 692.5
 flour (ingested) 693.1
  contact with skin 692.5
 food (ingested) 693.1
  in contact with skin 692.5
 fruit (ingested) 693.1
  contact with skin 692.5
 fungicides 692.3
 furs 692.89
 glycols 692.2
 greases NEC 692.1
 hair dyes 692.89
 hot
  objects and materials—*see* Burn, by site
  weather or places 692.89
 hydrocarbons 692.2
 infrared rays, except from sun 692.82
  solar NEC (*see* also Dermatitis, due to, sun)
    692.70
 ingested substance 693.9
  drugs and medicinals (*see also* Dermatitis,
    due to, drugs and medicinals) 693.0
  food 693.1
  specified substance NEC 693.8
 ingestion or injection of
  chemical 693.8
  drug (correct substance properly
    administered) 693.0
    wrong substance given or taken 977.9
      specified substance—*see* Table of drugs
        and chemicals
 insecticides 692.4
 internal agent 693.9
  drugs and medicinals (*see also* Dermatitis,
    due to, drugs and medicinals) 693.0
  food (ingested) 693.1
    in contact with skin 692.5
  specified agent NEC 693.8
 iodine 692.3
 iodoform 692.3

Dermatitis—*continued*
　irradiation 692.82
　jewelry 692.83
　keratolytics 692.3
　ketones 692.2
　lacquer tree (Rhus verniciflua) 692.6
　light (sun) NEC (*see also* Dermatitis, due to,
　　　sun) 692.70
　　other 692.82
　low temperature 692.89
　mascara 692.81
　meat (ingested) 693.1
　　contact with skin 692.5
　mercury, mercurials 692.3
　metals 692.83
　milk (ingested) 693.1
　　contact with skin 692.5
　Neomycin 692.3
　nylon 692.4
　oils NEC 692.1
　paint solvent 692.2
　pediculocides 692.3
　petroleum products (substances classifiable to
　　　981) 692.4
　phenol 692.3
　photosensitiveness, photosensitivity (sun)
　　　692.72
　　other light 692.82
　plants NEC 692.6
　plasters, medicated (any) 692.3
　plastic 692.4
　poison
　　ivy (Rhus toxicodendron) 692.6
　　oak (Rhus diversiloba) 692.6
　　plant or vine 692.6
　　sumac (Rhus venenata) 692.6
　　vine (Rhus radicans) 692.6
　preservatives 692.89
　primrose (primula) 692.6
　primula 692.6
　radiation 692.82
　　sun NEC (*see also* Dermatitis, due to, sun)
　　　692.70
　　tanning bed 692.82
　radioactive substance 692.82
　radium 692.82
　ragweed (Senecio jacobae) 692.6
　Rhus (diversiloba) (radicans) (toxicodendron)
　　　(venenata) (verniciflua) 692.6
　rubber 692.4
　scabicides 692.3
　Senecio jacobae 692.6
　solar radiation—*see* Dermatitis, due to, sun
　solvents (any) (substances classifiable to
　　　982.0-982.8) 692.2
　　chlorocompound group 692.2
　　cyclohexane group 692.2
　　ester group 692.2
　　glycol group 692.2
　　hydrocarbon group 692.2
　　ketone group 692.2
　　paint 692.2
　specified agent NEC 692.89
　sun 692.70
　　acute 692.72
　　chronic NEC 692.74
　　specified NEC 692.79
　sunburn (*see also* Sunburn) 692.71
　sunshine NEC (*see also* Dermatitis, due to,
　　　sun) 692.70
　tanning bed 692.82

Dermatitis—*continued*
　tetrachlorethylene 692.2
　toluene 692.2
　topical medications 692.3
　turpentine 692.2
　ultraviolet rays, except from sun 692.82
　　sun NEC (*see also* Dermatitis, due to, sun)
　　　692.70
　vaccine or vaccination (correct substance
　　　properly administered) 693.0
　　wrong substance given or taken
　　　bacterial vaccine 978.8
　　　　specified—*see* Table of drugs and
　　　　　chemicals
　　　other vaccines NEC 979.9
　　　　specified—*see* Table of drugs and
　　　　　chemicals
　varicose veins (*see also* Varicose, vein,
　　　inflamed or infected) 454.1
　x-rays 692.82
dyshydrotic 705.81
dysmenorrheica 625.8
eczematoid NEC 692.9
　infectious 690.8
eczematous NEC 692.9
epidemica 695.89
erysipelatosa 695.81
escharotica—*see* Burn, by site
exfoliativa, exfoliative 695.89
　generalized 695.89
　infantum 695.81
　neonatorum 695.81
eyelid 373.31
　allergic 373.32
　contact 373.32
　eczematous 373.31
　herpes (zoster) 053.20
　　simplex 054.41
　infective 373.5
　　due to
　　　actinomycosis 039.3 *[373.5]*
　　　herpes
　　　　simplex 054.41
　　　　zoster 053.20
　　　impetigo 684 *[373.5]*
　　　leprosy (*see also* Leprosy) 030.0 *[373.4]*
　　　lupus vulgaris (tuberculous) (*see also*
　　　　Tuberculosis) 017.0 *[373.4]*
　　　mycotic dermatitis (*see also*
　　　　Dermatomycosis) 111.9 *[373.5]*
　　　vaccinia 051.0 *[373.5]*
　　　　postvaccination 999.0 *[373.5]*
　　　yaws (*see also* Yaws) 102.9 *[373.4]*
facta, factitia 698.4
　psychogenic 316 *[698.4]*
ficta 698.4
　psychogenic 316 *[698.4]*
flexural 691.8
follicularis 704.8
friction 709.8
fungus 111.9
　specified type NEC 111.8
gangrenosa, gangrenous (infantum) (*see also*
　　Gangrene) 785.4
gestationis 646.8
gonococcal 098.89
gouty 274.89
harvest mite 133.8
heat 692.89
herpetiformis (bullous) (erythematous)
　　(pustular) (vesicular) 694.0

Dermatosis—*continued*
　hysterical 300.11
　linear IgA 694.8
　menstrual NEC 709.8
　neutrophilic, acute febrile 695.89
　occupational (*see also* Dermatitis) 692.9
　papulosa nigra 709.8
　pigmentary NEC 709.00
　　progressive 709.09
　　Schamberg's 709.09
　　Siemens-Bloch 757.33
　progressive pigmentary 709.09
　psychogenic 316
　pustular subcorneal 694.1
　Schamberg's (progressive pigmentary) 709.09
　senile NEC 709.3
　Unna's (seborrheic dermatitis) 690.10
Dermographia 708.3
Dermographism 708.3
Dermoid (cyst) (M9084/0)—*see also* Neoplasm,
　by site, benign
　with malignant transformation (M9084/3) 183.0
Dermopathy
　infiltrative, with thyrotoxicosis 242.0
　senile NEC 709.3
Dermophytosis —*see* Dermatophytosis
Descemet's membrane —*see* condition
Descemetocele 371.72
Descending —*see* condition
Descensus uteri (complete) (incomplete)
　　(partial) (without vaginal wall prolapse) 618.1
　with mention of vaginal wall prolapse—*see*
　　　Prolapse, uterovaginal
Desensitization to allergens V07.1
Desert
　rheumatism 114.0
　sore (*see also* Ulcer, skin) 707.9
Desertion (child) (newborn) 995.52
　adult 995.84
Desmoid (extra-abdominal) (tumor)
　　(M8821/1)—*see also* Neoplasm, connective
　　tissue, uncertain behavior
　abdominal (M8822/1)—*see* Neoplasm,
　　　connective tissue, uncertain behavior
Despondency 300.4
Desquamative dermatitis NEC 695.89
Destruction
　articular facet (*see also* Derangement, joint)
　　718.9
　　vertebra 724.9
　bone 733.90
　　syphilitic 095.5
　joint (*see also* Derangement, joint) 718.9
　　sacroiliac 724.6
　kidney 593.89
　live fetus to facilitate birth NEC 763.89
　ossicles (ear) 385.24
　rectal sphincter 569.49
　septum (nasal) 478.1
　tuberculous NEC (*see also* Tuberculosis) 011.9
　tympanic membrane 384.82
　tympanum 385.89
　vertebral disc—*see* Degeneration, intervertebral
　　disc .
Destructiveness (*see also* Disturbance, conduct)
　　312.9
　adjustment reaction 309.3
Detachment
　cartilage—*see also* Sprain, by site
　　knee—*see* Tear, meniscus
　cervix, annular 622.8

Detachment—*continued*
　complicating delivery 665.3
　choroid (old) (postinfectional) (simple)
　　(spontaneous) 363.70
　　hemorrhagic 363.72
　　serous 363.71
　knee, medial meniscus (old) 717.3
　　current injury 836.0
　ligament—*see* Sprain, by site
　placenta (premature)—*see* Placenta, separation
　retina (recent) 361.9
　　with retinal defect (rhegmatogenous) 361.00
　　　giant tear 361.03
　　　multiple 361.02
　　　partial
　　　　with
　　　　　giant tear 361.03
　　　　　multiple defects 361.02
　　　　　retinal dialysis (juvenile) 361.04
　　　　　single defect 361.01
　　　　retinal dialysis (juvenile) 361.04
　　　　single 361.01
　　　subtotal 361.05
　　　total 361.05
　　delimited (old) (partial) 361.06
　　old
　　　delimited 361.06
　　　partial 361.06
　　　total or subtotal 361.07
　　pigment epithelium (RPE) (serous) 362.42
　　　exudative 362.42
　　　hemorrhagic 362.43
　　rhegmatogenous (*see also* Detachment, retina,
　　　with retinal defect) 361.00
　　serous (without retinal defect) 361.2
　　specified type NEC 361.89
　　traction (with vitreoretinal organization)
　　　361.81
　vitreous humor 379.21
Detergent asthma 507.8
Deterioration
　epileptic
　　with behavioral disturbance 345.9 *[294.11]*
　　without behavioral disturbance 345.9 *[294.10]*
　heart, cardiac (*see also* Degeneration,
　　myocardial) 429.1
　mental (*see also* Psychosis) 298.9
　myocardium, myocardial (*see also*
　　Degeneration, myocardial) 429.1
　senile (simple) 797
　transplanted organ—*see* Complications,
　　transplant, organ, by site
de Toni-Fanconi syndrome (cystinosis) 270.0
Deuteranomaly 368.52
Deuteranopia (anomalous trichromat)
　　(complete) (incomplete) 368.52
Deutschländer's disease —*see* Fracture, foot
Development
　abnormal, bone 756.9
　arrested 783.40
　　bone 733.91
　　child 783.40
　　due to malnutrition (protein-calorie) 263.2
　　fetus or newborn 764.9
　　tracheal rings (congenital) 748.3
　defective, congenital—*see also* Anomaly
　　cauda equina 742.59
　　left ventricle 746.9
　　　with atresia or hypoplasia of aortic orifice or
　　　　valve with hypoplasia of ascending aorta
　　　　746.7

> *Note—Use the following fifth-digit subclassification with category 250:*
>
> 0 *type II [non-insulin dependent type] [NIDDM type] [adult-onset type] or unspecified type, not stated as uncontrolled*
> 1 *type I [insulin dependent type] [IDDM] [juvenile type], not stated as uncontrolled*
> 2 *type II [non-insulin dependent type] [NIDDM type] [adult-onset type] or unspecified type, uncontrolled*
> 3 *type I [insulin dependent type] [IDDM] [juvenile type], uncontrolled*

Diabetes, diabetic—*continued*
chemical 790.2
complicating pregnancy, childbirth, or
puerperium 648.8
coma (with ketoacidosis) 250.3
hyperglycemic 250.3
hyperosmolar (nonketotic) 250.2
hypoglycemic 250.3
insulin 250.3
complicating pregnancy, childbirth, or
puerperium (maternal) 648.0
affecting fetus or newborn 775.0
complication NEC 250.9
specified NEC 250.8
dorsal sclerosis 250.6 *[340]*
dwarfism-obesity syndrome 258.1
gangrene 250.7 *[785.4]*
gastroparesis 250.6 *[536.3]*
gestational 648.8
complicating pregnancy, childbirth, or
puerperium 648.8
glaucoma 240.5 *[365.44]*
glomerulosclerosis (intercapillary) 250.4
[581.81]
glycogenosis, secondary 250.8 *[259.8]*
hemochromatosis 275.0
hyperosmolar coma 250.2
hyperosmolarity 250.2
hypertension-nephrosis syndrome 250.4
[581.81]
hypoglycemia 250.8
hypoglycemic shock 250.8
insipidus 253.5
nephrogenic 588.1
pituitary 253.5
vasopressin-resistant 588.1
intercapillary glomerulosclerosis 250.4 *[581.81]*
iritis 250.5 *[364.42]*
ketosis, ketoacidosis 250.1
Kimmelstiel (-Wilson) disease or syndrome
(intercapillary glomerulosclerosis) 250.4
[581.81]
Lancereaux's (diabetes mellitus with marked
emaciation) 250.8 *[261]*
latent (chemical) 790.2
complicating pregnancy, childbirth, or
puerperium 648.8
lipoidosis 250.8 *[272.7]*
macular edema 250.5 *[362.01]*
maternal
with manifest disease in the infant 775.1
affecting fetus or newborn 775.0
microaneurysms, retinal 250.5 *[362.01]*
mononeuropathy 250.6 *[355.9]*
neonatal, transient 775.1
nephropathy 250.4 *[583.81]*
nephrosis (syndrome) 250.4 *[581.81]*
neuralgia 250.6 *[357.2]*
neuritis 250.6 *[357.2]*
neurogenic arthropathy 250.6 *[713.5]*
neuropathy 250.6 *[357.2]*
nonclinical 790.2
osteomyelitis 250.8 *[731.8]*
peripheral autonomic neuropathy 250.6 *[337.1]*
phosphate 275.3
polyneuropathy 250.6 *[357.2]*
renal (true) 271.4
retinal
edema 250.5 *[362.01]*
hemorrhage 250.5 *[362.01]*
microaneurysms 250.5 *[362.01]*

Diabetes, diabetic—*continued*
retinitis 250.5 *[362.01]*
retinopathy 250.5 *[362.01]*
background 250.5 *[362.01]*
proliferative 250.5 *[362.02]*
steroid induced
correct substance properly administered 251.8
overdose or wrong substance given or taken
962.0
stress 790.2
subclinical 790.2
subliminal 790.2
sugar 250.0
ulcer (skin) 250.8 *[707.9]*
lower extremity 250.8 *[707.10]*
ankle 250.8 *[707.13]*
calf 250.8 *[707.12]*
foot 250.8 *[707.15]*
heel 250.8 *[707.14]*
knee 250.8 *[707.19]*
specified site NEC 250.8 *[707.19]*
thigh 250.8 *[707.11]*
toes 250.8 *[707.15]*
specified site NEC 250.8 *[707.8]*
xanthoma 250.8 *[272.2]*
Diacyclothrombopathia 287.1
Diagnosis deferred 799.9
Dialysis (intermittent) (treatment)
anterior retinal (juvenile) (with detachment)
361.04
extracorporeal V56.0
peritoneal V56.8
renal V56.0
status only V45.1
specified type NEC V56.8
Diamond-Blackfan anemia or syndrome
(congenital hypoplastic anemia) 284.0
Diamond-Gardener syndrome (autoerythrocyte
sensitization) 287.2
Diaper rash 691.0
Diaphoresis (excessive) NEC 780.8
Diaphragm —*see* condition
Diaphragmalgia 786.52
Diaphragmitis 519.4
Diaphyseal aclasis 756.4
Diaphysitis 733.99
Diarrhea, diarrheal (acute) (autumn) (bilious)
(bloody) (catarrhal) (choleraic) (chronic)
(gravis) (green) (infantile) (lienteric)
(noninfectious) (presumed noninfectious)
(putrefactive) (secondary) (sporadic)
(summer) (symptomatic) (thermic) 787.91
achlorhydric 536.0
allergic 558.3
amebic (*see also* Amebiasis) 006.9
with abscess—*see* Abscess, amebic
acute 006.0
chronic 006.1
nondysenteric 006.2
bacillary—*see* Dysentery, bacillary
bacterial NEC 008.5
balantidial 007.0
bile salt-induced 579.8
cachectic NEC 787.91
chilomastix 007.8
choleriformis 001.1
coccidial 007.2
Cochin-China 579.1
anguilluliasis 127.2
psilosis 579.1
Dientamoeba 007.8

Diarrhea, diarrheal—*continued*
  dietetic 787.91
  due to
    achylia gastrica 536.8
    Aerobacter aerogenes 008.2
    Bacillus coli—*see* Enteritis, E. coli
    bacteria NEC 008.5
    bile salts 579.8
    Capillaria
      hepatica 128.8
      philippinensis 127.5
    Clostridium perfringens (C) (F) 008.46
    Enterobacter aerogenes 008.2
    enterococci 008.49
    Escherichia coli—*see* Enteritis, E. coli
    Giardia lamblia 007.1
    Heterophyes heterophyes 121.6
    irritating foods 787.91
    Metagonimus yokogawai 121.5
    Necator americanus 126.1
    Paracolobactrum arizonae 008.1
    Paracolon bacillus NEC 008.47
      Arizona 008.1
    Proteus (bacillus) (mirabilis) (Morganii) 008.3
    Pseudomonas aeruginosa 008.42
    S. japonicum 120.2
    specified organism NEC 008.8
      bacterial 008.49
      viral NEC 008.69
    Staphylococcus 008.41
    Streptococcus 008.49
      anaerobic 008.46
    Strongyloides stercoralis 127.2
    Trichuris trichiuria 127.3
    virus NEC (*see also* Enteritis, viral) 008.69
  dysenteric 009.2
    due to specified organism NEC 008.8
  dyspeptic 787.91
  endemic 009.3
  epidemic 009.3
  fermentative 787.91
  flagellate 007.9
  Flexner's (ulcerative) 004.1
  functional 564.5
    following gastrointestinal surgery 564.4
    psychogenic 306.4
  giardial 007.1
  Giardia lamblia 007.1
  hill 579.1
  hyperperistalsis (nervous) 306.4
  infectious 009.2
    presumed 009.3
  inflammatory 787.91
    due to specified organism NEC 008.8
  malarial (*see also* Malaria) 084.6
  mite 133.8
  mycotic 117.9
  nervous 306.4
  neurogenic 564.5
  parenteral NEC 009.2
  postgastrectomy 564.4
  postvagotomy 564.4
  prostaglandin induced 579.8
  protozoal NEC 007.9
  psychogenic 306.4
  septic 009.2
    due to specified organism NEC 008.8
  specified organism NEC 008.8
    bacterial 008.49
    viral NEC 008.69
  Staphylococcus 008.41

Diarrhea, diarrheal—*continued*
  Streptococcus 008.49
    anaerobic 088.46
  toxic 558.2
  travelers' 009.2
    due to specified organism NEC 008.8
  trichomonal 007.3
  tropical 579.1
  tuberculous 014.8
  ulcerative (chronic) (*see also* Colitis, ulcerative)
    556.9
  viral (*see also* Enteritis, viral) 008.8
  zymotic NEC 009.2
Diastasis
  cranial bones 733.99
    congenital 756.0
  joint (traumatic)—*see* Dislocation, by site
  muscle 728.84
    congenital 756.89
  recti (abdomen) 728.84
    complicating delivery 665.8
    congenital 756.79
Diastema, teeth, tooth 524.3
Diastematomyelia 742.51
Diataxia, cerebral, infantile 343.0
Diathesis
  allergic V15.09
  bleeding (familial) 287.9
  cystine (familial) 270.0
  gouty 274.9
  hemorrhagic (familial) 287.9
    newborn NEC 776.0
  oxalic 271.8
  scrofulous (*see also* Tuberculosis) 017.2
  spasmophilic (*see also* Tetany) 781.7
  ulcer 536.9
  uric acid 274.9
Diaz's disease or osteochondrosis 732.5
Dibothriocephaliasis 123.4
  larval 123.5
Dibothriocephalus (infection) (infestation)
    (latus) 123.4
  larval 123.5
Dicephalus 759.4
Dichotomy, teeth 520.2
Dichromat, dichromata (congenital) 368.59
Dichromatopsia (congenital) 368.59
Dichuchwa 104.0
Dicroceliasis 121.8
Didelphys, didelphic (*see also* Double uterus)
    752.2
Didymitis (*see also* Epididymitis) 604.90
Died —*see also* Death
  without
  medical attention (cause unknown) 798.9
  sign of disease 798.2
Dientamoeba diarrhea 007.8
Dietary
  inadequacy or deficiency 269.9
  surveillance and counseling V65.3
Dietl's crisis 593.4
Dieulafoy lesion (hemorrhagic)
  of
    duodenum 537.84
    intestine 569.86
    stomach 537.84
Dieulafoy's ulcer —*see* Ulcer, stomach
Difficult
  birth, affecting fetus or newborn 763.9
  delivery NEC 669.9

Difficulty
  feeding 783.3
    breast 676.8
  newborn 779.3
  nonorganic (infant) NEC 307.59
  mechanical, gastroduodenal stoma 537.89
  reading 315.00
  specific, spelling 315.09
  swallowing (*see also* Dysphagia) 787.2
  walking 719.7
Diffuse —*see* condition
Diffused ganglion 727.42
DiGeorge's syndrome (thymic hypoplasia) 279.11
Digestive —*see* condition
Di Guglielmo's disease or syndrome (M9841/3) 207.0
Diktyoma (M9051/3)—*see* Neoplasm, by site, malignant
Dilaceration, tooth 520.4
Dilatation
  anus 564.89
    venule—*see* Hemorrhoids
  aorta (focal) (general) (*see also* Aneurysm, aorta) 441.9
    congenital 747.29
    infectional 093.0
    ruptured 441.5
    syphilitic 093.0
  appendix (cystic) 543.9
  artery 447.8
  bile duct (common) (cystic) (congenital) 751.69
    acquired 576.8
  bladder (sphincter) 596.8
    congenital 753.8
    in pregnancy or childbirth 654.4
      causing obstructed labor 660.2
        affecting fetus or newborn 763.1
  blood vessel 459.89
  bronchus, bronchi 494.0
    with acute exacerbation 494.1
  calyx (due to obstruction) 593.89
  capillaries 448.9
  cardiac (acute) (chronic) (*see also* Hypertrophy, cardiac) 429.3
    congenital 746.89
      valve NEC 746.89
        pulmonary 746.09
    hypertensive (*see also* Hypertension, heart) 402.90
  cavum septi pellucidi 742.4
  cecum 564.89
    psychogenic 306.4
  cervix (uteri)—*see also* Incompetency, cervix
    incomplete, poor, slow
      affecting fetus or newborn 763.7
      complicating delivery 661.0
        affecting fetus or newborn 763.7
  colon 564.7
    congenital 751.3
    due to mechanical obstruction 560.89
    psychogenic 306.4
  common bile duct (congenital) 751.69
    acquired 576.8
      with calculus, choledocholithiasis, or stones—*see* Choledocholithiasis
  cystic duct 751.69
    acquired (any bile duct) 575.8
  duct, mammary 610.4
  duodenum 564.89
  esophagus 530.89

Dilatation—*continued*
  congenital 750.4
  due to
    achalasia 530.0
    cardiospasm 530.0
  Eustachian tube, congenital 744.24
  fontanel 756.0
  gallbladder 575.8
    congenital 751.69
  gastric 536.8
    acute 536.1
    psychogenic 306.4
  heart (acute) (chronic) (*see also* Hypertrophy, cardiac) 429.3
    congenital 746.89
    hypertensive (*see also* Hypertension, heart) 402.90
    valve—*see also* Endocarditis
      congenital 746.89
  ileum 564.89
    psychogenic 306.4
  inguinal rings—*see* Hernia, inguinal
  jejunum 564.89
    psychogenic 306.4
  kidney (calyx) (collecting structures) (cystic) (parenchyma) (pelvis) 593.89
  lacrimal passages 375.69
  lymphatic vessel 457.1
  mammary duct 610.4
  Meckel's diverticulum (congenital) 751.0
  meningeal vessels, congenital 742.8
  myocardium (acute) (chronic) (*see also* Hypertrophy, cardiac) 429.3
  organ or site, congenital NEC—*see* Distortion
  pancreatic duct 577.8
  pelvis, kidney 593.89
  pericardium—*see* Pericarditis
  pharynx 478.29
  prostate 602.8
  pulmonary
    artery (idiopathic) 417.8
      congenital 747.3
    valve, congenital 746.09
  pupil 379.43
  rectum 564.89
  renal 593.89
  saccule vestibularis, congenital 744.05
  salivary gland (duct) 527.8
  sphincter ani 564.89
  stomach 536.8
    acute 536.1
    psychogenic 306.4
  submaxillary duct 527.8
  trachea, congenital 748.3
  ureter (idiopathic) 593.89
    congenital 753.20
    due to obstruction 593.5
  urethra (acquired) 599.84
  vasomotor 443.9
  vein 459.89
  ventricular, ventricle (acute) (chronic) (*see also* Hypertrophy, cardiac) 429.3
    cerebral, congenital 742.4
    hypertensive (*see also* Hypertension, heart) 402.90
  venule 459.89
    anus—*see* Hemorrhoids
  vesical orifice 596.8
Dilated, dilation —*see* Dilatation

Diminished
  hearing (acuity) (*see also* Deafness) 389.9
  pulse pressure 785.9
  vision NEC 369.9
  vital capacity 794.2
Diminuta taenia 123.6
Diminution, sense or sensation (cold) (heat)
    (tactile) (vibratory) (*see also* Disturbance,
    sensation) 782.0
Dimitri-Sturge-Weber disease
    (encephalocutaneous angiomatosis) 759.6
Dimple
  parasacral 685.1
    with abscess 685.0
  pilonidal 685.1
    with abscess 685.0
  postanal 685.1
    with abscess 685.0
Dioctophyma renale (infection) (infestation)
    128.8
Dipetalonemiasis 125.4
Diphallus 752.69
Diphtheria, diphtheritic (gangrenous)
    (hemorrhagic) 032.9
  carrier (suspected) of V02.4
  cutaneous 032.85
  cystitis 032.84
  faucial 032.0
  infection of wound 032.85
  inoculation (anti) (not sick) V03.5
  laryngeal 032.3
  myocarditis 032.82
  nasal anterior 032.2
  nasopharyngeal 032.1
  neurological complication 032.89
  peritonitis 032.83
  specified site NEC 032.89
Diphyllobothriasis (intestine) 123.4
  larval 123.5
Diplacusis 388.41
Diplegia (upper limbs) 344.2
  brain or cerebral 437.8
  congenital 343.0
  facial 351.0
    congenital 352.6
  infantile or congenital (cerebral) (spastic)
    (spinal) 343.0
  lower limbs 344.1
  syphilitic, congenital 090.49
Diplococcus, diplococcal —*see* condition
Diplomyelia 742.59
Diplopia 368.2
  refractive 368.15
Dipsomania (*see also* Alcoholism) 303.9
  with psychosis (*see also* Psychosis, alcoholic)
    291.9
Dipylidiasis 123.8
  intestine 123.8
Direction, teeth, abnormal 524.3
Dirt-eating child 307.52
Disability
  heart—*see* Disease, heart
  learning NEC 315.2
  special spelling 315.09
Disarticulation (*see also* Derangement, joint)
    718.9
  meaning
    amputation
      status—*see* Absence, by site
      traumatic —*see* Amputation, traumatic
    dislocation, traumatic or congenital—*see*
      Dislocation

Disaster, cerebrovascular (*see also* Disease,
    cerebrovascular, acute) 436
Discharge
  anal NEC 787.99
  breast (female) (male) 611.79
  conjunctiva 372.89
  continued locomotor idiopathic (*see also*
    Epilepsy) 345.5
  diencephalic autonomic idiopathic (*see also*
    Epilepsy) 345.5
  ear 388.60
    blood 388.69
    cerebrospinal fluid 388.61
  excessive urine 788.42
  eye 379.93
  nasal 478.1
  nipple 611.79
  patterned motor idiopathic (*see also* Epilepsy)
    345.5
  penile 788.7
  postnasal—*see* Sinusitis
  sinus, from mediastinum 510.0
  umbilicus 789.9
  urethral 788.7
    bloody 599.84
  vaginal 623.5
Discitis 722.90
  cervical, cervicothoracic 722.91
  lumbar, lumbosacral 722.93
  thoracic, thoracolumbar 722.92
Discogenic syndrome —*see* Displacement,
    intervertebral disc
Discoid
  kidney 753.3
  meniscus, congenital 717.5
  semilunar cartilage 717.5
Discoloration
  mouth 528.9
  nails 703.8
  teeth 521.7
    due to
      drugs 521.7
        metals (copper) (silver) 521.7
        pulpal bleeding 521.7
      during formation 520.8
      posteruptive 521.7
Discomfort
  chest 786.59
  visual 368.13
Discomycosis —*see* Actinomycosis
Discontinuity, ossicles, ossicular chain 385.23
Discrepancy
  leg length (acquired) 736.81
    congenital 755.30
  uterine size-date 646.8
Discrimination
  political V62.4
  racial V62.4
  religious V62.4
  sex V62.4
Disease, diseased —*see also* Syndrome
  Abrami's (acquired hemolytic jaundice) 283.9
  absorbent system 459.89
  accumulation—*see* Thesaurismosis
  acid-peptic 536.8
  Acosta's 993.2
  Adams-Stokes (-Morgagni) (syncope with heart
    block) 426.9
  Addison's (bronze) (primary adrenal
    insufficiency) 255.4
    anemia (pernicious) 281.0

Disease, diseased—*continued*
  tuberculous (*see also* Tuberculosis) 017.6
  Addison-Gull—*see* Xanthoma
  adenoids (and tonsils) (chronic) 474.9
  adrenal (gland) (capsule) (cortex) 255.9
    hyperfunction 255.3
    hypofunction 255.4
    specified type NEC 255.8
  ainhum (dactylolysis spontanea) 136.0
  akamushi (scrub typhus) 081.2
  Akureyri (epidemic neuromyasthenia) 049.8
  Albarrán's (colibacilluria) 791.9
  Albers-Schönberg's (marble bones) 756.52
  Albert's 726.71
  Albright (-Martin) (-Bantam) 275.49
  Alibert's (mycosis fungoides) (M9700/3) 202.1
  Alibert-Bazin (M9700/3) 202.1
  alimentary canal 569.9
  alligator skin (ichthyosis congenital) 757.1
    acquired 701.1
  Almeida's (Brazilian blastomycosis) 116.1
  Alpers' 330.8
  alpine 993.2
  altitude 993.2
  alveoli, teeth 525.9
  Alzheimer's—*see* Alzheimer's
  amyloid (any site) 277.3
  anarthritic rheumatoid 446.5
  Anders' (adiposis tuberosa simplex) 272.8
  Andersen's (glycogenosis IV) 271.0
  Anderson's (angiokeratoma corporis diffusum) 272.7
  Andes 993.2
  Andrews' (bacterid) 686.8
  angiospastic, angiospasmodic 443.9
    cerebral 435.9
      with transient neurologic deficit 435.9
    vein 459.89
  anterior
    chamber 364.9
    horn cell 335.9
      specified type NEC 335.8
  antral (chronic) 473.0
    acute 461.0
  anus NEC 569.49
  aorta (nonsyphilitic) 447.9
    syphilitic NEC 093.89
  aortic (heart) (valve) (*see also* Endocarditis, aortic) 424.1
  apollo 077.4
  aponeurosis 726.90
  appendix 543.9
  aqueous (chamber) 364.9
  arc-welders' lung 503
  Armenian 277.3
  Arnold-Chiari (*see also* Spina bifida) 741.0
  arterial 447.9
    occlusive (*see also* Occlusion, by site) 444.22
      with embolus or thrombus—*see* Occlusion, by site
      due to stricture or stenosis 447.1
    specified type NEC 447.8
  arteriocardiorenal (*see also* Hypertension, cardiorenal) 404.90
  arteriolar (generalized) (obliterative) 447.9
    specified type NEC 447.8
  arteriorenal—*see* Hypertension, kidney
  arteriosclerotic—*see also* Arteriosclerosis
    cardiovascular 429.2
    coronary —*see* Arteriosclerosis, coronary
    heart —*see* Arteriosclerosis, coronary

Disease, diseased—*continued*
  vascular—*see* Arteriosclerosis
  artery 447.9
    cerebral 437.9
    coronary —*see* Arteriosclerosis, coronary
    specified type NEC 447.8
  arthropod-borne NEC 088.9
    specified type NEC 088.89
  Asboe-Hansen's (incontinentia pigmenti) 757.33
  atticoantral, chronic (with posterior or superior marginal perforation of ear drum) 382.2
  auditory canal, ear 380.9
  Aujeszky's 078.89
  auricle, ear NEC 380.30
  Australian X 062.4
  autoimmune NEC 279.4
    hemolytic (cold type) (warm type) 283.0
    parathyroid 252.1
    thyroid 245.2
  aviators' (*see also* Effect, adverse, high altitude) 993.2
  ax(e)-grinders' 502
  Ayala's 756.89
  Ayerza's (pulmonary artery sclerosis with pulmonary hypertension) 416.0
  Azorean (of the nervous system) 334.8
  Babington's (familial hemorrhagic telangiectasia) 448.0
  back bone NEC 733.90
  bacterial NEC 040.89
    zoonotic NEC 027.9
      specified type NEC 027.8
  Baehr-Schiffrin (thrombotic thrombocytopenic purpura) 446.6
  Baelz's (cheilitis glandularis apostematosa) 528.5
  Baerensprung's (eczema marginatum) 110.3
  Balfour's (chloroma) 205.3
  balloon (*see also* Effect, adverse, high altitude) 993.2
  Baló's 341.1
  Bamberger (-Marie) (hypertrophic pulmonary osteoarthropathy) 731.2
  Bang's (Brucella abortus) 023.1
  Bannister's 995.1
  Banti's (with cirrhosis) (with portal hypertension)—*see* Cirrhosis, liver
  Barcoo (*see also* Ulcer, skin) 707.9
  barium lung 503
  Barlow (-Möller) (infantile scurvy) 267
  barometer makers' 985.0
  Barraquer (-Simons) (progressive lipodystrophy) 272.6
  basal ganglia 333.90
    degenerative NEC 333.0
    specified NEC 333.89
  Basedow's (exophthalmic goiter) 242.0
  basement membrane NEC 583.89
    with
      pulmonary hemorrhage (Goodpasture's syndrome) 446.21 *[583.81]*
  Bateman's 078.0
    purpura (senile) 287.2
  Batten's 330.1 *[362.71]*
  Batten-Mayou (retina) 330.1 *[362.71]*
  Batten-Steinert 359.2
  Battey 031.0
  Baumgarten-Cruveilhier (cirrhosis of liver) 571.5
  bauxite-workers' 503
  Bayle's (dementia paralytica) 094.1

Disease, diseased—*continued*
  Bazin's (primary) (*see also* Tuberculosis) 017.1
  Beard's (neurasthenia) 300.5
  Beau's (*see also* Degeneration, myocardial)
    429.1
  Bechterew's (ankylosing spondylitis) 720.0
  Becker's (idiopathic mural endomyocardial
    disease) 425.2
  Begbie's (exophthalmic goiter) 242.0
  Behr's 362.50
  Beigel's (white piedra) 111.2
  Bekhterev's (ankylosing spondylitis) 720.0
  Bell's (*see also* Psychosis, affective) 296.0
  Bennett's (leukemia) 208.9
  Benson's 379.22
  Bergeron's (hysteroepilepsy) 300.11
  Berlin's 921.3
  Bernard-Soulier (thrombopathy) 287.1
  Bernhardt (-Roth) 355.1
  beryllium 503
  Besnier-Boeck (-Schaumann) (sarcoidosis) 135
  Best's 362.76
  Beurmann's (sporotrichosis) 117.1
  Bielschowsky (-Jansky) 330.1
  Biermer's (pernicious anemia) 281.0
  Biett's (discoid lupus erythematosus) 695.4
  bile duct (*see also* Disease, biliary) 576.9
  biliary (duct) (tract) 576.9
    with calculus, choledocholithiasis, or
      stones—*see* Choledocholithiasis
  Billroth's (meningocele) (*see also* Spina bifida)
    741.9
  Binswanger's 290.12
  Bird's (oxaluria) 271.8
  bird fanciers' 495.2
  black lung 500
  bladder 596.9
    specified NEC 596.8
  bleeder's 286.0
  Bloch-Sulzberger (incontinentia pigmenti)
    757.33
  Blocq's (astasia-abasia) 307.9
  blood (-forming organs) 289.9
    specified NEC 289.8
    vessel 459.9
  Bloodgood's 610.1
  Blount's (tibia vara) 732.4
  blue 746.9
  Bodechtel-Guttmann (subacute sclerosing
    panencephalitis) 046.2
  Boeck's (sarcoidosis) 135
  bone 733.90
    fibrocystic NEC 733.29
      jaw 526.2
    marrow 289.9
    Paget's (osteitis deformans) 731.0
    specified type NEC 733.99
    von Recklinghausen's (osteitis fibrosa cystica)
      252.0
  Bonfils'—*see* Disease, Hodgkin's
  Borna 062.9
  Bornholm (epidemic pleurodynia) 074.1
  Bostock's (*see also* Fever, hay) 477.9
  Bouchard's (myopathic dilatation of the
    stomach) 536.1
  Bouillaud's (rheumatic heart disease) 391.9
  Bourneville (-Brissaud) (tuberous sclerosis)
    759.5
  Bouveret (-Hoffmann) (paroxysmal
    tachycardia) 427.2

Disease, diseased—*continued*
  bowel 569.9
    functional 564.9
      psychogenic 306.4
  Bowen's (M8081/2)—*see* Neoplasm, skin, in
    situ
  Bozzolo's (multiple myeloma) (M9730/3) 203.0
  Bradley's (epidemic vomiting) 078.82
  Brailsford's 732.3
    radius, head 732.3
    tarsal, scaphoid 732.5
  Brailsford-Morquio (mucopolysaccharidosis
    IV) 277.5
  brain 348.9
    Alzheimer's 331.0
      with dementia—*see* Alzheimer's, dementia
    arterial, artery 437.9
    arteriosclerotic 437.0
    congenital 742.9
    degenerative—*see* Degeneration, brain
    inflammatory—*see also* Encephalitis
      late effect—*see* category 326
    organic 348.9
      arteriosclerotic 437.0
    parasitic NEC 123.9
    Pick's 331.1
      with dementia
        with behavioral disturbance 331.1 *[294.11]*
        without behavioral disturbance 331.1
          [294.10]
    senile 331.2
  braziers' 985.8
  breast 611.9
    cystic (chronic) 610.1
    fibrocystic 610.1
    inflammatory 611.0
    Paget's (M8540/3) 174.0
    puerperal, postpartum NEC 676.3
    specified NEC 611.8
  Breda's (*see also* Yaws) 102.9
  Breisky's (kraurosis vulvae) 624.0
  Bretonneau's (diphtheritic malignant angina)
    032.0
  Bright's (*see also* Nephritis) 583.9
    arteriosclerotic (*see also* Hypertension,
      kidney) 403.90
  Brill's (recrudescent typhus) 081.1
    flea-borne 081.0
    louse-borne 081.1
  Brill-Symmers (follicular lymphoma)
    (M9690/3) 202.0
  Brill-Zinsser (recrudescent typhus) 081.1
  Brinton's (leather bottle stomach) (M8142/3)
    151.9
  Brion-Kayser (*see also* Fever, paratyphoid)
    002.9
  broad
    beta 272.2
    ligament, noninflammatory 620.9
      specified NEC 620.8
  Brocq's 691.8
    meaning
      atopic (diffuse) neurodermatitis 691.8
      dermatitis herpetiformis 694.0
      lichen simplex chronicus 698.3
      parapsoriasis 696.2
      prurigo 698.2
  Brocq-Duhring (dermatitis herpetiformis) 694.0
  Brodie's (joint) (*see also* Osteomyelitis) 730.1
  bronchi 519.1
  bronchopulmonary 519.1

Disease, diseased—*continued*
  paralysis 335.22
  pseudohypertrophy, muscles 359.1
  Duchenne-Griesinger 359.1
  ductless glands 259.9
  Duhring's (dermatitis herpetiformis) 694.0
  Dukes (-Filatov) 057.8
  duodenum NEC 537.9
    specified NEC 537.89
  Duplay's 726.2
  Dupré's (meningism) 781.6
  Dupuytren's (muscle contracture) 728.6
  Durand-Nicolas-Favre (climatic bubo) 099.1
  Duroziez's (congenital mitral stenosis) 746.5
  Dutton's (trypanosomiasis) 086.9
  Eales' 362.18
  ear (chronic) (inner) NEC 388.9
    middle 385.9
      adhesive (*see also* Adhesions, middle ear)
        385.10
      specified NEC 385.89
  Eberth's (typhoid fever) 002.0
  Ebstein's
    heart 746.2
    meaning diabetes 250.4 *[581.81]*
  Echinococcus (*see also* Echinococcus) 122.9
  ECHO virus NEC 078.89
  Economo's (encephalitis lethargica) 049.8
  Eddowes' (brittle bones and blue sclera) 756.51
  Edsall's 992.2
  Eichstedt's (pityriasis versicolor) 111.0
  Ellis-van Creveld (chondroectodermal
    dysplasia) 756.55
  endocardium—*see* Endocarditis
  endocrine glands or system NEC 259.9
    specified NEC 259.8
  endomyocardial, idiopathic mural 425.2
  Engel-von Recklinghausen (osteitis fibrosa
    cystica) 252.0
  Engelmann's (diaphyseal sclerosis) 756.59
  English (rickets) 268.0
  Engman's (infectious eczematoid dermatitis)
    690.8
  enteroviral, enterovirus NEC 078.89
    central nervous system NEC 048
  epidemic NEC 136.9
  epididymis 608.9
  epigastric, functional 536.9
    psychogenic 306.4
  Erb (-Landouzy) 359.1
  Erb-Goldflam 358.0
  Erichsen's (railway spine) 300.16
  esophagus 530.9
    functional 530.5
    psychogenic 306.4
  Eulenburg's (congenital paramyotonia) 359.2
  Eustachian tube 381.9
  Evans' (thrombocytopenic purpura) 287.3
  external auditory canal 380.9
  extrapyramidal NEC 333.90
  eye 379.90
    anterior chamber 364.9
    inflammatory NEC 364.3
    muscle 378.9
  eyeball 360.9
  eyelid 374.9
  eyeworm of Africa 125.2
  Fabry's (angiokeratoma corporis diffusum)
    272.7
  facial nerve (seventh) 351.9
    newborn 767.5

Disease, diseased—*continued*
  Fahr-Volhard (malignant nephrosclerosis)
    403.00
  fallopian tube, noninflammatory 620.9
    specified NEC 620.8
  familial periodic 277.3
    paralysis 359.3
  Fanconi's (congenital pancytopenia) 284.0
  Farber's (disseminated lipogranulomatosis)
    272.8
  fascia 728.9
    inflammatory 728.9
  Fauchard's (periodontitis) 523.4
  Favre-Durand-Nicolas (climatic bubo) 099.1
  Favre-Racouchot (elastoidosis cutanea
    nodularis) 701.8
  Fede's 529.0
  Feer's 985.0
  Felix's (juvenile osteochondrosis, hip) 732.1
  Fenwick's (gastric atrophy) 537.89
  Fernels' (aortic aneurysm) 441.9
  fibrocaseous, of lung (*see also* Tuberculosis,
    pulmonary) 011.9
  fibrocystic—*see also* Fibrocystic, disease
    newborn 277.01
  Fiedler's (leptospiral jaundice) 100.0
  fifth 057.0
  Filatoff's (infectious mononucleosis) 075
  Filatov's (infectious mononucleosis) 075
  file-cutters' 984.9
    specified type of lead—*see* Table of drugs and
      chemicals
  filterable virus NEC 078.89
  fish skin 757.1
    acquired 701.1
  Flajani (-Basedow) (exophthalmic goiter) 242.0
  Flatau-Schilder 341.1
  flax-dressers' 504
  Fleischner's 732.3
  flint 502
  fluke—*see* Infestation, fluke
  Følling's (phenylketonuria) 270.1
  foot and mouth 078.4
  foot process 581.3
  Forbes' (glycogenosis III) 271.0
  Fordyce's (ectopic sebaceous glands) (mouth)
    750.26
  Fordyce-Fox (apocrine miliaria) 705.82
  Fothergill's
    meaning scarlatina anginosa 034.1
    neuralgia (*see also* Neuralgia, trigeminal)
      350.1
  Fournier's 608.83
  fourth 057.8
  Fox (-Fordyce) (apocrine miliaria) 705.82
  Francis' (*see also* Tularemia) 021.9
  Franklin's (heavy chain) 273.2
  Frei's (climatic bubo) 099.1
  Freiberg's (flattening metatarsal) 732.5
  Friedländer's (endarteritis obliterans)—*see*
    Arteriosclerosis
  Friedreich's
    combined systemic or ataxia 334.0
    facial hemihypertrophy 756.0
    myoclonia 333.2
  Fröhlich's (adiposogenital dystrophy) 253.8
  Frommel's 676.6
  frontal sinus (chronic) 473.1
    acute 461.1
  Fuller's earth 502
  fungus, fungous NEC 117.9

Disease, diseased—*continued*
  Gaisböck's (polycythemia hypertonica) 289.0
  gallbladder 575.9
    congenital 751.60
  Gamna's (siderotic splenomegaly) 289.51
  Gamstorp's (adynamia episodica hereditaria)
      359.3
  Gandy-Nanta (siderotic splenomegaly) 289.51
  gannister (occupational) 502
  Garré's (*see also* Osteomyelitis) 730.1
  gastric (*see also* Disease, stomach) 537.9
  gastrointestinal (tract) 569.9
    amyloid 277.3
    functional 536.9
      psychogenic 306.4
  Gaucher's (adult) (cerebroside lipidosis)
      (infantile) 272.7
  Gayet's (superior hemorrhagic
      polioencephalitis) 265.1
  Gee (-Herter) (-Heubner) (-Thaysen)
      (nontropical sprue) 579.0
  generalized neoplastic (M8000/6) 199.0
  genital organs NEC
    female 629.9
      specified NEC 629.8
    male 608.9
  Gerhardt's (erythromelalgia) 443.89
  Gerlier's (epidemic vertigo) 078.81
  Gibert's (pityriasis rosea) 696.3
  Gibney' s (perispondylitis) 720.9
  Gierke's (glycogenosis I) 271.0
  Gilbert's (familial nonhemolytic jaundice) 277.4
  Gilchrist's (North American blastomycosis)
      116.0
  Gilford (-Hutchinson) (progeria) 259.8
  Gilles de la Tourette's (motor-verbal tic) 307.23
  Giovannini's 117.9
  gland (lymph) 289.9
  Glanzmann's (hereditary hemorrhagic
      thrombasthenia) 287.1
  glassblowers' 527.1
  Glénard's (enteroptosis) 569.89
  Glisson's (*see also* Rickets) 268.0
  glomerular
    membranous, idiopathic 581.1
    minimal change 581.3
  glycogen storage (Andersen's) (Cori types 1-7)
      (Forbes') (McArdle-Schmid-Pearson)
      (Pompe's) (types I-VII) 271.0
    cardiac 271.0 *[425.7]*
    generalized 271.0
    glucose-6-phosphatase deficiency 271.0
    heart 271.0 *[425.7]*
    hepatorenal 271.0
    liver and kidneys 271.0
    myocardium 271.0 *[425.7]*
    von Gierke's (glycogenosis I) 271.0
  Goldflam-Erb 358.0
  Goldscheider's (epidermolysis bullosa) 757.39
  Goldstein's (familial hemorrhagic
      telangiectasia) 448.0
  gonococcal NEC 098.0
  Goodall's (epidemic vomiting) 078.82
  Gordon's (exudative enteropathy) 579.8
  Gougerot's (trisymptomatic) 709.1
  Gougerot-Carteaud (confluent reticulate
      papillomatosis) 701.8
  Gougerot-Hailey-Hailey (benign familial
      chronic pemphigus) 757.39

Disease, diseased—*continued*
  graft-versus-host (bone marrow) 996.85
    due to organ transplant NEC—*see*
        Complications, transplant, organ
  grain-handlers' 495.8
  Grancher's (splenopneumonia)—*see* Pneumonia
  granulomatous (childhood) (chronic) 288.1
  graphite lung 503
  Graves' (exophthalmic goiter) 242.0
  Greenfield's 330.0
  green monkey 078.89
  Griesinger's (*see also* Ancylostomiasis) 126.9
  grinders' 502
  Grisel's 723.5
  Gruby's (tinea tonsurans) 110.0
  Guertin's (electric chorea) 049.8
  Guillain-Barré 357.0
  Guinon's (motor-verbal tic) 307.23
  Gull's (thyroid atrophy with myxedema) 244.8
  Gull and Sutton's—*see* Hypertension, kidney
  gum NEC 523.9
  Günther's (congenital erythropoietic porphyria)
      277.1
  gynecological 629.9
    specified NEC 629.8
  H 270.0
  Haas' 732.3
  Habermann's (acute parapsoriasis varioliformis)
      696.2
  Haff 985.1
  Hageman (congenital factor XII deficiency) (*see
      also* Defect, congenital) 286.3
  Haglund's (osteochondrosis os tibiale
      externum) 732.5
  Hagner's (hypertrophic pulmonary
      osteoarthropathy) 731.2
  Hailey-Hailey (benign familial chronic
      pemphigus) 757.39
  hair (follicles) NEC 704.9
    specified type NEC 704.8
  Hallervorden-Spatz 333.0
  Hallopeau's (lichen sclerosus et atrophicus)
      701.0
  Hamman's (spontaneous mediastinal
      emphysema) 518.1
  hand, foot, and mouth 074.3
  Hand-Schüller-Christian (chronic histiocytosis
      X) 277.8
  Hanot's—*see* Cirrhosis, biliary
  Hansen's (leprosy) 030.9
    benign form 030.1
    malignant form 030.0
  Harada's 363.22
  Harley's (intermittent hemoglobinuria) 283.2
  Hart's (pellagra-cerebellar ataxia renal
      aminoaciduria) 270.0
  Hartnup (pellagra-cerebellar ataxia-renal
      aminoaciduria) 270.0
  Hashimoto's (struma lymphomatosa) 245.2
  Hb—*see* Disease, hemoglobin
  heart (organic) 429.9
    with
      acute pulmonary edema (*see also* Failure,
          ventricular, left) 428.1
        hypertensive 402.91
          with renal failure 404.92
          benign 402.11
            with renal failure 404.12
          malignant 402.01
            with renal failure 404.02

Disease, diseased—*continued*
   kidney disease—*see* Hypertension,
    cardiorenal
   rheumatic fever (conditions classifiable to
    390)
    active 391.9
     with chorea 392.0
    inactive or quiescent (with chorea) 398.90
   amyloid 277.3 *[425.7]*
   aortic (valve) (*see also* Endocarditis, aortic)
    424.1
   arteriosclerotic or sclerotic (minimal)
    (senile)—*see* Arteriosclerosis, coronary
   artery, arterial —*see* Arteriosclerosis, coronary
   atherosclerotic —*see* Arteriosclerosis,
    coronary
   beer drinkers' 425.5
   beriberi 265.0 *[425.7]*
   black 416.0
   congenital NEC 746.9
    cyanotic 746.9
    maternal, affecting fetus or newborn 760.3
    specified type NEC 746.89
   congestive (*see also* Failure, heart) 428.0
   coronary 414.9
   cryptogenic 429.9
   due to
    amyloidosis 277.3 *[425.7]*
    beriberi 265.0 *[425.7]*
    cardiac glycogenosis 271.0 *[425.7]*
    Friedreich's ataxia 334.0 *[425.8]*
    gout 274.82
    mucopolysaccharidosis 277.5 *[425.7]*
    myotonia atrophica 359.2 *[425.8]*
    progressive muscular dystrophy 359.1
     [425.8]
    sarcoidosis 135 *[425.8]*
   fetal 746.9
    inflammatory 746.89
   fibroid (*see also* Myocarditis) 429.0
   functional 427.9
    postoperative 997.1
    psychogenic 306.2
   glycogen storage 271.0 *[425.7]*
   gonococcal NEC 098.85
   gouty 274.82
   hypertensive (*see also* Hypertension, heart)
    402.90
    benign 402.10
    malignant 402.00
   hyperthyroid (*see also* Hyperthyroidism)
    242.9 *[425.7]*
   incompletely diagnosed—*see* Disease, heart
   ischemic (chronic) (*see also* Ischemia, heart)
    414.9
    acute (*see also* Infarct, myocardium) 410.9
     without myocardial infarction 411.89
      with coronary (artery) occlusion 411.81
    asymptomatic 412
    diagnosed on ECG or other special
     investigation but currently presenting no
     symptoms 412
   kyphoscoliotic 416.1
   mitral (*see also* Endocarditis, mitral) 394.9
   muscular (*see also* Degeneration, myocardial)
    429.1
   postpartum 674.8
   psychogenic (functional) 306.2
   pulmonary (chronic) 416.9
    acute 415.0

Disease, diseased—*continued*
   specified NEC 416.8
   rheumatic (chronic) (inactive) (old)
    (quiescent) (with chorea) 398.90
   active or acute 391.9
    with chorea (active) (rheumatic)
     (Sydenham's) 392.0
    specified type NEC 391.8
   maternal, affecting fetus or newborn 760.3
   rheumatoid—*see* Arthritis, rheumatoid
   sclerotic —*see* Arteriosclerosis, coronary
   senile (*see also* Myocarditis) 429.0
   specified type NEC 429.89
   syphilitic 093.89
    aortic 093.1
     aneurysm 093.0
    asymptomatic 093.89
    congenital 090.5
   thyroid (gland) (*see also* Hyperthyroidism)
    242.9 *[425.7]*
   thyrotoxic (*see also* Thyrotoxicosis) 242.9
    [425.7]
   tuberculous (*see also* Tuberculosis) 017.9
    [425.8]
   valve, valvular (obstructive)
    (regurgitant)—*see also* Endocarditis
    congenital NEC (*see also* Anomaly, heart,
     valve) 746.9
     pulmonary 746.00
     specified type NEC 746.89
   vascular—*see* Disease, cardiovascular
  heavy-chain (gamma G) 273.2
  Heberden's 715.04
  Hebra's
   dermatitis exfoliativa 695.89
   erythema multiforme exudativum 695.1
   pityriasis
    maculata et circinata 696.3
    rubra 695.89
     pilaris 696.4
   prurigo 698.2
  Heerfordt's (uveoparotitis) 135
  Heidenhain's 290.10
   with dementia 290.10
  Heilmeyer-Schöner (M9842/3) 207.1
  Heine-Medin (*see also* Poliomyelitis) 045.9
  Heller's (*see also* Psychosis, childhood) 299.1
  Heller-Döhle (syphilitic aortitis) 093.1
  hematopoietic organs 289.9
  hemoglobin (Hb) 282.7
   with thalassemia 282.4
   abnormal (mixed) NEC 282.7
    with thalassemia 282.4
   AS genotype 282.5
   Bart's 282.7
   C (Hb-C) 282.7
    with other abnormal hemoglobin NEC 282.7
    elliptocytosis 282.7
    Hb-S 282.63
    sickle-cell 282.63
    thalassemia 282.4
   constant spring 282.7
   D (Hb-D) 282.7
    with other abnormal hemoglobin NEC 282.7
    Hb-S 282.69
    sickle-cell 282.69
    thalassemia 282.4
   E (Hb-E) 282.7
    with other abnormal hemoglobin NEC 282.7
    Hb-S 282.69
    sickle-cell 282.69

Disease, diseased—*continued*
    thalassemia 282.4
    elliptocytosis 282.7
    F (Hb-F) 282.7
    G (Hb-G) 282.7
    H (Hb-H) 282.4
    hereditary persistence, fetal (HPFH) ("Swiss
        variety") 282.7
    high fetal gene 282.7
    I thalassemia 282.4
    M 289.7
    S—*see* Disease, sickle-cell, Hb-S
    spherocytosis 282.7
    unstable, hemolytic 282.7
    Zurich (Hb-Zurich) 282.7
  hemolytic (fetus) (newborn) 773.2
    autoimmune (cold type) (warm type) 283.0
    due to or with
      incompatibility
        ABO (blood group) 773.1
         blood (group) (Duffy) (Kell) (Kidd)
          (Lewis) (M) (S) NEC 773.2
         Rh (blood group) (factor) 773.0
        Rh negative mother 773.0
      unstable hemoglobin 282.7
  hemorrhagic 287.9
    newborn 776.0
  Henoch (-Schönlein) (purpura nervosa) 287.0
  hepatic—*see* Disease, liver
  hepatolenticular 275.1
  heredodegenerative NEC
    brain 331.89
    spinal cord 336.8
  Hers' (glycogenosis VI) 271.0
  Herter (-Gee) (-Heubner) (nontropical sprue)
    579.0
  Herxheimer's (diffuse idiopathic cutaneous
    atrophy) 701.8
  Heubner's 094.89
  Heubner-Herter (nontropical sprue) 579.0
  high fetal gene or hemoglobin thalassemia 282.4
  Hildenbrand's (typhus) 081.9
  hip (joint) NEC 719.95
    congenital 755.63
    suppurative 711.05
    tuberculous (*see also* Tuberculosis) 015.1
      [730.85]
  Hippel's (retinocerebral angiomatosis) 759.6
  Hirschfeld's (acute diabetes mellitus) (*see also*
    Diabetes) 250.0
  Hirschsprung's (congenital megacolon) 751.3
  His (-Werner) (trench fever) 083.1
  HIV 042
  Hodgkin's (M9650/3) 201.9

Note—Use the following fifth-digit subclassification with categories 201:

0 *unspecified site*
1 *lymph nodes of head, face, and neck*
2 *intrathoracic lymph nodes*
3 *intra-abdominal lymph nodes*
4 *lymph nodes of axilla and upper limb*
5 *lymph nodes of inguinal region and lower limb*
6 *intrapelvic lymph nodes*
7 *spleen*
8 *lymph nodes of multiple sites*

---

    lymphocytic
      depletion (M9653/3) 201.7
        diffuse fibrosis (M9654/3) 201.7

Disease, diseased—*continued*
    reticular type (M9655/3) 201.7
    predominance (M9651/3) 201.4
    lymphocytic-histiocytic predominance
      (M9651/3) 201.4
    mixed cellularity (M9652/3) 201.6
    nodular sclerosis (M9656/3) 201.5
      cellular phase (M9657/3) 201.5
  Hodgson's 441.9
    ruptured 441.5
  Hoffa (-Kastert) (liposynovitis prepatellaris)
    272.8
  Holla (*see also* Spherocytosis) 282.0
  homozygous-Hb-S 282.61
  hoof and mouth 078.4
  hookworm (*see also* Ancylostomiasis) 126.9
  Horton's (temporal arteritis) 446.5
  host-versus-graft (immune or nonimmune
    cause) 996.80
    bone marrow 996.85
    heart 996.83
    intestines 996.87
    kidney 996.81
    liver 996.82
    lung 996.84
    pancreas 996.86
    specified NEC 996.89
  HPFH (hereditary persistence of fetal
    hemoglobin) ("Swiss variety") 282.7
  Huchard's (continued arterial hypertension)
    401.9
  Huguier's (uterine fibroma) 218.9
  human immunodeficiency (virus) 042
  hunger 251.1
  Hunt's
    dyssynergia cerebellaris myoclonica 334.2
    herpetic geniculate ganglionitis 053.11
  Huntington's 333.4
  Huppert's (multiple myeloma) (M9730/3) 203.0
  Hurler's (mucopolysaccharidosis I) 277.5
  Hutchinson's, meaning
    angioma serpiginosum 709.1
    cheiropompholyx 705.81
    prurigo estivalis 692.72
  Hutchinson-Boeck (sarcoidosis) 135
  Hutchinson-Gilford (progeria) 259.8
  hyaline (diffuse) (generalized) 728.9
    membrane (lung) (newborn) 769
  hydatid (*see also* Echinococcus) 122.9
  Hyde's (prurigo nodularis) 698.3
  hyperkinetic (*see also* Hyperkinesia) 314.9
    heart 429.82
  hypertensive (*see also* Hypertension) 401.9
  hypophysis 253.9
    hyperfunction 253.1
    hypofunction 253.2
  Iceland (epidemic neuromyasthenia) 049.8
  I cell 272.7
  ill-defined 799.8
  immunologic NEC 279.9
  immunoproliferative 203.8
  inclusion 078.5
    salivary gland 078.5
  infancy, early NEC 779.9
  infective NEC 136.9
  inguinal gland 289.9
  internal semilunar cartilage, cystic 717.5
  intervertebral disc 722.90
    with myelopathy 722.70
    cervical, cervicothoracic 722.91
      with myelopathy 722.71

Disease, diseased—*continued*
  Kümmell's (-Verneuil) (spondylitis) 721.7
  Kundrat's (lymphosarcoma) 200.1
  kuru 046.0
  Kussmaul (-Meier) (polyarteritis nodosa) 446.0
  Kyasanur Forest 065.2
  Kyrle's (hyperkeratosis follicularis in cutem
      penetrans) 701.1
  labia
    inflammatory 616.9
      specified NEC 616.8
    noninflammatory 624.9
      specified NEC 624.8
  labyrinth, ear 386.8
  lacrimal system (apparatus) (passages) 375.9
    gland 375.00
    specified NEC 375.89
  Lafora's 333.2
  Lagleyze-von Hippel (retinocerebral
      angiomatosis) 759.6
  Lancereaux-Mathieu (leptospiral jaundice) 100.0
  Landry's 357.0
  Lane's 569.89
  lardaceous (any site) 277.3
  Larrey-Weil (leptospiral jaundice) 100.0
  Larsen (-Johansson) (juvenile osteopathia
      patellae) 732.4
  larynx 478.70
  Lasègue's (persecution mania) 297.9
  Leber's 377.16
  Lederer's (acquired infectious hemolytic
      anemia) 283.19
  Legg's (capital femoral osteochondrosis) 732.1
  Legg-Calvé-Perthes (capital femoral
      osteochondrosis) 732.1
  Legg-Calvé-Waldenström (femoral capital
      osteochondrosis) 732.1
  Legg-Perthes (femoral capital osteochondrosis)
      732.1
  Legionnaires' 482.84
  Leigh's 330.8
  Leiner's (exfoliative dermatitis) 695.89
  Leloir's (lupus erythematosus) 695.4
  Lenegre's 426.0
  lens (eye) 379.39
  Leriche's (osteoporosis, posttraumatic) 733.7
  Letterer-Siwe (acute histiocytosis X) (M9722/3)
      202.5
  Lev's (acquired complete heart block) 426.0
  Lewandowski's (*see also* Tuberculosis) 017.0
  Lewandowski-Lutz (epidermodysplasia
      verruciformis) 078.19
  Leyden's (periodic vomiting) 536.2
  Libman-Sacks (verrucous endocarditis) 710.0
      [424.91]
  Lichtheim's (subacute combined sclerosis with
      pernicious anemia) 281.0 *[336.2]*
  ligament 728.9
  light chain 203.0
  Lightwood's (renal tubular acidosis) 588.8
  Lignac's (cystinosis) 270.0
  Lindau's (retinocerebral angiomatosis) 759.6
  Lindau-von Hippel (angiomatosis
      retinocerebellosa) 759.6
  lip NEC 528.5
  lipidosis 272.7
  lipoid storage NEC 272.7
  Lipschültz's 616.50
  Little's—*see* Palsy, cerebral

Disease, diseased—*continued*
  liver 573.9
    alcoholic 571.3
      acute 571.1
      chronic 571.3
    chronic 571.9
      alcoholic 571.3
    cystic, congenital 751.62
    drug-induced 573.3
    due to
      chemicals 573.3
        fluorinated agents 573.3
        hypersensitivity drugs 573.3
        isoniazids 573.3
    fibrocystic (congenital) 751.62
    glycogen storage 271.0
    organic 573.9
    polycystic (congenital) 751.62
  Lobo's (keloid blastomycosis) 116.2
  Lobstein's (brittle bones and blue sclera) 756.61
  locomotor system 334.9
  Lorain's (pituitary dwarfism) 253.3
  Lou Gehrig's 335.20
  Lucas-Championnière (fibrinous bronchitis)
      466.0
  Ludwig's (submaxillary cellulitis) 528.3
  luetic—*see* Syphilis
  lumbosacral region 724.6
  lung NEC 518.89
    black 500
    congenital 748.60
    cystic 518.89
      congenital 748.4
    fibroid (chronic) (*see also* Fibrosis, lung) 515
    fluke 121.2
      Oriental 121.2
    in
      amyloidosis 277.3 *[517.8]*
      polymyositis 710.4 *[517.8]*
      sarcoidosis 135 *[517.8]*
      Sjögren's syndrome 710.2 *[517.8]*
      syphilis 095.1
      systemic lupus erythematosus 710.0 *[517.8]*
      systemic sclerosis 710.1 *[517.2]*
    interstitial (chronic) 515
      acute 136.3
    nonspecific, chronic 496
    obstructive (chronic) (COPD) 496
      with
        acute exacerbation NEC 491.21
        alveolitis, allergic (*see also* Alveolitis,
            allergic) 495.9
        asthma (chronic) (obstructive) 493.2
        bronchiectasis 494.0
          with acute exacerbation 494.1
        bronchitis (chronic) 491.20
          with acute exacerbation 491.21
        emphysema NEC 492.8
        diffuse (with fibrosis) 496
    polycystic 518.89
      asthma (chronic) (obstructive) 493.2
      congenital 748.4
    purulent (cavitary) 513.0
    restrictive 518.89
    rheumatoid 714.81
      diffuse interstitial 714.81
    specified NEC 518.89
  Lutembacher's (atrial septal defect with mitral
      stenosis) 745.5
  Lutz-Miescher (elastosis perforans serpiginosa)
      701.1

Disease, diseased—*continued*
  Lutz-Splendore-de Almeida (Brazilian
      blastomycosis) 116.1
  Lyell's (toxic epidermal necrolysis) 695.1
    due to drug
      correct substance properly administered
          695.1
        overdose or wrong substance given or taken
          977.9
          specific drug—*see* Table of drugs and
              chemicals
  Lyme 088.81
  lymphatic (gland) (system) 289.9
    channel (noninfective) 457.9
    vessel (noninfective) 457.9
      specified NEC 457.8
  lymphoproliferative (chronic) (M9970/1) 238.7
  Machado-Joseph 334.8
  Madelung's (lipomatosis) 272.8
  Madura (actinomycotic) 039.9
    mycotic 117.4
  Magitot's 526.4
  Majocchi's (purpura annularis telangiectodes)
      709.1
  malarial (*see also* Malaria) 084.6
  Malassez's (cystic) 608.89
  Malibu 919.8
    infected 919.9
  malignant (M8000/3)—*see also* Neoplasm, by
      site, malignant
    previous, affecting management of pregnancy
      V23.8
  Manson's 120.1
  maple bark 495.6
  maple syrup (urine) 270.3
  Marburg (virus) 078.89
  Marchiafava (-Bignami) 341.8
  Marfan's 090.49
    congenital syphilis 090.49
    meaning Marfan's syndrome 759.82
  Marie-Bamberger (hypertrophic pulmonary
      osteoarthropathy) (secondary) 731.2
    primary or idiopathic (acropachyderma)
      757.39
    pulmonary (hypertrophic osteoarthropathy)
      731.2
  Marie-Strümpell (ankylosing spondylitis) 720.0
  Marion's (bladder neck obstruction) 596.0
  Marsh's (exophthalmic goiter) 242.0
  Martin's 715.27
  mast cell 757.33
    systemic (M9741/3) 202.6
  mastoid (*see also* Mastoiditis) 383.9
    process 385.9
  maternal, unrelated to pregnancy NEC,
      affecting fetus or newborn 760.9
  Mathieu's (leptospiral jaundice) 100.0
  Mauclaire's 732.3
  Mauriac's (erythema nodosum syphiliticum)
      091.3
  Maxcy's 081.0
  McArdle (Schmid-Pearson) (glycogenosis V)
      271.0
  mediastinum NEC 519.3
  Medin's (*see also* Poliomyelitis) 045.9
  Mediterranean (with hemoglobinopathy) 282.4
  medullary center (idiopathic) (respiratory) 348.8
  Meige's (chronic hereditary edema) 757.0
  Meleda 757.39
  Ménétrier's (hypertrophic gastritis) 535.2

Disease, diseased—*continued*
  Ménière's (active) 386.00
    cochlear 386.02
    cochleovestibular 386.01
    inactive 386.04
    in remission 386.04
    vestibular 386.03
  meningeal—*see* Meningitis
  mental (*see also* Psychosis) 298.9
  Merzbacher-Pelizaeus 330.0
  mesenchymal 710.9
  mesenteric embolic 557.0
  metabolic NEC 277.9
  metal polishers' 502
  metastatic—*see* Metastasis
  Mibelli's 757.39
  microdrepanocytic 282.4
  Miescher's 709.3
  Mikulicz's (dryness of mouth, absent or
      decreased lacrimation) 527.1
  Milkman (-Looser) (osteomalacia with
      pseudofractures) 268.2
  Miller's (osteomalacia) 268.2
  Mills' 335.29
  Milroy's (chronic hereditary edema) 757.0
  Minamata 985.0
  Minor's 336.1
  Minot's (hemorrhagic disease, newborn) 776.0
  Minot-von Willebrand-Jürgens
      (angiohemophilia) 286.4
  Mitchell's (erythromelalgia) 443.89
  mitral—*see* Endocarditis, mitral
  Mljet (mal de Meleda) 757.39
  Möbius', Moebius' 346.8
  Moeller's 267
  Möller (-Barlow) (infantile scurvy) 267
  Mönckeberg's (*see also* arteriosclerosis,
      extremities) 440.20
  Mondor's (thrombophlebitis of breast) 451.89
  Monge's 993.2
  Morel-Kraepelin (*see also* Schizophrenia) 295.9
  Morgagni's (syndrome) (hyperostosis frontalis
      interna) 733.3
  Morgagni-Adams-Stokes (syncope with heart
      block) 426.9
  Morquio (-Brailsford) (-Ullrich)
      (mucopolysaccharidosis IV) 277.5
  Morton's (with metatarsalgia) 355.6
  Morvan's 336.0
  motor neuron (bulbar) (mixed type) 335.20
  Mouchet's (juvenile osteochondrosis, foot)
      732.5
  mouth 528.9
  Moyamoya 437.5
  Mucha's (acute parapsoriasis varioliformis)
      696.2
  mu-chain 273.2
  mucolipidosis (I) (II) (III) 272.7
  Münchmeyer's (exostosis luxurians) 728.11
  Murri's (intermittent hemoglobinuria) 283.2
  muscle 359.9
    inflammatory 728.9
    ocular 378.9
  musculoskeletal system 729.9
  mushroom workers' 495.5
  Myà's (congenital dilation, colon) 751.3
  mycotic 117.9
  myeloproliferative (chronic) (M9960/1) 238.7
  myocardium, myocardial (*see also*
      Degeneration, myocardial) 429.1

Disease, diseased—*continued*
  Pelizaeus-Merzbacher 330.0
    with dementia
      with behavioral disturbance 330.0 *[294.11]*
      without behavioral disturbance 330.0
        [294.10]
  Pellegrini-Stieda (calcification, knee joint)
    726.62
  pelvis, pelvic
    female NEC 629.9
      specified NEC 629.8
    gonococcal (acute) 098.19
      chronic or duration of 2 months or over
        098.39
    infection (*see also* Disease, pelvis,
      inflammatory) 614.9
    inflammatory (female) (PID) 614.9
      with
        abortion—*see* Abortion, by type, with
          sepsis
        ectopic pregnancy (*see also* categories
          633.0-633.9) 639.0
        molar pregnancy (*see also* categories
          630-632) 639.0
      acute 614.3
      chronic 614.4
      complicating pregnancy 646.6
        affecting fetus or newborn 760.8
      following
        abortion 639.0
        ectopic or molar pregnancy 639.0
      peritonitis (acute) 614.5
        chronic NEC 614.7
      puerperal, postpartum, childbirth 670
      specified NEC 614.8
    organ, female NEC 629.9
      specified NEC 629.8
    peritoneum, female NEC 629.9
      specified NEC 629.8
  penis 607.9
    inflammatory 607.2
  peptic NEC 536.9
    acid 536.8
  periapical tissues NEC 522.9
  pericardium 423.9
    specified type NEC 423.8
  perineum
    female
      inflammatory 616.9
        specified NEC 616.8
      noninflammatory 624.9
        specified NEC 624.8
    male (inflammatory) 682.2
  periodic (familial) (Reimann's) NEC 277.3
    paralysis 359.3
  periodontal NEC 523.9
    specified NEC 523.8
  periosteum 733.90
  peripheral
    arterial 443.9
    autonomic nervous system (*see also*
      Neuropathy, autonomic) 337.9
    nerve NEC (*see also* Neuropathy) 356.9
      multiple—*see* Polyneuropathy
    vascular 443.9
      specified type NEC 443.89
  peritoneum 568.9
    pelvic, female 629.9
      specified NEC 629.8
  Perrin-Ferraton (snapping hip) 719.65

Disease, diseased—*continued*
  persistent mucosal (middle ear) (with posterior
    or superior marginal perforation of ear
    drum) 382.2
  Perthes' (capital femoral osteochondrosis) 732.1
  Petit's (*see also* Hernia, lumbar) 553.8
  Peutz-Jeghers 759.6
  Peyronie's 607.89
  Pfeiffer's (infectious mononucleosis) 075
  pharynx 478.20
  Phocas' 610.1
  photochromogenic (acid-fast bacilli)
    (pulmonary) 031.0
    nonpulmonary 031.9
  Pick's
    brain 331.1
      with dementia
        with behavioral disturbance 331.1 *[294.11]*
        without behavioral disturbance 331.1
          [294.10]
    cerebral atrophy 331.1
      with dementia
        with behavioral disturbance 331.1 *[294.11]*
        without behavioral disturbance 331.1
          [294.10]
    lipid histiocytosis 272.7
    liver (pericardial pseudocirrhosis of liver)
      423.2
    pericardium (pericardial pseudocirrhosis of
      liver) 423.2
    polyserositis (pericardial pseudocirrhosis of
      liver) 423.2
  Pierson's (osteochondrosis) 732.1
  pigeon fancier's or breeders' 495.2
  pineal gland 259.8
  pink 985.0
  Pinkus' (lichen nitidus) 697.1
  pinworm 127.4
  pituitary (gland) 253.9
    hyperfunction 253.1
    hypofunction 253.2
  pituitary snuff-takers' 495.8
  placenta
    affecting fetus or newborn 762.2
    complicating pregnancy or childbirth 656.7
  pleura (cavity) (*see also* Pleurisy) 511.0
  Plummer's (toxic nodular goiter) 242.3
  pneumatic
    drill 994.9
    hammer 994.9
  policeman's 729.2
  Pollitzer's (hidradenitis suppurativa) 705.83
  polycystic (congenital) 759.89
    kidney or renal 753.12
      adult type (APKD) 753.13
      autosomal dominant 753.13
      autosomal recessive 753.14
      childhood type (CPKD) 753.14
      infantile type 753.14
    liver or hepatic 751.62
    lung or pulmonary 518.89
      congenital 748.4
    ovary, ovaries 256.4
    spleen 759.0
  Pompe's (glycogenosis II) 271.0
  Poncet's (tuberculous rheumatism) (*see also*
    Tuberculosis) 015.9
  Posada-Wernicke 114.9
  Potain's (pulmonary edema) 514

Disease, diseased—*continued*
   upper (acute) (infectious) NEC 465.9
     multiple sites NEC 465.8
     noninfectious NEC 478.9
     streptococcal 034.0
   retina, retinal NEC 362.9
    Batten's or Batten-Mayou 330.1 *[362.71]*
    degeneration 362.89
    vascular lesion 362.17
   rheumatic (*see also* Arthritis) 716.8
    heart—*see* Disease, heart, rheumatic
   rheumatoid (heart)—*see* Arthritis, rheumatoid
   rickettsial NEC 083.9
    specified type NEC 083.8
   Riedel's (ligneous thyroiditis) 245.3
   Riga (-Fede) (cachectic aphthae) 529.0
   Riggs' (compound periodontitis) 523.4
   Ritter's 695.81
   Rivalta's (cervicofacial actinomycosis) 039.3
   Robles' (onchocerciasis) 125.3 *[360.13]*
   Roger's (congenital interventricular septal
    defect) 745.4
   Rokitansky's (*see also* Necrosis, liver) 570
   Romberg's 349.89
   Rosenthal's (factor XI deficiency) 286.2
   Rossbach's (hyperchlorhydria) 536.8
    psychogenic 306.4
   Roth (-Bernhardt) 355.1
   Runeberg's (progressive pernicious anemia)
    281.0
   Rust's (tuberculous spondylitis) (*see also*
    Tuberculosis) 015.0 *[720.81]*
   Rustitskii's (multiple myeloma) (M9730/3)
    203.0
   Ruysch's (Hirschsprung's disease) 751.3
   Sachs (-Tay) 330.1
   sacroiliac NEC 724.6
   salivary gland or duct NEC 527.9
    inclusion 078.5
     streptococcal 034.0
    virus 078.5
   Sander's (paranoia) 297.1
   Sandhoff's 330.1
   sandworm 126.9
   Savill's (epidemic exfoliative dermatitis) 695.89
   Schamberg's (progressive pigmentary
    dermatosis) 709.09
   Schaumann's (sarcoidosis) 135
   Schenck's (sporotrichosis) 117.1
   Scheuermann's (osteochondrosis) 732.0
   Schilder (-Flatau) 341.1
   Schimmelbusch's 610.1
   Schlatter's tibia (tubercle) 732.4
   Schlatter-Osgood 732.4
   Schmorl's 722.30
    cervical 722.39
    lumbar, lumbosacral 722.32
    specified region NEC 722.39
    thoracic, thoracolumbar 722.31
   Scholz's 330.0
   Schönlein (-Henoch) (purpura rheumatica) 287.0
   Schottmüller's (*see also* Fever, paratyphoid)
    002.9
   Schüller-Christian (chronic histiocytosis X)
    277.8
   Schultz's (agranulocytosis) 288.0
   Schwalbe-Ziehen-Oppenheimer 333.6
   Schweninger-Buzzi (macular atrophy) 701.3
   sclera 379.19
   scrofulous (*see also* Tuberculosis) 017.2
   scrotum 608.9

Disease, diseased—*continued*
   sebaceous glands NEC 706.9
   Secretan's (posttraumatic edema) 782.3
   semilunar cartilage, cystic 717.5
   seminal vesicle 608.9
   Senear-Usher (pemphigus erythematosus) 694.4
   serum NEC 999.5
   Sever's (osteochondrosis calcaneum) 732.5
   Sézary's (reticulosis) (M9701/3) 202.2
   Shaver's (bauxite pneumoconiosis) 503
   Sheehan's (postpartum pituitary necrosis) 253.2
   shimamushi (scrub typhus) 081.2
   shipyard 077.1
   sickle-cell 282.60
    with
     crisis 282.62
     Hb-S disease 282.61
     other abnormal hemoglobin (Hb-D) (Hb-E)
      (Hb-G) (Hb-J) (Hb-K) (Hb-O) (Hb-P)
      (high fetal gene) 282.69
    elliptocytosis 282.60
    Hb-C 282.63
    Hb-S 282.61
     with
      crisis 282.62
      Hb-C 282.63
      other abnormal hemoglobin (Hb-D)
       (Hb-E) (Hb-G) (Hb-J) (Hb-K) (Hb-O)
       (Hb-P) (high fetal gene) 282.69
    spherocytosis 282.60
    thalassemia 282.4
   Siegal-Cattan-Mamou (periodic) 277.3
   silo fillers' 506.9
   Simian B 054.3
   Simmonds' (pituitary cachexia) 253.2
   Simons' (progressive lipodystrophy) 272.6
   Sinding-Larsen (juvenile osteopathia patellae)
    732.4
   sinus—*see also* Sinusitis
    brain 437.9
    specified NEC 478.1
   Sirkari's 085.0
   sixth 057.8
   Sjögren (-Gougerot) 710.2
    with lung involvement 710.2 *[517.8]*
   Skevas-Zerfus 989.5
   skin NEC 709.9
    due to metabolic disorder 277.9
    specified type NEC 709.8
   sleeping 347
    meaning sleeping sickness (*see also*
     Trypanosomiasis) 086.5
   small vessel 443.9
   Smith-Strang (oasthouse urine) 270.2
   Sneddon-Wilkinson (subcorneal pustular
    dermatosis) 694.1
   South African creeping 133.8
   Spencer's (epidemic vomiting) 078.82
   Spielmeyer-Stock 330.1
   Spielmeyer-Vogt 330.1
   spine, spinal 733.90
    combined system (*see also* Degeneration,
     combined) 266.2 *[336.2]*
     with pernicious anemia 281.0 *[336.2]*
    cord NEC 336.9
     congenital 742.9
    demyelinating NEC 341.8
    joint (*see also* Disease, joint, spine) 724.9
    tuberculous 015.0 *[730.8]*
   spinocerebellar 334.9
    specified NEC 334.8

Disease, diseased—*continued*
  spleen (organic) (postinfectional) 289.50
    amyloid 277.3
    lardaceous 277.3
    polycystic 759.0
    specified NEC 289.59
  sponge divers' 989.5
  Stanton's (melioidosis) 025
  Stargardt's 362.75
  Steinert's 359.2
  Sternberg's—*see* Disease, Hodgkin's
  Stevens-Johnson (erythema multiforme
    exudativum) 695.1
  Sticker's (erythema infectiosum) 057.0
  Stieda's (calcification, knee joint) 726.62
  Still's (juvenile rheumatoid arthritis) 714.30
  Stiller's (asthenia) 780.79
  Stokes' (exophthalmic goiter) 242.0
  Stokes-Adams (syncope with heart block) 426.9
  Stokvis (-Talma) (enterogenous cyanosis) 289.7
  stomach NEC (organic) 537.9
    functional 536.9
      psychogenic 306.4
    lardaceous 277.3
  stonemasons' 502
  storage
    glycogen (*see also* Disease, glycogen storage)
      271.0
    lipid 272.7
    mucopolysaccharide 277.5
  striatopallidal system 333.90
    specified NEC 333.89
  Strümpell-Marie (ankylosing spondylitis) 720.0
  Stuart's (congenital factor X deficiency) (*see*
    also Defect, coagulation) 286.3
  Stuart-Prower (congenital factor X deficiency)
    (*see also* Defect, coagulation) 286.3
  Sturge (-Weber) (-Dimitri) (encephalocutaneous
    angiomatosis) 759.6
  Stuttgart 100.89
  Sudeck's 733.7
  supporting structures of teeth NEC 525.9
  suprarenal (gland) (capsule) 255.9
    hyperfunction 255.3
    hypofunction 255.4
  Sutton's 709.09
  Sutton and Gull's—*see* Hypertension, kidney
  sweat glands NEC 705.9
    specified type NEC 705.89
  sweating 078.2
  Sweeley-Klionsky 272.4
  Swift (-Feer) 985.0
  swimming pool (bacillus) 031.1
  swineherd's 100.89
  Sylvest's (epidemic pleurodynia) 074.1
  Symmers (follicular lymphoma) (M9690/3)
    202.0
  sympathetic nervous system (*see also*
    Neuropathy, peripheral, autonomic) 337.9
  synovium 727.9
  syphilitic—*see* Syphilis
  systemic tissue mast cell (M9741/3) 202.6
  Taenzer's 757.4
  Takayasu's (pulseless) 446.7
  Talma's 728.85
  Tangier (familial high-density lipoprotein
    deficiency) 272.5
  Tarral-Besnier (pityriasis rubra pilaris) 696.4
  Tay-Sachs 330.1
  Taylor's 701.8
  tear duct 375.69

Disease, diseased—*continued*
  teeth, tooth 525.9
    hard tissues NEC 521.9
    pulp NEC 522.9
  tendon 727.9
    inflammatory NEC 727.9
  terminal vessel 443.9
  testis 608.9
  Thaysen-Gee (nontropical sprue) 579.0
  Thomsen's 359.2
  Thomson's (congenital poikiloderma) 757.33
  Thornwaldt's, Tornwaldt's (pharyngeal bursitis)
    478.29
  throat 478.20
    septic 034.0
  thromboembolic (*see also* Embolism) 444.9
  thymus (gland) 254.9
    specified NEC 254.8
  thyroid (gland) NEC 246.9
    heart (*see also* Hyperthyroidism) 242.9 [*425.7*]
    lardaceous 277.3
    specified NEC 246.8
  Tietze's 733.6
  Tommaselli's
    correct substance properly administered 599.7
    overdose or wrong substance given or taken
      961.4
  tongue 529.9
  tonsils, tonsillar (and adenoids) (chronic) 474.9
    specified NEC 474.8
  tooth, teeth 525.9
    hard tissues NEC 521.9
    pulp NEC 522.9
  Tornwaldt's (pharyngeal bursitis) 478.29
  Tourette's 307.23
  trachea 519.1
  tricuspid—*see* Endocarditis, tricuspid
  triglyceride-storage, type I, II, III 272.7
  triple vessel (coronary arteries) —*see*
    Arteriosclerosis, coronary
  trisymptomatic, Gougerot's 709.1
  trophoblastic (*see also* Hydatidiform mole) 630
    previous, affecting management of pregnancy
      V23.1
  tsutsugamushi (scrub typhus) 081.2
  tube (fallopian), noninflammatory 620.9
    specified NEC 620.8
  tuberculous NEC (*see also* Tuberculosis) 011.9
  tubo-ovarian
    inflammatory (*see also* Salpingo-oophoritis)
      614.2
    noninflammatory 620.9
      specified NEC 620.8
  tubotympanic, chronic (with anterior perforation
    of ear drum) 382.1
  tympanum 385.9
  Uhl's 746.84
  umbilicus (newborn) NEC 779.89
  Underwood's (sclerema neonatorum) 778.1
  undiagnosed 799.9
  Unna's (seborrheic dermatitis) 690.18
  unstable hemoglobin hemolytic 282.7
  Unverricht (-Lundborg) 333.2
  Urbach-Oppenheim (necrobiosis lipoidica
    diabeticorum) 250.8 [*709.3*]
  Urbach-Wiethe (lipoid proteinosis) 272.8
  ureter 593.9
  urethra 599.9
    specified type NEC 599.84
  urinary (tract) 599.9
    bladder 596.9

Disease, diseased—*continued*
  Weir Mitchell's (erythromelalgia) 443.89
  Werdnig-Hoffmann 335.0
  Werlhof's (*see also* Purpura, thrombocytopenic)
    287.3
  Wermer's 258.0
  Werner's (progeria adultorum) 259.8
  Werner-His (trench fever) 083.1
  Werner-Schultz (agranulocytosis) 288.0
  Wernicke's (superior hemorrhagic
    polioencephalitis) 265.1
  Wernicke-Posadas 114.9
  Whipple's (intestinal lipodystrophy) 040.2
  whipworm 127.3
  white
    blood cell 288.9
      specified NEC 288.8
    spot 701.0
  White's (congenital) (keratosis follicularis)
    757.39
  Whitmore's (melioidosis) 025
  Widal-Abrami (acquired hemolytic jaundice)
    283.9
  Wilkie's 557.1
  Wilkinson-Sneddon (subcorneal pustular
    dermatosis) 694.1
  Willis' (diabetes mellitus) (*see also* Diabetes)
    250.0
  Wilson's (hepatolenticular degeneration) 275.1
  Wilson-Brocq (dermatitis exfoliativa) 695.89
  winter vomiting 078.82
  Wise's 696.2
  Wohlfart-Kugelberg-Welander 335.11
  Woillez's (acute idiopathic pulmonary
    congestion) 518.5
  Wolman's (primary familial xanthomatosis)
    272.7
  wool-sorters' 022.1
  Zagari's (xerostomia) 527.7
  Zahorsky's (exanthem subitum) 057.8
  Ziehen-Oppenheim 333.6
  zoonotic, bacterial NEC 027.9
    specified type NEC 027.8
Disfigurement (due to scar) 709.2
  head V48.6
  limb V49.4
  neck V48.7
  trunk V48.7
Disgerminoma —*see* Dysgerminoma
Disinsertion, retina 361.04
Disintegration, complete, of the body 799.8
  traumatic 869.1
Disk kidney 753.3
Dislocatable hip, congenita l (*see also*
  Dislocation, hip, congenital) 754.30
Dislocation (articulation) (closed) (displacement)
  (simple) (subluxation) 839.8

Note—*"Closed" includes simple, complete,
partial, uncomplicated, and unspecified
dislocation. "Open" includes dislocation
specified as infected or compound and
dislocation with foreign body. "Chronic,"
"habitual," "old," or "recurrent" dislocations
should be coded as indicated under the entry
"Dislocation, recurrent"; and "pathological"
as indicated under the entry "Dislocation,
pathological." For late effect of dislocation see
Late, effect, dislocation.*

---

  with fracture—*see* Fracture, by site

Dislocation—*continued*
  acromioclavicular (joint) (closed) 831.04
    open 831.14
  anatomical site (closed)
    specified NEC 839.69
      open 839.79
    unspecified or ill-defined 839.8
      open 839.9
  ankle (scaphoid bone) (closed) 837.0
    open 837.1
  arm (closed) 839.8
    open 839.9
  astragalus (closed) 837.0
    open 837.1
  atlanto-axial (closed) 839.01
    open 839.11
  atlas (closed) 839.01
    open 839.11
  axis (closed) 839.02
    open 839.12
  back (closed) 839.8
    open 839.9
  Bell-Daly 723.8
  breast bone (closed) 839.61
    open 839.71
  capsule, joint—*see* Dislocation, by site
  carpal (bone)—*see* Dislocation, wrist
  carpometacarpal (joint) (closed) 833.04
    open 833.14
  cartilage (joint)—*see also* Dislocation, by site
    knee—*see* Tear, meniscus
  cervical, cervicodorsal, or cervicothoracic
    (spine) (vertebra)—*see* Dislocation,
    vertebra, cervical
  chiropractic (*see also* Lesion, nonallopathic)
    739.9
  chondrocostal—*see* Dislocation, costochondral
  chronic—*see* Dislocation, recurrent
  clavicle (closed) 831.04
    open 831.14
  coccyx (closed) 839.41
    open 839.51
  collar bone (closed) 831.04
    open 831.14
  compound (open) NEC 839.9
  congenital NEC 755.8
    hip (*see also* Dislocation, hip, congenital)
      754.30
    lens 743.37
    rib 756.3
    sacroiliac 755.69
    spine NEC 756.19
    vertebra 756.19
  coracoid (closed) 831.09
    open 831.19
  costal cartilage (closed) 839.69
    open 839.79
  costochondral (closed) 839.69
    open 839.79
  cricoarytenoid articulation (closed) 839.69
    open 839.79
  cricothyroid (cartilage) articulation (closed)
    839.69
    open 839.79
  dorsal vertebrae (closed) 839.21
    open 839.31
  ear ossicle 385.23
  elbow (closed) 832.00
    anterior (closed) 832.01
      open 832.11
    congenital 754.89

Dislocation—*continued*
  coccyx 839.41
    open 839.51
  congenital 756.19
  due to birth trauma 767.4
  open 839.50
  recurrent 724.9
  sacroiliac 839.42
    recurrent 724.6
  sacrum (sacrococcygeal) (sacroiliac) 839.42
    open 839.52
  spontaneous—*see* Dislocation, pathological
  sternoclavicular (joint) (closed) 839.61
    open 839.71
  sternum (closed) 839.61
    open 839.71
  subastragalar—*see* Dislocation, foot
  subglenoid (closed) 831.01
    open 831.11
  symphysis
    jaw (closed) 830.0
      open 830.1
    mandibular (closed) 830.0
      open 830.1
    pubis (closed) 839.69
      open 839.79
  tarsal (bone) (joint) 838.01
    open 838.11
  tarsometatarsal (joint) 838.03
    open 838.13
  temporomandibular (joint) (closed) 830.0
    open 830.1
    recurrent 524.69
  thigh
    distal end (*see also* Dislocation, femur, distal
      end) 836.50
    proximal end (*see also* Dislocation, hip)
      835.00
  thoracic (vertebrae) (closed) 839.21
    open 839.31
  thumb(s) (*see also* Dislocation, finger) 834.00
  thyroid cartilage (closed) 839.69
    open 839.79
  tibia
    distal end (closed) 837.0
      open 837.1
    proximal end (closed) 836.50
      anterior 836.51
        open 836.61
      lateral 836.54
        open 836.64
      medial 836.53
        open 836.63
      open 836.60
      posterior 836.52
        open 836.62
      rotatory 836.59
        open 836.69
  tibiofibular
    distal (closed) 837.0
      open 837.1
    superior (closed) 836.59
      open 836.69
  toe(s) (closed) 838.09
    open 838.19
  trachea (closed) 839.69
    open 839.79
  ulna
    distal end (closed) 833.09
      open 833.19
    proximal end—*see* Dislocation, elbow

Dislocation—*continued*
  vertebra (articular process) (body) (closed)
    839.40
    cervical, cervicodorsal or cervicothoracic
      (closed) 839.00
      first (atlas) 839.01
        open 839.11
      second (axis) 839.02
        open 839.12
      third 839.03
        open 839.13
      fourth 839.04
        open 839.14
      fifth 839.05
        open 839.15
      sixth 839.06
        open 839.16
      seventh 839.07
        open 839.17
      congenital 756.19
      multiple sites 839.08
        open 839.18
      open 839.10
    congenital 756.19
    dorsal 839.21
      open 839.31
      recurrent 724.9
    lumbar, lumbosacral 839.20
      open 839.30
    open NEC 839.50
    recurrent 724.9
    specified region NEC 839.49
      open 839.59
    thoracic 839.21
      open 839.31
  wrist (carpal bone) (scaphoid) (semilunar)
    (closed) 833.00
    carpometacarpal (joint) 833.04
      open 833.14
    metacarpal bone, proximal end 833.05
      open 833.15
    midcarpal (joint) 833.03
      open 833.13
    open 833.10
    radiocarpal (joint) 833.02
      open 833.12
    radioulnar (joint) 833.01
      open 833.11
    recurrent 718.33
    specified site NEC 833.09
      open 833.19
  xiphoid cartilage (closed) 839.61
    open 839.71
Dislodgement
  artificial skin graft 996.55
  decellularized allodermis graft 996.55
Disobedience, hostile (covert) (overt) (*see also*
  Disturbance, conduct) 312.0
Disorder —*see also* Disease
  academic underachievement, childhood and
    adolescence 313.83
  accommodation 367.51
    drug-induced 367.89
    toxic 367.89
  adjustment (*see also* Reaction, adjustment) 309.9
  adrenal (capsule) (cortex) (gland) 255.9
    specified type NEC 255.8
  adrenogenital 255.2
  affective (*see also* Psychosis, affective) 296.90
    atypical 296.81

Disorder—*continued*
  cornea NEC 371.89
    due to contact lens 371.82
  corticosteroid metabolism NEC 255.2
  cranial nerve—*see* Disorder, nerve, cranial
  cyclothymic 301.13
  degradation, branched-chain amino acid 270.3
  delusional 297.9
  dentition 520.6
  depressive NEC 311
    atypical 296.82
    major (*see also* Psychosis, affective) 296.2
      recurrent episode 296.3
      single episode 296.2
  development, specific 315.9
    associated with hyperkinesia 314.1
    language 315.31
    learning 315.2
      arithmetical 315.1
      reading 315.00
    mixed 315.5
    motor coordination 315.4
    specified type NEC 315.8
    speech 315.39
  diaphragm 519.4
  digestive 536.9
    fetus or newborn 777.9
      specified NEC 777.8
    psychogenic 306.4
  disintegrative (childhood) 299.1
  dissociative 300.14
    identity 300.14
  dysmorphic body 300.7
  dysthymic 300.4
  ear 388.9
    degenerative NEC 388.00
    external 380.9
      specified 380.89
    pinna 380.30
    specified type NEC 388.8
    vascular NEC 388.00
  eating NEC 307.50
  electrolyte NEC 276.9
    with
      abortion—*see* Abortion, by type, with
        metabolic disorder
      ectopic pregnancy (*see also* categories
        633.0-633.9) 639.4
      molar pregnancy (*see also* categories
        630-632) 639.4
    acidosis 276.2
      metabolic 276.2
      respiratory 276.2
    alkalosis 276.3
      metabolic 276.3
      respiratory 276.3
    following
      abortion 639.4
      ectopic or molar pregnancy 639.4
    neonatal, transitory NEC 775.5
  emancipation as adjustment reaction 309.22
  emotional (*see also* Disorder, mental,
    nonpsychotic) V40.9
  endocrine 259.9
    specified type NEC 259.8
  esophagus 530.9
    functional 530.5
    psychogenic 306.4
  explosive
    intermittent 312.34
    isolated 312.35

Disorder—*continued*
  expressive language 315.31
  eye 379.90
    globe—*see* Disorder, globe
    ill-defined NEC 379.99
    limited duction NEC 378.63
    specified NEC 379.8
  eyelid 374.9
    degenerative 374.50
    sensory 374.44
    specified type NEC 374.89
    vascular 374.85
  factitious —*see* Illness, factitious
  factor, coagulation (*see also* Defect,
    coagulation) 286.9
    VIII (congenital) (functional) 286.0
    IX (congenital) (functional) 286.1
  fascia 728.9
  feeding —*see* Feeding
  female sexual arousal 302.72
  fluid NEC 276.9
  gastric (functional) 536.9
    motility 536.8
    psychogenic 306.4
    secretion 536.8
  gastrointestinal (functional) NEC 536.9
    newborn (neonatal) 777.9
      specified NEC 777.8
    psychogenic 306.4
  gender (child) 302.6
    adult 302.85
  gender identity (childhood) 302.6
    adult-life 302.85
  genitourinary system, psychogenic 306.50
  globe 360.9
    degenerative 360.20
      specified NEC 360.29
    specified type NEC 360.89
  hearing—*see also* Deafness
    conductive type (air) (*see also* Deafness,
      conductive) 389.00
    mixed conductive and sensorineural 389.2
    nerve 389.12
    perceptive (*see also* Deafness, perceptive)
      389.10
    sensorineural type NEC (*see also* Deafness,
      perceptive) 389.10
  heart action 427.9
    postoperative 997.1
  hematological, transient neonatal 776.9
    specified type NEC 776.8
  hematopoietic organs 289.9
  hemorrhagic NEC 287.9
    due to circulating anticoagulants 286.5
    specified type NEC 287.8
  hemostasis (*see also* Defect, coagulation) 286.9
  homosexual conflict 302.0
  hypomanic (chronic) 301.11
  identity
    childhood and adolescence 313.82
      gender 302.6
    gender 302.6
  immune mechanism (immunity) 279.9
    single complement (C_1-C_9) 279.8
    specified type NEC 279.8
  impulse control (*see also* Disturbance, conduct,
    compulsive) 312.30
  infant sialic acid storage 271.8
  integument, fetus or newborn 778.9
    specified type NEC 778.8

Disorder—*continued*
  iron 275.0
  lactose 271.3
  lipid 272.9
    specified type NEC 272.8
    storage 272.7
  lipoprotein—*see also* Hyperlipemia
    deficiency (familial) 272.5
  lysine 270.7
  magnesium 275.2
  mannosidosis 271.8
  mineral 275.9
    specified type NEC 275.8
  mucopolysaccharide 277.5
  nitrogen 270.9
  ornithine 270.6
  oxalosis 271.8
  pentosuria 271.8
  phenylketonuria 270.1
  phosphate 275.3
  phosphorus 275.3
  plasma protein 273.9
    specified type NEC 273.8
  porphyrin 277.1
  purine 277.2
  pyrimidine 277.2
  serine 270.7
  sodium 276.9
  specified type NEC 277.8
  steroid 255.2
  threonine 270.7
  urea cycle 270.6
  xylose 271.8
micturition NEC 788.69
  psychogenic 306.53
misery and unhappiness, of childhood and
  adolescence 313.1
mitral valve 424.0
mood—*see* Psychosis, affective
motor tic 307.20
  chronic 307.22
  transient, childhood 307.21
movement NEC 333.90
  hysterical 300.11
  specified type NEC 333.99
  stereotypic 307.3
mucopolysaccharide 277.5
muscle 728.9
  psychogenic 306.0
  specified type NEC 728.3
muscular attachments, peripheral—*see also*
  Enthesopathy
  spine 720.1
musculoskeletal system NEC 729.9
  psychogenic 306.0
myeloproliferative (chronic) NEC (M9960/1)
  238.7
myoneural 358.9
  due to lead 358.2
  specified type NEC 358.8
  toxic 358.2
myotonic 359.2
neck region NEC 723.9
nerve 349.9
  abducens NEC 378.54
  accessory 352.4
  acoustic 388.5
  auditory 388.5
  auriculotemporal 350.8
  axillary 353.0
  cerebral—*see* Disorder, nerve, cranial

Disorder—*continued*
  cranial 352.9
    first 352.0
    second 377.49
    third
      partial 378.51
      total 378.52
    fourth 378.53
    fifth 350.9
    sixth 378.54
    seventh NEC 351.9
    eighth 388.5
    ninth 352.2
    tenth 352.3
    eleventh 352.4
    twelfth 352.5
    multiple 352.6
  entrapment—*see* Neuropathy, entrapment
  facial 351.9
    specified NEC 351.8
  femoral 355.2
  glossopharyngeal NEC 352.2
  hypoglossal 352.5
  iliohypogastric 355.79
  ilioinguinal 355.79
  intercostal 353.8
  lateral
    cutaneous of thigh 355.1
    popliteal 355.3
  lower limb NEC 355.8
  medial, popliteal 355.4
  median NEC 354.1
  obturator 355.79
  oculomotor
    partial 378.51
    total 378.52
  olfactory 352.0
  optic 377.49
    ischemic 377.41
    nutritional 377.33
    toxic 377.34
  peroneal 355.3
  phrenic 354.8
  plantar 355.6
  pneumogastric 352.3
  posterior tibial 355.5
  radial 354.3
  recurrent laryngeal 352.3
  root 353.9
    specified NEC 353.8
  saphenous 355.79
  sciatic NEC 355.0
  specified NEC 355.9
    lower limb 355.79
    upper limb 354.8
  spinal 355.9
  sympathetic NEC 337.9
  trigeminal 350.9
    specified NEC 350.8
  trochlear 378.53
  ulnar 354.2
  upper limb NEC 354.9
  vagus 352.3
nervous system NEC 349.9
  autonomic (peripheral) (*see also* Neuropathy,
    peripheral, autonomic) 337.9
  cranial 352.9
  parasympathetic (*see also* Neuropathy,
    peripheral, autonomic) 337.9
  specified type NEC 349.89

Disorder—*continued*
  hysterical 300.10
  intestinal 306.4
  joint 306.0
  learning 315.2
  limb 306.0
  lymphatic (system) 306.8
  menstrual 306.52
  micturition 306.53
  monoplegic NEC 306.0
  motor 307.9
  muscle 306.0
  musculoskeletal 306.0
  neurocirculatory 306.2
  obsessive 300.3
  occupational 300.89
  organ or part of body NEC 306.9
  organs of special sense 306.7
  paralytic NEC 306.0
  phobic 300.20
  physical NEC 306.9
  pruritic 306.3
  rectal 306.4
  respiratory (system) 306.1
  rheumatic 306.0
  sexual (function) 302.70
    specified type NEC 302.79
  skin (allergic) (eczematous) (pruritic) 306.3
  sleep 307.40
    initiation or maintenance 307.41
      persistent 307.42
      transient 307.41
    specified type NEC 307.49
  specified part of body NEC 306.8
  stomach 306.4
 psychomotor NEC 307.9
  hysterical 300.11
 psychoneurotic (*see also* Neurosis) 300.9
  mixed NEC 300.89
 psychophysiologic (*see also* Disorder,
    psychosomatic) 306.9
 psychosexual identity (childhood) 302.6
  adult-life 302.85
 psychosomatic NEC 306.9
  allergic NEC
    respiratory 306.1
  articulation, joint 306.0
  cardiovascular (system) 306.2
  cutaneous 306.3
  digestive (system) 306.4
  dysmenorrheic 306.52
  dyspneic 306.1
  endocrine (system) 306.6
  eye 306.7
  gastric 306.4
  gastrointestinal (system) 306.4
  genitourinary (system) 306.50
  heart (functional) (rhythm) 306.2
  hyperventilatory 306.1
  intestinal 306.4
  joint 306.0
  limb 306.0
  lymphatic (system) 306.8
  menstrual 306.52
  micturition 306.53
  monoplegic NEC 306.0
  muscle 306.0
  musculoskeletal 306.0
  neurocirculatory 306.2
  organs of special sense 306.7
  paralytic NEC 306.0

Disorder—*continued*
  pruritic 306.3
  rectal 306.4
  respiratory (system) 306.1
  rheumatic 306.0
  sexual (function) 302.70
    specified type NEC 302.79
  skin 306.3
  specified part of body NEC 306.8
  stomach 306.4
 psychotic—see Psychosis
 purine metabolism NEC 277.2
 pyrimidine metabolism NEC 277.2
 reactive attachment (of infancy or early
    childhood) 313.89
 reading, developmental 315.00
 reflex 796.1
 renal function, impaired 588.9
  specified type NEC 588.8
 renal transport NEC 588.8
 respiration, respiratory NEC 519.9
  due to
    aspiration of liquids or solids 508.9
    inhalation of fumes or vapors 506.9
  psychogenic 306.1
 retina 362.9
  specified type NEC 362.89
 sacroiliac joint NEC 724.6
 sacrum 724.6
 schizo-affective (*see also* Schizophrenia) 295.7
 schizoid, childhood or adolescence 313.22
 schizophreniform 295.4
 schizotypal personality 301.22
 secretion, thyrocalcitonin 246.0
 seizure 780.39
  recurrent 780.39
    epileptic—*see* Epilepsy
 sense of smell 781.1
  psychogenic 306.7
 separation anxiety 309.21
 sexual (*see also* Deviation, sexual) 302.9
  function, psychogenic 302.70
 shyness, of childhood and adolescence 313.21
 single complement (C_1-C_9) 279.8
 skin NEC 709.9
  fetus or newborn 778.9
    specified type 778.8
  psychogenic (allergic) (eczematous) (pruritic)
    306.3
  specified type NEC 709.8
  vascular 709.1
 sleep 780.50
  circadian rhythm 307.45
  initiation or maintenance (*see also* Insomnia)
    780.52
    nonorganic origin (transient) 307.41
      persistent 307.42
    nonorganic origin 307.40
      specified type NEC 307.49
  specified NEC 780.59
  with apnea—*see* Apnea, sleep
 social, of childhood and adolescence 313.22
  specified NEC 780.59
 soft tissue 729.9
 somatization 300.81
 somatoform (atypical) (undifferentiated) 300.82
  severe 300.81
 speech NEC 784.5
  nonorganic origin 307.9
 spine NEC 724.9

> *Note—For acquired displacement of bones, cartilage, joints, tendons, due to injury, see also Dislocation. Displacements at ages under one year should be considered congenital, provided there is no indication the condition was acquired after birth.*

Displacement, displaced—*continued*
  macula (congenital) 743.55
  Meckel's diverticulum (congenital) 751.0
  nail (congenital) 757.5
    acquired 703.8
  opening of Wharton's duct in mouth 750.26
  organ or site, congenital NEC—*see*
    Malposition, congenital
  ovary (acquired) 620.4
    congenital 752.0
    free in peritoneal cavity (congenital) 752.0
    into hernial sac 620.4
  oviduct (acquired) 620.4
    congenital 752.19
  parathyroid (gland) 252.8
  parotid gland (congenital) 750.26
  punctum lacrimale (congenital) 743.65
  sacroiliac (congenital) (joint) 755.69
    current injury—*see* Dislocation, sacroiliac
    old 724.6
  spine (congenital) 756.19
  spleen, congenital 759.0
  stomach (congenital) 750.7
    acquired 537.89
  subglenoid (closed) 831.01
  sublingual duct (congenital) 750.26
  teeth, tooth 524.3
  tongue (congenital) (downward) 750.19
  trachea (congenital) 748.3
  ureter or ureteric opening or orifice (congenital)
    753.4
  uterine opening of oviducts or fallopian tubes
    752.19
  uterus, uterine (*see also* Malposition, uterus)
    621.6
    congenital 752.3
  ventricular septum 746.89
    with rudimentary ventricle 746.89
  xyphoid bone (process) 738.3
Disproportion 653.9
  affecting fetus or newborn 763.1
  caused by
    conjoined twins 653.7
    contraction, pelvis (general) 653.1
      inlet 653.2
      midpelvic 653.8
      midplane 653.8
      outlet 653.3
    fetal
      ascites 653.7
      hydrocephalus 653.6
      hydrops 653.7
      meningomyelocele 653.7
      sacral teratoma 653.7
      tumor 653.7
    hydrocephalic fetus 653.6
    pelvis, pelvic, abnormality (bony) NEC 653.0
    unusually large fetus 653.5
  causing obstructed labor 660.1
  cephalopelvic, normally formed fetus 653.4
    causing obstructed labor 660.1
  fetal NEC 653.5
    causing obstructed labor 660.1
  fetopelvic, normally formed fetus 653.4
    causing obstructed labor 660.1
  mixed maternal and fetal origin, normally
    formed fetus 653.4
  pelvis, pelvic (bony) NEC 653.1
    causing obstructed labor 660.1
  specified type NEC 653.8

Disruption
  cesarean wound 674.1
  family V61.0
  gastrointestinal anastomosis 997.4
  ligament(s)—*see also* Sprain
    knee
      current injury—*see* Dislocation, knee
      old 717.89
        capsular 717.85
        collateral (medial) 717.82
          lateral 717.81
        cruciate (posterior) 717.84
          anterior 717.83
        specified site NEC 717.85
  marital V61.10
    involving divorce or estrangement V61.0
  operation wound (external) 998.32
    internal 998.31
  organ transplant, anastomosis site—*see*
    Complications, transplant, organ, by site
  ossicles, ossicular chain 385.23
    traumatic—*see* Fracture, skull, base
  parenchyma
    liver (hepatic)—*see* Laceration, liver, major
    spleen—*see* Laceration, spleen, parenchyma,
      massive
  phase-shift, of 24-hour sleep-wake cycle 780.55
    nonorganic origin 307.45
  sleep-wake cycle (24-hour) 780.55
    circadian rhythm 307.45
    nonorganic origin 307.45
  suture line (external) 998.32
    internal 998.31
  wound
    cesarean operation 674.1
    episiotomy 674.2
    operation 998.32
      cesarean 674.1
      internal 998.31
    perineal (obstetric) 674.2
    uterine 674.1
Disruptio uteri —*see also* Rupture, uterus
  complicating delivery—*see* Delivery,
    complicated, rupture, uterus
Dissatisfaction with
  employment V62.2
  school environment V62.3
Dissecting —*see* condition
Dissection
  aorta 441.00
    abdominal 441.02
    thoracic 441.01
    thoracoabdominal 441.03
  artery, arterial
    carotid 443.21
    coronary 414.12
    iliac 443.22
    renal 443.23
    specified NEC 443.29
    vertebral 443.24
    vascular 459.9
  wound—*see* Wound, open, by site
Disseminated —*see* condition
Dissociated personality NEC 300.15
Dissociation
  auriculoventricular or atrioventricular (any
    degree) (AV) 426.89
    with heart block 426.0
  interference 426.89
  isorhythmic 426.89

Distortion—*continued*
  peripheral vascular system NEC 747.60
    gastrointestinal 747.61
    lower limb 747.64
    renal 747.62
    spinal 747.82
    upper limb 747.63
  pituitary (gland) 759.2
  radius 755.59
  rectum 751.5
  rib 756.3
  sacroiliac joint 755.69
  sacrum 756.19
  scapula 755.59
  shoulder girdle 755.59
  site not listed—*see* Anomaly, specified type
    NEC
  skull bone(s) 756.0
    with
      anencephalus 740.0
      encephalocele 742.0
      hydrocephalus 742.3
        with spina bifida (*see also* Spina bifida)
          741.0
      microcephalus 742.1
  spinal cord 742.59
  spine 756.19
  spleen 759.0
  sternum 756.3
  thorax (wall) 756.3
  thymus (gland) 759.2
  thyroid (gland) 759.2
    cartilage 748.3
  tibia 755.69
  toe(s) 755.66
  tongue 750.19
  trachea (cartilage) 748.3
  ulna 755.59
  ureter 753.4
    causing obstruction 753.20
  urethra 753.8
    causing obstruction 753.6
  uterus 752.3
  vagina 752.49
  vein (peripheral) NEC (*see also* Distortion,
    peripheral vascular system) 747.60
    great 747.49
    portal 747.49
    pulmonary 747.49
  vena cava (inferior) (superior) 747.49
  vertebra 756.19
  visual NEC 368.15
    shape or size 368.14
  vulva 752.49
  wrist (bones) (joint) 755.59
Distress
  abdomen 789.0
  colon 789.0
  emotional V40.9
  epigastric 789.0
  fetal (syndrome) 768.4
    affecting management of pregnancy or
      childbirth 656.8
    liveborn infant 768.4
      first noted
        before onset of labor 768.2
        during labor or delivery 768.3
      stillborn infant (death before onset of labor)
        768.0
        death during labor 768.1
  gastrointestinal (functional) 536.9

Distress—*continued*
    psychogenic 306.4
  intestinal (functional) NEC 564.9
    psychogenic 306.4
  intrauterine (*see* Distress, fetal)
  leg 729.5
  maternal 669.0
  mental V40.9
  respiratory 786.09
    acute (adult) 518.82
    adult syndrome (following shock, surgery, or
      trauma) 518.5
      specified NEC 518.82
    fetus or newborn 770.89
    syndrome (idiopathic) (newborn) 769
  stomach 536.9
    psychogenic 306.4
Distribution vessel, atypical NEC 747.60
  coronary artery 746.85
  spinal 747.82
Districhiasis 704.2
Disturbance —*see also* Disease
  absorption NEC 579.9
    calcium 269.3
    carbohydrate 579.8
    fat 579.8
    protein 579.8
    specified type NEC 579.8
    vitamin (*see also* Deficiency, vitamin) 269.2
  acid-base equilibrium 276.9
  activity and attention, simple, with hyperkinesis
    314.01
  amino acid (metabolic) (*see also* Disorder,
    amino acid) 270.9
    imidazole 270.5
    maple syrup (urine) disease 270.3
    transport 270.0
  assimilation, food 579.9
  attention, simple 314.00
    with hyperactivity 314.01
  auditory, nerve, except deafness 388.5
  behavior (*see also* Disturbance, conduct) 312.9
  blood clotting (hypoproteinemia) (mechanism)
    (*see also* Defect, coagulation) 286.9
  central nervous system NEC 349.9
  cerebral nerve NEC 352.9
  circulatory 459.9
  conduct 312.9

> *Note—Use the following fifth-digit*
> *subclassification with categories 312.0-312.2:*
>
> *0 unspecified*
> *1 mild*
> *2 moderate*
> *3 severe*

    adjustment reaction 309.3
    adolescent onset type 312.82
    childhood onset type 312.81
    compulsive 312.30
      intermittent explosive disorder 312.34
      isolated explosive disorder 312.35
      kleptomania 312.32
      pathological gambling 312.31
      pyromania 312.33
    hyperkinetic 314.2
    intermittent explosive 312.34
    isolated explosive 312.35
    mixed with emotions 312.4
    socialized (type) 312.20
      aggressive 312.23

Diverticula, diverticulosis—*continued*
  laryngeal ventricle (congenital) 748.3
  Meckel's (displaced) (hypertrophic) 751.0
  midthoracic 530.6
  organ or site, congenital NEC—*see* Distortion
  pericardium (congenital) (cyst) 746.89
    acquired (true) 423.8
  pharyngoesophageal (pulsion) 530.6
  pharynx (congenital) 750.27
  pulsion (esophagus) 530.6
  rectosigmoid 562.10
    with
      diverticulitis 562.11
        with hemorrhage 562.13
      hemorrhage 562.12
    congenital 751.5
  rectum 562.10
    with
      diverticulitis 562.11
        with hemorrhage 562.13
      hemorrhage 562.12
  renal (calyces) (pelvis) 593.89
    with calculus 592.0
  Rokitansky's 530.6
  seminal vesicle 608.0
  sigmoid 562.10
    with
      diverticulitis 562.11
        with hemorrhage 562.13
      hemorrhage 562.12
    congenital 751.5
  small intestine 562.00
    with
      diverticulitis 562.01
        with hemorrhage 562.03
      hemorrhage 562.02
  stomach (cardia) (juxtacardia) (juxtapyloric)
    (acquired) 537.1
    congenital 750.7
  subdiaphragmatic 530.6
  trachea (congenital) 748.3
    acquired 519.1
  traction (esophagus) 530.6
  ureter (acquired) 593.89
    congenital 753.4
  ureterovesical orifice 593.89
  urethra (acquired) 599.2
    congenital 753.8
  ventricle, left (congenital) 746.89
  vesical (urinary) 596.3
    congenital 753.8
  Zenker's (esophagus) 530.6
Diverticulitis (acute) (*see also* Diverticula)
    562.11
  with hemorrhage 562.13
  bladder (urinary) 596.3
  cecum (perforated) 562.11
    with hemorrhage 562.13
  colon (perforated) 562.11
    with hemorrhage 562.13
  duodenum 562.01
    with hemorrhage 562.03
  esophagus 530.6
  ileum (perforated) 562.01
    with hemorrhage 562.03
  intestine (large) (perforated) 562.11
    with hemorrhage 562.13
    small 562.01
      with hemorrhage 562.03
  jejunum (perforated) 562.01
    with hemorrhage 562.03

Diverticulitis—*continued*
  Meckel's (perforated) 751.0
  pharyngoesophageal 530.6
  rectosigmoid (perforated) 562.11
    with hemorrhage 562.13
  rectum 562.11
    with hemorrhage 562.13
  sigmoid (old) (perforated) 562.11
    with hemorrhage 562.13
  small intestine (perforated) 562.01
    with hemorrhage 562.03
  vesical (urinary) 596.3
Diverticulosis —*see* Diverticula
Division
  cervix uteri 622.8
    external os into two openings by frenum
      752.49
  external (cervical) into two openings by frenum
    752.49
  glans penis 752.69
  hymen 752.49
  labia minora (congenital) 752.49
  ligament (partial or complete) (current)—*see*
    also Sprain, by site
    with open wound—*see* Wound, open, by site
  muscle (partial or complete) (current)—*see also*
    Sprain, by site
    with open wound—*see* Wound, open, by site
  nerve—*see* Injury, nerve, by site
  penis glans 752.69
  spinal cord—*see* Injury, spinal, by site
  vein 459.9
    traumatic—*see* Injury, vascular, by site
Divorce V61.0
Dix-Hallpike neurolabyrinthitis 386.12
Dizziness 780.4
  hysterical 300.11
  psychogenic 306.9
Doan-Wiseman syndrome (primary splenic
  neutropenia) 288.0
Dog bite —*see* Wound, open, by site
Döhle-Heller aortitis 093.1
Döhle body-panmyelopathic syndrome 288.2
Dolichocephaly, dolichocephalus 754.0
Dolichocolon 751.5
Dolichostenomelia 759.82
Donohue's syndrome (leprechaunism) 259.8
Donor
  blood V59.01
    other blood components V59.09
    stem cells V59.02
    whole blood V59.01
  bone V59.2
    marrow V59.3
  cornea V59.5
  heart V59.8
  kidney V59.4
  liver V59.6
  lung V59.8
  lymphocyte V59.8
  organ V59.9
    specified NEC V59.8
  potential, examination of V70.8
  skin V59.1
  specified organ or tissue NEC V59.8
  stem cells V59.02
  tissue V59.9
    specified type NEC V59.8
Donovanosis (granuloma venereum) 099.2
DOPS (diffuse obstructive pulmonary syndrome)
  496

Double
  albumin 273.8
  aortic arch 747.21
  auditory canal 744.29
  auricle (heart) 746.82
  bladder 753.8
  external (cervical) os 752.49
  kidney with double pelvis (renal) 753.3
  larynx 748.3
  meatus urinarius 753.8
  organ or site NEC—*see* Accessory
  orifice
    heart valve NEC 746.89
      pulmonary 746.09
  outlet, right ventricle 745.11
  pelvis (renal) with double ureter 753.4
  penis 752.69
  tongue 750.13
  ureter (one or both sides) 753.4
    with double pelvis (renal) 753.4
  urethra 753.8
  urinary meatus 753.8
  uterus (any degree) 752.2
    with doubling of cervix and vagina 752.2
    in pregnancy or childbirth 654.0
      affecting fetus or newborn 763.89
  vagina 752.49
    with doubling of cervix and uterus 752.2
  vision 368.2
  vocal cords 748.3
  vulva 752.49
  whammy (syndrome) 360.81
Douglas' pouch, cul-de-sac —*see* condition
Down's disease or syndrome (mongolism) 758.0
Down-growth, epithelial (anterior chamber)
    364.61
Dracontiasis 125.7
Dracunculiasis 125.7
Dracunculosis 125.7
Drainage
  abscess (spontaneous)—*see* Abscess
  anomalous pulmonary veins to hepatic veins or
      right atrium 747.41
  stump (amputation) (surgical) 997.62
  suprapubic, bladder 596.8
Dream state, hysterical 300.13
Drepanocytic anemia (*see also* Disease, sickle
    cell) 282.60
Dresbach's syndrome (elliptocytosis) 282.1
Dreschlera (infection) 118
  hawaiiensis 117.8
Dressler's syndrome (postmyocardial infarction)
    411.0
Dribbling (post-void) 788.35
Drift, ulnar 736.09
Drinking (alcohol)—*see also* Alcoholism
  excessive, to excess NEC (*see also* Abuse,
      drugs, nondependent) 305.0
    bouts, periodic 305.0
    continual 303.9
    episodic 305.0
    habitual 303.9
    periodic 305.0
Drip, postnasal (chronic)—*see* Sinusitis
Drivers' license examination V70.3
Droop
  Cooper's 611.8
  facial 781.99

Drop
  finger 736.29
  foot 736.79
  hematocrit (precipitous) 790.01
  toe 735.8
  wrist 736.05
Dropped
  dead 798.1
  heart beats 426.6
Dropsy, dropsical (*see also* Edema) 782.3
  abdomen 789.5
  amnion (*see also* Hydramnios) 657
  brain—*see* Hydrocephalus
  cardiac (*see also* Failure, heart) 428.0
  cardiorenal (*see also* Hypertension, cardiorenal)
    404.90
  chest 511.9
  fetus or newborn 778.0
    due to isoimmunization 773.3
  gangrenous (*see also* Gangrene) 785.4
  heart (*see also* Failure, heart) 428.0
  hepatic—*see* Cirrhosis, liver
  infantile—*see* Hydrops, fetalis
  kidney (*see also* Nephrosis) 581.9
  liver—*see* Cirrhosis, liver
  lung 514
  malarial (*see also* Malaria) 084.9
  neonatorum—*see* Hydrops, fetalis
  nephritic 581.9
  newborn—*see* Hydrops, fetalis
  nutritional 269.9
  ovary 620.8
  pericardium (*see also* Pericarditis) 423.9
  renal (*see also* Nephrosis) 581.9
  uremic—*see* Uremia
Drowned, drowning 994.1
  lung 518.5
Drowsiness 780.09
Drug —*see also* condition
  addiction (*see also* listing under Dependence)
    304.9
  adverse effect NEC, correct substance properly
    administered 995.2
  dependence (*see also* listing under Dependence)
    304.9
  habit (*see also* listing under Dependence) 304.9
  overdose—*see* Table of drugs and chemicals
  poisoning—*see* Table of drugs and chemicals
  therapy (maintenance) status NEC V58.1
    long-term (current) use V58.69
      antibiotics V58.62
      anticoagulant V58.61
  wrong substance given or taken in error—*see*
    Table of drugs and chemicals
Drunkenness (*see also* Abuse, drugs,
    nondependent) 305.0
  acute in alcoholism (*see also* Alcoholism) 303.0
  chronic (*see also* Alcoholism) 303.9
  pathologic 291.4
  simple (acute) 305.0
    in alcoholism 303.0
  sleep 307.47
Drusen
  optic disc or papilla 377.21
  retina (colloid) (hyaloid degeneration) 362.57
    hereditary 362.77
Drusenfieber 075
Dry, dryness —*see also* condition
  eye 375.15
    syndrome 375.15
  larynx 478.79

Dysfunction—*continued*
  gallbladder 575.8
  gastrointestinal 536.9
  gland, glandular NEC 259.9
  heart 427.9
    postoperative (immediate) 997.1
      long-term effect of cardiac surgery 429.4
  hemoglobin 288.8
  hepatic 573.9
  hepatocellular NEC 573.9
  hypophysis 253.9
    hyperfunction 253.1
    hypofunction 253.2
    posterior lobe 253.6
      hypofunction 253.5
  kidney (*see also* Disease, renal) 593.9
  labyrinthine 386.50
    specified NEC 386.58
  liver 573.9
    constitutional 277.4
  minimal brain (child) (*see also* Hyperkinesia) 314.9
  ovary, ovarian 256.9
    hyperfunction 256.1
      estrogen 256.0
    hypofunction 256.39
      postablative 256.2
    postablative 256.2
    specified NEC 256.8
  papillary muscle 429.81
    with myocardial infarction 410.8
  parathyroid 252.8
    hyperfunction 252.0
    hypofunction 252.1
  pineal gland 259.8
  pituitary (gland) 253.9
    hyperfunction 253.1
    hypofunction 253.2
    posterior 253.6
      hypofunction 253.5
  placental—*see* Placenta, insufficiency
  platelets (blood) 287.1
  polyglandular 258.9
    specified NEC 258.8
  psychosexual 302.70
    with
      dyspareunia (functional) (psychogenic) 302.76
      frigidity 302.72
      impotence 302.72
      inhibition
        orgasm
          female 302.73
          male 302.74
        sexual
          desire 302.71
          excitement 302.72
      premature ejaculation 302.75
      sexual aversion 302.79
      specified disorder NEC 302.79
      vaginismus 306.51
  pylorus 537.9
  rectum 564.9
    psychogenic 306.4
  segmental (*see also* Dysfunction, somatic) 739.9
  senile 797
  sinoatrial node 427.81
  somatic 739.9
    abdomen 739.9
    acromioclavicular 739.7
    cervical 739.1

Dysfunction—*continued*
    cervicothoracic 739.1
    costochondral 739.8
    costovertebral 739.8
    extremities
      lower 739.6
      upper 739.7
    head 739.0
    hip 739.5
    umbar, lumbosacral 739.3
    occipitocervical 739.0
    pelvic 739.5
    pubic 739.5
    rib cage 739.8
    sacral 739.4
    sacrococcygeal 739.4
    sacroiliac 739.4
    specified site NEC 739.9
    sternochondral 739.8
    sternoclavicular 739.7
    temporomandibular 739.0
    thoracic, thoracolumbar 739.2
  stomach 536.9
    psychogenic 306.4
  suprarenal 255.9
    hyperfunction 255.3
    hypofunction 255.4
  symbolic NEC 784.60
    specified type NEC 784.69
  temporomandibular (joint) (joint-pain-syndrome) NEC 524.60
    specified NEC 524.69
  testicular 257.9
    hyperfunction 257.0
    hypofunction 257.2
    specified type NEC 257.8
  thymus 254.9
  thyroid 246.9
    complicating pregnancy, childbirth, or puerperium 648.1
    hyperfunction—*see* Hyperthyroidism
    hypofunction—*see* Hypothyroidism
  uterus, complicating delivery 661.9
    affecting fetus or newborn 763.7
    hypertonic 661.4
    hypotonic 661.2
      primary 661.0
      secondary 661.1
  velopharyngeal (acquired) 528.9
    congenital 750.29
  ventricular 429.9
    with congestive heart failure (*see also* Failure, heart) 428.0
    due to
      cardiomyopathy—*see* Cardiomyopathy
      hypertension—*see* Hypertension, heart
  vesicourethral NEC 596.59
  vestibular 386.50
    specified type NEC 386.58
Dysgammaglobulinemia 279.06
Dysgenesis
  gonadal (due to chromosomal anomaly) 758.6
    pure 752.7
  kidney(s) 753.0
  ovarian 758.6
  renal 753.0
  reticular 279.2
  seminiferous tubules 758.6
  tidal platelet 287.3

Dysgerminoma (M9060/3)
  specified site—*see* Neoplasm, by site, malignant
  unspecified site
    female 183.0
    male 186.9
Dysgeusia 781.1
Dysgraphia 781.3
Dyshidrosis 705.81
Dysidrosis 705.81
Dysinsulinism 251.8
Dyskaryotic cervical smear 795.09
Dyskeratosis (*see also* Keratosis) 701.1
  bullosa hereditaria 757.39
  cervix 622.1
  congenital 757.39
  follicularis 757.39
    vitamin A deficiency 264.8
  gingiva 523.8
  oral soft tissue NEC 528.7
  tongue 528.7
  uterus NEC 621.8
Dyskinesia 781.3
  biliary 575.8
  esophagus 530.5
  hysterical 300.11
  intestinal 564.89
  nonorganic origin 307.9
  orofacial 333.82
  psychogenic 307.9
  tardive (oral) 333.82
Dyslalia 784.5
  developmental 315.39
Dyslexia 784.61
  developmental 315.02
  secondary to organic lesion 784.61
Dysmaturity (*see also* Immaturity) 765.1
  lung 770.4
  pulmonary 770.4
Dysmenorrhea (essential) (exfoliative)
    (functional) (intrinsic) (membranous)
    (primary) (secondary) 625.3
  psychogenic 306.52
Dysmetabolic syndrome X 277.7
Dysmetria 781.3
Dysmorodystrophia mesodermalis congenita
  759.82
Dysnomia 784.3
Dysorexia 783.0
  hysterical 300.11
Dysostosis
  cleidocranial, cleidocranialis 755.59
  craniofacial 756.0
  Fairbank's (idiopathic familial generalized
    osteophytosis) 756.50
  mandibularis 756.0
  mandibulofacial, incomplete 756.0
  multiplex 277.5
  orodigitofacial 759.89
Dyspareunia (female) 625.0
  male 608.89
  psychogenic 302.76
Dyspepsia (allergic) (congenital) (fermentative)
    (flatulent) (functional) (gastric)
    (gastrointestinal) (neurogenic) (occupational)
    (reflex) 536.8
  acid 536.8
  atonic 536.3
    psychogenic 306.4
  diarrhea 787.91
    psychogenic 306.4
  intestinal 564.89

Dyspepsia—*continued*
  psychogenic 306.4
  nervous 306.4
  neurotic 306.4
  psychogenic 306.4
Dysphagia 787.2
  functional 300.11
  hysterical 300.11
  nervous 300.11
  psychogenic 306.4
  sideropenic 280.8
  spastica 530.5
Dysphagocytosis, congenital 288.1
Dysphasia 784.5
Dysphonia 784.49
  clericorum 784.49
  functional 300.11
  hysterical 300.11
  psychogenic 306.1
  spastica 478.79
Dyspigmentation —*see also* Pigmentation
  eyelid (acquired) 374.52
Dyspituitarism 253.9
  hyperfunction 253.1
  hypofunction 253.2
  posterior lobe 253.6
Dysplasia —*see also* Anomaly
  artery
    fibromuscular NEC 447.8
      carotid 447.8
      renal 447.3
  bladder 596.8
  bone (fibrous) NEC 733.29
    diaphyseal, progressive 756.59
    jaw 526.89
    monostotic 733.29
    polyostotic 756.54
    solitary 733.29
  brain 742.9
  bronchopulmonary, fetus or newborn 770.7
  cervix (uteri) 622.1
    cervical intraepithelial neoplasia I [CIN 1]
      622.1
    cervical intraepithelial neoplasia II [CIN II]
      622.1
    cervical intraepithelial neoplasia III [CIN III]
      233.1
    CIN I 622.1
    CIN II 622.1
    CIN III 233.1
  chondroectodermal 756.55
  chondromatose 756.4
  craniocarpotarsal 759.89
  craniometaphyseal 756.89
  dentinal 520.5
  diaphyseal, progressive 756.59
  ectodermal (anhidrotic) (Bason) (Clouston's)
    (congenital) (Feinmesser) (hereditary)
    (hidrotic) (Marshall) (Robinson's) 757.31
  epiphysealis 756.9
    multiplex 756.56
    punctata 756.59
  epiphysis 756.9
    multiple 756.56
  epithelial
    epiglottis 478.79
    uterine cervix 622.1
  erythroid NEC 289.8
  eye (*see also* Microphthalmos) 743.10
  familial metaphyseal 756.89

Dysplasia—*continued*
 fibromuscular, artery NEC 447.8
  carotid 447.8
  renal 447.3
 fibrous
  bone NEC 733.29
  diaphyseal, progressive 756.59
  jaw 526.89
  monostotic 733.29
  polyostotic 756.54
  solitary 733.29
 high grade squamous intraepithelial (HGSIL)
   622.1
 hip (congenital) 755.63
  with dislocation (*see also* Dislocation, hip,
    congenital) 754.30
 hypohidrotic ectodermal 757.31
 joint 755.8
 kidney 753.15
 leg 755.69
 linguofacialis 759.89
 low grade squamous intraepithelial (LGSIL)
   622.1
 lung 748.5
 macular 743.55
 mammary (benign) (gland) 610.9
  cystic 610.1
  specified type NEC 610.8
 metaphyseal 756.9
  familial 756.89
 monostotic fibrous 733.29
 muscle 756.89
 myeloid NEC 289.8
 nervous system (general) 742.9
 neuroectodermal 759.6
 oculoauriculovertebral 756.0
 oculodentodigital 759.89
 olfactogenital 253.4
 osteo-onycho-arthro (hereditary) 756.89
 periosteum 733.99
 polyostotic fibrous 756.54
 progressive diaphyseal 756.59
 prostate 602.3
  intraepithelial neoplasia I [PIN I] 602.3
  intraepithelial neoplasia II [PIN II] 602.3
  intraepithelial neoplasia III [PIN III] 233.4
 renal 753.15
 renofacialis 753.0
 retinal NEC 743.56
 retrolental 362.21
 spinal cord 742.9
 thymic, with immunodeficiency 279.2
 vagina 623.0
 vocal cord 478.5
 vulva 624.8
  intraepithelial neoplasia I [VIN I] 624.8
  intraepithelial neoplasia II [VIN II] 624.8
  intraepithelial neoplasia III [VIN III] 233.3
  VIN I 624.8
  VIN II 624.8
  VIN III 233.3
Dyspnea (nocturnal) (paroxysmal) 786.09
 asthmatic (bronchial) (*see also* Asthma) 493.9
  with bronchitis (*see also* Asthma) 493.9
   chronic 493.2
  cardiac (*see also* Failure, ventricular, left)
    428.1
 cardiac (*see also* Failure, ventricular, left) 428.1
 functional 300.11
 hyperventilation 786.01
 hysterical 300.11

Dyspnea—*continued*
 Monday morning 504
 newborn 770.89
 psychogenic 306.1
 uremic—*see* Uremia
Dyspraxia 781.3
 syndrome 315.4
Dysproteinemia 273.8
 transient with copper deficiency 281.4
Dysprothrombinemia (constitutional) (*see also*
   Defect, coagulation) 286.3
Dysreflexia , autonomic 337.3
Dysrhythmia
 cardiac 427.9
  postoperative (immediate) 997.1
   long-term effect of cardiac surgery 429.4
  specified type NEC 427.89
 cerebral or cortical 348.3
Dyssecretosis, mucoserous 710.2
**Dyssocial reaction without manifest
   psychiatric disorder**
 adolescent V71.02
 adult V71.01
 child V71.02
Dyssomnia NEC 780.56
 nonorganic origin 307.47
Dyssplenism 289.4
Dyssynergia
 biliary (*see also* Disease, biliary) 576.8
 cerebellaris myoclonica 334.2
 detrusor sphincter (bladder) 596.55
 ventricular 429.89
Dystasia, hereditary areflexic 334.3
Dysthymia 300.4
Dysthymic disorder 300.4
Dysthyroidism 246.9
Dystocia 660.9
 affecting fetus or newborn 763.1
 cervical 661.0
  affecting fetus or newborn 763.7
 contraction ring 661.4
  affecting fetus or newborn 763.7
 fetal 660.9
  abnormal size 653.5
  affecting fetus or newborn 763.1
  deformity 653.7
 maternal 660.9
  affecting fetus or newborn 763.1
 positional 660.0
  affecting fetus or newborn 763.1
 shoulder (girdle) 660.4
  affecting fetus or newborn 763.1
 uterine NEC 661.4
  affecting fetus or newborn 763.7
Dystonia
 deformans progressiva 333.6
 due to drugs 333.7
 lenticularis 333.6
 musculorum deformans 333.6
 torsion (idiopathic) 333.6
  fragments (of) 333.89
  symptomatic 333.7
Dystonic
 movements 781.0
Dystopia kidney 753.3
Dystrophy, dystrophia 783.9
 adiposogenital 253.8
 asphyxiating thoracic 756.4
 Becker's type 359.1
 brevicollis 756.16
 Bruch's membrane 362.77

E

Eagle-Barrett syndrome 756.71
Eales' disease (syndrome) 362.18
Ear —*see also* condition
  ache 388.70
    otogenic 388.71
    referred 388.72
  lop 744.29
  piercing V50.3
  swimmers' acute 380.12
  tank 380.12
  tropical 111.8 *[380.15]*
  wax 380.4
Earache 388.70
  otogenic 388.71
  referred 388.72
Eaton-Lambert syndrome (*see also* Neoplasm,
    by site, malignant) 199.1 *[358.1]*
Eberth's disease (typhoid fever) 002.0
Ebstein's
  anomaly or syndrome (downward displacement,
      tricuspid valve into right ventricle) 746.2
  disease (diabetes) 250.4 *[581.81]*
Eccentro-osteochondrodysplasia 277.5
Ecchondroma (M9210/0)—*see* Neoplasm, bone,
    benign
Ecchondrosis (M9210/1) 238.0
Ecchordosis physaliphora 756.0
Ecchymosis (multiple) 459.89
  conjunctiva 372.72
  eye (traumatic) 921.0
  eyelids (traumatic) 921.1
  newborn 772.6
  spontaneous 782.7
  traumatic—*see* Contusion
Echinococciasis —*see* Echinococcus
Echinococcosis —*see* Echinococcus
Echinococcus (infection) 122.9
  granulosus 122.4
    liver 122.0
    lung 122.1
    orbit 122.3 *[376.13]*
    specified site NEC 122.3
    thyroid 122.2
  liver NEC 122.8
    granulosus 122.0
    multilocularis 122.5
  lung NEC 122.9
    granulosus 122.1
    multilocularis 122.6
  multilocularis 122.7
    liver 122.5
    specified site NEC 122.6
  orbit 122.9 *[376.13]*
    granulosus 122.3 *[376.13]*
    multilocularis 122.6 *[376.13]*
  specified site NEC 122.9
    granulosus 122.3
    multilocularis 122.6 *[376.13]*
  thyroid NEC 122.9
    granulosus 122.2
    multilocularis 122.6
Echinorhynchiasis 127.7
Echinostomiasis 121.8
Echolalia 784.69
ECHO virus infection NEC 079.1

Eclampsia, eclamptic (coma) (convulsions)
    (delirium) 780.39
  female, child-bearing age NEC—*see* Eclampsia,
      pregnancy
  gravidarum—*see* Eclampsia, pregnancy
  male 780.39
  not associated with pregnancy or childbirth
      780.39
  pregnancy, childbirth or puerperium 642.6
    with pre-existing hypertension 642.7
    affecting fetus or newborn 760.0
  uremic 586
Eclipse blindness (total) 363.31
Economic circumstance affecting care V60.9
  specified type NEC V60.8
Economo's disease (encephalitis lethargica)
    049.8
Ectasia, ectasis
  aorta (*see also* Aneurysm, aorta) 441.9
    ruptured 441.5
  breast 610.4
  capillary 448.9
  cornea (marginal) (postinfectional) 371.71
  duct (mammary) 610.4
  kidney 593.89
  mammary duct (gland) 610.4
  papillary 448.9
  renal 593.89
  salivary gland (duct) 527.8
  scar, cornea 371.71
  sclera 379.11
Ecthyma 686.8
  contagiosum 051.2
  gangrenosum 686.09
  infectiosum 051.2
Ectocardia 746.87
Ectodermal dysplasia, congenital 757.31
Ectodermosis erosiva pluriorificialis 695.1
Ectopic, ectopia (congenital) 759.89
  abdominal viscera 751.8
    due to defect in anterior abdominal wall
        756.79
  ACTH syndrome 255.0
  adrenal gland 759.1
  anus 751.5
  auricular beats 427.61
  beats 427.60
  bladder 753.5
  bone and cartilage in lung 748.69
  brain 742.4
  breast tissue 757.6
  cardiac 746.87
  cerebral 742.4
  cordis 746.87
  endometrium 617.9
  gallbladder 751.69
  gastric mucosa 750.7
  gestation—*see* Pregnancy, ectopic
  heart 746.87
  hormone secretion NEC 259.3
  hyperparathyroidism 259.3
  kidney (crossed) (intrathoracic) (pelvis) 753.3
    in pregnancy or childbirth 654.4
      causing obstructed labor 660.2
  lens 743.37
  lentis 743.37
  mole—*see* Pregnancy, ectopic

Ectopic, ectopia—*continued*
organ or site NEC—*see* Malposition, congenital
ovary 752.0
pancreas, pancreatic tissue 751.7
pregnancy—*see* Pregnancy, ectopic
pupil 364.75
renal 753.3
sebaceous glands of mouth 750.26
secretion
  ACTH 255.0
  adrenal hormone 259.3
  adrenalin 259.3
  adrenocorticotropin 255.0
  antidiuretic hormone (ADH) 259.3
  epinephrine 259.3
  hormone NEC 259.3
  norepinephrine 259.3
  pituitary (posterior) 259.3
spleen 759.0
testis 752.51
thyroid 759.2
ureter 753.4
ventricular beats 427.69
vesicae 753.5
Ectrodactyly 755.4
finger (*see also* Absence, finger, congenital) 755.29
toe (*see also* Absence, toe, congenital) 755.39
Ectromelia 755.4
lower limb 755.30
upper limb 755.20
Ectropion 374.10
anus 569.49
cervix 622.0
  with mention of cervicitis 616.0
cicatricial 374.14
congenital 743.62
eyelid 374.10
  cicatricial 374.14
  congenital 743.62
  mechanical 374.12
  paralytic 374.12
  senile 374.11
  spastic 374.13
iris (pigment epithelium) 364.54
lip (congenital) 750.26
  acquired 528.5
mechanical 374.12
paralytic 374.12
rectum 569.49
senile 374.11
spastic 374.13
urethra 599.84
uvea 364.54
Eczema (acute) (allergic) (chronic) (erythematous) (fissum) (occupational) (rubrum) (squamous) 692.9
asteatotic 706.8
atopic 691.8
contact NEC 692.9
dermatitis NEC 692.9
due to specified cause—*see* Dermatitis, due to
dyshidrotic 705.81
external ear 380.22
flexural 691.8
gouty 274.89
herpeticum 054.0
hypertrophicum 701.8
hypostatic—*see* Varicose, vein

Eczema—*continued*
impetiginous 684
infantile (acute) (chronic) (due to any substance) (intertriginous) (seborrheic) 690.12
intertriginous NEC 692.9
  infantile 690.12
intrinsic 691.8
lichenified NEC 692.9
marginatum 110.3
nummular 692.9
pustular 686.8
seborrheic 690.18
  infantile 690.12
solare 692.72
stasis (lower extremity) 454.1
  ulcerated 454.2
vaccination, vaccinatum 999.0
varicose (lower extremity)—*see* Varicose, vein
verrucosum callosum 698.3
Eczematoid, exudative 691.8
Eddowes' syndrome (brittle bones and blue sclera) 756.51
Edema, edematous 782.3
with nephritis (*see also* Nephrosis) 581.9
allergic 995.1
angioneurotic (allergic) (any site) (with urticaria) 995.1
  hereditary 277.6
angiospastic 443.9
Berlin's (traumatic) 921.3
brain 348.5
  due to birth injury 767.8
  fetus or newborn 767.8
cardiac (*see also* Failure, heart) 428.0
cardiovascular (*see also* Failure, heart) 428.0
cerebral—*see* Edema, brain
cerebrospinal vessel—*see* Edema, brain
cervix (acute) (uteri) 622.8
  puerperal, postpartum 674.8
chronic hereditary 757.0
circumscribed, acute 995.1
  hereditary 277.6
complicating pregnancy (gestational) 646.1
  with hypertension—*see* Toxemia, of pregnancy
conjunctiva 372.73
connective tissue 782.3
cornea 371.20
  due to contact lenses 371.24
  idiopathic 371.21
  secondary 371.22
due to
  lymphatic obstruction—*see* Edema, lymphatic
  salt retention 276.0
epiglottis—*see* Edema, glottis
essential, acute 995.1
  hereditary 277.6
extremities, lower—*see* Edema, legs
eyelid NEC 374.82
familial, hereditary (legs) 757.0
famine 262
fetus or newborn 778.5
genital organs
  female 629.8
  male 608.86
gestational 646.1
  with hypertension—*see* Toxemia, of pregnancy

Edema, edematous—*continued*
  glottis, glottic, glottides (obstructive) (passive) 478.6
    allergic 995.1
      hereditary 277.6
    due to external agent—*see* Condition, respiratory, acute, due to specified agent
  heart (*see also* Failure, heart) 428.0
    newborn 779.89
  heat 992.7
  hereditary (legs) 757.0
  inanition 262
  infectious 782.3
  intracranial 348.5
    due to injury at birth 767.8
  iris 364.8
  joint (*see also* Effusion, joint) 719.0
  larynx (*see also* Edema, glottis) 478.6
  legs 782.3
    due to venous obstruction 459.2
    hereditary 757.0
  localized 782.3
    due to venous obstruction 459.2
      lower extremity 459.2
  lower extremities—*see* Edema, legs
  lungs 514
    acute 518.4
      with heart disease or failure (*see also* Failure, ventricular, left) 428.1
        congestive 428.0
      chemical (due to fumes or vapors) 506.1
      due to
        external agent(s) NEC 508.9
          specified NEC 508.8
        fumes and vapors (chemical) (inhalation) 506.1
        radiation 508.0
    chemical (acute) 506.1
      chronic 506.4
    chronic 514
      chemical (due to fumes or vapors) 506.4
      due to
        external agent(s) NEC 508.9
          specified NEC 508.8
        fumes or vapors (chemical) (inhalation) 506.4
        radiation 508.1
    due to
      external agent 508.9
        specified NEC 508.8
      high altitude 993.2
      near drowning 994.1
    postoperative 518.4
    terminal 514
  lymphatic 457.1
    due to mastectomy operation 457.0
  macula 362.83
    cystoid 362.53
    diabetic 250.5 *[362.01]*
  malignant (*see also* Gangrene, gas) 040.0
  Milroy's 757.0
  nasopharynx 478.25
  neonatorum 778.5
  nutritional (newborn) 262
    with dyspigmentation, skin and hair 260
  optic disc or nerve—*see* Papilledema
  orbit 376.33
    circulatory 459.89
  palate (soft) (hard) 528.9
  pancreas 577.8
  penis 607.83

Edema, edematous—*continued*
  periodic 995.1
    hereditary 277.6
  pharynx 478.25
  pitting 782.3
  pulmonary—*see* Edema, lung
  Quincke's 995.1
    hereditary 277.6
  renal (*see also* Nephrosis) 581.9
  retina (localized) (macular) (peripheral) 362.83
    cystoid 362.53
    diabetic 250.5 *[362.01]*
  salt 276.0
  scrotum 608.86
  seminal vesicle 608.86
  spermatic cord 608.86
  spinal cord 336.1
  starvation 262
  stasis (*see also* Hypertension, venous) 459.30
  subconjunctival 372.73
  subglottic (*see also* Edema, glottis) 478.6
  supraglottic (*see also* Edema, glottis) 478.6
  testis 608.86
  toxic NEC 782.3
  traumatic NEC 782.3
  tunica vaginalis 608.86
  vas deferens 608.86
  vocal cord—*see* Edema, glottis
  vulva (acute) 624.8
Edentia (complete) (partial) (*see also* Absence, tooth) 520.0
  acquired 525.10
    due to
      caries 525.13
      extraction 525.10
      periodontal disease 525.12
      specified NEC 525.19
      trauma 525.11
  causing malocclusion 524.3
  congenital (deficiency of tooth buds) 520.0
Edentulism 525.10
Edsall's disease 992.2
Educational handicap V62.3
Edwards' syndrome 758.2
Effect, adverse NEC
  abnormal gravitational (G) forces or states 994.9
  air pressure—*see* Effect, adverse, atmospheric pressure
  altitude (high)—*see* Effect, adverse, high altitude
  anesthetic
    in labor and delivery NEC 668.9
      affecting fetus or newborn 763.5
  antitoxin—*see* Complications, vaccination
  atmospheric pressure 993.9
    due to explosion 993.4
    high 993.3
    low—*see* Effect, adverse, high altitude
    specified effect NEC 993.8
  biological, correct substance properly administered (*see also* Effect, adverse, drug) 995.2
  blood (derivatives) (serum) (transfusion)—*see* Complications, transfusion
  chemical substance NEC 989.9
    specified—*see* Table of drugs and chemicals
  cobalt, radioactive (*see also* Effect, adverse, radioactive substance) 990
  cold (temperature) (weather) 991.9
    chilblains 991.5
    frostbite—*see* Frostbite

Effect, adverse—*continued*
  specified effect NEC 991.8
  drugs and medicinals NEC 995.2
    correct substance properly administered 995.2
    overdose or wrong substance given or taken
      977.9
      specified drug—*see* Table of drugs and
        chemicals
  electric current (shock) 994.8
    burn—*see* Burn, by site
  electricity (electrocution) (shock) 994.8
    burn—*see* Burn, by site
  exertion (excessive) 994.5
  exposure 994.9
    exhaustion 994.4
  external cause NEC 994.9
  fallout (radioactive) NEC 990
  fluoroscopy NEC 990
  foodstuffs
    allergic reaction (*see also* Allergy, food) 693.1
      anaphylactic shock due to food NEC 995.60
    noxious 988.9
      specified type NEC (*see also* Poisoning, by
        name of noxious foodstuff) 988.8
  gases, fumes, or vapors—*see* Table of drugs
    and chemicals
  glue (airplane) sniffing 304.6
  heat—*see* Heat
  high altitude NEC 993.2
    anoxia 993.2
    on
      fears 993.0
      sinuses 993.1
    polycythemia 289.0
  hot weather—*see* Heat
  hunger 994.2
  immersion, foot 991.4
  immunization—*see* Complications, vaccination
  immunological agents—*see* Complications,
    vaccination
  implantation (removable) of isotope or radium
    NEC 990
  infrared (radiation) (rays) NEC 990
    burn—*see* Burn, by site
    dermatitis or eczema 692.82
  infusion—*see* Complications, infusion
  ingestion or injection of isotope (therapeutic)
    NEC 990
  irradiation NEC (*see also* Effect, adverse,
    radiation) 990
  isotope (radioactive) NEC 990
  lack of care (child) (infant) (newborn) 995.52
    adult 995.84
  lightning 994.0
    burn—*see* Burn, by site
  Lirugin—*see* Complications, vaccination
  medicinal substance, correct, properly
    administered (*see also* Effect, adverse,
    drugs) 995.2
  mesothorium NEC 990
  motion 994.6
  noise, inner ear 388.10
  overheated places—*see* Heat
  polonium NEC 990
  psychosocial, of work environment V62.1
  radiation (diagnostic) (fallout) (infrared)
    (natural source) (therapeutic) (tracer)
    (ultraviolet) (x-ray) NEC 990

Effect, adverse—*continued*
  with pulmonary manifestations
    acute 508.0
    chronic 508.1
    dermatitis or eczema 692.82
      due to sun NEC (*see also* Dermatitis, due to,
        sun) 692.70
    fibrosis of lungs 508.1
    maternal with suspected damage to fetus
      affecting management of pregnancy 655.6
    pneumonitis 508.0
  radioactive substance NEC 990
    dermatitis or eczema 692.82
  radioactivity NEC 990
  radiotherapy NEC 990
    dermatitis or eczema 692.82
  radium NEC 990
  reduced temperature 991.9
    frostbite—*see* Frostbite
    immersion, foot (hand) 991.4
    specified effect NEC 991.8
  roentgenography NEC 990
  roentgenoscopy NEC 990
  roentgen rays NEC 990
  serum (prophylactic) (therapeutic) NEC 999.5
  specified NEC 995.89
    external cause NEC 994.9
  strangulation 994.7
  submersion 994.1
  teletherapy NEC 990
  thirst 994.3
  transfusion—*see* Complications, transfusion
  ultraviolet (radiation) (rays) NEC 990
    burn—*see also* Burn, by site
      from sun (*see also* Sunburn) 692.71
    dermatitis or eczema 692.82
      due to sun NEC (*see also* Dermatitis, due to,
        sun) 692.70
  uranium NEC 990
  vaccine (any)—*see* Complications, vaccination
  weightlessness 994.9
  whole blood—*see also* Complications,
    transfusion
    overdose or wrong substance given (*see also*
      Table of drugs and chemicals) 964.7
  working environment V62.1
  x-rays NEC 990
    dermatitis or eczema 692.82
Effect, remote
  of cancer, —*see* condition
Effects, late —*see* Late, effect (of)
Effluvium, telogen 704.02
Effort
  intolerance 306.2
  syndrome (aviators) (psychogenic) 306.2
Effusion
  Amniotic fluid (*see also* Rupture, membranes,
    premature) 658.1
  brain (serous) 348.5
  bronchial (*see also* Bronchitis) 490
  cerebral 348.5
  cerebrospinal (*see also* Meningitis) 322.9
    vessel 348.5
  chest—*see* Effusion, pleura
  intracranial 348.5
  joint 719.00
    ankle 719.07
    elbow 719.02
    foot 719.07
    hand 719.04

Effusion—*continued*
  hip 719.05
  knee 719.06
  multiple sites 719.09
  pelvic region 719.05
  shoulder (region) 719.01
  specified site NEC 719.08
  wrist 719.03
 meninges (*see also* Meningitis) 322.9
 pericardium, pericardial (*see also* Pericarditis) 423.9
  acute 420.90
 peritoneal (chronic) 568.82
 pleura, pleurisy, pleuritic, pleuropericardial 511.9
  bacterial, nontuberculous 511.1
  fetus or newborn 511.9
  malignant 197.2
  nontuberculous 511.9
   bacterial 511.1
  pneumococcal 511.1
  staphylococcal 511.1
  streptococcal 511.1
  tuberculous (*see also* Tuberculosis, pleura) 012.0
   primary progressive 010.1
  traumatic 862.29
   with open wound 862.39
 pulmonary—*see* Effusion, pleura
 spinal (*see also* Meningitis) 322.9
 thorax, thoracic—*see* Effusion, pleura
Eggshell nails 703.8
 congenital 757.5
Ego-dystonic
 homosexuality 302.0
 lesbianism 302.0
Egyptian splenomegaly 120.1
Ehlers-Danlos syndrome 756.83
Ehrlichiosis 082.40
 chaffeensis 082.41
 specified type NEC 082.49
Eichstedt's disease (pityriasis versicolor) 111.0
Eisenmenger's complex or syndrome (ventricular septal defect) 745.4
Ejaculation, semen
 painful 608.89
  psychogenic 306.59
 premature 302.75
 retrograde 608.87
Ekbom syndrome (restless legs) 333.99
Ekman's syndrome (brittle bones and blue sclera) 756.51
Elastic skin 756.83
 acquired 701.8
Elastofibroma (M8820/0)—*see* Neoplasm, connective tissue, benign
Elastoidosis
 cutanea nodularis 701.8
 cutis cystica et comedonica 701.8
Elastoma 757.39
 juvenile 757.39
 Miescher's (elastosis perforans serpiginosa) 701.1
Elastomyofibrosis 425.3
Elastosis 701.8
 atrophicans 701.8
 perforans serpiginosa 701.1
 reactive perforating 701.1
 senilis 701.8
 solar (actinic) 692.74
Elbow —*see* condition

Electric
 current, electricity, effects (concussion) (fatal) (nonfatal) (shock) 994.8
  burn—*see* Burn, by site
 feet (foot) syndrome 266.2
Electrocution 994.8
Electrolyte imbalance 276.9
 with
  abortion—*see* Abortion, by type, with metabolic disorder
  ectopic pregnancy (*see also* categories 633.0-633.9) 639.4
  hyperemesis gravidarum (before 22 completed weeks gestation) 643.1
  molar pregnancy (*see also* categories 630-632) 639.4
 following
  abortion 639.4
  ectopic or molar pregnancy 639.4
Elephant man syndrome 237.71
Elephantiasis (nonfilarial) 457.1
 arabicum (*see also* Infestation, filarial) 125.9
 congenita hereditaria 757.0
 congenital (any site) 757.0
 due to
  Brugia (malayi) 125.1
  mastectomy operation 457.0
  Wuchereria (bancrofti) 125.0
   malayi 125.1
 eyelid 374.83
 filarial (*see also* Infestation, filarial) 125.9
 filariensis (*see also* Infestation, filarial) 125.9
 gingival 523.8
 glandular 457.1
 graecorum 030.9
 lymphangiectatic 457.1
 lymphatic vessel 457.1
  due to mastectomy operation 457.0
 neuromatosa 237.71
 postmastectomy 457.0
 scrotum 457.1
 streptococcal 457.1
 surgical 997.99
  postmastectomy 457.0
 telangiectodes 457.1
 vulva (nonfilarial) 624.8
Elevated —*see* Elevation
Elevation
 17-ketosteroids 791.9
 acid phosphatase 790.5
 alkaline phosphatase 790.5
 amylase 790.5
 antibody titers 795.79
 basal metabolic rate (BMR) 794.7
 blood pressure (*see also* Hypertension) 401.9
  reading (incidental) (isolated) (nonspecific), no diagnosis of hypertension 796.2
 body temperature (of unknown origin) (*see also* Pyrexia) 780.6
 conjugate, eye 378.81
 diaphragm, congenital 756.6
 immunoglobulin level 795.79
 indolacetic acid 791.9
 lactic acid dehydrogenase (LDH) level 790.4
 lipase 790.5
 prostate specific antigen (PSA) 790.93
 renin 790.99
  in hypertension (*see also* Hypertension, renovascular) 405.91
 Rh titer 999.7
 scapula, congenital 755.52

Elevation—*continued*
  sedimentation rate 790.1
  SGOT 790.4
  SGPT 790.4
  transaminase 790.4
  vanillylmandelic acid 791.9
  venous pressure 459.89
  VMA 791.9
Elliptocytosis (congenital) (hereditary) 282.1
  Hb-C (disease) 282.7
  hemoglobin disease 282.7
  sickle-cell (disease) 282.60
    trait 282.5
Ellis-van Creveld disease or syndrome
  (chondroectodermal dysplasia) 756.55
Ellison-Zollinger syndrome (gastric
  hypersecretion with pancreatic islet cell
  tumor) 251.5
Elongation, elongated (congenital)—*see also*
  Distortion
  bone 756.9
  cervix (uteri) 752.49
    acquired 622.6
    hypertrophic 622.6
  colon 751.5
  common bile duct 751.69
  cystic duct 751.69
  frenulum, penis 752.69
  labia minora, acquired 624.8
  ligamentum patellae 756.89
  petiolus (epiglottidis) 748.3
  styloid bone (process) 733.99
  tooth, teeth 520.2
  uvula 750.26
    acquired 528.9
Elschnig bodies or pearls 366.51
El Tor cholera 001.1
Emaciation (due to malnutrition) 261
Emancipation disorder 309.22
Embadomoniasis 007.8
Embarrassment heart, cardiac —*see* Disease,
  heart
Embedded tooth, teeth 520.6
  with abnormal position (same or adjacent tooth)
    524.3
  root only 525.3
Embolic —*see* condition
Embolism 444.9
  with
    abortion—*see* Abortion, by type, with
      embolism
    ectopic pregnancy (*see also* categories
      633.0-633.9) 639.6
    molar pregnancy (*see also* categories
      630-632) 639.6
  air (any site) 958.0
    with
      abortion—*see* Abortion, by type, with
        embolism
      ectopic pregnancy (*see also* categories
        633.0-633.9) 639.6
      molar pregnancy (*see also* categories
        630-632) 639.6
    due to implanted device—*see* Complications,
      due to (presence of) any device, implant,
      or graft classified to 996.0-996.5 NEC
    following
      abortion 639.6
      ectopic or molar pregnancy 639.6
    infusion, perfusion, or transfusion 999.1

Embolism—*continued*
    in pregnancy, childbirth, or puerperium 673.0
    traumatic 958.0
  amniotic fluid (pulmonary) 673.1
    with
      abortion—*see* Abortion, by type, with
        embolism
      ectopic pregnancy (*see also* categories
        633.0-633.9) 639.6
      molar pregnancy (*see also* categories
        630-632) 639.6
    following
      abortion 639.6
      ectopic or molar pregnancy 639.6
  aorta, aortic 444.1
    abdominal 444.0
    bifurcation 444.0
    saddle 444.0
    thoracic 444.1
  artery 444.9
    auditory, internal 433.8
    basilar (*see also* Occlusion, artery, basilar)
      433.0
    bladder 444.89
    carotid (common) (internal) (*see also*
      Occlusion, artery, carotid) 433.1
    cerebellar (anterior inferior) (posterior
      inferior) (superior) 433.8
    cerebral (*see also* Embolism, brain) 434.1
    choroidal (anterior) 433.8
    communicating posterior 433.8
    coronary (*see also* Infarct, myocardium) 410.9
      without myocardial infarction 411.81
    extremity 444.22
      lower 444.22
      upper 444.21
    hypophyseal 433.8
    mesenteric (with gangrene) 557.0
    ophthalmic (*see also* Occlusion, retina) 362.30
    peripheral 444.22
    pontine 433.8
    precerebral NEC—*see* Occlusion, artery,
      precerebral
    pulmonary—*see* Embolism, pulmonary
    renal 593.81
    retinal (*see also* Occlusion, retina) 362.30
    specified site NEC 444.89
    vertebral (*see also* Occlusion, artery,
      vertebral) 433.2
  auditory, internal 433.8
  basilar (artery) (*see also* Occlusion, artery,
    basilar) 433.0
  birth, mother—*see* Embolism, obstetrical
  blood-clot
    with
      abortion—*see* Abortion, by type, with
        embolism
      ectopic pregnancy (*see also* categories
        633.0-633.9) 639.6
      molar pregnancy (*see also* categories
        630-632) 639.6
    following
      abortion 639.6
      ectopic or molar pregnancy 639.6
    in pregnancy, childbirth, or puerperium 673.2
  brain 434.1
    with
      abortion—*see* Abortion, by type, with
        embolism
      ectopic pregnancy (*see also* categories
        633.0-633.9) 639.6

Embolism—*continued*
    molar pregnancy (*see also* categories
        630-632) 639.6
  following
    abortion 639.6
    ectopic or molar pregnancy 639.6
  late effect—*see* Late effect(s) (of)
    cerebrovascular disease
  puerperal, postpartum, childbirth 674.0
  capillary 448.9
  cardiac (*see also* Infarct, myocardium) 410.9
  carotid (artery) (common) (internal) (*see also*
    Occlusion, artery, carotid) 433.1
  cavernous sinus (venous)—*see* Embolism,
    intracranial venous sinus
  cerebral (*see also* Embolism, brain) 434.1
  cholesterol —*see* Atheroembolism
  choroidal (anterior) (artery) 433.8
  coronary (artery or vein) (systemic) (*see also*
    Infarct, myocardium) 410.9
  without myocardial infarction 411.81
  due to (presence of) any device, implant, or
    graft classifiable to 996.0-996.5 —*see*
    Complications, due to (presence of) any
    device, implant, or graft classified to
    996.0-996.5 NEC
  encephalomalacia (*see also* Embolism, brain)
    434.1
  extremities 444.22
    lower 444.22
    upper 444.21
  eye 362.30
  fat (cerebral) (pulmonary) (systemic) 958.1
    with
      abortion—*see* Abortion, by type, with
        embolism
      ectopic pregnancy (*see also* categories
        633.0-633.9) 639.6
      molar pregnancy (*see also* categories
        630-632) 639.6
    complicating delivery or puerperium 673.8
    following
      abortion 639.6
      ectopic or molar pregnancy 639.6
    in pregnancy, childbirth, or the puerperium
      673.8
  femoral (artery) 444.22
    vein 453.8
  following
    abortion 639.6
    ectopic or molar pregnancy 639.6
    infusion, perfusion, or transfusion
      air 999.1
      thrombus 999.2
  heart (fatty) (*see also* Infarct, myocardium)
    410.9
  hepatic (vein) 453.0
  iliac (artery) 444.81
  iliofemoral 444.81
  in pregnancy, childbirth, or puerperium
    (pulmonary)—*see* Embolism, obstetrical
  intestine (artery) (vein) (with gangrene) 557.0
  intracranial (*see also* Embolism, brain) 434.1
    venous sinus (any) 325
      late effect—*see* category 326

Embolism—*continued*
  nonpyogenic 437.6
    in pregnancy or puerperium 671.5
  kidney (artery) 593.81
  lateral sinus (venous)—*see* Embolism,
    intracranial venous sinus
  longitudinal sinus (venous)—*see* Embolism,
    intracranial venous sinus
  lower extremity 444.22
  lung (massive)—*see* Embolism, pulmonary
  meninges (*see also* Embolism, brain) 434.1
  mesenteric (artery) (with gangrene) 557.0
  multiple NEC 444.9
  obstetrical (pulmonary) 673.2
    air 673.0
    amniotic fluid (pulmonary) 673.1
    blood-clot 673.2
    cardiac 674.8
    fat 673.8
    heart 674.8
    pyemic 673.3
    septic 673.3
    specified NEC 674.8
  ophthalmic (*see also* Occlusion, retina) 362.30
  paradoxical NEC 444.9
  penis 607.82
  peripheral arteries NEC 444.22
    lower 444.22
    upper 444.21
  pituitary 253.8
  popliteal (artery) 444.22
  portal (vein) 452
  postoperative NEC 997.2
    cerebral 997.02
    mesenteric artery 997.71
    other vessels 997.79
    peripheral vascular 997.2
    pulmonary 415.11
    renal artery 997.72
  precerebral artery (*see also* Occlusion, artery,
    precerebral) 433.9
  puerperal—*see* Embolism, obstetrical
  pulmonary (artery) (vein) 415.1
    with
      abortion—*see* Abortion, by type, with
        embolism
      ectopic pregnancy (*see also* categories
        633.0-633.9) 639.6
      molar pregnancy (*see also* categories
        630-632) 639.6
    following
      abortion 639.6
      ectopic or molar pregnancy 639.6
    iatrogenic 415.11
    in pregnancy, childbirth, or puerperium—*see*
      Embolism, obstetrical
    postoperative 415.11
  pyemic (multiple) 038.9
    with
      abortion—*see* Abortion, by type, with
        embolism
      ectopic pregnancy (*see also* categories
        633.0-633.9) 639.6
      molar pregnancy (*see also* categories
        630-632) 639.6
    Aerobacter aerogenes 038.49
    enteric gram-negative bacilli 038.40
    Enterobacter aerogenes 038.49
    Escherichia coli 038.42

Embolism—*continued*
  following
    abortion 639.6
    ectopic or molar pregnancy 639.6
    Hemophilus influenzae 038.41
    pneumococcal 038.2
    Proteus vulgaris 038.49
    Pseudomonas (aeruginosa) 038.43
    puerperal, postpartum, childbirth (any
      organism) 673.3
    Serratia 038.44
    specified organism NEC 038.8
    staphylococcal 038.10
      aureus 038.11
      specified organism NEC 038.19
    streptococcal 038.0
  renal (artery) 593.81
    vein 453.3
  retina, retinal (*see also* Occlusion, retina) 362.30
  saddle (aorta) 444.0
  septicemic—*see* Embolism, pyemic
  sinus—*see* Embolism, intracranial venous sinus
  soap
    with
      abortion—*see* Abortion, by type, with
        embolism
      ectopic pregnancy (*see also* categories
        633.0-633.9) 639.6
      molar pregnancy (*see also* categories
        630-632) 639.6
    following
      abortion 639.6
      ectopic or molar pregnancy 639.6
  spinal cord (nonpyogenic) 336.1
    in pregnancy or puerperium 671.5
    pyogenic origin 324.1
      late effect—*see* category 326
  spleen, splenic (artery) 444.89
  thrombus (thromboembolism) following
    infusion, perfusion, or transfusion 999.2
  upper extremity 444.21
  vein 453.9
    with inflammation or phlebitis—*see*
      Thrombophlebitis
    cerebral (*see also* Embolism, brain) 434.1
    coronary (*see also* Infarct, myocardium) 410.9
      without myocardial infarction 411.81
    hepatic 453.0
    mesenteric (with gangrene) 557.0
    portal 452
    pulmonary—*see* Embolism, pulmonary
    renal 453.3
    specified NEC 453.8
      with inflammation or phlebitis—*see*
        Thrombophlebitis
  vena cava (inferior) (superior) 453.2
  vessels of brain (*see also* Embolism, brain)
    434.1
Embolization —*see* Embolism
Embolus —*see* Embolism
Embryoma (M9080/1)—*see also* Neoplasm, by
  site, uncertain behavior
  benign (M9080/0)—*see* Neoplasm, by site,
    benign
  kidney (M8960/3) 189.0
  liver (M8970/3) 155.0
  malignant (M9080/3)—*see also* Neoplasm, by
    site, malignant
    kidney (M8960/3) 189.0
    liver (M8970/3) 155.0
    testis (M9070/3) 186.9

Embryoma—*continued*
    undescended 186.0
  testis (M9070/3) 186.9
    undescended 186.0
Embryonic
  circulation 747.9
  heart 747.9
  vas deferens 752.8
Embryopathia NEC 759.9
Embryotomy, fetal 763.89
Embryotoxon 743.43
  interfering with vision 743.42
Emesis —*see* also Vomiting
  gravidarum—*see* Hyperemesis, gravidarum
Emissions, nocturnal (semen) 608.89
Emotional
  crisis—*see* Crisis, emotional
  disorder (*see also* Disorder, mental) 300.9
  instability (excessive) 301.3
  overlay—*see* Reaction, adjustment
  upset 300.9
Emotionality, pathological 301.3
Emotogenic disease (*see also* Disorder,
  psychogenic) 306.9
Emphysema (atrophic) (centriacinar)
    (centrilobular) (chronic) (diffuse) (essential)
    (hypertrophic) (interlobular) (lung)
    (obstructive) (panlobular) (paracicatricial)
    (paracinar) (postural) (pulmonary) (senile)
    (subpleural) (traction) (unilateral) (unilobular)
    (vesicular) 492.8
  with
    bronchitis
      acute and chronic 491.21
      chronic 491.20
        with acute bronchitis or acute
          exacerbation 491.21
  bullous (giant) 492.0
  cellular tissue 958.7
    surgical 998.81
  compensatory 518.2
  congenital 770.2
  conjunctiva 372.89
  connective tissue 958.7
    surgical 998.81
  due to fumes or vapors 506.4
  eye 376.89
  eyelid 374.85
    surgical 998.81
    traumatic 958.7
  fetus or newborn (interstitial) (mediastinal)
    (unilobular) 770.2
  heart 416.9
  interstitial 518.1
    congenital 770.2
    fetus or newborn 770.2
  laminated tissue 958.7
    surgical 998.81
  mediastinal 518.1
    fetus or newborn 770.2
  newborn (interstitial) (mediastinal) (unilobular)
    770.2
  obstructive diffuse with fibrosis 492.8
  orbit 376.89
  subcutaneous 958.7
    due to trauma 958.7
    nontraumatic 518.1
    surgical 998.81
  surgical 998.81
  thymus (gland) (congenital) 254.8
  traumatic 958.7

Emphysema—*continued*
  tuberculous (*see also* Tuberculosis, pulmonary) 011.9
Employment examination (certification) V70.5
Empty sella (turcica) syndrome 253.8
Empyema (chest) (diaphragmatic) (double) (encapsulated) (general) (interlobar) (lung) (medial) (necessitatis) (perforating chest wall) (pleura) (pneumococcal) (residual) (sacculated) (streptococcal) (supradiaphragmatic) 510.9
  with fistula 510.0
  accessory sinus (chronic) (*see also* Sinusitis) 473.9
  acute 510.9
    with fistula 510.0
  antrum (chronic) (*see also* Sinusitis, maxillary) 473.0
  brain (any part) (*see also* Abscess, brain) 324.0
  ethmoidal (sinus) (chronic) (*see also* Sinusitis, ethmoidal) 473.2
  extradural (*see also* Abscess, extradural) 324.9
  frontal (sinus) (chronic) (*see also* Sinusitis, frontal) 473.1
  gallbladder (*see also* Cholecystitis, acute) 575.0
  mastoid (process) (acute) (*see also* Mastoiditis, acute) 383.00
  maxilla, maxillary 526.4
    sinus (chronic) (*see also* Sinusitis, maxillary) 473.0
  nasal sinus (chronic) (*see also* Sinusitis) 473.9
  sinus (accessory) (nasal) (*see also* Sinusitis) 473.9
  sphenoidal (chronic) (sinus) (*see also* Sinusitis, sphenoidal) 473.3
  subarachnoid (*see also* Abscess, extradural) 324.9
  subdural (*see also* Abscess, extradural) 324.9
  tuberculous (*see also* Tuberculosis, pleura) 012.0
  ureter (*see also* Ureteritis) 593.89
  ventricular (*see also* Abscess, brain) 324.0
Enameloma 520.2
Encephalitis (bacterial) (chronic) (hemorrhagic) (idiopathic) (nonepidemic) (spurious) (subacute) 323.9
  acute—*see also* Encephalitis, viral
    disseminated (postinfectious) NEC 136.9 *[323.6]*
      postimmunization or postvaccination 323.5
    inclusional 049.8
    inclusion body 049.8
    necrotizing 049.8
  arboviral, arbovirus NEC 064
  arthropod-borne (*see also* Encephalitis, viral, arthropod-borne) 064
  Australian X 062.4
  Bwamba fever 066.3
  California (virus) 062.5
  Central European 063.2
  Czechoslovakian 063.2
  Dawson's (inclusion body) 046.2
  diffuse sclerosing 046.2
  due to
    actinomycosis 039.8 *[323.4]*
    cat-scratch disease 078.3 *[323.0]*
    infectious mononucleosis 075 *[323.0]*
    malaria (*see also* Malaria) 084.6 *[323.2]*
    Negishi virus 064
    ornithosis 073.7 *[323.0]*

Encephalitis—*continued*
  prophylactic inoculation against smallpox 323.5
  rickettsiosis (*see also* Rickettsiosis) 083.9 *[323.1]*
  rubella 056.01
  toxoplasmosis (acquired) 130.0
    congenital (active) 771.2 *[323.4]*
  typhus (fever) (*see also* Typhus) 081.9 *[323.1]*
  vaccination (smallpox) 323.5
  Eastern equine 062.2
  endemic 049.8
  epidemic 049.8
  equine (acute) (infectious) (viral) 062.9
    Eastern 062.2
    Venezuelan 066.2
    Western 062.1
  Far Eastern 063.0
  following vaccination or other immunization procedure 323.5
  herpes 054.3
  Ilheus (virus) 062.8
  inclusion body 046.2
  infectious (acute) (virus) NEC 049.8
  influenzal 487.8 *[323.4]*
    lethargic 049.8
  Japanese (B type) 062.0
  La Crosse 062.5
  Langat 063.8
  late effect—*see* Late, effect, encephalitis
  lead 984.9 *[323.7]*
  lethargic (acute) (infectious) (influenzal) 049.8
  lethargica 049.8
  louping ill 063.1
  lupus 710.0 *[323.8]*
  lymphatica 049.0
  Mengo 049.8
  meningococcal 036.1
  mumps 072.2
  Murray Valley 062.4
  myoclonic 049.8
  Negishi virus 064
  otitic NEC 382.4 *[323.4]*
  parasitic NEC 123.9 *[323.4]*
  periaxialis (concentrica) (diffusa) 341.1
  postchickenpox 052.0
  postexanthematous NEC 057.9 *[323.6]*
  postimmunization 323.5
  postinfectious NEC 136.9 *[323.6]*
  postmeasles 055.0
  posttraumatic 323.8
  postvaccinal (smallpox) 323.5
  postvaricella 052.0
  postviral NEC 079.99 *[323.6]*
    postexanthematous 057.9 *[323.6]*
      specified NEC 057.8 *[323.6]*
  Powassan 063.8
  progressive subcortical (Binswanger's) 290.12
  Rio Bravo 049.8
  rubella 056.01
  Russian
    autumnal 062.0
    spring-summer type (taiga) 063.0
  saturnine 984.9 *[323.7]*
  Semliki Forest 062.8
  serous 048
  slow-acting virus NEC 046.8
  specified cause NEC 323.8
  St. Louis type 062.3
  subacute sclerosing 046.2
  subcorticalis chronica 290.12

Encephalopathy—*continued*
  lead 984.9 *[323.7]*
  leukopolio 330.0
  metabolic (toxic)—*see* Delirium
  necrotizing, subacute 330.8
  pellagrous 265.2
  portal-systemic 572.2
  postcontusional 310.2
  posttraumatic 310.2
  saturnine 984.9 *[323.7]*
  spongioform, subacute (viral) 046.1
  subacute
    necrotizing 330.8
    spongioform 046.1
    viral, spongioform 046.1
  subcortical progressive (Schilder) 341.1
    chronic (Binswanger's) 290.12
  toxic 349.82
    metabolic—*see* Delirium
  traumatic (postconcussional) 310.2
    current (*see also* Concussion, brain) 850.9
      with skull fracture—*see* Fracture, skull, by
        site, with intracranial injury
  vitamin B deficiency NEC 266.9
  Wernicke's (superior hemorrhagic
    polioencephalitis) 265.1
Enchephalorrhagia (*see also* Hemorrhage,
  brain) 432.9
  healed or old V12.59
  late effect—*see* Late effect(s) (of)
    cerebrovascular disease
Encephalosis, posttraumatic 310.2
Enchondroma (M9220/0)—*see also* Neoplasm,
  bone, benign
  multiple, congenital 756.4
Enchondromatosis (cartilaginous) (congenital)
  (multiple) 756.4
Enchondroses, multiple (cartilaginous)
  (congenital) 756.4
Encopresis (*see also* Incontinence, feces) 787.6
  nonorganic origin 307.7
Encounter for —*see also* Admission for
  administrative purpose only V68.9
    referral of patient without examination or
      treatment V68.81
    specified purpose NEC V68.89
  chemotherapy V58.1
  end-of-life care V66.7
  hospice care V66.7
  palliative care V66.7
  radiotherapy V58.0
  screening mammogram NEC V76.12
    for high-risk patient V76.11
  paternity testing V70.4
  terminal care V66.7
Encystment —*see* Cyst
End-of-life care V66.7
Endamebiasis —*see* Amebiasis
Endamoeba —*see* Amebiasis
Endarteritis (bacterial, subacute) (infective)
  (septic) 447.6
  brain, cerebral or cerebrospinal 437.4
    late effect—*see* Late effect(s) (of)
      cerebrovascular disease
  coronary (artery) —*see* Arteriosclerosis,
    coronary
  deformans—*see* Arteriosclerosis
  embolic (*see also* Embolism) 444.9
  obliterans—*see also* Arteriosclerosis
    pulmonary 417.8
  pulmonary 417.8

Endarteritis—*continued*
  retina 362.18
  senile—*see* Arteriosclerosis
  syphilitic 093.89
    brain or cerebral 094.89
    congenital 090.5
    spinal 094.89
  tuberculous (*see also* Tuberculosis) 017.9
Endemic —*see* condition
Endocarditis (chronic) (indeterminate)
  (interstitial) (marantis) (nonbacterial
  thrombotic) (residual) (sclerotic) (sclerous)
  (senile) (valvular) 424.90
  with
    rheumatic fever (conditions classifiable to 390)
      active—*see* Endocarditis, acute, rheumatic
      inactive or quiescent (with chorea) 397.9
  acute or subacute 421.9
    rheumatic (aortic) (mitral) (pulmonary)
      (tricuspid) 391.1
      with chorea (acute) (rheumatic)
        (Sydenham's) 392.0
  aortic (heart) (nonrheumatic) (valve) 424.1
    with
      mitral (valve) disease 396.9
        active or acute 391.1
          with chorea (acute) (rheumatic)
            (Sydenham's) 392.0
      rheumatic fever (conditions classifiable to
        390)
        active—*see* Endocarditis, acute, rheumatic
        inactive or quiescent (with chorea) 395.9
          with mitral disease 396.9
  acute or subacute 421.9
  arteriosclerotic 424.1
  congenital 746.89
  hypertensive 424.1
  rheumatic (chronic) (inactive) 395.9
    with mitral (valve) disease 396.9
      active or acute 391.1
        with chorea (acute) (rheumatic)
          (Sydenham's) 392.0
      active or acute 391.1
        with chorea (acute) (rheumatic)
          (Sydenham's) 392.0
  specified cause, except rheumatic 424.1
  syphilitic 093.22
  arteriosclerotic or due to arteriosclerosis 424.99
  atypical verrucous (Libman-Sacks) 710.0
    [424.91]
  bacterial (acute) (any valve) (chronic)
    (subacute) 421.0
  blastomycotic 116.0 *[421.1]*
  candidal 112.81
  congenital 425.3
  constrictive 421.0
  Coxsackie 074.22
  due to
    blastomycosis 116.0 *[421.1]*
    candidiasis 112.81
    Coxsackie (virus) 074.22
    disseminated lupus erythematosus 710.0
      [424.91]
    histoplasmosis (*see also* Histoplasmosis)
      115.94
    hypertension (benign) 424.99
    moniliasis 112.81
    prosthetic cardiac valve 996.61
    Q fever 083.0 *[421.1]*
    serratia marcescens 421.0
    typhoid (fever) 002.0 *[421.1]*

Endocarditis—*continued*
  fetal 425.3
  gonococcal 098.84
  hypertensive 424.99
  infectious or infective (acute) (any valve)
    (chronic) (subacute) 421.0
  lenta (acute) (any valve) (chronic) (subacute)
    421.0
  Libman-Sacks 710.0 *[424.91]*
  Loeffler's (parietal fibroplastic) 421.0
  malignant (acute) (any valve) (chronic)
    (subacute) 421.0
  meningococcal 036.42
  mitral (chronic) (double) (fibroid) (heart)
    (inactive) (valve) (with chorea) 394.9
    with
      aortic (valve) disease 396.9
        active or acute 391.1
          with chorea (acute) (rheumatic)
            (Sydenham's) 392.0
        rheumatic fever (conditions classifiable to
          390)
          active—*see* Endocarditis, acute, rheumatic
          inactive or quiescent (with chorea) 394.9
            with aortic valve disease 396.9
    active or acute 391.1
      bacterial 421.0
      with chorea (acute) (rheumatic)
        (Sydenham's) 392.0
    arteriosclerotic 424.0
    congenital 746.89
    hypertensive 424.0
    nonrheumatic 424.0
      acute or subacute 421.9
    syphilitic 093.21
  monilial 112.81
  mycotic (acute) (any valve) (chronic) (subacute)
    421.0
  pneumococcic (acute) (any valve) (chronic)
    (subacute) 421.0
  pulmonary (chronic) (heart) (valve) 424.3
    with
      rheumatic fever (conditions classifiable to
        390)
        active—*see* Endocarditis, acute, rheumatic
        inactive or quiescent (with chorea) 397.1
    acute or subacute 421.9
      rheumatic 391.1
        with chorea (acute) (rheumatic)
          (Sydenham's) 392.0
    arteriosclerotic or due to arteriosclerosis 424.3
    congenital 746.09
    hypertensive or due to hypertension (benign)
      424.3
    rheumatic (chronic) (inactive) (with chorea)
      397.1
      active or acute 391.1
        with chorea (acute) (rheumatic)
          (Sydenham's) 392.0
    syphilitic 093.24
  purulent (acute) (any valve) (chronic)
    (subacute) 421.0
  rheumatic (chronic) (inactive) (with chorea)
    397.9
    active or acute (aortic) (mitral) (pulmonary)
      (tricuspid) 391.1
      with chorea (acute) (rheumatic)
        (Sydenham's) 392.0
  septic (acute) (any valve) (chronic) (subacute)
    421.0
  specified cause, except rheumatic 424.99

Endocarditis—*continued*
  streptococcal (acute) (any valve) (chronic)
    (subacute) 421.0
  subacute—*see* Endocarditis, acute
  suppurative (any valve) (acute) (chronic)
    (subacute) 421.0
  syphilitic NEC 093.20
  toxic (*see also* Endocarditis, acute) 421.9
  tricuspid (chronic) (heart) (inactive) (rheumatic)
    (valve) (with chorea) 397.0
    with
      rheumatic fever (conditions classifiable to
        390)
        active—*see* Endocarditis, acute, rheumatic
        inactive or quiescent (with chorea) 397.0
    active or acute 391.1
      with chorea (acute) (rheumatic)
        (Sydenham's) 392.0
    arteriosclerotic 424.2
    congenital 746.89
    hypertensive 424.2
    nonrheumatic 424.2
      acute or subacute 421.9
    specified cause, except rheumatic 424.2
    syphilitic 093.23
  tuberculous (*see also* Tuberculosis) 017.9
    [424.91]
  typhoid 002.0 *[421.1]*
  ulcerative (acute) (any valve) (chronic)
    (subacute) 421.0
  vegetative (acute) (any valve) (chronic)
    (subacute) 421.0
  verrucous (acute) (any valve) (chronic)
    (subacute) NEC 710.0 *[424.91]*
    nonbacterial 710.0 *[424.91]*
    nonrheumatic 710.0 *[424.91]*
Endocardium, endocardial —*see also* condition
  cushion defect 745.60
    specified type NEC 745.69
Endocervicitis (*see also* Cervicitis) 616.0
  due to
    intrauterine (contraceptive) device 996.65
  gonorrheal (acute) 098.15
    chronic or duration of 2 months or over 098.35
  hyperplastic 616.0
  syphilitic 095.8
  trichomonal 131.09
  tuberculous (*see also* Tuberculosis) 016.7
Endocrine —*see* condition
Endocrinopathy, pluriglandular 258.9
Endodontitis 522.0
Endomastoiditis (*see also* Mastoiditis) 383.9
Endometrioma 617.9
Endometriosis 617.9
  appendix 617.5
  bladder 617.8
  bowel 617.5
  broad ligament 617.3
  cervix 617.0
  colon 617.5
  cul-de-sac (Douglas') 617.3
  exocervix 617.0
  fallopian tube 617.2
  female genital organ NEC 617.8
  gallbladder 617.8
  in scar of skin 617.6
  internal 617.0
  intestine 617.5
  lung 617.8
  myometrium 617.0
  ovary 617.1

Enteritis (acute) (catarrhal) (choleraic) (chronic)
　　(congestive) (diarrheal) (exudative)
　　(follicular) (hemorrhagic) (infantile)
　　(lienteric) (noninfectious) (perforative)
　　(phlegmonous) (presumed noninfectious)
　　(pseudomembranous) 558.9
　adaptive 564.9
　aertrycke infection 003.0
　allergic 558.3
　amebic (*see also* Amebiasis) 006.9
　　with abscess—*see* Abscess, amebic
　　acute 006.0
　　　with abscess—*see* Abscess, amebic
　　　nondysenteric 006.2
　　chronic 006.1
　　　with abscess—*see* Abscess, amebic
　　　nondysenteric 006.2
　　nondysenteric 006.2
　anaerobic (cocci) (gram-negative)
　　(gram-positive) (mixed) NEC 008.46
　bacillary NEC 004.9
　bacterial NEC 008.5
　　specified NEC 008.49
　Bacteroides (fragilis) (melaninogeniscus)
　　(oralis) 008.46
　Butyrivibrio (fibriosolvens) 008.46
　Campylobacter 008.43
　Candida 112.85
　Chilomastix 007.8
　choleriformis 001.1
　chronic 558.9
　　ulcerative (*see also* Colitis, ulcerative) 556.9
　cicatrizing (chronic) 555.0
　Clostridium
　　botulinum 005.1
　　difficile 008.45
　　haemolyticum 008.46
　　novyi 008.46
　　perfringens (C) (F) 008.46
　　specified type NEC 008.46
　coccidial 007.2
　dietetic 558.9
　due to
　　achylia gastrica 536.8
　　adenovirus 008.62
　　Aerobacter aerogenes 008.2
　　anaerobes—*see* Enteritis, anaerobic 008.46
　　Arizona (bacillus) 008.1
　　astrovirus 008.66
　　Bacillus coli—*see* Enteritis, E. coli 008.0
　　bacteria NEC 008.5
　　　specified NEC 008.49
　　Bacteroides 008.46
　　Butyrivibrio (fibriosolvens) 008.46
　　Calcivirus 008.65
　　Campylobacter 008.43
　　Clostridium—*see* Enteritis, Clostridium
　　Cockle agent 008.64
　　Coxsackie (virus) 008.67
　　Ditchling agent 008.64
　　ECHO virus 008.67
　　Enterobacter aerogenes 008.2
　　enterococci 008.49
　　enterovirus NEC 008.67
　　Escherichia coli—*see* Enteritis, E. coli
　　Eubacterium 008.46
　　Fusobacterium (nucleatum) 008.46
　　gram-negative bacteria NEC 008.47
　　　anaerobic NEC 008.46

Enteritis—*continued*
　Hawaii agent 008.63
　irritating foods 558.9
　Klebsiella aerogenes 008.47
　Marin County agent 008.66
　Montgomery County agent 008.63
　Norwalk-like agent 008.63
　Norwalk virus 008.63
　Otofuke agent 008.63
　Paracolobactrum arizonae 008.1
　paracolon bacillus NEC 008.47
　　Arizona 008.1
　Paramatta agent 008.64
　Peptococcus 008.46
　Peptostreptococcus 008.46
　Propionibacterium 008.46
　Proteus (bacillus) (mirabilis) (morganii) 008.3
　Pseudomonas aeruginosa 008.42
　radiation 558.1
　Rotavirus 008.61
　Sapporo agent 008.63
　small round virus (SRV) NEC 008.64
　　featureless NEC 008.63
　　structured NEC 008.63
　Snow Mountain (SM) agent 008.63
　specified
　　bacteria NEC 008.49
　　organism, nonbacterial NEC 008.8
　　virus NEC 008.69
　Staphylococcus 008.41
　Streptococcus 008.49
　　anaerobic 008.46
　Taunton agent 008.63
　Torovirus 008.69
　Treponema 008.46
　Veillonella 008.46
　virus 008.8
　　specified type NEC 008.69
　Wollan (W) agent 008.64
　Yersinia enterocolitica 008.44
　dysentery—*see* Dysentery
　E. coli 008.00
　　enterohemorrhagic 008.04
　　enteroinvasive 008.03
　　enteropathogenic 008.01
　　enterotoxigenic 008.02
　　specified type NEC 008.09
　el tor 001.1
　embadomonial 007.8
　epidemic 009.0
　Eubacterium 008.46
　fermentative 558.9
　fulminant 557.0
　Fusobacterium (nucleatum) 008.46
　gangrenous (*see also* Enteritis, due to, by
　　organism) 009.0
　giardial 007.1
　gram-negative bacteria NEC 008.47
　　anaerobic NEC 008.46
　infectious NEC (*see also* Enteritis, due to, by
　　organism) 009.0
　　presumed 009.1
　influenzal 487.8
　ischemic 557.9
　　acute 557.0
　　chronic 557.1
　　due to mesenteric artery insufficiency 557.1
　membranous 564.9
　mucous 564.9
　myxomembranous 564.9

Enteritis—*continued*
  necrotic (*see also* Enteritis, due to, by organism)
    009.0
  necroticans 005.2
  necrotizing of fetus or newborn 777.5
  neurogenic 564.9
  newborn 777.8
    necrotizing 777.5
  parasitic NEC 129
  paratyphoid (fever) (*see also* Fever,
    paratyphoid) 002.9
  Peptococcus 008.46
  Peptostreptococcus 008.46
  Propionibacterium 008.46
  protozoal NEC 007.9
  regional (of) 555.9
    intestine
      large (bowel, colon, or rectum) 555.1
        with small intestine 555.2
      small (duodenum, ileum, or jejunum) 555.0
        with large intestine 555.2
  Salmonella infection 003.0
  salmonellosis 003.0
  segmental (*see also* Enteritis, regional) 555.9
  septic (*see also* Enteritis, due to, by organism)
    009.0
  Shigella 004.9
  simple 558.9
  spasmodic 564.9
  spastic 564.9
  staphylococcal 008.41
    due to food 005.0
  streptococcal 008.49
    anaerobic 008.46
  toxic 558.2
  Treponema (denticola) (macrodentium) 008.46
  trichomonal 007.3
  tuberculous (*see also* Tuberculosis) 014.8
  typhosa 002.0
  ulcerative (chronic) (*see also* Colitis, ulcerative)
    556.9
  Veillonella 008.46
  viral 008.8
    adenovirus 008.62
    enterovirus 008.67
    specified virus NEC 008.69
  Yersinia enterocolitica 008.44
  zymotic 009.0
Enteroarticular syndrome 099.3
Enterobiasis 127.4
Enterobius vermicularis 127.4
Enterocele (*see also* Hernia) 553.9
  pelvis, pelvic (acquired) (congenital) 618.6
  vagina, vaginal (acquired) (congenital) 618.6
Enterocolitis —*see also* Enteritis
  fetus or newborn 777.8
    necrotizing 777.5
  fulminant 557.0
  granulomatous 555.2
  hemorrhagic (acute) 557.0
    chronic 557.1
  necrotizing (acute) (membranous) 557.0
  primary necrotizing 777.5
  pseudomembranous 008.45
  radiation 558.1
    newborn 777.5
  ulcerative 556.0
Enterocystoma 751.5
Enterogastritis —*see* Enteritis
Enterogenous cyanosis 289.7

Enterolith, enterolithiasis (impaction) 560.39
  with hernia—*see also* Hernia, by site, with
    obstruction
    gangrenous—*see* Hernia, by site, with
      gangrene
Enteropathy 569.9
  exudative (of Gordon) 579.8
  gluten 579.0
  hemorrhagic, terminal 557.0
  protein-losing 579.8
Enteroperitonitis (*see also* Peritonitis) 567.9
Enteroptosis 569.89
Enterorrhagia 578.9
Enterospasm 564.9
  psychogenic 306.4
Enterostenosis (*see also* Obstruction, intestine)
  560.9
Enterostomy status V44.4
  with complication 569.60
Enthesopathy 726.39
  ankle and tarsus 726.70
  elbow region 726.30
    specified NEC 726.39
  hip 726.5
  knee 726.60
  peripheral NEC 726.8
  shoulder region 726.10
    adhesive 726.0
  spinal 720.1
  wrist and carpus 726.4
Entrance, air into vein —*see* Embolism, air
Entrapment, nerve —*see* Neuropathy,
  entrapment
Entropion (eyelid) 374.00
  cicatricial 374.04
  congenital 743.62
  late effect of trachoma (healed) 139.1
  mechanical 374.02
  paralytic 374.02
  senile 374.01
  spastic 374.03
Enucleation of eye (current) (traumatic) 871.3
Enuresis 788.30
  habit disturbance 307.6
  nocturnal 788.36
    psychogenic 307.6
  nonorganic origin 307.6
  psychogenic 307.6
Enzymopathy 277.9
Eosinopenia 288.0
Eosinophilia 288.3
  allergic 288.3
  hereditary 288.3
  idiopathic 288.3
  infiltrative 518.3
  Loeffler's 518.3
  myalgia syndrome 710.5
  pulmonary (tropical) 518.3
  secondary 288.3
  tropical 518.3
Eosinophilic —*see also* condition
  fasciitis 728.89
  granuloma (bone) 277.8
  infiltration lung 518.3
Ependymitis (acute) (cerebral) (chronic)
  (granular) (*see also* Meningitis) 322.9
Ependymoblastoma (M9392/3)
  specified site—*see* Neoplasm, by site, malignant
  unspecified site 191.9

Ependymoma (epithelial) (malignant) (M9391/3)
  anaplastic type (M9392/3)
    specified site—*see* Neoplasm, by site,
      malignant
    unspecified site 191.9
  benign (M9391/0)
    specified site—*see* Neoplasm, by site, benign
    unspecified site 225.0
  myxopapillary (M9394/1) 237.5
  papillary (M9393/1) 237.5
  specified site—*see* Neoplasm, by site, malignant
  unspecified site 191.9
Ependymopathy 349.2
  spinal cord 349.2
Ephelides, ephelis 709.09
Ephemeral fever (*see also* Pyrexia) 780.6
Epiblepharon (congenital) 743.62
Epicanthus, epicanthic fold (congenital)
  (eyelid) 743.63
Epicondylitis (elbow) (lateral) 726.32
  medial 726.31
Epicystitis (*see also* Cystitis) 595.9
Epidemic —*see* condition
Epidermidalization, cervix —*see* condition
Epidermidization, cervix *see* condition
Epidermis, epidermal —*see* condition
Epidermization, cervix —*see* condition
Epidermodysplasia verruciformis 078.19
Epidermoid
  cholesteatoma—*see* Cholesteatoma
  inclusion (*see also* Cyst, skin) 706.2
Epidermolysis
  acuta (combustiformis) (toxica) 695.1
  bullosa 757.39
  necroticans combustiformis 695.1
    due to drug
      correct substance properly administered
        695.1
      overdose or wrong substance given or taken
        977.9
      specified drug—*see* Table of drugs and
        chemicals
Epidermophytid —*see* Dermatophytosis
Epidermophytosis (infected)—*see*
  Dermatophytosis
Epidermosis, ear (middle) (*see also*
  Cholesteatoma) 385.30
Epididymis —*see* condition
Epididymitis (nonvenereal) 604.90
  with abscess 604.0
  acute 604.99
  blennorrhagic (acute) 098.0
    chronic or duration of 2 months or over 098.2
  caseous (*see also* Tuberculosis) 016.4
  chlamydial 099.54
  diphtheritic 032.89 *[604.91]*
  filarial 125.9 *[604.91]*
  gonococcal (acute) 098.0
    chronic or duration of 2 months or over 098.2
  recurrent 604.99
  residual 604.99
  syphilitic 095.8 *[604.91]*
  tuberculous (*see also* Tuberculosis) 016.4
Epididymo-orchitis (*see also* Epididymitis)
  604.90
  with abscess 604.0
  chlamydial 099.54
  gonococcal (acute) 098.13
    chronic or duration of 2 months or over 098.33
Epidural —*see* condition
Epigastritis (*see also* Gastritis) 535.5

Epigastrium, epigastric —*see* condition
Epigastrocele (*see also* Hernia, epigastric) 553.29
Epiglottiditis (acute) 464.30
  with obstruction 464.31
  chronic 476.1
  viral 464.30
    with obstruction 464.31
Epiglottis —*see* condition
Epiglottitis (acute) 464.30
  with obstruction 464.31
  chronic 476.1
  viral 464.30
    with obstruction 464.31
Epignathus 759.4
Epilepsia
  partialis continua (*see also* Epilepsy) 345.7
  procursiva (*see also* Epilepsy) 345.8
Epilepsy, epileptic (idiopathic) 345.9

---

*Note—use the following fifth-digit
subclassification with categories 345.0, 345.1,
345.4-345.9*

0   without mention of intractable epilepsy
1   with intractable epilepsy

---

  abdominal 345.5
  absence (attack) 345.0
  akinetic 345.0
    psychomotor 345.4
  automatism 345.4
  autonomic diencephalic 345.5
  brain 345.9
  Bravais-Jacksonian 345.5
  cerebral 345.9
  climacteric 345.9
  clonic 345.1
  clouded state 345.9
  coma 345.3
  communicating 345.4
  congenital 345.9
  convulsions 345.9
  cortical (focal) (motor) 345.5
  cursive (running) 345.8
  cysticercosis 123.1
  deterioration
    with behavioral disturbance 345.9 *[294.11]*
    without behavioral disturbance 345.9 *[294.10]*
  due to syphilis 094.89
  equivalent 345.5
  fit 345.9
  focal (motor) 345.5
  gelastic 345.8
  generalized 345.9
    convulsive 345.1
    flexion 345.1
    nonconvulsive 345.0
  grand mal (idiopathic) 345.1
  Jacksonian (motor) (sensory) 345.5
  Kojevnikoff's, Kojevnikov's, Kojewnikoff's
    345.7
  laryngeal 786.2
  limbic system 345.4
  major (motor) 345.1
  minor 345.0
  mixed (type) 345.9
  motor partial 345.5
  musicogenic 345.1
  myoclonus, myoclonic 345.1
    progressive (familial) 333.2
  nonconvulsive, generalized 345.0

Epilepsy, epileptic—*continued*
  parasitic NEC 123.9
  partial (focalized) 345.5
    with
      impairment of consciousness 345.4
      memory and ideational disturbances 345.4
    abdominal type 345.5
    motor type 345.5
    psychomotor type 345.4
    psychosensory type 345.4
    secondarily generalized 345.4
    sensory type 345.5
    somatomotor type 345.5
    somatosensory type 345.5
    temporal lobe type 345.4
    visceral type 345.5
    visual type 345.5
  peripheral 345.9
  petit mal 345.0
  photokinetic 345.8
  progressive myoclonic (familial) 333.2
  psychic equivalent 345.5
  psychomotor 345.4
  psychosensory 345.4
  reflex 345.1
  seizure 345.9
  senile 345.9
  sensory-induced 345.5
  sleep 347
  somatomotor type 345.5
  somatosensory 345.5
  specified type NEC 345.8
  status (grand mal) 345.3
    focal motor 345.7
    petit mal 345.2
    psychomotor 345.7
    temporal lobe 345.7
  symptomatic 345.9
  temporal lobe 345.4
  tonic (-clonic) 345.1
  traumatic (injury unspecified) 907.0
    injury specified—*see* Late, effect (of)
      specified injury
  twilight 293.0
  uncinate (gyrus) 345.4
  Unverricht (-Lundborg) (familial myoclonic)
    333.2
  visceral 345.5
  visual 345.5
Epileptiform
  convulsions 780.39
  seizure 780.39
Epiloia 759.5
Epimenorrhea 626.2
Epipharyngitis (*see also* Nasopharyngitis) 460
Epiphora 375.20
  due to
    excess lacrimation 375.21
    insufficient drainage 375.22
Epiphyseal arrest 733.91
  femoral head 732.2
Epiphyseolysis, epiphysiolysis (*see also*
  Osteochondrosis) 732.9
Epiphysitis (*see also* Osteochondrosis) 732.9
  juvenile 732.6
  marginal (Scheuermann's) 732.0
  os calcis 732.5
  syphilitic (congenital) 090.0
  vertebral (Scheuermann's) 732.0
Epiplocele (*see also* Hernia) 553.9
Epiploitis (*see also* Peritonitis) 567.9

Epiplosarcomphalocele (*see also* Hernia,
  umbilicus) 553.1
Episcleritis 379.00
  gouty 274.89 *[379.09]*
  nodular 379.02
  periodica fugax 379.01
    angioneurotic—*see* Edema, angioneurotic
  specified NEC 379.09
  staphylococcal 379.00
  suppurative 379.00
  syphilitic 095.0
  tuberculous (*see also* Tuberculosis) 017.3
    [379.09]
Episode
  brain (*see also* Disease, cerebrovascular, acute)
    436
  cerebral (*see also* Disease, cerebrovascular,
    acute) 436
  depersonalization (in neurotic state) 300.6
  hyporesponsive 780.09
  psychotic (*see also* Psychosis) 298.9
    organic, transient 293.9
  schizophrenic (acute) NEC (*see also*
    Schizophrenia) 295.4
Epispadias
  female 753.8
  male 752.62
Episplenitis 289.59
Epistaxis (multiple) 784.7
  hereditary 448.0
  vicarious menstruation 625.8
Epithelioma (malignant) (M8011/3)—*see also*
  Neoplasm, by site, malignant
  adenoides cysticum (M8100/0)—*see* Neoplasm,
    skin, benign
  basal cell (M8090/3)—*see* Neoplasm, skin,
    malignant
  benign (M8011/0)—*see* Neoplasm, by site,
    benign
  Bowen's (M8081/2)—*see* Neoplasm, skin, in
    situ
  calcifying (benign) (Malherbe's)
    (M8110/0)—*see* Neoplasm, skin, benign
  external site—*see* Neoplasm, skin, malignant
  intraepidermal, Jadassohn (M8096/0)—*see*
    Neoplasm, skin, benign
  squamous cell (M8070/3)—*see* Neoplasm, by
    site, malignant
Epitheliopathy
  pigment, retina 363.15
  posterior multifocal placoid (acute) 363.15
Epithelium, epithelial —*see* condition
Epituberculosis (allergic) (with atelectasis) (*see*
  also Tuberculosis) 010.8
Eponychia 757.5
Epstein's
  nephrosis or syndrome (*see also* Nephrosis)
    581.9
  pearl (mouth) 528.4
Epstein-Barr infection (viral) 075
  chronic 780.79 *[139.8]*
Epulis (giant cell) (gingiva) 523.8
Equinia 024
Equinovarus (congenital) 754.51
  acquired 736.71
Equivalent
  convulsive (abdominal) (*see also* Epilepsy)
    345.5
  epileptic (psychic) (*see also* Epilepsy) 345.5

Erb's
  disease 359.1
  palsy, paralysis (birth) (brachial) (newborn)
      767.6
    spinal (spastic) syphilitic 094.89
  pseudohypertrophic muscular dystrophy 359.1
Erb (-Duchenne) paralysis (birth injury)
      (newborn) 767.6
Erb-Goldflam disease or syndrome 358.0
Erdheim's syndrome (acromegalic
      macrospondylitis) 253.0
Erection, painful (persistent) 607.3
Ergosterol deficiency (vitamin D) 268.9
  with
      osteomalacia 268.2
      rickets (*see also* Rickets) 268.0
Ergotism (ergotized grain) 988.2
  from ergot used as drug (migraine therapy)
      correct substance properly administered
          349.82
      overdose or wrong substance given or taken
          975.0
Erichsen's disease (railway spine) 300.16
Erlacher-Blount syndrome (tibia vara) 732.4
Erosio interdigitalis blastomycetica 112.3
Erosion
  arteriosclerotic plaque—*see* Arteriosclerosis, by
      site
  artery NEC 447.2
    without rupture 447.8
  bone 733.99
  bronchus 519.1
  cartilage (joint) 733.99
  cervix (uteri) (acquired) (chronic) (congenital)
      622.0
    with mention of cervicitis 616.0
  cornea (recurrent) (*see also* Keratitis) 371.42
    traumatic 918.1
  dental (idiopathic) (occupational) 521.3
  duodenum, postpyloric—*see* Ulcer, duodenum
  esophagus 530.89
  gastric 535.4
  intestine 569.89
  lymphatic vessel 457.8
  pylorus, pyloric (ulcer) 535,4
  sclera 379.16
  spine, aneurysmal 094.89
  spleen 289.59
  stomach 535.4
  teeth (idiopathic) (occupational) 521.3
    due to
        medicine 521.3
        persistent vomiting 521.3
  urethra 599.84
  uterus 621.8
  vertebra 733.99
Erotomania 302.89
  Clérambault's 297.8
Error
  in diet 269.9
  refractive 367.9
    astigmatism (*see also* Astigmatism) 367.20
    drug-induced 367.89
    hypermetropia 367.0
    hyperopia 367.0
    myopia 367.1
    presbyopia 367.4
    toxic 367.89
Eructation 787.3
  nervous 306.4
  psychogenic 306.4

Eruption
  creeping 126.9
  drug—*see* Dermatitis, due to, drug
  Hutchinson, summer 692.72
  Kaposi's varicelliform 054.0
  napkin (psoriasiform) 691.0
  polymorphous
    light (sun) 692.72
      other source 692.82
  psoriasiform, napkin 691.0
  recalcitrant pustular 694.8
  ringed 695.89
  skin (*see also* Dermatitis) 782.1
    creeping (meaning hookworm) 126.9
    due to
        chemical(s) NEC 692.4
          internal use 693.8
        drug—*see* Dermatitis, due to, drug
        prophylactic inoculation or vaccination
            against disease—*see* Dermatitis, due to,
            vaccine
        smallpox vaccination NEC—*see* Dermatitis,
            due to, vaccine
    erysipeloid 027.1
    feigned 698.4
    Hutchinson, summer 692.72
    Kaposi's, varicelliform 054.0
      vaccinia 999.0
    lichenoid, axilla 698.3
    polymorphous, due to light 692.72
    toxic NEC 695.0
    vesicular 709.8
  teeth, tooth
    accelerated 520.6
    delayed 520.6
    difficult 520.6
    disturbance of 520.6
    in abnormal sequence 520.6
    incomplete 520.6
    late 520.6
    natal 520.6
    neonatal 520.6
    obstructed 520.6
    partial 520.6
    persistent primary 520.6
    premature 520.6
  vesicular 709.8
Erysipelas (gangrenous) (infantile) (newborn)
      (phlegmonous) (suppurative) 035
  external ear 035 *[380.13]*
  puerperal, postpartum, childbirth 670
Erysipelatoid (Rosenbach's) 027.1
Erysipeloid (Rosenbach's) 027.1
Erythema, erythematous (generalized) 695.9
  ab igne—*see* Burn, by site, first degree
  annulare (centrifugum) (rheumaticum) 695.0
  arthriticum epidemicum 026.1
  brucellum (*see also* Brucellosis) 023.9
  bullosum 695.1
  caloricum—*see* Burn, by site, first degree
  chronicum migrans 088.81
    chronicum 088.81
  circinatum 695.1
  diaper 691.0
  due to
    chemical (contact) NEC 692.4
      internal 693.8
    drug (internal use) 693.0
        contact 692.3

Erythema, erythematous—*continued*
  elevatum diutinum 695.89
  endemic 265.2
  epidemic, arthritic 026.1
  figuratum perstans 695.0
  gluteal 691.0
  gyratum (perstans) (repens) 695.1
  heat—*see* Burn, by site, first degree
  ichthyosiforme congenitum 757.1
  induratum (primary) (scrofulosorum) (*see also*
      Tuberculosis) 017.1
    nontuberculous 695.2
  infantum febrile 057.8
  infectional NEC 695.9
  infectiosum 057.0
  inflammation NEC 695.9
  intertrigo 695.89
  iris 695.1
  lupus (discoid) (localized) (*see also* Lupus,
      erythematosus) 695.4
  marginatum 695.0
    rheumaticum—*see* Fever, rheumatic
  medicamentosum—*see* Dermatitis, due to, drug
  migrans 529.1
  multiforme 695.1
    bullosum 695.1
    conjunctiva 695.1
    exudativum (Hebra) 695.1
    pemphigoides 694.5
  napkin 691.0
  neonatorum 778.8
  nodosum 695.2
    tuberculous (*see also* Tuberculosis) 017.1
  nummular, nummulare 695.1
  palmar 695.0
  palmaris hereditarium 695.0
  pernio 991.5
  perstans solare 692.72
  rash, newborn 778.8
  scarlatiniform (exfoliative) (recurrent) 695.0
  simplex marginatum 057.8
  solare (*see also* Sunburn) 692.71
  streptogenes 696.5
  toxic, toxicum NEC 695.0
    newborn 778.8
  tuberculous (primary) (*see also* Tuberculosis)
      017.0
  venenatum 695.0
Erythematosus —*see* condition
Erythematous —*see* condition
Erythermalgia (primary) 443.89
Erythralgia 443.89
Erythrasma 039.0
Erythredema 985.0
  polyneuritica 985.0
  polyneuropathy 985.0
Erythremia (acute) (M9841/3) 207.0
  chronic (M9842/3) 207.1
  secondary 289.0
Erythroblastopenia (acquired) 284.8
  congenital 284.0
Erythroblastophthisis 284.0
Erythroblastosis (fetalis) (newborn) 773.2
  due to
    ABO
      antibodies 773.1
      incompatibility, maternal/fetal 773.1
      isoimmunization 773.1
    Rh
      antibodies 773.0
      incompatibility, maternal/fetal 773.0
      isoimmunization 773.0

Erythrocyanosis (crurum) 443.89
Erythrocythemia —*see* Erythremia
Erythrocytopenia 285.9
Erythrocytosis (megalosplenic)
  familial 289.6
  oval, hereditary (*see also* Elliptocytosis) 282.1
  secondary 289.0
  stress 289.0
Erythroderma (*see also* Erythema) 695.9
  desquamativa (in infants) 695.89
  exfoliative 695.89
  ichthyosiform, congenital 757.1
  infantum 695.89
  maculopapular 696.2
  neonatorum 778.8
  psoriaticum 696.1
  secondary 695.9
Erythrogenesis imperfecta 284.0
Erythroleukemia (M9840/3) 207.0
Erythromelalgia 443.89
Erythromelia 701.8
Erythropenia 285.9
Erythrophagocytosis 289.9
Erythrophobia 300.23
Erythroplakia
  oral mucosa 528.7
  tongue 528.7
Erythroplasia (Queyrat) (M8080/2)
  specified site—*see* Neoplasm, skin, in situ
  unspecified site 233.5
Erythropoiesis, idiopathic ineffective 285.0
Escaped beats, heart 427.60
  postoperative 997.1
Esoenteritis —*see* Enteritis
Esophagalgia 530.89
Esophagectasis 530.89
  due to cardiospasm 530.0
Esophagismus 530.5
Esophagitis (alkaline) (chemical) (chronic)
    (infectional) (necrotic) (postoperative) 530.10
  acute 530.12
  candidal 112.84
  reflux 530.11
  specified NEC 530.19
  tuberculous (*see also* Tuberculosis) 017.8
  ulcerative 530.19
Esophagocele 530.6
Esophagodynia 530.89
Esophagomalacia 530.89
Esophagoptosis 530.89
Esophagospasm 530.5
Esophagostenosis 530.3
Esophagostomiasis 127.7
Esophagotracheal —*see* condition
Esophagus —*see* condition
Esophoria 378.41
  convergence, excess 378.84
  divergence, insufficiency 378.85
Esotropia (nonaccommodative) 378.00
  accommodative 378.35
  alternating 378.05
    with
      A pattern 378.06
      specified noncomitancy NEC 378.08
      V pattern 378.07
      X pattern 378.08
      Y pattern 378.08
    intermittent 378.22
  intermittent 378.20
    alternating 378.22

Examination—*continued*
    pill V25.41
      specified method NEC V25.49
  health (of)
    armed forces personnel V70.5
    checkup V70.0
    child, routine V20.2
    defined subpopulation NEC V70.5
    inhabitants of institutions V70.5
    occupational V70.5
    pre-employment screening V70.5
    preschool children V70.5
      for admission to school V70.3
    prisoners V70.5
      for entrance into prison V70.3
    prostitutes V70.5
    refugees V70.5
    school children V70.5
    students V70.5
  hearing V72.1
  infant V20.2
  laboratory V72.6
  lactating mother V24.1
  medical (for) (of) V70.9
    administrative purpose NEC V70.3
    admission to
      old age home V70.3
      prison V70.3
      school V70.3
    adoption V70.3
    armed forces personnel V70.5
    at health care facility V70.0
    camp V70.3
    child, routine V20.2
    clinical research investigation (control)
      (normal comparison) (participant) V70.7
    defined subpopulation NEC V70.5
    donor (potential) V70.8
    driving license V70.3
    general V70.9
      routine V70.0
      specified reason NEC V70.8
    immigration V70.3
    inhabitants of institutions V70.5
    insurance certification V70.3
    marriage V70.3
    medicolegal reasons V70.4
    naturalization V70.3
    occupational V70.5
    population survey V70.6
    pre-employment V70.5
    preschool children V70.5
      for admission to school V70.3
    prison V70.3
    prisoners V70.5
      for entrance into prison V70.3
    prostitutes V70.5
    refugees V70.5
    school children V70.5
    specified reason NEC V70.8
    sport competition V70.3
    students V70.5
  medicolegal reason V70.4
  pelvic (annual) (periodic) V72.3
  periodic (annual) (routine) V70.0
  postpartum
    immediately after delivery V24.0
    routine follow-up V24.2
  pregnancy (unconfirmed) (possible) V72.4
  prenatal V22.1
    first pregnancy V22.0

Examination—*continued*
  high-risk pregnancy V23.9
    specified problem NEC V23.8
  preoperative V72.84
    cardiovascular V72.81
    respiratory V72.82
    specified NEC V72.83
  psychiatric V70.2
    follow-up not needing further care V67.3
    requested by authority V70.1
  radiological NEC V72.5
  respiratory preoperative V72.82
  screening—*see* Screening
  sensitization V72.7
  skin V72.7
    hypersensitivity V72.7
  special V72.9
  specified type or reason NEC V72.85
    preoperative V72.83
      specified NEC V72.83
  teeth V72.2
  vaginal Papanicolaou smear V76.47
    following hysterectomy for malignant
      condition V67.01
  victim or culprit following
    alleged rape or seduction V71.5
    inflicted injury NEC V71.6
  vision V72.0
  well baby V20.2
Exanthem, exanthema (*see also* Rash) 782.1
  Boston 048
  epidemic, with meningitis 048
  lichenoid psoriasiform 696.2
  subitum 057.8
  viral, virus NEC 057.9
    specified type NEC 057.8
Excess, excessive, excessively
  alcohol level in blood 790.3
  carbohydrate tissue, localized 278.1
  carotene (dietary) 278.3
  cold 991.9
    specified effect NEC 991.8
  convergence 378.84
  crying of infant (baby) 780.92
  development, breast 611.1
  diaphoresis 780.8
  divergence 378.85
  drinking (alcohol) NEC (*see also* Abuse, drugs,
    nondependent) 305.0
    continual (*see also* Alcoholism) 303.9
    habitual (*see also* Alcoholism) 303.9
  eating 783.6
  eyelid fold (congenital) 743.62
  fat 278.00
    in heart (*see also* Degeneration, myocardial)
      429.1
    tissue, localized 278.1
  foreskin 605
  gas 787.3
  gastrin 251.5
  glucagon 251.4
  heat (*see also* Heat) 992.9
  large
    colon 564.7
      congenital 751.3
    fetus or infant 766.0
      with obstructed labor 660.1
        affecting management of pregnancy 656.6
      causing disproportion 653.5
    newborn (weight of 4500 grams or more)
      766.0

Excess, excessive, excessively— *continued*
   organ or site, congenital NEC—*see* Anomaly,
      specified type NEC
   lid fold (congenital) 743.62
   long
      colon 751.5
      organ or site, congenital NEC—*see* Anomaly,
         specified type NEC
      umbilical cord (entangled)
         affecting fetus or newborn 762.5
         in pregnancy or childbirth 663.3
            with compression 663.2
   menstruation 626.2
   number of teeth 520.1
      causing crowding 524.3
   nutrients (dietary) NEC 783.6
   potassium (K) 276.7
   salivation (*see also* Ptyalism) 527.7
   secretion—*see also* Hypersecretion
      milk 676.6
      sputum 786.4
      sweat 780.8
   short
      organ or site, congenital NEC—*see* Anomaly,
         specified type NEC
      umbilical cord
         affecting fetus or newborn 762.6
         in pregnancy or childbirth 663.4
   skin NEC 701.9
      eyelid 743.62
         acquired 374.30
   sodium (Na) 276.0
   sputum 786.4
   sweating 780.8
   tearing (ducts) (eye) (*see also* Epiphora) 375.20
   thirst 783.5
      due to deprivation of water 994.3
   vitamin
      A (dietary) 278.2
         administered as drug (chronic) (prolonged
            excessive intake) 278.2
            reaction to sudden overdose 963.5
      D (dietary) 278.4
         administered as drug (chronic) (prolonged
            excessive intake) 278.4
            reaction to sudden overdose 963.5
   weight 278.00
      gain 783.1
         of pregnancy 646.1
      loss 783.21
Excitability, abnormal , under minor stress
   309.29
Excitation
   catatonic (*see also* Schizophrenia) 295.2
   psychogenic 298.1
   reactive (from emotional stress, psychological
      trauma) 298.1
Excitement
   manic (*see also* Psychosis, affective) 296.0
      recurrent episode 296.1
      single episode 296.0
   mental, reactive (from emotional stress,
      psychological trauma) 298.1
   state, reactive (from emotional stress,
      psychological trauma) 298.1
Excluded pupils 364.76
Excoriation (traumatic) (*see also* Injury,
   superficial, by site) 919.8
   neurotic 698.4
Excyclophoria 378.44
Excyclotropia 378.33
Exencephalus, exencephaly 742.0

Exercise
   breathing V57.0
   remedial NEC V57.1
   therapeutic NEC V57.1
Exfoliation, teeth due to systemic causes 525.0
Exfoliative —*see also* condition
   dermatitis 695.89
Exhaustion, exhaustive (physical NEC) 780.79
   battle (*see also* Reaction, stress, acute) 308.9
   cardiac (*see also* Failure, heart) 428.9
   delirium (*see also* Reaction, stress, acute) 308.9
   due to
      cold 991.8
      excessive exertion 994.5
      exposure 994.4
   fetus or newborn 779.89
   heart (*see also* Failure, heart) 428.9
   heat 992.5
      due to
         salt depletion 992.4
         water depletion 992.3
   manic (*see also* Psychosis, affective) 296.0
      recurrent episode 296.1
      single episode 296.0
   maternal, complicating delivery 669.8
      affecting fetus or newborn 763.89
   mental 300.5
   myocardium, myocardial (*see also* Failure,
      heart) 428.9
   nervous 300.5
   old age 797
   postinfectional NEC 780.79
   psychogenic 300.5
   psychosis (*see also* Reaction, stress, acute) 308.9
   senile 797
      dementia 290.0
Exhibitionism (sexual) 302.4
Exomphalos 756.79
Exophoria 378.42
   convergence, insufficiency 378.83
   divergence, excess 378.85
Exophthalmic
   cachexia 242.0
   goiter 242.0
   ophthalmoplegia 242.0 *[376.22]*
Exophthalmos 376.30
   congenital 743.66
   constant 376.31
   endocrine NEC 259.9 *[376.22]*
   hyperthyroidism 242.0 *[376.21]*
   intermittent NEC 376.34
   malignant 242.0 *[376.21]*
   pulsating 376.35
      endocrine NEC 259.9 *[376.22]*
   thyrotoxic 242.0 *[376.21]*
Exostosis 726.91
   cartilaginous (M9210/0)—*see* Neoplasm, bone,
      benign
   congenital 756.4
   ear canal, external 380.81
   gonococcal 098.89
   hip 726.5
   intracranial 733.3
   jaw (bone) 526.81
   luxurians 728.11
   multiple (cancellous) (congenital) (hereditary)
      756.4
   nasal bones 726.91
   orbit, orbital 376.42
   osteocartilaginous (M9210/0)—*see* Neoplasm,
      bone, benign

Exostosis—*continued*
spine 721.8
with spondylosis—*see* Spondylosis
syphilitic 095.5
wrist 726.4
Exotropia 378.10
alternating 378.15
with
A pattern 378.16
specified noncomitancy 378.18
V pattern 378.17
X pattern 378.18
Y pattern 378.18
intermittent 378.24
intermittent 378.20
alternating 378.24
monocular 378.23
monocular 378.11
with
A pattern 378.12
specified noncomitancy NEC 378.14
V pattern 378.13
X pattern 378.14
Y pattern 378.14
intermittent 378.23
Explanation of
investigation finding V65.4
medication V65.4
Exposure 994.9
cold 991.9
specified effect NEC 991.8
effects of 994.9
exhaustion due to 994.4
to
AIDS virus V01.7
anthrax V01.81
asbestos V15.84
body fluids (hazardous) V15.85
cholera V01.0
communicable disease V01.9
specified type NEC V01.89
German measles V01.4
gonorrhea V01.6
hazardous body fluids V15.85
HIV V01.7
human immunodeficiency virus V01.7
lead V15.86
parasitic disease V01.89
poliomyelitis V01.2
potentially hazardous body fluids V15.85
rabies V01.5
rubella V01.4
smallpox V01.3
syphilis V01.6
tuberculosis V01.1
venereal disease V01.6
viral disease NEC V01.7
Exsanguination, fetal 772.0
Exstrophy
abdominal content 751.8
bladder (urinary) 753.5
Extensive —*see* condition
Extra —*see also* Accessory
rib 756.3
cervical 756.2
Extraction
with hook 763.89
breech NEC 669.6
affecting fetus or newborn 763.0
cataract postsurgical V45.61
manual NEC 669.8
affecting fetus or newborn 763.89

Extrasystole 427.60
atrial 427.61
postoperative 997.1
ventricular 427.69
Extrauterine gestation or pregnancy —*see*
Pregnancy, ectopic
Extravasation
blood 459.0
lower extremity 459.0
chyle into mesentery 457.8
pelvicalyceal 593.4
pyelosinus 593.4
urine 788.8
from ureter 788.8
Extremity —*see* condition
Extrophy —*see* Exstrophy
Extroversion
bladder 753.5
uterus 618.1
complicating delivery 665.2
affecting fetus or newborn 763.89
postpartal (old) 618.1
Extrusion
breast implant (prosthetic) 996.54
device, implant, or graft—*see* Complications,
mechanical
eye implant (ball) (globe) 996.59
intervertebral disc—*see* Displacement,
intervertebral disc
lacrimal gland 375.43
mesh (reinforcing) 996.59
ocular lens implant 996.53
prosthetic device NEC—*see* Complications,
mechanical
vitreous 379.26
Exudate, pleura —*see* Effusion, pleura
Exudates, retina 362.82
Exudative —*see* condition
Eye, eyeball, eyelid —*see* condition
Eyestrain 368.13
Eyeworm disease of Africa 125.2

F

Faber's anemia or syndrome (achlorhydric anemia) 280.9
Fabry's disease (angiokeratoma corporis diffusum) 272.7
Face, facial —*see* condition
Facet of cornea 371.44
Faciocephalalgia, autonomic (*see also* Neuropathy, peripheral, autonomic) 337.9
Facioscapulohumeral myopathy 359.1
Factitious disorder, illness —*see* Illness, factitious
Factor
deficiency—*see* Deficiency, factor
psychic, associated with diseases classified elsewhere 316
risk—*see* Problem
Fahr-Volhard disease (malignant nephrosclerosis) 403.00
Failure, failed
adenohypophyseal 253.2
attempted abortion (legal) (*see also* Abortion, failed) 638.9
bone marrow (anemia) 284.9
acquired (secondary) 284.8
congenital 284.0
idiopathic 284.9
cardiac (*see also* Failure, heart) 428.9
newborn 779.89
cardiorenal (chronic) 428.9
hypertensive (*see also* Hypertension, cardiorenal) 404.93
cardiorespiratory 799.1
specified during or due to a procedure 997.1
long-term effect of cardiac surgery 429.4
cardiovascular (chronic) 428.9
cerebrovascular 437.8
cervical dilatation in labor 661.0
affecting fetus or newborn 763.7
circulation, circulatory 799.8
fetus or newborn 779.89
peripheral 785.50
compensation—*see* Disease, heart
congestive (*see also* Failure, heart) 428.0
coronary (*see also* Insufficiency, coronary) 411.89
descent of head (at term) 652.5
affecting fetus or newborn 763.1
in labor 660.0
affecting fetus or newborn 763.1
device, implant, or graft—*see* Complications, mechanical
engagement of head NEC 652.5
in labor 660.0
extrarenal 788.9
fetal head to enter pelvic brim 652.5
affecting fetus or newborn 763.1
in labor 660.0
affecting fetus or newborn 763.1
forceps NEC 660.7
affecting fetus or newborn 763.1
fusion (joint) (spinal) 996.4
growth in childhood 783.43
heart (acute) (sudden) 428.9
with
abortion—*see* Abortion, by type, with specified complication NEC

Failure, failed—*continued*
acute pulmonary edema (*see also* Failure, ventricular, left) 428.1
with congestion (*see also* Failure, heart) 428.0
decompensation (*see also* Failure, heart) 428.0
dilation—*see* Disease, heart
ectopic pregnancy (*see also* categories 633.0-633.9) 639.8
molar pregnancy (*see also* categories 630-632) 639.8
arteriosclerotic 440.9
combined left-right sided 428.0
combined systolic and diastolic 428.40
acute 428.41
acute on chronic 428.43
chronic 428.42
compensated (*see also* Failure, heart) 428.0
complicating
abortion—*see* Abortion, by type, with specified complication NEC
delivery (cesarean) (instrumental) 669.4
ectopic pregnancy (*see also* categories 633.0-633.9) 639.8
molar pregnancy (*see also* categories 630-632) 639.8
obstetric anesthesia or sedation 668.1
surgery 997.1
congestive (compensated) (decompensated) (*see also* Failure, heart) 428.0
with rheumatic fever (conditions classifiable to 390)
active 391.8
inactive or quiescent (with chorea) 398.91
fetus or newborn 779.89
hypertensive (*see also* Hypertension, heart) 402.91
with renal disease (*see also* Hypertension, cardiorenal) 404.91
with renal failure 404.93
benign 402.11
malignant 402.01
rheumatic (chronic) (inactive) (with chorea) 398.91
active or acute 391.8
with chorea (Sydenham's) 392.0
decompensated (*see also* Failure, heart) 428.0
degenerative (*see also* Degeneration, myocardial) 429.1
diastolic 428.30
acute 428.31
actue on chronic 428.33
chronic 428.32
due to presence of (cardiac) prosthesis 429.4
fetus or newborn 779.89
following
abortion 639.8
cardiac surgery 429.4
ectopic or molar pregnancy 639.8
high output NEC 428.9
hypertensive (*see also* Hypertension, heart) 402.91
with renal disease (*see also* Hypertension, cardiorenal) 404.91
with renal failure 404.93
benign 402.11

Failure, failed—*continued*
    malignant 402.01
    left (ventricular) (*see also* Failure, ventricular,
       left) 428.1
       with right-sided failure (*see also* Failure,
         heart) 428.0
    low output (syndrome) NEC 428.9
    organic—*see* Disease, heart
    postoperative (immediate) 997.1
       long term effect of cardiac surgery 429.4
    rheumatic (chronic) (congestive) (inactive)
       398.91
    right (secondary to left heart failure,
       conditions classifiable to 428.1)
       (ventricular) (*see also* Failure, heart) 428.0
    senile 797
    specified during or due to a procedure 997.1
       long-term effect of cardiac surgery 429.4
    systolic 428.20
       acute 428.21
       acute on chronic 428.23
       chronic 428.22
    thyrotoxic (*see also* Thyrotoxicosis) 242.9
       [425.7]
    valvular—*see* Endocarditis
  hepatic 572.8
    acute 570
    due to a procedure 997.4
  hepatorenal 572.4
  hypertensive heart (*see also* Hypertension,
    heart) 402.91
    benign 402.11
    malignant 402.01
  induction (of labor) 659.1
    abortion (legal) (*see also* Abortion, failed)
       638.9
    affecting fetus or newborn 763.89
    by oxytocic drugs 659.1
    instrumental 659.0
    mechanical 659.0
    medical 659.1
    surgical 659.0
  initial alveolar expansion, newborn 770.4
  involution, thymus (gland) 254.8
  kidney—*see* Failure, renal
  lactation 676.4
  Leydig's cell, adult 257.2
  liver 572.8
    acute 570
  medullary 799.8
  mitral—*see* Endocarditis, mitral
  myocardium, myocardial (*see also* Failure,
    heart) 428.9
    chronic (*see also* Failure, heart) 428.0
    congestive (*see also* Failure, heart) 428.0
  ovarian (primary) 256.39
    iatrogenic 256.2
    postablative 256.2
    postirradiation 256.2
    postsurgical 256.2
  ovulation 628.0
  prerenal 788.9
  renal 586
    with
       abortion—*see* Abortion, by type, with renal
         failure
       ectopic pregnancy (*see also* categories
         633.0-633.9) 639.3
       edema (*see also* Nephrosis) 581.9
       hypertension (*see also* Hypertension,
         kidney) 403.91

Failure, failed—*continued*
    hypertensive heart disease (conditions
       classifiable to 402) 404.92
       with heart failure 404.93
       benign 404.12
         with heart failure 404.13
       malignant 404.02
         with heart failure 404.03
    molar pregnancy (*see also* categories
       630-632) 639.3
    tubular necrosis (acute) 584.5
  acute 584.9
    with lesion of
       necrosis
         cortical (renal) 584.6
         medullary (renal) (papillary) 584.7
         tubular 584.5
       specified pathology NEC 584.8
  chronic 585
    hypertensive or with hypertension (*see also*
       Hypertension, kidney) 403.91
  due to a procedure 997.5
  following
    abortion 639.3
    crushing 958.5
    ectopic or molar pregnancy 639.3
    labor and delivery (acute) 669.3
  hypertensive (*see also* Hypertension, kidney)
    403.91
  puerperal, postpartum 669.3
 respiration, respiratory 518.81
    acute 518.81
    acute and chronic 518.84
    center 348.8
       newborn 770.84
    chronic 518.83
    due to trauma, surgery or shock 518.5
    newborn 770.84
 rotation
    cecum 751.4
    colon 751.4
    intestine 751.4
    kidney 753.3
 segmentation—*see also* Fusion
    fingers (*see also* Syndactylism, fingers) 755.11
    toes (*see also* Syndactylism, toes) 755.13
 seminiferous tubule, adult 257.2
 senile (general) 797
    with psychosis 290.20
 testis, primary (seminal) 257.2
 to progress 661.2
 to thrive
    adult 783.7
    child 783.41
 transplant 996.80
    bone marrow 996.85
    organ (immune or nonimmune cause) 996.80
       bone marrow 996.85
       heart 996.83
       intestines 996.87
       kidney 996.81
       liver 996.82
       lung 996.84
       pancreas 996.86
       specified NEC 996.89
 skin 996.52
    artificial 996.55
    decellularized allodermis 996.55
    temporary allograft or pigskin graft—*omit
       code*

Fetishism 302.81
  transvestic 302.3
Fetomaternal hemorrhage
  affecting management of pregnancy 656.0
  fetus or newborn 772.0
Fetus, fetal —*see also* condition
  papyraceous 779.89
  type lung tissue 770.4
Fever 780.6
  with chills 780.6
    in malarial regions (*see also* Malaria) 084.6
  abortus NEC 023.9
  Aden 061
  African tick-borne 087.1
  American
    mountain tick 066.1
    spotted 082.0
  and ague (*see also* Malaria) 084.6
  aphthous 078.4
  arbovirus hemorrhagic 065.9
  Assam 085.0
  Australian A or Q 083.0
  Bangkok hemorrhagic 065.4
  biliary, Charcot's intermittent—*see*
    Choledocholithiasis
  bilious, hemoglobinuric 084.8
  blackwater 084.8
  blister 054.9
  Bonvale Dam 780.79
  boutonneuse 082.1
  brain 323.9
    late effect—*see* category 326
  breakbone 061
  Bullis 082.8
  Bunyamwera 066.3
  Burdwan 085.0
  Bwamba (encephalitis) 066.3
  Cameroon (*see also* Malaria) 084.6
  Canton 081.9
  catarrhal (acute) 460
    chronic 472.0
  cat-scratch 078.3
  cerebral 323.9
    late effect—*see* category 326
  cerebrospinal (meningococcal) (*see also*
    Meningitis, cerebrospinal) 036.0
  Chagres 084.0
  Chandipura 066.8
  changuinola 066.0
  Charcot's (biliary) (hepatic) (intermittent)—*see*
    Choledocholithiasis
  Chikungunya (viral) 066.3
    hemorrhagic 065.4
  childbed 670
  Chitral 066.0
  Colombo (*see also* Fever, paratyphoid) 002.9
  Colorado tick (virus) 066.1
  congestive
    malarial (*see also* Malaria) 084.6
    remittent (*see also* Malaria) 084.6
  Congo virus 065.0
  continued 780.6
    malarial 084.0
  Corsican (*see also* Malaria) 084.6
  Crimean hemorrhagic 065.0
  Cyprus (*see also* Brucellosis) 023.9
  dandy 061
  deer fly (*see also* Tularemia) 021.9
  dehydration, newborn 778.4
  dengue (virus) 061
    hemorrhagic 065.4

Fever—*continued*
  desert 114.0
  due to heat 992.0
  Dumdum 085.0
  enteric 002.0
  ephemeral (of unknown origin) (*see also*
    Pyrexia) 780.6
  epidemic, hemorrhagic of the Far East 065.0
  erysipelatous (*see also* Erysipelas) 035
  estivo-autumnal (malarial) 084.0
  etiocholanolone 277.3
  famine—*see also* Fever, relapsing
    meaning typhus—*see* Typhus
  Far Eastern hemorrhagic 065.0
  five day 083.1
  Fort Bragg 100.89
  gastroenteric 002.0
  gastromalarial (*see also* Malaria) 084.6
  Gibraltar (*see also* Brucellosis) 023.9
  glandular 075
  Guama (viral) 066.3
  Haverhill 026.1
  hay (allergic) (with rhinitis) 477.9
    with
      asthma (bronchial) (*see also* Asthma) 493.0
    due to
      dander 477.8
      dust 477.8
      fowl 477.8
      pollen, any plant or tree 477.0
      specified allergen other than pollen 477.8
  heat (effects) 992.0
  hematuric, bilious 084.8
  hemoglobinuric (malarial) 084.8
    bilious 084.8
  hemorrhagic (arthropod-borne) NEC 065.9
    with renal syndrome 078.6
    arenaviral 078.7
    Argentine 078.7
    Bangkok 065.4
    Bolivian 078.7
    Central Asian 065.0
    chikungunya 065.4
    Crimean 065.0
    dengue (virus) 065.4
    Ebola 065.8
    epidemic 078.6
      of Far East 065.0
    Far Eastern 065.0
    Junin virus 078.7
    Korean 078.6
    Kyasanur forest 065.2
    Machupo virus 078.7
    mite-borne NEC 065.8
    mosquito-borne 065.4
    Omsk 065.1
    Philippine 065.4
    Russian (Yaroslav) 078.6
    Singapore 065.4
    Southeast Asia 065.4
    Thailand 065.4
    tick-borne NEC 065.3
  hepatic (*see also* Cholecystitis) 575.8
    intermittent (Charcot's)—*see*
      Choledocholithiasis
  herpetic (*see also* Herpes) 054.9
  Hyalomma tick 065.0
  icterohemorrhagic 100.0
  inanition 780.6
    newborn 778.4
  infective NEC 136.9

Fibrosclerosis
  breast 610.3
  corpora cavernosa (penis) 607.89
  familial multifocal NEC 710.8
  multifocal (idiopathic) NEC 710.8
  penis (corpora cavernosa) 607.89
Fibrosis, fibrotic
  adrenal (gland) 255.8
  alveolar (diffuse) 516.3
  amnion 658.8
  anal papillae 569.49
  anus 569.49
  appendix, appendiceal, noninflammatory 543.9
  arteriocapillary—*see* Arteriosclerosis
  bauxite (of lung) 503
  biliary 576.8
    due to Clonorchis sinensis 121.1
  bladder 596.8
    interstitial 595.1
    localized submucosal 595.1
    panmural 595.1
  bone, diffuse 756.59
  breast 610.3
  capillary—*see also* Arteriosclerosis
    lung (chronic) (*see also* Fibrosis, lung) 515
  cardiac (*see also* Myocarditis) 429.0
  cervix 622.8
  chorion 658.8
  corpus cavernosum 607.89
  cystic (of pancreas) 277.00
    with
      manifestations
        gastrointestinal 277.03
        pulmonary 277.02
        specified NEC 277.09
      meconium ileus 277.01
      pulmonary exacerbation 277.02
  due to (presence of) any device, implant, or
    graft—*see* Complications, due to (presence
    of) any device, implant, or graft classified to
    996.0-996.5 NEC
  ejaculatory duct 608.89
  endocardium (*see also* Endocarditis) 424.90
  endomyocardial (African) 425.0
  epididymis 608.89
  eye muscle 378.62
  graphite (of lung) 503
  heart (*see also* Myocarditis) 429.0
  hepatic—*see also* Cirrhosis, liver
    due to Clonorchis sinensis 121.1
  hepatolienal—*see* Cirrhosis, liver
  hepatosplenic—*see* Cirrhosis, liver
  infrapatellar fat pad 729.31
  interstitial pulmonary, newborn 770.7
  intrascrotal 608.89
  kidney (*see also* Sclerosis, renal) 587
  liver—*see* Cirrhosis, liver
  lung (atrophic) (capillary) (chronic) (confluent)
      (massive) (perialveolar) (peribronchial) 515
    with
      anthracosilicosis (occupational) 500
      anthracosis (occupational) 500
      asbestosis (occupational) 501
      bagassosis (occupational) 495.1
      bauxite 503
      berylliosis (occupational) 503
      byssinosis (occupational) 504
      calcicosis (occupational) 502
      chalicosis (occupational) 502
      dust reticulation (occupational) 504
      farmers' lung 495.0

Fibrosis, fibrotic—*continued*
    gannister disease (occupational) 502
    graphite 503
    pneumonoconiosis (occupational) 505
    pneumosiderosis (occupational) 503
    siderosis (occupational) 503
    silicosis (occupational) 502
    tuberculosis (*see also* Tuberculosis) 011.4
  diffuse (idiopathic) (interstitial) 516.3
  due to
    bauxite 503
    fumes or vapors (chemical) (inhalation)
      506.4
    graphite 503
  following radiation 508.1
  postinflammatory 515
  silicotic (massive) (occupational) 502
  tuberculous (*see also* Tuberculosis) 011.4
  lymphatic gland 289.3
  median bar 600.9
  mediastinum (idiopathic) 519.3
  meninges 349.2
  muscle NEC 728.2
    iatrogenic (from injection) 999.9
  myocardium, myocardial (*see also* Myocarditis)
      429.0
  oral submucous 528.8
  ovary 620.8
  oviduct 620.8
  pancreas 577.8
    cystic 277.00
      with
        manifestations
          gastrointestinal 277.03
          pulmonary 277.02
          specified NEC 277.09
        meconium ileus 277.01
        pulmonary exacerbation 277.02
  penis 607.89
  periappendiceal 543.9
  periarticular (*see also* Ankylosis) 718.5
  pericardium 423.1
  perineum, in pregnancy or childbirth 654.8
    affecting fetus or newborn 763.89
    causing obstructed labor 660.2
      affecting fetus or newborn 763.1
  perineural NEC 355.9
    foot 355.6
  periureteral 593.89
  placenta—*see* Placenta, abnormal
  pleura 511.0
  popliteal fat pad 729.31
  preretinal 362.56
  prostate (chronic) 600.9
  pulmonary (chronic) (*see also* Fibrosis, lung)
      515
    alveolar capillary block 516.3
    interstitial
      diffuse (idiopathic) 516.3
      newborn 770.7
  radiation—*see* Effect, adverse, radiation
  rectal sphincter 569.49
  retroperitoneal, idiopathic 593.4
  scrotum 608.89
  seminal vesicle 608.89
  senile 797
  skin NEC 709.2
  spermatic cord 608.89
  spleen 289.59
    bilharzial (*see also* Schistosomiasis) 120.9

Findings, abnormal without diagnosis—*cont.*
  spinal fluid 792.0
  sputum 795.39
  stool 792.1
  throat 795.39
  urine 791.9
  viral
    human immunodeficiency V08
  wound 795.39
echocardiogram 793.2
echoencephalogram 794.01
echogram NEC—*see* Findings, abnormal,
  structure
electrocardiogram (ECG) (EKG) 794.31
electroencephalogram (EEG) 794.02
electrolyte level, urinary 791.9
electromyogram (EMG) 794.17
  ocular 794.14
electro-oculogram (EOG) 794.12
electroretinogram (ERG) 794.11
enzymes, serum NEC 790.5
fibrinogen titer coagulation study 790.92
filling defect—*see* Filling defect
function study NEC 794.9
  auditory 794.15
  bladder 794.9
  brain 794.00
  cardiac 794.30
  endocrine NEC 794.6
    thyroid 794.5
  kidney 794.4
  liver 794.8
  nervous system
    central 794.00
    peripheral 794.19
  oculomotor 794.14
  pancreas 794.9
  placenta 794.9
  pulmonary 794.2
  retina 794.11
  special senses 794.19
  spleen 794.9
  vestibular 794.16
gallbladder, nonvisualization 793.3
glucose 790.2
  tolerance test 790.2
glycosuria 791.5
heart
  shadow 793.2
  sounds 785.3
hematinuria 791.2
hematocrit
  drop (precipitous) 790.01
  elevated 282.7
  low 285.9
hematologic NEC 790.99
hematuria 599.7
hemoglobin
  elevated 282.7
  low 285.9
hemoglobinuria 791.2
histological NEC 795.4
hormones 259.9
immunoglobulins, elevated 795.79
indolacetic acid, elevated 791.9
iron 790.6
karyotype 795.2
ketonuria 791.6
lactic acid dehydrogenase (LDH) 790.4
lipase 790.5
lipids NEC 272.9

Findings, abnormal without diagnosis—*cont.*
lithium, blood 790.6
lung field (coin lesion) (shadow) 793.1
magnesium, blood 790.6
mammogram 793.80
  microcalcification 793.81
mediastinal shift 793.2
melanin, urine 791.9
microbiologic NEC 795.39
mineral, blood NEC 790.6
myoglobinuria 791.3
nasal swab, anthrax 795.31
nitrogen derivatives, blood 790.6
nonvisualization of gallbladder 793.3
nose culture, positive 795.39
odor of urine (unusual) NEC 791.9
oxygen saturation 790.91
Papanicolaou (smear) 795.1
  cervix 795.00
    atypical squamous cell changes of
      undetermined significance
      favor benign (ASCUS favor benign)
        795.01
        favor dysplasia (ASCUS favor dysplasia)
          795.02
      dyskaryotic 795.09
      nonspecific finding NEC 795.09
  other site 795.1
peritoneal fluid 792.9
phonocardiogram 794.39
phosphorus 275.3
pleural fluid 792.9
pneumoencephalogram 793.0
PO_2-oxygen ratio 790.91
poikilocytosis 790.09
potassium
  deficiency 276.8
  excess 276.7
PPD 795.5
prostate specific antigen (PSA) 790.93
protein, serum NEC 790.99
proteinuria 791.0
prothrombin time (partial) (prolonged) (PT)
  (PTT) 790.92
pyuria 791.9
radiologic (x-ray) 793.9
  abdomen 793.6
  biliary tract 793.3
  breast 793.89
    abnormal mammogram NOS 793.80
    mammographic microcalcification 793.81
  gastrointestinal tract 793.4
  genitourinary organs 793.5
  head 793.0
  intrathoracic organs NEC 793.2
  lung 793.1
  musculoskeletal 793.7
  placenta 793.9
  retroperitoneum 793.6
  skin 793.9
  skull 793.0
  subcutaneous tissue 793.9
red blood cell 790.09
  count 790.09
  morphology 790.09
  sickling 790.09
  volume 790.09
saliva 792.4
scan NEC 794.9
  bladder 794.9
  bone 794.9

Fissure, fissured—*continued*
spine (congenital) (*see also* Spina bifida) 741.9
sternum (congenital) 756.3
tongue (acquired) 529.5
congenital 750.13
Fistula (sinus) 686.9
abdomen (wall) 569.81
bladder 596.2
intestine 569.81
ureter 593.82
uterus 619.2
abdominorectal 569.81
abdominosigmoidal 569.81
abdominothoracic 510.0
abdominouterine 619.2
congenital 752.3
abdominovesical 596.2
accessory sinuses (*see also* Sinusitis) 473.9
actinomycotic—*see* Actinomycosis
alveolar
antrum (*see also* Sinusitis, maxillary) 473.0
process 522.7
anorectal 565.1
antrobuccal (*see also* Sinusitis, maxillary) 473.0
antrum (*see also* Sinusitis, maxillary) 473.0
anus, anal (infectional) (recurrent) 565.1
congenital 751.5
tuberculous (*see also* Tuberculosis) 014.8
aortic sinus 747.29
aortoduodenal 447.2
appendix, appendicular 543.9
arteriovenous (acquired) 447.0
brain 437.3
congenital 747.81
ruptured (*see also* Hemorrhage,
subarachnoid) 430
ruptured (*see also* Hemorrhage,
subarachnoid) 430
cerebral 437.3
congenital 747.81
congenital (peripheral) 747.60
brain—*see* Fistula, arteriovenous, brain,
congenital
coronary 746.85
gastrointestinal 747.61
lower limb 747.64
pulmonary 747.3
renal 747.62
specified NEC 747.69
upper limb 747.63
coronary 414.19
congenital 746.85
heart 414.19
pulmonary (vessels) 417.0
congenital 747.3
surgically created (for dialysis) V45.1
complication NEC 996.73
atherosclerosis —*see* Arteriosclerosis,
extremities
embolism 996.74
infection or inflammation 996.62
mechanical 996.1
occlusion NEC 996.74
thrombus 996.74
traumatic—*see* Injury, blood vessel, by site
artery 447.2
aural 383.81
congenital 744.49
auricle 383.81
congenital 744.49
Bartholin's gland 619.8

Fistula—*continued*
bile duct (*see also* Fistula, biliary) 576.4
biliary (duct) (tract) 576.4
congenital 751.69
bladder (neck) (sphincter) 596.2
into seminal vesicle 596.2
bone 733.99
brain 348.8
arteriovenous—*see* Fistula, arteriovenous,
brain
branchial (cleft) 744.41
branchiogenous 744.41
breast 611.0
puerperal, postpartum 675.1
bronchial 510.0
bronchocutaneous, bronchomediastinal,
bronchopleural, bronchopleuromediastinal
(infective) 510.0
tuberculous (*see also* Tuberculosis) 011.3
bronchoesophageal 530.89
congenital 750.3
buccal cavity (infective) 528.3
canal, ear 380.89
carotid-cavernous
congenital 747.81
with hemorrhage 430
traumatic 900.82
with hemorrhage (see also Hemorrhage,
brain, traumatic) 853.0
late effect 908.3
cecosigmoidal 569.81
cecum 569.81
cerebrospinal (fluid) 349.81
cervical, lateral (congenital) 744.41
cervicoaural (congenital) 744.49
cervicosigmoidal 619.1
cervicovesical 619.0
cervix 619.8
chest (wall) 510.0
cholecystocolic (*see also* Fistula, gallbladder)
575.5
cholecystocolonic (*see also* Fistula, gallbladder)
575.5
cholecystoduodenal (*see also* Fistula,
gallbladder) 575.5
cholecystoenteric (*see also* Fistula, gallbladder)
575.5
cholecystogastric (*see also* Fistula, gallbladder)
575.5
cholecystointestinal (*see also* Fistula,
gallbladder) 575.5
choledochoduodenal 576.4
cholocolic (*see also* Fistula, gallbladder) 575.5
coccyx 685.1
with abscess 685.0
colon 569.81
colostomy 569.69
colovaginal (acquired) 619.1
common duct (bile duct) 576.4
congenital, NEC—*see* Anomaly, specified type
NEC
cornea, causing hypotony 360.32
coronary, arteriovenous 414.19
congenital 746.85
costal region 510.0
cul-de-sac, Douglas' 619.8
cutaneous 686.9
cystic duct (*see also* Fistula, gallbladder) 575.5
congenital 751.69
dental 522.7

Fistula—*continued*
  pericardium (pleura) (sac) (*see also* Pericarditis) 423.8
  pericecal 569.81
  perineal—*see* Fistula, perineum
  perineorectal 569.81
  perineosigmoidal 569.81
  perineo-urethroscrotal 608.89
  perineum, perineal (with urethral involvement) NEC 599.1
    tuberculous (*see also* Tuberculosis) 017.9
    ureter 593.82
  perirectal 565.1
    tuberculous (*see also* Tuberculosis) 014.8
  peritoneum (*see also* Peritonitis) 567.2
  periurethral 599.1
  pharyngo-esophageal 478.29
  pharynx 478.29
    branchial cleft (congenital) 744.41
  pilonidal (infected) (rectum) 685.1
    with abscess 685.0
  pleura, pleural, pleurocutaneous, pleuroperitoneal 510.0
    stomach 510.0
    tuberculous (*see also* Tuberculosis) 012.0
  pleuropericardial 423.8
  postauricular 383.81
  postoperative, persistent 998.6
  preauricular (congenital) 744.46
  prostate 602.8
  pulmonary 510.0
    arteriovenous 417.0
      congenital 747.3
    tuberculous (*see also* Tuberculosis, pulmonary) 011.9
  pulmonoperitoneal 510.0
  rectolabial 619.1
  rectosigmoid (intercommunicating) 569.81
  rectoureteral 593.82
  rectourethral 599.1
    congenital 753.8
  rectouterine 619.1
    congenital 752.3
  rectovaginal 619.1
    congenital 752.49
    old, postpartal 619.1
    tuberculous (*see also* Tuberculosis) 014.8
  rectovesical 596.1
    congenital 753.8
  rectovesicovaginal 619.1
  rectovulvar 619.1
    congenital 752.49
  rectum (to skin) 565.1
    tuberculous (*see also* Tuberculosis) 014.8
  renal 593.89
  retroauricular 383.81
  round window (internal ear) 386.41
  salivary duct or gland 527.4
    congenital 750.24
  sclera 360.32
  scrotum (urinary) 608.89
    tuberculous (*see also* Tuberculosis) 016.5
  semicircular canals (internal ear) 386.43
  sigmoid 569.81
    vesicoabdominal 596.1
  sigmoidovaginal 619.1
    congenital 752.49
  skin 686.9
    ureter 593.82
    vagina 619.2

Fistula—*continued*
  sphenoidal sinus (*see also* Sinusitis, sphenoidal) 473.3
  splenocolic 289.59
  stercoral 569.81
  stomach 537.4
  sublingual gland 527.4
    congenital 750.24
  submaxillary
    gland 527.4
      congenital 750.24
    region 528.3
  thoracic 510.0
    duct 457.8
  thoracicoabdominal 510.0
  thoracicogastric 510.0
  thoracicointestinal 510.0
  thoracoabdominal 510.0
  thoracogastric 510.0
  thorax 510.0
  thyroglossal duct 759.2
  thyroid 246.8
  trachea (congenital) (external) (internal) 748.3
  tracheoesophageal 530.84
    congenital 750.3
    following tracheostomy 519.09
  traumatic
    arteriovenous (*see also* Injury, blood vessel, by site) 904.9
    brain—*see* Injury, intracranial
  tuberculous—*see* Tuberculosis, by site
  typhoid 002.0
  umbilical 759.89
  umbilico-urinary 753.8
  urachal, urachus 753.7
  ureter (persistent) 593.82
  ureteroabdominal 593.82
  ureterocervical 593.82
  ureterorectal 593.82
  ureterosigmoido-abdominal 593.82
  ureterovaginal 619.0
  ureterovesical 596.2
  urethra 599.1
    congenital 753.8
    tuberculous (*see also* Tuberculosis) 016.3
  urethroperineal 599.1
  urethroperineovesical 596.2
  urethrorectal 599.1
    congenital 753.8
  urethroscrotal 608.89
  urethrovaginal 619.0
  urethrovesical 596.2
  urethrovesicovaginal 619.0
  urinary (persistent) (recurrent) 599.1
  uteroabdominal (anterior wall) 619.2
    congenital 752.3
  uteroenteric 619.1
  uterofecal 619.1
  uterointestinal 619.1
    congenital 752.3
  uterorectal 619.1
    congenital 752.3
  uteroureteric 619.0
  uterovaginal 619.8
  uterovesical 619.0
    congenital 752.3
  uterus 619.8
  vagina (wall) 619.8
    postpartal, old 619.8
  vaginocutaneous (postpartal) 619.2
  vaginoileal (acquired) 619.1

Flat
chamber (anterior) (eye) 360.34
chest, congenital 754.89
electroencephalogram (EEG) 348.8
foot (acquired) (fixed type) (painful) (postural)
(spastic) 734
congenital 754.61
rocker bottom 754.61
vertical talus 754.61
rachitic 268.1
rocker bottom (congenital) 754.61
vertical talus, congenital 754.61
organ or site, congenital NEC—*see* Anomaly,
specified type NEC
pelvis 738.6
with disproportion (fetopelvic) 653.2
affecting fetus or newborn 763.1
causing obstructed labor 660.1
affecting fetus or newborn 763.1
congenital 755.69
Flatau-Schilder disease 341.1
Flattening
head, femur 736.39
hip 736.39
lip (congenital) 744.89
nose (congenital) 754.0
acquired 738.0
Flatulence 787.3
Flatus 787.3
vaginalis 629.8
Flax dressers' disease 504
Flea bite —*see* Injury, superficial, by site
Fleischer (-Kayser) ring (corneal pigmentation)
275.1 *[371.14]*
Fleischner's disease 732.3
Fleshy mole 631
Flexibilitas cerea (*see also* Catalepsy) 300.11
Flexion
cervix (*see also* Malposition, uterus) 621.6
contracture, joint (*see also* Contraction, joint)
718.4
deformity, joint (*see also* Contraction, joint)
718.4
hip, congenital (*see also* Subluxation,
congenital, hip) 754.32
uterus (*see also* Malposition, uterus) 621.6
Flexner's
bacillus 004.1
diarrhea (ulcerative) 004.1
dysentery 004.1
Flexner-Boyd dysentery 004.2
Flexure —*see* condition
Floater, vitreous 379.24
Floating
cartilage (joint) (*see also* Disorder, cartilage,
articular) 718.0
knee 717.6
gallbladder (congenital) 751.69
kidney 593.0
congenital 753.3
liver (congenital) 751.69
rib 756.3
spleen 289.59
Flooding 626.2
Floor —*see* condition
Floppy
infant NEC 781.99
valve syndrome (mitral) 424.0
Flu —*see also* Influenza
gastric NEC 008.8
Fluctuating blood pressure 796.4

Fluid
abdomen 789.5
chest (*see also* Pleurisy, with effusion) 511.9
heart (*see also* Failure, heart) 428.0
joint (*see also* Effusion, joint) 719.0
loss (acute) 276.5
with
hypernatremia 276.0
hyponatremia 276.1
lung—*see also* Edema, lung
encysted 511.8
peritoneal cavity 789.5
pleural cavity (*see also* Pleurisy, with effusion)
511.9
retention 276.6
Flukes NEC (*see also* Infestation, fluke) 121.9
blood NEC (*see also* Infestation, Schistosoma)
120.9
liver 121.3
Fluor (albus) (vaginalis) 623.5
trichomonal (Trichomonas vaginalis) 131.00
Fluorosis (dental) (chronic) 520.3
Flushing 782.62
menopausal 627.2
Flush syndrome 259.2
Flutter
atrial or auricular 427.32
heart (ventricular) 427.42
atrial 427.32
impure 427.32
postoperative 997.1
ventricular 427.42
Flux (bloody) (serosanguineous) 009.0
Focal —*see* condition
Fochier's abscess —*see* Abscess, by site
Focus, Assmann's (*see also* Tuberculosis) 011.0
Fogo selvagem 694.4
Foix-Alajouanine syndrome 336.1
Folds, anomalous —*see also* Anomaly, specified
type NEC
Bowman's membrane 371.31
Descemet's membrane 371.32
epicanthic 743.63
heart 746.89
posterior segment of eye, congenital 743.54
Folie à deux 297.3
Follicle
cervix (nabothian) (ruptured) 616.0
graafian, ruptured, with hemorrhage 620.0
nabothian 616.0
Folliclis (primary) (*see also* Tuberculosis) 017.0
Follicular —*see also* condition
cyst (atretic) 620.0
Folliculitis 704.8
abscedens et suffodiens 704.8
decalvans 704.09
gonorrheal (acute) 098.0
chronic or duration of 2 months or more 098.2
keloid, keloidalis 706.1
pustular 704.8
ulerythematosa reticulata 701.8
Folliculosis, conjunctival 372.02
Folling's disease (phenylketonuria) 270.1
Follow-up (examination) (routine) (following)
V67.9
cancer chemotherapy V67.2
chemotherapy V67.2
fracture V67.4
high-risk medication V67.51
injury NEC V67.59

Follow-up—*continued*
  postpartum
    immediately after delivery V24.0
    routine V24.2
  psychiatric V67.3
  psychotherapy V67.3
  radiotherapy V67.1
  specified condition NEC V67.59
  specified surgery NEC V67.09
  surgery V67.00
    vaginal pap smear V67.01
  treatment V67.9
    combined NEC V67.6
    fracture V67.4
    involving high-risk medication NEC V67.51
    mental disorder V67.3
    specified NEC V67.59
Fong's syndrome (hereditary
    osteoonychodysplasia) 756.89
Food
  allergy 693.1
  anaphylactic shock—*see* Anaphylactic shock,
      due to, food
  asphyxia (from aspiration or inhalation) (*see
      also* Asphyxia, food) 933.1
  choked on (*see also* Asphyxia, food) 933.1
  deprivation 994.2
    specified kind of food NEC 269.8
  intoxication (*see also* Poisoning, food) 005.9
  lack of 994.2
  poisoning (*see also* Poisoning, food) 005.9
  refusal or rejection NEC 307.59
  strangulation or suffocation (*see also* Asphyxia,
      food) 933.1
  toxemia (*see also* Poisoning, food) 005.9
Foot —*see also* condition
  and mouth disease 078.4
  process disease 581.3
Foramen ovale (nonclosure) (patent) (persistent)
    745.5
Forbes' (glycogen storage) disease 271.0
Forbes-Albright syndrome (nonpuerperal
    amenorrhea and lactation associated with
    pituitary tumor) 253.1
Forced birth or delivery NEC 669.8
  affecting fetus or newborn NEC 763.89
Forceps
  delivery NEC 669.5
    affecting fetus or newborn 763.2
Fordyce's disease (ectopic sebaceous glands)
    (mouth) 750.26
Fordyce-Fox disease (apocrine miliaria) 705.82
Forearm —*see* condition
Foreign body

> *Note—For foreign body with open wound or
> other injury, see Wound, open, or the type of
> injury specified.*

  accidentally left during a procedure 998.4
  anterior chamber (eye) 871.6
    magnetic 871.5
      retained or old 360.51
    retained or old 360.61
  ciliary body (eye) 871.6
    magnetic 871.5
      retained or old 360.52
    retained or old 360.62
  entering through orifice (current) (old)
    accessory sinus 932
    air passage (upper) 933.0
      lower 934.8

Foreign body—*continued*
  alimentary canal 938
  alveolar process 935.0
  antrum (Highmore) 932
  anus 937
  appendix 936
  asphyxia due to (*see also* Asphyxia, food)
      933.1
  auditory canal 931
  auricle 931
  bladder 939.0
  bronchioles 934.8
  bronchus (main) 934.1
  buccal cavity 935.0
  canthus (inner) 930.1
  cecum 936
  cervix (canal) uterine 939.1
  coil, ileocecal 936
  colon 936
  conjunctiva 930.1
  conjunctival sac 930.1
  cornea 930.0
  digestive organ or tract NEC 938
  duodenum 936
  ear (external) 931
  esophagus 935.1
  eye (external) 930.9
    combined sites 930.8
    intraocular—*see* Foreign body, by site
    specified site NEC 930.8
  eyeball 930.8
    intraocular—*see* Foreign body, intraocular
  eyelid 930.1
    retained or old 374.86
  frontal sinus 932
  gastrointestinal tract 938
  genitourinary tract 939.9
  globe 930.8
    penetrating 871.6
      magnetic 871.5
        retained or old 360.50
      retained or old 360.60
  gum 935.0
  Highmore's antrum 932
  hypopharynx 933.0
  ileocecal coil 936
  ileum 936
  inspiration (of) 933.1
  intestine (large) (small) 936
  lacrimal apparatus, duct, gland, or sac 930.2
  larynx 933.1
  lung 934.8
  maxillary sinus 932
  mouth 935.0
  nasal sinus 932
  nasopharynx 933.0
  nose (passage) 932
  nostril 932
  oral cavity 935.0
  palate 935.0
  penis 939.3
  pharynx 933.0
  pyriform sinus 933.0
  rectosigmoid 937
    junction 937
  rectum 937
  respiratory tract 934.9
    specified part NEC 934.8
  sclera 930.1
  sinus 932
    accessory 932

Foreign body—*continued*
   frontal 932
   maxillary 932
   nasal 932
   pyriform 933.0
  small intestine 936
  stomach (hairball) 935.2
  suffocation by (*see also* Asphyxia, food) 933.1
  swallowed 938
   tongue 933.0
  tear ducts or glands 930.2
  throat 933.0
  tongue 935.0
   swallowed 933.0
  tonsil, tonsillar 933.0
   fossa 933.0
  trachea 934.0
  ureter 939.0
  urethra 939.0
  uterus (any part) 939.1
  vagina 939.2
  vulva 939.2
  wind pipe 934.0
 granuloma (old) 728.82
  bone 733.99
  in operative wound (inadvertently left) 998.4
   due to surgical material intentionally
    left—*see* Complications, due to
    (presence of) any device, implant, or
    graft classified to 996.0-996.5 NEC
  muscle 728.82
  skin 709.4
  soft tissue 709.1
  subcutaneous tissue 709.4
 in
  bone (residual) 733.99
  open wound—*see* Wound, open, by site
   complicated
  soft tissue (residual) 729.6
 inadvertently left in operation wound (causing
  adhesions, obstruction, or perforation) 998.4
 ingestion, ingested NEC 938
 inhalation or inspiration (*see also* Asphyxia,
  food) 933.1
 internal organ, not entering through an
  orifice—*see* Injury, internal, by site, with
  open wound
 intraocular (nonmagnetic) 871.6
  combined sites 871.6
   magnetic 871.5
    retained or old 360.59
   retained or old 360.69
  magnetic 871.5
   retained or old 360.50
  retained or old 360.60
  specified site NEC 871.6
   magnetic 871.5
    retained or old 360.59
   retained or old 360.69
 iris (nonmagnetic) 871.6
  magnetic 871.5
   retained or old 360.52
  retained or old 360.62
 lens (nonmagnetic) 871.6
  magnetic 871.5
   retained or old 360.53
  retained or old 360.63
 lid, eye 930.1
 ocular muscle 870.4
  retained or old 376.6

Foreign body—*continued*
 old or residual
  bone 733.99
  eyelid 374.86
  middle ear 385.83
  muscle 729.6
   ocular 376.6
  retrobulbar 376.6
  skin 729.6
   with granuloma 709.4
  soft tissue 729.6
   with granuloma 709.4
  subcutaneous tissue 729.6
   with granuloma 709.4
 operation wound, left accidentally 998.4
 orbit 870.4
  retained or old 376.6
 posterior wall, eye 871.6
  magnetic 871.5
   retained or old 360.55
  retained or old 360.65
 respiratory tree 934.9
  specified site NEC 934.8
 retained (old) (nonmagnetic) (in)
  anterior chamber (eye) 360.61
   magnetic 360.51
  ciliary body 360.62
   magnetic 360.52
  eyelid 374.86
  globe 360.60
   magnetic 360.50
  intraocular 360.60
   magnetic 360.50
   specified site NEC 360.69
    magnetic 360.59
  iris 360.62
   magnetic 360.52
  lens 360.63
   magnetic 360.53
  muscle 729.6
  orbit 376.6
  posterior wall of globe 360.65
   magnetic 360.55
  retina 360.65
   magnetic 360.55
  retrobulbar 376.6
  skin 729.6
   with granuloma 709.4
  soft tissue 729.6
   with granuloma 709.4
  subcutaneous tissue 729.6
   with granuloma 709.4
  vitreous 360.64
   magnetic 360.54
 retina 871.6
  magnetic 871.5
   retained or old 360.55
  retained or old 360.65
 superficial, without major open wound (*see also*
  Injury, superficial, by site) 919.6
 swallowed NEC 938
 vitreous (humor) 871.6
  magnetic 871.5
   retained or old 360.54
  retained or old 360.64
Forking, aqueduct of Sylvius 742.3
 with spina bifida (*see also* Spina bifida) 741.0
Formation
 bone in scar tissue (skin) 709.3
 connective tissue in vitreous 379.25
 Elschnig pearls (postcataract extraction) 366.51

Formation—*continued*
  hyaline in cornea 371.49
  sequestrum in bone (due to infection) (*see also*
    Osteomyelitis) 730.1
  valve
    colon, congenital 751.5
    ureter (congenital) 753.29
Formication 782.0
Fort Bragg fever 100.89
Fossa —*see also* condition
  pyriform—*see* condition
Foster-Kennedy syndrome 377.04
Fothergill's
  disease, meaning scarlatina anginosa 034.1
  neuralgia (*see also* Neuralgia, trigeminal) 350.1
Foul breath 784.9
Found dead (cause unknown) 798.9
Foundling V20.0
Fournier's disease (idiopathic gangrene) 608.83
Fourth
  cranial nerve—*see* condition
  disease 057.8
  molar 520.1
Foville's syndrome 344.89
Fox's
  disease (apocrine miliaria) 705.82
  impetigo (contagiosa) 684
Fox-Fordyce disease (apocrine miliaria) 705.82
Fracture (abduction) (adduction) (avulsion)
  (compression) (crush) (dislocation) (oblique)
  (separation) (closed) 829.0

> *Note—For fracture of any of the following sites
> with fracture of other bones—see Fracture,
> multiple.*
>
> *"Closed" includes the following descriptions of
> fractures, with or without delayed healing,
> unless they are specified as open or compound:*
>
> > *comminuted*
> > *depressed*
> > *elevated*
> > *fissured*
> > *greenstick*
> > *impacted*
> > *linear*
> > *simple*
> > *slipped epiphysis*
> > *spiral*
> > *unspecified*
>
> *"Open" includes the following descriptions of
> fractures, with or without delayed healing:*
>
> > *compound*
> > *infected*
> > *missile*
> > *puncture*
> > *with foreign body*
>
> *For late effect of fracture, see Late, effect,
> fracture, by site.*

  with
    internal injuries in same region (conditions
      classifiable to 860-869)—*see also* Injury,
      internal, by site
     pelvic region—*see* Fracture, pelvis
  acetabulum (with visceral injury) (closed) 808.0
    open 808.1

Fracture—*continued*
  acromion (process) (closed) 811.01
    open 811.11
  alveolus (closed) 802.8
    open 802.9
  ankle (malleolus) (closed) 824.8
    bimalleolar (Dupuytren's) (Pott's) 824.4
      open 824.5
    bone 825.21
      open 825.31
    lateral malleolus only (fibular) 824.2
      open 824.3
    medial malleolus only (tibial) 824.0
      open 824.1
    open 824.9
    pathologic 733.16
    talus 825.21
      open 825.31
    trimalleolar 824.6
      open 824.7
  antrum—*see* Fracture, skull, base
  arm (closed) 818.0
    and leg(s) (any bones) 828.0
      open 828.1
    both (any bones) (with rib(s)) (with sternum)
      819.0
      open 819.1
    lower 813.80
      open 813.90
    open 818.1
    upper—*see* Fracture, humerus
  astragalus (closed) 825.21
    open 825.31
  atlas—*see* Fracture, vertebra, cervical, first
  axis—*see* Fracture, vertebra, cervical, second
  back—*see* Fracture, vertebra, by site
  Barton's—*see* Fracture, radius, lower end
  basal (skull)—*see* Fracture, skull, base
  Bennett's (closed) 815.01
    open 815.11
  bimalleolar (closed) 824.4
    open 824.5
  bone (closed) NEC 829.0
    birth injury NEC 767.3
    open 829.1
    pathologic NEC (*see also* Fracture,
      pathologic) 733.10
    stress NEC (*see also* Fracture, stress) 733.95
  boot top—*see* Fracture, fibula
  boxers'—*see* Fracture, metacarpal bone(s)
  breast bone—*see* Fracture, sternum
  bucket handle (semilunar cartilage)—*see* Tear,
    meniscus
  bursting—*see* Fracture, phalanx, hand, distal
  calcaneus (closed) 825.0
    open 825.1
  capitate (bone) (closed) 814.07
    open 814.17
  capitellum (humerus) (closed) 812.49
    open 812.59
  carpal bone(s) (wrist NEC) (closed) 814.00
    open 814.10
    specified site NEC 814.09
      open 814.19
  cartilage, knee (semilunar)—*see* Tear, meniscus
  cervical—*see* Fracture, vertebra, cervical
  chauffeur's—*see* Fracture, ulna, lower end
  chisel—*see* Fracture, radius, upper end
  clavicle (interligamentous part) (closed) 810.00
    acromial end 810.03
      open 810.13

Fracture—*continued*
  due to birth trauma 767.2
    open 810.10
    shaft (middle third) 810.02
      open 810.12
    sternal end 810.01
      open 810.11
  clayshovelers'—*see* Fracture, vertebra, cervical
  coccyx—*see also* Fracture, vertebra, coccyx
    complicating delivery 665.6
  collar bone—*see* Fracture, clavicle
  Colles' (reversed) (closed) 813.41
    open 813.51
  comminuted—*see* Fracture, by site
  compression—*see also* Fracture, by site
    nontraumatic—*see* Fracture, pathologic
  congenital 756.9
  coracoid process (closed) 811.02
    open 811.12
  coronoid process (ulna) (closed) 813.02
    mandible (closed) 802.23
      open 802.33
    open 813.12
  costochondral junction—*see* Fracture, rib
  costosternal junction—*see* Fracture, rib
  cranium—*see* Fracture, skull, by site
  cricoid cartilage (closed) 807.5
    open 807.6
  cuboid (ankle) (closed) 825.23
    open 825.33
  cuneiform
    foot (closed) 825.24
      open 825.34
    wrist (closed) 814.03
      open 814.13
  due to
    birth injury—*see* Birth injury, fracture
    gunshot—*see* Fracture, by site, open
    neoplasm—*see* Fracture, pathologic
    osteoporosis—*see* Fracture, pathologic
  Dupuytren's (ankle) (fibula) (closed) 824.4
    open 824.5
    radius 813.42
      open 813.52
  Duverney's—*see* Fracture, ilium
  elbow—*see also* Fracture, humerus, lower end
    olecranon (process) (closed) 813.01
      open 813.11
    supracondylar (closed) 812.41
      open 812.51
  ethmoid (bone) (sinus)—*see* Fracture, skull, base
  face bone(s) (closed) NEC 802.8
    with
      other bone(s)—*see also* Fracture, multiple, skull
      skull—*see also* Fracture, skull
        involving other bones—*see* Fracture, multiple, skull
    open 802.9
  fatigue—*see* Fracture, march
  femur, femoral (closed) 821.00
    cervicotrochanteric 820.03
      open 820.13
    condyles, epicondyles 821.21
      open 821.31
    distal end—*see* Fracture, femur, lower end
    epiphysis (separation)
      capital 820.01
        open 820.11
      head 820.01

Fracture—*continued*
      open 820.11
      lower 821.22
        open 821.32
      trochanteric 820.01
        open 820.11
      upper 820.01
        open 820.11
    head 820.09
      open 820.19
    lower end or extremity (distal end) (closed) 821.20
      condyles, epicondyles 821.21
        open 821.31
      epiphysis (separation) 821.22
        open 821.32
      multiple sites 821.29
        open 821.39
      open 821.30
      specified site NEC 821.29
        open 821.39
      supracondylar 821.23
        open 821.33
      T-shaped 821.21
        open 821.31
    neck (closed) 820.8
      base (cervicotrochanteric) 820.03
        open 820.13
      extracapsular 820.20
        open 820.30
      intertrochanteric (section) 820.21
        open 820.31
      intracapsular 820.00
        open 820.10
      intratrochanteric 820.21
        open 821.31
      midcervical 820.02
        open 820.12
      open 820.9
      pathologic 733.14
        specified part NEC 733.15
      specified site NEC 820.09
        open 820.19
      transcervical 820.02
        open 820.12
      transtrochanteric 820.20
        open 820.30
    open 821.10
    pathologic 733.14
      specified part NEC 733.15
    peritrochanteric (section) 820.20
      open 820.30
    shaft (lower third) (middle third) (upper third) 821.01
      open 821.11
    subcapital 820.09
      open 820.19
    subtrochanteric (region) (section) 820.22
      open 820.32
    supracondylar 821.23
      open 821.33
    transepiphyseal 820.01
      open 820.11
    trochanter (greater) (lesser) (*see also* Fracture, femur, neck, by site) 820.20
      open 820.30
    T-shaped, into knee joint 821.21
      open 821.31
    upper end 820.8
      open 820.9

Fracture—*continued*
  fibula (closed) 823.81
    with tibia 823.82
      open 823.92
    distal end 824.8
      open 824.9
    epiphysis
      lower 824.8
        open 824.9
      upper—*see* Fracture, fibula, upper end
    head—*see* Fracture, fibula, upper end
    involving ankle 824.2
      open 824.3
    lower end or extremity 824.8
      open 824.9
    malleolus (external) (lateral) 824.2
      open 824.3
    open NEC 823.91
    pathologic 733.16
    proximal end—*see* Fracture, fibula, upper end
    shaft 823.21
      with tibia 823.22
        open 823.32
      open 823.31
    stress 733.93
    torus 823.41
      with tibia 823.42
    upper end or extremity (epiphysis) (head)
      (proximal end) (styloid) 823.01
      with tibia 823.02
        open 823.12
      open 823.11
  finger(s), of one hand (closed) (*see also*
    Fracture, phalanx, hand) 816.00
    with
      metacarpal bone(s), of same hand 817.0
        open 817.1
      thumb of same hand 816.03
        open 816.13
    open 816.10
  foot, except toe(s) alone (closed) 825.20
    open 825.30
  forearm (closed) NEC 813.80
    lower end (distal end) (lower epiphysis)
      813.40
      open 813.50
    open 813.90
    shaft 813.20
      open 813.30
    upper end (proximal end) (upper epiphysis)
      813.00
      open 813.10
  fossa, anterior, middle, or posterior—*see*
    Fracture, skull, base
  frontal (bone)—*see also* Fracture, skull, vault
    sinus—*see* Fracture, skull base
  Galeazzi's—*see* Fracture, radius, lower end
  glenoid (cavity) (fossa) (scapula) (closed)
    811.03
    open 811.13
  Gosselin's—*see* Fracture, ankle
  greenstick—*see* Fracture, by site
  grenade-throwers'—*see* Fracture, humerus, shaft
  gutter—*see* Fracture, skull, vault
  hamate (closed) 814.08
    open 814.18
  hand, one (closed) 815.00
    carpals 814.00
      open 814.10
      specified site NEC 814.09
        open 814.19

Fracture—*continued*
  metacarpals 815.00
    open 815.10
  multiple, bones of one hand 817.0
    open 817.1
  open 815.10
  phalanges (*see also* Fracture, phalanx, hand)
    816.00
    open 816.10
  healing
    aftercare (*see also* Aftercare, fracture) V54.89
    change of cast V54.89
    complications—*see* condition
    convalescence V66.4
    removal of
      cast V54.89
      fixation device
        external V54.89
        internal V54.0
  heel bone (closed) 825.0
    open 825.1
  hip (closed) (*see also* Fracture, femur, neck)
    820.8
    open 820.9
    pathologic 733.14
  humerus (closed) 812.20
    anatomical neck 812.02
      open 812.12
    articular process (*see also* Fracture, humerus,
      condyle(s) 812.44
      open 812.54
    capitellum 812.49
      open 812.59
    condyle(s) 812.44
      lateral (external) 812.42
        open 812.52
      medial (internal epicondyle) 812.43
        open 812.53
      open 812.54
    distal end—*see* Fracture, humerus, lower end
    epiphysis
      lower (*see also* Fracture, humerus,
        condyle(s)) 812.44
        open 812.54
      upper 812.09
        open 812.19
    external condyle 812.42
      open 812.52
    great tuberosity 812.03
      open 812.13
    head 812.09
      open 812.19
    internal epicondyle 812.43
      open 812.53
    lesser tuberosity 812.09
      open 812.19
    lower end or extremity (distal end) (*see also*
      Fracture, humerus, by site) 812.40
      multiple sites NEC 812.49
        open 812.59
      open 812.50
      specified site NEC 812.49
        open 812.59
    neck 812.01
      open 812.11
    open 812.30
    pathologic 733.11
    proximal end—*see* Fracture, humerus, upper
      end
    shaft 812.21
      open 812.31

Fracture—*continued*
  shaft 815.03
    open 815.13
  metatarsus, metatarsal (bone(s)), of one foot
      (closed) 825.25
    with tarsal bone(s) 825.29
      open 825.39
    open 825.35
  Monteggia's (closed) 813.03
    open 813.13
  Moore's—*see* Fracture, radius, lower end
  multangular bone (closed)
    larger 814.05
      open 814.15
    smaller 814.06
      open 814.16
  multiple (closed) 829.0

Note—Multiple fractures of sites classifiable to the same three- or four-digit category are coded to that category, except for sites classifiable to 810-818 or 820-827 in different limbs.

Multiple fractures of sites classifiable to different fourth-digit subdivisions within the same three- digit category should be dealt with according to coding rules.

Multiple fractures of sites classifiable to different three-digit categories (identifiable from the listing under "Fracture"), and of sites classifiable to 810-818 or 820-827 in different limbs should be coded according to the following list, which should be referred to in the following priority order: skull or face bones, pelvis or vertebral column, legs, arms.

    arm (multiple bones in same arm except in
        hand alone) (sites classifiable to 810-817
        with sites classifiable to a different
        three-digit category in 810-817 in same
        arm) (closed) 818.0
      open 818.1
    arms, both or arm(s) with rib(s) or sternum
        (sites classifiable to 810-818 with sites
        classifiable to same range of categories in
        other limb or to 807) (closed) 819.0
      open 819.1
    bones of trunk NEC (closed) 809.0
      open 809.1
    hand, metacarpal bone(s) with phalanx or
        phalanges of same hand (sites classifiable
        to 815 with sites classifiable to 816 in
        same hand) (closed) 817.0
      open 817.1
    leg (multiple bones in same leg) (sites
        classifiable to 820-826 with sites
        classifiable to a different three-digit
        category in that range in same leg)
        (closed) 827.0
      open 827.1
    legs, both or leg(s) with arm(s), rib(s), or
        sternum (sites classifiable to 820-
        827 with sites classifiable to same range
        of categories in other leg or to 807 or
        810-819) (closed) 828.0
      open 828.1
    open 829.1
    pelvis with other bones except skull or face
        bones (sites classifiable to 808 with sites
        classifiable to 805-807 or 810-829)
        (closed) 809.0

Fracture—*continued*
  open 809.1
  skull, specified or unspecified bones, or face
      bone(s) with any other bone(s) (sites
      classifiable to 800-803 with sites
      classifiable to 805-829) (closed) 804.0

Note—Use the following fifth-digit subclassification with categories 800, 801, 803, and 804:

0 unspecified state of consciousness
1 with no loss of consciousness
2 with brief [less than one hour] loss of
     consciousness
3 with moderate [1-24 hours] loss of
     consciousness
4 with prolonged [more than 24 hours] loss of
     consciousness and return to pre-existing
     conscious level
5 with prolonged [more than 24 hours] loss of
     consciousness, without return to pre-existing
     conscious level
Use fifth-digit 5 to designate when a patient is unconcious and dies before regaining conciousness, regardless of the duration of the loss of conciousness
6 with loss of consciousness of unspecified
     duration
9 with concussion, unspecified

  with
    contusion, cerebral 804.1
    epidural hemorrhage 804.2
    extradural hemorrhage 804.2
    hemorrhage (intracranial) NEC 804.3
    intracranial injury NEC 804.4
    laceration, cerebral 804.1
    subarachnoid hemorrhage 804.2
    subdural hemorrhage 804.2
  open 804.5
    with
      contusion, cerebral 804.6
      epidural hemorrhage 804.7
      extradural hemorrhage 804.7
      hemorrhage (intracranial) NEC 804.8
      intracranial injury NEC 804.9
      laceration, cerebral 804.6
      subarachnoid hemorrhage 804.7
      subdural hemorrhage 804.7
  vertebral column with other bones, except
      skull or face bones (sites classifiable to
      805 or 806 with sites classifiable to
      807-808 or 810-829) (closed) 809.0
    open 809.1
  nasal (bone(s)) (closed) 802.0
    open 802.1
  sinus—Fracture, skull, base
  navicular
    carpal (wrist) (closed) 814.01
      open 814.11
    tarsal (ankle) (closed) 825.22
      open 825.32
  neck—*see* Fracture, vertebra, cervical
  neural arch—*see* Fracture, vertebra, by site
  nonunion 733.82
  nose, nasal, (bone) (septum) (closed) 802.0
    open 802.1
  occiput—*see* Fracture, skull, base
  odontoid process—*see* Fracture, vertebra,
      cervical

        (closed) 809.0

Fracture—*continued*
  olecranon (process) (ulna) (closed) 813.01
    open 813.11
  open 829.1
  orbit, orbital (bone) (region) (closed) 802.8
    floor (blow-out) 802.6
      open 802.7
    open 802.9
    roof—*see* Fracture, skull, base
    specified part NEC 802.8
      open 802.9
  os
    calcis (closed) 825.0
      open 825.1
    magnum (closed) 814.07
      open 814.17
    pubis (with visceral injury) (closed) 808.2
      open 808.3
    triquetrum (closed) 814.03
      open 814.13
  osseous
    auditory meatus—*see* Fracture, skull, base
    labyrinth—*see* Fracture, skull, base
  ossicles, auditory (incus) (malleus)
    (stapes)—*see* Fracture, skull, base
  osteoporotic—*see* Fracture, pathologic
  palate (closed) 802.8
    open 802.9
  paratrooper—*see* Fracture, tibia, lower end
  parietal bone—*see* Fracture, skull, vault
  parry—*see* Fracture, Monteggia's
  patella (closed) 822.0
    open 822.1
  pathologic (cause unknown) 733.10
    ankle 733.16
    femur (neck) 733.14
      specified NEC 733.15
    fibula 733.16
    hip 733.14
    humerus 733.11
    radius 733.12
    specified site NEC 733.19
    tibia 733.16
    ulna 733.12
    vertebrae (collapse) 733.13
    wrist 733.12
  pedicle (of vertebral arch)—*see* Fracture,
    vertebra, by site
  pelvis, pelvic (bone(s)) (with visceral injury)
    (closed) 808.8
    multiple (with disruption of pelvic circle)
      808.43
      open 808.53
    open 808.9
    rim (closed) 808.49
      open 808.59
  peritrochanteric (closed) 820.20
    open 820.30
  phalanx, phalanges, of one
    foot (closed) 826.0
      with bone(s) of same lower limb 827.0
        open 827.1
      open 826.1

Fracture—*continued*
  hand (closed) 816.00
    with metacarpal bone(s) of same hand 817.0
      open 817.1
    distal 816.02
      open 816.12
    middle 816.01
      open 816.11
    multiple sites NEC 816.03
      open 816.13
    open 816.10
    proximal 816.01
      open 816.11
  pisiform (closed) 814.04
    open 814.14
  pond—Fracture, skull, vault
  Pott's (closed) 824.4
    open 824.5
  prosthetic device, internal—*see* Complications,
    mechanical
  pubis (with visceral injury) (closed) 808.2
    open 808.3
  Quervain's (closed) 814.01
    open 814.11
  radius (alone) (closed) 813.81
    with ulna NEC 813.83
      open 813.93
    distal end—*see* Fracture, radius, lower end
    epiphysis
      lower—*see* Fracture, radius, lower end
      upper—*see* Fracture, radius, upper end
    head—*see* Fracture, radius, upper end
    lower end or extremity (distal end) (lower
      epiphysis) 813.42
      with ulna (lower end) 813.44
        open 813.54
      open 813.52
      torus 813.45
    neck—*see* Fracture, radius, upper end
    open NEC 813.91
    pathologic 733.12
    proximal end—*see* Fracture, radius, upper end
    shaft (closed) 813.21
      with ulna (shaft) 813.23
        open 813.33
      open 813.31
    upper end 813.07
      with ulna (upper end) 813.08
        open 813.18
      epiphysis 813.05
        open 813.15
      head 813.05
        open 813.15
      multiple sites 813.07
        open 813.17
      neck 813.06
        open 813.16
      open 813.17
      specified site NEC 813.07
        open 813.17
  ramus
    inferior or superior (with visceral injury)
      (closed) 808.2
      open 808.3
    ischium—*see* Fracture, ischium
    mandible 802.24
      open 802.34
  rib(s) (closed) 807.0

Fracture—*continued*

> *Note—Use the following fifth-digit*
> *subclassification with categories 807.0-807.1:*
>
> *0 rib(s), unspecified*
> *1 one rib*
> *2 two ribs*
> *3 three ribs*
> *4 four ribs*
> *5 five ribs*
> *6 six ribs*
> *7 seven ribs*
> *8 eight or more ribs*
> *9 multiple ribs, unspecified*

    with flail chest (open) 807.4
    open 807.1
  root, tooth 873.63
    complicated 873.73
  sacrum—*see* Fracture, vertebra, sacrum
  scaphoid
    ankle (closed) 825.22
      open 825.32
    wrist (closed) 814.01
      open 814.11
  scapula (closed) 811.00
    acromial, acromion (process) 811.01
      open 811.11
    body 811.09
      open 811.19
    coracoid process 811.02
      open 811.12
    glenoid (cavity) (fossa) 811.03
      open 811.13
    neck 811.03
      open 811.13
    open 811.10
  semilunar
    bone, wrist (closed) 814.02
      open 814.12
    cartilage (interior) (knee)—*see* Tear, meniscus
  sesamoid bone—*see* Fracture, by site
  Shepherd's (closed) 825.21
    open 825.31
  shoulder—*see also* Fracture, humerus, upper end
    blade—*see* Fracture, scapula
  silverfork—*see* Fracture, radius, lower end
  sinus (ethmoid) (frontal) (maxillary) (nasal)
    (sphenoidal)—*see* Fracture, skull, base
    maxillary—*see* Fracture, maxilla
  Skillern's—*see* Fracture, radius, shaft
  skull (multiple NEC) (with face bones) (closed)
    803.0

Fracture—*continued*

> *Note—Use the following fifth-digit*
> *subclassification with categories 800, 801, 803,*
> *and 804:*
>
> *0 unspecified state of consciousness*
> *1 with no loss of consciousness*
> *2 with brief [less than one hour] loss of*
> *consciousness*
> *3 with moderate [1-24 hours] loss of*
> *consciousness*
> *4 with prolonged [more than 24 hours] loss of*
> *consciousness and return to pre-existing*
> *conscious level*
> *5 with prolonged [more than 24 hours] loss of*
> *consciousness, without return to pre-existing*
> *conscious level*
> *Use fifth-digit 5 to designate when a patient is*
> *unconscious and dies before regaining*
> *consciousness, regardless of the duration of the*
> *loss of consciousness*
> *6 with loss of consciousness of unspecified*
> *duration*
> *9 with concussion, unspecified*

    with
      contusion, cerebral 803.1
      epidural hemorrhage 803.2
      extradural hemorrhage 803.2
      hemorrhage (intracranial) NEC 803.3
      intracranial injury NEC 803.4
      laceration, cerebral 803.1
      other bones—*see* Fracture, multiple, skull
      subarachnoid hemorrhage 803.2
      subdural hemorrhage 803.2
    base (antrum) (ethmoid bone) (fossa) (internal
      ear) (nasal sinus) (occiput) (sphenoid)
      (temporal bone) (closed) 801.0
    with
      contusion, cerebral 801.1
      epidural hemorrhage 801.2
      extradural hemorrhage 801.2
      hemorrhage (intracranial) NEC 801.3
      intracranial injury NEC 801.4
      laceration, cerebral 801.1
      subarachnoid hemorrhage 801.2
      subdural hemorrhage 801.2
    open 801.5
      with
        contusion, cerebral 801.6
        epidural hemorrhage 801.7
        extradural hemorrhage 801.7
        hemorrhage (intracranial) NEC 801.8
        intracranial injury NEC 801.9
        laceration, cerebral 801.6
        subarachnoid hemorrhage 801.7
        subdural hemorrhage 801.7
    birth injury 767.3
    face bones—*see* Fracture, face bones
    open 803.5
      with
        contusion, cerebral 803.6
        epidural hemorrhage 803.7
        extradural hemorrhage 803.7
        hemorrhage (intracranial) NEC 803.8
        intracranial injury NEC 803.9
        laceration, cerebral 803.6
        subarachnoid hemorrhage 803.7
        subdural hemorrhage 803.7
    vault (frontal bone) (parietal bone) (vertex)
      (closed) 800.0

Fracture—*continued*
with
contusion, cerebral 800.1
epidural hemorrhage 800.2
extradural hemorrhage 800.2
hemorrhage (intracranial) NEC 800.3
intracranial injury NEC 800.4
laceration, cerebral 800.1
subarachnoid hemorrhage 800.2
subdural hemorrhage 800.2
open 800.5
with
contusion, cerebral 800.6
epidural hemorrhage 800.7
extradural hemorrhage 800.7
hemorrhage (intracranial) NEC 800.8
intracranial injury NEC 800.9
laceration, cerebral 800.6
subarachnoid hemorrhage 800.7
subdural hemorrhage 800.7
Smith's 813.41
open 813.51
sphenoid (bone) (sinus)—*see* Fracture, skull, base
spine—*see also* Fracture, vertebra, by site
due to birth trauma 767.4
spinous process—*see* Fracture, vertebra, by site
spontaneous—*see* Fracture, pathologic
sprinters'—*see* Fracture, ilium
stapes—*see* Fracture, skull, base
stave—*see also* Fracture, metacarpus, metacarpal bone(s)
spine—*see* Fracture, tibia, upper end
sternum (closed) 807.2
with flail chest (open) 807.4
open 807.3
Stieda's—*see* Fracture, femur, lower end
stress 733.95
fibula 733.93
metatarsals 733.94
specified site NEC 733.95
tibia 733.93
styloid process
metacarpal (closed) 815.02
open 815.12
radius—*see* Fracture, radius, lower end
temporal bone—*see* Fracture, skull, base
ulna—*see* Fracture, ulna, lower end
supracondylar, elbow 812.41
open 812.51
symphysis pubis (with visceral injury) (closed) 808.2
open 808.3
talus (ankle bone) (closed) 825.21
open 825.31
tarsus, tarsal bone(s) (with metatarsus) of one foot (closed) NEC 825.29
open 825.39
temporal bone (styloid)—*see* Fracture, skull, base
tendon—*see* Sprain, by site
thigh—*see* Fracture, femur, shaft
thumb (and finger(s)) of one hand (closed) (*see also* Fracture, phalanx, hand) 816.00
with metacarpal bone(s) of same hand 817.0
open 817.1
metacarpal(s)—*see* Fracture, metacarpus
open 816.10
thyroid cartilage (closed) 807.5
open 807.6

Fracture—*continued*
tibia (closed) 823.80
with fibula 823.82
open 823.92
condyles—*see* Fracture, tibia, upper end
distal end 824.8
open 824.9
epiphysis
lower 824.8
open 824.9
upper—*see* Fracture, tibia, upper end
head (involving knee joint)—*see* Fracture, tibia, upper end
intercondyloid eminence—*see* Fracture, tibia, upper end
involving ankle 824.0
open 824.1
lower end or extremity (anterior lip) (posterior lip) 824.8
open 824.9
malleolus (internal) (medial) 824.0
open 824.1
open NEC 823.90
pathologic 733.16
proximal end—*see* Fracture, tibia, upper end
shaft 823.20
with fibula 823.22
open 823.32
open 823.30
spine—*see* Fracture, tibia, upper end
stress 733.93
torus 823.40
with tibia 823.42
tuberosity—*see* Fracture, tibia, upper end
upper end or extremity (condyle) (epiphysis) (head) (spine) (proximal end) (tuberosity) 823.00
with fibula 823.02
open 823.12
open 823.10
toe(s), of one foot (closed) 826.0
with bone(s) of same lower limb 827.0
open 827.1
open 826.1
tooth (root) 873.63
complicated 873.73
torus
fibula 823.41
with tibia 823.42
radius 813.45
tibia 823.40
with fibula 823.42
trachea (closed) 807.5
open 807.6
transverse process—*see* Fracture, vertebra, by site
trapezium (closed) 814.05
open 814.15
trapezoid bone (closed) 814.06
open 814.16
trimalleolar (closed) 824.6
open 824.7
triquetral (bone) (closed) 814.03
open 814.13
trochanter (greater) (lesser) (closed) (*see also* Fracture, femur, neck, by site) 820.20
open 820.30
trunk (bones) (closed) 809.0
open 809.1
tuberosity (external)—*see* Fracture, by site

Fracture—*continued*
  ulna (alone) (closed) 813.82
    with radius NEC 813.83
      open 813.93
    coronoid process (closed) 813.02
      open 813.12
    distal end—*see* Fracture, ulna, lower end
    epiphysis
      lower—*see* Fracture, ulna, lower end
      upper—*see* Fracture, ulna, upper, end
    head—*see* Fracture, ulna, lower end
    lower end (distal end) (head) (lower
      epiphysis) (styloid process) 813.43
      with radius (lower end) 813.44
        open 813.54
      open 813.53
    olecranon process (closed) 813.01
      open 813.11
    open NEC 813.92
    pathologic 733.12
    proximal end—*see* Fracture, ulna, upper end
    shaft 813.22
      with radius (shaft) 813.23
        open 813.33
      open 813.32
    styloid process—*see* Fracture, ulna, lower end
    transverse—*see* Fracture, ulna, by site
    upper end (epiphysis) 813.04
      with radius (upper end) 813.08
        open 813.18
      multiple sites 813.04
        open 813.14
      open 813.14
      specified site NEC 813.04
        open 813.14
  unciform (closed) 814.08
    open 814.18
  vertebra, vertebral (back) (body) (column)
    (neural arch) (pedicle) (spine) (spinous
    process) (transverse process) (closed) 805.8
    with
      hematomyelia—*see* Fracture, vertebra, by
        site, with spinal cord injury
      injury to
        cauda equina—*see* Fracture, vertebra,
          sacrum, with spinal cord injury
        nerve—*see* Fracture, vertebra, by site,
          with spinal cord injury
        paralysis—*see* Fracture, vertebra, by site,
          with spinal cord injury
        paraplegia—*see* Fracture, vertebra, by site,
          with spinal cord injury
        quadriplegia—*see* Fracture, vertebra, by
          site, with spinal cord injury
        spinal concussion—*see* Fracture, vertebra,
          by site, with spinal cord injury
      spinal cord injury (closed) NEC 806.8

Fracture—*continued*

> *Note—Use the following fifth-digit subclassification with categories 806.0-806.3:*
>
> *C_1-C_4 or unspecified level and D_1-D_6 (T_1-T_6) or unspecified level with:*
>
> *0 unspecified spinal cord injury*
> *1 complete lesion of cord*
> *2 anterior cord syndrome*
> *3 central cord syndrome*
> *4 specified injury NEC*
>
> *C_5-C_7 level and D_7-D_{12} level with:*
>
> *5 unspecified spinal cord injury*
> *6 complete lesion of cord*
> *7 anterior cord syndrome*
> *8 central cord syndrome*
> *9 specified injury NEC*

      cervical 806.0
        open 806.1
      dorsal, dorsolumbar 806.2
        open 806.3
      open 806.9
      thoracic, thoracolumbar 806.2
        open 806.3
    atlanto-axial—*see* Fracture, vertebra, cervical
    cervical (hangman) (teardrop) (closed) 805.00
      with spinal cord injury—*see* Fracture,
        vertebra, with spinal cord injury, cervical
      first (atlas) 805.01
        open 805.11
      second (axis) 805.02
        open 805.12
      third 805.03
        open 805.13
      fourth 805.04
        open 805.14
      fifth 805.05
        open 805.15
      sixth 805.06
        open 805.16
      seventh 805.07
        open 805.17
      multiple sites 805.08
        open 805.18
      open 805.10
    coccyx (closed) 805.6
      with spinal cord injury (closed) 806.60
        cauda equina injury 806.62
          complete lesion 806.61
            open 806.71
          open 806.72
        open 806.70
        specified type NEC 806.69
          open 806.79
      open 805.7
    collapsed 733.13
    compression, not due to trauma 733.13
    dorsal (closed) 805.2
      with spinal cord injury—*see* Fracture,
        vertebra, with spinal cord injury, dorsal
      open 805.3
    dorsolumbar (closed) 805.2
      with spinal cord injury—*see* Fracture,
        vertebra, with spinal cord injury, dorsal
      open 805.3
    due to osteoporosis 733.13
    fetus or newborn 767.4

Fulminant, fulminating —*see* condition
Functional —*see* condition
Fundus —*see also* condition
  flavimaculatus 362.76
Fungemia 117.9
Fungus, fungous
  cerebral 348.8
  disease NEC 117.9
  infection—*see* Infection, fungus
  testis (*see also* Tuberculosis) 016.5 *[608.81]*
Funiculitis (acute) 608.4
  chronic 608.4
  endemic 608.4
  gonococcal (acute) 098.14
    chronic or duration of 2 months or over 098.34
  tuberculous (*see also* Tuberculosis) 016.5
F.U.O. (*see also* Pyrexia) 780.6
Funnel
  breast (acquired) 738.3
    congenital 754.81
    late effect of rickets 268.1
  chest (acquired) 738.3
    congenital 754.81
    late effect of rickets 268.1
  pelvis (acquired) 738.6
    with disproportion (fetopelvic) 653.3
      affecting fetus or newborn 763.1
      causing obstructed labor 660.1
        affecting fetus or newborn 763.1
    congenital 755.69
    tuberculous (*see also* Tuberculosis) 016.9
Furfur 690.18
  microsporon 111.0
Furor, paroxysmal (idiopathic) (*see also*
    Epilepsy) 345.8
Furriers' lung 495.8
Furrowed tongue 529.5
  congenital 750.13
Furrowing nail (s) (transverse) 703.8
  congenital 757.5
Furuncle 680.9
  abdominal wall 680.2
  ankle 680.6
  anus 680.5
  arm (any part, above wrist) 680.3
  auditory canal, external 680.0
  axilla 680.3
  back (any part) 680.2
  breast 680.2
  buttock 680.5
  chest wall 680.2
  corpus cavernosum 607.2
  ear (any part) 680.0
  eyelid 373.13
  face (any part, except eye) 680.0
  finger (any) 680.4
  flank 680.2
  foot (any part) 680.7
  forearm 680.3
  gluteal (region) 680.5
  groin 680.2
  hand (any part) 680.4
  head (any part, except face) 680.8
  heel 680.7
  hip 680.6
  kidney (*see also* Abscess, kidney) 590.2
  knee 680.6
  labium (majus) (minus) 616.4
  lacrimal
    gland (*see also* Dacryoadenitis) 375.00

Furuncle—*continued*
  passages (duct) (sac) (see *also* Dacryocystitis)
    375.30
  leg, any part except foot 680.6
  malignant 022.0
  multiple sites 680.9
  neck 680.1
  nose (external) (septum) 680.0
  orbit 376.01
  partes posteriores 680.5
  pectoral region 680.2
  penis 607.2
  perineum 680.2
  pinna 680.0
  scalp (any part) 680.8
  scrotum 608.4
  seminal vesicle 608.0
  shoulder 680.3
  skin NEC 680.9
  specified site NEC 680.8
  spermatic cord 608.4
  temple (region) 680.0
  testis 604.90
  thigh 680.6
  thumb 680.4
  toe (any) 680.7
  trunk 680.2
  tunica vaginalis 608.4
  umbilicus 680.2
  upper arm 680.3
  vas deferens 608.4
  vulva 616.4
  wrist 680.4
Furunculosis (*see also* Furuncle) 680.9
  external auditory meatus 680.0 *[380.13]*
Fusarium (infection) 118
Fusion, fused (congenital)
  anal (with urogenital canal) 751.5
  aorta and pulmonary artery 745.0
  astragaloscaphoid 755.67
  atria 745.5
  atrium and ventricle 745.69
  auditory canal 744.02
  auricles, heart 745.5
  binocular, with defective stereopsis 368.33
  bone 756.9
  cervical spine—*see* Fusion, spine
  choanal 748.0
  commissure, mitral valve 746.5
  cranial sutures, premature 756.0
  cusps, heart valve NEC 746.89
    mitral 746.5
    tricuspid 746.89
  ear ossicles 744.04
  fingers (*see also* Syndactylism, fingers) 755.11
  hymen 752.42
  hymeno-urethral 599.89
    causing obstructed labor 660.1
      affecting fetus or newborn 763.1
  joint (acquired)—*see also* Ankylosis
    congenital 755.8
  kidneys (incomplete) 753.3
  labium (majus) (minus) 752.49
  larynx and trachea 748.3
  limb 755.8
    lower 755.69
    upper 755.59
  lobe, lung 748.5
  lumbosacral (acquired) 724.6
    congenital 756.15
    surgical V45.4

Fusion, fused—*continued*
  nares (anterior) (posterior) 748.0
  nose, nasal 748.0
  nostril(s) 748.0
  organ or site NEC—*see* Anomaly, specified
    type NEC
  ossicles 756.9
    auditory 744.04
  pulmonary valve segment 746.02
  pulmonic cusps 746.02
  ribs 756.3
  sacroiliac (acquired) (joint) 724.6
    congenital 755.69
    surgical V45.4
  skull, imperfect 756.0
  spine (acquired) 724.9
    arthrodesis status V45.4
    congenital (vertebra) 756.15
    postoperative status V45.4
  sublingual duct with submaxillary duct at
    opening in mouth 750.26
  talonavicular (bar) 755.67
  teeth, tooth 520.2
  testes 752.8
  toes (*see also* Syndactylism, toes) 755.13
  trachea and esophagus 750.3
  twins 759.4
  urethral-hymenal 599.89
  vagina 752.49
  valve cusps—*see* Fusion, cusps, heart valve
  ventricles, heart 745.4
  vertebra (arch)—*see* Fusion, spine
  vulva 752.49
Fusospirillosis (mouth) (tongue) (tonsil) 101
Fussy infant (baby) 780.91

G

Gafsa boil 085.1
Gain, weight (abnormal) (excessive) (*see also*
   Weight, gain) 783.1
Gaisböck's disease or syndrome (polycythemia
   hypertonica) 289.0
Gait
  abnormality 781.2
   hysterical 300.11
  ataxic 781.2
   hysterical 300.11
  disturbance 781.2
   hysterical 300.11
  paralytic 781.2
  scissor 781.2
  spastic 781.2
  staggering 781.2
   hysterical 300.11
Galactocele (breast) (infected) 611.5
  puerperal, postpartum 676.8
Galactophoritis 611.0
  puerperal, postpartum 675.2
Galactorrhea 676.6
  not associated with childbirth 611.6
Galactosemia (classic) (congenital) 271.1
Galactosuria 271.1
Galacturia 791.1
  bilharziasis 120.0
Galen's vein *—see* condition
Gallbladder *—see also* condition
  acute (*see also* Disease, gallbladder) 575.0
Gall duct *—see* condition
Gallop rhythm 427.89
Gallstone (cholemic) (colic) (impacted)*—see*
  also Cholelithiasis
  causing intestinal obstruction 560.31
Gambling, pathological 312.31
Gammaloidosis 277.3
Gammopathy 273.9
  macroglobulinemia 273.3
  monoclonal (benign) (essential) (idiopathic)
   (with lymphoplasmacytic dyscrasia) 273.1
Gamna's disease (siderotic splenomegaly)
  289.51
Gampsodactylia (congenital) 754.71
Gamstorp's disease (adynamia episodica
  hereditaria) 359.3
Gandy-Nanta disease (siderotic splenomegaly)
  289.51
**Gang activity without manifest psychiatric
  disorder** V71.09
  adolescent V71.02
  adult V71.01
  child V71.02
Gangliocytoma (M9490/0)*—see* Neoplasm,
  connective tissue, benign
Ganglioglioma (M9505/1)*—see* Neoplasm, by
  site, uncertain behavior
Ganglion 727.43
  joint 727.41
  of yaws (early) (late) 102.6
  periosteal (*see also* Periostitis) 730.3
  tendon sheath (compound) (diffuse) 727.42
  tuberculous (*see also* Tuberculosis) 015.9
Ganglioneuroblastoma (M9490/3)*—see*
  Neoplasm, connective tissue, malignant

Ganglioneuroma (M9490/0)*—see also*
  Neoplasm, connective tissue, benign
  malignant (M9490/3)*—see* Neoplasm,
   connective tissue, malignant
Ganglioneuromatosis (M9491/0)*—see*
  Neoplasm, connective tissue, benign
Ganglionitis
  fifth nerve (*see also* Neuralgia, trigeminal) 350.1
  gasserian 350.1
  geniculate 351.1
   herpetic 053.11
   newborn 767.5
  herpes zoster 053.11
  herpetic geniculate (Hunt's syndrome) 053.11
Gangliosidosis 330.1
Gangosa 102.5
Gangrene, gangrenous (anemia) (artery)
  (cellulitis) (dermatitis) (dry) (infective)
  (moist) (pemphigus) (septic) (skin) (stasis)
  (ulcer) 785.4
  with
   arteriosclerosis (native artery) 440.24
    bypass graft 440.30
     autologous vein 440.31
     nonautologous biological 440.32
   diabetes (mellitus) 250.7 *[785.4]*
  abdomen (wall) 785.4
   arteriosclerotic 440.29 *[785.4]*
  adenitis 683
  alveolar 526.5
  angina 462
   diphtheritic 032.0
  anus 569.49
  appendices epiploicae*—see* Gangrene,
   mesentery
  appendix*—see* Appendicitis, acute
  arteriosclerotic *—see* Arteriosclerosis, with,
   gangrene
  auricle 785.4
  Bacillus welchii (*see also* Gangrene, gas) 040.0
  bile duct (*see also* Cholangitis) 576.8
  bladder 595.89
  bowel*—see* Gangrene, intestine
  cecum*—see* Gangrene, intestine
  Clostridium perfringens or welchii (*see also*
   Gangrene, gas) 040.0
  colon*—see* Gangrene, intestine
  connective tissue 785.4
  cornea 371.40
  corpora cavernosa (infective) 607.2
   noninfective 607.89
  cutaneous, spreading 785.4
  decubital 707.0 *[785.4]*
  diabetic (any site) 250.7 *[785.4]*
  dropsical 785.4
  emphysematous (*see also* Gangrene, gas) 040.0
  epidemic (ergotized grain) 988.2
  epididymis (infectional) (*see also* Epididymitis)
   604.99
  erysipelas (*see also* Erysipelas) 035
  extremity (lower) (upper) 785.4
  gallbladder or duct (*see also* Cholecystitis,
   acute) 575.0
  gas (bacillus) 040.0

Gangrene, gangrenous—*continued*
  with
    abortion—*see* Abortion, by type, with sepsis
    ectopic pregnancy (*see also* categories
      633.0-633.9) 639.0
    molar pregnancy (*see also* categories
      630-632) 639.0
  following
    abortion 639.0
    ectopic or molar pregnancy 639.0
  puerperal, postpartum, childbirth 670
  glossitis 529.0
  gum 523.8
  hernia—*see* Hernia, by site, with gangrene
  hospital noma 528.1
  intestine, intestinal (acute) (hemorrhagic)
    (massive) 557.0
    with
      hernia—*see* Hernia, by site, with gangrene
      mesenteric embolism or infarction 557.0
      obstruction (*see also* Obstruction, intestine)
        560.9
  laryngitis 464.00
    with obstruction 464.01
  liver 573.8
  lung 513.0
    spirochetal 104.8
  lymphangitis 457.2
  Meleney's (cutaneous) 686.09
  mesentery 557.0
    with
      embolism or infarction 557.0
      intestinal obstruction (*see also* Obstruction,
        intestine) 560.9
  mouth 528.1
  noma 528.1
  orchitis 604.90
  ovary (*see also* Salpingo-oophoritis) 614.2
  pancreas 577.0
  penis (infectional) 607.2
    noninfective 607.89
  perineum 785.4
  pharynx 462
    septic 034.0
  pneumonia 513.0
  Pott's 440.24
  presenile 443.1
  pulmonary 513.0
  pulp, tooth 522.1
  quinsy 475
  Raynaud's (symmetric gangrene) 443.0 *[785.4]*
  rectum 569.49
  retropharyngeal 478.24
  rupture—*see* Hernia, by site, with gangrene
  scrotum 608.4
    noninfective 608.83
  senile 440.24
  sore throat 462
  spermatic cord 608.4
    noninfective 608.89
  spine 785.4
  spirochetal NEC 104.8
  spreading cutaneous 785.4
  stomach 537.89
  stomatitis 528.1
  symmetrical 443.0 *[785.4]*
  testis (infectional) (*see also* Orchitis) 604.99
    noninfective 608.89
  throat 462
    diphtheritic 032.0
  thyroid (gland) 246.8

Gangrene, gangrenous—*continued*
  tonsillitis (acute) 463
  tooth (pulp) 522.1
  tuberculous NEC (*see also* Tuberculosis) 011.9
  tunica vaginalis 608.4
    noninfective 608.89
  umbilicus 785.4
  uterus (*see also* Endometritis) 615.9
  uvulitis 528.3
  vas deferens 608.4
    noninfective 608.89
  vulva (*see also* Vulvitis) 616.10
Gannister disease (occupational) 502
  with tuberculosis—*see* Tuberculosis, pulmonary
Ganser's syndrome, hysterical 300.16
Gardner-Diamond syndrome (autoerythrocyte
  sensitization) 287.2
Gargoylism 277.5
Garré's
  disease (*see also* Osteomyelitis) 730.1
  osteitis (sclerosing) (*see also* Osteomyelitis)
    730.1
  osteomyelitis (*see also* Osteomyelitis) 730.1
Garrod's pads, knuckle 728.79
Gartner's duct
  cyst 752.11
  persistent 752.11
Gas
  asphyxia, asphyxiation, inhalation, poisoning,
    suffocation NEC 987.9
    specified gas—*see* Table of drugs and
      chemicals
  bacillus gangrene or infection—*see* Gas,
    gangrene
  cyst, mesentery 568.89
  excessive 787.3
  gangrene 040.0
    with
      abortion—*see* Abortion, by type, with sepsis
      ectopic pregnancy (*see also* categories
        633.0-633.9) 639.0
      molar pregnancy (*see also* categories
        630-632) 639.0
    following
      abortion 639.0
      ectopic or molar pregnancy 639.0
    puerperal, postpartum, childbirth 670
  on stomach 787.3
  pains 787.3
Gastradenitis 535.0
Gastralgia 536.8
  psychogenic 307.89
Gastrectasis, gastrectasia 536.1
  psychogenic 306.4
Gastric —*see* condition
Gastrinoma (M8153/1)
  malignant (M8153/3)
    pancreas 157.4
    specified site NEC—*see* Neoplasm, by site,
      malignant
    unspecified site 157.4
    specified site—*see* Neoplasm, by site,
      uncertain behavior
  unspecified site 235.5

Gastritis 535.5

> *Note—Use the following fifth-digit subclassification for category 535:*
>
> 0 *without mention of hemorrhage*
> 1 *with hemorrhage*

    acute 535.0
    alcoholic 535.3
    allergic 535.4
    antral 535.4
    atrophic 535.1
    atrophic-hyperplastic 535.1
    bile-induced 535.4
    catarrhal 535.0
    chronic (atrophic) 535.1
    cirrhotic 535.4
    corrosive (acute) 535.4
    dietetic 535.4
    due to diet deficiency 269.9 *[535.4]*
    eosinophilic 535.4
    erosive 535.4
    follicular 535.4
        chronic 535.1
    giant hypertrophic 535.2
    glandular 535.4
        chronic 535.1
    hypertrophic (mucosa) 535.2
        chronic giant 211.1
    irritant 535.4
    nervous 306.4
    phlegmonous 535.0
    psychogenic 306.4
    sclerotic 535.4
    spastic 536.8
    subacute 535.0
    superficial 535.4
    suppurative 535.0
    toxic 535.4
    tuberculous (*see also* Tuberculosis) 017.9
Gastrocarcinoma (M8010/3) 151.9
Gastrocolic —*see* condition
Gastrocolitis —*see* Enteritis
Gastrodisciasis 121.8
Gastroduodenitis (*see also* Gastritis) 535.5
    catarrhal 535.0
    infectional 535.0
    virus, viral 008.8
        specified type NEC 008.69
Gastrodynia 536.8
Gastroenteritis (acute) (catarrhal) (congestive) (hemorrhagic) (noninfectious) (*see also* Enteritis) 558.9
    aertrycke infection 003.0
    allergic 558.3
    chronic 558.9
        ulcerative (*see also* Colitis, ulcerative) 556.9
    dietetic 558.9
    due to
        food poisoning (*see also* Poisoning, food) 005.9
        radiation 558.1
    epidemic 009.0
    functional 558.9
    infectious (*see also* Enteritis, due to, by organism) 009.0
        presumed 009.1
    salmonella 003.0
    septic (*see also* Enteritis, due to, by organism) 009.0
    toxic 558.2

Gastroenteritis—*continued*
    tuberculous (*see also* Tuberculosis) 014.8
    ulcerative (*see also* Colitis, ulcerative) 556.9
    viral NEC 008.8
        specified type NEC 008.69
    zymotic 009.0
Gastroenterocolitis —*see* Enteritis
Gastroenteropathy, protein-losing 579.8
Gastroenteroptosis 569.89
Gastroesophageal laceration-hemorrhage syndrome 530.7
Gastroesophagitis 530.19
Gastrohepatitis (*see also* Gastritis) 535.5
Gastrointestinal —*see* condition
Gastrojejunal —*see* condition
Gastrojejunitis (*see also* Gastritis) 535.5
Gastrojejunocolic —*see* condition
Gastroliths 537.89
Gastromalacia 537.89
Gastroparalysis 536.8
    diabetic 250.6 *[337.1]*
Gastroparesis 536.3
    diabetic 250.6 *[536.3]*
Gastropathy, exudative 579.8
Gastroptosis 537.5
Gastrorrhagia 578.0
Gastrorrhea 536.8
    psychogenic 306.4
Gastroschisis (congenital) 756.79
    acquired 569.89
Gastrospasm (neurogenic) (reflex) 536.8
    neurotic 306.4
    psychogenic 306.4
Gastrostaxis 578.0
Gastrostenosis 537.89
Gastrostomy
    attention to V55.1
    complication 536.40
        specified type 536.49
    infection 536.41
    malfunctioning 536.42
    status V44.1
Gastrosuccorrhea (continuous) (intermittent) 536.8
    neurotic 306.4
    psychogenic 306.4
Gaucher's
    disease (adult) (cerebroside lipidosis) (infantile) 272.7
    hepatomegaly 272.7
    splenomegaly (cerebroside lipidosis) 272.7
Gayet's disease (superior hemorrhagic polioencephalitis) 265.1
Gayet-Wernicke's syndrome (superior hemorrhagic polioencephalitis) 265.1
Gee (-Herter) (-Heubner) (-Thaysen) disease or syndrome (nontropical sprue) 579.0
Gélineau's syndrome 347
Gemination, teeth 520.2
Gemistocytoma (M9411/3)
    specified site—*see* Neoplasm, by site, malignant
    unspecified site 191.9
General, generalized —*see* condition
Genital —*see* condition
Genito-anorectal syndrome 099.1
Genitourinary system —*see* condition
Genu
    congenital 755.64
    extrorsum (acquired) 736.42
        congenital 755.64
        late effects of rickets 268.1

Glomerulonephritis—*continued*
   chronic 582.4
    renal necrosis 583.9
     cortical 583.6
     medullary 583.7
    specified pathology NEC 583.89
     acute 580.89
     chronic 582.89
   necrosis, renal 583.9
    cortical 583.6
    medullary (papillary) 583.7
   specified pathology or lesion NEC 583.89
  acute 580.9
   with
    exudative nephritis 580.89
    interstitial nephritis (diffuse) (focal) 580.89
    necrotizing glomerulitis 580.4
   extracapillary with epithelial crescents 580.4
   poststreptococcal 580.0
   proliferative (diffuse) 580.0
   rapidly progressive 580.4
   specified pathology NEC 580.89
  arteriolar (*see also* Hypertension, kidney) 403.90
  arteriosclerotic (*see also* Hypertension, kidney)
   403.90
  ascending (*see also* Pyelitis) 590.80
  basement membrane NEC 583.89
   with
    pulmonary hemorrhage (Goodpasture's
     syndrome) 446.21 *[583.81]*
  chronic 582.9
   with
    exudative nephritis 582.89
    interstitial nephritis (diffuse) (focal) 582.89
    necrotizing glomerulitis 582.4
    specified pathology or lesion NEC 582.89
   endothelial 582.2
   extracapillary with epithelial crescents 582.4
   hypocomplementemic persistent 582.2
   lobular 582.2
   membranoproliferative 582.2
   membranous 582.1
    and proliferative (mixed) 582.2
    sclerosing 582.1
   mesangiocapillary 582.2
   mixed membranous and proliferative 582.2
   proliferative (diffuse) 582.0
   rapidly progressive 582.4
   sclerosing 582.1
  cirrhotic—*see* Sclerosis, renal
  desquamative—*see* Nephrosis
  due to or associated with
   amyloidosis 277.3 *[583.81]*
    with nephrotic syndrome 277.3 *[581.81]*
    chronic 277.3 *[582.81]*
   diabetes mellitus 250.4 *[583.81]*
    with nephrotic syndrome 250.4 *[581.81]*
   diphtheria 032.89 *[580.81]*
   gonococcal infection (acute) 098.19 *[583.81]*
    chronic or duration or 2 months or over
     098.39 *[583.81]*
   infectious hepatitis 070.9 *[580.81]*
   malaria (with nephrotic syndrome) 084.9
    [581.81]
   mumps 072.79 *[580.81]*
   polyarteritis (nodosa) (with nephrotic
    syndrome) 446.0 *[581.81]*
   specified pathology NEC 583.89
    acute 580.89
    chronic 582.89
   streptotrichosis 039.8 *[583.81]*

Glomerulonephritis—*continued*
  subacute bacterial endocarditis 421.0 *[580.81]*
  syphilis (late) 095.4
   congenital 090.5 *[583.81]*
   early 091.69 *[583.81]*
  systemic lupus erythematosus 710.0 *[583.81]*
   with nephrotic syndrome 710.0 *[581.81]*
   chronic 710.0 *[582.81]*
  tuberculosis (*see also* Tuberculosis) 016.0
   [583.81]
  typhoid fever 002.0 *[580.81]*
  extracapillary with epithelial crescents 583.4
   acute 580.4
   chronic 582.4
  exudative 583.89
   acute 580.89
   chronic 582.89
  focal (*see also* Nephritis) 583.9
   embolic 580.4
  granular 582.89
  granulomatous 582.89
  hydremic (*see also* Nephrosis) 581.9
  hypocomplementemic persistent 583.2
   with nephrotic syndrome 581.2
   chronic 582.2
  immune complex NEC 583.89
  infective (*see also* Pyelitis) 590.80
  interstitial (diffuse) (focal) 583.89
   with nephrotic syndrome 581.89
   acute 580.89
   chronic 582.89
  latent or quiescent 582.9
  lobular 583.2
   with nephrotic syndrome 581.2
   chronic 582.2
  membranoproliferative 583.2
   with nephrotic syndrome 581.2
   chronic 582.2
  membranous 583.1
   with nephrotic syndrome 581.1
   and proliferative (mixed) 583.2
    with nephrotic syndrome 581.2
    chronic 582.2
   chronic 582.1
   sclerosing 582.1
    with nephrotic syndrome 581.1
  mesangiocapillary 583.2
   with nephrotic syndrome 581.2
   chronic 582.2
  minimal change 581.3
  mixed membranous and proliferative 583.2
   with nephrotic syndrome 581.2
   chronic 582.2
  necrotizing 583.4
   acute 580.4
   chronic 582.4
  nephrotic (*see also* Nephrosis) 581.9
  old—*see* Glomerulonephritis, chronic
  parenchymatous 581.89
  poststreptococcal 580.0
  proliferative (diffuse) 583.0
   with nephrotic syndrome 581.0
   acute 580.0
   chronic 582.0
  purulent (*see also* Pyelitis) 590.80
  quiescent—*see* Nephritis, chronic
  rapidly progressive 583.4
   acute 580.4
   chronic 582.4
  sclerosing membranous (chronic) 582.1
   with nephrotic syndrome 581.1

Glomerulonephritis—*continued*
  septic (*see also* Pyelitis) 590.80
  specified pathology or lesion NEC 583.89
    with nephrotic syndrome 581.89
    acute 580.89
    chronic 582.89
  suppurative (acute) (disseminated) (*see also* Pyelitis) 590.80
  toxic—*see* Nephritis, acute
  tubal, tubular—*see* Nephrosis, tubular
  type II (Ellis)—*see* Nephrosis
  vascular—*see* Hypertension, kidney
Glomerulosclerosis (*see also* Sclerosis, renal) 587
  focal 582.1
    with nephrotic syndrome 581.1
  intercapillary (nodular) (with diabetes) 250.4 [581.81]
Glossagra 529.6
Glossalgia 529.6
Glossitis 529.0
  areata exfoliativa 529.1
  atrophic 529.4
  benign migratory 529.1
  gangrenous 529.0
  Hunter's 529.4
  median rhomboid 529.2
  Moeller's 529.4
  pellagrous 265.2
Glossocele 529.8
Glossodynia 529.6
  exfoliativa 529.4
Glossoncus 529.8
Glossophytia 529.3
Glossoplegia 529.8
Glossoptosis 529.8
Glossopyrosis 529.6
Glossotrichia 529.3
Glossy skin 701.9
Glottis —*see* condition
Glottitis —*see* Glossitis
Glucagonoma (M8152/0)
  malignant (M8152/3)
    pancreas 157.4
    specified site NEC—*see* Neoplasm, by site, malignant
    unspecified site 157.4
  pancreas 211.7
  specified site NEC—*see* Neoplasm, by site, benign
  unspecified site 211.7
Glucoglycinuria 270.7
Glue ear syndrome 381.20
Glue sniffing (airplane glue) (*see also* Dependence) 304.6
Glycinemia (with methylmalonic acidemia) 270.7
Glycinuria (renal) (with ketosis) 270.0
Glycogen
  infiltration (*see also* Disease, glycogen storage) 271.0
  storage disease (*see also* Disease, glycogen storage) 271.0
Glycogenosis (*see also* Disease, glycogen storage) 271.0
  cardiac 271.0 [425.7]
  Cori, types I–VII 271.0
  diabetic, secondary 250.8 [259.8]
  diffuse (with hepatic cirrhosis) 271.0
  generalized 271.0
  glucose-6-phosphatase deficiency 271.0
  hepatophosphorylase deficiency 271.0

Glycogenosis—*continued*
  hepatorenal 271.0
  myophosphorylase deficiency 271.0
Glycopenia 251.2
Glycoprolinuria 270.8
Glycosuria 791.5
  renal 271.4
Gnathostoma (spinigerum) (infection) (infestation) 128.1
  wandering swellings from 128.1
Gnathostomiasis 128.1
Goiter (adolescent) (colloid) (diffuse) (dipping) (due to iodine deficiency) (endemic) (euthyroid) (heart) (hyperplastic) (internal) (intrathoracic) (juvenile) (mixed type) (nonendemic) (parenchymatous) (plunging) (sporadic) (subclavicular) (substernal) 240.9
  with
    hyperthyroidism (recurrent) (*see also* Goiter, toxic) 242.0
    thyrotoxicosis (*see also* Goiter, toxic) 242.0
  adenomatous (*see also* Goiter, nodular) 241.9
  cancerous (M8000/3) 193
  complicating pregnancy, childbirth, or puerperium 648.1
  congenital 246.1
  cystic (*see also* Goiter, nodular) 241.9
  due to enzyme defect in synthesis of thyroid hormone (butane-insoluble iodine) (coupling) (deiodinase) (iodide trapping or organification) (iodotyrosine dehalogenase) (peroxidase) 246.1
  dyshormonogenic 246.1
  exophthalmic (*see also* Goiter, toxic) 242.0
  familial (with deaf-mutism) 243
  fibrous 245.3
  lingual 759.2
  lymphadenoid 245.2
  malignant (M8000/3) 193
  multinodular (nontoxic) 241.1
    toxic or with hyperthyroidism (*see also* Goiter, toxic) 242.2
  nodular (nontoxic) 241.9
    with
      hyperthyroidism (*see also* Goiter, toxic) 242.3
      thyrotoxicosis (*see also* Goiter, toxic) 242.3
    endemic 241.9
    exophthalmic (diffuse) (*see also* Goiter, toxic) 242.0
    multinodular (nontoxic) 241.1
    sporadic 241.9
    toxic (*see also* Goiter, toxic) 242.3
    uninodular (nontoxic) 241.0
  nontoxic (nodular) 241.9
    multinodular 241.1
    uninodular 241.0
  pulsating (*see also* Goiter, toxic) 242.0
  simple 240.0
  toxic 242.0

Note—Use the following fifth-digit subclassification with category 242:

0   *without mention of thyrotoxic crisis or storm*
1   *with mention of thyrotoxic crisis or storm*

  adenomatous 242.3
    multinodular 242.2
    uninodular 242.1
  multinodular 242.2

Goiter—*continued*
    nodular 242.3
       multinodular 242.2
       uninodular 242.1
     uninodular 242.1
    uninodular (nontoxic) 241.0
     toxic or with hyperthyroidism (*see also*
       Goiter, toxic) 242.1
Goldberg (-Maxwell) (-Morris) syndrome
    (testicular feminization) 257.8
Goldblatt's
  hypertension 440.1
  kidney 440.1
Goldenhar's syndrome (oculoauriculovertebral
    dysplasia) 756.0
Goldflam-Erb disease or syndrome 358.0
Goldscheider's disease (epidermolysis bullosa)
    757.39
Goldstein's disease (familial hemorrhagic
    telangiectasia) 448.0
Golfer's elbow 726.32
Goltz-Gorlin syndrome (dermal hypoplasia)
    757.39
Gonadoblastoma (M9073/1)
  specified site—*see* Neoplasm, by site uncertain
    behavior
  unspecified site
    female 236.2
    male 236.4
Gonecystitis (*see also* Vesiculitis) 608.0
Gongylonemiasis 125.6
  mouth 125.6
Goniosynechiae 364.73
Gonococcemia 098.89
Gonococcus, gonococcal (disease) (infection)
    (*see also* condition) 098.0
  anus 098.7
  bursa 098.52
  chronic NEC 098.2
  complicating pregnancy, childbirth, or
    puerperium 647.1
    affecting fetus or newborn 760.2
  conjunctiva, conjunctivitis (neonatorum) 098.40
  dermatosis 098.89
  endocardium 098.84
  epididymo-orchitis 098.13
    chronic or duration of 2 months or over 098.33
  eye (newborn) 098.40
  fallopian tube (chronic) 098.37
    acute 098.17
  genitourinary (acute) (organ) (system) (tract)
    (*see also* Gonorrhea) 098.0
    lower 098.0
     chronic 098.2
    upper 098.10
     chronic 098.30
  heart NEC 098.85
  joint 098.50
  keratoderma 098.81
  keratosis (blennorrhagica) 098.81
  lymphatic (gland) (node) 098.89
  meninges 098.82
  orchitis (acute) 098.13
    chronic or duration of 2 months or over 098.33
  pelvis (acute) 098.19
    chronic or duration of 2 months or over 098.39
  pericarditis 098.83
  peritonitis 098.86
  pharyngitis 098.6
  pharynx 098.6

Gonococcus, gonococcal—*continued*
  proctitis 098.7
  pyosalpinx (chronic) 098.37
    acute 098.17
  rectum 098.7
  septicemia 098.89
  skin 098.89
  specified site NEC 098.89
  synovitis 098.51
  tendon sheath 098.51
  throat 098.6
  urethra (acute) 098.0
    chronic of duration of 2 months or over 098.2
  vulva (acute) 098.0
    chronic or duration of 2 months or over 098.2
Gonocytoma (M9073/1)
  specified site—*see* Neoplasm, by site, uncertain
    behavior
  unspecified site
    female 236.2
    male 236.4
Gonorrhea 098.0
  acute 098.0
  Bartholin's gland (acute) 098.0
    chronic or duration of 2 months or over 098.2
  bladder (acute) 098.11
    chronic or duration of 2 months or over 098.31
  carrier (suspected of) V02.7
  cervix (acute) 098.15
    chronic or duration of 2 months or over 098.35
  chronic 098.2
  complicating pregnancy, childbirth, or
    puerperium 647.1
    affecting fetus or newborn 760.2
  conjunctiva, conjunctivitis (neonatorum) 098.40
  contact V01.6
  Cowper's gland (acute) 098.0
    chronic or duration of 2 months or over 098.2
  duration of two months or over 098.2
  exposure to V01.6
  fallopian tube (chronic) 098.37
    acute 098.17
  genitourinary (acute) (organ) (system) (tract)
    098.0
    chronic 098.2
    duration of two months or over 098.2
  kidney (acute) 098.19
    chronic or duration of 2 months or over 098.39
  ovary (acute) 098.19
    chronic or duration of 2 months or over 098.39
  pelvis (acute) 098.19
    chronic or duration of 2 months or over 098.39
  penis (acute) 098.0
    chronic or duration of 2 months or over 098.2
  prostate (acute) 098.12
    chronic or duration of 2 months or over 098.32
  seminal vesicle (acute) 098.14
    chronic or duration of 2 months or over 098.34
  specified site NEC—*see* Gonococcus
  spermatic cord (acute) 098.14
    chronic or duration of 2 months or over 098.34
  urethra (acute) 098.0
    chronic or duration of 2 months or over 098.2
  vagina (acute) 098.0
    chronic or duration of 2 months or over 098.2
  vas deferens (acute) 098.14
    chronic or duration of 2 months or over 098.34
  vulva (acute) 098.0
    chronic or duration of 2 months or over 098.2
Goodpasture's syndrome (pneumorenal) 446.21

Gopalan's syndrome (burning feet) 266.2
Gordon's disease (exudative enteropathy) 579.8
Gorlin-Chaudhry-Moss syndrome 759.89
Gougerot's syndrome (trisymptomatic) 709.1
Gougerot-Blum syndrome (pigmented purpuric
 lichenoid dermatitis) 709.1
Gougerot-Carteaud disease or syndrome
 (confluent reticulate papillomatosis) 701.8
Gougerot-Hailey-Hailey disease (benign
 familial chronic pemphigus) 757.39
Gougerot (-Houwer) -Sjögren syndrome
 (keratoconjunctivitis sicca) 710.2
Gouley's syndrome (constrictive pericarditis)
 423.2
Goundou 102.6
Gout, gouty 274.9
 with specified manifestations NEC 274.89
 arthritis (acute) 274.0
 arthropathy 274.0
 degeneration, heart 274.82
 diathesis 274.9
 eczema 274.89
 episcleritis 274.89 *[379.09]*
 external ear (tophus) 274.81
 glomerulonephritis 274.10
 iritis 274.89 *[364.11]*
 joint 274.0
 kidney 274.10
 lead 984.9
  specified type of lead—*see* Table of drugs and
   chemicals
 nephritis 274.10
 neuritis 274.89 *[357.4]*
 phlebitis 274.89 *[451.9]*
 rheumatic 714.0
 saturnine 984.9
  specified type of lead—*see* Table of drugs and
   chemicals
 spondylitis 274.0
 synovitis 274.0
 syphilitic 095.8
 tophi 274.0
  ear 274.81
  heart 274.82
  specified site NEC 274.82
Gowers'
 muscular dystrophy 359.1
 syndrome (vasovagal attack) 780.2
Gowers-Paton-Kennedy syndrome 377.04
Gradenigo's syndrome 383.02
Graft-versus-host disease (bone marrow) 996.85
 due to organ transplant NEC—*see*
  Complications, transplant, organ
Graham Steell's murmur (pulmonic
  regurgitation) (*see also* Endocarditis,
  pulmonary) 424.3
Grain-handlers' disease or lung 495.8
Grain mite (itch) 133.8
Grand
 mal (idiopathic) (*see also* Epilepsy) 345.1
  hysteria of Charcot 300.11
  nonrecurrent or isolated 780.39
 multipara
  affecting management of labor and delivery
   659.4
  status only (not pregnant) V61.5
Granite workers' lung 502

Granular —*see also* condition
 inflammation, pharynx 472.1
 kidney (contracting) (*see also* Sclerosis, renal)
  587
 liver—*see* Cirrhosis, liver
 nephritis—*see* Nephritis
Granulation tissue, abnormal —*see also*
  Granuloma
 abnormal or excessive 701.5
 postmastoidectomy cavity 383.33
 postoperative 701.5
 skin 701.5
Granulocytopenia, granulocytopenic (primary)
  288.0
 malignant 288.0
Granuloma NEC 686.1
 abdomen (wall) 568.89
  skin (pyogenicum) 686.1
   from residual foreign body 709.4
 annulare 695.89
 anus 569.49
 apical 522.6
 appendix 543.9
 aural 380.23
 beryllium (skin) 709.4
  lung 503
 bone (*see also* Osteomyelitis) 730.1
  eosinophilic 277.8
  from residual foreign body 733.99
 canaliculus lacrimalis 375.81
 cerebral 348.8
 cholesterin, middle ear 385.82
 coccidioidal (progressive) 114.3
  lung 114.4
  meninges 114.2
  primary (lung) 114.0
 colon 569.89
 conjunctiva 372.61
 dental 522.6
 ear, middle (cholesterin) 385.82
  with otitis media—*see* Otitis media
 eosinophilic 277.8
  bone 277.8
  lung 277.8
  oral mucosa 528.9
 exuberant 701.5
 eyelid 374.89
 facial
  lethal midline 446.3
  malignant 446.3
 faciale 701.8
 fissuratum (gum) 523.8
 foot NEC 686.1
 foreign body (in soft tissue) NEC 728.82
  bone 733.99
  in operative wound 998.4
  muscle 728.82
  skin 709.4
  subcutaneous tissue 709.4
 fungoides 202.1
 gangraenescens 446.3
 giant cell (central) (jaw) (reparative) 526.3
  gingiva 523.8
  peripheral (gingiva) 523.8
 gland (lymph) 289.3
 Hodgkin's (M9661/3) 201.1
 ileum 569.89
 infectious NEC 136.9
 inguinale (Donovan) 099.2
  venereal 099.2
 intestine 569.89

Growth (fungoid) (neoplastic) (new)
(M8000/1)—*see also* Neoplasm, by site,
unspecified nature
adenoid (vegetative) 474.12
benign (M8000/0)—*see* Neoplasm, by site,
benign
fetal, poor 764.9
affecting management of pregnancy 656.5
malignant (M8000/3)—*see* Neoplasm, by site
malignant
rapid, childhood V21.0
secondary (M8000/6)—*see* Neoplasm, by site,
malignant, secondary
Gruber's hernia —*see* Hernia, Gruber's
Gruby's disease (tinea tonsurans) 110.0
G-trisomy 758.0
Guama fever 066.3
Gubler (-Millard) paralysis or syndrome 344.89
Guérin-Stern syndrome (arthrogryposis
multiplex congenita) 754.89
Guertin's disease (electric chorea) 049.8
Guillain-Barré disease or syndrome 357.0
Guinea worms (infection) (infestation) 125.7
Guinon's disease (motor-verbal tic) 307.23
Gull's disease (thyroid atrophy with myxedema)
244.8
Gull and Sutton's disease —*see* Hypertension,
kidney
Gum —*see* condition
Gumboil 522.7
Gumma (syphilitic) 095.9
artery 093.89
cerebral or spinal 094.89
bone 095.5
of yaws (late) 102.6
brain 094.89
cauda equina 094.89
central nervous system NEC 094.9
ciliary body 095.8 *[364.11]*
congenital 090.5
testis 090.5
eyelid 095.8 *[373.5]*
heart 093.89
intracranial 094.89
iris 095.8 *[364.11]*
kidney 095.4
larynx 095.8
leptomeninges 094.2
liver 095.3
meninges 094.2
myocardium 093.82
nasopharynx 095.8
neurosyphilitic 094.9
nose 095.8
orbit 095.8
palate (soft) 095.8
penis 095.8
pericardium 093.81
pharynx 095.8
pituitary 095.8
scrofulous (*see also* Tuberculosis) 017.0
skin 095.8
specified site NEC 095.8
spinal cord 094.89
tongue 095.8
tonsil 095.8
trachea 095.8
tuberculous (*see also* Tuberculosis) 017.0

Gumma—*continued*
ulcerative due to yaws 102.4
ureter 095.8
yaws 102.4
bone 102.6
Gunn's syndrome (jaw-winking syndrome)
742.8
Gunshot wound —*see also* Wound, open, by site
fracture—*see* Fracture, by site, open
internal organs (abdomen, chest, or pelvis)—*see*
Injury, internal, by site, with open wound
intracranial—*see* Laceration, brain, with open
intracranial wound
Günther's disease or syndrome (congenital
erythropoietic porphyria) 277.1
Gustatory hallucination 780.1
Gynandrism 752.7
Gynandroblastoma (M8632/1)
specified site—*see* Neoplasm, by site, uncertain
behavior
unspecified site
female 236.2
male 236.4
Gynandromorphism 752.7
Gynatresia (congenital) 752.49
Gynecoid pelvis, male 738.6
Gynecological examination V72.3
for contraceptive maintenance V25.40
Gynecomastia 611.1
Gynephobia 300.29
Gyrate scalp 757.39

H

Haas' disease (osteochondrosis head of humerus) 732.3
Habermann's disease (acute parapsoriasis varioliformis) 696.2
Habit, habituation
chorea 307.22
disturbance, child 307.9
drug (*see also* Dependence) 304.9
laxative (*see also* Abuse, drugs, nondependent) 305.9
spasm 307.20
chronic 307.22
transient of childhood 307.21
tic 307.20
chronic 307.22
transient of childhood 307.21
use of
nonprescribed drugs (*see also* Abuse, drugs, nondependent) 305.9
patent medicines (*see also* Abuse, drugs, nondependent) 305.9
vomiting 536.2
Hadfield-Clarke syndrome (pancreatic infantilism) 577.8
Haff disease 985.1
Hageman factor defect, deficiency, or disease (*see also* Defect, coagulation) 286.3
Haglund's disease (osteochondrosis os tibiale externum) 732.5
Haglund-Läwen-Fründ syndrome 717.89
Hagner's disease (hypertrophic pulmonary osteoarthropathy) 731.2
Hag teeth, tooth 524.3
Hailey-Hailey disease (benign familial chronic pemphigus) 757.39
Hair —*see also* condition
plucking 307.9
Hairball in stomach 935.2
Hairy black tongue 529.3
Half vertebra 756.14
Halitosis 784.9
Hallermann-Streiff syndrome 756.0
Hallervorden-Spatz disease or syndrome 333.0
Hallopeau's
acrodermatitis (continua) 696.1
disease (lichen sclerosis et atrophicus) 701.0
Hallucination (auditory) (gustatory) (olfactory) (tactile) 780.1
alcoholic 291.3
drug-induced 292.12
visual 368.16
Hallucinosis 298.9
alcoholic (acute) 291.3
drug-induced 292.12
Hallus —*see* Hallux
Hallux 735.9
malleus (acquired) 735.3
rigidus (acquired) 735.2
congenital 755.66
late effects of rickets 268.1
valgus (acquired) 735.0
congenital 755.66
varus (acquired) 735.1
congenital 755.66
Halo, visual 368.15
Hamartoblastoma 759.6

Hamartoma 759.6
epithelial (gingival), odontogenic, central, or peripheral (M9321/0) 213.1
upper jaw (bone) 213.0
vascular 757.32
Hamartosis, hamartoses NEC 759.6
Hamman's disease or syndrome (spontaneous mediastinal emphysema) 518.1
Hamman-Rich syndrome (diffuse interstitial pulmonary fibrosis) 516.3
Hammer toe (acquired) 735.4
congenital 755.66
late effects of rickets 268.1
Hand —*see* condition
Hand-Schüller-Christian disease or syndrome (chronic histiocytosis x) 277.8
Hand-foot syndrome 282.61
Hanging (asphyxia) (strangulation) (suffocation) 994.7
Hangnail (finger) (with lymphangitis) 681.02
Hangover (alcohol) (*see also* Abuse, drugs, nondependent) 305.0
Hanot's cirrhosis or disease —*see* Cirrhosis, biliary
Hanot-Chauffard (-Troisier) syndrome (bronze diabetes) 275.0
Hansen's disease (leprosy) 030.9
benign form 030.1
malignant form 030.0
Harada's disease or syndrome 363.22
Hard chancre 091.0
Hard firm prostate 600.1
Hardening
artery—*see* Arteriosclerosis
brain 348.8
liver 571.8
Hare's syndrome (M8010/3) (carcinoma, pulmonary apex) 162.3
Harelip (*see also* Cleft, lip) 749.10
Harkavy's syndrome 446.0
Harlequin (fetus) 757.1
color change syndrome 779.89
Harley's disease (intermittent hemoglobinuria) 283.2
Harris'
lines 733.91
syndrome (organic hyperinsulinism) 251.1
Hart's disease or syndrome (pellagra-cerebellar ataxia-renal aminoaciduria) 270.0
Hartmann's pouch (abnormal sacculation of gallbladder neck) 575.8
of intestine V44.3
attention to V55.3
Hartnup disease (pellagra-cerebellar ataxia-renal aminoaciduria) 270.0
Harvester lung 495.0
Hashimoto's disease or struma (struma lymphomatosa) 245.2
Hassall-Henle bodies (corneal warts) 371.41
Haut mal (*see also* Epilepsy) 345.1
Haverhill fever 026.1
Hawaiian wood rose dependence 304.5
Hawkins' keloid 701.4
Hay
asthma (*see also* Asthma) 493.0
fever (allergic) (with rhinitis) 477.9
with asthma (bronchial) (*see also* Asthma) 493.0

Hay —*continued*
  allergic, due to grass, pollen, ragweed, or tree 477.0
  conjunctivitis 372.05
  due to
    dander 477.8
    dust 477.8
    fowl 477.8
    pollen 477.0
    specified allergen other than pollen 477.8
Hayem-Faber syndrome (achlorhydric anemia) 280.9
Hayem-Widal syndrome (acquired hemolytic jaundice) 283.9
Haygarth's nodosities 715.04
Hazard-Crile tumor (M8350/3) 193
Hb (abnormal)
  disease—*see* Disease, hemoglobin
  trait—*see* Trait
H disease 270.0
Head —*see also* condition
  banging 307.3
Headache 784.0
  allergic 346.2
  cluster 346.2
  due to
    loss, spinal fluid 349.0
    lumbar puncture 349.0
    saddle block 349.0
  emotional 307.81
  histamine 346.2
  lumbar puncture 349.0
  menopausal 627.2
  migraine 346.9
  nonorganic origin 307.81
  postspinal 349.0
  psychogenic 307.81
  psychophysiologic 307.81
  sick 346.1
  spinal 349.0
    complicating labor and delivery 668.8
      postpartum 668.8
  spinal fluid loss 349.0
  tension 307.81
  vascular 784.0
    migraine type 346.9
  vasomotor 346.9
Health
  advice V65.4
  audit V70.0
  checkup V70.0
  education V65.4
  hazard (*see also* History of) V15.9
    specified cause NEC V15.89
  instruction V65.4
  services provided because (of)
    boarding school residence V60.6
    holiday relief for person providing home care V60.5
    inadequate
      housing V60.1
      resources V60.2
    lack of housing V60.0
    no care available in home V60.4
    person living alone V60.3
    poverty V60.3
    residence in institution V60.6
    specified cause NEC V60.8
    vacation relief for person providing home care V60.5

Healthy
  donor (*see also* Donor) V59.9
  infant or child
    accompanying sick mother V65.0
    receiving care V20.1
  person
    accompanying sick relative V65.0
    admitted for sterilization V25.2
    receiving prophylactic inoculation or vaccination (*see also* Vaccination, prophylactic) V05.9
Hearing examination V72.1
Heart —*see* condition
Heartburn 787.1
  psychogenic 306.4
Heat (effects) 992.9
  apoplexy 992.0
  burn—*see also* Burn, by site
    from sun (*see also* Sunburn) 692.71
  collapse 992.1
  cramps 992.2
  dermatitis or eczema 692.89
  edema 992.7
  erythema—*see* Burn, by site
  excessive 992.9
    specified effect NEC 992.8
  exhaustion 992.5
    anhydrotic 992.3
    due to
      salt (and water) depletion 992.4
      water depletion 992.3
  fatigue (transient) 992.6
  fever 992.0
  hyperpyrexia 992.0
  prickly 705.1
  prostration—*see* Heat, exhaustion
  pyrexia 992.0
  rash 705.1
  specified effect NEC 992.8
  stroke 992.0
  sunburn (*see also* Sunburn) 692.71
  syncope 992.1
Heavy-chain disease 273.2
Heavy-for-dates (fetus or infant) 766.1
  4500 grams or more 766.0
  exceptionally 766.0
Hebephrenia, hebephrenic (acute) (*see also* Schizophrenia) 295.1
  dementia (praecox) (*see also* Schizophrenia) 295.1
  schizophrenia (*see also* Schizophrenia) 295.1
Heberden's
  disease or nodes 715.04
  syndrome (angina pectoris) 413.9
Hebra's disease
  dermatitis exfoliativa 695.89
  erythema multiforme exudativum 695.1
  pityriasis 695.89
    maculata et circinata 696.3
    rubra 695.89
      pilaris 696.4
  prurigo 698.2
Hebra, nose 040.1
Hedinger's syndrome (malignant carcinoid) 259.2
Heel —*see* condition
Heerfordt's disease or syndrome (uveoparotitis) 135
Hegglin's anomaly or syndrome 288.2
Heidenhain's disease 290.10
  with dementia 290.10

Hematocephalus 742.4
Hematochezia (*see also* Melena) 578.1
Hematochyluria (*see also* Infestation, filarial) 125.9
Hematocolpos 626.8
Hematocornea 371.12
Hematogenous —*see* condition
Hematoma (skin surface intact) (traumatic)—*see also* Contusion

> *Note—Hematomas are coded according to origin and the nature and site of the hematoma or the accompanying injury. Hematomas of unspecified origin are coded as injuries of the sites involved, except:*
> *(a) hematomas of genital organs which are coded as diseases of the organ involved unless they complicate pregnancy or delivery*
> *(b) hematomas of the eye which are coded as diseases of the eye.*
>
> *For late effect of hematoma classifiable to 920-924 see Late, effect, contusion*

with
  crush injury—*see* Crush
  fracture—*see* Fracture, by site
  injury of internal organs—*see also* Injury, internal, by site
    kidney—*see* Hematoma, kidney, traumatic
    liver—*see* Hematoma, liver, traumatic
    spleen—*see* Hematoma, spleen
  nerve injury—*see* Injury, nerve
  open wound—*see* Wound, open, by site
  skin surface intact—*see* Contusion
abdomen (wall)—*see* Contusion, abdomen
amnion 658.8
aorta, dissecting 441.00
  abdominal 441.02
  thoracic 441.01
  thoracoabdominal 441.03
arterial (complicating trauma) 904.9
  specified site—*see* Injury, blood vessel, by site
auricle (ear) 380.31
birth injury 767.8
  skull 767.1
brain (traumatic) 853.0

> *Note—Use the following fifth-digit subclassification with categories 851-854:*
>
> *0 unspecified state of consciousness*
> *1 with no loss of consciousness*
> *2 with brief [less than one hour] loss of consciousness*
> *3 with moderate [1-24 hours] loss of consciousness*
> *4 with prolonged [more than 24 hours] loss of consciousness and return to pre-existing conscious level*
> *5 with prolonged [more than 24 hours] loss of consciousness, without return to pre-existing conscious level*
> *Use fifth-digit 5 to designate when a patient is unconscious and dies before regaining consciousness, regardless of the duration of the loss of consciousness*
> *6 with loss of consciousness of unspecified duration*
> *9 with concussion, unspecified*

Hematoma— *continued*
with
  cerebral
    contusion—*see* Contusion, brain
    laceration—*see* Laceration, brain
   open intracranial wound 853.1
   skull fracture—*see* Fracture, skull, by site
  extradural or epidural 852.4
   with open intracranial wound 852.5
   fetus or newborn 767.0
   nontraumatic 432.0
  fetus or newborn NEC 767.0
  nontraumatic (*see also* Hemorrhage, brain) 431
   epidural or extradural 432.0
   newborn NEC 772.8
   subarachnoid, arachnoid, or meningeal (*see also* Hemorrhage, subarachnoid) 430
   subdural (*see also* Hemorrhage, subdural) 432.1
  subarachnoid, arachnoid, or meningeal 852.0
   with open intracranial wound 852.1
   fetus or newborn 772.2
   nontraumatic (*see also* Hemorrhage, subarachnoid) 430
  subdural 852.2
   with open intracranial wound 852.3
   fetus or newborn (localized) 767.0
   nontraumatic (*see also* Hemorrhage, subdural) 432.1
breast (nontraumatic) 611.8
broad ligament (nontraumatic) 620.7
  complicating delivery 665.7
  traumatic—*see* Injury, internal, broad ligament
calcified NEC 959.9
capitis 920
  due to birth injury 767.1
  newborn 767.1
cerebral—*see* Hematoma, brain
cesarean section wound 674.3
chorion—*see* Placenta, abnormal
complicating delivery (perineum) (vulva) 664.5
  pelvic 665.7
  vagina 665.7
corpus
  cavernosum (nontraumatic) 607.82
  luteum (nontraumatic) (ruptured) 620.1
dura (mater)—*see* Hematoma, brain, subdural
epididymis (nontraumatic) 608.83
epidural (traumatic)—*see also* Hematoma, brain, extradural
  spinal—*see* Injury, spinal, by site
episiotomy 674.3
external ear 380.31
extradural—*see also* Hematoma, brain, extradural
  fetus or newborn 767.0
  nontraumatic 432.0
   fetus or newborn 767.0
fallopian tube 620.8
genital organ (nontraumatic)
  female NEC 629.8
  male NEC 608.83
  traumatic (external site) 922.4
   internal—*see* Injury, internal, genital organ
graafian follicle (ruptured) 620.0
internal organs (abdomen, chest, or pelvis)—*see also* Injury, internal, by site
  kidney—*see* Hematoma, kidney, traumatic
  liver—*see* Hematoma, liver, traumatic
  spleen—*see* Hematoma, spleen

Hematoma—*continued*
  intracranial—*see* Hematoma, brain
  kidney, cystic 593.81
    traumatic 866.01
      with open wound into cavity 866.11
  labia (nontraumatic) 624.5
  lingual (and other parts of neck, scalp, or face, except eye) 920
  liver (subcapsular) 573.8
    birth injury 767.8
    fetus or newborn 767.8
    traumatic NEC 864.01
      with
        laceration—*see* Laceration, liver
        open wound into cavity 864.11
  mediastinum—*see* Injury, internal, mediastinum
  meninges, meningeal (brain)—*see also* Hematoma, brain, subarachnoid
    spinal—*see* Injury, spinal, by site
  mesosalpinx (nontraumatic) 620.8
    traumatic—*see* Injury, internal, pelvis
  muscle (traumatic)—*see* Contusion, by site
  nasal (septum) (and other part(s) of neck, scalp, or face, except eye) 920
  obstetrical surgical wound 674.3
  orbit, orbital (nontraumatic) 376.32
    traumatic 921.2
  ovary (corpus luteum) (nontraumatic) 620.1
    traumatic—*see* Injury, internal, ovary
  pelvis (female) (nontraumatic) 629.8
    complicating delivery 665.7
    male 608.83
    traumatic—*see also* Injury, internal, pelvis
      specified organ NEC (*see also* Injury, internal, pelvis) 867.6
  penis (nontraumatic) 607.82
  pericranial (and neck, or face any part, except eye) 920
    due to injury at birth 767.1
  perineal wound (obstetrical) 674.3
    complicating delivery 664.5
  perirenal, cystic 593.81
  pinna 380.31
  placenta—*see* Placenta, abnormal
  postoperative 998.12
  retroperitoneal (nontraumatic) 568.81
    traumatic—*see* Injury, internal, retroperitoneum
  retropubic, male 568.81
  scalp (and neck, or face any part, except eye) 920
    fetus or newborn 767.1
  scrotum (nontraumatic) 608.83
    traumatic 922.4
  seminal vesicle (nontraumatic) 608.83
    traumatic—*see* Injury, internal, seminal vesicle
  spermatic cord—*see also* Injury, internal, spermatic cord
    nontraumatic 608.83
  spinal (cord) (meninges)—*see also* Injury, spinal, by site
    fetus or newborn 767.4
    nontraumatic 336.1
  spleen 865.01
    with
      laceration—*see* Laceration, spleen
      open wound into cavity 865.11
  sternocleidomastoid, birth injury 767.8

Hematoma—*continued*
  sternomastoid, birth injury 767.8
  subarachnoid—*see also* Hematoma, brain, subarachnoid
    fetus or newborn 772.2
    nontraumatic (*see also* Hemorrhage, subarachnoid) 430
      newborn 772.2
  subdural—*see also* Hematoma, brain, subdural
    fetus or newborn (localized) 767.0
    nontraumatic (*see also* Hemorrhage, subdural) 432.1
  subperiosteal (syndrome) 267
    traumatic—*see* Hematoma, by site
  superficial, fetus or newborn 772.6
  syncytium—*see* Placenta, abnormal
  testis (nontraumatic) 608.83
    birth injury 767.8
    traumatic 922.4
  tunica vaginalis (nontraumatic) 608.83
  umbilical cord 663.6
    affecting fetus or newborn 762.6
  uterine ligament (nontraumatic) 620.7
    traumatic—*see* Injury, internal, pelvis
  uterus 621.4
    traumatic—*see* Injury, internal, pelvis
  vagina (nontraumatic) (ruptured) 623.6
    complicating delivery 665.7
    traumatic 922.4
  vas deferens (nontraumatic) 608.83
    traumatic—*see* Injury, internal, vas deferens
  vitreous 379.23
  vocal cord 920
  vulva (nontraumatic) 624.5
    complicating delivery 664.5
    fetus or newborn 767.8
    traumatic 922.4
Hematometra 621.4
Hematomyelia 336.1
  with fracture of vertebra (*see also* Fracture, vertebra, by site, with spinal cord injury) 806.8
  fetus or newborn 767.4
Hematomyelitis 323.9
  late effect—*see* category 326
Hematoperitoneum (*see also* Hemoperitoneum) 568.81
Hematopneumothorax (*see also* Hemothorax) 511.8
Hematoporphyria (acquired) (congenital) 277.1
Hematoporphyrinuria (acquired) (congenital) 277.1
Hematorachis, hematorrhachis 336.1
  fetus or newborn 767.4
Hematosalpinx 620.8
  with
    ectopic pregnancy (*see also* categories 633.0-633.9) 639.2
    molar pregnancy (*see also* categories 630-632) 639.2
  infectional (*see also* Salpingo-oophoritis) 614.2
Hematospermia 608.82
Hematothorax (*see also* Hemothorax) 511.8
Hematotympanum 381.03
Hematuria (benign) (essential) (idiopathic) 599.7
  due to S. hematobium 120.0
  endemic 120.0
  intermittent 599.7
  malarial 084.8
  paroxysmal 599.7

Hematuria—*continued*
  sulfonamide
    correct substance properly administered 599.7
    overdose or wrong substance given or taken
      961.0
  tropical (bilharziasis) 120.0
  tuberculous (*see also* Tuberculosis) 016.9
Hematuric bilious fever 084.8
Hemeralopia 368.10
Hemiabiotrophy 799.8
Hemi-akinesia 781.8
Hemianalgesia (*see also* Disturbance, sensation)
  782.0
Hemianencephaly 740.0
Hemianesthesia (*see also* Disturbance,
  sensation) 782.0
Hemianopia, hemianopsia (altitudinal)
  (homonymous) 368.46
  binasal 368.47
  bitemporal 368.47
  heteronymous 368.47
  syphilitic 095.8
Hemiasomatognosia 307.9
Hemiathetosis 781.0
Hemiatrophy 799.8
  cerebellar 334.8
  face 349.89
    progressive 349.89
  fascia 728.9
  leg 728.2
  tongue 529.8
Hemiballism (us) 333.5
Hemiblock (cardiac) (heart) (left) 426.2
Hemicardia 746.89
Hemicephalus, hemicephaly 740.0
Hemichorea 333.5
Hemicrania 346.9
  congenital malformation 740.0
Hemidystrophy —*see* Hemiatrophy
Hemiectromelia 755.4
Hemihypalgesia (*see also* Disturbance,
  sensation) 782.0
Hemihypertrophy (congenital) 759.89
  cranial 756.0
Hemihypesthesia (*see also* Disturbance,
  sensation) 782.0
Hemi-inattention 781.8
Hemimelia 755.4
  lower limb 755.30
    paraxial (complete) (incomplete) (intercalary)
      (terminal) 755.32
      fibula 755.37
      tibia 755.36
    transverse (complete) (partial) 755.31
  upper limb 755.20
    paraxial (complete) (incomplete) (intercalary)
      (terminal) 755.22
      radial 755.26
      ulnar 755.27
    transverse (complete) (partial) 755.21
Hemiparalysis (*see also* Hemiplegia) 342.9
Hemiparesis (*see also* Hemiplegia) 342.9
Hemiparesthesia (*see also* Disturbance,
  sensation) 782.0

Hemiplegia 342.9
  acute (*see also* Disease, cerebrovascular, acute)
    436
  alternans facialis 344.89
  apoplectic (*see also* Disease, cerebrovascular,
    acute) 436
    late effect or residual
      affecting
        dominant side 438.21
        nondominant side 438.22
        unspecfied side 438.20
  arteriosclerotic 437.0
    late effect or residual
      affecting
        dominant side 438.21
        nondominant side 438.22
        unspecified side 438.20
  ascending (spinal) NEC 344.89
  attack (*see also* Disease, cerebrovascular, acute)
    436
  brain, cerebral (current episode) 437.8
    congenital 343.1
  cerebral—*see* Hemiplegia, brain
  congenital (cerebral) (spastic) (spinal) 343.1
  conversion neurosis (hysterical) 300.11
  cortical—*see* Hemiplegia, brain
  due to
    arteriosclerosis 437.0
      late effect or residual
        affecting
          dominant side 438.21
          nondominant side 438.22
          unspecified side 438.20
    cerebrovascular lesion (*see also* Disease,
      cerebrovascular, acute) 436
      late effect
        affecting
          dominant side 438.21
          nondominant side 438.22
          unspecified side 438.20
  embolic (current) (*see also* Embolism, brain)
    434.1
    late effect
      affecting
        dominant side 438.21
        nondominant side 438.22
        unspecified side 438.20
  flaccid 342.0
  hypertensive (current episode) 437.8
  infantile (postnatal) 343.4
  late effect
    birth injury, intracranial or spinal 343.4
    cerebrovascular lesion—*see* Late effect(s) (of)
      cerebrovascular disease
    viral encephalitis 139.0
  middle alternating NEC 344.89
  newborn NEC 767.0
  seizure (current episode) (*see also* Disease,
    cerebrovascular, acute) 436
  spastic 342.1
    congenital or infantile 343.1
  specified NEC 342.8
  thrombotic (current) (*see also* Thrombosis,
    brain) 434.0
    late effect—*see* late effect(s) (of)
      cerebrovascular disease
Hemisection, spinal cord —*see* Fracture,
  vertebra, by site, with spinal cord injury
Hemispasm 781.0
  facial 781.0
Hemispatial neglect 781.8

Hemorrhage, hemorrhagic—*continued*
 blood dyscrasia 289.9
 bowel 578.9
  newborn 772.4
 brain (miliary) (nontraumatic) 431
  with
   birth injury 767.0
  arachnoid—*see* Hemorrhage, subarachnoid
  due to
   birth injury 767.0
   rupture of aneurysm (congenital) (*see also*
    Hemorrhage, subarachnoid) 430
    mycotic 431
   syphilis 094.89
  epidural or extradural—*see* Hemorrhage,
   extradural
  fetus or newborn (anoxic) (hypoxic) (due to
   birth trauma) (nontraumatic) 767.0
   intraventricular 772.10
    grade I 772.11
    grade II 772.12
    grade III 772.13
    grade IV 772.14
  iatrogenic 997.02
  postoperative 997.02
  puerperal, postpartum, childbirth 674.0
  stem 431
  subarachnoid, arachnoid or meningeal—*see*
   Hemorrhage, subarachnoid
  subdural—*see* Hemorrhage, subdural
  traumatic NEC 853.0

---

*Note—Use the following fifth-digit
subclassification with categories 851-854:*

0 unspecified state of consciousness
1 with no loss of consciousness
*2 with brief [less than one hour] loss of
consciousness*
*3 with moderate [1-24 hours] loss of
consciousness*
*4 with prolonged [more than 24 hours] loss of
consciousness and return to pre-existing
conscious level*
*5 with prolonged [more than 24 hours] loss of
consciousness, without return to pre-existing
conscious level*
*Use fifth-digit 5 to designate when a patient is
unconscious and dies before regaining
consciousness, regardless of the duration of the
loss of consciousness*
*6 with loss of consciousness of unspecified
duration*
9 with concussion, unspecified

---

   with
    cerebral
     contusion—*see* Contusion, brain
     laceration—*see* Laceration, brain
    open intracranial wound 853.1
    skull fracture—*see* Fracture, skull, by site
   extradural or epidural 852.4
    with open intracranial wound 852.5
   subarachnoid 852.0
    with open intracranial wound 852.1
   subdural 852.2
    with open intracranial wound 852.3
 breast 611.79
 bronchial tube—*see* Hemorrhage, lung
 bronchopulmonary—*see* Hemorrhage, lung
 bronchus (cause unknown) (*see also*
  Hemorrhage, lung) 786.3

Hemorrhage, hemorrhagic—*continued*
 bulbar (*see also* Hemorrhage, brain) 431
 bursa 727.89
 capillary 448.9
  primary 287.8
 capsular—*see* Hemorrhage, brain
 cardiovascular 429.89
 cecum 578.9
 cephalic (*see also* Hemorrhage, brain) 431
 cerebellar (*see also* Hemorrhage, brain) 431
 cerebellum (*see also* Hemorrhage, brain) 431
 cerebral (*see also* Hemorrhage, brain) 431
  fetus or newborn (anoxic) (traumatic) 767.0
 cerebromeningeal (*see also* Hemorrhage, brain)
  431
 cerebrospinal (*see also* Hemorrhage, brain) 431
 cerebrum (*see also* Hemorrhage, brain) 431
 cervix (stump) (uteri) 622.8
 cesarean section wound 674.3
 chamber, anterior (eye) 364.41
 childbirth—*see* Hemorrhage, complicating,
  delivery
 choroid 363.61
  expulsive 363.62
 ciliary body 364.41
 cochlea 386.8
 colon—*see* Hemorrhage, intestine
 complicating
  delivery 641.9
   affecting fetus or newborn 762.1
   associated with
    afibrinogenemia 641.3
     affecting fetus or newborn 763.89
    coagulation defect 641.3
     affecting fetus or newborn 763.89
    hyperfibrinolysis 641.3
     affecting fetus or newborn 763.89
    hypofibrinogenemia 641.3
     affecting fetus or newborn 763.89
   due to
    low-lying placenta 641.1
     affecting fetus or newborn 762.0
    placenta previa 641.1
     affecting fetus or newborn 762.0
    premature separation of placenta 641.2
     affecting fetus or newborn 762.1
    retained
     placenta 666.0
     secundines 666.2
    trauma 641.8
     affecting fetus or newborn 763.89
    uterine leiomyoma 641.8
     affecting fetus or newborn 763.89
  surgical procedure 998.11
 concealed NEC 459.0
 congenital 772.9
 conjunctiva 372.72
  newborn 772.8
 cord, newborn 772.0
  slipped ligature 772.3
  stump 772.3
 corpus luteum (ruptured) 620.1
 cortical (*see also* Hemorrhage, brain) 431
 cranial 432.9
 cutaneous 782.7
  newborn 772.6
 cyst, pancreas 577.2
 cystitis—*see* Cystitis
 delayed
  with

Hemorrhage, hemorrhagic—*continued*
  intrauterine 621.4
    complicating delivery—*see* Hemorrhage,
      complicating, delivery
    in pregnancy or childbirth—*see* Hemorrhage,
      pregnancy
    postpartum (*see also* Hemorrhage,
      postpartum) 666.1
  intraventricular (*see also* Hemorrhage, brain)
    431
    fetus or newborn (anoxic) (traumatic) 772.10
      grade I 772.11
      grade II 772.12
      grade III 772.13
      grade IV 772.14
  intravesical 596.7
  iris (postinfectional) (postinflammatory) (toxic)
    364.41
  joint (nontraumatic) 719.10
    ankle 719.17
    elbow 719.12
    foot 719.17
    forearm 719.13
    hand 719.14
    hip 719.15
    knee 719.16
    lower leg 719.16
    multiple sites 719.19
    pelvic region 719.15
    shoulder (region) 719.11
    specified site NEC 719.18
    thigh 719.15
    upper arm 719.12
    wrist 719.13
  kidney 593.81
  knee (joint) 719.16
  labyrinth 386.8
  leg NEC 459.0
  lenticular striate artery (*see also* Hemorrhage,
    brain) 431
  ligature, vessel 998.11
  liver 573.8
  lower extremity NEC 459.0
  lung 786.3
    newborn 770.3
    tuberculous (*see also* Tuberculosis,
      pulmonary) 011.9
  malaria 084.8
  marginal sinus 641.2
  massive subaponeurotic, birth injury 767.1
  maternal, affecting fetus or newborn 762.1
  mediastinum 786.3
  medulla (*see also* Hemorrhage, brain) 431
  membrane (brain) (*see also* Hemorrhage,
    subarachnoid) 430
    spinal cord—*see* Hemorrhage, spinal cord
  meninges, meningeal (brain) (middle) (*see also*
    Hemorrhage, subarachnoid) 430
    spinal cord—*see* Hemorrhage, spinal cord
  mesentery 568.81
  metritis 626.8
  midbrain (*see also* Hemorrhage, brain) 431
  mole 631
  mouth 528.9
  mucous membrane NEC 459.0
    newborn 772.8
  muscle 728.89
  nail (subungual) 703.8
  nasal turbinate 784.7
    newborn 772.8
  nasopharynx 478.29

Hemorrhage, hemorrhagic—*continued*
  navel, newborn 772.3
  newborn 772.9
    adrenal 772.5
    alveolar (lung) 770.3
    brain (anoxic) (hypoxic) (due to birth trauma)
      767.0
    cerebral (anoxic) (hypoxic) (due to birth
      trauma) 767.0
    conjunctiva 772.8
    cutaneous 772.6
    diathesis 776.0
    due to vitamin K deficiency 776.0
    gastrointestinal 772.4
    internal (organs) 772.8
    intestines 772.4
    intra-alveolar (lung) 770.3
    intracranial (from any perinatal cause) 767.0
    intraventricular (from any perinatal cause)
      772.10
      grade I 772.11
      grade II 772.12
      grade III 772.13
      grade IV 772.14
    lung 770.3
    pulmonary (massive) 770.3
    spinal cord, traumatic 767.4
    stomach 772.4
    subaponeurotic (massive) 767.1
    subarachnoid (from any perinatal cause) 772.2
    subconjunctival 772.8
    umbilicus 772.0
      slipped ligature 772.3
      vasa previa 772.0
  nipple 611.79
  nose 784.7
    newborn 772.8
  obstetrical surgical wound 674.3
  omentum 568.89
    newborn 772.4
  optic nerve (sheath) 377.42
  orbit 376.32
  ovary 620.1
  oviduct 620.8
  pancreas 577.8
  parathyroid (gland) (spontaneous) 252.8
  parturition—*see* Hemorrhage, complicating,
    delivery
  penis 607.82
  pericardium, pericarditis 423.0
  perineal wound (obstetrical) 674.3
  peritoneum, peritoneal 459.0
  peritonsillar tissue 474.8
    after operation on tonsils 998.11
    due to infection 475
  petechial 782.7
  pituitary (gland) 253.8
  placenta NEC 641.9
    affecting fetus or newborn 762.1
    from surgical or instrumental damage 641.8
      affecting fetus or newborn 762.1
    previa 641.1
      affecting fetus or newborn 762.0
  pleura—*see* Hemorrhage, lung
  polioencephalitis, superior 265.1
  polymyositis—*see* Polymyositis
  pons (*see also* Hemorrhage, brain) 431
  pontine (*see also* Hemorrhage, brain) 431
  popliteal 459.0
  postcoital 626.7
  postextraction (dental) 998.11

> *Note—Use the following fifth-digit subclassification with category 550:*
>
> *0 unilateral or unspecified (not specified as recurrent)*
> *1 unilateral or unspecified, recurrent*
> *2 bilateral (not specified as recurrent)*
> *3 bilateral, recurrent*

Hernia, hernial—*continued*
  ventral 553.20
    with
      gangrene (obstructed) 551.20
      obstruction 552.20
        and gangrene 551.20
    recurrent 553.21
      with
        gangrene (obstructed) 551.21
        obstruction 552.21
          and gangrene 551.21
  vesical
    congenital (female) (male) 756.71
    female 618.0
    male 596.8
  vitreous (into anterior chamber) 379.21
    traumatic 871.1
Herniation —*see also* Hernia
  brain (stem) 348.4
  cerebral 348.4
  gastric mucosa (into duodenal bulb) 537.89
  mediastinum 519.3
  nucleus pulposus—*see* Displacement,
    intervertebral disc
Herpangina 074.0
Herpes, herpetic 054.9
  auricularis (zoster) 053.71
    simplex 054.73
  blepharitis (zoster) 053.20
    simplex 054.41
  circinate 110.5
  circinatus 110.5
    bullous 694.5
  conjunctiva (simplex) 054.43
    zoster 053.21
  cornea (simplex) 054.43
    disciform (simplex) 054.43
    zoster 053.21
  encephalitis 054.3
  eye (zoster) 053.29
    simplex 054.40
  eyelid (zoster) 053.20
    simplex 054.41
  febrilis 054.9
  fever 054.9
  geniculate ganglionitis 053.11
  genital, genitalis 054.10
    specified site NEC 054.19
  gestationis 646.8
  gingivostomatitis 054.2
  iridocyclitis (simplex) 054.44
    zoster 053.22
  iris (any site) 695.1
  iritis (simplex) 054.44
  keratitis (simplex) 054.43
    dendritic 054.42
    disciform 054.43
    interstitial 054.43
      zoster 053.21
  keratoconjunctivitis (simplex) 054.43
    zoster 053.21
  labialis 054.9
    meningococcal 036.89
  lip 054.9
  meningitis (simplex) 054.72
    zoster 053.0
  ophthalmicus (zoster) 053.20
    simplex 054.40
  otitis externa (zoster) 053.71
    simplex 054.73
  penis 054.13

Herpes, herpetic—*continued*
  perianal 054.10
  pharyngitis 054.79
  progenitalis 054.10
  scrotum 054.19
  septicemia 054.5
  simplex 054.9
    complicated 054.8
      ophthalmic 054.40
        specified NEC 054.49
      specified NEC 054.79
    congenital 771.2
    external ear 054.73
    keratitis 054.43
      dendritic 054.42
    meningitis 054.72
    neuritis 054.79
    specified complication NEC 054.79
      ophthalmic 054.49
    visceral 054.71
  stomatitis 054.2
  tonsurans 110.0
    maculosus (of Hebra) 696.3
  visceral 054.71
  vulva 054.12
  vulvovaginitis 054.11
  whitlow 054.6
  zoster 053.9
    auricularis 053.71
    complicated 053.8
      specified NEC 053.79
    conjunctiva 053.21
    cornea 053.21
    ear 053.71
    eye 053.29
    geniculate 053.11
    keratitis 053.21
      interstitial 053.21
    neuritis 053.10
    ophthalmicus(a) 053.20
    oticus 053.71
    otitis externa 053.71
    specified complication NEC 053.79
    specified site NEC 053.9
  zosteriform, intermediate type 053.9
Herrick's
  anemia (hemoglobin S disease) 282.61
  syndrome (hemoglobin S disease) 282.61
Hers' disease (glycogenosis VI) 271.0
Herter's infantilism (nontropical sprue) 579.0
Herter (-Gee) disease or syndrome (nontropical
  sprue) 579.0
Herxheimer's disease (diffuse idiopathic
  cutaneous atrophy) 701.8
Herxheimer's reaction 995.0
Hesselbach's hernia —*see* Hernia, Hesselbach's
Heterochromia (congenital) 743.46
  acquired 364.53
  cataract 366.33
  cyclitis 364.21
  hair 704.3
  iritis 364.21
  retained metallic foreign body 360.62
    magnetic 360.52
  uveitis 364.21
Heterophoria 378.40
  alternating 378.45
  vertical 378.43
Heterophyes, small intestine 121.6
Heterophyiasis 121.6
Heteropsia 368.8

Heterotopia, heterotopic —*see also*
   Malposition, congenital
  cerebralis 742.4
  pancreas, pancreatic 751.7
  spinalis 742.59
Heterotropia 378.30
  intermittent 378.20
    vertical 378.31
  vertical (constant) (intermittent) 378.31
Heubner's disease 094.89
Heubner-Herter disease or syndrome
   (nontropical sprue) 579.0
Hexadactylism 755.00
Heyd's syndrome (hepatorenal) 572.4
HGSIL (high grade squamous intraepithelial
   dysplasia) 622.1
Hibernoma (M8880/0)—*see* Lipoma
Hiccough 786.8
  epidemic 078.89
  psychogenic 306.1
Hiccup (*see also* Hiccough) 786.8
Hicks (-Braxton) contractures 644.1
Hidden penis 752.65
Hidradenitis (axillaris) (suppurative) 705.83
Hidradenoma (nodular) (M8400/0)—*see also*
   Neoplasm, skin, benign
  clear cell (M8402/0)—*see* Neoplasm, skin,
    benign
  papillary (M8405/0)—*see* Neoplasm, skin,
    benign
Hidrocystoma (M8404/0)—*see* Neoplasm, skin,
   benign
High
  A$_2$ anemia 282.4
  altitude effects 993.2
    anoxia 993.2
    on
      ears 993.0
      sinuses 993.1
    polycythemia 289.0
  arch
    foot 755.67
    palate 750.26
  artery (arterial) tension (*see also* Hypertension)
    401.9
    without diagnosis of hypertension 796.2
  basal metabolic rate (BMR) 794.7
  blood pressure (*see also* Hypertension) 401.9
    incidental reading (isolated) (nonspecific), no
      diagnosis of hypertension 796.2
  compliance bladder 596.4
  diaphragm (congenital) 756.6
  frequency deafness (congenital) (regional) 389.8
  head at term 652.5
  output failure (cardiac) (*see also* Failure, heart)
    428.9
  oxygen-affinity hemoglobin 289.0
  palate 750.26
  risk
    behavior —*see* Problem
    family situation V61.9
      specified circumstance NEC V61.8
    individual NEC V62.89
    infant NEC V20.1
    patient taking drugs (prescribed) V67.51
      nonprescribed (*see also* Abuse, drugs,
       nondependent) 305.9
    pregnancy V23.9
      inadequate prenatal care V23.7
      specified problem NEC V23.8

High—*continued*
  temperature (of unknown origin) (*see also*
    Pyrexia) 780.6
  thoracic rib 756.3
Hildenbrand's disease (typhus) 081.9
Hilger's syndrome 337.0
Hill diarrhea 579.1
Hilliard's lupus (*see also* Tuberculosis) 017.0
Hilum —*see* condition
Hip —*see* condition
Hippel's disease (retinocerebral angiomatosis)
   759.6
Hippus 379.49
Hirschfeld's disease (acute diabetes mellitus)
   (*see also* Diabetes) 250.0
Hirschsprung's disease or megacolon
   (congenital) 751.3
Hirsuties (*see also* Hypertrichosis) 704.1
Hirsutism (*see also* Hypertrichosis) 704.1
Hirudiniasis (external) (internal) 134.2
His-Werner disease (trench fever) 083.1
Hiss-Russell dysentery 004.1
Histamine cephalgia 346.2
Histidinemia 270.5
Histidinuria 270.5
Histiocytoma (M8832/0)—*see also* Neoplasm,
   skin, benign
  fibrous (M8830/0)—*see also* Neoplasm, skin,
    benign
    atypical (M8830/1)—*see* Neoplasm,
      connective tissue, uncertain behavior
    malignant (M8830/0)—*see* Neoplasm,
      connective tissue, malignant
Histiocytosis (acute) (chronic) (subacute) 277.8
  acute differentiated progressive (M9722/3) 202.5
  cholesterol 277.8
  essential 277.8
  lipid, lipoid (essential) 272.7
  lipochrome (familial) 288.1
  malignant (M9720/3) 202.3
  X (chronic) 277.8
    acute (progressive) (M9722/3) 202.5
Histoplasmosis 115.90
  with
    endocarditis 115.94
    meningitis 115.91
    pericarditis 115.93
    pneumonia 115.95
    retinitis 115.92
    specified manifestation NEC 115.99
  African (due to Histoplasma duboisii) 115.10
    with
      endocarditis 115.14
      meningitis 115.11
      pericarditis 115.13
      pneumonia 115.15
      retinitis 115.12
      specified manifestation NEC 115.19
  American (due to Histoplasma capsulatum)
    115.00
    with
      endocarditis 115.04
      meningitis 115.01
      pericarditis 115.03
      pneumonia 115.05
      retinitis 115.02
      specified manifestation NEC 115.09
  Darling's—*see* Histoplasmosis, American
  large form (*see also* Histoplasmosis, African)
    115.10

Hyperactive, hyperactivity—*continued*
 nasal mucous membrane 478.1
 stomach 536.8
 thyroid (gland) (*see also* Thyrotoxicosis) 242.9
Hyperacusis 388.42
Hyperadrenalism (cortical) 255.3
 medullary 255.6
Hyperadrenocorticism 255.3
 congenital 255.2
 iatrogenic
  correct substance properly administered 255.3
  overdose or wrong substance given or taken
   962.0
Hyperaffectivity 301.11
Hyperaldosteronism (atypical) (hyperplastic)
  (normoaldosteronal) (normotensive) (primary)
  (secondary) 255.1
Hyperalgesia (*see also* Disturbance, sensation)
  782.0
Hyperalimentation 783.6
 carotene 278.3
 specified NEC 278.8
 vitamin A 278.2
 vitamin D 278.4
Hyperaminoaciduria 270.9
 arginine 270.6
 citrulline 270.6
 cystine 270.0
 glycine 270.0
 lysine 270.7
 ornithine 270.6
 renal (types I, II, III) 270.0
Hyperammonemia (congenital) 270.6
Hyperamnesia 780.99
Hyperamylasemia 790.5
Hyperaphia 782.0
Hyperazotemia 791.9
Hyperbetalipoproteinemia (acquired)
  (essential) (familial) (hereditary) (primary)
  (secondary) 272.0
 with prebetalipoproteinemia 272.2
Hyperbilirubinemia 782.4
 congenital 277.4
 constitutional 277.4
 neonatal (transient) (*see also* Jaundice, fetus or
  newborn) 774.6
 of prematurity 774.2
Hyperbilirubinemica encephalopathia, new-
 born 774.7
 due to isoimmunization 773.4
Hypercalcemia, hypercalcemic (idiopathic)
  275.42
 nephropathy 588.8
Hypercalcinuria 275.40
Hypercapnia 786.09
 with mixed acid-base disorder 276.4
 fetal, affecting newborn 770.89
Hypercarotinemia 278.3
Hypercementosis 521.5
Hyperchloremia 276.9
Hyperchlorhydria 536.8
 neurotic 306.4
 psychogenic 306.4
Hypercholesterinemia —*see*
  Hypercholesterolemia
Hypercholesterolemia 272.0
 with hyperglyceridemia, endogenous 272.2
 essential 272.0
 familial 272.0
 hereditary 272.0
 primary 272.0
 pure 272.0

Hypercholesterolosis 272.0
Hyperchylia gastricsa 536.8
 psychogenic 306.4
Hyperchylomicronemia (familial) (with
  hyperbetalipoproteinemia) 272.3
Hypercoagulation syndrome 289.8
Hypercorticosteronism
 correct substance properly administered 255.3
 overdose or wrong substance given or taken
  962.0
Hypercortisonism
 correct substance properly administered 255.3
 overdose or wrong substance given or taken
  962.0
Hyperdynamic beta-adrenergic state or syn-
 drome (circulatory) 429.82
Hyperelectrolytemia 276.9
Hyperemesis 536.2
 arising during pregnancy—*see* Hyperemesis,
  gravidarum
 gravidarum (mild) (before 22 completed weeks
  gestation) 643.0
  with
   carbohydrate depletion 643.1
   dehydration 643.1
   electrolyte imbalance 643.1
   metabolic disturbance 643.1
  affecting fetus or newborn 761.8
  severe (with metabolic disturbance) 643.1
 psychogenic 306.4
Hyperemia (acute) 780.99
 anal mucosa 569.49
 bladder 596.7
 cerebral 437.8
 conjunctiva 372.71
 ear, internal, acute 386.30
 enteric 564.89
 eye 372.71
 eyelid (active) (passive) 374.82
 intestine 564.89
 iris 364.41
 kidney 593.81
 labyrinth 386.30
 liver (active) (passive) 573.8
 lung 514
 ovary 620.8
 passive 780.99
 pulmonary 514
 renal 593.81
 retina 362.89
 spleen 289.59
 stomach 537.89
Hyperesthesia (body surface) (*see also*
  Disturbance, sensation) 782.0
 larynx (reflex) 478.79
  hysterical 300.11
 pharynx (reflex) 478.29
Hyperestrinism 256.0
Hyperestrogenism 256.0
Hyperestrogenosis 256.0
Hyperextension, joint 718.80
 ankle 718.87
 elbow 718.82
 foot 718.87
 hand 718.84
 hip 718.85
 knee 718.86
 multiple sites 718.89
 pelvic region 718.85
 shoulder (region) 718.81
 specified site NEC 718.88
 wrist 718.83

Hyperplasia, hyperplastic—*continued*
  medulla, adrenal 255.8
  myometrium, myometrial 621.2
  nose (lymphoid) (polypoid) 478.1
  oral soft tissue (inflammatory) (irritative)
    (mucosa) NEC 528.9
    gingiva 523.8
    tongue 529.8
  organ or site, congenital NEC—*see* Anomaly,
    specified type NEC
  ovary 620.8
  palate, papillary 528.9
  pancreatic islet cells 251.9
    alpha
      with excess
        gastrin 251.5
        glucagon 251.4
    beta 251.1
  parathyroid (gland) 252.0
  persistent, vitreous (primary) 743.51
  pharynx (lymphoid) 478.29
  prostate 600.9
    adenofibromatous 600.2
    nodular 600.1
  renal artery (fibromuscular) 447.3
  reticuloendothelial (cell) 289.9
  salivary gland (any) 527.1
  Schimmelbusch's 610.1
  suprarenal (capsule) (gland) 255.8
  thymus (gland) (persistent) 254.0
  thyroid (*see also* Goiter) 240.9
    primary 242.0
    secondary 242.2
  tonsil (lymphoid tissue) 474.11
    and adenoids 474.10
  urethrovaginal 599.89
  uterus, uterine (myometrium) 621.2
    endometrium 621.3
  vitreous (humor), primary persistent 743.51
  vulva 624.3
  zygoma 738.11
Hyperpnea (*see also* Hyperventilation) 786.01
Hyperpotassemia 276.7
Hyperprebetalipoproteinemia 272.1
  with chylomicronemia 272.3
  familial 272.1
Hyperprolactinemia 253.1
Hyperprolinemia 270.8
Hyperproteinemia 273.8
Hyperprothrombinemia 289.8
Hyperpselaphesia 782.0
Hyperpyrexia 780.6
  heat (effects of) 992.0
  malarial (*see also* Malaria) 084.6
  malignant, due to anesthetic 995.86
  rheumatic—*see* Fever, rheumatic
  unknown origin (*see also* Pyrexia) 780.6
Hyperreactor, vascular 780.2
Hyperreflexia 796.1
  bladder, autonomic 596.54
    with cauda equina 344.61
  detrusor 344.61
Hypersalivation (*see also* Ptyalism) 527.7
Hypersarcosinemia 270.8
Hypersecretion
  ACTH 255.3
  androgens (ovarian) 256.1
  calcitonin 246.0
  corticoadrenal 255.3
  cortisol 255.0
  estrogen 256.0

Hypersecretion—*continued*
  gastric 536.8
    psychogenic 306.4
  gastrin 251.5
  glucagon 251.4
  hormone
    ACTH 255.3
    anterior pituitary 253.1
    growth NEC 253.0
    ovarian androgen 256.1
    testicular 257.0
    thyroid stimulating 242.8
  insulin—*see* Hyperinsulinism
  lacrimal glands (*see also* Epiphora) 375.20
  medulloadrenal 255.6
  milk 676.6
  ovarian androgens 256.1
  pituitary (anterior) 253.1
  salivary gland (any) 527.7
  testicular hormones 257.0
  thyrocalcitonin 246.0
  upper respiratory 478.9
Hypersegmentation, hereditary 288.2
  eosinophils 288.2
  neutrophil nuclei 288.2
Hypersensitive, hypersensitiveness
  hypersensitivity —*see also* Allergy
  angiitis 446.20
    specified NEC 446.29
  carotid sinus 337.0
  colon 564.9
    psychogenic 306.4
  DNA (deoxyribonucleic acid) NEC 287.2
  drug (*see also* Allergy, drug) 995.2
  esophagus 530.89
  insect bites—*see* Injury, superficial, by site
  labyrinth 386.58
  pain (*see also* Disturbance, sensation) 782.0
  pneumonitis NEC 495.9
  reaction (*see also* Allergy) 995.3
    upper respiratory tract NEC 478.8
  stomach (allergic) (nonallergic) 536.8
    psychogenic 306.4
Hypersomatotropism (classic) 253.0
Hypersomnia 780.54
  with sleep apnea 780.53
  nonorganic origin 307.43
    persistent (primary) 307.44
    transient 307.43
Hypersplenia 289.4
Hypersplenism 289.4
Hypersteatosis 706.3
Hyperstimulation, ovarian 256.1
Hypersuprarenalism 255.3
Hypersusceptibility —*see* Allergy
Hyper-TBG-nemia 246.8
Hypertelorism 756.0
  orbit, orbital 376.41

— "H" listing resumes after
Hypertension table...

Hypertension, hypertensive

	Malignant	Benign	Unspecified
(arterial) (arteriolar) (crisis) (degeneration) (disease) (essential) (fluctuating) (idiopathic) (intermittent) (labile) (low renin) (orthostatic) (paroxysmal) (primary) (systemic) (uncontrolled) (vascular)	401.0	401.1	401.9
with			
heart involvement (conditions classifiable to 425.8, 428, 429.0-429.3, 429.8, 429.9 due to hypertension) (*see also* Hypertension, heart)	402.00	402.10	402.90
with kidney involvement—*see* Hypertension, cardiorenal			
renal involvement (only conditions classifiable to 585, 586, 587) (excludes conditions classifiable to 584) (*see also* Hypertension, kidney)	403.00	403.10	403.90
with heart involvement—*see* Hypertension, cardiorenal			
failure (and sclerosis) (*see also* Hypertension, kidney)	403.01	403.11	403.91
sclerosis without failure (*see also* Hypertension, kidney)	403.00	403.10	403.90
accelerated (*see also* Hypertension, by type, malignant)	401.0	—	—
antepartum—*see* Hypertension complicating pregnancy, childbirth, or the puerperium			
cardiorenal (disease)	404.00	404.10	404.90
with			
heart failure	404.01	404.11	404.91
and renal failure	404.03	404.13	404.93
renal failure	404.02	404.12	404.92
and heart failure	404.03	404.13	404.93
cardiovascular disease (arteriosclerotic) (sclerotic)	402.00	402.10	402.90
with			
heart failure	402.01	402.11	402.91
renal involvement (conditions classifiable to 403) (*see also* Hypertension, cardiorenal)	404.00	404.10	404.90
cardiovascular renal (disease) (sclerosis) (*see also* Hypertension cardiorenal)	404.00	404.10	404.90
cerebrovascular disease NEC	437.2	437.2	437.2
complicating pregnancy, childbirth, or the puerperium	642.2	642.0	642.9
with			
albuminuria (and edema) (mild)	—	—	642.4
severe	—	—	642.5
edema (mild)	—	—	642.4
severe	—	—	642.5
heart disease	642.2	642.2	642.2
and renal disease	642.2	642.2	642.2
renal disease	642.2	642.2	642.2
and heart disease	642.2	642.2	642.2
chronic	642.2	642.0	642.0
with pre-eclampsia or eclampsia	642.7	642.7	642.7
fetus or newborn	760.0	760.0	760.0
essential	—	642.0	642.0
with pre-eclampsia or eclampsia	—	642.7	642.7
fetus or newborn	760.0	760.0	760.0
fetus or newborn	760.0	760.0	760.0
gestational	—	—	642.3
pre-existing	642.2	642.0	642.0
with pre-eclampsia or eclampsia	642.7	642.7	642.7
fetus or newborn	760.0	760.0	760.0
secondary to renal disease	642.1	642.1	642.1
with pre-eclampsia or eclampsia	642.7	642.7	642.7
fetus or newborn	760.0	760.0	760.0
transient	—	—	642.3
due to			
aldosteronism, primary	405.09	405.19	405.99
brain tumor	405.09	405.19	405.99
bulbar poliomyelitis	405.09	405.19	405.99
calculus			
kidney	405.09	405.19	405.99
ureter	405.09	405.19	405.99
coarctation, aorta	405.09	405.19	405.99
Cushing's disease	405.09	405.19	405.99
glomerulosclerosis (*see also* Hypertension, kidney)	403.00	403.10	403.90
periarteritis nodosa	405.09	405.19	405.99
pheochromocytoma	405.09	405.19	405.99
polycystic kidney(s)	405.09	405.19	405.99
polycythemia	405.09	405.19	405.99
porphyria	405.09	405.19	405.99
pyelonephritis	405.09	405.19	405.99

	Malignant	Benign	Unspecified
renal (artery)			
aneurysm	405.01	405.11	405.91
anomaly	405.01	405.11	405.91
embolism	405.01	405.11	405.91
fibromuscular hyperplasia	405.01	405.11	405.91
occlusion	405.01	405.11	405.91
stenosis	405.01	405.11	405.91
thrombosis	405.01	405.11	405.91
encephalopathy	437.2	437.2	437.2
gestational (transient) NEC	—	—	642.3
Goldblatt's	440.1	440.1	440.1
heart (disease) (conditions classifiable to 425.8, 428, 429.0-429.3, 429.8, 429.9 due to hypertension)	402.00	402.10	402.90
with			
heart failure	402.01	402.11	402.91
of newborn	—	—	747.83
hypertensive kidney disease (conditions classifiable to 403)			
(*see also* Hypertension, cardiorenal)	404.00	404.10	404.90
renal sclerosis (*see also* Hypertension, cardiorenal)	404.00	404.10	404.90
intracranial, benign	—	348.2	—
intraocular	—	—	365.04
kidney	403.00	403.10	403.90
with			
heart involvement (conditions classifiable to 425.8, 428, 429.0-429.3, 429.8, 429.9 due to hypertension) (*see also* Hypertension cardiorenal)	404.00	404.10	404.90
hypertensive heart (disease) (conditions classifiable to 402)			
(*see also* Hypertension, cardiorenal)	404.00	404.10	404.90
lesser circulation	—	—	416.0
necrotizing	401.0	—	—
ocular	—	—	365.04
portal (due to chronic liver disease)	—	—	572.3
postoperative 997.91			
psychogenic	—	—	306.2
puerperal, postpartum—*see* Hypertension, complicating pregnancy, childbirth, or the puerperium			
pulmonary (artery)	—	—	416.8
idiopathic	—	—	416.0
primary	—	—	416.0
with cor pulmonale (chronic)	—	—	416.8
acute	—	—	415.0
secondary	—	—	416.8
renal (disease) (*see also* Hypertension, kidney)	403.00	403.10	403.90
renovascular NEC	405.01	405.11	405.91
secondary NEC	405.09	405.19	405.99
due to			
aldosteronism, primary	405.09	405.19	405.99
brain tumor	405.09	405.19	405.99
bulbar poliomyelitis	405.09	405.19	405.99
calculus			
kidney	405.09	405.19	405.99
ureter	405.09	405.19	405.99
coarctation, aorta	405.09	405.19	405.99
Cushing's disease	405.09	405.19	405.99
glomerulosclerosis (*see also* Hypertension, kidney)	403.00	403.10	403.90
periarteritis nodosa	405.09	405.19	405.99
pheochromocytoma	405.09	405.19	405.99
polycystic kidney(s)	405.09	405.19	405.99
polycythemia	405.09	405.19	405.99
porphyria	405.09	405.19	405.99
pyelonephritis	405.09	405.19	405.99
renal (artery)			
aneurysm	405.01	405.11	405.91
anomaly	405.01	405.11	405.91
embolism	405.01	405.11	405.91
fibromuscular hyperplasia	405.01	405.11	405.91
occlusion	405.01	405.11	405.91
stenosis	405.01	405.11	405.91
thrombosis	405.01	405.11	405.91
transient	—	—	796.2
of pregnancy	—	—	642.3
venous, chronic (asymptomatic) (idiopathic)	—	—	459.30
due to			
deep vein thrombosis (*see also* Syndrome, postphlebetic)	—	—	459.10
with			
complication NEC	—	—	459.39
inflammation	—	—	459.32

	Malignant	Benign	Unspecified
with ulcer	—	—	459.33
ulcer	—	—	459.31
with inflammation	—	—	459.33

This page intentionally left blank

Hypertrophy, hypertrophic—*continued*
  frenum 529.8
    papillae (foliate) 529.3
  tonsil (faucial) (infective) (lingual) (lymphoid)
      474.11
    and adenoids 474.10
    with
        adenoiditis 474.01
        tonsillitis 474.00
          and adenoiditis 474.02
  tunica vaginalis 608.89
  turbinate (mucous membrane) 478.0
  ureter 593.89
  urethra 599.84
  uterus 621.2
    puerperal, postpartum 674.8
  uvula 528.9
  vagina 623.8
  vas deferens 608.89
  vein 459.89
  ventricle, ventricular (heart) (left) (right)—*see
      also* Hypertrophy, cardiac
    congenital 746.89
    due to hypertension (left) (right) (*see also*
        Hypertension, heart) 402.90
      benign 402.10
      malignant 402.00
    right with ventricular septal defect, pulmonary
        stenosis or atresia, and dextraposition of
        aorta 745.2
  verumontanum 599.89
  vesical 596.8
  vocal cord 478.5
  vulva 624.3
    stasis (nonfilarial) 624.3
Hypertropia (intermittent) (periodic) 378.31
Hypertyrosinemia 270.2
Hyperuricemia 790.6
Hypervalinemia 270.3
Hyperventilation (tetany) 786.01
  hysterical 300.11
  psychogenic 306.1
  syndrome 306.1
Hyperviscidosis 277.00
Hyperviscosity (of serum) (syndrome) NEC
    273.3
  polycythemic 289.0
  sclerocythemic 282.8
Hypervitaminosis (dietary) NEC 278.8
  A (dietary) 278.2
  D (dietary) 278.4
  from excessive administration or use of vitamin
      preparations (chronic) 278.8
    reaction to sudden overdose 963.5
    vitamin A 278.2
      reaction to sudden overdose 963.5
    vitamin D 278.4
      reaction to sudden overdose 963.5
    vitamin K
      correct substance properly administered
          278.8
      overdose or wrong substance given or taken
          964.3
Hypervolemia 276.6
Hypesthesia (*see also* Disturbance, sensation)
    782.0
  cornea 371.81
Hyphema (anterior chamber) (ciliary body) (iris)
    364.41
  traumatic 921.3
Hyphemia —*see* Hyphema

Hypoacidity, gastric 536.8
  psychogenic 306.4
Hypoactive labyrinth (function)—*see*
  Hypofunction, labyrinth
Hypoadrenalism 255.4
  tuberculous (*see also* Tuberculosis) 017.6
Hypoadrenocorticism 255.4
  pituitary 253.4
Hypoalbuminemia 273.8
Hypoalphalipoproteinemia 272.5
Hypobarism 993.2
Hypobaropathy 993.2
Hypobetalipoproteinemia (familial) 272.5
Hypocalcemia 275.41
  cow's milk 775.4
  dietary 269.3
  neonatal 775.4
  phosphate-loading 775.4
Hypocalcification, teeth 520.4
Hypochloremia 276.9
Hypochlorhydria 536.8
  neurotic 306.4
  psychogenic 306.4
Hypocholesteremia 272.5
Hypochondria (reaction) 300.7
Hypochondriac 300.7
Hypochondriasis 300.7
Hypochromasia blood cells 280.9
Hypochromic anemia 280.9
  due to blood loss (chronic) 280.0
    acute 285.1
  microcytic 280.9
Hypocoagulability (*see also* Defect, coagulation)
    286.9
Hypocomplementemia 279.8
Hypocythemia (progressive) 284.9
Hypodontia (*see also* Anodontia) 520.0
Hypoeosinophilia 288.8
Hypoesthesia (*see also* Disturbance, sensation)
    782.0
  cornea 371.81
  tactile 782.0
Hypoestrinism 256.39
Hypoestrogenism 256.39
Hypoferremia 280.9
  due to blood loss (chronic) 280.0
Hypofertility
  female 628.9
  male 606.1
Hypofibrinogenemia) 286.3
  acquired 286.6
  congenital 286.3
Hypofunction
  adrenal (gland) 255.4
    cortex 255.4
    medulla 255.5
    specified NEC 255.5
  cerebral 331.9
  corticoadrenal NEC 255.4
  intestinal 564.89
  labyrinth (unilateral) 386.53
    with loss of labyrinthine reactivity 386.55
    bilateral 386.54
      with loss of labyrinthine reactivity 386.56
  Leydig cell 257.2
  ovary 256.39
    postablative 256.2
  pituitary (anterior) (gland) (lobe) 253.2
    posterior 253.5
  testicular 257.2
    iatrogenic 257.1

Hypofunction—*continued*
   postablative 257.1
    postirradiation 257.1
    postsurgical 257.1
Hypogammaglobulinemia 279.00
  acquired primary 279.06
  non-sex-linked, congenital 279.06
  sporadic 279.06
  transient of infancy 279.09
Hypogenitalism (congenital) (female) (male)
   752.8
  penis 752.69
Hypoglycemia (spontaneous) 251.2
  coma 251.0
   diabetic 250.3
  diabetic 250.8
  due to insulin 251.0
   therapeutic misadventure 962.3
  familial (idiopathic) 251.2
  following gastrointestinal surgery 579.3
  infantile (idiopathic) 251.2
  in infant of diabetic mother 775.0
  leucine-induced 270.3
  neonatal 775.6
  reactive 251.2
  specified NEC 251.1
Hypoglycemic shock 251.0
  diabetic 250.8
  due to insulin 251.0
  functional (syndrome) 251.1
Hypogonadism
  female 256.39
  gonadotrophic (isolated) 253.4
  hypogonadotropic (isolated) (with anosmia)
   253.4
  isolated 253.4
  male 257.2
  ovarian (primary) 256.39
  pituitary (secondary) 253.4
  testicular (primary) (secondary) 257.2
Hypohidrosis 705.0
Hypohidrotic ectodermal dysplasia 757.31
Hypoidrosis 705.0
Hypoinsulinemia, postsurgical 251.3
  postpancreatectomy (complete) (partial) 251.3
Hypokalemia 276.8
Hypokinesia 780.99
Hypoleukia splenica 289.4
Hypoleukocytosis 288.8
Hypolipidemia 272.5
Hypolipoproteinemia 272.5
Hypomagnesemia 275.2
  neonatal 775.4
Hypomania, hypomanic reaction (*see also*
   Psychosis, affective) 296.0
  recurrent episode 296.1
  single episode 296.0
Hypomastia (congenital) 757.6
Hypomenorrhea 626.1
Hypometabolism 783.9
Hypomotility
  gastrointestinal tract 536.8
   psychogenic 306.4
  intestine 564.89
   psychogenic 306.4
  stomach 536.8
   psychogenic 306.4
Hyponasality 784.49
Hyponatremia 276.1
Hypo-ovarianism 256.39
Hypo-ovarism 256.39

Hypoparathyroidism (idiopathic) (surgically
   induced) 252.1
  neonatal 775.4
Hypopharyngitis 462
Hypophoria 378.40
Hypophosphatasia 275.3
Hypophosphatemia (acquired) (congenital)
   (familial) 275.3
  renal 275.3
Hypophyseal, hypophysis —*see also* condition
  dwarfism 253.3
  gigantism 253.0
  syndrome 253.8
Hypophyseothalamic syndrome 253.8
Hypopiesis —*see* Hypotension
Hypopigmentation 709.00
  eyelid 374.53
Hypopinealism 259.8
Hypopituitarism (juvenile) (syndrome) 253.2
  due to
   hormone therapy 253.7
   hypophysectomy 253.7
   radiotherapy 253.7
  postablative 253.7
  postpartum hemorrhage 253.2
Hypoplasia, hypoplasis 759.89
  adrenal (gland) 759.1
  alimentary tract 751.8
   lower 751.2
   upper 750.8
  anus, anal (canal) 751.2
  aorta 747.22
  aortic
   arch (tubular) 747.10
   orifice or valve with hypoplasia of ascending
    aorta and defective development of left
    ventricle (with mitral valve atresia) 746.7
  appendix 751.2
  areola 757.6
  arm (*see also* Absence, arm, congenital) 755.20
  artery (congenital) (peripheral) NEC 747.60
   brain 747.81
   cerebral 747.81
   coronary 746.85
   gastrointestinal 747.61
   lower limb 747.64
   pulmonary 747.3
   renal 747.62
   retinal 743.58
   specified NEC 747.69
   spinal 747.82
   umbilical 747.5
   upper limb 747.63
  auditory canal 744.29
   causing impairment of hearing 744.02
  biliary duct (common) or passage 751.61
  bladder 753.8
  bone NEC 756.9
   face 756.0
   malar 756.0
   mandible 524.04
    alveolar 524.74
   marrow 284.9
    acquired (secondary) 284.8
    congenital 284.0
    idiopathic 284.9
   maxilla 524.03
    alveolar 524.73
   skull (*see also* Hypoplasia, skull) 756.0
  brain 742.1
   gyri 742.2

Hypothyroidism—*continued*
  postablative NEC 244.1
  postsurgical 244.0
  primary 244.9
  secondary NEC 244.8
  specified cause NEC 244.8
  sporadic goitrous 246.1
Hypotonia, hypotonicity, hypotony 781.3
  benign congenital 358.8
  bladder 596.4
  congenital 779.89
    benign 358.8
  eye 360.30
    due to
      fistula 360.32
      ocular disorder NEC 360.33
    following loss of aqueous or vitreous 360.33
    primary 360.31
  infantile muscular (benign) 359.0
  muscle 728.9
  uterus, uterine (contractions)—*see* Inertia, uterus
Hypotrichosis 704.09
  congenital 757.4
  lid (congenital) 757.4
    acquired 374.55
  postinfectional NEC 704.09
Hypotropia 378.32
Hypoventilation 786.09
Hypovitaminosis (*see also* Deficiency, vitamin)
  269.2
Hypovolemia 276.5
  surgical shock 998.0
  traumatic (shock) 958.4
Hypoxemia (*see also* Anoxia) 799.0
Hypoxia (*see also* Anoxia) 799.0
  cerebral 348.1
    during or resulting from a procedure 997.01
    newborn 768.9
      mild or moderate 768.6
      severe 768.5
  fetal, affecting newborn 768.9
  intrauterine—*see* Distress, fetal
  myocardial (*see also* Insufficiency, coronary)
    411.89
    arteriosclerotic —*see* Arteriosclerosis,
      coronary
  newborn 768.9
Hypsarrhythmia (*see also* Epilepsy) 345.6
Hysteralgia, pregnant uterus 646.8
Hysteria, hysterical 300.10
  anxiety 300.20
  Charcot's gland 300.11
  conversion (any manifestation) 300.11
  dissociative type NEC 300.15
  psychosis, acute 298.1
Hysteroepilepsy 300.11
Hysterotomy , affecting fetus or newborn
  763.89

I

Iatrogenic syndrome of excess cortisol 255.0
Iceland disease (epidemic neuromyasthenia)
  049.8
Ichthyosis (congenita) 757.1
  acquired 701.1
  fetalis gravior 757.1
  follicularis 757.1
  hystrix 757.39
  lamellar 757.1
  lingual 528.6
  palmaris and plantaris 757.39
  simplex 757.1
  vera 757.1
  vulgaris 757.1
Ichthyotoxism 988.0
  bacterial (*see also* Poisoning, food) 005.9
Icteroanemia, hemolytic (acquired) 283.9
  congenital (*see also* Spherocytosis) 282.0
Icterus (*see also* Jaundice) 782.4
  catarrhal—*see* Icterus, infectious
  conjunctiva 782.4
    newborn 774.6
  epidemic—*see* Icterus, infectious
  febrilis—*see* Icterus, infectious
  fetus or newborn—*see* Jaundice, fetus or
    newborn
  gravis (*see also* Necrosis, liver) 570
    complicating pregnancy 646.7
      affecting fetus or newborn 760.8
    fetus or newborn NEC 773.0
    obstetrical 646.7
      affecting fetus or newborn 760.8
  hematogenous (acquired) 283.9
  hemolytic (acquired) 283.9
    congenital (*see also* Spherocytosis) 282.0
  hemorrhagic (acute) 100.0
    leptospiral 100.0
    newborn 776.0
    spirochetal 100.0
  infectious 070.1
    with hepatic coma 070.0
    leptospiral 100.0
    spirochetal 100.0
  intermittens juvenilis 277.4
  malignant (*see also* Necrosis, liver) 570
  neonatorum (*see also* Jaundice, fetus or
    newborn) 774.6
  pernicious (*see also* Necrosis, liver) 570
  spirochetal 100.0
Ictus solaris, solis 992.0
Identity disorder 313.82
  dissociative 300.14
  gender role (child) 302.6
    adult 302.85
  psychosexual (child) 302.6
    adult 302.85
Idioglossia 307.9
Idiopathic —*see* condition
Idiosyncrasy (*see also* Allergy) 995.3
  drug, medicinal substance, and biological—*see*
    Allergy, drug
Idiot, idiocy (congenital) 318.2
  amaurotic (Bielschowsky) (-Jansky) (family)
    (infantile (late)) (juvenile (late))
    (Vogt-Spielmeyer) 330.1
  microcephalic 742.1
  Mongolian 758.0
  oxycephalic 756.0
Id reaction (due to bacteria) 692.89

IgE asthma 493.0
Ileitis (chronic) (*see also* Enteritis) 558.9
  infectious 009.0
  noninfectious 558.9
  regional (ulcerative) 555.0
    with large intestine 555.2
  segmental 555.0
    with large intestine 555.2
  terminal (ulcerative) 555.0
    with large intestine 555.2
Ileocolitis (*see also* Enteritis) 558.9
  infectious 009.0
  regional 555.2
  ulcerative 556.1
Ileostomy status V44.2
  with complication 569.60
Ileotyphus 002.0
Ileum —*see* condition
Ileus (adynamic) (bowel) (colon) (inhibitory)
    (intestine) (neurogenic) (paralytic) 560.1
  arteriomesenteric duodenal 537.2
  due to gallstone (in intestine) 560.31
  duodenal, chronic 537.2
  following gastrointestinal surgery 997.4
  gallstone 560.31
  mechanical (*see also* Obstruction, intestine)
    560.9
  meconium 777.1
    due to cystic fibrosis 277.01
  myxedema 564.89
  postoperative 997.4
  transitory, newborn 777.4
Iliac —*see* condition
Iliotibial band friction syndrome 728.89
Ill, louping 063.1
Illegitimacy V61.6
Illness —*see also* Disease
  factitious 300.19
    with
      combined physical and psychological
        symptoms 300.19
      physical symptoms 300.19
      psychological symptoms 300.16
    chronic (with physical symptoms) 301.51
  heart—*see* Disease, heart
  manic-depressive (*see also* Psychosis, affective)
    296.80
  mental (*see also* Disorder, mental) 300.9
Imbalance 781.2
  autonomic (*see also* Neuropathy, peripheral,
    autonomic) 337.9
  electrolyte 276.9
    with
      abortion—*see* Abortion, by type, with
        metabolic disorder
      ectopic pregnancy (*see also* categories
        633.0-633.9) 639.4
      hyperemesis gravidarum (before 22
        completed weeks gestation) 643.1
      molar pregnancy (*see also* categories
        630-632) 639.4
    following
      abortion 639.4
      ectopic or molar pregnancy 639.4
    neonatal, transitory NEC 775.5
  endocrine 259.9
  eye muscle NEC 378.9
    heterophoria—*see* Heterophoria

Imbalance—*continued*
  glomerulotubular NEC 593.89
  hormone 259.9
  hysterical (*see also* Hysteria) 300.10
  labyrinth NEC 386.50
  posture 729.9
  sympathetic (*see also* Neuropathy, peripheral,
    autonomic) 337.9
Imbecile, imbecility 318.0
  moral 301.7
  old age 290.9
  senile 290.9
  specified IQ—*see* IQ
  unspecified IQ 318.0
Imbedding, intrauterine device 996.32
Imbibition, cholesterol (gallbladder) 575.6
Imerslund (-Gräsbeck) syndrome (anemia due to
    familial selective vitamin B_{12} malabsorption)
    281.1
Iminoacidopathy 270.8
Iminoglycinuria, familial 270.8
Immature —*see also* Immaturity
  personality 301.89
Immaturity 765.1
  extreme 765.0
  fetus or infant light-for-dates—*see*
    Light-for-dates
  lung, fetus or newborn 770.4
  organ or site NEC—*see* Hypoplasia
  pulmonary, fetus or newborn 770.4
  reaction 301.89
  sexual (female) (male) 259.0
Immersion 994.1
  foot 991.4
  hand 991.4
Immobile, immobility
  intestine 564.89
  joint—*see* Ankylosis
  syndrome (paraplegic) 728.3
Immunization
  ABO
    affecting management of pregnancy 656.2
      fetus or newborn 773.1
  complication—*see* Complications, vaccination
  Rh factor
    affecting management of pregnancy 656.1
      fetus or newborn 773.0
    from transfusion 999.7
Immunodeficiency 279.3
  with
    adenosine-deaminase deficiency 279.2
    defect, predominant
      B-cell 279.00
      T-cell 279.10
    hyperimmunoglobulinemia 279.2
    lymphopenia, hereditary 279.2
    thrombocytopenia and eczema 279.12
    thymic
      aplasia 279.2
      dysplasia 279.2
  autosomal recessive, Swiss-type 279.2
  common variable 279.06
  severe combined (SCID) 279.2
  to Rh factor
    affecting management of pregnancy 656.1
      fetus or newborn 773.0
  X-linked, with increased IgM 279.05
Immunotherapy, prophylactic V07.2

Impaction, impacted
  bowel, colon, rectum 560.30
    with hernia—*see also* Hernia, by site, with
      obstruction
      gangrenous—*see* Hernia, by site, with
        gangrene
    by
      calculus 560.39
      gallstone 560.31
    fecal 560.39
    specified type NEC 560.39
  calculus—*see* Calculus
  cerumen (ear) (external) 380.4
  cuspid 520.6
    with abnormal position (same or adjacent
      tooth) 524.3
  dental 520.6
    with abnormal position (same or adjacent
      tooth) 524.3
  fecal, feces 560.39
    with hernia—*see also* Hernia, by site, with
      obstruction
      gangrenous—*see* Hernia, by site, with
        gangrene
  fracture—*see* Fracture, by site
  gallbladder—*see* Cholelithiasis
  gallstone(s)—*see* Cholelithiasis
    in intestine (any part) 560.31
  intestine(s) 560.30
    with hernia—*see also* Hernia, by site, with
      obstruction
      gangrenous—*see* Hernia, by site, with
        gangrene
    by
      calculus 560.39
      gallstone 560.31
    fecal 560.39
    specified type NEC 560.39
  intrauterine device (IUD) 996.32
  molar 520.6
    with abnormal position (same or adjacent
      tooth) 524.3
  shoulder 660.4
    affecting fetus or newborn 763.1
  tooth, teeth 520.6
    with abnormal position (same or adjacent
      tooth) 524.3
  turbinate 733.99
Impaired, impairment (function)
  arm V49.1
    movement, involving
      musculoskeletal system V49.1
      nervous system V49.2
  auditory discrimination 388.43
  back V48.3
  body (entire) V49.89
  hearing (*see also* Deafness) 389.9
  heart—*see* Disease, heart
  kidney (*see also* Disease, renal) 593.9
    disorder resulting from 588.9
      specified NEC 588.8
  leg V49.1
    movement, involving
      musculoskeletal system V49.1
      nervous system V49.2
  limb V49.1
    movement, involving
      musculoskeletal system V49.1
      nervous system V49.2
  liver 573.8
  mastication 524.9

Impaired, impairment—*continued*
  mobility
    ear ossicles NEC 385.22
    incostapedial joint 385.22
    malleus 385.21
  myocardium, myocardial (*see also*
      Insufficiency, myocardial) 428.0
  neuromusculoskeletal NEC V49.89
    back V48.3
    head V48.2
    limb V49.2
    neck V48.3
    spine V48.3
    trunk V48.3
  rectal sphincter 787.99
  renal (*see also* Disease, renal) 593.9
    disorder resulting from 588.9
      specified NEC 588.8
  spine V48.3
  vision NEC 369.9
    both eyes NEC 369.3
    moderate 369.74
      both eyes 369.25
        with impairment of lesser eye (specified
            as)
          blind, not further specified 369.15
          low vision, not further specified 369.23
          near-total 369.17
          profound 369.18
          severe 369.24
          total 369.16
      one eye 369.74
        with vision of other eye (specified as)
          near-normal 369.75
          normal 369.76
    near-total 369.64
      both eyes 369.04
        with impairment of lesser eye (specified
            as)
          blind, not further specified 369.02
          total 369.03
      one eye 369.64
        with vision of other eye (specified as)
          near-normal 369.65
          normal 369.66
    one eye 369.60
      with low vision of other eye 369.10
    profound 369.67
      both eyes 369.08
        with impairment of lesser eye (specified
            as)
          blind, not further specified 369.05
          near-total 369.07
          total 369.06
      one eye 369.67
        with vision of other eye (specified as)
          near-normal 369.68
          normal 369.69
    severe 369.71
      both eyes 369.22
        with impairment of lesser eye (specified
            as)
          blind, not further specified 369.11
          low vision, not further specified 369.21
          near-total 369.13
          profound 369.14
          total 369.12
      one eye 369.71
        with vision of other eye (specified as)
          near-normal 369.72
          normal 369.73

Impaired, impairment—*continued*
  total
    both eyes 369.01
    one eye 369.61
      with vision of other eye (specified as)
        near-normal 369.62
        normal 369.63
Impaludism —*see* Malaria
Impediment, speech NEC 784.5
  psychogenic 307.9
  secondary to organic lesion 784.5
Impending
  cerebrovascular accident or attack 435.9
  coronary syndrome 411.1
  delirium tremens 291.0
  myocardial infarction 411.1
Imperception, auditory (acquired) (congenital)
    389.9
Imperfect
  aeration, lung (newborn) 770.5
  closure (congenital)
    alimentary tract NEC 751.8
      lower 751.5
      upper 750.8
    atrioventricular ostium 745.69
    atrium (secundum) 745.5
      primum 745.61
    branchial cleft or sinus 744.41
    choroid 743.59
    cricoid cartilage 748.3
    cusps, heart valve NEC 746.89
      pulmonary 746.09
    ductus
      arteriosus 747.0
      Botalli 747.0
    ear drum 744.29
      causing impairment of hearing 744.03
    endocardial cushion 745.60
    epiglottis 748.3
    esophagus with communication to bronchus
        or trachea 750.3
    Eustachian valve 746.89
    eyelid 743.62
    face, facial (*see also* Cleft, lip) 749.10
    foramen
      Botalli 745.5
      ovale 745.5
    genitalia, genital organ(s) or system
      female 752.8
        external 752.49
        internal NEC 752.8
        uterus 752.3
      male 752.8
        penis 752.69
    glottis 748.3
    heart valve (cusps) NEC 746.89
    interatrial ostium or septum 745.5
    interauricular ostium or septum 745.5
    interventricular ostium or septum 745.4
    iris 743.46
    kidney 753.3
    larynx 748.3
    lens 743.36
    lip (*see also* Cleft, lip) 749.10
    nasal septum or sinus 748.1
    nose 748.1
    omphalomesenteric duct 751.0
    optic nerve entry 743.57
    organ or site NEC—*see* Anomaly, specified
        type, by site

Incompetency, Incompetence—*continued*
  pulmonary valve (heart) (*see also*
     Endocarditis, pulmonary) 424.3
  aortic (valve) (*see also* Insufficiency, aortic)
     424.1
    syphilitic 093.22
  cardiac (orifice) 530.0
    valve—*see* Endocarditis
  cervix, cervical (os) 622.5
    in pregnancy 654.5
      affecting fetus or newborn 761.0
  esophagogastric (junction) (sphincter) 530.0
  heart valve, congenital 746.89
  mitral (valve)—*see* Insufficiency, mitral
  papillary muscle (heart) 429.81
  pelvic fundus 618.8
  pulmonary valve (heart) (*see also* Endocarditis,
     pulmonary) 424.3
    congenital 746.09
  tricuspid (annular) (rheumatic) (valve) (*see also*
     Endocarditis, tricuspid) 397.0
  valvular—*see* Endocarditis
  vein, venous (saphenous) (varicose) (*see also*
     Varicose, vein) 454.9
  velopharyngeal (closure)
    acquired 528.9
    congenital 750.29
Incomplete —*see also* condition
  bladder emptying 788.21
  expansion lungs (newborn) 770.5
  gestation (liveborn)—*see* Immaturity
  rotation—*see* Malrotation
Incontinence 788.30
  without sensory awareness 788.34
  anal sphincter 787.6
  continuous leakage 788.37
  feces 787.6
    due to hysteria 300.11
    nonorganic origin 307.7
  hysterical 300.11
  mixed (male) (female) (urge and stress) 788.33
  overflow 788.39
  paradoxical 788.39
  rectal 787.6
  specified NEC 788.39
  stress (female) 625.6
    male NEC 788.32
  urethral sphincter 599.84
  urge 788.31
    and stress (male) (female) 788.33
  urine 788.30
    active 788.30
    male 788.30
      stress 788.32
        and urge 788.33
      neurogenic 788.39
      nonorganic origin 307.6
      stress (female) 625.6
        male NEC 788.32
      urge 788.31
        and stress 788.33
Incontinentia pigmenti 757.33
Incoordinate
  uterus (action) (contractions) 661.4
    affecting fetus or newborn 763.7
Incoordination
  esophageal-pharyngeal (newborn) 787.2
  muscular 781.3
  papillary muscle 429.81

Increase, increased
  abnormal, in development 783.9
  androgens (ovarian) 256.1
  anticoagulants (antithrombin) (anti-VIIIa)
     (anti-IXa) (anti-Xa) (anti-XIa) 286.5
    postpartum 666.3
  cold sense (*see also* Disturbance, sensation)
    782.0
  estrogen 256.0
  function
    adrenal (cortex) 255.3
      medulla 255.6
    pituitary (anterior) (gland) (lobe) 253.1
      posterior 253.6
  heat sense (*see also* Disturbance, sensation)
    782.0
  intracranial pressure 781.99
    injury at birth 767.8
  light reflex of retina 362.13
  permeability, capillary 448.9
  pressure
    intracranial 781.99
      injury at birth 767.8
    intraocular 365.00
  pulsations 785.9
  pulse pressure 785.9
  sphericity, lens 743.36
  splenic activity 289.4
  venous pressure 459.89
    portal 572.3
Incrustation, cornea, lead or zinc 930.0
Incyclophoria 378.44
Incyclotropia 378.33
Indeterminate sex 752.7
India rubber skin 756.83
Indicanuria 270.2
Indigestion (bilious) (functional) 536.8
  acid 536.8
  catarrhal 536.8
  due to decomposed food NEC 005.9
  fat 579.8
  nervous 306.4
  psychogenic 306.4
Indirect —*see* condition
Indolent bubo NEC 099.8
Induced
  abortion—*see* Abortion, induced
  birth, affecting fetus or newborn 763.89
  delivery—*see* Delivery
  labor—*see* Delivery
Induration, indurated
  brain 348.8
  breast (fibrous) 611.79
    puerperal, postpartum 676.3
  broad ligament 620.8
  chancre 091.0
    anus 091.1
    congenital 090.0
    extragenital NEC 091.2
  corpora cavernosa (penis) (plastic) 607.89
  liver (chronic) 573.8
    acute 573.8
  lung (black) (brown) (chronic) (fibroid) (*see*
    also Fibrosis, lung) 515
    essential brown 275.0 *[516.1]*
  penile 607.89
  phlebitic—*see* Phlebitis
  skin 782.8
  stomach 537.89
Induratio penis plastica 607.89
Industrial —*see* condition

Inebriety (*see also* Abuse, drugs, nondependent) 305.0
Inefficiency
　kidney (*see also* Disease, renal) 593.9
　thyroid (acquired) (gland) 244.9
Inelasticity, skin 782.8
Inequality, leg (acquired) (length) 736.81
　congenital 755.30
Inertia
　bladder 596.4
　　neurogenic 596.54
　　　with cauda equina syndrome 344.61
　stomach 536.8
　　psychogenic 306.4
　uterus, uterine 661.2
　　affecting fetus or newborn 763.7
　　primary 661.0
　　secondary 661.1
　vesical 596.4
　　neurogenic 596.54
　　　with cauda equina 344.61
Infant —*see also* condition
　excessive crying of 780.92
　fussy (baby) 780.91
　held for adoption V68.89
　newborn—*see* Newborn
　syndrome of diabetic mother 775.0
"Infant Hercules" syndrome 255.2
Infantile —*see also* condition
　genitalia, genitals 259.0
　　in pregnancy or childbirth NEC 654.4
　　　affecting fetus or newborn 763.89
　　　causing obstructed labor 660.2
　　　　affecting fetus or newborn 763.1
　heart 746.9
　kidney 753.3
　lack of care 995.52
　macula degeneration 362.75
　melanodontia 521.05
　os, uterus (*see also* Infantile, genitalia) 259.0
　pelvis 738.6
　　with disproportion (fetopelvic) 653.1
　　　affecting fetus or newborn 763.1
　　　causing obstructed labor 660.1
　　　　affecting fetus or newborn 763.1
　penis 259.0
　testis 257.2
　uterus (*see also* Infantile, genitalia) 259.0
　vulva 752.49
Infantilism 259.9
　with dwarfism (hypophyseal) 253.3
　Brissaud's (infantile myxedema) 244.9
　celiac 579.0
　Herter's (nontropical sprue) 579.0
　hypophyseal 253.3
　hypothalamic (with obesity) 253.8
　idiopathic 259.9
　intestinal 579.0
　pancreatic 577.8
　pituitary 253.3
　renal 588.0
　sexual (with obesity) 259.0
Infants, healthy liveborn —*see* Newborn
Infarct, infarction
　adrenal (capsule) (gland) 255.4
　amnion 658.8
　anterior (with contiguous portion of
　　intraventricular septum) NEC (*see also*
　　Infarct, myocardium) 410.1
　appendices epiploicae 557.0
　bowel 557.0

Infarct, infarction—*continued*
　brain (stem) 434.91
　　embolic (*see also* Embolism, brain) 434.11
　　healed or old, without residuals V12.59
　　　iatrogenic 997.02
　　　postoperative 997.02
　　puerperal, postpartum, childbirth 674.0
　　thrombotic (*see also* Thrombosis, brain)
　　　434.01
　breast 611.8
　Brewer's (kidney) 593.81
　cardiac (*see also* Infarct, myocardium) 410.9
　cerebellar (*see also* Infarct, brain) 434.91
　　embolic (*see also* Embolism, brain) 434.11
　cerebral (*see also* Infarct, brain) 434.91
　　embolic (*see also* Embolism, brain) 434.11
　chorion 658.8
　colon (acute) (agnogenic) (embolic)
　　(hemorrhagic) (nonocclusive)
　　(nonthrombotic) (occlusive) (segmental)
　　(thrombotic) (with gangrene) 557.0
　coronary artery (*see also* Infarct, myocardium)
　　410.9
　embolic (*see also* Embolism) 444.9
　fallopian tube 620.8
　gallbladder 575.8
　heart (*see also* Infarct, myocardium) 410.9
　hepatic 573.4
　hypophysis (anterior lobe) 253.8
　impending (myocardium) 411.1
　intestine (acute) (agnogenic) (embolic)
　　(hemorrhagic) (nonocclusive)
　　(nonthrombotic) (occlusive) (thrombotic)
　　(with gangrene) 557.0
　kidney 593.81
　liver 573.4
　lung (embolic) (thrombotic) 415.19
　　with
　　　abortion—*see* Abortion, by type, with,
　　　　embolism
　　　ectopic pregnancy (*see also* categories
　　　　633.0-633.9) 639.6
　　　molar pregnancy (*see also* categories
　　　　630-632) 639.6
　　following
　　　abortion 639.6
　　　ectopic or molar pregnancy 639.6
　　iatrogenic 415.11
　　in pregnancy, childbirth, or puerperium—*see*
　　　Embolism, obstetrical
　　postoperative 415.11
　lymph node or vessel 457.8
　medullary (brain)—*see* Infarct, brain
　meibomian gland (eyelid) 374.85
　mesentery, mesenteric (embolic) (thrombotic)
　　(with gangrene) 557.0
　midbrain—*see* Infarct, brain
　myocardium, myocardial (acute or with a stated
　　duration of 8 weeks or less) (with
　　hypertension) 410.9

<table>
<tr><td>Note—use the following fifth-digit subclassification with category 410

0　episode unspecified
1　initial episode
2　subsequent episode without recurrence</td></tr>
</table>

Infection, infected, infective—*continued*
    chronic 006.1
    free-living 136.2
    hartmanni 007.8
    specified
        site NEC 006.8
        type NEC 007.8
    amniotic fluid or cavity 658.4
        affecting fetus or newborn 762.7
    anaerobes (cocci) (gram-negative) (gram
        positive) (mixed) NEC 041.84
    anal canal 569.49
    Ancylostoma braziliense 126.2
    Angiostrongylus cantonensis 128.8
    anisakiasis 127.1
    Anisakis larva 127.1
    anthrax (*see also* Anthrax) 022.9
    antrum (chronic) (*see also* Sinusitis, maxillary)
        473.0
    anus (papillae) (sphincter) 569.49
    arbor virus NEC 066.9
    arbovirus NEC 066.9
    argentophil-rod 027.0
    Ascaris lumbricoides 127.0
    ascomycetes 117.4
    Aspergillus (flavus) (fumigatus) (terreus) 117.3
    atypical
        acid-fast (bacilli) (*see also* Mycobacterium,
            atypical) 031.9
        mycobacteria (*see also* Mycobacterium,
            atypical) 031.9
    auditory meatus (circumscribed) (diffuse)
        (external) (*see also* Otitis, externa) 380.10
    auricle (ear) (*see also* Otitis, externa) 380.10
    axillary gland 683
    Babesiasis 088.82
    Babesiosis 088.82
    Bacillus NEC 041.89
        abortus 023.1
        anthracis (*see also* Anthrax) 022.9
        cereus (food poisoning) 005.89
        coli—*see* Infection, Escherichia coli
        coliform NEC 041.85
        Ducrey's (any location) 099.0
        Flexner's 004.1
        fragilis NEC 041.82
        Friedländer's NEC 041.3
        fusiformis 101
        gas (gangrene) (*see also* Gangrene, gas) 040.0
        mallei 024
        melitensis 023.0
        paratyphoid, paratyphosus 002.9
            A 002.1
            B 002.2
            C 002.3
        Schmorl's 040.3
        Shiga 004.0
        suipestifer (*see also* Infection, Salmonella)
            003.9
        swimming pool 031.1
        typhosa 002.0
        welchii (*see also* Gangrene, gas) 040.0
        Whitmore's 025
    bacterial NEC 041.9
        specified NEC 041.89
            anaerobic NEC 041.84
            gram-negative NEC 041.85
                anaerobic NEC 041.84
    Bacterium
        paratyphosum 002.9
            A 002.1

Infection, infected, infective—*continued*
        B 002.2
        C 002.3
        typhosum 002.0
    Bacteroides (fragilis) (melaninogenicus) (oralis)
        NEC 041.84
    balantidium coli 007.0
    Bartholin's gland 616.8
    Basidiobolus 117.7
    Bedsonia 079.98
        specified NEC 079.88
    bile duct 576.1
    bladder (*see also* Cystitis) 595.9
    Blastomyces, blastomycotic 116.0
        brasiliensis 116.1
        dermatitidis 116.0
        European 117.5
        Loboi 116.2
        North American 116.0
        South American 116.1
    blood stream—*see* Septicemia
    bone 730.9
        specified—*see* Osteomyelitis
    Bordetella 033.9
        bronchiseptica 033.8
        parapertussis 033.1
        pertussis 033.0
    Borrelia
        bergdorfi 088.81
        vincentii (mouth) (pharynx) (tonsil) 101
    brain (*see also* Encephalitis) 323.9
        late effect—*see* category 326
        membranes—(*see also* Meningitis) 322.9
        septic 324.0
            late effect—*see* category 326
            meninges (*see also* Meningitis) 320.9
    branchial cyst 744.42
    breast 611.0
        puerperal, postpartum 675.2
            with nipple 675.9
                specified type NEC 675.8
            nonpurulent 675.2
            purulent 675.1
    bronchus (*see also* Bronchitis) 490
        fungus NEC 117.9
    Brucella 023.9
        abortus 023.1
        canis 023.3
        melitensis 023.0
        mixed 023.8
        suis 023.2
    Brugia (Wuchereria) malayi 125.1
    bursa—*see* Bursitis
    buttocks (skin) 686.9
    Candida (albicans) (tropicalis) (*see also*
        Candidiasis) 112.9
        congenital 771.7
    Candiru 136.8
    Capillaria
        hepatica 128.8
        philippinensis 127.5
    cartilage 733.99
    cat liver fluke 121.0
    cellulitis—*see* Cellulitis, by site
    Cephalosporum falciforme 117.4
    Cercomonas hominis (intestinal) 007.3
    cerebrospinal (*see also* Meningitis) 322.9
        late effect—*see* category 326
    cervical gland 683
    cervix (*see also* Cervicitis) 616.0
    cesarean section wound 674.3

Infection, infected, infective—*continued*
duboisii (*see also* Histoplasmosis, African)
115.10
HIV V08
with symptoms, symptomatic 042
hookworm (*see also* Ancylostomiasis) 126.9
human immunodeficiency virus V08
with symptoms, symptomatic 042
human papillomavirus 079.4
hydrocele 603.1
hydronephrosis 591
Hymenolepis 123.6
hypopharynx 478.29
inguinal glands 683
due to soft chancre 099.0
intestine, intestinal (*see also* Enteritis, due to, by
organism) 009.0
intrauterine (*see also* Endometritis) 615.9
complicating delivery 646.6
isospora belli or hominis 007.2
Japanese B encephalitis 062.0
jaw (bone) (acute) (chronic) (lower) (subacute)
(upper) 526.4
joint—*see* Arthritis, infectious or infective
kidney (cortex) (hematogenous) 590.9
with
abortion—*see* Abortion, by type, with
urinary tract infection
calculus 592.0
ectopic pregnancy (*see also* categories
633.0-633.9) 639.8
molar pregnancy (*see also* categories
630-632) 639.8
complicating pregnancy or puerperium 646.6
affecting fetus or newborn 760.1
following
abortion 639.8
ectopic or molar pregnancy 639.8
pelvis and ureter 590.3
Klebsiella pneumoniae NEC 041.3
knee (skin) NEC 686.9
joint—*see* Arthritis, infectious
Koch's (*see also* Tuberculosis, pulmonary)
011.9
labia (majora) (minora) (*see also* Vulvitis)
616.10
lacrimal
gland (*see also* Dacryoadenitis) 375.00
passages (duct) (sac) (*see also* Dacryocystitis)
375.30
larynx NEC 478.79
leg (skin) NEC 686.9
Leishmania (*see also* Leishmaniasis) 085.9
braziliensis 085.5
donovani 085.0
Ethiopica 085.3
furunculosa 085.1
infantum 085.0
mexicana 085.4
tropica (minor) 085.1
major 085.2
Leptosphaeria senegalensis 117.4
leptospira (*see also* Leptospirosis) 100.9
Australis 100.89
Bataviae 100.89
pyrogenes 100.89
specified type NEC 100.89
leptospirochetal NEC (*see also* Leptospirosis)
100.9
Leptothrix—*see* Actinomycosis

Infection, infected, infective—*continued*
Listeria monocytogenes (listeriosis) 027.0
congenital 771.2
liver fluke—*see* Infestation, fluke, liver
Loa loa 125.2
eyelid 125.2 *[373.6]*
Loboa loboi 116.2
local, skin (staphylococcal) (streptococcal) NEC
686.9
abscess—*see* Abscess, by site
cellulitis—*see* Cellulitis, by site
ulcer (*see also* Ulcer, skin) 707.9
Loefflerella
mallei 024
whitmori 025
lung 518.89
atypical Mycobacterium 031.0
tuberculous (*see also* Tuberculosis,
pulmonary) 011.9
basilar 518.89
chronic 518.89
fungus NEC 117.9
spirochetal 104.8
virus—*see* Pneumonia, virus
lymph gland (axillary) (cervical) (inguinal) 683
mesenteric 289.2
lymphoid tissue, base of tongue or posterior
pharynx, NEC 474.00
madurella
grisea 117.4
mycetomii 117.4
major
with
abortion—*see* Abortion, by type, with sepsis
ectopic pregnancy (*see also* categories
633.0-633.9) 639.0
molar pregnancy (*see also* categories
630-632) 639.0
following
abortion 639.0
ectopic or molar pregnancy 639.0
puerperal, postpartum, childbirth 670
malarial—*see* Malaria
Malassezia furfur 111.0
Malleomyces
mallei 024
pseudomallei 025
mammary gland 611.0
puerperal, postpartum 675.2
Mansonella (ozzardi) 125.5
mastoid (suppurative)—*see* Mastoiditis
maxilla, maxillary 526.4
sinus (chronic) (*see also* Sinusitis, maxillary)
473.0
mediastinum 519.2
medina 125.7
meibomian
cyst 373.12
gland 373.12
melioidosis 025
meninges (*see also* Meningitis) 320.9
meningococcal (*see also* condition) 036.9
brain 036.1
cerebrospinal 036.0
endocardium 036.42
generalized 036.2
meninges 036.0
meningococcemia 036.2
specified site NEC 036.89
mesenteric lymph nodes or glands NEC 289.2
Metagonimus 121.5

Infection, infected, infective—*continued*
  metatarsophalangeal 711.97
  microorganism resistant to drugs—*see*
      Resistance (to), drugs by microorganisms
  Microsporidia 136.8
  microsporum, microsporic—*see*
      Dermatophytosis
  Mima polymorpha NEC 041.85
  mixed flora NEC 041.89
  Monilia (*see also* Candidiasis) 112.9
    neonatal 771.7
  Monosporium apiospermum 117.6
  mouth (focus) NEC 528.9
    parasitic 112.0
  Mucor 117.7
  muscle NEC 728.89
  mycelium NEC 117.9
  mycetoma
    actinomycotic NEC (*see also* Actinomycosis)
        039.9
    mycotic NEC 117.4
  Mycobacterium, mycobacterial (*see also*
      Mycobacterium) 031.9
  mycoplasma NEC 041.81
  mycotic NEC 117.9
    pathogenic to compromised host only 118
    skin NEC 111.9
    systemic 117.9
  myocardium NEC 422.90
  nail (chronic) (with lymphangitis) 681.9
    finger 681.02
      fungus 110.1
    ingrowing 703.0
    toe 681.11
      fungus 110.1
  nasal sinus (chronic) (*see also* Sinusitis) 473.9
  nasopharynx (chronic) 478.29
    acute 460
  navel 686.9
    newborn 771.4
  Neisserian—*see* Gonococcus
  Neotestudina rosatii 117.4
  newborn, generalized 771.89
  nipple 611.0
    puerperal, postpartum 675.0
      with breast 675.9
        specified type NEC 675.8
  Nocardia—*see* Actinomycosis
  nose 478.1
  nostril 478.1
  obstetrical surgical wound 674.3
  Oesophagostomum (apiostomum) 127.7
  Oestrus ovis 134.0
  Oidium albicans (*see also* Candidiasis) 112.9
  Onchocerca (volvulus) 125.3
    eye 125.3 *[360.13]*
    eyelid 125.3 *[373.6]*
  operation wound 998.59
  Opisthorchis (felineus) (tenuicollis) (viverrini)
      121.0
  orbit 376.00
    chronic 376.10
  ovary (*see also* Salpingo-oophoritis) 614.2
  Oxyuris vermicularis 127.4
  pancreas 577.0
  Paracoccidioides brasiliensis 116.1
  Paragonimus (westermani) 121.2
  parainfluenza virus 079.89
  parameningococcus NEC 036.9
    with meningitis 036.0
  parasitic NEC 136.9

Infection, infected, infective—*continued*
  paratyphoid 002.9
    Type A 002.1
    Type B 002.2
    Type C 002.3
  paraurethral ducts 597.89
  parotid gland 527.2
  Pasteurella NEC 027.2
    multocida (cat-bite) (dog-bite) 027.2
    pestis (*see also* Plague) 020.9
    pseudotuberculosis 027.2
    septica (cat-bite) (dog-bite) 027.2
    tularensis (*see also* Tularemia) 021.9
  pelvic, female (*see also* Disease, pelvis,
      inflammatory) 614.9
  penis (glans) (retention) NEC 607.2
    herpetic 054.13
  Peptococcus 041.84
  Peptostreptococcus 041.84
  periapical (pulpal origin) 522.4
  peridental 523.3
  perineal wound (obstetrical) 674.3
  periodontal 523.3
  periorbital 376.00
    chronic 376.10
  perirectal 569.49
  perirenal (*see also* Infection, kidney) 590.9
  peritoneal (*see also* Peritonitis) 567.9
  periureteral 593.89
  periurethral 597.89
  Petriellidium boydii 117.6
  pharynx 478.29
    Coxsackie virus 074.0
    phlegmonous 462
    posterior, lymphoid 474.00
  Phialophora
    gougerotii 117.8
    jeanselmei 117.8
    verrucosa 117.2
  Piedraia hortai 111.3
  pinna, acute 380.11
  pinta 103.9
    intermediate 103.1
    late 103.2
    mixed 103.3
    primary 103.0
  pinworm 127.4
  pityrosporum furfur 111.0
  pleuropneumonia-like organisms NEC (PPLO)
      041.81
  pneumococcal NEC 041.2
    generalized (purulent) 038.2
  Pneumococcus NEC 041.2
  postoperative wound 998.59
  posttraumatic NEC 958.3
  postvaccinal 999.3
  prepuce NEC 607.1
  Propionibacterium 041.84
  prostate (capsule) (*see also* Prostatitis) 601.9
  Proteus (mirabilis) (morganii) (vulgaris) NEC
      041.6
    enteritis 008.3
  protozoal NEC 136.8
    intestinal NEC 007.9
  Pseudomonas NEC 041.7
    mallei 024
    pneumonia 482.1
    pseudomallei 025
  psittacosis 073.9
  puerperal, postpartum (major) 670
    minor 646.6

Infertility—*continued*
    cervical anomaly 628.4
    fallopian tube anomaly 628.2
    ovarian failure 256.39 *[628.0]*
    Stein-Leventhal syndrome 256.4 *[628.0]*
    uterine anomaly 628.3
    vaginal anomaly 628.4
  nonimplantation 628.3
  origin
    cervical 628.4
    pituitary-hypothalamus NEC 253.8 *[628.1]*
      anterior pituitary NEC 253.4 *[628.1]*
        hyperfunction NEC 253.1 *[628.1]*
      dwarfism 253.3 *[628.1]*
      panhypopituitarism 253.2 *[628.1]*
    specified NEC 628.8
    tubal (block) (occlusion) (stenosis) 628.2
      adhesions 614.6 *[628.2]*
    uterine 628.3
    vaginal 628.4
  previous, requiring supervision of pregnancy
    V23.0
  male 606.9
    absolute 606.0
    due to
      azoospermia 606.0
      drug therapy 606.8
      extratesticular cause NEC 606.8
      germinal cell
        aplasia 606.0
        desquamation 606.1
      hypospermatogenesis 606.1
      infection 606.8
      obstruction, afferent ducts 606.8
      oligospermia 606.1
      radiation 606.8
      spermatogenic arrest (complete) 606.0
        incomplete 606.1
      systemic disease 606.8

Infestation 134.9
  Acanthocheilonema (perstans) 125.4
    streptocerca 125.6
  Acariasis 133.9
    demodex folliculorum 133.8
    Sarcoptes scabiei 133.0
    trombiculae 133.8
  Agamofilaria streptocerca 125.6
  Ancylostoma, Ankylostoma 126.9
    americanum 126.1
    braziliense 126.2
    canium 126.8
    ceylanicum 126.3
    duodenale 126.0
    new world 126.1
    old world 126.0
  Angiostrongylus cantonensis 128.8
  anisakiasis 127.1
  Anisakis larva 127.1
  arthropod NEC 134.1
  Ascaris lumbricoides 127.0
  Bacillus fusiformis 101
  Balantidium coli 007.0
  beef tapeworm 123.2
  Bothriocephalus (latus) 123.4
    larval 123.5
  broad tapeworm 123.4
    larval 123.5
  Brugia malayi 125.1
  Candiru 136.8
  Capillaria
    hepatica 128.8

Infestation—*continued*
    philippinensis 127.5
  cat liver fluke 121.0
  Cercomonas hominis (intestinal) 007.3
  cestodes 123.9
    specified type NEC 123.8
  chigger 133.8
  chigoe 134.1
  Chilomastix 007.8
  Clonorchis (sinensis) (liver) 121.1
  coccidia 007.2
  complicating pregnancy, childbirth, or
    puerperium 647.9
    affecting fetus or newborn 760.8
  Cysticercus cellulosae 123.1
  Demodex folliculorum 133.8
  Dermatobia (hominis) 134.0
  Dibothriocephalus (latus) 123.4
    larval 123.5
  Dicrocoelium dendriticum 121.8
  Diphyllobothrium (adult) (intestinal) (latum)
    (pacificum) 123.4
    larval 123.5
  Diplogonoporus (grandis) 123.8
  Dipylidium (caninum) 123.8
  Distoma hepaticum 121.3
  dog tapeworm 123.8
  Dracunculus medinensis 125.7
  dragon worm 125.7
  dwarf tapeworm 123.6
  Echinococcus (*see also* Echinococcus) 122.9
  Echinostoma ilocanum 121.8
  Embadomonas 007.8
  Endamoeba (histolytica)—*see* Infection, ameba
  Entamoeba (histolytica)—*see* Infection, ameba
  Enterobius vermicularis 127.4
  Epidermophyton—*see* Dermatophytosis
  eyeworm 125.2
  Fasciola
    gigantica 121.3
    hepatica 121.3
  Fasciolopsis (buski) (small intestine) 121.4
  filarial 125.9
    due to
      Acanthocheilonema (perstans) 125.4
        streptocerca 125.6
      Brugia (Wuchereria) malayi 125.1
      Dracunculus medinensis 125.7
      guinea worms 125.7
      Mansonella (ozzardi) 125.5
      Onchocerca volvulus 125.3
        eye 125.3 *[360.13]*
        eyelid 125.3 *[373.6]*
      Wuchereria (bancrofti) 125.0
        malayi 125.1
    specified type NEC 125.6
  fish tapeworm 123.4
    larval 123.5
  fluke 121.9
    blood NEC (*see also* Schistosomiasis) 120.9
    cat liver 121.0
    intestinal (giant) 121.4
    liver (sheep) 121.3
      cat 121.0
      Chinese 121.1
      clonorchiasis 121.1
      fascioliasis 121.3
      Oriental 121.1
    lung (oriental) 121.2
    sheep liver 121.3
  fly larva 134.0

Injury—*continued*
  diaphragm—*see* Injury, internal, diaphragm
  duodenum—*see* Injury, internal, duodenum
  ear (auricle) (canal) (drum) (external) 959.09
  elbow (and forearm) (and wrist) 959.3
  epididymis 959.1
  epigastric region 959.1
  epiglottis 959.09
  epiphyseal, current—*see* Fracture, by site
  esophagus—*see* Injury, internal, esophagus
  Eustachian tube 959.09
  extremity (lower) (upper) NEC 959.8
  eye 921.9
    penetrating eyeball—*see* Injury, eyeball,
        penetrating
    superficial 918.9
  eyeball 921.3
    penetrating 871.7
      with
        partial loss (of intraocular tissue) 871.12
        prolapse or exposure (of intraocular
            tissue) 871.1
        without prolapse 871.0
      foreign body (nonmagnetic) 871.6
        magnetic 871.5
    superficial 918.9
  eyebrow 959.09
  eyelid(s) 921.1
    laceration—*see* Laceration, eyelid
    superficial 918.0
  face (and neck) 959.09
  fallopian tube—*see* Injury, internal, fallopian
      tube
  finger(s) (nail) 959.5
  flank 959.1
  foot (and ankle) (and knee) (and leg except
      thigh) 959.7
  forceps NEC 767.9
    scalp 767.1
  forearm (and elbow) (and wrist) 959.3
  forehead 959.09
  gallbladder—*see* Injury, internal, gallbladder
  gasserian ganglion 951.2
  gastrointestinal tract—*see* Injury, internal,
      gastrointestinal tract
  genital organ(s)
    with
      abortion—*see* Abortion, by type, with,
          damage to pelvic organs
      ectopic pregnancy (*see also* categories
          633.0-633.9) 639.2
      molar pregnancy (*see also* categories
          630-632) 639.2
    external 959.1
    following
      abortion 639.2
      ectopic or molar pregnancy 639.2
    internal—*see* Injury, internal, genital organs
    obstetrical trauma NEC 665.9
      affecting fetus or newborn 763.89
  gland
    lacrimal 921.1
      laceration 870.8
    parathyroid 959.09
    salivary 959.09
    thyroid 959.09
  globe (eye) (*see also* Injury, eyeball) 921.3
  grease gun—*see* Wound, open, by site,
      complicated
  groin 959.1

Injury—*continued*
  gum 959.09
  hand(s) (except fingers) 959.4
  head NEC 959.01
    with
      loss of consciousness 850.5
      skull fracture—*see* Fracture, skull, by site
  heart—*see* Injury, internal, heart
  heel 959.7
  hip (and thigh) 959.6
  hymen 959.1
  hyperextension (cervical) (vertebra) 847.0
  ileum—*see* Injury, internal, ileum
  iliac region 959.1
  infrared rays NEC 990
  instrumental (during surgery) 998.2
    birth injury—*see* Birth, injury
    nonsurgical (*see also* Injury, by site) 959.9
    obstetrical 665.9
      affecting fetus or newborn 763.89
      bladder 665.5
      cervix 665.3
      high vaginal 665.4
      perineal NEC 664.9
      urethra 665.5
      uterus 665.5
  internal 869.0

> *Note—For injury of internal organ(s) by foreign
> body entering through a natural orifice (e.g.,
> inhaled, ingested, or swallowed)—see Foreign
> body, entering through orifice.*
>
> *For internal injury of any of the following sites
> with internal injury of any other of the sites—
> see Injury, internal, multiple.*

    with
      fracture
        pelvis—*see* Fracture, pelvis
        specified site, except pelvis—*see* Injury,
            internal, by site
      open wound into cavity 869.1
    abdomen, abdominal (viscera) NEC 868.00
      with
        fracture, pelvis—*see* Fracture, pelvis
        open wound into cavity 868.10
      specified site NEC 868.09
        with open wound into cavity 868.19
    adrenal (gland) 868.01
      with open wound into cavity 868.11
    aorta (thoracic) 901.0
      abdominal 902.0
    appendix 863.85
      with open wound into cavity 863.95
    bile duct 868.02
      with open wound into cavity 868.12
    bladder (sphincter) 867.0
      with
        abortion—*see* Abortion, by type, with,
            damage to pelvic organs
        ectopic pregnancy (*see also* categories
            633.0-633.9) 639.2
        molar pregnancy (*see also* categories
            630-632) 639.2
        open wound into cavity 867.1
      following
        abortion 639.2
        ectopic or molar pregnancy 639.2
      obstetrical trauma 665.5
        affecting fetus or newborn 763.89
    blood vessel—*see* Injury, blood vessel, by site

Injury—*continued*
   multiple 869.0

> *Note—Multiple internal injuries of sites*
> *classifiable to the same three- or four- digit*
> *category should be classified to that category.*
> *Multiple injuries classifiable to different*
> *fourth-digit subdivisions of 861 (heart and lung*
> *injuries) should be dealt with according to*
> *coding rules.*

     with open wound into cavity 869.1
     intra-abdominal organ (sites classifiable to
       863-868)
      with
       intrathoracic organ(s) (sites classifiable
        to 861-862) 869.0
        with open wound into cavity 869.1
       other intra-abdominal organ(s) (sites
        classifiable to 863-868, except
        where classifiable to the same
        three-digit category) 868.09
        with open wound into cavity 868.19
     intrathoracic organ (sites classifiable to
       861-862)
      with
       intra-abdominal organ(s) (sites
        classifiable to 863-868) 869.0
        with open wound into cavity 869.1
       other intrathoracic organ(s) (sites
        classifiable to 861-862, except
        where classifiable to the same
        three-digit category) 862.8
        with open wound into cavity 862.9
   myocardium—*see* Injury, internal, heart
   ovary 867.6
    with open wound into cavity 867.7
   pancreas (multiple sites) 863.84
    with open wound into cavity 863.94
    body 863.82
     with open wound into cavity 863.92
    head 863.81
     with open wound into cavity 863.91
    tail 863.83
     with open wound into cavity 863.93
   pelvis, pelvic (organs) (viscera) 867.8
    with
     fracture, pelvis—*see* Fracture, pelvis
     open wound into cavity 867.9
    specified site NEC 867.6
     with open wound into cavity 867.7
   peritoneum 868.03
    with open wound into cavity 868.13
   pleura 862.29
    with open wound into cavity 862.39
   prostate 867.6
   with open wound into cavity 867.7
   rectum 863.45
    with
     colon 863.46
      with open wound into cavity 863.56
     open wound into cavity 863.55
   retroperitoneum 868.04
    with open wound into cavity 868.14
   round ligament 867.6
    with open wound into cavity 867.7
   seminal vesicle 867.6
    with open wound into cavity 867.7
   spermatic cord 867.6
    with open wound into cavity 867.7
   scrotal—*see* Wound, open, spermatic cord

Injury—*continued*
   spleen 865.00
    with
     disruption of parenchyma (massive)
      865.04
      with open wound into cavity 865.14
     hematoma (without rupture of capsule)
      865.01
      with open wound into cavity 865.11
     open wound into cavity 865.10
     tear, capsular 865.02
      with open wound into cavity 865.12
      extending into parenchyma 865.03
       with open wound into cavity 865.13
   stomach 863.0
    with open wound into cavity 863.1
   suprarenal gland (multiple) 868.01
    with open wound into cavity 868.11
   thorax, thoracic (cavity) (organs) (multiple)
    (*see also* Injury, internal, intrathoracic
    organs) 862.8
    with open wound into cavity 862.9
   thymus (gland) 862.29
    with open wound into cavity 862.39
   trachea (intrathoracic) 862.29
    with open wound into cavity 862.39
    cervical region (*see also* Wound, open,
     trachea) 874.02
   ureter 867.2
    with open wound into cavity 867.3
   urethra (sphincter) 867.0
    with
     abortion—*see* Abortion, by type, with,
      damage to pelvic organs
     ectopic pregnancy (*see also* categories
      633.0-633.9) 639.2
     molar pregnancy (*see also* categories
      630-632) 639.2
     open wound into cavity 867.1
    following
     abortion 639.2
     ectopic or molar pregnancy 639.2
    obstetrical trauma 665.5
     affecting fetus or newborn 763.89
   uterus 867.4
    with
     abortion—*see* Abortion, by type, with,
      damage to pelvic organs
     ectopic pregnancy (*see also* categories
      633.0-633.9) 639.2
     molar pregnancy (*see also* categories
      630-632) 639.2
     open wound into cavity 867.5
    following
     abortion 639.2
     ectopic or molar pregnancy 639.2
    obstetrical trauma NEC 665.5
     affecting fetus or newborn 763.89
   vas deferens 867.6
    with open wound into cavity 867.7
   vesical (sphincter) 867.0
    with open wound into cavity 867.1
   viscera (abdominal) (*see also* Injury, internal,
    multiple) 868.00
    with
     fracture, pelvis—*see* Fracture, pelvis
     open wound into cavity 868.10
    thoracic NEC (*see also* Injury, internal,
     intrathoracic organs) 862.8
     with open wound into cavity 862.9

Injury—*continued*
  interscapular region 959.1
  intervertebral disc 959.1
  intestine—*see* Injury, internal, intestine
  intra-abdominal (organs) NEC—*see* Injury,
    internal, intra-abdominal
  intracranial 854.0

> *Note—Use the following fifth-digit*
> *subclassification with categories 851-854:*
>
> *0 unspecified state of consciousness*
> *1 with no loss of consciousness*
> *2 with brief [less than one hour] loss of*
> *   consciousness*
> *3 with moderate [1-24 hours] loss of*
> *   consciousness*
> *4 with prolonged [more than 24 hours] loss of*
> *   consciousness and return to pre-existing*
> *   conscious level*
> *5 with prolonged [more than 24 hours] loss of*
> *   consciousness, without return to pre-existing*
> *   conscious level*
> *Use fifth-digit 5 to designate when a patient is*
> *unconscious and dies before regaining*
> *consciousness, regardless of the duration of the*
> *loss of consciousness*
> *6 with loss of consciousness of unspecified*
> *   duration*
> *9 with concussion, unspecified*

    with
      open intracranial wound 854.1
      skull fracture—*see* Fracture, skull, by site
    contusion 851.8
      with open intracranial wound 851.9
      brain stem 851.4
        with open intracranial wound 851.5
      cerebellum 851.4
        with open intracranial wound 851.5
      cortex (cerebral) 851.0
        with open intracranial wound 851.2
    hematoma—*see* Injury, intracranial,
      hemorrhage
    hemorrhage 853.0
      with
        laceration—*see* Injury, intracranial,
          laceration
        open intracranial wound 853.1
      extradural 852.4
        with open intracranial wound 852.5
      subarachnoid 852.0
        with open intracranial wound 852.1
      subdural 852.2
        with open intracranial wound 852.3
    laceration 851.8
      with open intracranial wound 851.9
      brain stem 851.6
        with open intracranial wound 851.7
      cerebellum 851.6
        with open intracranial wound 851.7
      cortex (cerebral) 851.2
        with open intracranial wound 851.3
  intraocular—*see* Injury, eyeball, penetrating
  intrathoracic organs (multiple)—*see* Injury,
    internal, intrathoracic organs
  intrauterine—*see* Injury, internal, intrauterine
  iris 921.3
    penetrating—*see* Injury, eyeball, penetrating
  jaw 959.09
  jejunum—*see* Injury, internal, jejunum

Injury—*continued*
  joint NEC 959.9
    old or residual 718.80
      ankle 718.87
      elbow 718.82
      foot 718.87
      hand 718.84
      hip 718.85
      knee 718.86
      multiple sites 718.89
      pelvic region 718.85
      shoulder (region) 718.81
      specified site NEC 718.88
      wrist 718.83
  kidney—*see* Injury, internal, kidney
  knee (and ankle) (and foot) (and leg, except
    thigh) 959.7
  labium (majus) (minus) 959.1
  labyrinth, ear 959.09
  lacrimal apparatus, gland, or sac 921.1
    laceration 870.8
  larynx 959.09
  late effect—*see* Late, effects (of), injury
  leg except thigh (and ankle) (and foot) (and
    knee) 959.7
    upper or thigh 959.6
  lens, eye 921.3
    penetrating—*see* Injury, eyeball, penetrating
  lid, eye—*see* Injury, eyelid
  lip 959.09
  liver—*see* Injury, internal, liver
  lobe, parietal—*see* Injury, intracranial
  lumbar (region) 959.1
    plexus 953.5
  lumbosacral (region) 959.1
    plexus 953.5
  lung—*see* Injury, internal, lung
  malar region 959.09
  mastoid region 959.09
  maternal, during pregnancy, affecting fetus or
    newborn 760.5
  maxilla 959.09
  mediastinum—*see* Injury, internal, mediastinum
  membrane
    brain (*see also* Injury, intracranial) 854.0
    tympanic 959.09
  meningeal artery—*see* Hemorrhage, brain,
    traumatic, subarachnoid
  meninges (cerebral)—*see* Injury, intracranial
  mesenteric
    artery—*see* Injury, blood vessel, mesenteric,
      artery
    plexus, inferior 954.1
    vein—*see* Injury, blood vessel, mesenteric,
      vein
  mesentery—*see* Injury, internal, mesentery
  mesosalpinx—*see* Injury, internal, mesosalpinx
  middle ear 959.09
  midthoracic region 959.1
  mouth 959.09
  multiple (sites not classifiable to the same
    four-digit category in 959.0-959.7) 959.8
    internal 869.0
      with open wound into cavity 869.1
  musculocutaneous nerve 955.4
  nail
    finger 959.5
    toe 959.7
  nasal (septum) (sinus) 959.09
  nasopharynx 959.09

Injury—*continued*
  neck (and face) 959.09
  nerve 957.9
    abducens 951.3
    abducent 951.3
    accessory 951.6
    acoustic 951.5
    ankle and foot 956.9
    anterior crural, femoral 956.1
    arm (*see also* Injury, nerve, upper limb) 955.9
    auditory 951.5
    axillary 955.0
    brachial plexus 953.4
    cervical sympathetic 954.0
    cranial 951.9
      first or olfactory 951.8
      second or optic 950.0
      third or oculomotor 951.0
      fourth or trochlear 951.1
      fifth or trigeminal 951.2
      sixth or abducens 951.3
      seventh or facial 951.4
      eighth, acoustic, or auditory 951.5
      ninth or glossopharyngeal 951.8
      tenth, pneumogastric, or vagus 951.8
      eleventh or accessory 951.6
      twelfth or hypoglossal 951.7
      newborn 767.7
    cutaneous sensory
      lower limb 956.4
      upper limb 955.5
    digital (finger) 955.6
      toe 956.5
    facial 951.4
      newborn 767.5
    femoral 956.1
    finger 955.9
    foot and ankle 956.9
    forearm 955.9
    glossopharyngeal 951.8
    hand and wrist 955.9
    head and neck, superficial 957.0
    hypoglossal 951.7
    involving several parts of body 957.8
    leg (*see also* Injury, nerve, lower limb) 956.9
    lower limb 956.9
      multiple 956.8
      specified site NEC 956.5
    lumbar plexus 953.5
    lumbosacral plexus 953.5
    median 955.1
      forearm 955.1
      wrist and hand 955.1
    multiple (in several parts of body) (sites not
      classifiable to the same three-digit
      category) 957.8
    musculocutaneous 955.4
    musculospiral 955.3
      upper arm 955.3
    oculomotor 951.0
    olfactory 951.8
    optic 950.0
    pelvic girdle 956.9
      multiple sites 956.8
      specified site NEC 956.5
    peripheral 957.9
      multiple (in several regions) (sites not
        classifiable to the same three-digit
        category) 957.8
      specified site NEC 957.1

Injury—*continued*
    peroneal 956.3
      ankle and foot 956.3
      lower leg 956.3
    plantar 956.5
    plexus 957.9
      celiac 954.1
      mesenteric, inferior 954.1
      spinal 953.9
        brachial 953.4
        lumbosacral 953.5
        multiple sites 953.8
      sympathetic NEC 954.1
    pneumogastric 951.8
    radial 955.3
      wrist and hand 955.3
    sacral plexus 953.5
    sciatic 956.0
      thigh 956.0
    shoulder girdle 955.9
      multiple 955.8
      specified site NEC 955.7
    specified site NEC 957.1
    spinal 953.9
      plexus—*see* Injury, nerve, plexus, spinal
      root 953.9
        cervical 953.0
        dorsal 953.1
        lumbar 953.2
        multiple sites 953.8
        sacral 953.3
    splanchnic 954.1
    sympathetic NEC 954.1
      cervical 954.0
    thigh 956.9
    tibial 956.5
      ankle and foot 956.2
      lower leg 956.5
      posterior 956.2
    toe 956.9
    trigeminal 951.2
    trochlear 951.1
    trunk, excluding shoulder and pelvic girdles
      954.9
      specified site NEC 954.8
      sympathetic NEC 954.1
    ulnar 955.2
      forearm 955.2
      wrist (and hand) 955.2
    upper limb 955.9
      multiple 955.8
      specified site NEC 955.7
    vagus 951.8
    wrist and hand 955.9
  nervous system, diffuse 957.8
  nose (septum) 959.09
  obstetrical NEC 665.9
    affecting fetus or newborn 763.89
  occipital (region) (scalp) 959.09
    lobe (*see also* Injury, intracranial) 854.0
  optic 950.9
    chiasm 950.1
    cortex 950.3
    nerve 950.0
    pathways 950.2
  orbit, orbital (region) 921.2
    penetrating 870.3
      with foreign body 870.4
  ovary—*see* Injury, internal, ovary

Injury—*continued*
  paint-gun—*see* Wound, open, by site,
      complicated
  palate (soft) 959.09
  pancreas—*see* Injury, internal, pancreas
  parathyroid (gland) 959.09
  parietal (region) (scalp) 959.09
    lobe—*see* Injury, intracranial
  pelvic
    floor 959.1
      complicating delivery 664.1
        affecting fetus or newborn 763.89
    joint or ligament, complicating delivery 665.6
      affecting fetus or newborn 763.89
    organs—*see also* Injury, internal, pelvis
      with
        abortion—*see* Abortion, by type, with
          damage to pelvic organs
        ectopic pregnancy (*see also* categories
          633.0-633.9) 639.2
        molar pregnancy (*see also* categories
          633.0-633.9) 639.2
      following
        abortion 639.2
        ectopic or molar pregnancy 639.2
      obstetrical trauma 665.5
        affecting fetus or newborn 763.89
  pelvis 959.1
  penis 959.1
  perineum 959.1
  peritoneum—*see* Injury, internal, peritoneum
  periurethral tissue
    with
      abortion—*see* Abortion, by type, with
        damage to pelvic organs
      ectopic pregnancy (*see also* categories
        633.0-633.9) 639.2
      molar pregnancy (*see also* categories
        630-632) 639.2
    complicating delivery 665.5
      affecting fetus or newborn 763.89
    following
      abortion 639.2
      ectopic or molar pregnancy 639.2
  phalanges
    foot 959.7
    hand 959.5
  pharynx 959.09
  pleura—*see* Injury, internal, pleura
  popliteal space 959.7
  prepuce 959.1
  prostate—*see* Injury, internal, prostate
  pubic region 959.1
  pudenda 959.1
  radiation NEC 990
  radioactive substance or radium NEC 990
  rectovaginal septum 959.1
  rectum—*see* Injury, internal, rectum
  retina 921.3
    penetrating—*see* Injury, eyeball, penetrating
  retroperitoneal—*see* Injury, internal,
    retroperitoneum
  roentgen rays NEC 990
  round ligament—*see* Injury, internal, round
    ligament
  sacral (region) 959.1
    plexus 953.5
  sacroiliac ligament NEC 959.1
  sacrum 959.1

Injury—*continued*
  salivary ducts or glands 959.09
  scalp 959.09
    due to birth trauma 767.1
    fetus or newborn 767.1
  scapular region 959.2
  sclera 921.3
    penetrating—*see* Injury, eyeball, penetrating
    superficial 918.2
  scrotum 959.1
  seminal vesicle—*see* Injury, internal, seminal
    vesicle
  shoulder (and upper arm) 959.2
  sinus
    cavernous (*see also* Injury, intracranial) 854.0
    nasal 959.09
  skeleton NEC, birth injury 767.3
  skin NEC 959.9
  skull—*see* Fracture, skull, by site
  soft tissue (of external sites) (severe)—*see*
    Wound, open, by site
  specified site NEC 959.8
  spermatic cord—*see* Injury, internal, spermatic
    cord
  spinal (cord) 952.9
    with fracture, vertebra—*see* Fracture,
      vertebra, by site, with spinal cord injury
    cervical (C_1-C_4) 952.00
      with
        anterior cord syndrome 952.02
        central cord syndrome 952.03
        complete lesion of cord 952.01
        incomplete lesion NEC 952.04
        posterior cord syndrome 952.04
      C_5-C_7 level 952.05
        with
          anterior cord syndrome 952.07
          central cord syndrome 952.08
          complete lesion of cord 952.06
          incomplete lesion NEC 952.09
          posterior cord syndrome 952.09
        specified type NEC 952.09
      specified type NEC 952.04
    dorsal (D_1-D_6) (T_1-T_6) (thoracic) 952.10
      with
        anterior cord syndrome 952.12
        central cord syndrome 952.13
        complete lesion of cord 952.11
        incomplete lesion NEC 952.14
        posterior cord syndrome 952.14
      D_7-D_{12} level (T_7-T_{12}) 952.15
        with
          anterior cord syndrome 952.17
          central cord syndrome 952.18
          complete lesion of cord 952.16
          incomplete lesion NEC 952.19
          posterior cord syndrome 952.19
        specified type NEC 952.19
      specified type NEC 952.14
    lumbar 952.2
    multiple sites 952.8
    nerve (root) NEC—*see* Injury, nerve, spinal,
      root
    plexus 953.9
      brachial 953.4
      lumbosacral 953.5
      multiple sites 953.8
    sacral 952.3
    thoracic (*see also* Injury, spinal, dorsal) 952.10

> *Note—Use the following fourth-digit subdivisions with categories 910-919:*
>
> *.0 Abrasion or friction burn without mention of infection*
> *.1 Abrasion or friction burn, infected*
> *.2 Blister without mention of infection*
> *.3 Blister, infected*
> *.4 Insect bite, nonvenomous, without mention of infection*
> *.5 Insect bite, nonvenomous, infected*
> *.6 Superficial foreign body (splinter) without major open wound and without mention of infection*
> *.7 Superficial foreign body (splinter) without major open wound, infected*
> *.8 Other and unspecified superficial injury without mention of infection*
> *.9 Other and unspecified superficial injury, infected*
>
> For late effects of superficial injury, *see* category 906.2.

Inspiration
food or foreign body (*see also* Asphyxia, food or foreign body) 933.1
mucus (*see also* Asphyxia, mucus) 933.1
Inspissated bile syndrome, newborn 774.4
Instability
detrusor 596.59
emotional (excessive) 301.3
joint (posttraumatic) 718.80
ankle 718.87
elbow 718.82
foot 718.87
hand 718.84
hip 718.85
knee 718.86
lumbosacral 724.6
multiple sites 718.89
pelvic region 718.85
sacroiliac 724.6
shoulder (region) 718.81
specified site NEC 718.88
wrist 718.83
lumbosacral 724.6
nervous 301.89
personality (emotional) 301.59
thyroid, paroxysmal 242.9
urethral 599.83
vasomotor 780.2
Insufficiency, insufficient
accommodation 367.4
adrenal (gland) (acute) (chronic) 255.4
medulla 255.5
primary 255.4
specified NEC 255.5
adrenocortical 255.4
anus 569.49
aortic (valve) 424.1
with
mitral (valve) disease 396.1
insufficiency, incompetence, or regurgitation 396.3
stenosis or obstruction 396.1
stenosis or obstruction 424.1
with mitral (valve) disease 396.8
congenital 746.4
rheumatic 395.1
with
mitral (valve) disease 396.1
insufficiency, incompetence, or regurgitation 396.3
stenosis or obstruction 396.1
stenosis or obstruction 395.2
with mitral (valve) disease 396.8
specified cause NEC 424.1
syphilitic 093.22
arterial 447.1
basilar artery 435.0
carotid artery 435.8
cerebral 437.1
coronary (acute or subacute) 411.89
mesenteric 557.1
peripheral 443.9
precerebral 435.9
vertebral artery 435.1
vertibrobasilar 435.3
arteriovenous 459.9
basilar artery 435.0
biliary 575.8

Insufficiency, insufficient—*continued*
cardiac (*see also* Insufficiency, myocardial) 428.0
complicating surgery 997.1
due to presence of (cardiac) prosthesis 429.4
postoperative 997.1
long-term effect of cardiac surgery 429.4
specified during or due to a procedure 997.1
long-term effect of cardiac surgery 429.4
cardiorenal (*see also* Hypertension, cardiorenal) 404.90
cardiovascular (*see also* Disease, cardiovascular) 429.2
renal (*see also* Hypertension, cardiorenal) 404.90
carotid artery 435.8
cerebral (vascular) 437.9
cerebrovascular 437.9
with transient focal neurological signs and symptoms 435.9
acute 437.1
with transient focal neurological signs and symptoms 435.9
circulatory NEC 459.9
fetus or newborn 779.89
convergence 378.83
coronary (acute or subacute) 411.89
chronic or with a stated duration of over 8 weeks 414.8
corticoadrenal 255.4
dietary 269.9
divergence 378.85
food 994.2
gastroesophageal 530.89
gonadal
ovary 256.39
testis 257.2
gonadotropic hormone secretion 253.4
heart—*see also* Insufficiency, myocardial
fetus or newborn 779.89
valve (*see also* Endocarditis) 424.90
congenital NEC 746.89
hepatic 573.8
idiopathic autonomic 333.0
kidney (acute) (chronic) 593.9
labyrinth, labyrinthine (function) 386.53
bilateral 386.54
unilateral 386.53
lacrimal 375.15
liver 573.8
lung (acute) (*see also* Insufficiency, pulmonary) 518.82
following trauma, surgery, or shock 518.5
newborn 770.89
mental (congenital) (*see also* Retardation, mental) 319
mesenteric 557.1
mitral (valve) 424.0
with
aortic (valve) disease 396.3
insufficiency, incompetence, or regurgitation 396.3
stenosis or obstruction 396.2
obstruction or stenosis 394.2
with aortic valve disease 396.8
congenital 746.6

Insufficiency, insufficient—*continued*
- rheumatic 394.1
  - with
    - aortic (valve) disease 396.3
      - insufficiency, incompetence, or regurgitation 396.3
      - stenosis or obstruction 396.2
    - obstruction or stenosis 394.2
      - with aortic valve disease 396.8
    - active or acute 391.1
      - with chorea, rheumatic (Sydenham's) 392.0
  - specified cause, except rheumatic 424.0
- muscle
  - heart—*see* Insufficiency, myocardial
  - ocular (*see also* Strabismus) 378.9
- myocardial, myocardium (with arteriosclerosis) 428.0
  - with rheumatic fever (conditions classifiable to 390)
    - active, acute, or subacute 391.2
      - with chorea 392.0
    - inactive or quiescent (with chorea) 398.0
  - congenital 746.89
  - due to presence of (cardiac) prosthesis 429.4
  - fetus or newborn 779.89
  - following cardiac surgery 429.4
  - hypertensive (*see also* Hypertension, heart) 402.91
    - benign 402.11
    - malignant 402.01
  - postoperative 997.1
    - long-term effect of cardiac surgery 429.4
  - rheumatic 398.0
    - active, acute, or subacute 391.2
      - with chorea (Sydenham's) 392.0
  - syphilitic 093.82
- nourishment 994.2
- organic 799.8
- ovary 256.39
  - postablative 256.2
- pancreatic 577.8
- parathyroid (gland) 252.1
- peripheral vascular (arterial) 443.9
- pituitary (anterior) 253.2
  - posterior 253.5
- placental—*see* Placenta, insufficiency
- platelets 287.5
- prenatal care in current pregnancy V23.7
- progressive pluriglandular 258.9
- pseudocholinesterase 289.8
- pulmonary (acute) 518.82
  - following
    - shock 518.5
    - surgery 518.5
    - trauma 518.5
  - newborn 770.89
  - valve (*see also* Endocarditis, pulmonary) 424.3
    - congenital 746.09
- pyloric 537.0
- renal (acute) (chronic) 593.9
  - due to a procedure 997.5
- respiratory 786.09
  - acute 518.82
    - following shock, surgery, or trauma 518.5
  - newborn 770.89
- rotation—*see* Malrotation
- suprarenal 255.4
  - medulla 255.5
- tarso-orbital fascia, congenital 743.66

Insufficiency, insufficient—*continued*
- tear film 375.15
- testis 257.2
- thyroid (gland) (acquired)—*see also* Hypothyroidism
  - congenital 243
- tricuspid (*see also* Endocarditis, tricuspid) 397.0
  - congenital 746.89
  - syphilitic 093.23
- urethral sphincter 599.84
- valve, valvular (heart) (*see also* Endocarditis) 424.90
- vascular 459.9
  - intestine NEC 557.9
  - mesenteric 557.1
  - peripheral 443.9
  - renal (*see also* Hypertension, kidney) 403.90
- velopharyngeal
  - acquired 528.9
  - congenital 750.29
- venous (peripheral) 459.81
- ventricular—*see* Insufficiency, myocardial
- vertebral artery 435.1
- vertibrobasilar artery 435.3
- weight gain during pregnancy 646.8
- zinc 269.3

Insufflation
- fallopian
  - fertility testing V26.21
  - following sterilization reversal V26.22
- meconium 770.1

Insular —*see* condition

Insulinoma (M8151/0)
- malignant (M8151/3)
  - pancreas 157.4
  - specified site—*see* Neoplasm, by site, malignant
  - unspecified site 157.4
- pancreas 211.7
- specified site—*see* Neoplasm, by site, benign
- unspecified site 211.7

Insuloma —*see* Insulinoma

Insult
- brain 437.9
  - acute 436
- cerebral 437.9
  - acute 436
- cerebrovascular 437.9
  - acute 436
- vascular NEC 437.9
  - acute 436

Insurance examination (certification) V70.3

Intemperance (*see also* Alcoholism) 303.9

Interception of pregnancy (menstrual extraction) V25.3

Intermenstrual
- bleeding 626.6
  - irregular 626.6
  - regular 626.5
- hemorrhage 626.6
  - irregular 626.6
  - regular 626.5
- pain(s) 625.2

Intermittent— *see* condition

Internal —*see* condition

Interproximal wear 521.1

Interruption
- aortic arch 747.11
- bundle of His 426.50
- fallopian tube (for sterilization) V25.2

Interruption—*continued*
  phase-shift, sleep cycle 307.45
  repeated REM-sleep 307.48
  sleep
    due to perceived environmental disturbances 307.48
    phase-shift, of 24-hour sleep-wake cycle 307.45
    repeated REM-sleep type 307.48
  vas deferens (for sterilization) V25.2
Intersexuality 752.7
Interstitial —*see* condition
Intertrigo 695.89
  labialis 528.5
Intervertebral disc —*see* condition
Intestine, intestinal —*see also* condition
  flu 487.8
Intolerance
  carbohydrate NEC 579.8
  cardiovascular exercise, with pain (at rest) (with less than ordinary activity) (with ordinary activity) V47.2
  cold 780.99
  disaccharide (hereditary) 271.3
  drug
    correct substance properly administered 995.2
    wrong substance given or taken in error 977.9
      specified drug—*see* Table of drugs and chemicals
  effort 306.2
  fat NEC 579.8
  foods NEC 579.8
  fructose (hereditary) 271.2
  glucose (-galactose) (congenital) 271.3
  gluten 579.0
  lactose (hereditary) (infantile) 271.3
  lysine (congenital) 270.7
  milk NEC 579.8
  protein (familial) 270.7
  starch NEC 579.8
  sucrose (-isomaltose) (congenital) 271.3
Intoxicated NEC (*see also* Alcoholism) 305.0
Intoxication
  acid 276.2
  acute
    alcoholic 305.0
      with alcoholism 303.0
      hangover effects 305.0
    caffeine 305.9
    hallucinogenic (*see also* Abuse, drugs, nondependent) 305.3
  alcohol (acute) 305.0
    with alcoholism 303.0
    hangover effects 305.0
    idiosyncratic 291.4
    pathological 291.4
  alimentary canal 558.2
  ammonia (hepatic) 572.2
  chemical—*see also* Table of drugs and chemicals
    via placenta or breast milk 760.70
      alcohol 760.71
      anti-infective agents 760.74
      cocaine 760.75
      "crack" 760.75
      hallucinogenic agents NEC 760.73
      medicinal agents NEC 760.79
      narcotics 760.72
      obstetric anesthetic or analgesic drug 763.5
      specified agent NEC 760.79

Intoxication—*continued*
    suspected, affecting management of pregnancy 655.5
  cocaine, through placenta or breast milk 760.75
  delirium
    alcohol 291.0
    drug 292.81
  drug
    with delirium 292.81
    correct substance properly administered (*see also* Allergy, drug) 995.2
    newborn 779.4
    obstetric anesthetic or sedation 668.9
      affecting fetus or newborn 763.5
    overdose or wrong substance given or taken—*see* Table of drugs and chemicals
    pathologic 292.2
    specific to newborn 779.4
    via placenta or breast milk 760.70
      alcohol 760.71
      anti-infective agents 760.74
      cocaine 760.75
      "crack" 760.75
      hallucinogenic agents 760.73
      medicinal agents NEC 760.79
      narcotics 760.72
      obstetric anesthetic or analgesic drug 763.5
      specified agent NEC 760.79
      suspected, affecting management of pregnancy 655.5
  enteric—*see* Intoxication, intestinal
  fetus or newborn, via placenta or breast milk 760.70
    alcohol 760.71
    anti-infective agents 760.74
    cocaine 760.75
    "crack" 760.75
    hallucinogenic agents 760.73
    medicinal agents NEC 760.79
    narcotics 760.72
    obstetric anesthetic or analgesic drug 763.5
    specified agent NEC 760.79
    suspected, affecting management of pregnancy 655.5
  food—*see* Poisoning, food
  gastrointestinal 558.2
  hallucinogenic (acute) 305.3
  hepatocerebral 572.2
  idiosyncratic alcohol 291.4
  intestinal 569.89
    due to putrefaction of food 005.9
  methyl alcohol (*see also* Alcoholism) 305.0
    with alcoholism 303.0
  pathologic 291.4
    drug 292.2
  potassium (K) 276.7
  septic
    with
      abortion—*see* Abortion, by type, with sepsis
      ectopic pregnancy (*see also* categories 633.0-633.9) 639.0
      molar pregnancy (*see also* categories 630-632) 639.0
    during labor 659.3
    following
      abortion 639.0
      ectopic or molar pregnancy 639.0
    generalized—*see* Septicemia
    puerperal, postpartum, childbirth 670
  serum (prophylactic) (therapeutic) 999.5
  uremic—*see* Uremia
  water 276.6

Intracranial —*see* condition
Intrahepatic gallbladder 751.69
Intraligamentous —*see also* condition
  pregnancy—*see* Pregnancy, cornual
Intraocular —*see also* condition
  sepsis 360.00
Intrathoracic —*see also* condition
  kidney 753.3
  stomach—*see* Hernia, diaphragm
Intrauterine contraceptive device
  checking V25.42
  insertion V25.1
  in situ V45.51
  management V25.42
  prescription V25.02
    repeat V25.42
  reinsertion V25.42
  removal V25.42
Intraventricular —*see* condition
Intrinsic deformity —*see* Deformity
Intrusion, repetitive, of sleep (due to
    environmental disturbances) (with atypical
    polysomnographic features) 307.48
Intumescent, lens (eye) NEC 366.9
  senile 366.12
Intussusception (colon) (enteric) (intestine)
    (rectum) 560.0
  appendix 543.9
  congenital 751.5
  fallopian tube 620.8
  ileocecal 560.0
  ileocolic 560.0
  ureter (with obstruction) 593.4
Invagination
  basilar 756.0
  colon or intestine 560.0
Invalid (since birth) 799.8
Invalidism (chronic) 799.8
Inversion
  albumin-globulin (A-G) ratio 273.8
  bladder 596.8
  cecum (*see also* Intussusception) 560.0
  cervix 622.8
  nipple 611.79
    congenital 757.6
    puerperal, postpartum 676.3
  optic papilla 743.57
  organ or site, congenital NEC—*see* Anomaly,
    specified type NEC
  sleep rhythm 780.55
    nonorganic origin 307.45
  testis (congenital) 752.51
  uterus (postinfectional) (postpartal, old) 621.7
    chronic 621.7
    complicating delivery 665.2
      affecting fetus or newborn 763.89
  vagina—*see* Prolapse, vagina
Investigation
  allergens V72.7
  clinical research (control) (normal comparison)
    (participant) V70.7
Inviability —*see* Immaturity
Involuntary movement, abnormal 781.0
Involution, involutional —*see also* condition
  breast, cystic or fibrocystic 610.1
  depression (*see also* Psychosis, affective) 296.2
    recurrent episode 296.3
    single episode 296.2
  melancholia (*see also* Psychosis, affective)
    296.2
    recurrent episode 296.3

Involution, involutional— *continued*
    single episode 296.2
  ovary, senile 620.3
  paranoid state (reaction) 297.2
  paraphrenia (climacteric) (menopause) 297.2
  psychosis 298.8
  thymus failure 254.8
IQ
  under 20 318.2
  20-34 318.1
  35-49 318.0
  50-70 317
IRDS 769
Irideremia 743.45
Iridis rubeosis 364.42
  diabetic 250.5 *[364.42]*
Iridochoroiditis (panuveitis) 360.12
Iridocyclitis NEC 364.3
  acute 364.00
    primary 364.01
    recurrent 364.02
  chronic 364.10
    in
      lepromatous leprosy 030.0 *[364.11]*
      sarcoidosis 135 *[364.11]*
      tuberculosis (*see also* Tuberculosis) 017.3
        [364.11]
  due to allergy 364.04
  endogenous 364.01
  gonococcal 098.41
  granulomatous 364.10
  herpetic (simplex) 054.44
    zoster 053.22
  hypopyon 364.05
  lens induced 364.23
  nongranulomatous 364.00
  primary 364.01
  recurrent 364.02
  rheumatic 364.10
  secondary 364.04
    infectious 364.03
    noninfectious 364.04
  subacute 364.00
    primary 364.01
    recurrent 364.02
  sympathetic 360.11
  syphilitic (secondary) 091.52
  tuberculous (chronic) (*see also* Tuberculosis)
    017.3 *[364.11]*
Iridocyclochoroiditis (panuveitis) 360.12
Iridodialysis 364.76
Iridodonesis 364.8
Iridoplegia (complete) (partial) (reflex) 379.49
Iridoschisis 364.52
Iris —*see* condition
Iritis 364.3
  acute 364.00
    primary 364.01
    recurrent 364.02
  chronic 364.10
    in
      sarcoidosis 135 *[364.11]*
      tuberculosis (*see also* Tuberculosis) 017.3
        [364.11]
  diabetic 250.5 *[364.42]*
  due to
    allergy 364.04
    herpes simplex 054.44
    leprosy 030.0 *[364.11]*
  endogenous 364.01
  gonococcal 098.41

Iritis—*continued*
  gouty 274.89 *[364.11]*
  granulomatous 364.10
  hypopyon 364.05
  lens induced 364.23
  nongranulomatous 364.00
  papulosa 095.8 *[364.11]*
  primary 364.01
  recurrent 364.02
  rheumatic 364.10
  secondary 364.04
    infectious 364.03
    noninfectious 364.04
  subacute 364.00
    primary 364.01
    recurrent 364.02
  sympathetic 360.11
  syphilitic (secondary) 091.52
    congenital 090.0 *[364.11]*
    late 095.8 *[364.11]*
  tuberculous (*see also* Tuberculosis) 017.3
    [364.11]
  uratic 274.89 *[364.11]*
Iron
  deficiency anemia 280.9
  metabolism disease 275.0
  storage disease 275.0
Iron-miners' lung 503
Irradiated enamel (tooth, teeth) 521.8
Irradiation
  burn—*see* Burn, by site
  effects, adverse 990
Irreducible, irreducibility —*see* condition
Irregular, irregularity
  action, heart 427.9
  alveolar process 525.8
  bleeding NEC 626.4
  breathing 786.09
  colon 569.89
  contour of cornea 743.41
    acquired 371.70
  dentin in pulp 522.3
  eye movements NEC 379.59
  menstruation (cause unknown) 626.4
  periods 626.4
  prostate 602.9
  pupil 364.75
  respiratory 786.09
  septum (nasal) 470
  shape, organ or site, congenital NEC—*see*
    Distortion
  sleep-wake rhythm (non-24-hour) 780.55
    nonorganic origin 307.45
  vertebra 733.99
Irritability (nervous) 799.2
  bladder 596.8
    neurogenic 596.54
      with cauda equina syndrome 344.61
  bowel (syndrome) 564.1
  bronchial (*see also* Bronchitis) 490
  cerebral, newborn 779.1
  colon 564.1
    psychogenic 306.4
  duodenum 564.89
  heart (psychogenic) 306.2
  ileum 564.89
  jejunum 564.89
  myocardium 306.2
  rectum 564.89
  stomach 536.9
    psychogenic 306.4

Irritability—*continued*
  sympathetic (nervous system) (*see also*
    Neuropathy, peripheral, autonomic) 337.9
  urethra 599.84
  ventricular (heart) (psychogenic) 306.2
Irritable —*see* Irritability
Irritation
  anus 569.49
  axillary nerve 353.0
  bladder 596.8
  brachial plexus 353.0
  brain (traumatic) (*see also* Injury, intracranial)
    854.0
    nontraumatic—*see* Encephalitis
  bronchial (*see also* Bronchitis) 490
  cerebral (traumatic) (*see also* Injury,
    intracranial) 854.0
    nontraumatic—*see* Encephalitis
  cervical plexus 353.2
  cervix (*see also* Cervicitis) 616.0
  choroid, sympathetic 360.11
  cranial nerve—*see* Disorder, nerve, cranial
  digestive tract 536.9
    psychogenic 306.4
  gastric 536.9
    psychogenic 306.4
  gastrointestinal (tract) 536.9
    functional 536.9
    psychogenic 306.4
  globe, sympathetic 360.11
  intestinal (bowel) 564.9
  labyrinth 386.50
  lumbosacral plexus 353.1
  meninges (traumatic) (*see also* Injury,
    intracranial) 854.0
    nontraumatic—*see* Meningitis
  myocardium 306.2
  nerve—*see* Disorder, nerve
  nervous 799.2
  nose 478.1
  penis 607.89
  perineum 709.9
  peripheral
    autonomic nervous system (*see also*
      Neuropathy, peripheral, autonomic) 337.9
    nerve—*see* Disorder, nerve
  peritoneum (*see also* Peritonitis) 567.9
  pharynx 478.29
  plantar nerve 355.6
  spinal (cord) (traumatic)—*see also* Injury,
    spinal, by site
    nerve—*see also* Disorder, nerve
      root NEC 724.9
      traumatic—*see* Injury, nerve, spinal
    nontraumatic—*see* Myelitis
  stomach 536.9
    psychogenic 306.4
  sympathetic nerve NEC (*see also* Neuropathy,
    peripheral, autonomic) 337.9
  ulnar nerve 354.2
  vagina 623.9
Isambert's disease 012.3
Ischemia, ischemic 459.9
  basilar artery (with transient neurologic deficit)
    435.0
  bone NEC 733.40
  bowel (transient) 557.9
    acute 557.0
    chronic 557.1
    due to mesenteric artery insufficiency 557.1

J

Jaccoud's nodular fibrositis, chronic
(Jaccoud's syndrome) 714.4
Jackson's
membrane 751.4
paralysis or syndrome 344.89
veil 751.4
Jacksonian
epilepsy (*see also* Epilepsy) 345.5
seizures (focal) (*see also* Epilepsy) 345.5
Jacob's ulcer (M8090/3)—*see* Neoplasm, skin,
malignant, by site
Jacquet's dermatitis (diaper dermatitis) 691.0
Jadassohn's
blue nevus (M8780/0)—*see* Neoplasm, skin,
benign
disease (maculopapular erythroderma) 696.2
intraepidermal epithelioma (M8096/0)—*see*
Neoplasm, skin, benign
Jadassohn-Lewandowski syndrome
(pachyonychia congenita) 757.5
Jadassohn-Pellizari's disease (anetoderma)
701.3
Jadassohn-Tièche nevus (M8780/0)—*see*
Neoplasm, skin, benign
Jaffe-Lichtenstein (-Uehlinger) syndrome 252.0
Jahnke's syndrome (encephalocutaneous
angiomatosis) 759.6
Jakob-Creutzfeldt disease or syndrome 046.1
with dementia
with behavioral disturbance 046.1 *[294.11]*
without behavioral disturbance 046.1 *[294.10]*
Jaksch (-Luzet) disease or syndrome
(pseudoleukemia infantum) 285.8
Jamaican
neuropathy 349.82
paraplegic tropical ataxic-spastic syndrome
349.82
Janet's disease (psychasthenia) 300.89
Janiceps 759.4
Jansky-Bielschowsky amaurotic familial idiocy
330.1
Japanese
B type encephalitis 062.0
river fever 081.2
seven-day fever 100.89
Jaundice (yellow) 782.4
acholuric (familial) (splenomegalic) (*see also*
Spherocytosis) 282.0
acquired 283.9
breast milk 774.39
catarrhal (acute) 070.1
with hepatic coma 070.0
chronic 571.9
epidemic—*see* Jaundice, epidemic
cholestatic (benign) 782.4
chronic idiopathic 277.4
epidemic (catarrhal) 070.1
with hepatic coma 070.0
leptospiral 100.0
spirochetal 100.0
febrile (acute) 070.1
with hepatic coma 070.0
leptospiral 100.0
spirochetal 100.0

Jaundice—*continued*
fetus or newborn 774.6
due to or associated with
ABO
antibodies 773.1
incompatibility, maternal/fetal 773.1
isoimmunization 773.1
absence or deficiency of enzyme system for
bilirubin conjugation (congenital) 774.39
blood group incompatibility NEC 773.2
breast milk inhibitors to conjugation 774.39
associated with preterm delivery 774.2
bruising 774.1
Crigler-Najjar syndrome 277.4 *[774.31]*
delayed conjugation 774.30
associated with preterm delivery 774.2
development 774.39
drugs or toxins transmitted from mother
774.1
G-6-PD deficiency 282.2 *[774.0]*
galactosemia 271.1 *[774.5]*
Gilbert's syndrome 277.4 *[774.31]*
hepatocellular damage 774.4
hereditary hemolytic anemia (*see also*
Anemia, hemolytic) 282.9 *[774.0]*
hypothyroidism, congenital 243 *[774.31]*
incompatibility, maternal/fetal NEC 773.2
infection 774.1
inspissated bile syndrome 774.4
isoimmunization NEC 773.2
mucoviscidosis 277.01 *[774.5]*
obliteration of bile duct, congenital 751.61
[774.5]
polycythemia 774.1
preterm delivery 774.2
red cell defect 282.9 *[774.0]*
Rh
antibodies 773.0
incompatibility, maternal/fetal 773.0
isoimmunization 773.0
spherocytosis (congenital) 282.0 *[774.0]*
swallowed maternal blood 774.1
physiological NEC 774.6
from injection, inoculation, infusion, or
transfusion (blood) (plasma) (serum) (other
substance) (onset within 8 months after
administration)—*see* Hepatitis, viral
Gilbert's (familial nonhemolytic) 277.4
hematogenous 283.9
hemolytic (acquired) 283.9
congenital (*see also* Spherocytosis) 282.0
hemorrhagic (acute) 100.0
leptospiral 100.0
newborn 776.0
spirochetal 100.0
hepatocellular 573.8
homologous (serum)—*see* Hepatitis, viral
idiopathic, chronic 277.4
infectious (acute) (subacute) 070.1
with hepatic coma 070.0
leptospiral 100.0
spirochetal 100.0
leptospiral 100.0
malignant (*see also* Necrosis, liver) 570
newborn (physiological) (*see also* Jaundice,
fetus or newborn) 774.6

Jaundice—*continued*
nonhemolytic, congenital familial (Gilbert's)
277.4
nuclear, newborn (*see also* Kernicterus of
newborn) 774.7
obstructive NEC (*see also* Obstruction, biliary)
576.8
postimmunization—*see* Hepatitis, viral
posttransfusion—*see* Hepatitis, viral
regurgitation (*see also* Obstruction, biliary)
576.8
serum (homologous) (prophylactic)
(therapeutic)—*see* Hepatitis, viral
spirochetal (hemorrhagic) 100.0
symptomatic 782.4
newborn 774.6
Jaw —*see* condition
Jaw-blinking 374.43
congenital 742.8
Jaw-winking phenomenon or syndrome 742.8
Jealousy
alcoholic 291.5
childhood 313.3
sibling 313.3
Jejunitis (*see also* Enteritis) 558.9
Jejunostomy status V44.4
Jejunum, jejunal —*see* condition
Jensen's disease 363.05
Jericho boil 085.1
Jerks, myoclonic 333.2
Jeune's disease or syndrome (asphyxiating
thoracic dystrophy) 756.4
Jigger disease 134.1
Job's syndrome (chronic granulomatous disease)
288.1
Jod-Basedow phenomenon 242.8
Johnson-Stevens disease (erythema multiforme
exudativum) 695.1
Joint —*see also* condition
Charcot's 094.0 *[713.5]*
false 733.82
flail—*see* Flail, joint
mice—*see* Loose, body, joint, by site
sinus to bone 730.9
von Gies' 095.8
Jordan's anomaly or syndrome 288.2
Josephs-Diamond-Blackfan anemia (congenital
hypoplastic) 284.0
Joubert syndrome 759.89
Jumpers' knee 727.2
Jungle yellow fever 060.0
Jüngling's disease (sarcoidosis) 135
Junin virus hemorrhagic fever 078.7
Juvenile —*see also* condition
delinquent 312.9
group (*see also* Disturbance, conduct) 312.2
neurotic 312.4

K

Kahler (-Bozzolo) disease (multiple myeloma) (M9730/3) 203.0
Kakergasia 300.9
Kakke 265.0
Kala-azar (Indian) (infantile) (Mediterranean) (Sudanese) 085.0
Kalischer's syndrome (encephalocutaneous angiomatosis) 759.6
Kallmann's syndrome (hypogonadotropic hypogonadism with anosmia) 253.4
Kanner's syndrome (autism) (*see also* Psychosis, childhood) 299.0
Kaolinosis 502
Kaposi's
disease 757.33
lichen ruber 696.4
acuminatus 696.4
moniliformis 697.8
xeroderma pigmentosum 757.33
sarcoma (M9140/3) 176.9
adipose tissue 176.1
aponeurosis 176.1
artery 176.1
blood vessel 176.1
bursa 176.1
connective tissue 176.1
external genitalia 176.8
fascia 176.1
fatty tissue 176.1
fibrous tissue 176.1
gastrointestinal tract NEC 176.3
ligament 176.1
lung 176.4
lymph
gland(s) 176.5
node(s) 176.5
lymphatic(s) NEC 176.1
muscle (skeletal) 176.1
oral cavity NEC 176.8
palate 176.2
scrotum 176.8
skin 176.0
soft tissue 176.1
specified site NEC 176.8
subcutaneous tissue 176.1
synovia 176.1
tendon (sheath) 176.1
vein 176.1
vessel 176.1
viscera NEC 176.9
vulva 176.8
varicelliform eruption 054.0
vaccinia 999.0
Kartagener's syndrome or triad (sinusitis, bronchiectasis, situs inversus) 759.3
Kasabach-Merritt syndrome (capillary hemangioma associated with thrombocytopenic purpura) 287.3
Kaschin-Beck disease (endemic polyarthritis)—*see* Disease, Kaschin-Beck
Kast's syndrome (dyschondroplasia with hemangiomas) 756.4
Katatonia (*see also* Schizophrenia) 295.2
Katayama disease or fever 120.2
Kathisophobia 781.0
Kawasaki disease 446.1
Kayser-Fleischer ring (cornea) (pseudosclerosis) 275.1 *[371.14]*

Kaznelson's syndrome (congenital hypoplastic anemia) 284.0
Kedani fever 081.2
Kelis 701.4
Kelly (-Patterson) syndrome (sideropenic dysphagia) 280.8
Keloid, cheloid 701.4
Addison's (morphea) 701.0
cornea 371.00
Hawkins' 701.4
scar 701.4
Keloma 701.4
Kenya fever 082.1
Keratectasia 371.71
congenital 743.41
Keratitis (nodular) (nonulcerative) (simple) (zonular) NEC 370.9
with ulceration (*see also* Ulcer, cornea) 370.00
actinic 370.24
arborescens 054.42
areolar 370.22
bullosa 370.8
deep—*see* Keratitis, interstitial
dendritic(a) 054.42
desiccation 370.34
diffuse interstitial 370.52
disciform(is) 054.43
varicella 052.7 *[370.44]*
epithelialis vernalis 372.13 *[370.32]*
exposure 370.34
filamentary 370.23
gonococcal (congenital) (prenatal) 098.43
herpes, herpetic (simplex) NEC 054.43
zoster 053.21
hypopyon 370.04
in
chickenpox 052.7 *[370.44]*
exanthema (*see also* Exanthem) 057.9 *[370.44]*
paravaccinia (*see also* Paravaccinia) 051.9 *[370.44]*
smallpox (*see also* Smallpox) 050.9 *[370.44]*
vernal conjunctivitis 372.13 *[370.32]*
interstitial (nonsyphilitic) 370.50
with ulcer (*see also* Ulcer, cornea) 370.00
diffuse 370.52
herpes, herpetic (simplex) 054.43
zoster 053.21
syphilitic (congenital) (hereditary) 090.3
tuberculous (*see also* Tuberculosis) 017.3 *[370.59]*
lagophthalmic 370.34
macular 370.22
neuroparalytic 370.35
neurotrophic 370.35
nummular 370.22
oyster-shuckers' 370.8
parenchymatous—*see* Keratitis, interstitial
petrificans 370.8
phlyctenular 370.31
postmeasles 055.71
punctata, punctate 370.21
leprosa 030.0 *[370.21]*
profunda 090.3
superficial (Thygeson's) 370.21
purulent 370.8
pustuliformis profunda 090.3

Kidney —*see* condition
Kienböck's
  disease 732.3
    adult 732.8
  osteochondrosis 732.3
Kimmelstiel (-Wilson) disease or syndrome
    (intercapillary glomerulosclerosis) 250.4
    [581.81]
Kink, kinking
  appendix 543.9
  artery 447.1
  cystic duct, congenital 751.61
  hair (acquired) 704.2
  ileum or intestine (*see also* Obstruction,
    intestine) 560.9
  Lane's (*see also* Obstruction, intestine) 560.9
  organ or site, congenital NEC—*see* Anomaly,
    specified type NEC, by site
  ureter (pelvic junction) 593.3
    congenital 753.20
  vein(s) 459.2
    caval 459.2
    peripheral 459.2
Kinnier Wilson's disease (hepatolenticular
    degeneration) 275.1
Kissing
  osteophytes 721.5
  spine 721.5
  vertebra 721.5
Klauder's syndrome (erythema multiforme
    exudativum) 695.1
Kleb's disease (*see also* Nephritis) 583.9
Klein-Waardenburg syndrome
    (ptosisepicanthus) 270.2
Kleine-Levin syndrome 349.89
Kleptomania 312.32
Klinefelter's syndrome 758.7
Klinger's disease 446.4
Klippel's disease 723.8
Klippel-Feil disease or syndrome (brevicollis)
    756.16
Klippel-Trenaunay syndrome 759.89
Klumpke (-Déjérine) palsy, paralysis (birth)
    (newborn) 767.6
Klüver-Bucy (-Terzian) syndrome 310.0
Knee —*see* condition
Knifegrinders' rot (*see also* Tuberculosis) 011.4
Knock-knee (acquired) 736.41
  congenital 755.64
Knot
  intestinal, syndrome (volvulus) 560.2
  umbilical cord (true) 663.2
    affecting fetus or newborn 762.5
Knots, surfer 919.8
  infected 919.9
Knotting (of)
  hair 704.2
  intestine 560.2
Knuckle pads (Garrod's) 728.79
Köbner's disease (epidermolysis bullosa) 757.39
Koch's
  infection (*see also* Tuberculosis, pulmonary)
    011.9
  relapsing fever 087.9
Koch-Weeks conjunctivitis 372.03
Koenig-Wichman disease (pemphigus) 694.4

Köhler's disease (osteochondrosis) 732.5
  first (osteochondrosis juvenilis) 732.5
  second (Freiburg's infarction, metatarsal head)
    732.5
  patellar 732.4
  tarsal navicular (bone) (osteoarthosis juvenilis)
    732.5
Köhler-Mouchet disease (osteoarthrosis
    juvenilis) 732.5
Köhler-Pellegrini-Stieda disease or syndrome
    (calcification, knee joint) 726.62
Koilonychia 703.8
  congenital 757.5
Kojevnikov's, Kojewnikoff's epilepsy (*see also*
    Epilepsy) 345.7
König's
  disease (osteochondritis dissecans) 732.7
  syndrome 564.89
Koniophthisis (*see also* Tuberculosis) 011.4
Koplik's spots 055.9
Kopp's asthma 254.8
Korean hemorrhagic fever 078.6
Korsakoff (-Wernicke) disease, psychosis, or
    syndrome (nonalcoholic) 294.0
  alcoholic 291.1
Korsakov's disease —*see* Korsakoff's disease
Korsakow's disease —*see* Korsakoff's disease
Kostmann's disease or syndrome (infantile
    genetic agranulocytosis) 288.0
Krabbe's
  disease (leukodystrophy) 330.0
  syndrome
    congenital muscle hypoplasia 756.89
    cutaneocerebral angioma 759.6
Kraepelin-Morel disease (*see also*
    Schizophrenia) 295.9
Kraft-Weber-Dimitri disease 759.6
Kraurosis
  ani 569.49
  penis 607.0
  vagina 623.8
  vulva 624.0
Kreotoxism 005.9
Krukenberg's
  spindle 371.13
  tumor (M8490/6) 198.6
Kufs' disease 330.1
Kugelberg-Welander disease 335.11
Kuhnt-Junius degeneration or disease 362.52
Kulchitsky's cell carcinoma (carcinoid tumor of
    intestine) 259.2
Kümmell's disease or spondylitis 721.7
Kundrat's disease (lymphosarcoma) 200.1
Kunekune —*see* Dermatophytosis
Kunkel syndrome (lupoid hepatitis) 571.49
Kupffer cell sarcoma (M9124/3) 155.0
Kuru 046.0
Kussmaul's
  coma (diabetic) 250.3
  disease (polyarteritis nodosa) 446.0
  respiration (air hunger) 786.09
Kwashiorkor (marasmus type) 260
Kyasanur Forest disease 065.2
Kyphoscoliosis, kyphoscoliotic (acquired) (*see
    also* Scoliosis) 737.30
  congenital 756.19
  due to radiation 737.33
  heart (disease) 416.1

Kyphoscoliosis, kyphoscoliotic—*continued*
  idiopathic 737.30
    infantile
      progressive 737.32
      resolving 737.31
  late effect of rickets 268.1 *[737.43]*
  specified NEC 737.39
  thoracogenic 737.34
  tuberculous (*see also* Tuberculosis) 015.0
    [737.43]
Kyphosis, kyphotic (acquired) (postural) 737.10
  adolescent postural 737.0
  congenital 756.19
  dorsalis juvenilis 732.0
  due to or associated with
    Charcot-Marie-Tooth disease 356.1 *[737.41]*
    mucopolysaccharidosis 277.5 *[737.41]*
    neurofibromatosis 237.71 *[737.41]*
    osteitis
      deformans 731.0 *[737.41]*
      fibrosa cystica 252.0 *[737.41]*
    osteoporosis (*see also* Osteoporosis) 733.0
      [737.41]
    poliomyelitis (*see also* Poliomyelitis) 138
      [737.41]
    radiation 737.11
    tuberculosis (*see also* Tuberculosis) 015.0
      [737.41]
  Kümmell's 721.7
  late effect of rickets 268.1 *[737.41]*
  Morquio-Brailsford type (spinal) 277.5 *[737.41]*
  pelvis 738.6
  postlaminectomy 737.12
  specified cause NEC 737.19
  syphilitic, congenital 090.5 *[737.41]*
  tuberculous (*see also* Tuberculosis) 015.0
    [737.41]
Kyrle's disease (hyperkeratosis follicularis in
  cutem penetrans) 701.1

L

Labia, labium —*see* condition
Labiated hymen 752.49
Labile
  blood pressure 796.2
  emotions, emotionality 301.3
  vasomotor system 443.9
Labioglossal paralysis 335.22
Labium leporinum (*see also* Cleft, lip) 749.10
Labor (*see also* Delivery)
  with complications—*see* Delivery, complicated
  abnormal NEC 661.9
    affecting fetus or newborn 763.7
  arrested active phase 661.1
    affecting fetus or newborn 763.7
  desultory 661.2
    affecting fetus or newborn 763.7
  dyscoordinate 661.4
    affecting fetus or newborn 763.7
  early onset (22-36 weeks gestation) 644.2
  failed
    induction 659.1
      mechanical 659.0
      medical 659.1
      surgical 659.0
    trial (vaginal delivery) 660.6
  false 644.1
  forced or induced, affecting fetus or newborn
    763.89
  hypertonic 661.4
    affecting fetus or newborn 763.7
  hypotonic 661.2
    affecting fetus or newborn 763.7
    primary 661.0
      affecting fetus or newborn 763.7
    secondary 661.1
      affecting fetus or newborn 763.7
  incoordinate 661.4
    affecting fetus or newborn 763.7
  irregular 661.2
    affecting fetus or newborn 763.7
  long—*see* Labor, prolonged
  missed (at or near term) 656.4
  obstructed NEC 660.9
    affecting fetus or newborn 763.1
    specified cause NEC 660.8
      affecting fetus or newborn 763.1
  pains, spurious 644.1
  precipitate 661.3
    affecting fetus or newborn 763.6
  premature 644.2
    threatened 644.0
  prolonged or protracted 662.1
    affecting fetus or newborn 763.89
    first stage 662.0
      affecting fetus or newborn 763.89
    second stage 662.2
      affecting fetus or newborn 763.89
  threatened NEC 644.1
  undelivered 644.1

Labored breathing (*see also* Hyperventilation)
  786.09
Labyrinthitis (inner ear) (destructive) (latent)
  386.30
  circumscribed 386.32
  diffuse 386.31
  focal 386.32
  purulent 386.33
  serous 386.31
  suppurative 386.33
  syphilitic 095.8
  toxic 386.34
  viral 386.35
Laceration —*see also* Wound, open, by site
  accidental, complicating surgery 998.2
  Achilles tendon 845.09
    with open wound 892.2
  anus (sphincter) 863.89
    with
      abortion—*see* Abortion, by type, with
        damage to pelvic organs
      ectopic pregnancy (*see also* categories
        633.0-633.9) 639.2
      molar pregnancy (*see also* categories
        630-632) 639.2
    complicating delivery 664.2
      with laceration of anal or rectal mucosa
        664.3
    following
      abortion 639.2
      ectopic or molar pregnancy 639.2
    nontraumatic, nonpuerperal 565.0
  bladder (urinary)
    with
      abortion—*see* Abortion, by type, with
        damage to pelvic organs
      ectopic pregnancy (*see also* categories
        633.0-633.9) 639.2
      molar pregnancy (*see also* categories
        630-632) 639.2
    following
      abortion 639.2
      ectopic or molar pregnancy 639.2
    obstetrical trauma 665.5
  blood vessel—*see* Injury, blood vessel, by site
  bowel
    with
      abortion—*see* Abortion, by type, with
        damage to pelvic organs
      ectopic pregnancy (*see also* categories
        633.0-633.9) 639.2
      molar pregnancy (*see also* categories
        630-632) 639.2
    following
      abortion 639.2
      ectopic or molar pregnancy 639.2
    obstetrical trauma 665.5

Laceration—*continued*
  brain (with hemorrhage) (cerebral) (membrane)
    851.8

---

*Note—Use the following fifth-digit
subclassification with categories 851-854:*

0 unspecified state of consciousness
1 with no loss of consciousness
*2 with brief [less than one hour] loss of
    consciousness*
*3 with moderate [1-24 hours] loss of
    consciousness*
*4 with prolonged [more than 24 hours] loss of
    consciousness and return to pre-existing
    conscious level*
*5 with prolonged [more than 24 hours] loss of
    consciousness, without return to pre-existing
    conscious level*
*Use fifth-digit 5 to designate when a patient is
unconscious and dies before regaining
consciousness, regardless of the duration of the
loss of consciousness*
*6 with loss of consciousness of unspecified
    duration*
9 with concussion, unspecified

---

  with
    open intracranial wound 851.9
    skull fracture—see Fracture, skull, by site
  cerebellum 851.6
    with open intracranial wound 851.7
  cortex 851.2
    with open intracranial wound 851.3
  during birth 767.0
  stem 851.6
    with open intracranial wound 851.7
broad ligament
  with
    abortion—see Abortion, by type, with
      damage to pelvic organs
    ectopic pregnancy (see also categories
      633.0-633.9) 639.2
    molar pregnancy (see also categories
      630-632) 639.2
  following
    abortion 639.2
    ectopic or molar pregnancy 639.2
  nontraumatic 620.6
  obstetrical trauma 665.6
  syndrome (nontraumatic) 620.6
capsule, joint—see Sprain, by site
cardiac—see Laceration, heart
causing eversion of cervix uteri (old) 622.0
central, complicating delivery 664.4
cerebellum—see Laceration, brain, cerebellum
cerebral—see also Laceration, brain
  during birth 767.0
cervix (uteri)
  with
    abortion—see Abortion, by type, with
      damage to pelvic organs
    ectopic pregnancy (see also categories
      633.0-633.9) 639.2
    molar pregnancy (see also categories
      630-632) 639.2
  following
    abortion 639.2
    ectopic or molar pregnancy 639.2
  nonpuerperal, nontraumatic 622.3
  obstetrical trauma (current) 665.3
  old (postpartal) 622.3

Laceration—*continued*
  traumatic—see Injury, internal, cervix
chordae heart 429.5
complicated 879.9
cornea—see Laceration, eyeball
  superficial 918.1
cortex (cerebral)—see Laceration, brain, cortex
esophagus 530.89
eye(s)—see Laceration, ocular
eyeball NEC 871.4
  with prolapse or exposure of intraocular tissue
    871.1
  penetrating—see Penetrating wound, eyeball
  specified as without prolapse of intraocular
    tissue 871.0
eyelid NEC 870.8
  full thickness 870.1
    involving lacrimal passages 870.2
  skin (and periocular area) 870.0
    penetrating—see Penetrating wound, orbit
fourchette
  with
    abortion—see Abortion, by type, with
      damage to pelvic organs
    ectopic pregnancy (see also categories
      633.0-633.9) 639.2
    molar pregnancy (see also categories
      630-632) 639.2
  complicating delivery 664.0
  following
    abortion 639.2
    ectopic or molar pregnancy 639.2
heart (without penetration of heart chambers)
    861.02
  with
    open wound into thorax 861.12
    penetration of heart chambers 861.03
      with open wound into thorax 861.13
hernial sac—see Hernia, by site
internal organ (abdomen) (chest) (pelvis)
    NEC—see Injury, internal, by site
kidney (parenchyma) 866.02
  with
    complete disruption of parenchyma
      (rupture) 866.03
      with open wound into cavity 866.13
    open wound into cavity 866.12
labia
  complicating delivery 664.0
ligament—see also Sprain, by site
  with open wound—see Wound, open, by site
liver 864.05
  with open wound into cavity 864.15
  major (disruption of hepatic parenchyma)
    864.04
    with open wound into cavity 864.14
  minor (capsule only) 864.02
    with open wound into cavity 864.12
  moderate (involving parenchyma without
    major disruption) 864.03
    with open wound into cavity 864.13
  multiple 864.04
    with open wound into cavity 864.14
  stellate 864.04
    with open wound into cavity 864.14
lung 861.22
  with open wound into thorax 861.32
meninges—see Laceration, brain
meniscus (knee) (see also Tear, meniscus) 836.2
  old 717.5
  site other than knee—see also Sprain, by site

Laceration—*continued*
   old NEC (*see also* Disorder, cartilage,
      articular) 718.0
  muscle—*see also* Sprain, by site
  with open wound—*see* Wound, open, by site
  myocardium—*see* Laceration, heart
  nerve—*see* Injury, nerve, by site
  ocular NEC (*see also* Laceration, eyeball) 871.4
   adnexa NEC 870.8
    penetrating 870.3
     with foreign body 870.4
  orbit (eye) 870.8
   penetrating 870.3
    with foreign body 870.4
  pelvic
   floor (muscles)
    with
     abortion—*see* Abortion, by type, with
      damage to pelvic organs
     ectopic pregnancy (*see also* categories
      633.0-633.9) 639.2
     molar pregnancy (*see also* categories
      630-632) 639.2
    complicating delivery 664.1
    following
     abortion 639.2
     ectopic or molar pregnancy 639.2
    nonpuerperal 618.7
    old (postpartal) 618.7
   organ NEC
    with
     abortion—*see* Abortion, by type, with
      damage to pelvic organs
     ectopic pregnancy (*see also* categories
      633.0-633.9) 639.2
     molar pregnancy (*see also* categories
      630-632) 639.2
    complicating delivery 665.5
     affecting fetus or newborn 763.89
    following
     abortion 639.2
     ectopic or molar pregnancy 639.2
    obstetrical trauma 665.5
  perineum, perineal (old) (postpartal) 618.7
   with
    abortion—*see* Abortion, by type, with
     damage to pelvic floor
    ectopic pregnancy (*see also* categories
     633.0-633.9) 639.2
    molar pregnancy (*see also* categories
     630-632) 639.2
   complicating delivery 664.4
    first degree 664.0
    second degree 664.1
    third degree 664.2
    fourth degree 664.3
    central 664.4
    involving
     anal sphincter 664.2
     fourchette 664.0
     hymen 664.0
     labia 664.0
     pelvic floor 664.1
     perineal muscles 664.1
     rectovaginal septum 664.2
      with anal mucosa 664.3
     skin 664.0
     sphincter (anal) 664.2
      with anal mucosa 664.3
     vagina 664.0
     vaginal muscles 664.1

Laceration—*continued*
  vulva 664.0
   secondary 674.2
   following
    abortion 639.2
    ectopic or molar pregnancy 639.2
  male 879.6
   complicated 879.7
  muscles, complicating delivery 664.1
  nonpuerperal, current injury 879.6
   complicated 879.7
  secondary (postpartal) 674.2
  peritoneum
   with
    abortion—*see* Abortion, by type, with
     damage to pelvic organs
    ectopic pregnancy (*see also* categories
     633.0-633.9) 639.2
    molar pregnancy (*see also* categories
     630-632) 639.2
   following
    abortion 639.2
    ectopic or molar pregnancy 639.2
   obstetrical trauma 665.5
  periurethral tissue
   with
    abortion—*see* Abortion, by type, with
     damage to pelvic organs
    ectopic pregnancy (*see also* categories
     633.0-633.9) 639.2
    molar pregnancy (*see also* categories
     630-632) 639.2
   following
    abortion 639.2
    ectopic or molar pregnancy 639.2
   obstetrical trauma 665.5
  rectovaginal (septum)
   with
    abortion—*see* Abortion, by type, with
     damage to pelvic organs
    ectopic pregnancy (*see also* categories
     633.0-633.9) 639.2
    molar pregnancy (*see also* categories
     630-632) 639.2
   complicating delivery 665.4
    with perineum 664.2
     involving anal or rectal mucosa 664.3
   following
    abortion 639.2
    ectopic or molar pregnancy 639.2
   nonpuerperal 623.4
   old (postpartal) 623.4
  spinal cord (meninges)—*see also* Injury, spinal,
   by site
   due to injury at birth 767.4
   fetus or newborn 767.4
  spleen 865.09
   with
    disruption of parenchyma (massive) 865.04
     with open wound into cavity 865.14
    open wound into cavity 865.19
   capsule (without disruption of parenchyma)
    865.02
    with open wound into cavity 865.12
   parenchyma 865.03
    with open wound into cavity 865.13
    massive disruption (rupture) 865.04
     with open wound into cavity 865.14

Late —*continued*

internal organ NEC (injury classifiable to 867 and 869) 908.2

abdomen (injury classifiable to 863-866 and 868) 908.1

thorax (injury classifiable to 860-862) 908.0

intracranial (injury classifiable to 850-854) 907.0

with skull fracture (injury classifiable to 800-801 and 803-804) 905.0

nerve NEC (injury classifiable to 957) 907.9

cranial (injury classifiable to 950-951) 907.1

peripheral NEC (injury classifiable to 957) 907.9

lower limb and pelvic girdle (injury classifiable to 956) 907.5

upper limb and shoulder girdle (injury classifiable to 955) 907.4

roots and plexus(es), spinal (injury classifiable to 953) 907.3

trunk (injury classifiable to 954) 907.3

pregnancy complication(s) 677

puerperal complication(s) 677

spinal

cord (injury classifiable to 806 and 952) 907.2

nerve root(s) and plexus(es) (injury classifiable to 953) 907.3

superficial (injury classifiable to 910-919) 906.2

tendon (tendon injury classifiable to 840-848, 880-884 with .2, and 890-894 with .2) 905.8

meningitis

bacterial (conditions classifiable to 320)—*see* category 326

unspecified cause (conditions classifiable to 322)—*see* category 326

myelitis (*see also* Late, effect(s) (of), encephalitis)—*see* category 326

parasitic diseases (conditions classifiable to 001-136 NEC) 139.8

phlebitis or thrombophlebitis of intracranial venous sinuses (conditions classifiable to 325)—*see* category 326

poisoning due to drug, medicinal or biological substance (conditions classifiable to 960-979) 909.0

poliomyelitis, acute (conditions classifiable to 045) 138

radiation (conditions classifiable to 990) 909.2

rickets 268.1

sprain and strain without mention of tendon injury (injury classifiable to 840-848, except tendon injury) 905.7

tendon involvement 905.8

toxic effect of

drug, medicinal or biological substance (conditions classifiable to 960-979) 909.0

nonmedical substance (conditions classifiable to 980-989) 909.1

trachoma (conditions classifiable to 076) 139.1

tuberculosis 137.0

bones and joints (conditions classifiable to 015) 137.3

central nervous system (conditions classifiable to 013) 137.1

Late —*continued*

genitourinary (conditions classifiable to 016) 137.2

pulmonary (conditions classifiable to 010-012) 137.0

specified organs NEC (conditions classifiable to 014, 017-018) 137.4

viral encephalitis (conditions classifiable to 049.8, 049.9, 062-064) 139.0

wound, open

extremity (injury classifiable to 880-884 and 890-894, except .2) 906.1

tendon (injury classifiable to 880-884 with .2 and 890-894 with .2) 905.8

head, neck, and trunk (injury classifiable to 870-879) 906.0

Latent —*see* condition

Lateral —*see* condition

Laterocession —*see* Lateroversion

Lateroflexion —*see* Lateroversion

Lateroversion

cervix—*see* Lateroversion, uterus

uterus, uterine (cervix) (postinfectional) (postpartal, old) 621.6

congenital 752.3

in pregnancy or childbirth 654.4

affecting fetus or newborn 763.89

Lathyrism 988.2

Launois' syndrome (pituitary gigantism) 253.0

Launois-Bensaude's lipomatosis 272.8

Launois-Cléret syndrome (adiposogenital dystrophy) 253.8

Laurence-Moon-Biedl syndrome (obesity, polydactyly, and mental retardation) 759.89

LAV (disease) (illness) (infection)—*see* Human immunodeficiency virus (disease) (illness) (infection)

LAV/HTLV-III (disease) (illness) (infection)—*see* Human immunodeficiency virus (disease) (illness) (infection)

Lawford's syndrome (encephalocutaneous angiomatosis) 759.6

Lax, laxity —*see also* Relaxation

ligament 728.4

skin (acquired) 701.8

congenital 756.83

Laxative habit (*see also* Abuse, drugs, nondependent) 305.9

Lazy leukocyte syndrome 288.0

Lead —*see also* condition

exposure to V15.86

incrustation of cornea 371.15

poisoning 984.9

specified type of lead—*see* Table of drugs and chemicals

Lead miner's lung 503

Leakage

amniotic fluid 658.1

with delayed delivery 658.2

affecting fetus or newborn 761.1

bile from drainage tube (T tube) 997.4

blood (microscopic), fetal, into maternal circulation 656.0

affecting management of pregnancy or puerperium 656.0

device, implant, or graft—*see* Complications, mechanical

spinal fluid at lumbar puncture site 997.09

urine, continuous 788.37

Leaky heart —*see* Endocarditis

Learning defect, specific NEC (strephosymbolia) 315.2

Leather bottle stomach (M8142/3) 151.9
Leber's
  congenital amaurosis 362.76
  optic atrophy (hereditary) 377.16
Lederer's anemia or disease (acquired
    infectious hemolytic anemia) 283.19
Lederer-Brill syndrome (acquired infectious
    hemolytic anemia) 283.19
Leeches (aquatic) (land) 134.2
Left-sided neglect 781.8
Leg —*see* condition
Legal investigation V62.5
Legg (-Calvé) -Perthes disease or syndrome
    (osteochondrosis, femoral capital) 732.1
Legionnaires' disease 482.84
Leigh's disease 330.8
Leiner's disease (exfoliative dermatitis) 695.89
Leiofibromyoma (M8890/0)—*see also*
    Leiomyoma
  uterus (cervix) (corpus) (*see also* Leiomyoma,
    uterus) 218.9
Leiomyoblastoma (M8891/1)—*see* Neoplasm,
    connective tissue, uncertain behavior
Leiomyofibroma (M8890/0)—*see also*
    Neoplasm, connective tissue, benign
  uterus (cervix) (corpus) (*see also* Leiomyoma,
    uterus) 218.9
Leiomyoma (M8890/0)—*see also* Neoplasm,
    connective tissue, benign
  bizarre (M8893/0)—*see* Neoplasm, connective
    tissue, benign
  cellular (M8892/1)—*see* Neoplasm, connective
    tissue, uncertain behavior
  epithelioid (M8891/1)—*see* Neoplasm,
    connective tissue, uncertain behavior
  prostate (polypoid) 600.2
  uterus (cervix) (corpus) 218.9
    interstitial 218.1
    intramural 218.1
    submucous 218.0
    subperitoneal 218.2
    subserous 218.2
    vascular (M8894/0)—*see* Neoplasm,
      connective tissue, benign
Leiomyomatosis (intravascular) (M8890/1)—*see*
    Neoplasm, connective tissue, uncertain
    behavior
Leiomyosarcoma (M8890/3)—*see also*
    Neoplasm, connective tissue, malignant
  epithelioid (M8891/3)—*see* Neoplasm,
    connective tissue, malignant
Leishmaniasis 085.9
  American 085.5
    cutaneous 085.4
    mucocutaneous 085.5
  Asian desert 085.2
  Brazilian 085.5
  cutaneous 085.9
    acute necrotizing 085.2
    American 085.4
    Asian desert 085.2
    diffuse 085.3
    dry form 085.1
    Ethiopian 085.3
    eyelid 085.5 *[373.6]*
    late 085.1
    lepromatous 085.3
    recurrent 085.1
    rural 085.2
    ulcerating 085.1
    urban 085.1

Leishmaniasis—*continued*
    wet form 085.2
    zoonotic form 085.2
  dermal—*see also* Leishmaniasis, cutaneous
    post kala-azar 085.0
  eyelid 085.5 *[373.6]*
  infantile 085.0
  Mediterranean 085.0
  mucocutaneous (American) 085.5
  naso-oral 085.5
  nasopharyngeal 085.5
  Old World 085.1
  tegumentaria diffusa 085.4
  vaccination, prophylactic (against) V05.2
  visceral (Indian) 085.0
Leishmanoid, dermal —*see also* Leishmaniasis,
    cutaneous
  post kala-azar 085.0
Leloir's disease 695.4
Lenegre's disease 426.0
Lengthening, leg 736.81
Lennox's syndrome (*see also* Epilepsy) 345.0
Lens —*see* condition
Lenticonus (anterior) (posterior) (congenital)
    743.36
Lenticular degeneration, progressive 275.1
Lentiglobus (posterior) (congenital) 743.36
Lentigo (congenital) 709.09
  juvenile 709.09
  Maligna (M8742/2)—*see also* Neoplasm, skin,
    in situ
    melanoma (M8742/3)—*see* Melanoma
  senile 709.09
Leonine leprosy 030.0
Leontiasis
  ossium 733.3
  syphilitic 095.8
    congenital 090.5
Léopold-Lévi's syndrome (paroxysmal thyroid
    instability) 242.9
Lepore hemoglobin syndrome 282.4
Lepothrix 039.0
Lepra 030.9
  Willan's 696.1
Leprechaunism 259.8
Lepromatous leprosy 030.0
Leprosy 030.9
  anesthetic 030.1
  beriberi 030.1
  borderline (group B) (infiltrated) (neuritic) 030.3
  cornea (*see also* Leprosy, by type) 030.9
    [371.89]
  dimorphous (group B) (infiltrated)
    (lepromatous) (neuritic) (tuberculoid) 030.3
  eyelid 030.0 *[373.4]*
  indeterminate (group I) (macular) (neuritic)
    (uncharacteristic) 030.2
  leonine 030.0
  lepromatous (diffuse) (infiltrated) (macular)
    (neuritic) (nodular) (type L) 030.0
  macular (early) (neuritic) (simple) 030.2
  maculoanesthetic 030.1
  mixed 030.0
  neuro 030.1
  nodular 030.0
  primary neuritic 030.3
  specified type or group NEC 030.8
  tubercular 030.1
  tuberculoid (macular) (maculoanesthetic)
    (major) (minor) (neuritic) (type T) 030.1
Leptocytosis, hereditary 282.4

Leptomeningitis (chronic) (circumscribed) (hemorrhagic) (nonsuppurative) (*see also* Meningitis) 322.9
  aseptic 047.9
    adenovirus 049.1
    Coxsackie virus 047.0
    ECHO virus 047.1
    enterovirus 047.9
    lymphocytic choriomeningitis 049.0
  epidemic 036.0
  late effect—*see* category 326
  meningococcal 036.0
  pneumococcal 320.1
  syphilitic 094.2
  tuberculous (*see also* Tuberculosis, meninges) 013.0
Leptomeningopathy (*see also* Meningitis) 322.9
Leptospiral —*see* condition
Leptospirochetal —*see* condition
Leptospirosis 100.9
  autumnalis 100.89
  canicula 100.89
  grippotyphosa 100.89
  hebdomidis 100.89
  icterohemorrhagica 100.0
  nanukayami 100.89
  pomona 100.89
  Weil's disease 100.0
Leptothricosis —*see* Actinomycosis
Leptothrix infestation —*see* Actinomycosis
Leptotricosis —*see* Actinomycosis
Leptus dermatitis 133.8
Léri's pleonosteosis 756.89
Léri-Weill syndrome 756.59
Leriche syndrome (aortic bifurcation occlusion) 444.0
Lermoyez's syndrome (*see also* Disease, Ménière's) 386.00
Lesbianism —*omit code*
  egodystonic 302.0
  problems with 302.0
Lesch-Nyhan syndrome (hypoxanthine-guanine-phosphoribosyltransferase deficiency) 277.2
Lesion
  abducens nerve 378.54
  alveolar process 525.8
  anorectal 569.49
  aortic (valve)—*see* Endocarditis, aortic
  auditory nerve 388.5
  basal ganglion 333.90
  bile duct (*see also* Disease, biliary) 576.8
  bladder 596.9
  bone 733.90
  brachial plexus 353.0
  brain 348.8
    congenital 742.9
    vascular (*see also* Lesion, cerebrovascular) 437.9
      degenerative 437.1
      healed or old without residuals V12.59
      hypertensive 437.2
      late effect—*see* Late effect(s) (of) cerebrovascular disease
  buccal 528.9
  calcified—*see* Calcification
  canthus 373.9
  carate—*see* Pinta, lesions
  cardia 537.89
  cardiac—*see also* Disease, heart congenital 746.9
    valvular—*see* Endocarditis

Lesion—*continued*
  cauda equina 344.60
    with neurogenic bladder 344.61
  cecum 569.89
  cerebral—*see* Lesion, brain
  cerebrovascular (*see also* Disease, cerebrovascular NEC) 437.9
    degenerative 437.1
    healed or old without residuals V12.59
    hypertensive 437.2
    specified type NEC 437.8
  cervical root (nerve) NEC 353.2
  chiasmal 377.54
    associated with
      inflammatory disorders 377.54
      neoplasm NEC 377.52
      pituitary 377.51
      pituitary disorders 377.51
      vascular disorders 377.53
  chorda tympani 351.8
  coin, lung 793.1
  colon 569.89
  congenital—*see* Anomaly
  conjunctiva 372.9
  coronary artery (*see also* Ischemia, heart) 414.9
  cranial nerve 352.9
    first 352.0
    second 377.49
    third
      partial 378.51
      total 378.52
    fourth 378.53
    fifth 350.9
    sixth 378.54
    seventh 351.9
    eighth 388.5
    ninth 352.2
    tenth 352.3
    eleventh 352.4
    twelfth 352.5
  cystic—*see* Cyst
  degenerative—*see* Degeneration
  dermal (skin) 709.9
  Dieulafoy (hemorrhagic)
    of
      duodenum 537.84
      intestine 569.86
      stomach 537.84
  duodenum 537.89
    with obstruction 537.3
  eyelid 373.9
  gasserian ganglion 350.8
  gastric 537.89
  gastroduodenal 537.89
  gastrointestinal 569.89
  glossopharyngeal nerve 352.2
  heart (organic)—*see also* Disease, heart
    vascular—*see* Disease, cardiovascular
  helix (ear) 709.9
  hyperchromic, due to pinta (carate) 103.1
  hyperkeratotic (*see also* Hyperkeratosis) 701.1
  hypoglossal nerve 352.5
  hypopharynx 478.29
  hypothalamic 253.9
  ileocecal coil 569.89
  ileum 569.89
  iliohypogastric nerve 355.79
  ilioinguinal nerve 355.79
  in continuity—*see* Injury, nerve, by site
  inflammatory—*see* Inflammation
  intestine 569.89

Leukoencephalitis
  acute hemorrhagic (postinfectious) NEC 136.9
      [323.6]
    postimmunization or postvaccinal 323.5
  subacute sclerosing 046.2
    van Bogaert's 046.2
  van Bogaert's (sclerosing) 046.2
Leukoencephalopathy (*see also* Encephalitis)
    323.9
  acute necrotizing hemorrhagic (postinfectious)
      136.9 *[323.6]*
    postimmunization or postvaccinal 323.5
  metachromatic 330.0
  multifocal (progressive) 046.3
  progressive multifocal 046.3
Leukoerythroblastosis 289.0
Leukoerythrosis 289.0
Leukokeratosis (*see also* Leukoplakia) 702.8
  mouth 528.6
  nicotina palati 528.7
  tongue 528.6
Leukokoria 360.44
Leukokoraurosis vulva, vulvae 624.0
Leukolymphosarcoma (M9850/3) 207.8
Leukoma (cornea) (interfering with central
    vision) 371.03
  adherent 371.04
Leukomalacia, periventricular 779.7
Leukomelanopathy, hereditary 288.2
Leukonychia (punctata) (striata) 703.8
  congenital 757.5
Leukopathia
  unguium 703.8
    congenital 757.5
Leukopenia 288.0
  cyclic 288.0
  familial 288.0
  malignant 288.0
  periodic 288.0
  transitory neonatal 776.7
Leukopenic —*see* condition
Leukoplakia 702.8
  anus 569.49
  bladder (postinfectional) 596.8
  buccal 528.6
  cervix (uteri) 622.2
  esophagus 530.83
  gingiva 528.6
  kidney (pelvis) 593.89
  larynx 478.79
  lip 528.6
  mouth 528.6
  oral soft tissue (including tongue) (mucosa)
    528.6
  palate 528.6
  pelvis (kidney) 593.89
  penis (infectional) 607.0
  rectum 569.49
  syphilitic 095.8
  tongue 528.6
  tonsil 478.29
  ureter (postinfectional) 593.89
  urethra (postinfectional) 599.84
  uterus 621.8
  vagina 623.1
  vesical 596.8
  vocal cords 478.5
  vulva 624.0
Leukopolioencephalopathy 330.0
Leukorrhea (vagina) 623.5
  due to trichomonas (vaginalis) 131.00
  trichomonal (Trichomonas vaginalis) 131.00

Leukosarcoma (M9850/3) 207.8
Leukosis (M9800/3)—*see* Leukemia
Lev's disease or syndrome (acquired complete
    heart block) 426.0
Levi's syndrome (pituitary dwarfism) 253.3
Levocardia (isolated) 746.87
  with situs inversus 759.3
Levulosuria 271.2
Lewandowski's disease (primary) (*see also*
    Tuberculosis) 017.0
Lewandowski-Lutz disease (epidermodysplasia
    verruciformis) 078.19
Leyden's disease (periodic vomiting) 536.2
Leyden's-Möbius dystrophy 359.1
Leydig cell
  carcinoma (M8650/3)
    specified site—*see* Neoplasm, by site,
      malignant
    unspecified site
      female 183.0
      male 186.9
  tumor (M8650/1)
    benign (M8650/0)
      specified site—*see* Neoplasm, by site,
        benign
      unspecified site
        female 220
        male 222.0
    malignant (M8650/3)
      specified site—*see* Neoplasm, by site,
        malignant
      unspecified site
        female 183.0
        male 186.9
    specified site—*see* Neoplasm, by site,
      uncertain behavior
    unspecified site
      female 236.2
      male 236.4
Leydig-Sertoli cell tumor (M8631/0)
  specified site—*see* Neoplasm, by site, benign
  unspecified site
    female 220
    male 222.0
LGSIL (low grade squamous intraepithelial
    dysplasia) 622.1
Liar, pathologic 301.7
Libman-Sacks disease or syndrome 710.0
    [424.91]
Lice (infestation) 132.9
  body (pediculus corporis) 132.1
  crab 132.2
  head (pediculus capitis) 132.0
  mixed (classifiable to more than one of the
    categories 132.0-132.2) 132.3
  pubic (pediculus pubis) 132.2
Lichen 697.9
  albus 701.0
  annularis 695.89
  atrophicus 701.0
  corneus obtusus 698.3
  myxedematous 701.8
  nitidus 697.1
  pilaris 757.39
    acquired 701.1
  planopilaris 697.0
  planus (acute) (chronicus) (hypertrophic)
    (verrucous) 697.0
    morphoeicus 701.0
    sclerosus (et atrophicus) 701.0
  ruber 696.4

Lipomatosis (dolorosa) 272.8
  epidural 214.8
  fetal (M8881/0)—*see* Lipoma, by site
  Launois-Bensaude's 272.8
Lipomyohemangioma (M8860/0)
  specified site—*see* Neoplasm, connective
    tissue, benign
  unspecified site 223.0
Lipomyoma (M8860/0)
  specified site—*see* Neoplasm, connective
    tissue, benign
  unspecified site 223.0
Lipomyxoma (M8852/0)—*see* Lipoma, by site
Lipomyxosarcoma (M8852/3)—*see* Neoplasm,
  connective tissue, malignant
Lipophagocytosis 289.8
Lipoproteinemia (alpha) 272.4
  broad-beta 272.2
  floating-beta 272.2
  hyper-pre-beta 272.1
Lipoproteinosis (Rössle-Urbach-Wiethe) 272.8
Liposarcoma (M8850/3)—*see also* Neoplasm,
  connective tissue, malignant
  differentiated type (M8851/3)—*see* Neoplasm,
    connective tissue, malignant
  embryonal (M8852/3)—*see* Neoplasm,
    connective tissue, malignant
  mixed type (M8855/3)—*see* Neoplasm,
    connective tissue, malignant
  myxoid (M8852/3)—*see* Neoplasm, connective
    tissue, malignant
  pleomorphic (M8854/3)—*see* Neoplasm,
    connective tissue, malignant
  round cell (M8853/3)—*see* Neoplasm,
    connective tissue, malignant
  well differentiated type (M8851/3)—*see*
    Neoplasm, connective tissue, malignant
Liposynovitis prepatellaris 272.8
Lipping
  cervix 622.0
  spine (*see also* Spondylosis) 721.90
  vertebra (*see also* Spondylosis) 721.90
Lip pits (mucus), congenital 750.25
Lipschütz disease or ulcer 616.50
Lipuria 791.1
  bilharziasis 120.0
Liquefaction, vitreous humor 379.21
Lisping 307.9
Lissauer's paralysis 094.1
Lissencephalia, lissencephaly 742.2
Listerellose 027.0
Listeriose 027.0
Listeriosis 027.0
  congenital 771.2
  fetal 771.2
  suspected fetal damage affecting management
    of pregnancy 655.4
Listlessness 780.79
Lithemia 790.6
Lithiasis —*see also* Calculus
  hepatic (duct)—*see* Choledocholithiasis
  urinary 592.9
Lithopedion 779.9
  affecting management of pregnancy 656.8
Lithosis (occupational) 502
  with tuberculosis—*see* Tuberculosis, pulmonary
Lithuria 791.9
Litigation V62.5
Little
  league elbow 718.82
  stroke syndrome 435.9
Little's disease —*see* Palsy, cerebral

Littre's
  gland—*see* condition
  hernia—*see* Hernia, Littre's
Littritis (*see also* Urethritis) 597.89
Livedo 782.61
  annularis 782.61
  racemose 782.61
  reticularis 782.61
Live flesh 781.0
Liver —*see also* condition
  donor V59.6
Livida, asphyxia
  newborn 768.6
Living
  alone V60.3
    with handicapped person V60.4
Lloyd's syndrome 258.1
Loa loa 125.2
Loasis 125.2
Lobe, lobar —*see* condition
Lobo's disease or blastomycosis 116.2
Lobomycosis 116.2
Lobotomy syndrome 310.0
Lobstein's disease (brittle bones and blue sclera)
  756.51
Lobster-claw hand 755.58
Lobulation (congenital)—*see also* Anomaly,
  specified type NEC, by site
  kidney, fetal 753.3
  liver, abnormal 751.69
  spleen 759.0
Lobule, lobular —*see* condition
Local, localized —*see* condition
Locked bowel or intestine (*see also* Obstruction,
  intestine) 560.9
Locked twins 660.5
  affecting fetus or newborn 763.1
Locked-in state 344.81
Locking
  joint (*see also* Derangement, joint) 718.90
  knee 717.9
Lockjaw (*see also* Tetanus) 037
Locomotor ataxia (progressive) 094.0
Löffler's
  endocarditis 421.0
  eosinophilia or syndrome 518.3
  pneumonia 518.3
  syndrome (eosinophilic pneumonitis) 518.3
Löfgren's syndrome (sarcoidosis) 135
Loiasis 125.2
  eyelid 125.2 *[373.6]*
Loneliness V62.89
Lone star fever 082.8
Long labor 662.1
  affecting fetus or newborn 763.89
  first stage 662.0
  second stage 662.2
Long-term (current) drug use V58.69
  antibiotics V58.62
  anticoagulants V58.61
Longitudinal stripes or grooves, nails 703.8
  congenital 757.5
Loop
  intestine (*see also* Volvulus) 560.2
  intrascleral nerve 379.29
  vascular on papilla (optic) 743.57
Loose —*see also* condition
  body
    in tendon sheath 727.82
    joint 718.10
      ankle 718.17

Loose—*continued*
　　elbow 718.12
　　foot 718.17
　　hand 718.14
　　hip 718.15
　　knee 717.6
　　multiple sites 718.19
　　pelvic region 718.15
　　prosthetic implant—*see* Complications,
　　　　mechanical
　　shoulder (region) 718.11
　　specified site NEC 718.18
　　wrist 718.13
　cartilage (joint) (*see also* Loose, body, joint)
　　718.1
　　knee 717.6
　facet (vertebral) 724.9
　prosthetic implant—*see* Complications,
　　mechanical
　sesamoid, joint (*see also* Loose, body, joint)
　　718.1
　tooth, teeth 525.8
Loosening epiphysis 732.9
Looser (-Debray) -Milkman syndrome
　　(osteomalacia with pseudofractures) 268.2
Lop ear (deformity) 744.29
Lorain's disease or syndrome (pituitary
　　dwarfism) 253.3
Lorain-Levi syndrome (pituitary dwarfism)
　　253.3
Lordosis (acquired) (postural) 737.20
　congenital 754.2
　due to or associated with
　　Charcot-Marie-Tooth disease 356.1 *[737.42]*
　　mucopolysaccharidosis 277.5 *[737.42]*
　　neurofibromatosis 237.71 *[737.42]*
　　osteitis
　　　deformans 731.0 *[737.42]*
　　　fibrosa cystica 252.0 *[737.42]*
　　osteoporosis (*see also* Osteoporosis) 733.00
　　　[737.42]
　　poliomyelitis (*see also* Poliomyelitis) 138
　　　[737.42]
　　tuberculosis (*see also* Tuberculosis) 015.0
　　　[737.42]
　late effect of rickets 268.1 *[737.42]*
　postlaminectomy 737.21
　postsurgical NEC 737.22
　rachitic 268.1 *[737.42]*
　specified NEC 737.29
　tuberculous (*see also* Tuberculosis) 015.0
　　[737.42]

Loss
　appetite 783.0
　　hysterical 300.11
　　nonorganic origin 307.59
　　psychogenic 307.59
　blood—*see* Hemorrhage
　central vision 368.41
　consciousness 780.09
　　transient 780.2
　control, sphincter, rectum 787.6
　　nonorganic origin 307.7
　ear ossicle, partial 385.24
　elasticity, skin 782.8
　extremity or member, traumatic, current—*see*
　　Amputation, traumatic
　fluid (acute) 276.5
　　with
　　　hypernatremia 276.0
　　　hyponatremia 276.1

Loss —*continued*
　fetus or newborn 775.5
　hair 704.00
　hearing—*see also* Deafness
　　central 389.14
　　conductive (air) 389.00
　　　with sensorineural hearing loss 389.2
　　　combined types 389.08
　　　external ear 389.01
　　　inner ear 389.04
　　　middle ear 389.03
　　　multiple types 389.08
　　　tympanic membrane 389.02
　　mixed type 389.2
　　nerve 389.12
　　neural 389.12
　　noise-induced 388.12
　　perceptive NEC (*see also* Loss, hearing,
　　　sensorineural) 389.10
　　sensorineural 389.10
　　　with conductive hearing loss 389.2
　　　central 389.14
　　　combined types 389.18
　　　multiple types 389.18
　　　neural 389.12
　　　sensory 389.11
　　sensory 389.11
　　specified type NEC 389.8
　　sudden NEC 388.2
　height 781.91
　labyrinthine reactivity (unilateral) 386.55
　　bilateral 386.56
　memory (*see also* Amnesia) 780.99
　　mild, following organic brain damage 310.1
　mind (*see also* Psychosis) 298.9
　organ or part—*see* Absence, by site, acquired
　sensation 782.0
　sense of
　　smell (*see also* Disturbance, sensation) 781.1
　　taste (*see also* Disturbance, sensation) 781.1
　　touch (*see also* Disturbance, sensation) 781.1
　sight (acquired) (complete) (congenital)—*see*
　　Blindness
　spinal fluid
　　headache 349.0
　substance of
　　bone (*see also* Osteoporosis) 733.00
　　cartilage 733.99
　　　ear 380.32
　　vitreous (humor) 379.26
　tooth, teeth
　　acquired 525.10
　　　due to
　　　　caries 525.13
　　　　extraction 525.10
　　　　periodontal disease 525.12
　　　　specified NEC 525.19
　　　　trauma 525.11
　vision, visual (*see also* Blindness) 369.9
　　both eyes (*see also* Blindness, both eyes) 369.3
　　complete (*see also* Blindness, both eyes)
　　　369.00
　　one eye 369.8
　　sudden 368.11
　　transient 368.12
　vitreous 379.26
　voice (*see also* Aphonia) 784.41
　weight (cause unknown) 783.21
Lou Gehrig's disease 335.20
Louis-Bar syndrome (ataxia-telangiectasia)
　　334.8
Louping ill 063.1

> *Note—Use the following fifth-digit subclassification with categories 200-202:*
>
> *0 unspecified site*
> *1 lymph nodes of head, face and neck*
> *2 intrathoracic lymph nodes*
> *3 intra-abdominal lymph nodes*
> *4 lymph nodes of axilla and upper limb*
> *5 lymph nodes of inguinal region and*
>   *lower limb*
> *6 intrapelvic lymph nodes*
> *7 spleen*
> *8 lymph nodes of multiple sites*

M

Macacus ear 744.29
Maceration
  fetus (cause not stated) 779.9
  wet feet, tropical (syndrome) 991.4
Machado-Joseph disease 334.8
Machupo virus hemorrhagic fever 078.7
Macleod's syndrome (abnormal transradiancy,
    one lung) 492.8
Macrocephalia, macrocephaly 756.0
Macrocheilia (congenital) 744.81
Macrochilia (congenital) 744.81
Macrocolon (congenital) 751.3
Macrocornea 743.41
  associated with buphthalmos 743.22
Macrocytic *—see* condition
Macrocytosis 289.8
Macrodactylia, macrodactylism (fingers)
    (thumbs) 755.57
  toes 755.65
Macrodontia 520.2
Macroencephaly 742.4
Macrogenia 524.05
Macrogenitosomia (female) (male) (praecox)
    255.2
Macrogingivae 523.8
Macroglobulinemia (essential) (idiopathic)
    (monoclonal) (primary) (syndrome)
    (Waldenström's) 273.3
Macroglossia (congenital) 750.15
  acquired 529.8
Macrognathia, macrognathism (congenital)
    524.00
  mandibular 524.02
    alveolar 524.72
  maxillary 524.01
    alveolar 524.71
Macrogyria (congenital) 742.4
Macrohydrocephalus (*see also* Hydrocephalus)
    331.4
Macromastia (*see also* Hypertrophy, breast)
    611.1
Macropsia 368.14
Macrosigmoid 564.7
  congenital 751.3
Macrospondylitis, acromegalic 253.0
Macrostomia (congenital) 744.83
Macrotia (external ear) (congenital) 744.22
Macula
  cornea, corneal
    congenital 743.43
      interfering with vision 743.42
    interfering with central vision 371.03
    not interfering with central vision 371.02
  degeneration (*see also* Degeneration, macula)
    362.50
    hereditary (*see also* Dystrophy, retina) 362.70
  edema, cystoid 362.53
Maculae ceruleae 132.1
Macules and papules 709.8
Maculopathy, toxic 362.55
Madarosis 374.55
Madelung's
  deformity (radius) 755.54
  disease (lipomatosis) 272.8
  lipomatosis 272.8
Madness (*see also* Psychosis) 298.9
  myxedema (acute) 293.0
    subacute 293.1

Madura
  disease (actinomycotic) 039.9
    mycotic 117.4
  foot (actinomycotic) 039.4
    mycotic 117.4
Maduromycosis (actinomycotic) 039.9
  mycotic 117.4
Maffucci's syndrome (dyschondroplasia with
    hemangiomas) 756.4
Magenblase syndrome 306.4
Main en griffe (acquired) 736.06
  congenital 755.59
Maintenance
  chemotherapy regimen or treatment V58.1
  dialysis regimen or treatment
    extracorporeal (renal) V56.0
    peritoneal V56.8
    renal V56.0
  drug therapy or regimen V58.1
  external fixation NEC V54.89
  radiotherapy V58.0
  traction NEC V54.89
Majocchi's
  disease (purpura annularis telangiectodes) 709.1
  granuloma 110.6
Major *—see* condition
Mal
  cerebral (idiopathic) (*see also* Epilepsy) 345.9
  comital (*see also* Epilepsy) 345.9
  de los pintos (*see also* Pinta) 103.9
  de Meleda 757.39
  de mer 994.6
  lie—*see* Presentation, fetal
  perforant (*see also* Ulcer, lower extremity)
    707.15
Malabar itch 110.9
  beard 110.0
  foot 110.4
  scalp 110.0
Malabsorption 579.9
  calcium 579.8
  carbohydrate 579.8
  disaccharide 271.3
  drug-induced 579.8
  due to bacterial overgrowth 579.8
  fat 579.8
  folate, congenital 281.2
  galactose 271.1
  glucose-galactose (congenital) 271.3
  intestinal 579.9
  isomaltose 271.3
  lactose (hereditary) 271.3
  methionine 270.4
  monosaccharide 271.8
  postgastrectomy 579.3
  postsurgical 579.3
  protein 579.8
  sucrose (-isomaltose) (congenital) 271.3
  syndrome 579.9
    postgastrectomy 579.3
    postsurgical 579.3
Malacia, bone 268.2
  juvenile (*see also* Rickets) 268.0
  Kienböck's (juvenile) (lunate) (wrist) 732.3
    adult 732.8

Malformation—*continued*
respiratory organs 748.9
specified type NEC 748.8
Rieger's 743.44
sense organs NEC 742.9
specified type NEC 742.8
skin 757.9
specified type NEC 757.8
spinal cord 742.9
teeth, tooth NEC 520.9
tendon 756.9
throat 750.9
umbilical cord (complicating delivery) 663.9
affecting fetus or newborn 762.6
umbilicus 759.9
urinary system NEC 753.9
specified type NEC 753.8
Malfunction —*see also* Dysfunction
arterial graft 996.1
cardiac pacemaker 996.01
catheter device—*see* Complications,
mechanical, catheter
colostomy 569.62
cystostomy 997.5
device, implant, or graft NEC—*see*
Complications, mechanical
enteric stoma 569.62
enterostomy 569.62
gastroenteric 536.8
gastrostomy 536.42
nephrostomy 997.5
pacemaker—*see* Complications, mechanical,
pacemaker
prosthetic device, internal—*see* Complications,
mechanical
tracheostomy 519.02
vascular graft or shunt 996.1
Malgaigne's fracture (closed) 808.43
open 808.53
Malherbe's
calcifying epithelioma (M8110/0)—*see*
Neoplasm, skin, benign
tumor (M8110/0)—*see* Neoplasm, skin, benign
Malibu disease 919.8
infected 919.9
Malignancy (M8000/3)—*see* Neoplasm, by site,
malignant
Malignant —*see* condition
Malingerer, malingering V65.2
Mallet, finger (acquired) 736.1
congenital 755.59
late effect of rickets 268.1
Malleus 024
Mallory's bodies 034.1
Mallory-Weiss syndrome 530.7
Malnutrition (calorie) 263.9
complicating pregnancy 648.9
degree
first 263.1
second 263.0
third 262
mild 263.1
moderate 263.0
severe 261
protein-calorie 262
fetus 764.2
"light-for-dates" 764.1
following gastrointestinal surgery 579.3
intrauterine or fetal 764.2
fetus or infant "light-for-dates" 764.1

Malnutrition—*continued*
lack of care, or neglect (child) (infant) 995.52
adult 995.84
malignant 260
mild 263.1
moderate 263.0
protein 260
protein-calorie 263.9
severe 262
specified type NEC 263.8
severe 261
protein-calorie NEC 262
Malocclusion (teeth) 524.4
due to
abnormal swallowing 524.5
accessory teeth (causing crowding) 524.3
dentofacial abnormality NEC 524.8
impacted teeth (causing crowding) 524.3
missing teeth 524.3
mouth breathing 524.5
supernumerary teeth (causing crowding) 524.3
thumb sucking 524.5
tongue, lip, or finger habits 524.5
temporomandibular (joint) 524.69
Malposition
cardiac apex (congenital) 746.87
cervix—*see* Malposition, uterus
congenital
adrenal (gland) 759.1
alimentary tract 751.8
lower 751.5
upper 750.8
aorta 747.21
appendix 751.5
arterial trunk 747.29
artery (peripheral) NEC (*see also* Malposition,
congenital, peripheral vascular system)
747.60
coronary 746.85
pulmonary 747.3
auditory canal 744.29
causing impairment of hearing 744.02
auricle (ear) 744.29
causing impairment of hearing 744.02
cervical 744.43
biliary duct or passage 751.69
bladder (mucosa) 753.8
exteriorized or extroverted 753.5
brachial plexus 742.8
brain tissue 742.4
breast 757.6
bronchus 748.3
cardiac apex 746.87
cecum 751.5
clavicle 755.51
colon 751.5
digestive organ or tract NEC 751.8
lower 751.5
upper 750.8
ear (auricle) (external) 744.29
ossicles 744.04
endocrine (gland) NEC 759.2
epiglottis 748.3
Eustachian tube 744.24
eye 743.8
facial features 744.89
fallopian tube 752.19
finger(s) 755.59
supernumerary 755.01

Maltreatment—*continued*
  psychological 995.82
  sexual 995.83
  child 995.50
    emotional 995.51
    multiple forms 995.59
    neglect (nutritional) 995.52
    psychological 995.51
    physical 995.54
      shaken infant syndrome 995.55
    sexual 995.53
  spouse 995.80—*(see also* Maltreatment, adult)
Malt workers' lung 495.4
Malum coxae senilis 715.25
Malunion, fracture 733.81
Mammillitis (*see also* Mastitis) 611.0
  puerperal, postpartum 675.2
Mammitis (*see also* Mastitis) 611.0
  puerperal, postpartum 675.2
Mammographic microcalcification 793.81
Mammoplasia 611.1
Management
  contraceptive V25.9
    specified type NEC V25.8
  procreative V26.9
    specified type NEC V26.8
Mangled NEC (*see also* nature and site of injury) 959.9
Mania (monopolar) (*see also* Psychosis, affective) 296.0
  alcoholic (acute) (chronic) 291.9
  Bell's—*see* Mania, chronic
  chronic 296.0
    recurrent episode 296.1
    single episode 296.0
  compulsive 300.3
  delirious (acute) 296.0
    recurrent episode 296.1
    single episode 296.0
  epileptic (*see also* Epilepsy) 345.4
  hysterical 300.10
  inhibited 296.89
  puerperal (after delivery) 296.0
    recurrent episode 296.1
    single episode 296.0
  recurrent episode 296.1
  senile 290.8
  single episode 296.0
  stupor 296.89
  stuporous 296.89
  unproductive 296.89
Manic-depressive insanity, psychosis reaction, or syndrome (*see also* Psychosis, affective) 296.80
  circular (alternating) 296.7
    currently
      depressed 296.5
      episode unspecified 296.7
      hypomanic, previously depressed 296.4
      manic 296.4
    mixed 296.6
  depressed (type), depressive 296.2
    atypical 296.82
    recurrent episode 296.3
    single episode 296.2
  hypomanic 296.0
    recurrent episode 296.1
    single episode 296.0
  manic 296.0
    atypical 296.81
    recurrent episode 296.1

Manic-depressive...—*continued*
    single episode 296.0
    mixed NEC 296.89
    perplexed 296.89
    stuporous 296.89
Manifestations, rheumatoid
  lungs 714.81
  pannus—*see* Arthritis, rheumatoid
  subcutaneous nodules—*see* Arthritis, rheumatoid
Mankowsky's syndrome (familial dysplastic osteopathy) 731.2
Mannoheptulosuria 271.8
Mannosidosis 271.8
Manson's
  disease (schistosomiasis) 120.1
  pyosis (pemphigus contagiosus) 684
  schistosomiasis 120.1
Mansonellosis 125.5
Manual —*see* condition
Maple bark disease 495.6
Maple bark-strippers' lung 495.6
Maple syrup (urine) disease or syndrome 270.3
Marable's syndrome (celiac artery compression) 447.4
Marasmus 261
  brain 331.9
  due to malnutrition 261
  intestinal 569.89
  nutritional 261
  senile 797
  tuberculous NEC (*see also* Tuberculosis) 011.9
Marble
  bones 756.52
  skin 782.61
Marburg disease (virus) 078.89
March
  foot 733.94
  hemoglobinuria 283.2
Marchand multiple nodular hyperplasia (liver) 571.5
Marchesani (-Weill) syndrome (brachymorphism and ectopia lentis) 759.89
Marchiafava (-Bignami) disease or syndrome 341.8
Marchiafava-Micheli syndrome (paroxysmal nocturnal hemoglobinuria) 283.2
Marcus Gunn's syndrome (jaw-winking syndrome) 742.8
Marfan's
  congenital syphilis 090.49
  disease 090.49
  syndrome (arachnodactyly) 759.82
    meaning congenital syphilis 090.49
      with luxation of lens 090.49 *[379.32]*
Marginal
  implantation, placenta—*see* Placenta, previa
  placenta—*see* Placenta, previa
  sinus (hemorrhage) (rupture) 641.2
    affecting fetus or newborn 762.1
Marie's
  cerebellar ataxia 334.2
  syndrome (acromegaly) 253.0
Marie-Bamberger disease or syndrome (hypertrophic) (pulmonary) (secondary) 731.2
  idiopathic (acropachyderma) 757.39
  primary (acropachyderma) 757.39
Marie-Charcot-Tooth neuropathic atrophy, muscle 356.1
Marie-Strümpell arthritis or disease (ankylosing spondylitis) 720.0

Marihuana, marijuana
  abuse (*see also* Abuse, drugs, nondependent)
    305.2
  dependence (*see also* Dependence) 304.3
Marion's disease (bladder neck obstruction)
  596.0
Marital conflict V61.10
Mark
  port wine 757.32
  raspberry 757.32
  strawberry 757.32
  stretch 701.3
  tattoo 709.09
Maroteaux-Lamy syndrome
  (mucopolysaccharidosis VI) 277.5
Marriage license examination V70.3
Marrow (bone)
  arrest 284.9
  megakaryocytic 287.3
  poor function 289.9
Marseilles fever 082.1
Marsh's disease (exophthalmic goiter) 242.0
Marshall's (hidrotic) ectodermal dysplasia 757.31
Marsh fever (*see also* Malaria) 084.6
Martin's disease 715.27
Martin-Albright syndrome
  (pseudohypoparathyroidism) 275.49
Martorell-Fabre syndrome (pulseless disease)
  446.7
Masculinization, female with adrenal
  hyperplasia 255.2
Masculinovoblastoma (M8670/0) 220
Masochism 302.83
Masons' lung 502
Mass
  abdominal 789.3
  anus 787.99
  bone 733.90
  breast 611.72
  cheek 784.2
  chest 786.6
  cystic—*see* Cyst
  ear 388.8
  epigastric 789.3
  eye 379.92
  female genital organ 625.8
  gum 784.2
  head 784.2
  intracranial 784.2
  joint 719.60
    ankle 719.67
    elbow 719.62
    foot 719.67
    hand 719.64
    hip 719.65
    knee 719.66
    multiple sites 719.69
    pelvic region 719.65
    shoulder (region) 719.61
    specified site NEC 719.68
    wrist 719.63
  kidney (*see also* Disease, kidney) 593.9
  lung 786.6
  lymph node 785.6
  malignant (M8000/3)—*see* Neoplasm, by site,
    malignant
  mediastinal 786.6
  mouth 784.2
  muscle (limb) 729.89
  neck 784.2
  nose or sinus 784.2

Mass—*continued*
  palate 784.2
  pelvis, pelvic 789.3
  penis 607.89
  perineum 625.8
  rectum 787.99
  scrotum 608.89
  skin 782.2
  specified organ NEC—*see* Disease of specified
    organ or site
  splenic 789.2
  substernal 786.6
    thyroid (*see also* Goiter) 240.9
  superficial (localized) 782.2
  testes 608.89
  throat 784.2
  tongue 784.2
  umbilicus 789.3
  uterus 625.8
  vagina 625.8
  vulva 625.8
Massive —*see* condition
Mastalgia 611.71
  psychogenic 307.89
Mast cell
  disease 757.33
    systemic (M9741/3) 202.6
  leukemia (M9900/3) 207.8
  sarcoma (M9742/3) 202.6
  tumor (M9740/1) 238.5
    malignant (M9740/3) 202.6
Masters-Allen syndrome 620.6
Mastitis (acute) (adolescent) (diffuse)
    (interstitial) (lobular) (nonpuerperal)
    (nonsuppurative) (parenchymatous)
    (phlegmonous) (simple) (subacute)
    (suppurative) 611.0
  chronic (cystic) (fibrocystic) 610.1
  cystic 610.1
    Schimmelbusch's type 610.1
  fibrocystic 610.1
  infective 611.0
  lactational 675.2
  lymphangitis 611.0
  neonatal (noninfective) 778.7
    infective 771.5
  periductal 610.4
  plasma cell 610.4
  puerperal, postpartum, (interstitial)
    (nonpurulent) (parenchymatous) 675.2
    purulent 675.1
    stagnation 676.2
  puerperalis 675.2
  retromammary 611.0
    puerperal, postpartum 675.1
  submammary 611.0
    puerperal, postpartum 675.1
Mastocytoma (M9740/1) 238.5
  malignant (M9740/3) 202.6
Mastocytosis 757.33
  malignant (M9741/3) 202.6
  systemic (M9741/3) 202.6
Mastodynia 611.71
  psychogenic 307.89
Mastoid —*see* condition
Mastoidalgia (*see also* Otalgia) 388.70
Mastoiditis (coalescent) (hemorrhagic)
    (pneumococcal) (streptococcal) (suppurative)
    383.9
  acute or subacute 383.00

Mastoiditis—*continued*
　with
　　Gradenigo's syndrome 383.02
　　petrositis 383.02
　　specified complication NEC 383.02
　　subperiosteal abscess 383.01
　chronic (necrotic) (recurrent) 383.1
　tuberculous (*see also* Tuberculosis) 015.6
Mastopathy, mastopathia 611.9
　chronica cystica 610.1
　diffuse cystic 610.1
　estrogenic 611.8
　ovarian origin 611.8
Mastoplasia 611.1
Masturbation 307.9
Maternal condition, affecting fetus or newborn
　acute yellow atrophy of liver 760.8
　albuminuria 760.1
　anesthesia or analgesia 763.5
　blood loss 762.1
　chorioamnionitis 762.7
　circulatory disease, chronic (conditions
　　classifiable to 390-459, 745-747) 760.3
　congenital heart disease (conditions classifiable
　　to 745-746) 760.3
　cortical necrosis of kidney 760.1
　death 761.6
　diabetes mellitus 775.0
　　manifest diabetes in the infant 775.1
　disease NEC 760.9
　　circulatory system, chronic (conditions
　　　classifiable to 390-459, 745-747) 760.3
　　genitourinary system (conditions classifiable
　　　to 580-599) 760.1
　　respiratory (conditions classifiable to 490-519,
　　　748) 760.3
　eclampsia 760.0
　hemorrhage NEC 762.1
　hepatitis acute, malignant, or subacute 760.8
　hyperemesis (gravidarum) 761.8
　hypertension (arising during pregnancy)
　　(conditions classifiable to 642) 760.0
　infection
　　disease classifiable to 001-136 760.2
　　genital tract NEC 760.8
　　urinary tract 760.1
　influenza 760.2
　　manifest influenza in the infant 771.2
　injury (conditions classifiable to 800-996) 760.5
　malaria 760.2
　　manifest malaria in infant or fetus 771.2
　malnutrition 760.4
　necrosis of liver 760.8
　nephritis (conditions classifiable to 580-583)
　　760.1
　nephrosis (conditions classifiable to 581) 760.1
　noxious substance transmitted via breast milk or
　　placenta 760.70
　　alcohol 760.71
　　anti-infective agents 760.74
　　cocaine 760.75
　　"crack" 760.75
　　diethylstilbestrol [DES] 760.76
　　hallucinogenic agents 760.73
　　medicinal agents NEC 760.79
　　narcotics 760.72
　　obstetric anesthetic or analgesic drug 760.72
　　specified agent NEC 760.79
　nutritional disorder (conditions classifiable to
　　260-269) 760.4
　operation unrelated to current delivery 760.6

Maternal condition, affecting fetus. . .—*cont.*
　pre-eclampsia 760.0
　pyelitis or pyelonephritis, arising during
　　pregnancy (conditions classifiable to 590)
　　760.1
　renal disease or failure 760.1
　respiratory disease, chronic (conditions
　　classifiable to 490-519, 748) 760.3
　rheumatic heart disease (chronic) (conditions
　　classifiable to 393-398) 760.3
　rubella (conditions classifiable to 056) 760.2
　　manifest rubella in the infant or fetus 771.0
　surgery unrelated to current delivery 760.6
　　to uterus or pelvic organs 763.89
　syphilis (conditions classifiable to 090-097)
　　760.2
　　manifest syphilis in the infant or fetus 090.0
　thrombophlebitis 760.3
　toxemia (of pregnancy) 760.0
　　pre-eclamptic 760.0
　toxoplasmosis (conditions classifiable to 130)
　　760.2
　　manifest toxoplasmosis in the infant or fetus
　　　771.2
　transmission of chemical substance through the
　　placenta 760.70
　　alcohol 760.71
　　anti-infective 760.74
　　cocaine 760.75
　　"crack" 760.75
　　diethylstilbestrol [DES] 760.76
　　hallucinogenic agents 760.73
　　narcotics 760.72
　　specified substance NEC 760.79
　uremia 760.1
　urinary tract conditions (conditions classifiable
　　to 580-599) 760.1
　vomiting (pernicious) (persistent) (vicious)
　　761.8
Maternity —*see* Delivery
Matheiu's disease (leptospiral jaundice) 100.0
Mauclaire's disease or osteochondrosis 732.3
Maxcy's disease 081.0
Maxilla, maxillary —*see* condition
May (-Hegglin) anomaly or syndrome 288.2
Mayaro fever 066.3
Mazoplasia 610.8
MBD (minimal brain dysfunction), child (*see
　also* Hyperkinesia) 314.9
McArdle (-Schmid-Pearson) disease or
　syndrome (glycogenosis V) 271.0
McCune-Albright syndrome (osteitis fibrosa
　disseminata) 756.59
MCLS (mucocutaneous lymph node syndrome)
　446.1
McQuarrie's syndrome (idiopathic familial
　hypoglycemia) 251.2
Measles (black) (hemorrhagic) (suppressed) 055.9
　with
　　encephalitis 055.0
　　keratitis 055.71
　　keratoconjunctivitis 055.71
　　otitis media 055.2
　　pneumonia 055.1
　complication 055.8
　　specified type NEC 055.79
　encephalitis 055.0
　French 056.9
　German 056.9
　keratitis 055.71
　keratoconjunctivitis 055.71

Meningismus (infectional) (pneumococcal) 781.6
  due to serum or vaccine 997.09 *[321.8]*
  influenzal NEC 487.8
Meningitis (basal) (basic) (basilar) (brain)
    (cerebral) (cervical) (congestive) (diffuse)
    (hemorrhagic) (infantile) (membranous)
    (metastatic) (nonspecific) (pontine)
    (progressive) (simple) (spinal) (subacute)
    (sympathetica) (toxic) 322.9
  abacterial NEC (*see also* Meningitis, aseptic)
    047.9
  actinomycotic 039.8 *[320.7]*
  adenoviral 049.1
  Aerobacter aerogenes 320.82
  anaerobes (cocci) (gram-negative)
    (gram-positive) (mixed) (NEC) 320.81
  arbovirus NEC 066.9 *[321.2]*
    specified type NEC 066.8 *[321.2]*
  aseptic (acute) NEC 047.9
    adenovirus 049.1
    Coxsackie virus 047.0
    due to
      adenovirus 049.1
      Coxsackie virus 047.0
      ECHO virus 047.1
      enterovirus 047.9
      mumps 072.1
      poliovirus (*see also* Poliomyelitis) 045.2
        [321.2]
    ECHO virus 047.1
    herpes (simplex) virus 054.72
      zoster 053.0
    leptospiral 100.81
    lymphocytic choriomeningitis 049.0
    noninfective 322.0
  Bacillus pyocyaneus 320.89
  bacterial NEC 320.9
    anaerobic 320.81
    gram-negative 320.82
      anaerobic 320.81
  Bacteroides (fragilis) (oralis) (melaninogenicus)
    320.81
  cancerous (M8000/6) 198.4
  candidal 112.83
  carcinomatous (M8010/6) 198.4
  caseous (*see also* Tuberculosis, meninges) 013.0
  cerebrospinal (acute) (chronic) (diplococcal)
    (endemic) (epidemic) (fulminant)
    (infectious) (malignant) (meningococcal)
    (sporadic) 036.0
    carrier (suspected) of V02.59
  chronic NEC 322.2
  clear cerebrospinal fluid NEC 322.0
  Clostridium (haemolyticum) (novyi) NEC
    320.81
  coccidioidomycosis 114.2
  Coxsackie virus 047.0
  cryptococcal 117.5 *[321.0]*
  diplococcal 036.0
    gram-negative 036.0
    gram-positive 320.1
  Diplococcus pneumoniae 320.1
  due to
    actinomycosis 039.8 *[320.7]*
    adenovirus 049.1
    coccidiomycosis 114.2
    enterovirus 047.9
      specified NEC 047.8
    histoplasmosis (*see also* Histoplasmosis)
      115.91
    Listerosis 027.0 *[320.7]*

Meningitis—*continued*
  Lyme disease 088.81 *[320.7]*
  moniliasis 112.83
  mumps 072.1
  neurosyphilis 094.2
  nonbacterial organisms NEC 321.8
  oidiomycosis 112.83
  poliovirus (*see also* Poliomyelitis) 045.2
    [321.2]
  preventive immunization, inoculation, or
    vaccination 997.09 *[321.8]*
  sarcoidosis 135 *[321.4]*
  sporotrichosis 117.1 *[321.1]*
  syphilis 094.2
    acute 091.81
    congenital 090.42
    secondary 091.81
  trypanosomiasis (*see also* Trypanosomiasis)
    086.9 *[321.3]*
  whooping cough 033.9 *[320.7]*
  E. coli 320.82
  ECHO virus 047.1
  endothelial-leukocytic, benign, recurrent 047.9
  Enterobacter aerogenes 320.82
  enteroviral 047.9
    specified type NEC 047.8
  enterovirus 047.9
    specified NEC 047.8
  eosinophilic 322.1
  epidemic NEC 036.0
  Escherichia coli (E. coli) 320.82
  Eubacterium 320.81
  fibrinopurulent NEC 320.9
    specified type NEC 320.89
  Friedländer (bacillus) 320.82
  fungal NEC 117.9 *[321.1]*
  Fusobacterium 320.81
  gonococcal 098.82
  gram-negative bacteria NEC 320.82
    anaerobic 320.81
    cocci 036.0
      specified NEC 320.82
  gram-negative cocci NEC 036.0
    specified NEC 320.82
  gram-positive cocci NEC 320.9
  H. influenzae 320.0
  herpes (simplex) virus 054.72
    zoster 053.0
  infectious NEC 320.9
  influenzal 320.0
  Klebsiella pneumoniae 320.82
  late effect—*see* Late, effect, meningitis
  leptospiral (aseptic) 100.81
  Listerella (monocytogenes) 027.0 *[320.7]*
  Listeria monocytogenes 027.0 *[320.7]*
  lymphocytic (acute) (benign) (serous) 049.0
    choriomeningitis virus 049.0
  meningococcal (chronic) 036.0
  Mima polymorpha 320.82
  Mollaret's 047.9
  monilial 112.83
  mumps (virus) 072.1
  mycotic NEC 117.9 *[321.1]*
  Neisseria 036.0
  neurosyphilis 094.2
  nonbacterial NEC (*see also* Meningitis, aseptic)
    047.9
  nonpyogenic NEC 322.0
  oidiomycosis 112.83
  ossificans 349.2
  Peptococcus 320.81

Meningomyelitis (*see also* Meningoencephalitis) 323.9
　blastomycotic NEC (*see also* Blastomycosis) 116.0 *[323.4]*
　due to
　　actinomycosis 039.8 *[320.7]*
　　blastomycosis (*see also* Blastomycosis) 116.0 *[323.4]*
　　Meningococcus 036.0
　　sporotrichosis 117.1 *[323.4]*
　　torula 117.5 *[323.4]*
　late effect—*see* category 326
　lethargic 049.8
　meningococcal 036.0
　syphilitic 094.2
　tuberculous (*see also* Tuberculosis, meninges) 013.0
Meningomyelocele (*see also* Spina bifida) 741.9
　syphilitic 094.89
Meningomyeloneuritis —*see* Meningoencephalitis
Meningoradiculitis —*see* Meningitis
Meningovascular —*see* condition
Meniscocytosis 282.60
Menkes' syndrome —*see* Syndrome, Menkes'
Menolipsis 626.0
Menometrorrhagia 626.2
Menopause, menopausal (symptoms) (syndrome) 627.2
　arthritis (any site) NEC 716.3
　artificial 627.4
　bleeding 627.0
　crisis 627.2
　depression (*see also* Psychosis, affective) 296.2
　　agitated 296.2
　　　recurrent episode 296.3
　　　single episode 296.2
　　psychotic 296.2
　　　recurrent episode 296.3
　　　single episode 296.2
　　recurrent episode 296.3
　　single episode 296.2
　melancholia (*see also* Psychosis, affective) 296.2
　　recurrent episode 296.3
　　single episode 296.2
　paranoid state 297.2
　paraphrenia 297.2
　postsurgical 627.4
　premature 256.31
　　postirradiation 256.2
　　postsurgical 256.2
　psychoneurosis 627.2
　psychosis NEC 298.8
　surgical 627.4
　toxic polyarthritis NEC 716.39
Menorrhagia (primary) 626.2
　climacteric 627.0
　menopausal 627.0
　postclimacteric 627.1
　postmenopausal 627.1
　preclimacteric 627.0
　premenopausal 627.0
　puberty (menses retained) 626.3
Menorrhalgia 625.3
Menoschesis 626.8
Menostaxis 626.2
Menses, retention 626.8
Menstrual —*see* Menstruation
　cycle, irregular 626.4
　disorders NEC 626.9

Menstrual—*continued*
　extraction V25.3
　fluid, retained 626.8
　molimen 625.4
　period, normal V65.5
　regulation V25.3
Menstruation
　absent 626.0
　anovulatory 628.0
　delayed 626.8
　difficult 625.3
　disorder 626.9
　　psychogenic 306.52
　　specified NEC 626.8
　during pregnancy 640.8
　excessive 626.2
　frequent 626.2
　infrequent 626.1
　irregular 626.4
　latent 626.8
　membranous 626.8
　painful (primary) (secondary) 625.3
　　psychogenic 306.52
　passage of clots 626.2
　precocious 626.8
　protracted 626.8
　retained 626.8
　retrograde 626.8
　scanty 626.1
　suppression 626.8
　vicarious (nasal) 625.8
Mentagra (*see also* Sycosis) 704.8
Mental —*see also* condition
　deficiency (*see also* Retardation, mental) 319
　deterioration (*see also* Psychosis) 298.9
　disorder (*see also* Disorder, mental) 300.9
　exhaustion 300.5
　insufficiency (congenital) (*see also* Retardation, mental) 319
　observation without need for further medical care NEC V71.09
　retardation (*see also* Retardation, mental) 319
　subnormality (*see also* Retardation, mental) 319
　　mild 317
　　moderate 318.0
　　profound 318.2
　　severe 318.1
　upset (*see also* Disorder, mental) 300.9
Meralgia paresthetica 355.1
Mercurial —*see* condition
Mercurialism NEC 985.0
Merergasia 300.9
MERFF 758.89
Merkel cell tumor —*see* Neoplasm, by site, malignant
Merocele (*see also* Hernia, femoral) 553.00
Meromelia 755.4
　lower limb 755.30
　　intercalary 755.32
　　　femur 755.34
　　　　tibiofibular (complete) (incomplete) 755.33
　　　fibula 755.37
　　　metatarsal(s) 755.38
　　　tarsal(s) 755.38
　　　tibia 755.36
　　　tibiofibular 755.35
　　terminal (complete) (partial) (transverse) 755.31
　　　longitudinal 755.32
　　　　metatarsal(s) 755.38
　　　　phalange(s) 755.39

Milk
  crust 690.11
  excess secretion 676.6
  fever, female 672
  poisoning 988.8
  retention 676.2
  sickness 988.8
  spots 423.1
Milkers' nodes 051.1
Milk-leg (deep vessels) 671.4
  complicating pregnancy 671.3
  nonpuerperal 451.19
  puerperal, postpartum, childbirth 671.4
Milkman (-Looser) disease or syndrome
      (osteomalacia with pseudofractures) 268.2
Milky urine (see also Chyluria) 791.1
Millar's asthma (laryngismus stridulus) 478.75
Millard-Gubler paralysis or syndrome 344.89
Millard-Gubler-Foville paralysis 344.89
Miller's disease (osteomalacia) 268.2
Miller Fisher's syndrome 357.0
Milles' syndrome (encephalocutaneous
      angiomatosis) 759.6
Mills' disease 335.29
Millstone makers' asthma or lung 502
Milroy's disease (chronic hereditary edema)
      757.0
Miners' —see also condition
  asthma 500
  elbow 727.2
  knee 727.2
  lung 500
  nystagmus 300.89
  phthisis (see also Tuberculosis) 011.4
  tuberculosis (see also Tuberculosis) 011.4
Minkowski-Chauffard syndrome (see also
      Spherocytosis) 282.0
Minor —see condition
Minor's disease 336.1
Minot's disease (hemorrhagic disease, newborn)
      776.0
Minot-von Willebrand (-Jürgens) disease or
      syndrome (angiohemophilia) 286.4
Minus (and plus) hand (intrinsic) 736.09
Miosis (persistent) (pupil) 379.42
Mirizzi's syndrome (hepatic duct stenosis) (see
      also Obstruction, biliary) 576.2
  with calculus, cholelithiasis, or stones—see
      Choledocholithiasis
Mirror writing 315.09
  secondary to organic lesion 784.69
Misadventure (prophylactic) (therapeutic) (see
      also Complications) 999.9
  administration of insulin 962.3
  infusion—see Complications, infusion
  local applications (of fomentations, plasters,
      etc.) 999.9
    burn or scald—see Burn, by site
  medical care (early) (late) NEC 999.9
    adverse effect of drugs or chemicals—see
        Table of drugs and chemicals
    burn or scald—see Burn, by site
  radiation NEC 990
  radiotherapy NEC 990
  surgical procedure (early) (late)—see
      Complications, surgical procedure
  transfusion—see Complications, transfusion
  vaccination or other immunological
      procedure—see Complications, vaccination
Misanthropy 301.7
Miscarriage —see Abortion, spontaneous

Mischief, malicious, child (see also Disturbance,
      conduct) 312.0
Misdirection , aqueous 365.83
Mismanagement, feeding 783.3
Misplaced, misplacement
  kidney (see also Disease, renal) 593.0
    congenital 753.3
  organ or site, congenital NEC—see
      Malposition, congenital
Missed
  abortion 632
  delivery (at or near term) 656.4
  labor (at or near term) 656.4
Missing —see also Absence
  teeth (acquired) 525.10
    congenital (see also Anodontia) 520.0
    due to
      caries 525.13
      extraction 525.10
      periodontal disease 525.12
      specified NEC 525.19
      trauma 525.11
  vertebrae (congenital) 756.13
Misuse of drugs NEC (see also Abuse, drug,
      nondependent) 305.9
Mitchell's disease (erythromelalgia) 443.89
Mite (s)
  diarrhea 133.8
  grain (itch) 133.8
  hair follicle (itch) 133.8
  in sputum 133.8
Mitral —see condition
Mittelschmerz 625.2
Mixed —see condition
Mljet disease (mal de Meleda) 757.39
Mobile, mobility
  cecum 751.4
  coccyx 733.99
  excessive—see Hypermobility
  gallbladder 751.69
  kidney 593.0
    congenital 753.3
  organ or site, congenital NEC—see
      Malposition, congenital
  spleen 289.59
Mobitz heart block (atrioventricular) 426.10
  type I (Wenckebach's) 426.13
  type II 426.12
Möbius'
  disease 346.8
  syndrome
    congenital oculofacial paralysis 352.6
    ophthalmoplegic migraine 346.8
Moeller (-Barlow) disease (infantile scurvy) 267
  glossitis 529.4
Mohr's syndrome (Types I and II) 759.89
Mola destruens (M9100/1) 236.1
Molarization, premolars 520.2
Molar pregnancy 631
  hydatidiform (delivered) (undelivered) 630
Mold (s) in vitreous 117.9
Molding, head (during birth) 767.3
Mole (pigmented) (M8720/0)—see also
      Neoplasm, skin, benign
  blood 631
  Breus' 631
  cancerous (M8720/3)—see Melanoma
  carneous 631
  destructive (M9100/1) 236.1
  ectopic—see Pregnancy, ectopic
  fleshy 631

Mole—*continued*
　hemorrhagic 631
　hydatid, hydatidiform (benign) (complicating
　　　pregnancy) (delivered) (undelivered) (*see*
　　　also Hydatidiform mole) 630
　　　invasive (M9100/1) 236.1
　　　malignant (M9100/1) 236.1
　　　previous, affecting management of pregnancy
　　　　V23.1
　　invasive (hydatidiform) (M9100/1) 236.1
　　malignant
　　　meaning
　　　　malignant hydatidiform mole (M9100/1)
　　　　　236.1
　　　　melanoma (M8720/3)—*see* Melanoma
　　nonpigmented (M8730/0)—*see* Neoplasm, skin,
　　　benign
　　pregnancy NEC 631
　　skin (M8720/0)—*see* Neoplasm, skin, benign
　　tubal—*see* Pregnancy, tubal
　　vesicular (*see also* Hydatidiform mole) 630
Molimen, molimina (menstrual) 625.4
Mollaret's meningitis 047.9
Mollities (cerebellar) (cerebral) 437.8
　ossium 268.2
Molluscum
　contagiosum 078.0
　epitheliale 078.0
　fibrosum (M8851/0)—*see* Lipoma, by site
　pendulum (M8851/0)—*see* Lipoma, by site
**Mönckeberg's arteriosclerosis, degeneration
　　disease, or sclerosis** (*see also*
　　Arteriosclerosis, extremities) 440.20
Monday fever 504
Monday morning dyspnea or asthma 504
Mondini's malformation (cochlea) 744.05
Mondor's disease (thrombophlebitis of breast)
　　451.89
**Mongolian, mongolianism, mongolism
　　mongoloid** 758.0
　spot 757.33
Monilethrix (congenital) 757.4
Monilia infestation —*see* Candidiasis
Moniliasis —*see also* Candidiasis
　neonatal 771.7
　vulvovaginitis 112.1
Monoarthritis 716.60
　ankle 716.67
　arm 716.62
　　lower (and wrist) 716.63
　　upper (and elbow) 716.62
　foot (and ankle) 716.67
　forearm (and wrist) 716.63
　hand 716.64
　leg 716.66
　　lower 716.66
　　upper 716.65
　pelvic region (hip) (thigh) 716.65
　shoulder (region) 716.61
　specified site NEC 716.68
Monoblastic —*see* condition
Monochromatism (cone) (rod) 368.54
Monocytic —*see* condition
Monocytosis (symptomatic) 288.8
Monofixation syndrome 378.34
Monomania (*see also* Psychosis) 298.9
Mononeuritis 355.9
　cranial nerve—*see* Disorder, nerve, cranial
　femoral nerve 355.2
　lateral
　　cutaneous nerve of thigh 355.1

Mononeuritis—*continued*
　popliteal nerve 355.3
　lower limb 355.8
　　specified nerve NEC 355.79
　medial popliteal nerve 355.4
　median nerve 354.1
　multiplex 354.5
　plantar nerve 355.6
　posterior tibial nerve 355.5
　radial nerve 354.3
　sciatic nerve 355.0
　ulnar nerve 354.2
　upper limb 354.9
　　specified nerve NEC 354.8
　vestibular 388.5
Mononeuropathy (*see also* Mononeuritis) 355.9
　diabetic NEC 250.6 *[355.9]*
　　lower limb 250.6 *[355.8]*
　　upper limb 250.6 *[354.9]*
　iliohypogastric nerve 355.79
　ilioinguinal nerve 355.79
　obturator nerve 355.79
　saphenous nerve 355.79
Mononucleosis, infectious 075
　with hepatitis 075 *[573.1]*
Monoplegia 344.5
　brain (current episode) (*see also* Paralysis,
　　brain) 437.8
　　fetus or newborn 767.8
　cerebral (current episode) (*see also* Paralysis,
　　brain) 437.8
　congenital or infantile (cerebral) (spastic)
　　(spinal) 343.3
　embolic (current) (*see also* Embolism, brain)
　　434.1
　　late effect—*see* Late effect(s) (of)
　　　cerebrovascular disease
　infantile (cerebral) (spastic) (spinal) 343.3
　lower limb 344.30
　　affecting
　　　dominant side 344.31
　　　nondominant side 344.32
　　due to late effect of cerebrovascular accident
　　　—*see* Late effect(s) (of) cerebrovascular
　　　accident
　newborn 767.8
　psychogenic 306.0
　　specified as conversion reaction 300.11
　thrombotic (current) (*see also* Thrombosis,
　　brain) 434.0
　　late effect—*see* Late effect(s) (of)
　　　cerebrovascular disease
　transient 781.4
　upper limb 344.40
　　affecting
　　　dominant side 344.41
　　　nondominant side 344.42
　　due to late effect of cerebrovascular accident
　　　—*see* Late effect(s) (of) cerebrovascular
　　　accident
Monorchism, monorchidism 752.8
Monteggia's fracture (closed) 813.03
　open 813.13
Mood swings
　brief compensatory 296.99
　rebound 296.99
Moore's syndrome (*see also* Epilepsy) 345.5
Mooren's ulcer (cornea) 370.07
Mooser-Neill reaction 081.0
Mooser bodies 081.0

Moral
 deficiency 301.7
 imbecility 301.7
Morax-Axenfeld conjunctivitis 372.03
Morbilli (*see also* Measles) 055.9
Morbus
 anglicus, anglorum 268.0
 Beigel 111.2
 caducus (*see also* Epilepsy) 345.9
 caeruleus 746.89
 celiacus 579.0
 comitialis (*see also* Epilepsy) 345.9
 cordis—*see also* Disease, heart
  valvulorum—*see* Endocarditis
 coxae 719.95
  tuberculous (*see also* Tuberculosis) 015.1
 hemorrhagicus neonatorum 776.0
 maculosus neonatorum 772.6
 renum 593.0
 senilis (*see also* Osteoarthrosis) 715.9
Morel-Kraepelin disease (*see also*
  Schizophrenia) 295.9
Morel-Moore syndrome (hyperostosis frontalis
  interna) 733.3
Morel-Morgagni syndrome (hyperostosis
  frontalis interna) 733.3
Morgagni
 cyst, organ, hydatid, or appendage 752.8
  fallopian tube 752.11
 disease or syndrome (hyperostosis frontalis
  interna) 733.3
Morgagni-Adams-Stokes syndrome (syncope
  with heart block) 426.9
Morgagni-Stewart-Morel syndrome
  (hyperostosis frontalis interna) 733.3
Moria (*see also* Psychosis) 298.9
Morning sickness 643.0
Moron 317
Morphea (guttate) (linear) 701.0
Morphine dependence (*see also* Dependence)
  304.0
Morphinism (*see also* Dependence) 304.0
Morphinomania (*see also* Dependence) 304.0
Morphoea 701.0
Morquio (-Brailsford) (-Ullrich) disease or
  syndrome (mucopolysaccharidosis IV) 277.5
 kyphosis 277.5
Morris syndrome (testicular feminization) 257.8
Morsus humanus (open wound)—*see also*
  Wound, open, by site
 skin surface intact—*see* Contusion
Mortification (dry) (moist) (*see also* Gangrene)
  785.4
Morton's
 disease 355.6
 foot 355.6
 metatarsalgia (syndrome) 355.6
 neuralgia 355.6
 neuroma 355.6
 syndrome (metatarsalgia) (neuralgia) 355.6
 toe 355.6
Morvan's disease 336.0
Mosaicism, mosaic (chromosomal) 758.9
 autosomal 758.5
 sex 758.81
Moschcowitz's syndrome (thrombotic
  thrombocytopenic purpura) 446.6
Mother yaw 102.0
Motion sickness (from travel, any vehicle) (from
  roundabouts or swings) 994.6
Mottled teeth (enamel) (endemic) (nonendemic)
  520.3

Mottling enamel (endemic) (nonendemic) (teeth)
  520.3
Mouchet's disease 732.5
Mould (s) (in vitreous) 117.9
Moulders'
 bronchitis 502
 tuberculosis (*see also* Tuberculosis) 011.4
Mounier-Kuhn syndrome 494.0
 with acute exacerbation 494.1
Mountain
 fever—*see* Fever, mountain
 sickness 993.2
  with polycythemia, acquired 289.0
  acute 289.0
 tick fever 066.1
Mouse, joint (*see also* Loose, body, joint) 718.1
 knee 717.6
Mouth —*see* condition
Movable
 coccyx 724.71
 kidney (*see also* Disease, renal) 593.0
  congenital 753.3
 organ or site, congenital NEC—*see*
   Malposition, congenital
 spleen 289.59
Movement
 abnormal (dystonic) (involuntary) 781.0
 decreased fetal 655.7
 paradoxical facial 374.43
Moya Moya disease 437.5
Mozart's ear 744.29
Mucha's disease (acute parapsoriasis
  varioliformis) 696.2
Mucha-Haberman syndrome (acute
  parapsoriasis varioliformis) 696.2
Mu-chain disease 273.2
Mucinosis (cutaneous) (papular) 701.8
Mucocele
 appendix 543.9
 buccal cavity 528.9
 gallbladder (*see also* Disease, gallbladder) 575.3
 lacrimal sac 375.43
 orbit (eye) 376.81
 salivary gland (any) 527.6
 sinus (accessory) (nasal) 478.1
 turbinate (bone) (middle) (nasal) 478.1
 uterus 621.8
Mucocutaneous lymph node syndrome (acute)
  (febrile) (infantile) 446.1
Mucoenteritis 564.9
Mucolipidosis I, II, III 272.7
Mucopolysaccharidosis (types 1-6) 277.5
 cardiopathy 277.5 [425.7]
Mucormycosis (lung) 117.7
Mucositis —*see also* Inflammation by site
 necroticans agranulocytica 288.0
Mucous —*see also* condition
 patches (syphilitic) 091.3
  congenital 090.0
Mucoviscidosis 277.00
 with meconium obstruction 277.01
Mucus
 asphyxia or suffocation (*see also* Asphyxia,
   mucus) 933.1
  newborn 770.1
 in stool 792.1
 plug (*see also* Asphyxia, mucus) 933.1
  aspiration, of newborn 770.1
  tracheobronchial 519.1
   newborn 770.1
Muguet 112.0
Mulberry molars 090.5

Mullerian mixed tumor (M8950/3)—*see*
  Neoplasm, by site, malignant
Multicystic kidney 753.19
Multilobed placenta —*see* Placenta, abnormal
Multinodular prostate 600.1
Multiparity V61.5
  affecting
    fetus or newborn 763.89
    management of
      labor and delivery 659.4
      pregnancy V23.3
  requiring contraceptive management (*see also*
      Contraception) V25.9
Multipartita placenta —*see* Placenta, abnormal
Multiple, multiplex —*see also* condition
  birth
    affecting fetus or newborn 761.5
    healthy liveborn—*see* Newborn, multiple
  digits (congenital) 755.00
    fingers 755.01
    toes 755.02
  organ or site NEC—*see* Accessory
  personality 300.14
  renal arteries 747.62
Mumps 072.9
  with complication 072.8
    specified type NEC 072.79
  encephalitis 072.2
  hepatitis 072.71
  meningitis (aseptic) 072.1
  meningoencephalitis 072.2
  oophoritis 072.79
  orchitis 072.0
  pancreatitis 072.3
  polyneuropathy 072.72
  vaccination, prophylactic (against) V04.6
Mumu (*see also* Infestation, filarial) 125.9
Münchausen syndrome 301.51
Münchmeyer's disease or syndrome (exostosis
    luxurians) 728.11
Mural —*see* condition
Murmur (cardiac) (heart) (nonorganic) (organic)
    785.2
  abdominal 787.5
  aortic (valve) (*see also* Endocarditis, aortic)
    424.1
  benign—*omit code*
  cardiorespiratory 785.2
  diastolic—*see* condition
  Flint (*see also* Endocarditis, aortic) 424.1
  functional—*omit code*
  Graham Steell (pulmonic regurgitation) (*see
      also* Endocarditis, pulmonary) 424.3
  innocent—*omit code*
  insignificant—*omit code*
  midsystolic 785.2
  mitral (valve)—*see* stenosis, mitral
  physiologic—*see* condition
  presystolic, mitral—*see* Insufficiency, mitral
  pulmonic (valve) (*see also* Endocarditis,
      pulmonary) 424.3
  Still's (vibratory)—*omit code*
  systolic (valvular)—*see* condition
  tricuspid (valve)—*see* Endocarditis, tricuspid
  valvular—*see* condition
  vibratory—*omit code*
  undiagnosed 785.2
Murri's disease (intermittent hemoglobinuria)
    283.2
Muscae volitantes 379.24
Muscle, muscular —*see* condition
Musculoneuralgia 729.1

Mushrooming hip 718.95
Mushroom workers' (pickers') lung 495.5
Mutism (*see also* Aphasia) 784.3
  akinetic 784.3
  deaf (acquired) (congenital) 389.7
  elective (selective) 313.23
    adjustment reaction 309.83
  hysterical 300.11
Myà's disease (congenital dilation, colon) 751.3
Myalgia (intercostal) 729.1
  eosinophilia syndrome 710.5
  epidemic 074.1
    cervical 078.89
  psychogenic 307.89
  traumatic NEC 959.9
Myasthenia, myasthenic 358.0
  cordis—*see* Failure, heart
  gravis 358.0
    neonatal 775.2
    pseudoparalytica 358.0
  stomach 536.8
    psychogenic 306.4
  syndrome in
    botulism 005.1 *[358.1]*
    diabetes mellitus 250.6 *[358.1]*
    hypothyroidism (*see also* Hypothyroidism)
        244.9 *[358.1]*
    malignant neoplasm NEC 199.1 *[358.1]*
    pernicious anemia 281.0 *[358.1]*
    thyrotoxicosis (*see also* Thyrotoxicosis) 242.9
        [358.1]
Mycelium infection NEC 117.9
Mycetismus 988.1
Mycetoma (actinomycotic) 039.9
  bone 039.8
    mycotic 117.4
  foot 039.4
    mycotic 117.4
  madurae 039.9
    mycotic 117.4
  maduromycotic 039.9
    mycotic 117.4
  mycotic 117.4
  nocardial 039.9
Mycobacteriosis —*see* Mycobacterium
Mycobacterium, mycobacterial (infection)
    031.9
  acid-fast (bacilli) 031.9
  anonymous (*see also* Mycobacterium, atypical)
    031.9
  atypical (acid-fast bacilli) 031.9
    cutaneous 031.1
    pulmonary 031.0
      tuberculous (*see also* Tuberculosis,
          pulmonary) 011.9
    specified site NEC 031.8
  avium 031.0
    intracellulare complex bacteremia (MAC)
        031.2
  balnei 031.1
  Battey 031.0
  cutaneous 031.1
  disseminated 031.2
    avium-intracellulare complex (DMAC) 031.2
  fortuitum 031.0
  intracellulare (battey bacillus) 031.0
  kakerifu 031.8
  kansasii 031.0
  kasongo 031.8
  leprae—*see* Leprosy
  luciflavum 031.0

Mycobacterium, mycobacterial—*continued*
  marinum 031.1
  pulmonary 031.0
    tuberculous (*see also* Tuberculosis,
        pulmonary) 011.9
  scrofulaceum 031.1
  tuberculosis (human, bovine)—*see also*
      Tuberculosis
    avian type 031.0
  ulcerans 031.1
  xenopi 031.0
Mycosis, mycotic 117.9
  cutaneous NEC 111.9
  ear 111.8 *[380.15]*
  fungoides (M9700/3) 202.1
  mouth 112.0
  pharynx 117.9
  skin NEC 111.9
  stomatitis 112.0
  systemic NEC 117.9
  tonsil 117.9
  vagina, vaginitis 112.1
Mydriasis (persistent) (pupil) 379.43
Myelatelia 742.59
Myelinoclasis, perivascular, acute
    (postinfectious) NEC 136.9 *[323.6]*
  postimmunization or postvaccinal 323.5
Myelinosis, central pontine 341.8
Myelitis (acute) (ascending) (cerebellar)
    (childhood) (chronic) (descending) (diffuse)
    (disseminated) (pressure) (progressive) (spinal
    cord) (subacute) (transverse) (*see also*
    Encephalitis) 323.9
  late effect—*see* category 326
  optic neuritis in 341.0
  postchickenpox 052.7
  postvaccinal 323.5
  syphilitic (transverse) 094.89
  tuberculous (*see also* Tuberculosis) 013.6
  virus 049.9
Myeloblastic —*see* condition
Myelocele (*see also* Spina bifida) 741.9
  with hydrocephalus 741.0
Myelocystocele (*see also* Spina bifida) 741.9
Myelocytic —*see* condition
Myelocytoma 205.1
Myelodysplasia (spinal cord) 742.59
  meaning myelodysplastic syndrome—*see*
      Syndrome, myelodysplastic
Myeloencephalitis —*see* Encephalitis
Myelofibrosis (osteosclerosis) 289.8
Myelogenous —*see* condition
Myeloid —*see* condition
Myelokathexis 288.0
Myeloleukodystrophy 330.0
Myelolipoma (M8870/0)—*see* Neoplasm, by
    site, benign
Myeloma (multiple) (plasma cell) (plasmacytic)
    (M9730/3) 203.0
  monostotic (M9731/1) 238.6
  solitary (M9731/1) 238.6
Myelomalacia 336.8
Myelomata, multiple (M9730/3) 203.0
Myelomatosis (M9730/3) 203.0
Myelomeningitis —*see* Meningoencephalitis
Myelomeningocele (spinal cord) (*see also* Spina
    bifida) 741.9
  fetal, causing fetopelvic disproportion 653.7
Myelo-osteo-musculodysplasia hereditaria
    756.89
Myelopathic —*see* condition

Myelopathy (spinal cord) 336.9
  cervical 721.1
  diabetic 250.6 *[336.3]*
  drug-induced 336.8
  due to or with
    carbon tetrachloride 987.8 *[323.7]*
    degeneration or displacement, intervertebral
        disc 722.70
      cervical, cervicothoracic 722.71
      lumbar, lumbosacral 722.73
      thoracic, thoracolumbar 722.72
    hydroxyquinoline derivatives 961.3 *[323.7]*
    infection—*see* Encephalitis
    intervertebral disc disorder 722.70
      cervical, cervicothoracic 722.71
      lumbar, lumbosacral 722.73
      thoracic, thoracolumbar 722.72
    lead 984.9 *[323.7]*
    mercury 985.0 *[323.7]*
    neoplastic disease (*see also* Neoplasm, by
        site) 239.9 *[336.3]*
    pernicious anemia 281.0 *[336.3]*
    spondylosis 721.91
      cervical 721.1
      lumbar, lumbosacral 721.42
      thoracic 721.41
    thallium 985.8 *[323.7]*
  lumbar, lumbosacral 721.42
  necrotic (subacute) 336.1
  radiation-induced 336.8
  spondylogenic NEC 721.91
    cervical 721.1
    lumbar, lumbosacral 721.42
    thoracic 721.41
  thoracic 721.41
  toxic NEC 989.9 *[323.7]*
  transverse (*see also* Encephalitis) 323.9
  vascular 336.1
Myeloproliferative disease (M9960/1) 238.7
Myeloradiculitis (*see also* Polyneuropathy) 357.0
Myeloradiculodysplasia (spinal) 742.59
Myelosarcoma (M9930/3) 205.3
Myelosclerosis 289.8
  with myeloid metaplasia (M9961/1) 238.7
  disseminated, of nervous system 340
  megakaryocytic (M9961/1) 238.7
Myelosis (M9860/3) (*see also* Leukemia,
    myeloid) 205.9
  acute (M9861/3) 205.0
  aleukemic (M9864/3) 205.8
  chronic (M9863/3) 205.1
  erythremic (M9840/3) 207.0
    acute (M9841/3) 207.0
  megakaryocytic (M9920/3) 207.2
  nonleukemic (chronic) 288.8
  subacute (M9862/3) 205.2
Myesthenia —*see* Myasthenia
Myiasis (cavernous) 134.0
  orbit 134.0 *[376.13]*
Myoadenoma, prostate 600.2
Myoblastoma
  granular cell (M9580/0)—*see also* Neoplasm,
      connective tissue, benign
    malignant (M9580/3)—*see* Neoplasm,
      connective tissue, malignant
  tongue (M9580/0) 210.1
Myocardial —*see* condition

Myxochondrosarcoma (M9220/3)—*see*
   Neoplasm, cartilage, malignant
Myxofibroma (M8811/0)—*see also* Neoplasm,
   connective tissue, benign
  odontogenic (M9320/0) 213.1
   upper jaw (bone) 213.0
Myxofibrosarcoma (M8811/3)—*see* Neoplasm,
   connective tissue, malignant
Myxolipoma (M8852/0) (*see also* Lipoma, by
   site) 214.9
Myxoliposarcoma (M8852/3)—*see* Neoplasm,
   connective tissue, malignant
Myxoma (M8840/0)—*see also* Neoplasm,
   connective tissue, benign
  odontogenic (M9320/0) 213.1
   upper jaw (bone) 213.0
Myxosarcoma (M8840/3)—*see* Neoplasm,
   connective tissue, malignant

N

Necrobiosis 799.8
  brain or cerebral (*see also* Softening, brain)
    437.8
  lipoidica 709.3
    diabeticorum 250.8 *[709.3]*
Necrodermolysis 695.1
Necrolysis, toxic epidermal 695.1
  due to drug
    correct substance properly administered 695.1
    overdose or wrong substance given or taken
      977.9
      specified drug—*see* Table of drugs and
        chemicals
Necrophilia 302.89
Necrosis, necrotic
  adrenal (capsule) (gland) 255.8
  antrum, nasal sinus 478.1
  aorta (hyaline) (*see also* Aneurysm, aorta) 441.9
    cystic medial 441.00
      abdominal 441.02
      thoracic 441.01
      thoracoabdominal 441.03
    ruptured 441.5
  arteritis 446.0
  artery 447.5
  aseptic, bone 733.40
    femur (head) (neck) 733.42
      medial condyle 733.43
    humoral head 733.41
    medial femoral condyle 733.43
    specified site NEC 733.49
    talus 733.44
  avascular, bone NEC (*see also* Necrosis,
    aseptic, bone) 733.40
  bladder (aseptic) (sphincter) 596.8
  bone (*see also* Osteomyelitis) 730.1
    acute 730.0
    aseptic or avascular 733.40
      femur (head) (neck) 733.42
        medial condyle 733.43
      humoral head 733.41
      medial femoral condyle 733.43
      specified site NEC 733.49
      talus 733.44
    ethmoid 478.1
    ischemic 733.40
    jaw 526.4
    marrow 289.8
    Paget's (osteitis deformans) 731.0
    tuberculous—*see* Tuberculosis, bone
  brain (softening) (*see also* Softening, brain)
    437.8
  breast (aseptic) (fat) (segmental) 611.3
  bronchus, bronchi 519.1
  central nervous system NEC (*see also*
    Softening, brain) 437.8
  cerebellar (*see also* Softening, brain) 437.8
  cerebral (softening) (*see also* Softening, brain)
    437.8
  cerebrospinal (softening) (*see also* Softening,
    brain) 437.8
  cornea (*see also* Keratitis) 371.40
  cortical, kidney 583.6
  cystic medial (aorta) 441.00
    abdominal 441.02
    thoracic 441.01
    thoracoabdominal 441.03
  dental 521.09
    pulp 522.1

Necrosis, necrotic—*continued*
  due to swallowing corrosive substance—*see*
    Burn, by site
  ear (ossicle) 385.24
  esophagus 530.89
  ethmoid (bone) 478.1
  eyelid 374.50
  fat, fatty (generalized) (*see also* Degeneration,
    fatty) 272.8
    breast (aseptic) (segmental) 611.3
    intestine 569.89
    localized—*see* Degeneration, by site, fatty
    mesentery 567.8
    omentum 567.8
    pancreas 577.8
    peritoneum 567.8
    skin (subcutaneous) 709.3
      newborn 778.1
  femur (aseptic) (avascular) 733.42
    head 733.42
    medial condyle 733.43
    neck 733.42
  gallbladder (*see also* Cholecystitis, acute) 575.0
  gangrenous 785.4
  gastric 537.89
  glottis 478.79
  heart (myocardium)—*see* Infarct, myocardium
  hepatic (*see also* Necrosis, liver) 570
  hip (aseptic) (avascular) 733.42
  intestine (acute) (hemorrhagic) (massive) 557.0
  ischemic 785.4
  jaw 526.4
  kidney (bilateral) 583.9
    acute 584.9
    cortical 583.6
      acute 584.6
        with
          abortion—*see* Abortion, by type, with
            renal failure
          ectopic pregnancy (*see also* categories
            633.0-633.9) 639.3
          molar pregnancy (*see also* categories
            630-632) 639.3
        complicating pregnancy 646.2
          affecting fetus or newborn 760.1
        following labor and delivery 669.3
    medullary (papillary) (*see also* Pyelitis) 590.80
      in
        acute renal failure 584.7
        nephritis, nephropathy 583.7
    papillary (*see also* Pyelitis) 590.80
      in
        acute renal failure 584.7
        nephritis, nephropathy 583.7
    tubular 584.5
      with
        abortion—*see* Abortion, by type, with
          renal failure
        ectopic pregnancy (*see also* categories
          633.0-633.9) 639.3
        molar pregnancy (*see also* categories
          630-632) 639.3
      complicating
        abortion 639.3
        ectopic or molar pregnancy 639.3
        pregnancy 646.2
          affecting fetus or newborn 760.1
      following labor and delivery 669.3
      traumatic 958.5
  larynx 478.79

Necrosis, necrotic—*continued*
  liver (acute) (congenital) (diffuse) (massive)
    (subacute) 570
    with
      abortion—*see* Abortion, by type, with
        specified complication NEC
      ectopic pregnancy (*see also* categories
        633.0-633.9) 639.8
      molar pregnancy (*see also* categories
        630-632) 639.8
      complicating pregnancy 646.7
        affecting fetus or newborn 760.8
      following
        abortion 639.8
        ectopic or molar pregnancy 639.8
      obstetrical 646.7
      postabortal 639.8
      puerperal, postpartum 674.8
      toxic 573.3
  lung 513.0
  lymphatic gland 683
  mammary gland 611.3
  mastoid (chronic) 383.1
  mesentery 557.0
    fat 567.8
  mitral valve—*see* Insufficiency, mitral
  myocardium, myocardial—*see* Infarct,
    myocardium
  nose (septum) 478.1
  omentum 557.0
    with mesenteric infarction 557.0
    fat 567.8
  orbit, orbital 376.10
  ossicles, ear (aseptic) 385.24
  ovary (*see also* Salpingo-oophoritis) 614.2
  pancreas (aseptic) (duct) (fat) 577.8
    acute 577.0
    infective 577.0
  papillary, kidney (*see also* Pyelitis) 590.80
  peritoneum 557.0
    with mesenteric infarction 557.0
    fat 567.8
  pharynx 462
    in granulocytopenia 288.0
  phosphorus 983.9
  pituitary (gland) (postpartum) (Sheehan) 253.2
  placenta (*see also* Placenta, abnormal) 656.7
  pneumonia 513.0
  pulmonary 513.0
  pulp (dental) 522.1
  pylorus 537.89
  radiation—*see* Necrosis, by site
  radium—*see* Necrosis, by site
  renal—*see* Necrosis, kidney
  sclera 379.19
  scrotum 608.89
  skin or subcutaneous tissue 709.8
    due to burn—*see* Burn, by site
    gangrenous 785.4
  spine, spinal (column) 730.18
    acute 730.18
    cord 336.1
  spleen 289.59
  stomach 537.89
  stomatitis 528.1
  subcutaneous fat 709.3
    fetus or newborn 778.1
  subendocardial—*see* Infarct, myocardium
  suprarenal (capsule) (gland) 255.8

Necrosis, necrotic—*continued*
  teeth, tooth 521.09
  testis 608.89
  thymus (gland) 254.8
  tonsil 474.8
  trachea 519.1
  tuberculous NEC—*see* Tuberculosis
  tubular (acute) (anoxic) (toxic) 584.5
    due to a procedure 997.5
  umbilical cord, affecting fetus or newborn 762.6
  vagina 623.8
  vertebra (lumbar) 730.18
    acute 730.18
    tuberculous (*see also* Tuberculosis) 015.0
      [730.8]
  vesical (aseptic) (bladder) 596.8
  x-ray—*see* Necrosis, by site
Necrospermia 606.0
Necrotizing angiitis 446.0
Negativism 301.7
Neglect (child) (newborn) NEC 995.52
  adult 995.84
  after or at birth 995.52
  hemispatial 781.8
  left-sided 781.8
  sensory 781.8
  visuospatial 781.8
Negri bodies 071
Neill-Dingwall syndrome (microcephaly and
  dwarfism) 759.89
Neisserian infection NEC—*see* Gonococcus
Nematodiasis NEC (*see also* Infestation,
  Nematode) 127.9
  ancylostoma (*see also* Ancylostomiasis) 126.9
Neoformans cryptococcus infection 117.5
Neonatal —*see also* condition
  teeth, tooth 520.6
Neonatorum —*see* condition

*"N" listing resumes after
"Neoplasm, neoplastic" table…*

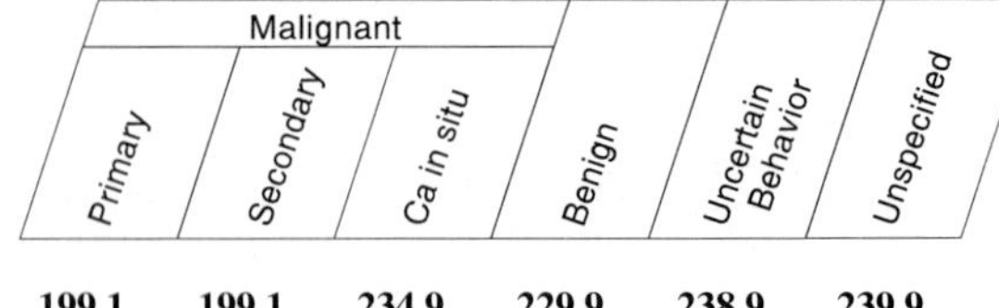

	Malignant					
	Primary	Secondary	Ca in situ	Benign	Uncertain Behavior	Unspecified
Neoplasm, neoplastic	**199.1**	**199.1**	**234.9**	**229.9**	**238.9**	**239.9**

> *Note—1. The list below gives the code numbers for neoplasms by anatomical site. For each site there are six possible code numbers according to whether the neoplasm in question is malignant, benign, in situ, of uncertain behavior, or of unspecified nature. The description of the neoplasm will often indicate which of the six columns is appropriate; e.g., malignant melanoma of skin, benign fibroadenoma of breast, carcinoma in situ of cervix uteri.*
>
> *Where such descriptors are not present, the remainder of the Index should be consulted where guidance is given to the appropriate column for each morphological (histological) variety listed; e.g., Mesonephroma—see Neoplasm, malignant; Embryoma—see also Neoplasm, uncertain behavior; Disease, Bowen's—see Neoplasm, skin, in situ. However, the guidance in the Index can be overridden if one of the descriptors mentioned above is present; e.g., malignant adenoma of colon is coded to 153.9 and not to 211.3 as the adjective "malignant" overrides the Index entry "Adenoma—see also Neoplasm, benign."*
>
> *Note—2. Sites marked with the sign * (e.g., face NEC*) should be classified to malignant neoplasm of skin of these sites if the variety of neoplasm is a squamous cell carcinoma or an epidermoid carcinoma and to benign neoplasm of skin of these sites if the variety of neoplasm is a papilloma (any type).*

	Primary	Secondary	Ca in situ	Benign	Uncertain Behavior	Unspecified
abdomen, abdominal	195.2	198.89	234.8	229.8	238.8	239.8
cavity	195.2	198.89	234.8	229.8	238.8	239.8
organ	195.2	198.89	234.8	229.8	238.8	239.8
viscera	195.2	198.89	234.8	229.8	238.8	239.8
wall	173.5	198.2	232.5	216.5	238.2	239.2
connective tissue	171.5	198.89	—	215.5	238.1	239.2
abdominopelvic	195.8	198.89	234.8	229.8	238.8	239.8
accessory sinus—*see* Neoplasm, sinus						
acoustic nerve	192.0	198.4	—	225.1	237.9	239.7
acromion (process)	170.4	198.5	—	213.4	238.0	239.2
adenoid (pharynx) (tissue)	147.1	198.89	230.0	210.7	235.1	239.0
adipose tissue *(see also* Neoplasm,						
connective tissue)	171.9	198.89	—	215.9	238.1	239.2
adnexa (uterine)	183.9	198.82	233.3	221.8	236.3	239.5
adrenal (cortex) (gland) (medulla)	194.0	198.7	234.8	227.0	237.2	239.7
ala nasi (external)	173.3	198.2	232.3	216.3	238.2	239.2
alimentary canal or tract NEC	159.9	197.8	230.9	211.9	235.5	239.0
alveolar	143.9	198.89	230.0	210.4	235.1	239.0
mucosa	143.9	198.89	230.0	210.4	235.1	239.0
lower	143.1	198.89	230.0	210.4	235.1	239.0
upper	143.0	198.89	230.0	210.4	235.1	239.0
ridge or process	170.1	198.5	—	213.1	238.0	239.2
carcinoma	143.9	—	—	—	—	—
lower	143.1	—	—	—	—	—
upper	143.0	—	—	—	—	—
lower	170.1	198.5	—	213.1	238.0	239.2
mucosa	143.9	198.89	230.0	210.4	235.1	239.0
lower	143.1	198.89	230.0	210.4	235.1	239.0
upper	143.0	198.89	230.0	210.4	235.1	239.0
upper	170.0	198.5	—	213.0	238.0	239.2
sulcus	145.1	198.89	230.0	210.4	235.1	239.0
alveolus	143.9	198.89	230.0	210.4	235.1	239.0
lower	143.1	198.89	230.0	210.4	235.1	239.0
upper	143.0	198.89	230.0	210.4	235.1	239.0
ampulla of Vater	156.2	197.8	230.8	211.5	235.3	239.0
ankle NEC*	195.5	198.89	232.7	229.8	238.8	239.8
anorectum, anorectal (junction)	154.8	197.5	230.7	211.4	235.2	239.0
antecubital fossa or space*	195.4	198.89	232.6	229.8	238.8	239.8
antrum (Highmore) (maxillary)	160.2	197.3	231.8	212.0	235.9	239.1
pyloric	151.2	197.8	230.2	211.1	235.2	239.0
tympanicum	160.1	197.3	231.8	212.0	235.9	239.1
anus, anal	154.3	197.5	230.6	211.4	235.5	239.0
canal	154.2	197.5	230.5	211.4	235.5	239.0

	Malignant					
	Primary	Secondary	Ca in situ	Benign	Uncertain Behavior	Unspecified

anus, anal—*continued*

	Primary	Secondary	Ca in situ	Benign	Uncertain Behavior	Unspecified
contiguous sites with rectosigmoid junction or rectum	154.8	—	—	—	—	—
margin	173.5	198.2	232.5	216.5	238.2	239.2
skin	173.5	198.2	232.5	216.5	238.2	239.2
sphincter	154.2	197.5	230.5	211.4	235.5	239.0
aorta (thoracic)	171.4	198.89	—	215.4	238.1	239.2
abdominal	171.5	198.89	—	215.5	238.1	239.2
aortic body	194.6	198.89	—	227.6	237.3	239.7
aponeurosis	171.9	198.89	—	215.9	238.1	239.2
palmar	171.2	198.89	—	215.2	238.1	239.2
plantar	171.3	198.89	—	215.3	238.1	239.2
appendix	153.5	197.5	230.3	211.3	235.2	239.0
arachnoid (cerebral)	192.1	198.4	—	225.2	237.6	239.7
spinal	192.3	198.4	—	225.4	237.6	239.7
areola (female)	174.0	198.81	233.0	217	238.3	239.3
male	175.0	198.81	233.0	217	238.3	239.3
arm NEC*	195.4	198.89	232.6	229.8	238.8	239.8
artery—*see* Neoplasm, connective tissue						
aryepiglottic fold	148.2	198.89	230.0	210.8	235.1	239.0
hypopharyngeal aspect	148.2	198.89	230.0	210.8	235.1	239.0
laryngeal aspect	161.1	197.3	231.0	212.1	235.6	239.1
marginal zone	148.2	198.89	230.0	210.8	235.1	239.0
arytenoid (cartilage)	161.3	197.3	231.0	212.1	235.6	239.1
fold—*see* Neoplasm, aryepiglottic						
atlas	170.2	198.5	—	213.2	238.0	239.2
atrium, cardiac	164.1	198.89	—	212.7	238.8	239.8
auditory						
canal (external) (skin)	173.2	198.2	232.2	216.2	238.2	239.2
internal	160.1	197.3	231.8	212.0	235.9	239.1
nerve	192.0	198.4	—	225.1	237.9	239.7
tube	160.1	197.3	231.8	212.0	235.9	239.1
opening	147.2	198.89	230.0	210.7	235.1	239.0
auricle, ear	173.2	198.2	232.2	216.2	238.2	239.2
cartilage	171.0	198.89	—	215.0	238.1	239.2
auricular canal (external)	173.2	198.2	232.2	216.2	238.2	239.2
internal	160.1	197.3	231.8	212.0	235.9	239.1
autonomic nerve or nervous system NEC	171.9	198.89	—	215.9	238.1	239.2
axilla, axillary	195.1	198.89	234.8	229.8	238.8	239.8
fold	173.5	198.2	232.5	216.5	238.2	239.2
back NEC*	195.8	198.89	232.5	229.8	238.8	239.8
Bartholin's gland	184.1	198.82	233.3	221.2	236.3	239.5
basal ganglia	191.0	198.3	—	225.0	237.5	239.6
basis pedunculi	191.7	198.3	—	225.0	237.5	239.6
bile or biliary (tract)	156.9	197.8	230.8	211.5	235.3	239.0
canaliculi (biliferi) (intrahepatic)	155.1	197.8	230.8	211.5	235.3	239.0
canals, interlobular	155.1	197.8	230.8	211.5	235.3	239.0
contiguous sites	156.8	—	—	—	—	—
duct or passage (common) (cyst) (extrahepatic)	156.1	197.8	230.8	211.5	235.3	239.0
contiguous sites with gallbladder	156.8	—	—	—	—	—
interlobular	155.1	197.8	230.8	211.5	235.3	239.0
intrahepatic	155.1	197.8	230.8	211.5	235.3	239.0
and extrahepatic	156.9	197.8	230.8	211.5	235.3	239.0
bladder (urinary)	188.9	198.1	233.7	223.3	236.7	239.4
contiguous sites	188.8	—	—	—	—	—
dome	188.1	198.1	233.7	223.3	236.7	239.4
neck	188.5	198.1	233.7	223.3	236.7	239.4
orifice	188.9	198.1	233.7	223.3	236.7	239.4
ureteric	188.6	198.1	233.7	223.3	236.7	239.4
urethral	188.5	198.1	233.7	223.3	236.7	239.4
sphincter	188.8	198.1	233.7	223.3	236.7	239.4
trigone	188.0	198.1	233.7	223.3	236.7	239.4

| | Malignant | | | | | |
	Primary	Secondary	Ca in situ	Benign	Uncertain Behavior	Unspecified
urachus	188.7	—	233.7	223.3	236.7	239.4
wall	188.9	198.1	233.7	223.3	236.7	239.4
anterior	188.3	198.1	233.7	223.3	236.7	239.4
lateral	188.2	198.1	233.7	223.3	236.7	239.4
posterior	188.4	198.1	233.7	223.3	236.7	239.4

blood vessel—*see* Neoplasm, connective tissue

> *Note—Carcinomas and adenocarcinomas, of any type other than intraosseous or odontogenic, of the sites listed under "Neoplasm, bone" should be considered as constituting metastatic spread from an unspecified primary site and coded to 198.5 for morbidity coding and to 199.1 for underlying cause of death coding.*

	Primary	Secondary	Ca in situ	Benign	Uncertain Behavior	Unspecified
bone (periosteum)	170.9	198.5	—	213.9	238.0	239.2
acetabulum	170.6	198.5	—	213.6	238.0	239.2
acromion (process)	170.4	198.5	—	213.4	238.0	239.2
ankle	170.8	198.5	—	213.8	238.0	239.2
arm NEC	170.4	198.5	—	213.4	238.0	239.2
astragalus	170.8	198.5	—	213.8	238.0	239.2
atlas	170.2	198.5	—	213.2	238.0	239.2
axis	170.2	198.5	—	213.2	238.0	239.2
back NEC	170.2	198.5	—	213.2	238.0	239.2
calcaneus	170.8	198.5	—	213.8	238.0	239.2
calvarium	170.0	198.5	—	213.0	238.0	239.2
carpus (any)	170.5	198.5	—	213.5	238.0	239.2
cartilage NEC	170.9	198.5	—	213.9	238.0	239.2
clavicle	170.3	198.5	—	213.3	238.0	239.2
clivus	170.0	198.5	—	213.0	238.0	239.2
coccygeal vertebra	170.6	198.5	—	213.6	238.0	239.2
coccyx	170.6	198.5	—	213.6	238.0	239.2
costal cartilage	170.3	198.5	—	213.3	238.0	239.2
costovertebral joint	170.3	198.5	—	213.3	238.0	239.2
cranial	170.0	198.5	—	213.0	238.0	239.2
cuboid	170.8	198.5	—	213.8	238.0	239.2
cuneiform	170.9	198.5	—	213.9	238.0	239.2
ankle	170.8	198.5	—	213.8	238.0	239.2
wrist	170.5	198.5	—	213.5	238.0	239.2
digital	170.9	198.5	—	213.9	238.0	239.2
finger	170.5	198.5	—	213.5	238.0	239.2
toe	170.8	198.5	—	213.8	238.0	239.2
elbow	170.4	198.5	—	213.4	238.0	239.2
ethmoid (labyrinth)	170.0	198.5	—	213.0	238.0	239.2
face	170.0	198.5	—	213.0	238.0	239.2
lower jaw	170.1	198.5	—	213.1	238.0	239.2
femur (any part)	170.7	198.5	—	213.7	238.0	239.2
fibula (any part)	170.7	198.5	—	213.7	238.0	239.2
finger (any)	170.5	198.5	—	213.5	238.0	239.2
foot	170.8	198.5	—	213.8	238.0	239.2
forearm	170.4	198.5	—	213.4	238.0	239.2
frontal	170.0	198.5	—	213.0	238.0	239.2
hand	170.5	198.5	—	213.5	238.0	239.2
heel	170.8	198.5	—	213.8	238.0	239.2
hip	170.6	198.5	—	213.6	238.0	239.2
humerus (any part)	170.4	198.5	—	213.4	238.0	239.2
hyoid	170.0	198.5	—	213.0	238.0	239.2
ilium	170.6	198.5	—	213.6	238.0	239.2
innominate	170.6	198.5	—	213.6	238.0	239.2
intervertebral cartilage or disc	170.2	198.5	—	213.2	238.0	239.2
ischium	170.6	198.5	—	213.6	238.0	239.2
jaw (lower)	170.1	198.5	—	213.1	238.0	239.2
upper	170.0	198.5	—	213.0	238.0	239.2
knee	170.7	198.5	—	213.7	238.0	239.2
leg NEC	170.7	198.5	—	213.7	238.0	239.2
limb NEC	170.9	198.5	—	213.9	238.0	239.2
lower (long bones)	170.7	198.5	—	213.7	238.0	239.2

| | Malignant | | | | | |
---	Primary	Secondary	Ca in situ	Benign	Uncertain Behavior	Unspecified
bone—*continued*						
short bones	170.8	198.5	—	213.8	238.0	239.2
upper (long bones)	170.4	198.5	—	213.4	238.0	239.2
short bones	170.5	198.5	—	213.5	238.0	239.2
long	170.9	198.5	—	213.9	238.0	239.2
lower limbs NEC	170.7	198.5	—	213.7	238.0	239.2
upper limbs NEC	170.4	198.5	—	213.4	238.0	239.2
malar	170.0	198.5	—	213.0	238.0	239.2
mandible	170.1	198.5	—	213.1	238.0	239.2
marrow NEC	202.9	198.5	—	—	—	238.7
mastoid	170.0	198.5	—	213.0	238.0	239.2
maxilla, maxillary (superior)	170.0	198.5	—	213.0	238.0	239.2
inferior	170.1	198.5	—	213.1	238.0	239.2
metacarpus (any)	170.5	198.5	—	213.5	238.0	239.2
metatarsus (any)	170.8	198.5	—	213.8	238.0	239.2
navicular (ankle)	170.8	198.5	—	213.8	238.0	239.2
hand	170.5	198.5	—	213.5	238.0	239.2
nose, nasal	170.0	198.5	—	213.0	238.0	239.2
occipital	170.0	198.5	—	213.0	238.0	239.2
orbit	170.0	198.5	—	213.0	238.0	239.2
parietal	170.0	198.5	—	213.0	238.0	239.2
patella	170.8	198.5	—	213.8	238.0	239.2
pelvic	170.6	198.5	—	213.6	238.0	239.2
phalanges	170.9	198.5	—	213.9	238.0	239.2
foot	170.8	198.5	—	213.8	238.0	239.2
hand	170.5	198.5	—	213.5	238.0	239.2
pubic	170.6	198.5	—	213.6	238.0	239.2
radius (any part)	170.4	198.5	—	213.4	238.0	239.2
rib	170.3	198.5	—	213.3	238.0	239.2
sacral vertebra	170.6	198.5	—	213.6	238.0	239.2
sacrum	170.6	198.5	—	213.6	238.0	239.2
scaphoid (of hand)	170.5	198.5	—	213.5	238.0	239.2
of ankle	170.8	198.5	—	213.8	238.0	239.2
scapula (any part)	170.4	198.5	—	213.4	238.0	239.2
sella turcica	170.0	198.5	—	213.0	238.0	239.2
short	170.9	198.5	—	213.9	238.0	239.2
lower limb	170.8	198.5	—	213.8	238.0	239.2
upper limb	170.5	198.5	—	213.5	238.0	239.2
shoulder	170.4	198.5	—	213.4	238.0	239.2
skeleton, skeletal NEC	170.9	198.5	—	213.9	238.0	239.2
skull	170.0	198.5	—	213.0	238.0	239.2
sphenoid	170.0	198.5	—	213.0	238.0	239.2
spine, spinal (column)	170.2	198.5	—	213.2	238.0	239.2
coccyx	170.6	198.5	—	213.6	238.0	239.2
sacrum	170.6	198.5	—	213.6	238.0	239.2
sternum	170.3	198.5	—	213.3	238.0	239.2
tarsus (any)	170.8	198.5	—	213.8	238.0	239.2
temporal	170.0	198.5	—	213.0	238.0	239.2
thumb	170.5	198.5	—	213.5	238.0	239.2
tibia (any part)	170.7	198.5	—	213.7	238.0	239.2
toe (any)	170.8	198.5	—	213.8	238.0	239.2
trapezium	170.5	198.5	—	213.5	238.0	239.2
trapezoid	170.5	198.5	—	213.5	238.0	239.2
turbinate	170.0	198.5	—	213.0	238.0	239.2
ulna (any part)	170.4	198.5	—	213.4	238.0	239.2
unciform	170.5	198.5	—	213.5	238.0	239.2
vertebra (column)	170.2	198.5	—	213.2	238.0	239.2
coccyx	170.6	198.5	—	213.6	238.0	239.2
sacrum	170.6	198.5	—	213.6	238.0	239.2
vomer	170.0	198.5	—	213.0	238.0	239.2
wrist	170.5	198.5	—	213.5	238.0	239.2
xiphoid process	170.3	198.5	—	213.3	238.0	239.2
zygomatic	170.0	198.5	—	213.0	238.0	239.2

| | Malignant | | | | | |
	Primary	Secondary	Ca in situ	Benign	Uncertain Behavior	Unspecified
book-leaf (mouth)	145.8	198.89	230.0	210.4	235.1	239.0
bowel—*see* Neoplasm, intestine						
brachial plexus	171.2	198.89	—	215.2	238.1	239.2
brain NEC	191.9	198.3	—	225.0	237.5	239.6
basal ganglia	191.0	198.3	—	225.0	237.5	239.6
cerebellopontine angle	191.6	198.3	—	225.0	237.5	239.6
cerebellum NOS	191.6	198.3	—	225.0	237.5	239.6
cerebrum	191.0	198.3	—	225.0	237.5	239.6
choroid plexus	191.5	198.3	—	225.0	237.5	239.6
contiguous sites	191.8	—	—	—	—	—
corpus callosum	191.8	198.3	—	225.0	237.5	239.6
corpus striatum	191.0	198.3	—	225.0	237.5	239.6
cortex (cerebral)	191.0	198.3	—	225.0	237.5	239.6
frontal lobe	191.1	198.3	—	225.0	237.5	239.6
globus pallidus	191.0	198.3	—	225.0	237.5	239.6
hippocampus	191.2	198.3	—	225.0	237.5	239.6
hypothalamus	191.0	198.3	—	225.0	237.5	239.6
internal capsule	191.0	198.3	—	225.0	237.5	239.6
medulla oblongata	191.7	198.3	—	225.0	237.5	239.6
meninges	192.1	198.4	—	225.2	237.6	239.7
midbrain	191.7	198.3	—	225.0	237.5	239.6
occipital lobe	191.4	198.3	—	225.0	237.5	239.6
parietal lobe	191.3	198.3	—	225.0	237.5	239.6
peduncle	191.7	198.3	—	225.0	237.5	239.6
pons	191.7	198.3	—	225.0	237.5	239.6
stem	191.7	198.3	—	225.0	237.5	239.6
tapetum	191.8	198.3	—	225.0	237.5	239.6
temporal lobe	191.2	198.3	—	225.0	237.5	239.6
thalamus	191.0	198.3	—	225.0	237.5	239.6
uncus	191.2	198.3	—	225.0	237.5	239.6
ventricle (floor)	191.5	198.3	—	225.0	237.5	239.6
branchial (cleft) (vestiges)	146.8	198.89	230.0	210.6	235.1	239.0
breast (connective tissue) (female)						
(glandular tissue) (soft parts)	174.9	198.81	233.0	217	238.3	239.3
areola	174.0	198.81	233.0	217	238.3	239.3
male	175.0	198.81	233.0	217	238.3	239.3
axillary tail	174.6	198.81	233.0	217	238.3	239.3
central portion	174.1	198.81	233.0	217	238.3	239.3
contiguous sites	174.8	—	—	—	—	—
ectopic sites	174.8	198.81	233.0	217	238.3	239.3
inner	174.8	198.81	233.0	217	238.3	239.3
lower	174.8	198.81	233.0	217	238.3	239.3
lower-inner quadrant	174.3	198.81	233.0	217	238.3	239.3
lower-outer quadrant	174.5	198.81	233.0	217	238.3	239.3
male	175.9	198.81	233.0	217	238.3	239.3
areola	175.0	198.81	233.0	217	238.3	239.3
ectopic tissue	175.9	198.81	233.0	217	238.3	239.3
nipple	175.0	198.81	233.0	217	238.3	239.3
mastectomy site (skin)	173.5	198.2	—	—	—	—
specified as breast tissue	174.8	198.81	—	—	—	—
midline	174.8	198.81	233.0	217	238.3	239.3
nipple	174.0	198.81	233.0	217	238.3	239.3
male	175.0	198.81	233.0	217	238.3	239.3
outer	174.8	198.81	233.0	217	238.3	239.3
skin	173.5	198.2	232.5	216.5	238.2	239.2
tail (axillary)	174.6	198.81	233.0	217	238.3	239.3
upper	174.8	198.81	233.0	217	238.3	239.3
upper-inner quadrant	174.2	198.81	233.0	217	238.3	239.3
upper-outer quadrant	174.4	198.81	233.0	217	238.3	239.3
broad ligament	183.3	198.82	233.3	221.0	236.3	239.5
bronchiogenic, bronchogenic (lung)	162.9	197.0	231.2	212.3	235.7	239.1
bronchiole	162.9	197.0	231.2	212.3	235.7	239.1

	Malignant					
	Primary	Secondary	Ca in situ	Benign	Uncertain Behavior	Unspecified
bronchus	162.9	197.0	231.2	212.3	235.7	239.1
carina	162.2	197.0	231.2	212.3	235.7	239.1
contiguous sites with lung or trachea	162.8	—	—	—	—	—
lower lobe of lung	162.5	197.0	231.2	212.3	235.7	239.1
main	162.2	197.0	231.2	212.3	235.7	239.1
middle lobe of lung	162.4	197.0	231.2	212.3	235.7	239.1
upper lobe of lung	162.3	197.0	231.2	212.3	235.7	239.1
brow	173.3	198.2	232.3	216.3	238.2	239.2
buccal (cavity)	145.9	198.89	230.0	210.4	235.1	239.0
commissure	145.0	198.89	230.0	210.4	235.1	239.0
groove (lower) (upper)	145.1	198.89	230.0	210.4	235.1	239.0
mucosa	145.0	198.89	230.0	210.4	235.1	239.0
sulcus (lower) (upper)	145.1	198.89	230.0	210.4	235.1	239.0
bulbourethral gland	189.3	198.1	233.9	223.81	236.99	239.5
bursa—*see* Neoplasm, connective tissue						
buttock NEC*	195.3	198.89	232.5	229.8	238.8	239.8
calf*	195.5	198.89	232.7	229.8	238.8	239.8
calvarium	170.0	198.5	—	213.0	238.0	239.2
calyx, renal	189.1	198.0	233.9	223.1	236.91	239.5
canal						
anal	154.2	197.5	230.5	211.4	235.5	239.0
auditory (external)	173.2	198.2	232.2	216.2	238.2	239.2
auricular (external)	173.2	198.2	232.2	216.2	238.2	239.2
canaliculi, biliary (biliferi) (intrahepatic)	155.1	197.8	230.8	211.5	235.3	239.0
canthus (eye) (inner) (outer)	173.1	198.2	232.1	216.1	238.2	239.2
capillary—*see* Neoplasm, connective tissue						
caput coli	153.4	197.5	230.3	211.3	235.2	239.0
cardia (gastric)	151.0	197.8	230.2	211.1	235.2	239.0
cardiac orifice (stomach)	151.0	197.8	230.2	211.1	235.2	239.0
cardio-esophageal junction	151.0	197.8	230.2	211.1	235.2	239.0
cardio-esophagus	151.0	197.8	230.2	211.1	235.2	239.0
carina (bronchus)	162.2	197.0	231.2	212.3	235.7	239.1
carotid (artery)	171.0	198.89	—	215.0	238.1	239.2
body	194.5	198.89	—	227.5	237.3	239.7
carpus (any bone)	170.5	198.5	—	213.5	238.0	239.2
cartilage (articular) (joint) NEC—*see also*						
Neoplasm, bone	170.9	198.5	—	213.9	238.0	239.2
arytenoid	161.3	197.3	231.0	212.1	235.6	239.1
auricular	171.0	198.89	—	215.0	238.1	239.2
bronchi	162.2	197.3	—	212.3	235.7	239.1
connective tissue—*see* Neoplasm, connective tissue						
costal	170.3	198.5	—	213.3	238.0	239.2
cricoid	161.3	197.3	231.0	212.1	235.6	239.1
cuneiform	161.3	197.3	231.0	212.1	235.6	239.1
ear (external)	171.0	198.89	—	215.0	238.1	239.2
ensiform	170.3	198.5	—	213.3	238.0	239.2
epiglottis	161.1	197.3	231.0	212.1	235.6	239.1
anterior surface	146.4	198.89	230.0	210.6	235.1	239.0
eyelid	171.0	198.89	—	215.0	238.1	239.2
intervertebral	170.2	198.5	—	213.2	238.0	239.2
larynx, laryngeal	161.3	197.3	231.0	212.1	235.6	239.1
nose, nasal	160.0	197.3	231.8	212.0	235.9	239.1
pinna	171.0	198.89	—	215.0	238.1	239.2
rib	170.3	198.5	—	213.3	238.0	239.2
semilunar (knee)	170.7	198.5	—	213.7	238.0	239.2
thyroid	161.3	197.3	231.0	212.1	235.6	239.1
trachea	162.0	197.3	231.1	212.2	235.7	239.1
cauda equina	192.2	198.3	—	225.3	237.5	239.7
cavity						
buccal	145.9	198.89	230.0	210.4	235.1	239.0
nasal	160.0	197.3	231.8	212.0	235.9	239.1
oral	145.9	198.89	230.0	210.4	235.1	239.0

| | Malignant | | | | |
	Primary	Secondary	Ca in situ	Benign	Uncertain Behavior	Unspecified
cavity—*continued*						
peritoneal	158.9	197.6	—	211.8	235.4	239.0
tympanic	160.1	197.3	231.8	212.0	235.9	239.1
cecum	153.4	197.5	230.3	211.3	235.2	239.0
central						
nervous system—*see* Neoplasm, nervous system						
white matter	191.0	198.3	—	225.0	237.5	239.6
cerebellopontine (angle)	191.6	198.3	—	225.0	237.5	239.6
cerebellum, cerebellar	191.6	198.3	—	225.0	237.5	239.6
cerebrum, cerebral (cortex) (hemisphere) (white matter)	191.0	198.3	—	225.0	237.5	239.6
meninges	192.1	198.4	—	225.2	237.6	239.7
peduncle	191.7	198.3	—	225.0	237.5	239.6
ventricle (any)	191.5	198.3	—	225.0	237.5	239.6
cervical region	195.0	198.89	234.8	229.8	238.8	239.8
cervix (cervical) (uteri) (uterus)	180.9	198.82	233.1	219.0	236.0	239.5
canal	180.0	198.82	233.1	219.0	236.0	239.5
contiguous sites	180.8	—	—	—	—	—
endocervix (canal) (gland)	180.0	198.82	233.1	219.0	236.0	239.5
exocervix	180.1	198.82	233.1	219.0	236.0	239.5
external os	180.1	198.82	233.1	219.0	236.0	239.5
internal os	180.0	198.82	233.1	219.0	236.0	239.5
nabothian gland	180.0	198.82	233.1	219.0	236.0	239.5
squamocolumnar junction	180.8	198.82	233.1	219.0	236.0	239.5
stump	180.8	198.82	233.1	219.0	236.0	239.5
cheek	195.0	198.89	234.8	229.8	238.8	239.8
external	173.3	198.2	232.3	216.3	238.2	239.2
inner aspect	145.0	198.89	230.0	210.4	235.1	239.0
internal	145.0	198.89	230.0	210.4	235.1	239.0
mucosa	145.0	198.89	230.0	210.4	235.1	239.0
chest (wall) NEC	195.1	198.89	234.8	229.8	238.8	239.8
chiasma opticum	192.0	198.4	—	225.1	237.9	239.7
chin	173.3	198.2	232.3	216.3	238.2	239.2
choana	147.3	198.89	230.0	210.7	235.1	239.0
cholangiole	155.1	197.8	230.8	211.5	235.3	239.0
choledochal duct	156.1	197.8	230.8	211.5	235.3	239.0
choroid	190.6	198.4	234.0	224.6	238.8	239.8
plexus	191.5	198.3	—	225.0	237.5	239.6
ciliary body	190.0	198.4	234.0	224.0	238.8	239.8
clavicle	170.3	198.5	—	213.3	238.0	239.2
clitoris	184.3	198.82	233.3	221.2	236.3	239.5
clivus	170.0	198.5	—	213.0	238.0	239.2
cloacogenic zone	154.8	197.5	230.7	211.4	235.5	239.0
coccygeal						
body or glomus	194.6	198.89	—	227.6	237.3	239.7
vertebra	170.6	198.5	—	213.6	238.0	239.2
coccyx	170.6	198.5	—	213.6	238.0	239.2
colon—*see also* Neoplasm, intestine, large and rectum	154.0	197.5	230.4	211.4	235.2	239.0
column, spinal—*see* Neoplasm, spine						
columnella	173.3	198.2	232.3	216.3	238.2	239.2
commissure						
labial, lip	140.6	198.89	230.0	210.4	235.1	239.0
laryngeal	161.0	197.3	231.0	212.1	235.6	239.1
common (bile) duct	156.1	197.8	230.8	211.5	235.3	239.0
concha	173.2	198.2	232.2	216.2	238.2	239.2
nose	160.0	197.3	231.8	212.0	235.9	239.1
conjunctiva	190.3	198.4	234.0	224.3	238.8	239.8

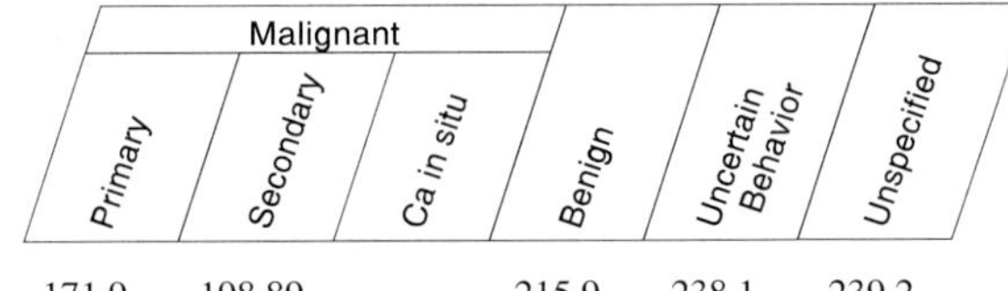

	Primary	Secondary	Ca in situ	Benign	Uncertain Behavior	Unspecified
connective tissue NEC	171.9	198.89	—	215.9	238.1	239.2

> *Note—For neoplasms of connective tissue (blood vessel, bursa, fasica, ligament, muscle, peripheral nerves, sympathetic and parasympathetic nerves, and ganglia, synovia, tendon, etc.) or of morphological types that indicate connective tissue, code according to the list under "Neoplasm, connective tissue;" for sites that do not appear in this list, code to neoplasm of that site; e.g.: liposarcoma, shoulder 171.2; leiomyosarcoma,stomach 151.9; neurofibroma,chest wall 215.4.*
>
> *Morphological types that indicate connective tissue appear in their proper place in the alphabetic index with the instruction "see Neoplasm, connective tissue..."*

	Primary	Secondary	Ca in situ	Benign	Uncertain Behavior	Unspecified
abdomen	171.5	198.89	—	215.5	238.1	239.2
abdominal wall	171.5	198.89	—	215.5	238.1	239.2
ankle	171.3	198.89	—	215.3	238.1	239.2
antecubital fossa or space	171.2	198.89	—	215.2	238.1	239.2
arm	171.2	198.89	—	215.2	238.1	239.2
auricle (ear)	171.0	198.89	—	215.0	238.1	239.2
axilla	171.4	198.89	—	215.4	238.1	239.2
back	171.7	198.89	—	215.7	238.1	239.2
breast (female) *(see also* Neoplasm, breast)	174.9	198.81	233.0	217	238.3	239.3
male	175.9	198.81	233.0	217	238.3	239.3
buttock	171.6	198.89	—	215.6	238.1	239.2
calf	171.3	198.89	—	215.3	238.1	239.2
cervical region	171.0	198.89	—	215.0	238.1	239.2
cheek	171.0	198.89	—	215.0	238.1	239.2
chest (wall)	171.4	198.89	—	215.4	238.1	239.2
chin	171.0	198.89	—	215.0	238.1	239.2
contiguous sites	171.8	—	—	—	—	—
diaphragm	171.4	198.89	—	215.4	238.1	239.2
ear (external)	171.0	198.89	—	215.0	238.1	239.2
elbow	171.2	198.89	—	215.2	238.1	239.2
extrarectal	171.6	198.89	—	215.6	238.1	239.2
extremity	171.8	198.89	—	215.8	238.1	239.2
lower	171.3	198.89	—	215.3	238.1	239.2
upper	171.2	198.89	—	215.2	238.1	239.2
eyelid	171.0	198.89	—	215.0	238.1	239.2
face	171.0	198.89	—	215.0	238.1	239.2
finger	171.2	198.89	—	215.2	238.1	239.2
flank	171.7	198.89	—	215.7	238.1	239.2
foot	171.3	198.89	—	215.3	238.1	239.2
forearm	171.2	198.89	—	215.2	238.1	239.2
forehead	171.0	198.89	—	215.0	238.1	239.2
gluteal region	171.6	198.89	—	215.6	238.1	239.2
great vessels NEC	171.4	198.89	—	215.4	238.1	239.2
groin	171.6	198.89	—	215.6	238.1	239.2
hand	171.2	198.89	—	215.2	238.1	239.2
head	171.0	198.89	—	215.0	238.1	239.2
heel	171.3	198.89	—	215.3	238.1	239.2
hip	171.3	198.89	—	215.3	238.1	239.2
hypochondrium	171.5	198.89	—	215.5	238.1	239.2
iliopsoas muscle	171.6	198.89	—	215.5	238.1	239.2
infraclavicular region	171.4	198.89	—	215.4	238.1	239.2
inguinal (canal) (region)	171.6	198.89	—	215.6	238.1	239.2
intrathoracic	171.4	198.89	—	215.4	238.1	239.2
ischorectal fossa	171.6	198.89	—	215.6	238.1	239.2
jaw	143.9	198.89	230.0	210.4	235.1	239.0
knee	171.3	198.89	—	215.3	238.1	239.2
leg	171.3	198.89	—	215.3	238.1	239.2

| | Malignant | | | | | |
	Primary	Secondary	Ca in situ	Benign	Uncertain Behavior	Unspecified
connective tissue—*continued*						
limb NEC	171.9	198.89	—	215.8	238.1	239.2
lower	171.3	198.89	—	215.3	238.1	239.2
upper	171.2	198.89	—	215.2	238.1	239.2
nates	171.6	198.89	—	215.6	238.1	239.2
neck	171.0	198.89	—	215.0	238.1	239.2
orbit	190.1	198.4	234.0	224.1	238.8	239.8
pararectal	171.6	198.89	—	215.6	238.1	239.2
para-urethral	171.6	198.89	—	215.6	238.1	239.2
paravaginal	171.6	198.89	—	215.6	238.1	239.2
pelvis (floor)	171.6	198.89	—	215.6	238.1	239.2
pelvo-abdominal	171.8	198.89	—	215.8	238.1	239.2
perineum	171.6	198.89	—	215.6	238.1	239.2
perirectal (tissue)	171.6	198.89	—	215.6	238.1	239.2
periurethral (tissue)	171.6	198.89	—	215.6	238.1	239.2
popliteal fossa or space	171.3	198.89	—	215.3	238.1	239.2
presacral	171.6	198.89	—	215.6	238.1	239.2
psoas muscle	171.5	198.89	—	215.5	238.1	239.2
pterygoid fossa	171.0	198.89	—	215.0	238.1	239.2
rectovaginal septum or wall	171.6	198.89	—	215.6	238.1	239.2
rectovesical	171.6	198.89	—	215.6	238.1	239.2
retroperitoneum	158.0	197.6	—	211.8	235.4	239.0
sacrococcygeal region	171.6	198.89	—	215.6	238.1	239.2
scalp	171.0	198.89	—	215.0	238.1	239.2
scapular region	171.4	198.89	—	215.4	238.1	239.2
shoulder	171.2	198.89	—	215.2	238.1	239.2
skin (dermis) NEC	173.9	198.2	232.9	216.9	238.2	239.2
submental	171.0	198.89	—	215.0	238.1	239.2
supraclavicular region	171.0	198.89	—	215.0	238.1	239.2
temple	171.0	198.89	—	215.0	238.1	239.2
temporal region	171.0	198.89	—	215.0	238.1	239.2
thigh	171.3	198.89	—	215.3	238.1	239.2
thoracic (duct) (wall)	171.4	198.89	—	215.4	238.1	239.2
thorax	171.4	198.89	—	215.4	238.1	239.2
thumb	171.2	198.89	—	215.2	238.1	239.2
toe	171.3	198.89	—	215.3	238.1	239.2
trunk	171.7	198.89	—	215.7	238.1	239.2
umbilicus	171.5	198.89	—	215.5	238.1	239.2
vesicorectal	171.6	198.89	—	215.6	238.1	239.2
wrist	171.2	198.89	—	215.2	238.1	239.2
conus medullaris	192.2	198.3	—	225.3	237.5	239.7
cord (true) (vocal)	161.0	197.3	231.0	212.1	235.6	239.1
false	161.1	197.3	231.0	212.1	235.6	239.1
spermatic	187.6	198.82	233.6	222.8	236.6	239.5
spinal (cervical) (lumbar) (thoracic)	192.2	198.3	—	225.3	237.5	239.7
cornea (limbus)	190.4	198.4	234.0	224.4	238.8	239.8
corpus						
albicans	183.0	198.6	233.3	220	236.2	239.5
callosum, brain	191.8	198.3	—	225.0	237.5	239.6
cavernosum	187.3	198.82	233.5	222.1	236.6	239.5
gastric	151.4	197.8	230.2	211.1	235.2	239.0
penis	187.3	198.82	233.5	222.1	236.6	239.5
striatum, cerebrum	191.0	198.3	—	225.0	237.5	239.6
uteri	182.0	198.82	233.2	219.1	236.0	239.5
isthmus	182.1	198.82	233.2	219.1	236.0	239.5
cortex						
adrenal	194.0	198.7	234.8	227.0	237.2	239.7
cerebral	191.0	198.3	—	225.0	237.5	239.6
costal cartilage	170.3	198.5	—	213.3	238.0	239.2
costovertebral joint	170.3	198.5	—	213.3	238.0	239.2

	Malignant					
	Primary	Secondary	Ca in situ	Benign	Uncertain Behavior	Unspecified
Cowper's gland	189.3	198.1	233.9	223.81	236.99	239.5
cranial (fossa, any)	191.9	198.3	—	225.0	237.5	239.6
meninges	192.1	198.4	—	225.2	237.6	239.7
nerve (any)	192.0	198.4	—	225.1	237.9	239.7
craniobuccal pouch	194.3	198.89	234.8	227.3	237.0	239.7
craniopharyngeal (duct) (pouch)	194.3	198.89	234.8	227.3	237.0	239.7
cricoid	148.0	198.89	230.0	210.8	235.1	239.0
cartilage	161.3	197.3	231.0	212.1	235.6	239.1
cricopharynx	148.0	198.89	230.0	210.8	235.1	239.0
crypt of Morgagni	154.8	197.5	230.7	211.4	235.2	239.0
crystalline lens	190.0	198.4	234.0	224.0	238.8	239.8
cul-de-sac (Douglas')	158.8	197.6	—	211.8	235.4	239.0
cuneiform cartilage	161.3	197.3	231.0	212.1	235.6	239.1
cutaneous—*see* Neoplasm, skin						
cutis—*see* Neoplasm, skin						
cystic (bile) duct (common)	156.1	197.8	230.8	211.5	235.3	239.0
dermis—*see* Neoplasm, skin						
diaphragm	171.4	198.89	—	215.4	238.1	239.2
digestive organs, system, tube, tract NEC	159.9	197.8	230.9	211.9	235.5	239.0
contiguous sites with peritoneum	159.8	—	—	—	—	—
disc, intervertebral	170.2	198.5	—	213.2	238.0	239.2
disease, generalized	199.0	199.0	234.9	229.9	238.9	199.0
disseminated	199.0	199.0	234.9	229.9	238.9	199.0
Douglas' cul-de-sac or pouch	158.8	197.6	—	211.8	235.4	239.0
duodenojejunal junction	152.8	197.4	230.7	211.2	235.2	239.0
duodenum	152.0	197.4	230.7	211.2	235.2	239.0
dura (cranial) (mater)	192.1	198.4	—	225.2	237.6	239.7
cerebral	192.1	198.4	—	225.2	237.6	239.7
spinal	192.3	198.4	—	225.4	237.6	239.7
ear (external)	173.2	198.2	232.2	216.2	238.2	239.2
auricle or auris	173.2	198.2	232.2	216.2	238.2	239.2
canal, external	173.2	198.2	232.2	216.2	238.2	239.2
cartilage	171.0	198.89	—	215.0	238.1	239.2
external meatus	173.2	198.2	232.2	216.2	238.2	239.2
inner	160.1	197.3	231.8	212.0	235.9	239.8
lobule	173.2	198.2	232.2	216.2	238.2	239.2
middle	160.1	197.3	231.8	212.0	235.9	239.8
contiguous sites with accessory sinuses or nasal cavities	160.8	—	—	—	—	—
skin	173.2	198.2	232.2	216.2	238.2	239.2
earlobe	173.2	198.2	232.2	216.2	238.2	239.2
ejaculatory duct	187.8	198.82	233.6	222.8	236.6	239.5
elbow NEC*	195.4	198.89	232.6	229.8	238.8	239.8
endocardium	164.1	198.89	—	212.7	238.8	239.8
endocervix (canal) (gland)	180.0	198.82	233.1	219.0	236.0	239.5
endocrine gland NEC	194.9	198.89	—	227.9	237.4	239.7
pluriglandular NEC	194.8	198.89	234.8	227.8	237.4	239.7
endometrium (gland) (stroma)	182.0	198.82	233.2	219.1	236.0	239.5
ensiform cartilage	170.3	198.5	—	213.3	238.0	239.2
enteric—*see* Neoplasm, intestine						
ependyma (brain)	191.5	198.3	—	225.0	237.5	239.6
epicardium	164.1	198.89		212.7	238.8	239.8
epididymis	187.5	198.82	233.6	222.3	236.6	239.5
epidural	192.9	198.4	—	225.9	237.9	239.7
epiglottis	161.1	197.3	231.0	212.1	235.6	239.1
anterior aspect or surface	146.4	198.89	230.0	210.6	235.1	239.0
cartilage	161.3	197.3	231.0	212.1	235.6	239.1
free border (margin)	146.4	198.89	230.0	210.6	235.1	239.0
junctional region	146.5	198.89	230.0	210.6	235.1	239.0
posterior (laryngeal) surface	161.1	197.3	231.0	212.1	235.6	239.1
suprahyoid portion	161.1	197.3	231.0	212.1	235.6	239.1

	Malignant					
	Primary	Secondary	Ca in situ	Benign	Uncertain Behavior	Unspecified
esophagogastric junction	151.0	197.8	230.2	211.1	235.2	239.0
esophagus	150.9	197.8	230.1	211.0	235.5	239.0
abdominal	150.2	197.8	230.1	211.0	235.5	239.0
cervical	150.0	197.8	230.1	211.0	235.5	239.0
contiguous sites	150.8	—	—	—	—	—
distal (third)	150.5	197.8	230.1	211.0	235.5	239.0
lower (third)	150.5	197.8	230.1	211.0	235.5	239.0
middle (third)	150.4	197.8	230.1	211.0	235.5	239.0
proximal (third)	150.3	197.8	230.1	211.0	235.5	239.0
specified part NEC	150.8	197.8	230.1	211.0	235.5	239.0
thoracic	150.1	197.8	230.1	211.0	235.5	239.0
upper (third)	150.3	197.8	230.1	211.0	235.5	239.0
ethmoid (sinus)	160.3	197.3	231.8	212.0	235.9	239.1
bone or labyrinth	170.0	198.5	—	213.0	238.0	239.2
Eustachian tube	160.1	197.3	231.8	212.0	235.9	239.1
exocervix	180.1	198.82	233.1	219.0	236.0	239.5
external						
meatus (ear)	173.2	198.2	232.2	216.2	238.2	239.2
os, cervix uteri	180.1	198.82	233.1	219.0	236.0	239.5
extradural	192.9	198.4	—	225.9	237.9	239.7
extrahepatic (bile) duct	156.1	197.8	230.8	211.5	235.3	239.0
contiguous sites with gallbladder	156.8	—	—	—	—	—
extraocular muscle	190.1	198.4	234.0	224.1	238.8	239.8
extrarectal	195.3	198.89	234.8	229.8	238.8	239.8
extremity*	195.8	198.89	232.8	229.8	238.8	239.8
lower*	195.5	198.89	232.7	229.8	238.8	239.8
upper*	195.4	198.89	232.6	229.8	238.8	239.8
eye NEC	190.9	198.4	234.0	224.9	238.8	239.8
contiguous sites	190.8	—	—	—	—	—
specified sites NEC	190.8	198.4	234.0	224.8	238.8	239.8
eyeball	190.0	198.4	234.0	224.0	238.8	239.8
eyebrow	173.3	198.2	232.3	216.3	238.2	239.2
eyelid (lower) (skin) (upper)	173.1	198.2	232.1	216.1	238.2	239.2
cartilage	171.0	198.89	—	215.0	238.1	239.2
face NEC*	195.0	198.89	232.3	229.8	238.8	239.8
fallopian tube (accessory)	183.2	198.82	233.3	221.0	236.3	239.5
falx (cerebelli) (cerebri)	192.1	198.4	—	225.2	237.6	239.7
fascia—*see also* Neoplasm, connective tissue						
palmar	171.2	198.89	—	215.2	238.1	239.2
plantar	171.3	198.89	—	215.3	238.1	239.2
fatty tissue—*see* Neoplasm, connective tissue						
fauces, faucial NEC	146.9	198.89	230.0	210.6	235.1	239.0
pillars	146.2	198.89	230.0	210.6	235.1	239.0
tonsil	146.0	198.89	230.0	210.5	235.1	239.0
femur (any part)	170.7	198.5	—	213.7	238.0	239.2
fetal membrane	181	198.82	233.2	219.8	236.1	239.5
fibrous tissue—*see* Neoplasm, connective tissue						
fibula (any part)	170.7	198.5	—	213.7	238.0	239.2
filum terminale	192.2	198.3	—	225.3	237.5	239.7
finger NEC*	195.4	198.89	232.6	229.8	238.8	239.8
flank NEC*	195.8	198.89	232.5	229.8	238.8	239.8
follicle, nabothian	180.0	198.82	233.1	219.0	236.0	239.5
foot NEC*	195.5	198.89	232.7	229.8	238.8	239.8
forearm NEC*	195.4	198.89	232.6	229.8	238.8	239.8
forehead (skin)	173.3	198.2	232.3	216.3	238.2	239.2
foreskin	187.1	198.82	233.5	222.1	236.6	239.5

	Malignant					
	Primary	Secondary	Ca in situ	Benign	Uncertain Behavior	Unspecified
fornix						
pharyngeal	147.3	198.89	230.0	210.7	235.1	239.0
vagina	184.0	198.82	233.3	221.1	236.3	239.5
fossa (of)						
anterior (cranial)	191.9	198.3	—	225.0	237.5	239.6
cranial	191.9	198.3	—	225.0	237.5	239.6
ischiorectal	195.3	198.89	234.8	229.8	238.8	239.8
middle (cranial)	191.9	198.3	—	225.0	237.5	239.6
pituitary	194.3	198.89	234.8	227.3	237.0	239.7
posterior (cranial)	191.9	198.3	—	225.0	237.5	239.6
pterygoid	171.0	198.89	—	215.0	238.1	239.2
pyriform	148.1	198.89	230.0	210.8	235.1	239.0
Rosenmüller	147.2	198.89	230.0	210.7	235.1	239.0
tonsillar	146.1	198.89	230.0	210.6	235.1	239.0
fourchette	184.4	198.82	233.3	221.2	236.3	239.5
frenulum						
labii—*see* Neoplasm, lip, internal						
linguae	141.3	198.89	230.0	210.1	235.1	239.0
frontal						
bone	170.0	198.5	—	213.0	238.0	239.2
lobe, brain	191.1	198.3	—	225.0	237.5	239.6
meninges	192.1	198.4	—	225.2	237.6	239.7
pole	191.1	198.3	—	225.0	237.5	239.6
sinus	160.4	197.3	231.8	212.0	235.9	239.1
fundus						
stomach	151.3	197.8	230.2	211.1	235.2	239.0
uterus	182.0	198.82	233.2	219.1	236.0	239.5
gall duct (extrahepatic)	156.1	197.8	230.8	211.5	235.3	239.0
intrahepatic	155.1	197.8	230.8	211.5	235.3	239.0
gallbladder	156.0	197.8	230.8	211.5	235.3	239.0
contiguous sites with extrahepatic bile ducts	156.8	—	—	—	—	—
ganglia (*see also* Neoplasm, connective tissue)	171.9	198.89	—	215.9	238.1	239.2
basal	191.0	198.3	—	225.0	237.5	239.6
ganglion (*see also* Neoplasm, connective tissue)	171.9	198.89	—	215.9	238.1	239.2
cranial nerve	192.0	198.4	—	225.1	237.9	239.7
Gartner's duct	184.0	198.82	233.3	221.1	236.3	239.5
gastric—*see* Neoplasm, stomach						
gastrocolic	159.8	197.8	230.9	211.9	235.5	239.0
gastroesophageal junction	151.0	197.8	230.2	211.1	235.2	239.0
gastrointestinal (tract) NEC	159.9	197.8	230.9	211.9	235.5	239.0
generalized	199.0	199.0	234.9	229.9	238.9	199.0
genital organ or tract						
female NEC	184.9	198.82	233.3	221.9	236.3	239.5
contiguous sites	184.8	—	—	—	—	—
specified site NEC	184.8	198.82	233.3	221.8	236.3	239.5
male NEC	187.9	198.82	233.6	222.9	236.6	239.5
contiguous sites	187.8	—	—	—	—	—
specified site NEC	187.8	198.82	233.6	222.8	236.6	239.5
genitourinary tract						
female	184.9	198.82	233.3	221.9	236.3	239.5
male	187.9	198.82	233.6	222.9	236.6	239.5
gingiva (alveolar) (marginal)	143.9	198.89	230.0	210.4	235.1	239.0
lower	143.1	198.89	230.0	210.4	235.1	239.0
mandibular	143.1	198.89	230.0	210.4	235.1	239.0
maxillary	143.0	198.89	230.0	210.4	235.1	239.0
upper	143.0	198.89	230.0	210.4	235.1	239.0

	Malignant					
	Primary	Secondary	Ca in situ	Benign	Uncertain Behavior	Unspecified
gland, glandular (lymphatic) (system)— *see also* Neoplasm, lymph gland						
endocrine NEC	194.9	198.89	—	227.9	237.4	239.7
salivary—*see* Neoplasm, salivary, gland						
glans penis	187.2	198.82	233.5	222.1	236.6	239.5
globus pallidus	191.0	198.3	—	225.0	237.5	239.6
glomus						
coccygeal	194.6	198.89	—	227.6	237.3	239.7
jugularis	194.6	198.89	—	227.6	237.3	239.7
glosso-epiglottic fold(s)	146.4	198.89	230.0	210.6	235.1	239.0
glossopalatine fold	146.2	198.89	230.0	210.6	235.1	239.0
glossopharyngeal sulcus	146.1	198.89	230.0	210.6	235.1	239.0
glottis	161.0	197.3	231.0	212.1	235.6	239.1
gluteal region*	195.3	198.89	232.5	229.8	238.8	239.8
great vessels NEC	171.4	198.89	—	215.4	238.1	239.2
groin NEC*	195.3	198.89	232.5	229.8	238.8	239.8
gum	143.9	198.89	230.0	210.4	235.1	239.0
contiguous sites	143.8	—	—	—	—	—
lower	143.1	198.89	230.0	210.4	235.1	239.0
upper	143.0	198.89	230.0	210.4	235.1	239.0
hand NEC*	195.4	198.89	232.6	229.8	238.8	239.8
head NEC*	195.0	198.89	232.4	229.8	238.8	239.8
heart	164.1	198.89	—	212.7	238.8	239.8
contiguous sites with mediastinum or thymus	164.8	—	—	—	—	—
heel NEC*	195.5	198.89	232.7	229.8	238.8	239.8
helix	173.2	198.2	232.2	216.2	238.2	239.2
hematopoietic, hemopoietic tissue NEC	202.8	198.89	—	—	—	238.7
hemisphere, cerebral	191.0	198.3	—	225.0	237.5	239.6
hemorrhoidal zone	154.2	197.5	230.5	211.4	235.5	239.0
hepatic	155.2	197.7	230.8	211.5	235.3	239.0
duct (bile)	156.1	197.8	230.8	211.5	235.3	239.0
flexure (colon)	153.0	197.5	230.3	211.3	235.2	239.0
primary	155.0	—	—	—	—	—
hilus of lung	162.2	197.0	231.2	212.3	235.7	239.1
hip NEC*	195.5	198.89	232.7	229.8	238.8	239.8
hippocampus, brain	191.2	198.3	—	225.0	237.5	239.6
humerus (any part)	170.4	198.5	—	213.4	238.0	239.2
hymen	184.0	198.82	233.3	221.1	236.3	239.5
hypopharynx, hypopharyngeal NEC	148.9	198.89	230.0	210.8	235.1	239.0
contiguous sites	148.8	—	—	—	—	—
postcricoid region	148.0	198.89	230.0	210.8	235.1	239.0
posterior wall	148.3	198.89	230.0	210.8	235.1	239.0
pyriform fossa (sinus)	148.1	198.89	230.0	210.8	235.1	239.0
specified site NEC	148.8	198.89	230.0	210.8	235.1	239.0
wall	148.9	198.89	230.0	210.8	235.1	239.0
posterior	148.3	198.89	230.0	210.8	235.1	239.0
hypophysis	194.3	198.89	234.8	227.3	237.0	239.7
hypothalamus	191.0	198.3	—	225.0	237.5	239.6
ileocecum, ileocecal (coil, junction, valve)	153.4	197.5	230.3	211.3	235.2	239.0
ileum	152.2	197.4	230.7	211.2	235.2	239.0
ilium	170.6	198.5	—	213.6	238.0	239.2
immunoproliferative NEC	203.8	—	—	—	—	—
infraclavicular (region)*	195.1	198.89	232.5	229.8	238.8	239.8
inguinal (region)*	195.3	198.89	232.5	229.8	238.8	239.8
insula	191.0	198.3	—	225.0	237.5	239.6
insular tissue (pancreas)	157.4	197.8	230.9	211.7	235.5	239.0
brain	191.0	198.3	—	225.0	237.5	239.6

	Malignant					
	Primary	Secondary	Ca in situ	Benign	Uncertain Behavior	Unspecified
interarytenoid fold	148.2	198.89	230.0	210.8	235.1	239.0
hypopharyngeal aspect	148.2	198.89	230.0	210.8	235.1	239.0
laryngeal aspect	161.1	197.3	231.0	212.1	235.6	239.1
marginal zone	148.2	198.89	230.0	210.8	235.1	239.0
interdental papillae	143.9	198.89	230.0	210.4	235.1	239.0
lower	143.1	198.89	230.0	210.4	235.1	239.0
upper	143.0	198.89	230.0	210.4	235.1	239.0
internal						
capsule	191.0	198.3	—	225.0	237.5	239.6
os (cervix)	180.0	198.82	233.1	219.0	236.0	239.5
intervertebral cartilage or disc	170.2	198.5	—	213.2	238.0	239.2
intestine, intestinal	159.0	197.8	230.7	211.9	235.2	239.0
large	153.9	197.5	230.3	211.3	235.2	239.0
appendix	153.5	197.5	230.3	211.3	235.2	239.0
caput coli	153.4	197.5	230.3	211.3	235.2	239.0
cecum	153.4	197.5	230.3	211.3	235.2	239.0
colon	153.9	197.5	230.3	211.3	235.2	239.0
and rectum	154.0	197.5	230.4	211.4	235.2	239.0
ascending	153.6	197.5	230.3	211.3	235.2	239.0
caput	153.4	197.5	230.3	211.3	235.2	239.0
contiguous sites	153.8	—	—	—	—	—
descending	153.2	197.5	230.3	211.3	235.2	239.0
distal	153.2	197.5	230.3	211.3	235.2	239.0
left	153.2	197.5	230.3	211.3	235.2	239.0
pelvic	153.3	197.5	230.3	211.3	235.2	239.0
right	153.6	197.5	230.3	211.3	235.2	239.0
sigmoid (flexure)	153.3	197.5	230.3	211.3	235.2	239.0
transverse	153.1	197.5	230.3	211.3	235.2	239.0
contiguous sites	153.8	—	—	—	—	—
hepatic flexure	153.0	197.5	230.3	211.3	235.2	239.0
ileocecum,ileocecal (coil, valve)	153.4	197.5	230.3	211.3	235.2	239.0
sigmoid flexure (lower) (upper)	153.3	197.5	230.3	211.3	235.2	239.0
splenic flexure	153.7	197.5	230.3	211.3	235.2	239.0
small	152.9	197.4	230.7	211.2	235.2	239.0
contiguous sites	152.8	—	—	—	—	—
duodenum	152.0	197.4	230.7	211.2	235.2	239.0
ileum	152.2	197.4	230.7	211.2	235.2	239.0
jejunum	152.1	197.4	230.7	211.2	235.2	239.0
tract NEC	159.0	197.8	230.7	211.9	235.2	239.0
intra-abdominal	195.2	198.89	234.8	229.8	238.8	239.8
intracranial NEC	191.9	198.3	—	225.0	237.5	239.6
intrahepatic (bile) duct	155.1	197.8	230.8	211.5	235.3	239.0
intraocular	190.0	198.4	234.0	224.0	238.8	239.8
intraorbital	190.1	198.4	234.0	224.1	238.8	239.8
intrasellar	194.3	198.89	234.8	227.3	237.0	239.7
intrathoracic (cavity) (organs NEC)	195.1	198.89	234.8	229.8	238.8	239.8
contiguous sites with respiratory						
organs	165.8	—	—	—	—	—
iris	190.0	198.4	234.0	224.0	238.8	239.8
ischiorectal (fossa)	195.3	198.89	234.8	229.8	238.8	239.8
ischium	170.6	198.5	—	213.6	238.0	239.2
island of Reil	191.0	198.3		225.0	237.5	239.6
islands or islets of Langerhans	157.4	197.8	230.9	211.7	235.5	239.0
isthmus uteri	182.1	198.82	233.2	219.1	236.0	239.5
jaw	195.0	198.89	234.8	229.8	238.8	239.8
bone	170.1	198.5	—	213.1	238.0	239.2
carcinoma	143.9	—	—	—	—	—
lower	143.1	—	—	—	—	—
upper	143.0	—	—	—	—	—
lower	170.1	198.5	—	213.1	238.0	239.2
upper	170.0	198.5	—	213.0	238.0	239.2

| | Malignant | | | | | |
	Primary	Secondary	Ca in situ	Benign	Uncertain Behavior	Unspecified
jaw—*continued*						
carcinoma (any type) (lower) (upper)	195.0	—	—	—	—	—
skin	173.3	198.2	232.3	216.3	238.2	239.2
soft tissues	143.9	198.89	230.0	210.4	235.1	239.0
lower	143.1	198.89	230.0	210.4	235.1	239.0
upper	143.0	198.89	230.0	210.4	235.1	239.0
jejunum	152.1	197.4	230.7	211.2	235.2	239.0
joint NEC (*see also* Neoplasm, bone)	170.9	198.5	—	213.9	238.0	239.2
acromioclavicular	170.4	198.5	—	213.4	238.0	239.2
bursa or synovial membrane—*see* Neoplasm, connective tissue						
costovertebral	170.3	198.5	—	213.3	238.0	239.2
sternocostal	170.3	198.5	—	213.3	238.0	239.2
temporomandibular	170.1	198.5	—	213.1	238.0	239.2
junction						
anorectal	154.8	197.5	230.7	211.4	235.5	239.0
cardioesophageal	151.0	197.8	230.2	211.1	235.2	239.0
esophagogastric	151.0	197.8	230.2	211.1	235.2	239.0
gastroesophageal	151.0	197.8	230.2	211.1	235.2	239.0
hard and soft palate	145.5	198.89	230.0	210.4	235.1	239.0
ileocecal	153.4	197.5	230.3	211.3	235.2	239.0
pelvirectal	154.0	197.5	230.4	211.4	235.2	239.0
pelviureteric	189.1	198.0	233.9	223.1	236.91	239.5
rectosigmoid	154.0	197.5	230.4	211.4	235.2	239.0
squamocolumnar, of cervix	180.8	198.82	233.1	219.0	236.0	239.5
kidney (parenchyma)	189.0	198.0	233.9	223.0	236.91	239.5
calyx	189.1	198.0	233.9	223.1	236.91	239.5
hilus	189.1	198.0	233.9	223.1	236.91	239.5
pelvis	189.1	198.0	233.9	223.1	236.91	239.5
knee NEC*	195.5	198.89	232.7	229.8	238.8	239.8
labia (skin)	184.4	198.82	233.3	221.2	236.3	239.5
majora	184.1	198.82	233.3	221.2	236.3	239.5
minora	184.2	198.82	233.3	221.2	236.3	239.5
labial—*see also* Neoplasm, lip						
sulcus (lower) (upper)	145.1	198.89	230.0	210.4	235.1	239.0
labium (skin)	184.4	198.82	233.3	221.2	236.3	239.5
majus	184.1	198.82	233.3	221.2	236.3	239.5
minus	184.2	198.82	233.3	221.2	236.3	239.5
lacrimal						
canaliculi	190.7	198.4	234.0	224.7	238.8	239.8
duct (nasal)	190.7	198.4	234.0	224.7	238.8	239.8
gland	190.2	198.4	234.0	224.2	238.8	239.8
punctum	190.7	198.4	234.0	224.7	238.8	239.8
sac	190.7	198.4	234.0	224.7	238.8	239.8
Langerhans, islands or islets	157.4	197.8	230.9	211.7	235.5	239.0
laryngopharynx	148.9	198.89	230.0	210.8	235.1	239.0
larynx, laryngeal NEC	161.9	197.3	231.0	212.1	235.6	239.1
aryepiglottic fold	161.1	197.3	231.0	212.1	235.6	239.1
cartilage (arytenoid) (cricoid) (cuneiform) (thyroid)	161.3	197.3	231.0	212.1	235.6	239.1
commissure (anterior) (posterior)	161.0	197.3	231.0	212.1	235.6	239.1
contiguous sites	161.8	—	—	—	—	—
extrinsic NEC	161.1	197.3	231.0	212.1	235.6	239.1
meaning hypopharynx	148.9	198.89	230.0	210.8	235.1	239.0
interarytenoid fold	161.1	197.3	231.0	212.1	235.6	239.1
intrinsic	161.0	197.3	231.0	212.1	235.6	239.1
ventricular band	161.1	197.3	231.0	212.1	235.6	239.1
leg NEC*	195.5	198.89	232.7	229.8	238.8	239.8
lens, crystalline	190.0	198.4	234.0	224.0	238.8	239.8

	Malignant					
	Primary	Secondary	Ca in situ	Benign	Uncertain Behavior	Unspecified
lid (lower) (upper)	173.1	198.2	232.1	216.1	238.2	239.2
ligament—*see also* Neoplasm, connective tissue						
broad	183.3	198.82	233.3	221.0	236.3	239.5
Mackenrodt's	183.8	198.82	233.3	221.8	236.3	239.5
non-uterine—*see* Neoplasm, connective tissue						
round	183.5	198.82	—	221.0	236.3	239.5
sacro-uterine	183.4	198.82	—	221.0	236.3	239.5
uterine	183.4	198.82	—	221.0	236.3	239.5
utero-ovarian	183.8	198.82	233.3	221.8	236.3	239.5
uterosacral	183.4	198.82	—	221.0	236.3	239.5
limb*	195.8	198.89	232.8	229.8	238.8	239.8
lower*	195.5	198.89	232.7	229.8	238.8	239.8
upper*	195.4	198.89	232.6	229.8	238.8	239.8
limbus of cornea	190.4	198.4	234.0	224.4	238.8	239.8
lingual NEC *(see also* Neoplasm, tongue)	141.9	198.89	230.0	210.1	235.1	239.0
lingula, lung	162.3	197.0	231.2	212.3	235.7	239.1
lip (external) (lipstick area) (vermillion border)	140.9	198.89	230.0	210.0	235.1	239.0
buccal aspect—*see* Neoplasm, lip, internal						
commissure	140.6	198.89	230.0	210.4	235.1	239.0
contiguous sites	140.8	—	—	—	—	—
with oral cavity or pharynx	149.8	—	—	—	—	—
frenulum—*see* Neoplasm, lip, internal						
inner aspect—*see* Neoplasm, lip, internal						
internal (buccal) (frenulum) (mucosa) (oral)	140.5	198.89	230.0	210.0	235.1	239.0
lower	140.4	198.89	230.0	210.0	235.1	239.0
upper	140.3	198.89	230.0	210.0	235.1	239.0
lower	140.1	198.89	230.0	210.0	235.1	239.0
internal (buccal) (frenulum) (mucosa) (oral)	140.4	198.89	230.0	210.0	235.1	239.0
mucosa—*see* Neoplasm, lip, internal						
oral aspect—*see* Neoplasm, lip, internal						
skin (commissure) (lower) (upper) . .	173.0	198.2	232.0	216.0	238.2	239.2
upper	140.0	198.89	230.0	210.0	235.1	239.0
internal (buccal) (frenulum) (mucosa) (oral)	140.3	198.89	230.0	210.0	235.1	239.0
liver	155.2	197.7	230.8	211.5	235.3	239.0
primary	155.0	—	—	—	—	—
lobe						
azygos	162.3	197.0	231.2	212.3	235.7	239.1
frontal	191.1	198.3	—	225.0	237.5	239.6
lower	162.5	197.0	231.2	212.3	235.7	239.1
middle	162.4	197.0	231.2	212.3	235.7	239.1
occipital	191.4	198.3	—	225.0	237.5	239.6
parietal	191.3	198.3	—	225.0	237.5	239.6
temporal	191.2	198.3	—	225.0	237.5	239.6
upper	162.3	197.0	231.2	212.3	235.7	239.1
lumbosacral plexus	171.6	198.4	—	215.6	238.1	239.2
lung	162.9	197.0	231.2	212.3	235.7	239.1
azygos lobe	162.3	197.0	231.2	212.3	235.7	239.1
carina	162.2	197.0	231.2	212.3	235.7	239.1
contiguous sites with bronchus or trachea	162.8	—	—	—	—	—
hilus	162.2	197.0	231.2	212.3	235.7	239.1

	Malignant					
	Primary	Secondary	Ca in situ	Benign	Uncertain Behavior	Unspecified
lung—*continued*						
lingula	162.3	197.0	231.2	212.3	235.7	239.1
lobe NEC	162.9	197.0	231.2	212.3	235.7	239.1
lower lobe	162.5	197.0	231.2	212.3	235.7	239.1
main bronchus	162.2	197.0	231.2	212.3	235.7	239.1
middle lobe	162.4	197.0	231.2	212.3	235.7	239.1
upper lobe	162.3	197.0	231.2	212.3	235.7	239.1
lymph, lymphatic						
channel NEC *(see also* Neoplasm, connective tissue)	171.9	198.89	—	215.9	238.1	239.2
gland (secondary)	—	196.9	—	229.0	238.8	239.8
abdominal	—	196.2	—	229.0	238.8	239.8
aortic	—	196.2	—	229.0	238.8	239.8
arm	—	196.3	—	229.0	238.8	239.8
auricular (anterior) (posterior)	—	196.0	—	229.0	238.8	239.8
axilla, axillary	—	196.3	—	229.0	238.8	239.8
brachial	—	196.3	—	229.0	238.8	239.8
bronchial	—	196.1	—	229.0	238.8	239.8
bronchopulmonary	—	196.1	—	229.0	238.8	239.8
celiac	—	196.2	—	229.0	238.8	239.8
cervical	—	196.0	—	229.0	238.8	239.8
cervicofacial	—	196.0	—	229.0	238.8	239.8
Cloquet	—	196.5	—	229.0	238.8	239.8
colic	—	196.2	—	229.0	238.8	239.8
common duct	—	196.2	—	229.0	238.8	239.8
cubital	—	196.3	—	229.0	238.8	239.8
diaphragmatic	—	196.1	—	229.0	238.8	239.8
epigastric, inferior	—	196.6	—	229.0	238.8	239.8
epitrochlear	—	196.3	—	229.0	238.8	239.8
esophageal	—	196.1	—	229.0	238.8	239.8
face	—	196.0	—	229.0	238.8	239.8
femoral	—	196.5	—	229.0	238.8	239.8
gastric	—	196.2	—	229.0	238.8	239.8
groin	—	196.5	—	229.0	238.8	239.8
head	—	196.0	—	229.0	238.8	239.8
hepatic	—	196.2	—	229.0	238.8	239.8
hilar (pulmonary)	—	196.1	—	229.0	238.8	239.8
splenic	—	196.2	—	229.0	238.8	239.8
hypogastric	—	196.6	—	229.0	238.8	239.8
ileocolic	—	196.2	—	229.0	238.8	239.8
iliac	—	196.6	—	229.0	238.8	239.8
infraclavicular	—	196.3	—	229.0	238.8	239.8
inguina, inguinal	—	196.5	—	229.0	238.8	239.8
innominate	—	196.1	—	229.0	238.8	239.8
intercostal	—	196.1	—	229.0	238.8	239.8
intestinal	—	196.2	—	229.0	238.8	239.8
intrabdominal	—	196.2	—	229.0	238.8	239.8
intrapelvic	—	196.6	—	229.0	238.8	239.8
intrathoracic	—	196.1	—	229.0	238.8	239.9
jugular	—	196.0	—	229.0	238.8	239.8
leg	—	196.5	—	229.0	238.8	239.8
limb						
lower	—	196.5	—	229.0	238.8	239.8
upper	—	196.3	—	229.0	238.8	239.8
lower limb	—	196.5	—	229.0	238.8	238.9
lumbar	—	196.2	—	229.0	238.8	239.8
mandibular	—	196.0	—	229.0	238.8	239.8
mediastinal	—	196.1	—	229.0	238.8	239.8
mesenteric (inferior) (superior)	—	196.2	—	229.0	238.8	239.8
midcolic	—	196.2	—	229.0	238.8	239.8

| | Malignant | | | | | |
	Primary	Secondary	Ca in situ	Benign	Uncertain Behavior	Unspecified
lymph, lymphatic—*continued*						
multiple sites in categories						
196.0-196.6	—	196.8	—	229.0	238.8	239.8
neck	—	196.0	—	229.0	238.8	239.8
obturator	—	196.6	—	229.0	238.8	239.8
occipital	—	196.0	—	229.0	238.8	239.8
pancreatic	—	196.2	—	229.0	238.8	239.8
para-aortic	—	196.2	—	229.0	238.8	239.8
paracervical	—	196.6	—	229.0	238.8	239.8
parametrial	—	196.6	—	229.0	238.8	239.8
parasternal	—	196.1	—	229.0	238.8	239.8
parotid	—	196.0	—	229.0	238.8	239.8
pectoral	—	196.3	—	229.0	238.8	239.8
pelvic	—	196.6	—	229.0	238.8	239.8
peri-aortic	—	196.2	—	229.0	238.8	239.8
peripancreatic	—	196.2	—	229.0	238.8	239.8
popliteal	—	196.5	—	229.0	238.8	239.8
porta hepatis	—	196.2	—	229.0	238.8	239.8
portal	—	196.2	—	229.0	238.8	239.8
preauricular	—	196.0	—	229.0	238.8	239.8
prelaryngeal	—	196.0	—	229.0	238.8	239.8
presymphysial	—	196.6	—	229.0	238.8	239.8
pretracheal	—	196.0	—	229.0	238.8	239.8
primary (any site) NEC	202.9	—	—	—	—	—
pulmonary (hiler)	—	196.1	—	229.0	238.8	239.8
pyloric	—	196.2	—	229.0	238.8	239.8
retroperitoneal	—	196.2	—	229.0	238.8	239.8
retropharyngeal	—	196.0	—	229.0	238.8	239.8
Rosenmüller's	—	196.5	—	229.0	238.8	239.8
sacral	—	196.6	—	229.0	238.8	239.8
scalene	—	196.0	—	229.0	238.8	239.8
site NEC	—	196.9	—	229.0	238.8	239.8
splenic (hilar)	—	196.2	—	229.0	238.8	239.8
subclavicular	—	196.3	—	229.0	238.8	239.8
subinguinal	—	196.5	—	229.0	238.8	239.8
sublingual	—	196.0	—	229.0	238.8	239.8
submandibular	—	196.0	—	229.0	238.8	239.8
submaxillary	—	196.0	—	229.0	238.8	239.8
submental	—	196.0	—	229.0	238.8	239.8
subscapular	—	196.3	—	229.0	238.8	239.8
supraclavicular	—	196.0	—	229.0	238.8	239.8
thoracic	—	196.1	—	229.0	238.8	239.8
tibial	—	196.5	—	229.0	238.8	239.8
tracheal	—	196.1	—	229.0	238.8	239.8
tracheobronchial	—	196.1	—	229.0	238.8	239.8
upper limb	—	196.3	—	229.0	238.8	239.8
Virchow's	—	196.0	—	229.0	238.8	239.8
node—*see also* Neoplasm, lymph gland						
primary NEC	202.9	—	—	—	—	—
vessel (*see also* Neoplasm, connective						
tissue)	171.9	198.89	—	215.9	238.1	239.2
Mackenrodt's ligament	183.8	198.82	233.3	221.8	236.3	239.5
malar	170.0	198.5	—	213.0	238.0	239.2
region—*see* Neoplasm, cheek						
mammary gland—*see* Neoplasm, breast						
mandible	170.1	198.5	—	213.1	238.0	239.2
alveolar						
mucose	143.1	198.89	230.0	210.4	235.1	239.0
ridge or process	170.1	198.5	—	213.1	238.0	239.2
carcinoma	143.1	—	—	—	—	—
carcinoma	143.1	—	—	—	—	—

	Malignant					
	Primary	Secondary	Ca in situ	Benign	Uncertain Behavior	Unspecified
marrow (bone) NEC	202.9	198.5	—	—	—	238.7
mastectomy site (skin)	173.5	198.2	—	—	—	—
specified as breast tissue	174.8	198.81	—	—	—	—
mastoid (air cells) (antrum) (cavity)	160.1	197.3	231.8	212.0	235.9	239.1
bone or process	170.0	198.5	—	213.0	238.0	239.2
maxilla, maxillary (superior)	170.0	198.5	—	213.0	238.0	239.2
alveolar						
mucosa	143.0	198.89	230.0	210.4	235.1	239.0
ridge or process	170.0	198.5	—	213.0	238.0	239.2
carcinoma	143.0	—	—	—	—	—
antrum	160.2	197.3	231.8	212.0	235.9	239.1
carcinoma	143.0	—	—	—	—	—
inferior—*see* Neoplasm, mandible						
sinus	160.2	197.3	231.8	212.0	235.9	239.1
meatus						
external (ear)	173.2	198.2	232.2	216.2	238.2	239.2
Meckel's diverticulum	152.3	197.4	230.7	211.2	235.2	239.0
mediastinum, mediastinal	164.9	197.1	—	212.5	235.8	239.8
anterior	164.2	197.1	—	212.5	235.8	239.8
contiguous sites with heart and						
thymus	164.8	—	—	—	—	—
posterior	164.3	197.1	—	212.5	235.8	239.8
medulla						
adrenal	194.0	198.7	234.8	227.0	237.2	239.7
oblongata	191.7	198.3	—	225.0	237.5	239.6
meibomian gland	173.1	198.2	232.1	216.1	238.2	239.2
melanoma —*see* Melanoma						
meninges (brain) (cerebral) (cranial)						
(intracranial)	192.1	198.4	—	225.2	237.6	239.7
spinal (cord)	192.3	198.4	—	225.4	237.6	239.7
meniscus, knee joint (lateral) (medial)	170.7	198.5	—	213.7	238.0	239.2
mesentery, mesenteric	158.8	197.6	—	211.8	235.4	239.0
mesoappendix	158.8	197.6	—	211.8	235.4	239.0
mesocolon	158.8	197.6	—	211.8	235.4	239.0
mesopharynx—*see* Neoplasm, oropharynx						
mesosalpinx	183.3	198.82	233.3	221.0	236.3	239.5
mesovarium	183.3	198.82	233.3	221.0	236.3	239.5
metacarpus (any bone)	170.5	198.5	—	213.5	238.0	239.2
metastatic NEC—*see also* Neoplasm,						
by site, secondary	—	199.1	—	—	—	—
metatarsus (any bone)	170.8	198.5	—	213.8	238.0	239.2
midbrain	191.7	198.3	—	225.0	237.5	239.6
milk duct—*see* Neoplasm, breast						
mons						
pubis	184.4	198.82	233.3	221.2	236.3	239.5
veneris	184.4	198.82	233.3	221.2	236.3	239.5
motor tract	192.9	198.4	—	225.9	237.9	239.7
brain	191.9	198.3	—	225.0	237.5	239.6
spinal	192.2	198.3	—	225.3	237.5	239.7
mouth	145.9	198.89	230.0	210.4	235.1	239.0
contiguous sites	145.8	—	—	—	—	—
floor	144.9	198.89	230.0	210.3	235.1	239.0
anterior portion	144.0	198.89	230.0	210.3	235.1	239.0
contiguous sites	144.8	—	—	—	—	—
lateral portion	144.1	198.89	230.0	210.3	235.1	239.0
roof	145.5	198.89	230.0	210.4	235.1	239.0
specified part NEC	145.8	198.89	230.0	210.4	235.1	239.0
vestibule	145.1	198.89	230.0	210.4	235.1	239.0
mucosa						
alveolar (ridge or process)	143.9	198.89	230.0	210.4	235.1	239.0
lower	143.1	198.89	230.0	210.4	235.1	239.0
upper	143.0	198.89	230.0	210.4	235.1	239.0

	Malignant					
	Primary	Secondary	Ca in situ	Benign	Uncertain Behavior	Unspecified
mucosa—*continued*						
buccal	145.0	198.89	230.0	210.4	235.1	239.0
cheek	145.0	198.89	230.0	210.4	235.1	239.0
lip—*see* Neoplasm, lip, internal						
nasal	160.0	197.3	231.8	212.0	235.9	239.1
oral	145.0	198.89	230.0	210.4	235.1	239.0
Müllerian duct						
female	184.8	198.82	233.3	221.8	236.3	239.5
male	187.8	198.82	233.6	222.8	236.6	239.5
multiple sites NEC	199.0	199.0	234.9	229.9	238.9	199.0
muscle—*see also* Neoplasm, connective tissue						
extraocular	190.1	198.4	234.0	224.1	238.8	239.8
myocardium	164.1	198.89	—	212.7	238.8	239.8
myometrium	182.0	198.82	233.2	219.1	236.0	239.5
myopericardium	164.1	198.89	—	212.7	238.8	239.8
nabothian gland (follicle)	180.0	198.82	233.1	219.0	236.0	239.5
nail	173.9	198.2	232.9	216.9	238.2	239.2
finger	173.6	198.2	232.6	216.6	238.2	239.2
toe	173.7	198.2	232.7	216.7	238.2	239.2
nares, naris (anterior) (posterior)	160.0	197.3	231.8	212.0	235.9	239.1
nasal—*see* Neoplasm, nose						
nasolabial groove	173.3	198.2	232.3	216.3	238.2	239.2
nasolacrimal duct	190.7	198.4	234.0	224.7	238.8	239.8
nasopharynx, nasopharyngeal	147.9	198.89	230.0	210.7	235.1	239.0
contiguous sites	147.8	—	—	—	—	—
floor	147.3	198.89	230.0	210.7	235.1	239.0
roof	147.0	198.89	230.0	210.7	235.1	239.0
specified site NEC	147.8	198.89	230.0	210.7	235.1	239.0
wall	147.9	198.89	230.0	210.7	235.1	239.0
anterior	147.3	198.89	230.0	210.7	235.1	239.0
lateral	147.2	198.89	230.0	210.7	235.1	239.0
posterior	147.1	198.89	230.0	210.7	235.1	239.0
superior	147.0	198.89	230.0	210.7	235.1	239.0
nates	173.5	198.2	232.5	216.5	238.2	239.2
neck NEC*	195.0	198.89	234.8	229.8	238.8	239.8
nerve (autonomic) (ganglion) (parasympathetic) (peripheral) (sympathetic)—*see also* Neoplasm, connective tissue						
abducens	192.0	198.4	—	225.1	237.9	239.7
accessory (spinal)	192.0	198.4	—	225.1	237.9	239.7
acoustic	192.0	198.4	—	225.1	237.9	239.7
auditory	192.0	198.4	—	225.1	237.9	239.7
brachial	171.2	198.89	—	215.2	238.1	239.2
cranial (any)	192.0	198.4	—	225.1	237.9	239.7
facial	192.0	198.4	—	225.1	237.9	239.7
femoral	171.3	198.89	—	215.3	238.1	239.2
glossopharyngeal	192.0	198.4	—	225.1	237.9	239.7
hypoglossal	192.0	198.4	—	225.1	237.9	239.7
intercostal	171.4	198.89	—	215.4	238.1	239.2
lumbar	171.7	198.89	—	215.7	238.1	239.2
median	171.2	198.89	—	215.2	238.1	239.2
obturator	171.3	198.89	—	215.3	238.1	239.2
oculomotor	192.0	198.4	—	225.1	237.9	239.7
olfactory	192.0	198.4	—	225.1	237.9	239.7
optic	192.0	198.4	—	225.1	237.9	239.7
peripheral NEC	171.9	198.89	—	215.9	238.1	239.2
radial	171.2	198.89	—	215.2	238.1	239.2
sacral	171.6	198.89	—	215.6	238.1	239.2
sciatic	171.3	198.89	—	215.3	238.1	239.2
spinal NEC	171.9	198.89	—	215.9	238.1	239.2

| | Malignant | | | | | |
	Primary	Secondary	Ca in situ	Benign	Uncertain Behavior	Unspecified
nerve—*continued*						
trigeminal	192.0	198.4	—	225.1	237.9	239.7
trochlear	192.0	198.4	—	225.1	237.9	239.7
ulnar	171.2	198.89	—	215.2	238.1	239.2
vagus	192.0	198.4	—	225.1	237.9	239.7
nervous system (central) NEC	192.9	198.4	—	225.9	237.9	239.7
autonomic NEC	171.9	198.89	—	215.9	238.1	239.2
brain—*see also* Neoplasm, brain						
membrane or meninges	192.1	198.4	—	225.2	237.6	239.7
contiguous sites	192.8	—	—	—	—	—
parasympathetic NEC	171.9	198.89	—	215.9	238.1	239.2
sympathetic NEC	171.9	198.89	—	215.9	238.1	239.2
nipple (female)	174.0	198.81	233.0	217	238.3	239.3
male	175.0	198.81	233.0	217	238.3	239.3
nose, nasal	195.0	198.89	234.8	229.8	238.8	239.8
ala (external)	173.3	198.2	232.3	216.3	238.2	239.2
bone	170.0	198.5	—	213.0	238.0	239.2
cartilage	160.0	197.3	231.8	212.0	235.9	239.1
cavity	160.0	197.3	231.8	212.0	235.9	239.1
contiguous sites with accessory						
sinuses or middle ear	160.8	—	—	—	—	—
choana	147.3	198.89	230.0	210.7	235.1	239.0
external (skin)	173.3	198.2	232.3	216.3	238.2	239.2
fossa	160.0	197.3	231.8	212.0	235.9	239.1
internal	160.0	197.3	231.8	212.0	235.9	239.1
mucosa	160.0	197.3	231.8	212.0	235.9	239.1
septum	160.0	197.3	231.8	212.0	235.9	239.1
posterior margin	147.3	198.89	230.0	210.7	235.1	239.0
sinus—*see* Neoplasm, sinus						
skin	173.3	198.2	232.3	216.3	238.2	239.2
turbinate (mucosa)	160.0	197.3	231.8	212.0	235.9	239.1
bone	170.0	198.5	—	213.0	238.0	239.2
vestibule	160.0	197.3	231.8	212.0	235.9 .	239.1
nostril	160.0	197.3	231.8	212.0	235.9	239.1
nucleus pulposus	170.2	198.5	—	213.2	238.0	239.2
occipital						
bone	170.0	198.5	—	213.0	238.0	239.2
lobe or pole, brain	191.4	198.3	—	225.0	237.5	239.6
odontogenic—*see* Neoplasm, jaw bone						
oesophagus—*see* Neoplasm, esophagus						
olfactory nerve or bulb	192.0	198.4	—	225.1	237.9	239.7
olive (brain)	191.7	198.3	—	225.0	237.5	239.6
omentum	158.8	197.6	—	211.8	235.4	239.0
operculum (brain)	191.0	198.3	—	225.0	237.5	239.6
optic nerve, chiasm, or tract	192.0	198.4	—	225.1	237.9	239.7
oral (cavity)	145.9	198.89	230.0	210.4	235.1	239.0
contiguous sites with lip or pharynx	149.8	—	—	—	—	—
ill-defined	149.9	198.89	230.0	210.4	235.1	239.0
mucosa	145.9	198.89	230.0	210.4	235.1	239.0
orbit	190.1	198.4	234.0	224.1	238.8	239.8
bone	170.0	198.5	—	213.0	238.0	239.2
eye	190.1	198.4	234.0	224.1	238.8	239.8
soft parts	190.1	198.4	234.0	224.1	238.8	239.8
organ of Zuckerkandl	194.6	198.89	—	227.6	237.3	239.7
oropharynx	146.9	198.89	230.0	210.6	235.1	239.0
branchial cleft (vestige)	146.8	198.89	230.0	210.6	235.1	239.0
contiguous sites	146.8	—	—	—	—	—
junctional region	146.5	198.89	230.0	210.6	235.1	239.0
lateral wall	146.6	198.89	230.0	210.6	235.1	239.0
pillars of fauces	146.2	198.89	230.0	210.6	235.1	239.0

| | Malignant | | | | | |
	Primary	Secondary	Ca in situ	Benign	Uncertain Behavior	Unspecified
oropharynx—*continued*						
posterior wall	146.7	198.89	230.0	210.6	235.1	239.0
specified part NEC	146.8	198.89	230.0	210.6	235.1	239.0
vallecula	146.3	198.89	230.0	210.6	235.1	239.0
os						
external	180.1	198.82	233.1	219.0	236.0	239.5
internal	180.0	198.82	233.1	219.0	236.0	239.5
ovary	183.0	198.6	233.3	220	236.2	239.5
oviduct	183.2	198.82	233.3	221.0	236.3	239.5
palate	145.5	198.89	230.0	210.4	235.1	239.0
hard	145.2	198.89	230.0	210.4	235.1	239.0
junction of hard and soft palate	145.5	198.89	230.0	210.4	235.1	239.0
soft	145.3	198.89	230.0	210.4	235.1	239.0
nasopharyngeal surface	147.3	198.89	230.0	210.7	235.1	239.0
posterior surface	147.3	198.89	230.0	210.7	235.1	239.0
superior surface	147.3	198.89	230.0	210.7	235.1	239.0
palatoglossal arch	146.2	198.89	230.0	210.6	235.1	239.0
palatopharyngeal arch	146.2	198.89	230.0	210.6	235.1	239.0
pallium	191.0	198.3	—	225.0	237.5	239.6
palpebra	173.1	198.2	232.1	216.1	238.2	239.2
pancreas	157.9	197.8	230.9	211.6	235.5	239.0
body	157.1	197.8	230.9	211.6	235.5	239.0
contiguous sites	157.8	—	—	—	—	—
duct (of Santorini) (of Wirsung)	157.3	197.8	230.9	211.6	235.5	239.0
ectopic tissue	157.8	197.8	230.9	211.6	235.5	239.0
head	157.0	197.8	230.9	211.6	235.5	239.0
islet cells	157.4	197.8	230.9	211.7	235.5	239.0
neck	157.8	197.8	230.9	211.6	235.5	239.0
tail	157.2	197.8	230.9	211.6	235.5	239.0
para-aortic body	194.6	198.89	—	227.6	237.3	239.7
paraganglion NEC	194.6	198.89	—	227.6	237.3	239.7
parametrium	183.4	198.82	—	221.0	236.3	239.5
paranephric	158.0	197.6	—	211.8	235.4	239.0
pararectal	195.3	198.89	—	229.8	238.8	239.8
parasagittal (region)	195.0	198.89	234.8	229.8	238.8	239.8
parasellar	192.9	198.4	—	225.9	237.9	239.7
parathyroid (gland)	194.1	198.89	234.8	227.1	237.4	239.7
paraurethral	195.3	198.89	—	229.8	238.8	239.8
gland	189.4	198.1	233.9	223.89	236.99	239.5
paravaginal	195.3	198.89	—	229.8	238.8	239.8
parenchyma, kidney	189.0	198.0	233.9	223.0	236.91	239.5
parietal						
bone	170.0	198.5	—	213.0	238.0	239.2
lobe, brain	191.3	198.3	—	225.0	237.5	239.6
paroophoron	183.3	198.82	233.3	221.0	236.3	239.5
parotid (duct) (gland)	142.0	198.89	230.0	210.2	235.0	239.0
parovarium	183.3	198.82	233.3	221.0	236.3	239.5
patella	170.8	198.5	—	213.8	238.0	239.2
peduncle, cerebral	191.7	198.3	—	225.0	237.5	239.6
pelvirectal junction	154.0	197.5	230.4	211.4	235.2	239.0
pelvis, pelvic	195.3	198.89	234.8	229.8	238.8	239.8
bone	170.6	198.5		213.6	238.0	239.2
floor	195.3	198.89	234.8	229.8	238.8	239.8
renal	189.1	198.0	233.9	223.1	236.91	239.5
viscera	195.3	198.89	234.8	229.8	238.8	239.8
wall	195.3	198.89	234.8	229.8	238.8	239.8
pelvo-abdominal	195.8	198.89	234.8	229.8	238.8	239.8
penis	187.4	198.82	233.5	222.1	236.6	239.5
body	187.3	198.82	233.5	222.1	236.6	239.5
corpus (cavernosum)	187.3	198.82	233.5	222.1	236.6	239.5
glans	187.2	198.82	233.5	222.1	236.6	239.5
skin NEC	187.4	198.82	233.5	222.1	236.6	239.5

	Malignant					
	Primary	Secondary	Ca in situ	Benign	Uncertain Behavior	Unspecified
periadrenal (tissue)	158.0	197.6	—	211.8	235.4	239.0
perianal (skin)	173.5	198.2	232.5	216.5	238.2	239.2
pericardium	164.1	198.89	—	212.7	238.8	239.8
perinephric	158.0	197.6	—	211.8	235.4	239.0
perineum	195.3	198.89	234.8	229.8	238.8	239.8
periodontal tissue NEC	143.9	198.89	230.0	210.4	235.1	239.0
periosteum—*see* Neoplasm, bone						
peripancreatic	158.0	197.6	—	211.8	235.4	239.0
peripheral nerve NEC	171.9	198.89	—	215.9	238.1	239.2
perirectal (tissue)	195.3	198.89	—	229.8	238.8	239.8
perirenal (tissue)	158.0	197.6	—	211.8	235.4	239.0
peritoneum, peritoneal (cavity)	158.9	197.6	—	211.8	235.4	239.0
contiguous sites	158.8	—	—	—	—	—
with digestive organs	159.8	—	—	—	—	—
parietal	158.8	197.6	—	211.8	235.4	239.0
pelvic	158.8	197.6	—	211.8	235.4	239.0
specified part NEC	158.8	197.6	—	211.8	235.4	239.0
peritonsillar (tissue)	195.0	198.89	234.8	229.8	238.8	239.8
periurethral tissue	195.3	198.89	—	229.8	238.8	239.8
phalanges	170.9	198.5	—	213.9	238.0	239.2
foot	170.8	198.5	—	213.8	238.0	239.2
hand	170.5	198.5	—	213.5	238.0	239.2
pharynx, pharyngeal	149.0	198.89	230.0	210.9	235.1	239.0
bursa	147.1	198.89	230.0	210.7	235.1	239.0
fornix	147.3	198.89	230.0	210.7	235.1	239.0
recess	147.2	198.89	230.0	210.7	235.1	239.0
region	149.0	198.89	230.0	210.9	235.1	239.0
tonsil	147.1	198.89	230.0	210.7	235.1	239.0
wall (lateral) (posterior)	149.0	198.89	230.0	210.9	235.1	239.0
pia mater (cerebral) (cranial)	192.1	198.4	—	225.2	237.6	239.7
spinal	192.3	198.4	—	225.4	237.6	239.7
pillars of fauces	146.2	198.89	230.0	210.6	235.1	239.0
pineal (body) (gland)	194.4	198.89	234.8	227.4	237.1	239.7
pinna (ear) NEC	173.2	198.2	232.2	216.2	238.2	239.2
cartilage	171.0	198.89	—	215.0	238.1	239.2
piriform fossa or sinus	148.1	198.89	230.0	210.8	235.1	239.0
pituitary (body) (fossa) (gland) (lobe)	194.3	198.89	234.8	227.3	237.0	239.7
placenta	181	198.82	233.2	219.8	236.1	239.5
pleura, pleural (cavity)	163.9	197.2	—	212.4	235.8	239.1
contiguous sites	163.8	—	—	—	—	—
parietal	163.0	197.2	—	212.4	235.8	239.1
visceral	163.1	197.2	—	212.4	235.8	239.1
plexus						
brachial	171.2	198.89	—	215.2	238.1	239.2
cervical	171.0	198.89	—	215.0	238.1	239.2
choroid	191.5	198.3	—	225.0	237.5	239.6
lumbosacral	171.6	198.89	—	215.6	238.1	239.2
sacral	171.6	198.89	—	215.6	238.1	239.2
pluri-endocrine	194.8	198.89	234.8	227.8	237.4	239.7
pole						
frontal	191.1	198.3	—	225.0	237.5	239.6
occipital	191.4	198.3	—	225.0	237.5	239.6
pons (varolii)	191.7	198.3	—	225.0	237.5	239.6
popliteal fossa or space*	195.5	198.89	234.8	229.8	238.8	239.8
postcricoid (region)	148.0	198.89	230.0	210.8	235.1	239.0
posterior fossa (cranial)	191.6	198.3	—	225.0	237.5	239.6
postnasal space	147.9	198.89	230.0	210.7	235.1	239.0
prepuce	187.1	198.82	233.5	222.1	236.6	239.5
prepylorus	151.1	197.8	230.2	211.1	235.2	239.0
presacral (region)	195.3	198.89	—	229.8	238.8	239.8

	Malignant					
	Primary	Secondary	Ca in situ	Benign	Uncertain Behavior	Unspecified
prostate (gland)	185	198.82	233.4	222.2	236.5	239.5
utricle	189.3	198.1	233.9	223.81	236.99	239.5
pterygoid fossa	171.0	198.89	—	215.0	238.1	239.2
pubic bone	170.6	198.5	—	213.6	238.0	239.2
pudenda, pudendum (female)	184.4	198.82	233.3	221.2	236.3	239.5
pulmonary	162.9	197.0	231.2	212.3	235.7	239.1
putamen	191.0	198.3	—	225.0	237.5	239.6
pyloric						
antrum	151.2	197.8	230.2	211.1	235.2	239.0
canal	151.1	197.8	230.2	211.1	235.2	239.0
pylorus	151.1	197.8	230.2	211.1	235.2	239.0
pyramid (brain)	191.7	198.3	—	225.0	237.5	239.6
pyriform fossa or sinus	148.1	198.89	230.0	210.8	235.1	239.0
radius (any part)	170.4	198.5	—	213.4	238.0	239.2
Rathke's pouch	194.3	198.89	234.8	227.3	237.0	239.7
rectosigmoid (colon) (junction)	154.0	197.5	230.4	211.4	235.2	239.0
contiguous sites with anus or rectum	154.8	—	—	—	—	—
rectouterine pouch	158.8	197.6	—	211.8	235.4	239.0
rectovaginal septum or wall	195.3	198.89	234.8	229.8	238.8	239.8
rectovesical septum	195.3	198.89	234.8	229.8	238.8	239.8
rectum (ampulla)	154.1	197.5	230.4	211.4	235.2	239.0
and colon	154.0	197.5	230.4	211.4	235.2	239.0
contiguous sites with anus or rectosigmoid junction	154.8	—	—	—	—	—
renal	189.0	198.0	233.9	223.0	236.91	239.5
calyx	189.1	198.0	233.9	223.1	236.91	239.5
hilus	189.1	198.0	233.9	223.1	236.91	239.5
parenchyma	189.0	198.0	233.9	223.0	236.91	239.5
pelvis	189.1	198.0	233.9	223.1	236.91	239.5
respiratory						
organs or system NEC	165.9	197.3	231.9	212.9	235.9	239.1
contiguous sites with intrathoracic organs	165.8	—	—	—	—	—
specified sites NEC	165.8	197.3	231.8	212.8	235.9	239.1
tract NEC	165.9	197.3	231.9	212.9	235.9	239.1
upper	165.0	197.3	231.9	212.9	235.9	239.1
retina	190.5	198.4	234.0	224.5	238.8	239.8
retrobulbar	190.1	198.4	—	224.1	238.8	239.8
retrocecal	158.0	197.6	—	211.8	235.4	239.0
retromolar (area) (triangle) (trigone)	145.6	198.89	230.0	210.4	235.1	239.0
retro-orbital	195.0	198.89	234.8	229.8	238.8	239.8
retroperitoneal (space) (tissue)	158.0	197.6	—	211.8	235.4	239.0
contiguous sites	158.8	—	—	—	—	—
retroperitoneum	158.0	197.6	—	211.8	235.4	239.0
contiguous sites	158.8	—	—	—	—	—
retropharyngeal	149.0	198.89	230.0	210.9	235.1	239.0
retrovesical (septum)	195.3	198.89	234.8	229.8	238.8	239.8
rhinencephalon	191.0	198.3	—	225.0	237.5	239.6
rib	170.3	198.5	—	213.3	238.0	239.2
Rosenmüller's fossa	147.2	198.89	230.0	210.7	235.1	239.0
round ligament	183.5	198.82	—	221.0	236.3	239.5
sacrococcyx, sacrococcygeal	170.6	198.5	—	213.6	238.0	239.2
region	195.3	198.89	234.8	229.8	238.8	239.8
sacrouterine ligament	183.4	198.82	—	221.0	236.3	239.5
sacrum, sacral (vertebra)	170.6	198.5	—	213.6	238.0	239.2
salivary gland or duct (major)	142.9	198.89	230.0	210.2	235.0	239.0
contiguous sites	142.8	—	—	—	—	—
minor NEC	145.9	198.89	230.0	210.4	235.1	239.0
parotid	142.0	198.89	230.0	210.2	235.0	239.0
pluriglandular	142.8	198.89	230.0	210.2	235.0	239.0

	Malignant					
	Primary	Secondary	Ca in situ	Benign	Uncertain Behavior	Unspecified
salivary gland or duct (major)—*continued*						
sublingual	142.2	198.89	230.0	210.2	235.0	239.0
submandibular	142.1	198.89	230.0	210.2	235.0	239.0
submaxillary	142.1	198.89	230.0	210.2	235.0	239.0
salpinx (uterine)	183.2	198.82	233.3	221.0	236.3	239.5
Santorini's duct	157.3	197.8	230.9	211.6	235.5	239.0
scalp	173.4	198.2	232.4	216.4	238.2	239.2
scapula (any part)	170.4	198.5	—	213.4	238.0	239.2
scapular region	195.1	198.89	234.8	229.8	238.8	239.8
scar NEC (*see also* Neoplasm, skin)	173.9	198.2	232.9	216.9	238.2	239.2
sciatic nerve	171.3	198.89	—	215.3	238.1	239.2
sclera	190.0	198.4	234.0	224.0	238.8	239.8
scrotum (skin)	187.7	198.82	233.6	222.4	236.6	239.5
sebaceous gland—*see* Neoplasm, skin						
sella turcica	194.3	198.89	234.8	227.3	237.0	239.7
bone	170.0	198.5	—	213.0	238.0	239.2
semilunar cartilage (knee)	170.7	198.5	—	213.7	238.0	239.2
seminal vesicle	187.8	198.82	233.6	222.8	236.6	239.5
septum						
nasal	160.0	197.3	231.8	212.0	235.9	239.1
posterior margin	147.3	198.89	230.0	210.7	235.1	239.0
rectovaginal	195.3	198.89	234.8	229.8	238.8	239.8
rectovesical	195.3	198.89	234.8	229.8	238.8	239.8
urethrovaginal	184.9	198.82	233.3	221.9	236.3	239.5
vesicovaginal	184.9	198.82	233.3	221.9	236.3	239.5
shoulder NEC*	195.4	198.89	232.6	229.8	238.8	239.8
sigmoid flexure (lower) (upper)	153.3	197.5	230.3	211.3	235.2	239.0
sinus (accessory)	160.9	197.3	231.8	212.0	235.9	239.1
bone (any)	170.0	198.5	—	213.0	238.0	239.2
contiguous sites with middle ear or nasal cavities	160.8	—	—	—	—	—
ethmoidal	160.3	197.3	231.8	212.0	235.9	239.1
frontal	160.4	197.3	231.8	212.0	235.9	239.1
maxillary	160.2	197.3	231.8	212.0	235.9	239.1
nasal, paranasal NEC	160.9	197.3	231.8	212.0	235.9	239.1
pyriform	148.1	198.89	230.0	210.8	235.1	239.0
sphenoidal	160.5	197.3	231.8	212.0	235.9	239.1
skeleton, skeletal NEC	170.9	198.5	—	213.9	238.0	239.2
Skene's gland	189.4	198.1	233.9	223.89	236.99	239.5
skin NEC	173.9	198.2	232.9	216.9	238.2	239.2
abdominal wall	173.5	198.2	232.5	216.5	238.2	239.2
ala nasi	173.3	198.2	232.3	216.3	238.2	239.2
ankle	173.7	198.2	232.7	216.7	238.2	239.2
antecubital space	173.6	198.2	232.6	216.6	238.2	239.2
anus	173.5	198.2	232.5	216.5	238.2	239.2
arm	173.6	198.2	232.6	216.6	238.2	239.2
auditory canal (external)	173.2	198.2	232.2	216.2	238.2	239.2
auricle (ear)	173.2	198.2	232.2	216.2	238.2	239.2
auricular canal (external)	173.2	198.2	232.2	216.2	238.2	239.2
axilla, axillary fold	173.5	198.2	232.5	216.5	238.2	239.2
back	173.5	198.2	232.5	216.5	238.2	239.2
breast	173.5	198.2	232.5	216.5	238.2	239.2
brow	173.3	198.2	232.3	216.3	238.2	239.2
buttock	173.5	198.2	232.5	216.5	238.2	239.2
calf	173.7	198.2	232.7	216.7	238.2	239.2
canthus (eye) (inner) (outer)	173.1	198.2	232.1	216.1	238.2	239.2
cervical region	173.4	198.2	232.4	216.4	238.2	239.2
cheek (external)	173.3	198.2	232.3	216.3	238.2	239.2
chest (wall)	173.5	198.2	232.5	216.5	238.2	239.2
chin	173.3	198.2	232.3	216.3	238.2	239.2

	Malignant					
	Primary	Secondary	Ca in situ	Benign	Uncertain Behavior	Unspecified
skin NEC—*continued*						
clavicular area	173.5	198.2	232.5	216.5	238.2	239.2
clitoris	184.3	198.82	233.3	221.2	236.3	239.5
columnella	173.3	198.2	232.3	216.3	238.2	239.2
concha	173.2	198.2	232.2	216.2	238.2	239.2
contiguous sites	173.8	—	—	—	—	—
ear (external)	173.2	198.2	232.2	216.2	238.2	239.2
elbow	173.6	198.2	232.6	216.6	238.2	239.2
eyebrow	173.3	198.2	232.3	216.3	238.2	239.2
eyelid	173.1	198.2	232.1	216.1	238.2	239.2
face NEC	173.3	198.2	232.3	216.3	238.2	239.2
female genital organs (external)	184.4	198.82	233.3	221.2	236.3	239.5
clitoris	184.3	198.82	233.3	221.2	236.3	239.5
labium NEC	184.4	198.82	233.3	221.2	236.3	239.5
majus	184.1	198.82	233.3	221.2	236.3	239.5
minus	184.2	198.82	233.3	221.2	236.3	239.5
pudendum	184.4	198.82	233.3	221.2	236.3	239.5
vulva	184.4	198.82	233.3	221.2	236.3	239.5
finger	173.6	198.2	232.6	216.6	238.2	239.2
flank	173.5	198.2	232.5	216.5	238.2	239.2
foot	173.7	198.2	232.7	216.7	238.2	239.2
forearm	173.6	198.2	232.6	216.6	238.2	239.2
forehead	173.3	198.2	232.3	216.3	238.2	239.2
glabella	173.3	198.2	232.3	216.3	238.2	239.2
gluteal region	173.5	198.2	232.5	216.5	238.2	239.2
groin	173.5	198.2	232.5	216.5	238.2	239.2
hand	173.6	198.2	232.6	216.6	238.2	239.2
head NEC	173.4	198.2	232.4	216.4	238.2	239.2
heel	173.7	198.2	232.7	216.7	238.2	239.2
helix	173.2	198.2	232.2	216.2	238.2	239.2
hip	173.7	198.2	232.7	216.7	238.2	239.2
infraclavicular region	173.5	198.2	232.5	216.5	238.2	239.2
inguinal region	173.5	198.2	232.5	216.5	238.2	239.2
jaw	173.3	198.2	232.3	216.3	238.2	239.2
knee	173.7	198.2	232.7	216.7	238.2	239.2
labia						
majora	184.1	198.82	233.3	221.2	236.3	239.5
minora	184.2	198.82	233.3	221.2	236.3	239.5
leg	173.7	198.2	232.7	216.7	238.2	239.2
lid (lower) (upper)	173.1	198.2	232.1	216.1	238.2	239.2
limb NEC	173.9	198.2	232.9	216.9	238.2	239.5
lower	173.7	198.2	232.7	216.7	238.2	239.2
upper	173.6	198.2	232.6	216.6	238.2	239.2
lip (lower) (upper)	173.0	198.2	232.0	216.0	238.2	239.2
male genital organs	187.9	198.82	233.6	222.9	236.6	239.5
penis	187.4	198.82	233.5	222.1	236.6	239.5
prepuce	187.1	198.82	233.5	222.1	236.6	239.5
scrotum	187.7	198.82	233.6	222.4	236.6	239.5
mastectomy site	173.5	198.2	—	—	—	—
specified as breast tissue	174.8	198.81	—	—	—	
meatus, acoustic (external)	173.2	198.2	232.2	216.2	238.2	239.2
melanoma —*see* Melanoma						
nates	173.5	198.2	232.5	216.5	238.2	239.2
neck	173.4	198.2	232.4	216.4	238.2	239.2
nose (external)	173.3	198.2	232.3	216.3	238.2	239.2
palm	173.6	198.2	232.6	216.6	238.2	239.2
palpebra	173.1	198.2	232.1	216.1	238.2	239.2
penis NEC	187.4	198.82	233.5	222.1	236.6	239.5
perianal	173.5	198.2	232.5	216.5	238.2	239.2
perineum	173.5	198.2	232.5	216.5	238.2	239.2

| | Malignant | | | | | |
	Primary	Secondary	Ca in situ	Benign	Uncertain Behavior	Unspecified
skin NEC—*continued*						
pinna	173.2	198.2	232.2	216.2	238.2	239.2
plantar	173.7	198.2	232.7	216.7	238.2	239.2
popliteal fossa or space	173.7	198.2	232.7	216.7	238.2	239.2
prepuce	187.1	198.82	233.5	222.1	236.6	239.5
pubes	173.5	198.2	232.5	216.5	238.2	239.2
sacrococcygeal region	173.5	198.2	232.5	216.5	238.2	239.2
scalp	173.4	198.2	232.4	216.4	238.2	239.2
scapular region	173.5	198.2	232.5	216.5	238.2	239.2
scrotum	187.7	198.82	233.6	222.4	236.6	239.5
shoulder	173.6	198.2	232.6	216.6	238.2	239.2
sole (foot)	173.7	198.2	232.7	216.7	238.2	239.2
specified sites NEC	173.8	198.2	232.8	216.8	232.8	239.2
submammary fold	173.5	198.2	232.5	216.5	238.2	239.2
supraclavicular region	173.4	198.2	232.4	216.4	238.2	239.2
temple	173.3	198.2	232.3	216.3	238.2	239.2
thigh	173.7	198.2	232.7	216.7	238.2	239.2
thoracic wall	173.5	198.2	232.5	216.5	238.2	239.2
thumb	173.6	198.2	232.6	216.6	238.2	239.2
toe	173.7	198.2	232.7	216.7	238.2	239.2
tragus	173.2	198.2	232.2	216.2	238.2	239.2
trunk	173.5	198.2	232.5	216.5	238.2	239.2
umbilicus	173.5	198.2	232.5	216.5	238.2	239.2
vulva	184.4	198.82	233.3	221.2	236.3	239.5
wrist	173.6	198.2	232.6	216.6	238.2	239.2
skull	170.0	198.5	—	213.0	238.0	239.2
soft parts or tissues—*see* Neoplasm, connective tissue						
specified site NEC	195.8	198.89	234.8	229.8	238.8	239.8
spermatic cord	187.6	198.82	233.6	222.8	236.6	239.5
sphenoid	160.5	197.3	231.8	212.0	235.9	239.1
bone	170.0	198.5	—	213.0	238.0	239.2
sinus	160.5	197.3	231.8	212.0	235.9	239.1
sphincter						
anal	154.2	197.5	230.5	211.4	235.5	239.0
of Oddi	156.1	197.8	230.8	211.5	235.3	239.0
spine, spinal (column)	170.2	198.5	—	213.2	238.0	239.2
bulb	191.7	198.3	—	225.0	237.5	239.6
coccyx	170.6	198.5	—	213.6	238.0	239.2
cord (cervical) (lumbar) (sacral) (thoracic)	192.2	198.3	—	225.3	237.5	239.7
dura mater	192.3	198.4	—	225.4	237.6	239.7
lumbosacral	170.2	198.5	—	213.2	238.0	239.2
membrane	192.3	198.4	—	225.4	237.6	239.7
meninges	192.3	198.4	—	225.4	237.6	239.7
nerve (root)	171.9	198.89	—	215.9	238.1	239.2
pia mater	192.3	198.4	—	225.4	237.6	239.7
root	171.9	198.89	—	215.9	238.1	239.2
sacrum	170.6	198.5	—	213.6	238.0	239.2
spleen, splenic NEC	159.1	197.8	230.9	211.9	235.5	239.0
flexure (colon)	153.7	197.5	230.3	211.3	235.2	239.0
stem, brain	191.7	198.3	—	225.0	237.5	239.6
Stensen's duct	142.0	198.89	230.0	210.2	235.0	239.0
sternum	170.3	198.5	—	213.3	238.0	239.2
stomach	151.9	197.8	230.2	211.1	235.2	239.0
antrum (pyloric)	151.2	197.8	230.2	211.1	235.2	239.0
body	151.4	197.8	230.2	211.1	235.2	239.0
cardia	151.0	197.8	230.2	211.1	235.2	239.0
cardiac orifice	151.0	197.8	230.2	211.1	235.2	239.0
contiguous sites	151.8	—	—	—	—	—
corpus	151.4	197.8	230.2	211.1	235.2	239.0

| | Malignant | | | | | |
	Primary	Secondary	Ca in situ	Benign	Uncertain Behavior	Unspecified
stomach—*continued*						
fundus	151.3	197.8	230.2	211.1	235.2	239.0
greater curvature NEC	151.6	197.8	230.2	211.1	235.2	239.0
lesser curvature NEC	151.5	197.8	230.2	211.1	235.2	239.0
prepylorus	151.1	197.8	230.2	211.1	235.2	239.0
pylorus	151.1	197.8	230.2	211.1	235.2	239.0
wall NEC	151.9	197.8	230.2	211.1	235.2	239.0
anterior NEC	151.8	197.8	230.2	211.1	235.2	239.0
posterior NEC	151.8	197.8	230.2	211.1	235.2	239.0
stroma, endometrial	182.0	198.82	233.2	219.1	236.0	239.5
stump, cervical	180.8	198.82	233.1	219.0	236.0	239.5
subcutaneous (nodule) (tissue) NEC—*see* Neoplasm, connective tissue						
subdural	192.1	198.4	—	225.2	237.6	239.7
subglottis, subglottic	161.2	197.3	231.0	212.1	235.6	239.1
sublingual	144.9	198.89	230.0	210.3	235.1	239.0
gland or duct	142.2	198.89	230.0	210.2	235.0	239.0
submandibular gland	142.1	198.89	230.0	210.2	235.0	239.0
submaxillary gland or duct	142.1	198.89	230.0	210.2	235.0	239.0
submental	195.0	198.89	234.8	229.8	238.8	239.8
subpleural	162.9	197.0	—	212.3	235.7	239.1
substernal	164.2	197.1	—	212.5	235.8	239.8
sudoriferous, sudoriparous gland, site unspecified.	173.9	198.2	232.9	216.9	238.2	239.2
specified site—*see* Neoplasm, skin						
supraclavicular region	195.0	198.89	234.8	229.8	238.8	239.8
supraglottis	161.1	197.3	231.0	212.1	235.6	239.1
suprarenal (capsule) (cortex) (gland) (medulla)	194.0	198.7	234.8	227.0	237.2	239.7
suprasellar (region)	191.9	198.3	—	225.0	237.5	239.6
sweat gland (apocrine) (eccrine), site unspecified	173.9	198.2	232.9	216.9	238.2	239.2
specified site—*see* Neoplasm, skin						
sympathetic nerve or nervous system NEC	171.9	198.89	—	215.9	238.1	239.2
symphysis pubis	170.6	198.5	—	213.6	238.0	239.2
synovial membrane—*see* Neoplasm, connective tissue						
tapetum, brain	191.8	198.3	—	225.0	237.5	239.6
tarsus (any bone)	170.8	198.5	—	213.8	238.0	239.2
temple (skin)	173.3	198.2	232.3	216.3	238.2	239.2
temporal						
bone	170.0	198.5	—	213.0	238.0	239.2
lobe or pole	191.2	198.3	—	225.0	237.5	239.6
region	195.0	198.89	234.8	229.8	238.8	239.8
skin	173.3	198.2	232.3	216.3	238.2	239.2
tendon (sheath)—*see* Neoplasm, connective tissue						
tentorium (cerebelli)	192.1	198.4	—	225.2	237.6	239.7
testis, testes (descended) (scrotal)	186.9	198.82	233.6	222.0	236.4	239.5
ectopic	186.0	198.82	233.6	222.0	236.4	239.5
retained	186.0	198.82	233.6	222.0	236.4	239.5
undescended	186.0	198.82	233.6	222.0	236.4	239.5
thalamus	191.0	198.3	—	225.0	237.5	239.6
thigh NEC*	195.5	198.89	234.8	229.8	238.8	239.8
thorax, thoracic (cavity) (organs NEC)	195.1	198.89	234.8	229.8	238.8	239.8
duct	171.4	198.89	—	215.4	238.1	239.2
wall NEC	195.1	198.89	234.8	229.8	238.8	239.8
throat	149.0	198.89	230.0	210.9	235.1	239.0
thumb NEC*	195.4	198.89	232.6	229.8	238.8	239.8

	Malignant			Benign	Uncertain Behavior	Unspecified
	Primary	Secondary	Ca in situ	Benign	Uncertain Behavior	Unspecified
thymus (gland)	164.0	198.89	—	212.6	235.8	239.8
contiguous sites with heart and						
mediastinum	164.8	—	—	—	—	—
thyroglossal duct	193	198.89	234.8	226	237.4	239.7
thyroid (gland)	193	198.89	234.8	226	237.4	239.7
cartilage	161.3	197.3	231.0	212.1	235.6	239.1
tibia (any part)	170.7	198.5	—	213.7	238.0	239.2
toe NEC*	195.5	198.89	232.7	229.8	238.8	239.8
tongue	141.9	198.89	230.0	210.1	235.1	239.0
anterior (two-thirds) NEC	141.4	198.89	230.0	210.1	235.1	239.0
dorsal surface	141.1	198.89	230.0	210.1	235.1	239.0
ventral surface	141.3	198.89	230.0	210.1	235.1	239.0
base (dorsal surface)	141.0	198.89	230.0	210.1	235.1	239.0
border (lateral)	141.2	198.89	230.0	210.1	235.1	239.0
contiguous sites	141.8	—	—	—	—	—
dorsal surface NEC	141.1	198.89	230.0	210.1	235.1	239.0
fixed part NEC	141.0	198.89	230.0	210.1	235.1	239.0
foramen cecum	141.1	198.89	230.0	210.1	235.1	239.0
frenulum linguae	141.3	198.89	230.0	210.1	235.1	239.0
junctional zone	141.5	198.89	230.0	210.1	235.1	239.0
margin (lateral)	141.2	198.89	230.0	210.1	235.1	239.0
midline NEC	141.1	198.89	230.0	210.1	235.1	239.0
mobile part NEC	141.4	198.89	230.0	210.1	235.1	239.0
posterior (third)	141.0	198.89	230.0	210.1	235.1	239.0
root	141.0	198.89	230.0	210.1	235.1	239.0
surface (dorsal)	141.1	198.89	230.0	210.1	235.1	239.0
base	141.0	198.89	230.0	210.1	235.1	239.0
ventral	141.3	198.89	230.0	210.1	235.1	239.0
tip	141.2	198.89	230.0	210.1	235.1	239.0
tonsil	141.6	198.89	230.0	210.1	235.1	239.0
tonsil	146.0	198.89	230.0	210.5	235.1	239.0
fauces, faucial	146.0	198.89	230.0	210.5	235.1	239.0
lingual	141.6	198.89	230.0	210.1	235.1	239.0
palatine	146.0	198.89	230.0	210.5	235.1	239.0
pharyngeal	147.1	198.89	230.0	210.7	235.1	239.0
pillar (anterior) (posterior)	146.2	198.89	230.0	210.6	235.1	239.0
tonsillar fossa	146.1	198.89	230.0	210.6	235.1	239.0
tooth socket NEC	143.9	198.89	230.0	210.4	235.1	239.0
trachea (cartilage) (mucosa)	162.0	197.3	231.1	212.2	235.7	239.1
contiguous sites with bronchus or lung	162.8	—	—	—	—	—
tracheobronchial	162.8	197.3	231.1	212.2	235.7	239.1
contiguous sites with lung	162.8	—	—	—	—	—
tragus	173.2	198.2	232.2	216.2	238.2	239.2
trunk NEC*	195.8	198.89	232.5	229.8	238.8	239.8
tubo-ovarian	183.8	198.82	233.3	221.8	236.3	239.5
tunica vaginalis	187.8	198.82	233.6	222.8	236.6	239.5
turbinate (bone)	170.0	198.5	—	213.0	238.0	239.2
nasal	160.0	197.3	231.8	212.0	235.9	239.1
tympanic cavity	160.1	197.3	231.8	212.0	235.9	239.1
ulna (any part)	170.4	198.5	—	213.4	238.0	239.2
umbilicus, umbilical	173.5	198.2	232.5	216.5	238.2	239.2
uncus, brain	191.2	198.3	—	225.0	237.5	239.6
unknown site or unspecified	199.1	199.1	234.9	229.9	238.9	239.9
urachus	188.7	198.1	233.7	223.3	236.7	239.4
ureter, ureteral	189.2	198.1	233.9	223.2	236.91	239.5
orifice (bladder)	188.6	198.1	233.7	223.3	236.7	239.4
ureter-bladder (junction)	188.6	198.1	233.7	223.3	236.7	239.4
urethra, urethral (gland)	189.3	198.1	233.9	223.81	236.99	239.5
orifice, internal	188.5	198.1	233.7	223.3	236.7	239.4
urethrovaginal (septum)	184.9	198.82	233.3	221.9	236.3	239.5

	Malignant			Benign	Uncertain Behavior	Unspecified
	Primary	Secondary	Ca in situ			
urinary organ or system NEC	189.9	198.1	233.9	223.9	236.99	239.5
bladder—*see* Neoplasm, bladder						
contiguous sites	189.8	—	—	—	—	—
specified sites NEC	189.8	198.1	233.9	223.89	236.99	239.5
utero-ovarian	183.8	198.82	233.3	221.8	236.3	239.5
ligament	183.3	198.82	—	221.0	236.3	239.5
uterosacral ligament	183.4	198.82	—	221.0	236.3	239.5
uterus, uteri, uterine	179	198.82	233.2	219.9	236.0	239.5
adnexa NEC	183.9	198.82	233.3	221.8	236.3	239.5
contiguous sites	183.8	—	—	—	—	—
body	182.0	198.82	233.2	219.1	236.0	239.5
contiguous sites	182.8	—	—	—	—	—
cervix	180.9	198.82	233.1	219.0	236.0	239.5
cornu	182.0	198.82	233.2	219.1	236.0	239.5
corpus	182.0	198.82	233.2	219.1	236.0	239.5
endocervix (canal) (gland)	180.0	198.82	233.1	219.0	236.0	239.5
endometrium	182.0	198.82	233.2	219.1	236.0	239.5
exocervix	180.1	198.82	233.1	219.0	236.0	239.5
external os	180.1	198.82	233.1	219.0	236.0	239.5
fundus	182.0	198.82	233.2	219.1	236.0	239.5
internal os	180.0	198.82	233.1	219.0	236.0	239.5
isthmus	182.1	198.82	233.2	219.1	236.0	239.5
ligament	183.4	198.82	—	221.0	236.3	239.5
broad	183.3	198.82	233.3	221.0	236.3	239.5
round	183.5	198.82	—	221.0	236.3	239.5
lower segment	182.1	198.82	233.2	219.1	236.0	239.5
myometrium	182.0	198.82	233.2	219.1	236.0	239.5
squamocolumnar junction	180.8	198.82	233.1	219.0	236.0	239.5
tube	183.2	198.82	233.3	221.0	236.3	239.5
utricle, prostatic	189.3	198.1	233.9	223.81	236.99	239.5
uveal tract	190.0	198.4	234.0	224.0	238.8	239.8
uvula	145.4	198.89	230.0	210.4	235.1	239.0
vagina, vaginal (fornix) (vault) (wall)	184.0	198.82	233.3	221.1	236.3	239.5
vaginovesical	184.9	198.82	233.3	221.9	236.3	239.5
septum	194.9	198.82	233.3	221.9	236.3	239.5
vallecula (epiglottis)	146.3	198.89	230.0	210.6	235.1	239.0
vascular—*see* Neoplasm, connective tissue						
vas deferens	187.6	198.82	233.6	222.8	236.6	239.5
Vater's ampulla	156.2	197.8	230.8	211.5	235.3	239.0
vein, venous—*see* Neoplasm, connective tissue						
vena cava (abdominal) (inferior)	171.5	198.89	—	215.5	238.1	239.2
superior	171.4	198.89	—	215.4	238.1	239.2
ventricle (cerebral) (floor) (fourth) (lateral) (third)	191.5	198.3	—	225.0	237.5	239.6
cardiac (left) (right)	164.1	198.89	—	212.7	238.8	239.8
ventricular band of larynx	161.1	197.3	231.0	212.1	235.6	239.1
ventriculus—*see* Neoplasm, stomach						
vermillion border—*see* Neoplasm, lip						
vermis, cerebellum	191.6	198.3	—	225.0	237.5	239.6
vertebra (column)	170.2	198.5	—	213.2	238.0	239.2
coccyx	170.6	198.5	—	213.6	238.0	239.2
sacrum	170.6	198.5	—	213.6	238.0	239.2
vesical—*see* Neoplasm, bladder						
vesicle, seminal	187.8	198.82	233.6	222.8	236.6	239.5
vesicocervical tissue	184.9	198.82	233.3	221.9	236.3	239.5
vesicorectal	195.3	198.89	234.8	229.8	238.8	239.8
vesicovaginal	184.9	198.82	233.3	221.9	236.3	239.5
septum	184.9	198.82	233.3	221.9	236.3	239.5
vessel (blood)—*see* Neoplasm, connective tissue						

	Malignant					
	Primary	Secondary	Ca in situ	Benign	Uncertain Behavior	Unspecified
vestibular gland, greater	184.1	198.82	233.3	221.2	236.3	239.5
vestibule						
mouth	145.1	198.89	230.0	210.4	235.1	239.0
nose	160.0	197.3	231.8	212.0	235.9	239.1
Virchow's gland	—	196.0	—	229.0	238.8	239.8
viscera NEC	195.8	198.89	234.8	229.8	238.8	239.8
vocal cords (true)	161.0	197.3	231.0	212.1	235.6	239.1
false	161.1	197.3	231.0	212.1	235.6	239.1
vomer	170.0	198.5	—	213.0	238.0	239.2
vulva	184.4	198.82	233.3	221.2	236.3	239.5
vulvovaginal gland	184.4	198.82	233.3	221.2	236.3	239.5
Waldeyer's ring	149.1	198.89	230.0	210.9	235.1	239.0
Wharton's duct	142.1	198.89	230.0	210.2	235.0	239.0
white matter (central) (cerebral)	191.0	198.3	—	225.0	237.5	239.6
windpipe	162.0	197.3	231.1	212.2	235.7	239.1
Wirsung's duct	157.3	197.8	230.9	211.6	235.5	239.0
wolffian (body) (duct)						
female	184.8	198.82	233.3	221.8	236.3	239.5
male	187.8	198.82	233.6	222.8	236.6	239.5
womb—*see* Neoplasm, uterus						
wrist NEC*	195.4	198.89	232.6	229.8	238.8	239.8
xiphoid process	170.3	198.5	—	213.3	238.0	239.2
Zuckerkandl's organ	194.6	198.89	—	227.6	237.3	239.7

Neovascularization
choroid 362.16
ciliary body 364.42
cornea 370.60
deep 370.63
localized 370.61
iris 364.42
retina 362.16
subretinal 362.16
Nephralgia 788.0
Nephritis, nephritic (albuminuric) (azotemic)
(congenital) (degenerative) (diffuse)
(disseminated) (epithelial) (familial) (focal)
(granulomatous) (hemorrhagic) (infantile)
(nonsuppurative, excretory) (uremic) 583.9
with
edema—*see* Nephrosis
lesion of
glomerulonephritis
hypocomplementemic persistent 583.2
with nephrotic syndrome 581.2
chronic 582.2
lobular 583.2
with nephrotic syndrome 581.2
chronic 582.2
membranoproliferative 583.2
with nephrotic syndrome 581.2
chronic 582.2
membranous 583.1
with nephrotic syndrome 581.1
chronic 582.1
mesangiocapillary 583.2
with nephrotic syndrome 581.2
chronic 582.2
mixed membranous and proliferative 583.2
with nephrotic syndrome 581.2
chronic 582.2
proliferative (diffuse) 583.0
with nephrotic syndrome 581.0
acute 580.0
chronic 582.0
rapidly progressive 583.4
acute 580.4
chronic 582.4
interstitial nephritis (diffuse) (focal) 583.89
with nephrotic syndrome 581.89
acute 580.89
chronic 582.89
necrotizing glomerulitis 583.4
acute 580.4
chronic 582.4
renal necrosis 583.9
cortical 583.6
medullary 583.7
specified pathology NEC 583.89
with nephrotic syndrome 581.89
acute 580.89
chronic 582.89
necrosis, renal 583.9
cortical 583.6
medullary (papillary) 583.7
nephrotic syndrome (*see also* Nephrosis) 581.9
papillary necrosis 583.7
specified pathology NEC 583.89
acute 580.9
extracapillary with epithelial crescents 580.4
hypertensive (*see also* Hypertension, kidney)
403.90
necrotizing 580.4
poststreptococcal 580.0
proliferative (diffuse) 580.0

Nephritis, nephritic—*continued*
rapidly progressive 580.4
specified pathology NEC 580.89
amyloid 277.3 *[583.81]*
chronic 277.3 *[582.81]*
arteriolar (*see also* Hypertension, kidney) 403.90
arteriosclerotic (*see also* Hypertension, kidney)
403.90
ascending (*see also* Pyelitis) 590.80
atrophic 582.9
basement membrane NEC 583.89
with
pulmonary hemorrhage (Goodpasture's
syndrome) 446.21 *[583.81]*
calculous, calculus 592.0
cardiac (*see also* Hypertension, kidney) 403.90
cardiovascular (*see also* Hypertension, kidney)
403.90
chronic 582.9
arteriosclerotic (*see also* Hypertension,
kidney) 403.90
hypertensive (*see also* Hypertension, kidney)
403.90
cirrhotic (*see also* Sclerosis, renal) 587
complicating pregnancy, childbirth, or
puerperium 646.2
with hypertension 642.1
affecting fetus or newborn 760.0
affecting fetus or newborn 760.1
croupous 580.9
desquamative—*see* Nephrosis
due to
amyloidosis 277.3 *[583.81]*
chronic 277.3 *[582.81]*
arteriosclerosis (*see also* Hypertension,
kidney) 403.90
diabetes mellitus 250.4 *[583.81]*
with nephrotic syndrome 250.4 *[581.81]*
diphtheria 032.89 *[580.81]*
gonococcal infection (acute) 098.19 *[583.81]*
chronic or duration of 2 months or over
098.39 *[583.81]*
gout 274.10
infectious hepatitis 070.9 *[580.81]*
mumps 072.79 *[580.81]*
specified kidney pathology NEC 583.89
acute 580.89
chronic 582.89
streptotrichosis 039.8 *[583.81]*
subacute bacterial endocarditis 421.0 *[580.81]*
systemic lupus erythematosus 710.0 *[583.81]*
chronic 710.0 *[582.81]*
typhoid fever 002.0 *[580.81]*
endothelial 582.2
end stage (chronic) (terminal) NEC 585
epimembranous 581.1
exudative 583.89
with nephrotic syndrome 581.89
acute 580.89
chronic 582.89
gonococcal (acute) 098.19 *[583.81]*
chronic or duration of 2 months or over
098.39 *[583.81]*
gouty 274.10
hereditary (Alport's syndrome) 759.89
hydremic—*see* Nephrosis
hypertensive (*see also* Hypertension, kidney)
403.90
hypocomplementemic persistent 583.2
with nephrotic syndrome 581.2
chronic 582.2

Nephrosis, nephrotic (Epstein's) (syndrome) 581.9
  with
    lesion of
      focal glomerulosclerosis 581.1
      glomerulonephritis
        endothelial 581.2
        hypocomplementemic persistent 581.2
        lobular 581.2
        membranoproliferative 581.2
        membranous 581.1
        mesangiocapillary 581.2
        minimal change 581.3
        mixed membranous and proliferative 581.2
        proliferative 581.0
      segmental hyalinosis 581.1
      specified pathology NEC 581.89
  acute—*see* Nephrosis, tubular
  anoxic—*see* Nephrosis, tubular
  arteriosclerotic (*see also* Hypertension, kidney) 403.90
  chemical—*see* Nephrosis, tubular
  cholemic 572.4
  complicating pregnancy, childbirth, or puerperium—*see* Nephritis, complicating pregnancy
  diabetic 250.4 *[581.81]*
  hemoglobinuric—*see* Nephrosis, tubular
  in
    amyloidosis 277.3 *[581.81]*
    diabetes mellitus 250.4 *[581.81]*
    epidemic hemorrhagic fever 078.6
    malaria 084.9 *[581.81]*
    polyarteritis 446.0 *[581.81]*
    systemic lupus erythematosus 710.0 *[581.81]*
  ischemic—*see* Nephrosis, tubular
  lipoid 581.3
  lower nephron—*see* Nephrosis, tubular
  lupoid 710.0 *[581.81]*
  lupus 710.0 *[581.81]*
  malarial 084.9 *[581.81]*
  minimal change 581.3
  necrotizing—*see* Nephrosis, tubular
  osmotic (sucrose) 588.8
  polyarteritic 446.0 *[581.81]*
  radiation 581.9
  specified lesion or cause NEC 581.89
  syphilitic 095.4
  toxic—*see* Nephrosis, tubular
  tubular (acute) 584.5
    due to a procedure 997.5
    radiation 581.9
Nephrosonephritis hemorrhagic (endemic) 078.6
Nephrostomy status V44.6
  with complication 997.5
Nerve —*see* condition
Nerves 799.2
Nervous (*see also* condition) 799.2
  breakdown 300.9
  heart 306.2
  stomach 306.4
  tension 799.2
Nervousness 799.2
Nesidioblastoma (M8150/0)
  pancreas 211.7
  specified site NEC—*see* Neoplasm, by site, benign
  unspecified site 211.7
Netherton's syndrome (ichthyosiform erythroderma) 757.1
Nettle rash 708.8

Nettleship's disease (urticaria pigmentosa) 757.33
Neumann's disease (pemphigus vegetans) 694.4
Neuralgia, neuralgic (acute) (*see also* Neuritis) 729.2
  accessory (nerve) 352.4
  acoustic (nerve) 388.5
  ankle 355.8
  anterior crural 355.8
  anus 787.99
  arm 723.4
  auditory (nerve) 388.5
  axilla 353.0
  bladder 788.1
  brachial 723.4
  brain—*see* Disorder, nerve, cranial
  broad ligament 625.9
  cerebral—*see* Disorder, nerve, cranial
  ciliary 346.2
  cranial nerve—*see also* Disorder, nerve, cranial
    fifth or trigeminal (*see also* Neuralgia, trigeminal) 350.1
  ear 388.71
    middle 352.1
  facial 351.8
  finger 354.9
  flank 355.8
  foot 355.8
  forearm 354.9
  Fothergill's (*see also* Neuralgia, trigeminal) 350.1
    postherpetic 053.12
  glossopharyngeal (nerve) 352.1
  groin 355.8
  hand 354.9
  heel 355.8
  Horton's 346.2
  Hunt's 053.11
  hypoglossal (nerve) 352.5
  iliac region 355.8
  infraorbital (*see also* Neuralgia, trigeminal) 350.1
  inguinal 355.8
  intercostal (nerve) 353.8
    postherpetic 053.19
  jaw 352.1
  kidney 788.0
  knee 355.8
  loin 355.8
  malarial (*see also* Malaria) 084.6
  mastoid 385.89
  maxilla 352.1
  median thenar 354.1
  metatarsal 355.6
  middle ear 352.1
  migrainous 346.2
  Morton's 355.6
  nerve, cranial—*see* Disorder, nerve, cranial
  nose 352.0
  occipital 723.8
  olfactory (nerve) 352.0
  ophthalmic 377.30
    postherpetic 053.19
  optic (nerve) 377.30
  penis 607.9
  perineum 355.8
  pleura 511.0
  postherpetic NEC 053.19
    geniculate ganglion 053.11
    ophthalmic 053.19
    trifacial 053.12

Neuritis—*continued*
  rheumatic (chronic) 729.2
  sacral region 355.8
  sciatic (nerve) 724.3
    due to displacement of intervertebral disc
      722.10
  serum 999.5
  specified nerve NEC—*see* Disorder, nerve
  spinal (nerve) 355.9
    root (*see also* Radiculitis) 729.2
  subscapular (nerve) 723.4
  suprascapular (nerve) 723.4
  syphilitic 095.8
  thenar (median) 354.1
  thoracic NEC 724.4
  toxic NEC 357.7
  trochlear (nerve) 378.53
  ulnar (nerve) 723.4
  vagus (nerve) 352.3
Neuroangiomatosis, encephalofacial 759.6
Neuroastrocytoma (M9505/1)—*see* Neoplasm,
  by site, uncertain behavior
Neuro-avitaminosis 269.2
Neuroblastoma (M9500/3)
  olfactory (M9522/3) 160.0
  specified site—*see* Neoplasm, by site, malignant
  unspecified site 194.0
Neurochorioretinitis (*see also* Chorioretinitis)
  363.20
Neurocirculatory asthenia 306.2
Neurocytoma (M9506/0)—*see* Neoplasm, by
  site, benign
Neurodermatitis (circumscribed) (circumscripta)
  (local) 698.3
  atopic 691.8
  diffuse (Brocq) 691.8
  disseminated 691.8
  nodulosa 698.3
Neuroencephalomyelopathy, optic 341.0
Neuroepithelioma (M9503/3)—*see also*
  Neoplasm, by site, malignant
  olfactory (M9521/3) 160.0
Neurofibroma (M9540/0)—*see also* Neoplasm,
  connective tissue, benign
  melanotic (M9541/0)—*see* Neoplasm,
    connective tissue, benign
  multiple (M9540/1) 237.70
    Type 1 237.71
    Type 2 237.72
  plexiform (M9550/0)—*see* Neoplasm,
    connective tissue, benign
Neurofibromatosis (multiple) (M9540/1) 237.70
  acoustic 237.72
  malignant (M9540/3)—*see* Neoplasm,
    connective tissue, malignant
  Type 1 237.71
  Type 2 237.72
  von Recklinghausen's 237.71
Neurofibrosarcoma (M9540/3)—*see* Neoplasm,
  connective tissue, malignant
Neurogenic —*see also* condition
  bladder (atonic) (automatic) (autonomic)
    (flaccid) (hypertonic) (hypotonic) (inertia)
    (infranuclear) (irritable) (motor) (nonreflex)
    (nuclear) (paralysis) (reflex) (sensory)
    (spastic) (supranuclear) (uninhibited) 596.54
    with cauda equina syndrome 344.61
  bowel 564.81
  heart 306.2
Neuroglioma (M9505/1)—*see* Neoplasm, by
  site, uncertain behavior
Neurolabyrinthitis (of Dix and Hallpike) 386.12

Neurolathyrism 988.2
Neuroleprosy 030.1
Neuroleptic malignant syndrome 333.92
Neurolipomatosis 272.8
Neuroma (M9570/0)—*see also* Neoplasm,
  connective tissue, benign
  acoustic (nerve) (M9560/0) 225.1
  amputation (traumatic)—*see also* Injury, nerve,
    by site
    surgical complication (late) 997.61
  appendix 211.3
  auditory nerve 225.1
  digital 355.6
    toe 355.6
  interdigital (toe) 355.6
  intermetatarsal 355.6
  Morton's 355.6
  multiple 237.70
    Type 1 237.71
    Type 2 237.72
  nonneoplastic 355.9
    arm NEC 354.9
    leg NEC 355.8
    lower extremity NEC 355.8
    specified site NEC—*see* Mononeuritis, by site
    upper extremity NEC 354.9
  optic (nerve) 225.1
  plantar 355.6
  plexiform (M9550/0)—*see* Neoplasm,
    connective tissue, benign
  surgical (nonneoplastic) 355.9
    arm NEC 354.9
    leg NEC 355.8
    lower extremity NEC 355.8
    upper extremity NEC 354.9
  traumatic—*see also* Injury, nerve, by site
    old—*see* Neuroma, nonneoplastic
Neuromyalgia 729.1
Neuromyasthenia (epidemic) 049.8
Neuromyelitis 341.8
  ascending 357.0
  optica 341.0
Neuromyopathy NEC 358.9
Neuromyositis 729.1
Neuronevus (M8725/0)—*see* Neoplasm, skin,
  benign
Neuronitis 357.0
  ascending (acute) 355.2
  vestibular 386.12
Neuroparalytic —*see* condition
Neuropathy, neuropathic (*see also* Disorder,
  nerve) 355.9
  acute motor 357.82
  alcoholic 357.5
    with psychosis 291.1
  arm NEC 354.9
  autonomic (peripheral)—*see* Neuropathy,
    peripheral, autonomic
  axillary nerve 353.0
  brachial plexus 353.0
  cervical plexus 353.2
  chronic
    progressive segmentally demyelinating 357.89
    relapsing demyelinating 357.89
  congenital sensory 356.2
  Déjérine-Sottas 356.0
  diabetic 250.6 *[357.2]*
  entrapment 355.9
    iliohypogastric nerve 355.79
    ilioinguinal nerve 355.79
    lateral cutaneous nerve of thigh 355.1

Nevus—*continued*
 pilosus (M8720/0)
 port wine 757.32
 sanguineous 757.32
 sebaceous (senile) 702.8
 senile 448.1
 spider 448.1
 spindle cell (and epithelioid cell) (M8770/0)
 stellar 448.1
 strawberry 757.32
 syringocystadenomatous papilliferous
  (M8406/0)
 unius lateris 757.33
 Unna's 757.32
 vascular 757.32
 verrucous 757.33
 white sponge (oral mucosa) 750.26
Newborn (infant) (liveborn)
 gestation
  24 completed weeks 765.22
  25-26 completed weeks 765.23
  27-28 completed weeks 765.24
  29-30 completed weeks 765.25
  31-32 completed weeks 765.26
  33-34 completed weeks 765.27
  35-36 completed weeks 765.28
  37 or more completed weeks 765.29
  less than 24 completed weeks 765.21
  unspecified completed weeks 765.20
 multiple NEC
  born in hospital (without mention of cesarean
    delivery or section) V37.00
   with cesarean delivery or section V37.01
  born outside hospital
   hospitalized V37.1
   not hospitalized V37.2
  mates all liveborn
   born in hospital (without mention of
     cesarean delivery or section) V34.00
    with cesarean delivery or section V34.01
   born outside hospital
    hospitalized V34.1
    not hospitalized V34.2
  mates all stillborn
   born in hospital (without mention of
     cesarean delivery or section) V35.00
    with cesarean delivery or section V35.01
   born outside hospital
    hospitalized V35.1
    not hospitalized V35.2
  mates liveborn and stillborn
   born in hospital (without mention of
     cesarean delivery or section) V36.00
    with cesarean delivery or section V36.01
   born outside hospital
    hospitalized V36.1
    not hospitalized V36.2
 single
  born in hospital (without mention of cesarean
    delivery or section) V30.00
   with cesarean delivery or section V30.01
  born outside hospital
   hospitalized V30.1
   not hospitalized V30.2
 twin NEC
  born in hospital (without mention of cesarean
    delivery or section) V33.00
   with cesarean delivery or section V33.01
  born outside hospital
   hospitalized V33.1
   not hospitalized V33.2

Newborn—*continued*
 mate liveborn
  born in hospital V31.0
  born outside hospital
   hospitalized V31.1
   not hospitalized V31.2
 mate stillborn
  born in hospital V32.0
  born outside hospital
   hospitalized V32.1
   not hospitalized V32.2
 unspecified as to single or multiple birth
  born in hospital (without mention of cesarean
    delivery or section) V39.00
   with cesarean delivery or section V39.01
  born outside hospital
   hospitalized V39.1
   not hospitalized V39.2
Newcastle's conjunctivitis or disease 077.8
Nezelof's syndrome (pure alymphocytosis)
 279.13
Niacin (amide) deficiency 265.2
Nicolas-Durand-Favre disease (climatic bubo)
 099.1
Nicolas-Favre disease (climatic bubo) 099.1
Nicotinic acid (amide) deficiency 265.2
Niemann-Pick disease (lipid histiocytosis)
 (splenomegaly) 272.7
Night
 blindness (*see also* Blindness, night) 368.60
  congenital 368.61
  vitamin A deficiency 264.5
 cramps 729.82
 sweats 780.8
 terrors, child 307.46
Nightmare 307.47
 REM-sleep type 307.47
Nipple —*see* condition
Nisbet's chancre 099.0
Nishimoto (-Takeuchi) disease 437.5
Nitritoid crisis or reaction —*see* Crisis, nitritoid
Nitrogen retention, extrarenal 788.9
Nitrosohemoglobinemia 289.8
Njovera 104.0
No
 diagnosis 799.9
 disease (found) V71.9
 room at the inn V65.0
Nocardiasis —*see* Nocardiosis
Nocardiosis 039.9
 with pneumonia 039.1
 lung 039.1
 specified type NEC 039.8
Nocturia 788.43
 psychogenic 306.53
Nocturnal —*see also* condition
 dyspnea (paroxysmal) 786.09
 emissions 608.89
 enuresis 788.36
  psychogenic 307.6
 frequency (micturition) 788.43
  psychogenic 306.53
Nodal rhythm disorder 427.89
Nodding of head 781.0
Node (s)—*see also* Nodule
 Heberden's 715.04
 larynx 478.79
 lymph—*see* condition
 milkers' 051.1
 Osler's 421.0
 rheumatic 729.89

O

Oasthouse urine disease 270.2
Obermeyer's relapsing fever (European) 087.0
Obesity (constitutional) (exogenous) (familial)
      (nutritional) (simple) 278.00
   adrenal 255.8
   due to hyperalimentation 278.00
   endocrine NEC 259.9
   endogenous 259.9
   Fröhlich's (adiposogenital dystrophy) 253.8
   glandular NEC 259.9
   hypothyroid (*see also* Hypothyroidism) 244.9
   morbid 278.01
   of pregnancy 646.1
   pituitary 253.8
   thyroid (*see also* Hypothyroidism) 244.9
Oblique —*see also* condition
   lie before labor, affecting fetus or newborn 761.7
Obliquity, pelvis 738.6
Obliteration
   abdominal aorta 446.7
   appendix (lumen) 543.9
   artery 447.1
   ascending aorta 446.7
   bile ducts 576.8
      with calculus, choledocholithiasis, or
            stones—*see* Choledocholithiasis
      congenital 751.61
         jaundice from 751.61 *[774.5]*
   common duct 576.8
      with calculus, choledocholithiasis, or
            stones—*see* Choledocholithiasis
      congenital 751.61
   cystic duct 575.8
      with calculus, choledocholithiasis, or
            stones—*see* Choledocholithiasis
   disease, arteriolar 447.1
   endometrium 621.8
   eye, anterior chamber 360.34
   fallopian tube 628.2
   lymphatic vessel 457.1
      postmastectomy 457.0
   organ or site, congenital NEC—*see* Atresia
   placental blood vessels—*see* Placenta, abnormal
   supra-aortic branches 446.7
   ureter 593.89
   urethra 599.84
   vein 459.9
   vestibule (oral) 525.8
Observation (for) V71.9
   without need for further medical care V71.9
   accident NEC V71.4
      at work V71.3
   criminal assault V71.6
   deleterious agent ingestion V71.89
   disease V71.9
      cardiovascular V71.7
      heart V71.7
      mental V71.09
      specified condition NEC V71.89
   foreign body ingestion V71.89
   growth and development variations V21.8
   injuries (accidental) V71.4
      inflicted NEC V71.6
         during alleged rape or seduction V71.5
   malignant neoplasm, suspected V71.1
   postpartum
      immediately after delivery V24.0
      routine follow-up V24.2

Observation—*continued*
   pregnancy
      high-risk V23.9
         specified problem NEC V23.8
      normal (without complication) V22.1
         with nonobstetric complication V22.2
         first V22.0
   rape or seduction, alleged V71.5
      injury during V71.5
   suicide attempt, alleged V71.89
   suspected (undiagnosed) (unproven)
      abuse V71.81
      cardiovascular disease V71.7
      child or wife battering victim V71.6
      concussion (cerebral) V71.6
      condition NEC V71.89
         infant—*see* Observation, suspected,
               condition, newborn
         newborn V29.9
            cardiovascular disease V29.8
            congenital anomaly V29.8
            genetic V29.3
            infectious V29.0
            ingestion foreign object V29.8
            injury V29.8
            metabolic V29.3
            neoplasm V29.8
            neurological V29.1
            poison, poisoning V29.8
            respiratory V29.2
            specified NEC V29.8
      exposure
         anthrax V71.82
         biologic agent NEC V71.83
      infectious disease not requiring isolation
            V71.89
      malignant neoplasm V71.1
      mental disorder V71.09
      neglect V71.81
      neoplasm
         benign V71.89
         malignant V71.1
      specified condition NEC V71.89
      tuberculosis V71.2
   tuberculosis, suspected V71.2
Obsession, obsessional 300.3
   ideas and mental images 300.3
   impulses 300.3
   neurosis 300.3
   phobia 300.3
   psychasthenia 300.3
   ruminations 300.3
   state 300.3
   syndrome 300.3
Obsessive-compulsive 300.3
   neurosis 300.3
   reaction 300.3
Obstetrical trauma NEC (complicating
      delivery) 665.9
   with
      abortion—*see* Abortion, by type, with damage
            to pelvic organs
      ectopic pregnancy (*see also* categories
            633.0-633.9) 639.2
      molar pregnancy (*see also* categories
            630-632) 639.2
   affecting fetus or newborn 763.89

Obstruction, obstructed, . . .—*continued*
  glottis 478.79
  hepatic 573.8
    duct (*see also* Obstruction, biliary) 576.2
      congenital 751.61
  icterus (*see also* Obstruction, biliary) 576.8
    congenital 751.61
  ileocecal coil (*see also* Obstruction, intestine)
      560.9
  ileum (*see also* Obstruction, intestine) 560.9
  iliofemoral (artery) 444.81
  internal anastomosis—*see* Complications,
      mechanical, graft
  intestine (mechanical) (neurogenic)
      (paroxysmal) (postinfectional) (reflex) 560.9
    with
      adhesions (intestinal) (peritoneal) 560.81
      hernia—*see also* Hernia, by site, with
          obstruction
        gangrenous—*see* Hernia, by site, with
            gangrene
    adynamic (*see also* Ileus) 560.1
    by gallstone 560.31
    congenital or infantile (small) 751.1
      large 751.2
    due to
      Ascaris lumbricoides 127.0
      mural thickening 560.89
      procedure 997.4
        involving urinary tract 997.5
    impaction 560.39
    infantile—*see* Obstruction, intestine,
        congenital
    newborn
      due to
        fecaliths 777.1
        inspissated milk 777.2
        meconium (plug) 777.1
          in mucoviscidosis 277.01
        transitory 777.4
      specified cause NEC 560.89
      transitory, newborn 777.4
    volvulus 560.2
  intracardiac ball valve prosthesis 996.02
  jaundice (*see also* Obstruction, biliary) 576.8
    congenital 751.61
  jejunum (*see also* Obstruction, intestine) 560.9
  kidney 593.89
  labor 660.9
    affecting fetus or newborn 763.1
    by
      bony pelvis (conditions classifiable to
          653.0-653.9) 660.1
      deep transverse arrest 660.3
      impacted shoulder 660.4
      locked twins 660.5
      malposition (fetus) (conditions classifiable
          to 652.0-652.9) 660.0
        head during labor 660.3
      persistent occipitoposterior position 660.3
      soft tissue, pelvic (conditions classifiable to
          654.0-654.9) 660.2
  lacrimal
    canaliculi 375.53
    congenital 743.65
    punctum 375.52
    sac 375.54
  lacrimonasal duct 375.56
    congenital 743.65
    neonatal 375.55
  lacteal, with steatorrhea 579.2

Obstruction, obstructed, . . .—*continued*
  laryngitis (*see also* Laryngitis) 464.01
  larynx 478.79
    congenital 748.3
  liver 573.8
    cirrhotic (*see also* Cirrhosis, liver) 571.5
  lung 518.89
    with
      asthma—*see* Asthma
      bronchitis (chronic) 491.2
      emphysema NEC 492.8
    airway, chronic 496
    chronic NEC 496
      with
        asthma (chronic) (obstructive) 493.2
    disease, chronic 496
      with
        asthma (chronic) (obstructive) 493.2
    emphysematous 492.8
  lymphatic 457.1
  meconium
    fetus or newborn 777.1
      in mucoviscidosis 277.01
    newborn due to fecaliths 777.1
  mediastinum 519.3
  mitral (rheumatic)—*see* Stenosis, mitral
  nasal 478.1
    duct 375.56
      neonatal 375.55
    sinus—*see* Sinusitis
  nasolacrimal duct 375.56
    congenital 743.65
    neonatal 375.55
  nasopharynx 478.29
  nose 478.1
  organ or site, congenital NEC—*see* Atresia
  pancreatic duct 577.8
  parotid gland 527.8
  pelviureteral junction (*see also* Obstruction,
      ureter) 593.4
  pharynx 478.29
  portal (circulation) (vein) 452
  prostate 600.9
    valve (urinary) 596.0
  pulmonary
    valve (heart) (*see also* Endocarditis,
        pulmonary) 424.3
    vein, isolated 747.49
  pyemic—*see* Septicemia
  pylorus (acquired) 537.0
    congenital 750.5
    infantile 750.5
  rectosigmoid (*see also* Obstruction, intestine)
      560.9
  rectum 569.49
  renal 593.89
  respiratory 519.8
    chronic 496
  retinal (artery) (vein) (central) (*see also*
      Occlusion, retina) 362.30
  salivary duct (any) 527.8
    with calculus 527.5
  sigmoid (*see also* Obstruction, intestine) 560.9
  sinus (accessory) (nasal) (*see also* Sinusitis)
      473.9
  Stensen's duct 527.8
  stomach 537.89
    acute 536.1
    congenital 750.7
  submaxillary gland 527.8
    with calculus 527.5

> *Note—Use the following fifth-digit
> subclassification with category 715:*
>
> *0 site unspecified*
> *1 shoulder region*
> *2 upper arm*
> *3 forearm*
> *4 hand*
> *5 pelvic region and thigh*
> *6 lower leg*
> *7 ankle and foot*
> *8 other specified sites except spine*
> *9 multiple sites*

> *Note—Use the following fifth-digit subclassification with category 730:*
>
> *0   site unspecified*
> *1   shoulder region*
> *2   upper arm*
> *3   forearm*
> *4   hand*
> *5   pelvic region and thigh*
> *6   lower leg*
> *7   ankle and foot*
> *8   other specified sites*
> *9   multiple sites*

P

Pacemaker syndrome 429.4
Pachyderma, pachydermia 701.8
  laryngis 478.5
  laryngitis 478.79
  larynx (verrucosa) 478.79
Pachydermatitis 701.8
Pachydermatocele (congenital) 757.39
  acquired 701.8
Pachydermatosis 701.8
Pachydermoperiostitis
  secondary 731.2
Pachydermoperiostosis
  primary idiopathic 757.39
  secondary 731.2
Pachymeningitis (adhesive) (basal) (brain)
    (cerebral) (cervical) (chronic) (circumscribed)
    (external) (fibrous) (hemorrhagic)
    (hypertrophic) (internal) (purulent) (spinal)
    (suppurative) (*see also* Meningitis) 322.9
  gonococcal 098.82
Pachyonychia (congenital) 757.5
  acquired 703.8
Pachyperiosteodermia
  primary or idiopathic 757.39
  secondary 731.2
Pachyperiostosis
  primary or idiopathic 757.39
  secondary 731.2
Pacinian tumor (M9507/0)—*see* Neoplasm,
    skin, benign
Pads, knuckle or Garrod's 728.79
Paget's disease (osteitis deformans) 731.0
  with infiltrating duct carcinoma of the breast
    (M8541/3)—*see* Neoplasm, breast,
    malignant
  bone 731.0
    osteosarcoma in (M9184/3)—*see* Neoplasm,
      bone, malignant
  breast (M8540/3) 174.0
  extramammary (M8542/3)—*see also* Neoplasm,
    skin, malignant
    anus 154.3
      skin 173.5
  malignant (M8540/3)
    breast 174.0
    specified site NEC (M8542/3)—*see*
      Neoplasm, skin, malignant
    unspecified site 174.0
  mammary (M8540/3) 174.0
  necrosis of bone 731.0
  nipple (M8540/3) 174.0
  osteitis deformans 731.0
Paget-Schroetter syndrome (intermittent venous
    claudication) 453.8
Pain(s)
  abdominal 789.0
  adnexa (uteri) 625.9
  alimentary, due to vascular insufficiency 557.9
  anginoid (*see also* Pain, precordial) 786.51
  anus 569.42
  arch 729.5
  arm 729.5
  back (postural) 724.5
    low 724.2
    psychogenic 307.89
  bile duct 576.9
  bladder 788.9

Pain(s)—*continued*
  bone 733.90
  breast 611.71
    psychogenic 307.89
  broad ligament 625.9
  cartilage NEC 733.90
  cecum 789.0
  cervicobrachial 723.3
  chest (central) 786.50
    atypical 786.59
    midsternal 786.51
    musculoskeletal 786.59
    noncardiac 786.59
    substernal 786.51
    wall (anterior) 786.52
  coccyx 724.79
  colon 789.0
  common duct 576.9
  coronary—*see* Angina
  costochondral 786.52
  diaphragm 786.52
  due to (presence of) any device, implant, or
    graft classifiable to 996.0-996.5—*see*
    Complications, due to (presence of) any
    device, implant, or graft classified to
    996.0-996.5 NEC
  ear (*see also* Otalgia) 388.70
  epigastric, epigastrium 789.0
  extremity (lower) (upper) 729.5
  eye 379.91
  face, facial 784.0
    atypical 350.2
    nerve 351.8
  false (labor) 644.1
  female genital organ NEC 625.9
    psychogenic 307.89
  finger 729.5
  flank 789.0
  foot 729.5
  gallbladder 575.9
  gas (intestinal) 787.3
  gastric 536.8
  generalized 780.99
  genital organ
    female 625.9
    male 608.9
    psychogenic 307.89
  groin 789.0
  growing 781.99
  hand 729.5
  head (*see also* Headache) 784.0
  heart (*see also* Pain, precordial) 786.51
  infraorbital (*see also* Neuralgia, trigeminal)
    350.1
  intermenstrual 625.2
  jaw 526.9
  joint 719.40
    ankle 719.47
    elbow 719.42
    foot 719.47
    hand 719.44
    hip 719.45
    knee 719.46
    multiple sites 719.49
    pelvic region 719.45
    psychogenic 307.89
    shoulder (region) 719.41
    specified site NEC 719.48

Panneuritis endemica 265.0 *[357.4]*
Panniculitis 729.30
  back 724.8
  knee 729.31
  neck 723.6
  nodular, nonsuppurative 729.30
  sacral 724.8
  specified site NEC 729.39
Panniculus adiposus (abdominal) 278.1
Pannus 370.62
  allergic eczematous 370.62
  degenerativus 370.62
  keratic 370.62
  rheumatoid—*see* Arthritis, rheumatoid
  trachomatosus, trachomatous (active) 076.1
    [370.62]
    late effect 139.1
Panophthalmitis 360.02
Panotitis —*see* Otitis media
Pansinusitis (chronic) (hyperplastic)
    (nonpurulent) (purulent) 473.8
  acute 461.8
  due to fungus NEC 117.9
  tuberculous (*see also* Tuberculosis) 012.8
Panuveitis 360.12
  sympathetic 360.11
Panvalvular disease —*see* Endocarditis, mitral
Papageienkrankheit 073.9
Papanicolaou smear
  cervix (screening test) V76.2
    as part of gynecological examination V72.3
    for suspected malignant neoplasm V76.2
      no disease found V71.1
    nonspecific abnormal finding 795.00
      atypical squamous cell changes of
          undetermined significance
        favor benign (ASCUS favor benign)
          795.01
        favor dysplasia (ASCUS favor dysplasia)
          795.02
      nonspecific finding NEC 795.09
      unsatisfactory 795.09
  other specified site—*see also* Screening,
      malignant neoplasm
    for suspected malignant neoplasm—*see also*
        Screening, malignant neoplasm
      no disease found V71.1
    nonspecific abnormal finding 795.1
  vagina V76.47
    following hysterectomy for malignant
        condition V67.01
Papilledema 377.00
  associated with
    decreased ocular pressure 377.02
    increased intracranial pressure 377.01
    retinal disorder 377.03
  choked disc 377.00
  infectional 377.00
Papillitis 377.31
  anus 569.49
  chronic lingual 529.4
  necrotizing, kidney 584.7
  optic 377.31
  rectum 569.49
  renal, necrotizing 584.7
  tongue 529.0

Papilloma (M8050/0)—*see also* Neoplasm, by
  site, benign

> *Note—Except where otherwise indicated, the
> morphological varieties of papilloma in the list
> below should be coded by site as for
> "Neoplasm, benign."*

  acuminatum (female) (male) 078.11
  bladder (urinary) (transitional cell) (M8120/1)
    236.7
    benign (M8120/0) 223.3
  choroid plexus (M9390/0) 225.0
    anaplastic type (M9390/3) 191.5
    malignant (M9390/3) 191.5
  ductal (M8503/0)
  dyskeratotic (M8052/0)
  epidermoid (M8052/0)
  hyperkeratotic (M8052/0)
  intracystic (M8504/0)
  intraductal (M8503/0)
  inverted (M8053/0)
  keratotic (M8052/0)
  parakeratotic (M8052/0)
  pinta (primary) 103.0
  renal pelvis (transitional cell) (M8120/1) 236.99
    benign (M8120/0) 223.1
  Schneiderian (M8121/0)
    specified site—*see* Neoplasm, by site, benign
    unspecified site 212.0
  serous surface (M8461/0)
    borderline malignancy (M8461/1)
      specified site—*see* Neoplasm, by site,
        uncertain behavior
      unspecified site 236.2
    specified site—*see* Neoplasm, by site, benign
    unspecified site 220
  squamous (cell) (M8052/0)
  transitional (cell) (M8120/0)
    bladder (urinary) (M8120/1) 236.7
    inverted type (M8121/1)—*see* Neoplasm, by
      site, uncertain behavior
    renal pelvis (M8120/1) 236.91
    ureter (M8120/1) 236.91
  ureter (transitional cell) (M8120/1) 236.91
    benign (M8120/0) 223.2
  urothelial (M8120/1)—*see* Neoplasm, by site,
    uncertain behavior
  verrucous (M8051/0)
  villous (M8261/1)—*see* Neoplasm, by site,
    uncertain behavior
  yaws, plantar or palmar 102.1
Papillomata, multiple, of yaws 102.1
Papillomatosis (M8060/0)—*see also* Neoplasm,
  by site, benign
  confluent and reticulate 701.8
  cutaneous 701.8
  ductal, breast 610.1
  Gougerot-Carteaud (confluent reticulate) 701.8
  intraductal (diffuse) (M8505/0)—*see* Neoplasm,
    by site, benign
  subareolar duct (M8506/0) 217
Papillon-Léage and Psaume syndrome
    (orodigitofacial dysostosis) 759.89
Papule 709.8
  carate (primary) 103.0
  fibrous, of nose (M8724/0) 216.3
  pinta (primary) 103.0
Papulosis, malignant 447.8
Papyraceous fetus 779.89
  complicating pregnancy 646.0
Paracephalus 759.7
Parachute mitral valve 746.5

Paracoccidioidomycosis 116.1
  mucocutaneous-lymphangitic 116.1
  pulmonary 116.1
  visceral 116.1
Paracoccidiomycosis —*see*
  Paracoccidioidomycosis
Paracusis 388.40
Paradentosis 523.5
Paradoxical facial movements 374.43
Paraffinoma 999.9
Paraganglioma (M8680/1)
  adrenal (M8700/0) 227.0
    malignant (M8700/3) 194.0
  aortic body (M8691/1) 237.3
    malignant (M8691/3) 194.6
  carotid body (M8692/1) 237.3
    malignant (M8692/3) 194.5
  chromaffin (M8700/0)—*see also* Neoplasm, by
    site, benign
    malignant (M8700/3)—*see* Neoplasm, by site,
      malignant
  extra-adrenal (M8693/1)
    malignant (M8693/3)
      specified site—*see* Neoplasm, by site,
        malignant
      unspecified site 194.6
    specified site—*see* Neoplasm, by site,
      uncertain behavior
    unspecified site 237.3
  glomus jugulare (M8690/1) 237.3
    malignant (M8690/3) 194.6
  jugular (M8690/1) 237.3
    malignant (M8680/3)
      specified site—*see* Neoplasm, by site,
        malignant
      unspecified site 194.6
  nonchromaffin (M8693/1)
    malignant (M8693/3)
      specified site—*see* Neoplasm, by site,
        malignant
      unspecified site 194.6
    specified site—*see* Neoplasm, by site,
      uncertain behavior
    unspecified site 237.3
  parasympathetic (M8682/1)
    specified site—*see* Neoplasm, by site,
      uncertain behavior
    unspecified site 237.3
  specified site—*see* Neoplasm, by site, uncertain
    behavior
  sympathetic (M8681/1)
    specified site—*see* Neoplasm, by site,
      uncertain behavior
    unspecified site 237.3
  unspecified site 237.3
Parageusia 781.1
  psychogenic 306.7
Paragonimiasis 121.2
Paragranuloma, Hodgkin's (M9660/3) 201.0
Parahemophilia (*see also* Defect, coagulation)
  286.3
Parakeratosis 690.8
  psoriasiformis 696.2
  variegata 696.2
Paralysis, paralytic (complete) (incomplete)
  344.9
  with
    broken
      back—*see* Fracture, vertebra, by site, with
        spinal cord injury

Paralysis, paralytic—*continued*
    neck—*see* Fracture, vertebra, cervical, with
      spinal cord injury
    fracture, vertebra—*see* Fracture, vertebra, by
      site, with spinal cord injury
    syphilis 094.89
  abdomen and back muscles 355.9
  abdominal muscles 355.9
  abducens (nerve) 378.54
  abductor 355.9
    lower extremity 355.8
    upper extremity 354.9
  accessory nerve 352.4
  accommodation 367.51
    hysterical 300.11
  acoustic nerve 388.5
  agitans 332.0
    arteriosclerotic 332.0
  alternating 344.89
    oculomotor 344.89
  amyotrophic 335.20
  ankle 355.8
  anterior serratus 355.9
  anus (sphincter) 569.49
  apoplectic (current episode) (*see also* Disease,
      cerebrovascular, acute) 436
    late effect—*see* Late effect(s) (of)
      cerebrovascular disease
    category 438
  arm 344.40
    affecting
      dominant side 344.41
      nondominant side 344.42
    both 344.2
    due to old CVA—*see* category 438
    hysterical 300.11
    late effect—*see* Late effect(s) (of)
      cerebrovascular disease
    psychogenic 306.0
    transient 781.4
      traumatic NEC (*see also* Injury, nerve,
        upper limb) 955.9
  arteriosclerotic (current episode) 437.0
    late effect—*see* Late effect(s) (of)
      cerebrovascular disease
  ascending (spinal), acute 357.0
  associated, nuclear 344.89
  asthenic bulbar 358.0
  ataxic NEC 334.9
    general 094.1
  athetoid 333.7
  atrophic 356.9
    infantile, acute (*see also* Poliomyelitis, with
      paralysis) 045.1
    muscle NEC 355.9
    progressive 335.21
    spinal (acute) (*see also* Poliomyelitis, with
      paralysis) 045.1
  attack (*see also* Disease, cerebrovascular, acute)
    436
  axillary 353.0
  Babinski-Nageotte's 344.89
  Bell's 351.0
    newborn 767.5
  Benedikt's 344.89
  birth (injury) 767.7
    brain 767.0
    intracranial 767.0
    spinal cord 767.4
  bladder (sphincter) 596.53
    neurogenic 596.54

Paralysis, paralytic—*continued*
  hypoglossal (nerve) 352.5
  hypokalemic periodic 359.3
  Hyrtl's sphincter (rectum) 569.49
  hysterical 300.11
  ileus (*see also* Ileus) 560.1
  infantile (*see also* Poliomyelitis) 045.9
    atrophic acute 045.1
    bulbar 045.0
    cerebral—*see* Palsy, cerebral
    paralytic 045.1
    progressive acute 045.9
    spastic—*see* Palsy, cerebral
    spinal 045.9
  infective (*see also* Poliomyelitis) 045.9
  inferior nuclear 344.9
  insane, general or progressive 094.1
  internuclear 378.86
  interosseous 355.9
  intestine (*see also* Ileus) 560.1
  intracranial (current episode) (*see also*
     Paralysis, brain) 437.8
    due to birth injury 767.0
  iris 379.49
    due to diphtheria (toxin) 032.81 *[379.49]*
  ischemic, Volkmann's (complicating trauma)
     958.6
  Jackson's 344.89
  jake 357.7
  Jamaica ginger (jake) 357.7
  juvenile general 090.40
  Klumpke (-Déjérine) (birth) (newborn) 767.6
  labioglossal (laryngeal) (pharyngeal) 335.22
  Landry's 357.0
  laryngeal nerve (recurrent) (superior) (*see also*
     Paralysis, vocal cord) 478.30
  larynx (*see also* Paralysis, vocal cord) 478.30
    due to diphtheria (toxin) 032.3
  late effect
    due to
      birth injury, brain or spinal (cord)—*see*
        Palsy, cerebral
      edema, brain or cerebral—*see* Paralysis,
        brain
      lesion
        cerebrovascular—*see* category 438
        late effect—*see* Late effect(s) (of)
          cerebrovascular disease
        spinal (cord)—*see* Paralysis, spinal
  lateral 335.24
  lead 984.9
    specified type of lead—*see* Table of drugs and
     chemicals
  left side—*see* Hemiplegia
  leg 344.30
    affecting
      dominant side 344.31
      nondominant side 344.32
    both (*see also* Paraplegia) 344.1
    crossed 344.89
    hysterical 300.11
    psychogenic 306.0
    transient or transitory 781.4
      traumatic NEC (*see also* Injury, nerve,
        lower limb) 956.9
  levator palpebrae superioris 374.31
  limb NEC 344.5
    all four—*see* Quadriplegia
    quadriplegia—*see* Quadriplegia
  lip 528.5
  Lissauer's 094.1

Paralysis, paralytic—*continued*
  local 355.9
  lower limb—*see also* Paralysis, leg
    both (*see also* Paraplegia) 344.1
  lung 518.89
    newborn 770.89
  median nerve 354.1
  medullary (tegmental) 344.89
  mesencephalic NEC 344.89
    tegmental 344.89
  middle alternating 344.89
  Millard-Gubler-Foville 344.89
  monoplegic—*see* Monoplegia
  motor NEC 344.9
    cerebral—*see* Paralysis, brain
    spinal—*see* Paralysis, spinal
  multiple
    cerebral—*see* Paralysis, brain
    spinal—*see* Paralysis, spinal
  muscle (flaccid) 359.9
    due to nerve lesion NEC 355.9
    eye (extrinsic) 378.55
      intrinsic 367.51
      oblique 378.51
    iris sphincter 364.8
    ischemic (complicating trauma) (Volkmann's)
     958.6
    pseudohypertrophic 359.1
  muscular (atrophic) 359.9
    progressive 335.21
  musculocutaneous nerve 354.9
  musculospiral 354.9
  nerve—*see also* Disorder, nerve
    third or oculomotor (partial) 378.51
      total 378.52
    fourth or trochlear 378.53
    sixth or abducens 378.54
    seventh or facial 351.0
      birth injury 767.5
      due to
        injection NEC 999.9
        operation NEC 997.09
      newborn 767.5
    accessory 352.4
    auditory 388.5
    birth injury 767.7
    cranial or cerebral (*see also* Disorder, nerve,
     cranial) 352.9
    facial 351.0
      birth injury 767.5
      newborn 767.5
    laryngeal (*see also* Paralysis, vocal cord)
     478.30
    newborn 767.7
    phrenic 354.8
      newborn 767.7
    radial 354.3
      birth injury 767.6
      newborn 767.6
    syphilitic 094.89
    traumatic NEC (*see also* Injury, nerve, by
     site) 957.9
    trigeminal 350.9
    ulnar 354.2
  newborn NEC 767.0
  normokalemic periodic 359.3
  obstetrical, newborn 767.7
  ocular 378.9
  oculofacial, congenital 352.6
  oculomotor (nerve) (partial) 378.51
    alternating 344.89

Paralysis, paralytic—*continued*
  external bilateral 378.55
    total 378.52
  olfactory nerve 352.0
  palate 528.9
  palatopharyngolaryngeal 352.6
  paratrigeminal 350.9
  periodic (familial) (hyperkalemic)
    (hypokalemic) (normokalemic) (secondary)
    359.3
  peripheral
    autonomic nervous system—*see* Neuropathy,
      peripheral, autonomic
    nerve NEC 355.9
  peroneal (nerve) 355.3
  pharynx 478.29
  phrenic nerve 354.8
  plantar nerves 355.6
  pneumogastric nerve 352.3
  poliomyelitis (current) (*see also* Poliomyelitis,
    with paralysis) 045.1
    bulbar 045.0
  popliteal nerve 355.3
  pressure (*see also* Neuropathy, entrapment)
    355.9
  progressive 335.21
    atrophic 335.21
    bulbar 335.22
    general 094.1
    hemifacial 349.89
    infantile, acute (*see also* Poliomyelitis) 045.9
    multiple 335.20
  pseudobulbar 335.23
  pseudohypertrophic 359.1
    muscle 359.1
  psychogenic 306.0
  pupil, pupillary 379.49
  quadriceps 355.8
  quadriplegic (*see also* Quadriplegia) 344.0
  radial nerve 354.3
    birth injury 767.6
  rectum (sphincter) 569.49
  rectus muscle (eye) 378.55
  recurrent laryngeal nerve (*see also* Paralysis,
    vocal cord) 478.30
  respiratory (muscle) (system) (tract) 786.09
    center NEC 344.89
      fetus or newborn 770.89
    congenital 768.9
    newborn 768.9
  right side—*see* Hemiplegia
  Saturday night 354.3
  saturnine 984.9
    specified type of lead—*see* Table of drugs and
      chemicals
  sciatic nerve 355.0
  secondary—*see* Paralysis, late effect
  seizure (cerebral) (current episode) (*see also*
    Disease, cerebrovascular, acute) 436
    late effect—*see* Late effect(s) (of)
      cerebrovascular disease
  senile NEC 344.9
  serratus magnus 355.9
  shaking (*see also* Parkinsonism) 332.0
  shock (*see also* Disease, cerebrovascular, acute)
    436
    late effect—*see* Late effect(s) (of)
      cerebrovascular disease
  shoulder 354.9
  soft palate 528.9
  spasmodic—*see* Paralysis, spastic

Paralysis, paralytic—*continued*
  spastic 344.9
    cerebral infantile—*see* Palsy, cerebral
    congenital (cerebral)—*see* Palsy, cerebral
    familial 334.1
    hereditary 334.1
    infantile 343.9
    noncongenital or noninfantile, cerebral 344.9
    syphilitic 094.0
      spinal 094.89
  sphincter, bladder (*see also* Paralysis, bladder)
    596.53
  spinal (cord) NEC 344.1
    accessory nerve 352.4
    acute (*see also* Poliomyelitis) 045.9
    ascending acute 357.0
    atrophic (acute) (*see also* Poliomyelitis, with
      paralysis) 045.1
      spastic, syphilitic 094.89
    congenital NEC 343.9
    hemiplegic —*see* Hemiplegia
    hereditary 336.8
    infantile (*see also* Poliomyelitis) 045.9
    late effect NEC 344.89
    monoplegic—*see* Monoplegia
    nerve 355.9
    progressive 335.10
    quadriplegic —*see* Quadriplegia
    spastic NEC 343.9
    traumatic—*see* Injury, spinal, by site
  sternomastoid 352.4
  stomach 536.3
    nerve 352.3
  stroke (current episode) (*see also* Disease,
    cerebrovascular, acute) 436
    late effect—*see* Late effect(s) (of)
      cerebrovascular disease
  subscapularis 354.8
  superior nuclear NEC 334.9
  supranuclear 356.8
  sympathetic
    cervical NEC 337.0
    nerve NEC (*see also* Neuropathy, peripheral,
      autonomic) 337.9
    nervous system—*see* Neuropathy, peripheral,
      autonomic
  syndrome 344.9
    specified NEC 344.89
  syphilitic spastic spinal (Erb's) 094.89
  tabetic general 094.1
  thigh 355.8
  throat 478.29
    diphtheritic 032.0
    muscle 478.29
  thrombotic (current episode) (*see also*
    Thrombosis, brain) 434.0
    late effect—*see* Late effect(s) (of)
      cerebrovascular disease
  thumb NEC 354.9
  tick (-bite) 989.5
  Todd's (postepileptic transitory paralysis)
    344.89
  toe 355.6
  tongue 529.8
  transient
    arm or leg NEC 781.4
    traumatic NEC (*see also* Injury, nerve, by
      site) 957.9
  trapezius 352.4
  traumatic, transient NEC (*see also* Injury, nerve,
    by site) 957.9

Parasitic —*see also* condition
  disease NEC (*see also* Infestation, parasitic)
    136.9
    contact V01.89
    exposure to V01.89
    intestinal NEC 129
    skin NEC 134.9
  stomatitis 112.0
  sycosis 110.0
    beard 110.0
    scalp 110.0
  twin 759.4
Parasitism NEC 136.9
  intestinal NEC 129
  skin NEC 134.9
  specified—*see* Infestation
Parasitophobia 300.29
Parasomnia 780.59
  nonorganic origin 307.47
Paraspadias 752.69
Paraspasm facialis 351.8
Parathyroid gland —*see* condition
Parathyroiditis (autoimmune) 252.1
Parathyroprival tetany 252.1
Paratrachoma 077.0
Paratyphilitis (*see also* Appendicitis) 541
Paratyphoid (fever)—*see* Fever, paratyphoid
Paratyphus —*see* Fever, paratyphoid
Paraurethral duct 753.8
Para-urethritis 597.89
  gonococcal (acute) 098.0
    chronic or duration of 2 months or over 098.2
Paravaccinia NEC 051.9
  milkers' node 051.1
Paravaginitis (*see also* Vaginitis) 616.10
Parencephalitis (*see also* Encephalitis) 323.9
  late effect—*see* category 326
Parergasia 298.9
Paresis (*see also* Paralysis) 344.9
  accommodation 367.51
  bladder (spastic) (sphincter) (*see also* Paralysis,
    bladder) 596.53
    tabetic 094.0
  bowel, colon, or intestine (*see also* Ileus) 560.1
  brain or cerebral—*see* Paralysis, brain
  extrinsic muscle, eye 378.55
  general 094.1
    arrested 094.1
    brain 094.1
    cerebral 094.1
    insane 094.1
    juvenile 090.40
      remission 090.49
    progressive 094.1
    remission (sustained) 094.1
    tabetic 094.1
  heart (*see also* Failure, heart) 428.9
  infantile (*see also* Poliomyelitis) 045.9
  insane 094.1
  juvenile 090.40
  late effect—*see* Paralysis, late effect
  luetic (general) 094.1
  peripheral progressive 356.9
  pseudohypertrophic 359.1
  senile NEC 344.9
  stomach 536.3
  syphilitic (general) 094.1
    congenital 090.40
  transient, limb 781.4
  vesical (sphincter) NEC 596.53

Paresthesia (*see also* Disturbance, sensation)
  782.0
  Berger's (paresthesia of lower limb) 782.0
  Bernhardt 355.1
  Magnan's 782.0
Paretic —*see* condition
Parinaud's
  conjunctivitis 372.02
  oculoglandular syndrome 372.02
  ophthalmoplegia 378.81
  syndrome (paralysis of conjugate upward gaze)
    378.81
Parkes Weber and Dimitri syndrome
  (encephalocutaneous angiomatosis) 759.6
Parkinson's disease, syndrome, or tremor
  —*see* Parkinsonism
Parkinsonism (arteriosclerotic) (idiopathic)
  (primary) 332.0
  associated with orthostatic hypotension
    (idiopathic) (symptomatic) 333.0
  due to drugs 332.1
  secondary 332.1
  syphilitic 094.82
Parodontitis 523.4
Parodontosis 523.5
Paronychia (with lymphangitis) 681.9
  candidal (chronic) 112.3
  chronic 681.9
    candidal 112.3
    finger 681.02
    toe 681.11
  finger 681.02
  toe 681.11
  tuberculous (primary) (*see also* Tuberculosis)
    017.0
Parorexia NEC 307.52
  hysterical 300.11
Parosmia 781.1
  psychogenic 306.7
Parotid gland —*see* condition
Parotiditis (*see also* Parotitis) 527.2
  epidemic 072.9
  infectious 072.9
Parotitis 527.2
  allergic 527.2
  chronic 527.2
  epidemic (*see also* Mumps) 072.9
  infectious (*see also* Mumps) 072.9
  noninfectious 527.2
  nonspecific toxic 527.2
  not mumps 527.2
  postoperative 527.2
  purulent 527.2
  septic 527.2
  suppurative (acute) 527.2
  surgical 527.2
  toxic 527.2
Paroxysmal —*see also* condition
  dyspnea (nocturnal) 786.09
Parrot's disease (syphilitic osteochondritis) 090.0
Parrot fever 073.9
Parry's disease or syndrome (exophthalmic
  goiter) 242.0
Parry-Romberg syndrome 349.89
Parson's disease (exophthalmic goiter) 242.0
Parsonage-Aldren-Turner syndrome 353.5
Parsonage-Turner syndrome 353.5
Pars planitis 363.21
Particolored infant 757.39
Parturition —*see* Delivery

Perforation, perforative—*continued*
  foreign body (external site)—*see also* Wound,
       open, by site, complicated
     internal site, by ingested object—*see* Foreign
       body
  frontal sinus (*see also* Sinusitis, frontal) 473.1
  gallbladder or duct (*see also* Disease,
       gallbladder) 575.4
  gastric (ulcer)—*see* Ulcer, stomach, with
       perforation
  heart valve—*see* Endocarditis
  ileum (*see also* Perforation, intestine) 569.83
  instrumental
     external—*see* Wound, open, by site
     pregnant uterus, complicating delivery 665.9
     surgical (accidental) (blood vessel) (nerve)
       (organ) 998.2
  intestine 569.83
     with
        abortion—*see* Abortion, by type, with
          damage to pelvic organs
        ectopic pregnancy (*see also* categories
          633.0-633.9) 639.2
        molar pregnancy (*see also* categories
          630-632) 639.2
     fetus or newborn 777.6
     obstetrical trauma 665.5
     ulcerative NEC 569.83
  jejunum, jejunal 569.83
     ulcer—*see* Ulcer, gastrojejunal, with
       perforation
  mastoid (antrum) (cell) 383.89
  maxillary sinus (*see also* Sinusitis, maxillary)
       473.0
  membrana tympani—*see* Perforation, tympanum
  nasal
     septum 478.1
        congenital 748.1
        syphilitic 095.8
     sinus (*see also* Sinusitis) 473.9
        congenital 748.1
  palate (hard) 526.89
     soft 528.9
        syphilitic 095.8
     syphilitic 095.8
  palatine vault 526.89
     syphilitic 095.8
        congenital 090.5
  pelvic
     floor
        with
           abortion—*see* Abortion, by type, with
             damage to pelvic organs
           ectopic pregnancy (*see also* categories
             633.0-633.9) 639.2
           molar pregnancy (*see also* categories
             630-632) 639.2
        obstetrical trauma 664.1
     organ
        with
           abortion—*see* Abortion, by type, with
             damage to pelvic organs
           ectopic pregnancy (*see also* categories
             633.0-633.9) 639.2
           molar pregnancy (*see also* categories
             630-632) 639.2
        following
           abortion 639.2
           ectopic or molar pregnancy 639.2
        obstetrical trauma 665.5
  perineum—*see* Laceration, perineum

Perforation, perforative—*continued*
  periurethral tissue
     with
        abortion—*see* Abortion, by type, with
          damage to pelvic organs
        ectopic pregnancy (*see also* categories
          630-632) 639.2
        molar pregnancy (*see also* categories
          630-632) 639.2
  pharynx 478.29
  pylorus, pyloric (ulcer)—*see* Ulcer, stomach,
       with perforation
  rectum 569.49
  sigmoid 569.83
  sinus (accessory) (chronic) (nasal) (*see also*
       Sinusitis) 473.9
  sphenoidal sinus (*see also* Sinusitis, sphenoidal)
       473.3
  stomach (due to ulcer)—*see* Ulcer, stomach,
       with perforation
  surgical (accidental) (by instrument) (blood
       vessel) (nerve) (organ) 998.2
  traumatic
     external—*see* Wound, open, by site
     eye (*see also* Penetrating wound, ocular) 871.7
     internal organ—*see* Injury, internal, by site
  tympanum (membrane) (persistent
       posttraumatic) (postinflammatory) 384.20
     with
        otitis media—*see* Otitis media
     attic 384.22
     central 384.21
     healed 384.81
     marginal NEC 384.23
     multiple 384.24
     pars flaccida 384.22
     total 384.25
     traumatic—*see* Wound, open, ear, drum
  typhoid, gastrointestinal 002.0
  ulcer—*see* Ulcer, by site, with perforation
  ureter 593.89
  urethra
     with
        abortion—*see* Abortion, by type, with
          damage to pelvic organs
        ectopic pregnancy (*see also* categories
          633.0-633.9) 639.2
        molar pregnancy (*see also* categories
          630-632) 639.2
     following
        abortion 639.2
        ectopic or molar pregnancy 639.2
     obstetrical trauma 665.5
  uterus—*see also* Injury, internal, uterus
     with
        abortion—*see* Abortion, by type, with
          damage to pelvic organs
        ectopic pregnancy (*see also* categories
          633.0-633.9) 639.2
        molar pregnancy (*see also* categories
          630-632) 639.2
     by intrauterine contraceptive device 996.32
     following
        abortion 639.2
        ectopic or molar pregnancy 639.2
     obstetrical trauma—*see* Injury, internal,
       uterus, obstetrical trauma
  uvula 528.9
     syphilitic 095.8
  vagina—*see* Laceration, vagina
  viscus NEC 799.8

Perifolliculitis—*continued*
scalp 704.8
superficial pustular 704.8
Perigastritis (acute) 535.0
Perigastrojejunitis (acute) 535.0
Perihepatitis (acute) 573.3
chlamydial 099.56
gonococcal 098.86
Peri-ileitis (subacute) 569.89
Perilabyrinthitis (acute)—*see* Labyrinthitis
Perimeningitis —*see* Meningitis
Perimetritis (*see also* Endometritis) 615.9
Perimetrosalpingitis (*see also*
Salpingo-oophoritis) 614.2
Perinephric —*see* condition
Perinephritic —*see* condition
Perinephritis (*see also* Infection, kidney) 590.9
purulent (*see also* Abscess, kidney) 590.2
Perineum, perineal —*see* condition
Perineuritis NEC 729.2
Periodic —*see also* condition
disease (familial) 277.3
edema 995.1
hereditary 277.6
fever 277.3
paralysis (familial) 359.3
peritonitis 277.3
polyserositis 277.3
somnolence 347
Periodontal
cyst 522.8
pocket 523.8
Periodontitis (chronic) (complex) (compound)
(local) (simplex) 523.4
acute 523.3
apical 522.6
acute (pulpal origin) 522.4
Periodontoclasia 523.5
Periodontosis 523.5
Periods —*see also* Menstruation
heavy 626.2
irregular 626.4
Perionychia (with lymphangitis) 681.9
finger 681.02
toe 681.11
Perioophoritis (*see also* Salpingo-oophoritis)
614.2
Periorchitis (*see also* Orchitis) 604.90
Periosteum, periosteal —*see* condition
Periostitis (circumscribed) (diffuse) (infective)
730.3

---

*Note—Use the following fifth-digit
subclassification with category 730:*

0 site unspecified
1 shoulder region
2 upper arm
3 forearm
4 hand
5 pelvic region and thigh
6 lower leg
7 ankle and foot
8 other specified sites
9 multiple sites

---

with osteomyelitis (*see also* Osteomyelitis)
730.2
acute or subacute 730.0
chronic or old 730.1
albuminosa, albuminosus 730.3
alveolar 526.5

Periostitis—*continued*
alveolodental 526.5
dental 526.5
gonorrheal 098.89
hyperplastica, generalized 731.2
jaw (lower) (upper) 526.4
monomelic 733.99
orbital 376.02
syphilitic 095.5
congenital 090.0 *[730.8]*
secondary 091.61
tuberculous (*see also* Tuberculosis, bone) 015.9
[730.8]
yaws (early) (hypertrophic) (late) 102.6
Periostosis (*see also* Periostitis) 730.3
with osteomyelitis (*see also* Osteomyelitis)
730.2
acute or subacute 730.0
chronic or old 730.1
hyperplastic 756.59
Periphlebitis (*see also* Phlebitis) 451.9
lower extremity 451.2
deep (vessels) 451.19
superficial (vessels) 451.0
portal 572.1
retina 362.18
superficial (vessels) 451.0
tuberculous (*see also* Tuberculosis) 017.9
retina 017.3 *[362.18]*
Peripneumonia —*see* Pneumonia
Periproctitis 569.49
Periprostatitis (*see also* Prostatitis) 601.9
Perirectal —*see* condition
Perirenal —*see* condition
Perisalpingitis (*see also* Salpingo-oophoritis)
614.2
Perisigmoiditis 569.89
Perisplenitis (infectional) 289.59
Perispondylitis —*see* Spondylitis
Peristalsis reversed or visible 787.4
Peritendinitis (*see also* Tenosynovitis) 726.90
adhesive (shoulder) 726.0
Perithelioma (M9150/1)—*see* Pericytoma
Peritoneum, peritoneal —*see also* condition
equilibration test V56.32
Peritonitis (acute) (adhesive) (fibrinous)
(hemorrhagic) (idiopathic) (localized)
(perforative) (primary) (with adhesions) (with
effusion) 567.9
with or following
abortion—*see* Abortion, by type, with sepsis
abscess 567.2
appendicitis 540.0
with peritoneal abscess 540.1
ectopic pregnancy (*see also* categories
633.0-633.9) 639.0
molar pregnancy (*see also* categories
630-632) 639.0
aseptic 998.7
bacterial 567.2
bile, biliary 567.8
chemical 998.7
chlamydial 099.56
chronic proliferative 567.8
congenital NEC 777.6
diaphragmatic 567.2
diffuse NEC 567.2
diphtheritic 032.83
disseminated NEC 567.2
due to
bile 567.8

Pneumonia—*continued*
    pneumoniae 481
    virus (*see also* Pneumonia, viral) 480.9
  Eaton's agent 483.0
  embolic, embolism (*see also* Embolism,
    pulmonary) 415.1
  eosinophilic 518.3
  Escherichia coli (E. coli) 482.82
  Eubacterium 482.81
  fibrinous—*see* Pneumonia, lobar
  fibroid (chronic) (*see also* Fibrosis, lung) 515
  fibrous (*see also* Fibrosis, lung) 515
  Friedländer's bacillus 482.0
  Fusobacterium (nucleatum) 482.81
  gangrenous 513.0
  giant cell (*see also* Pneumonia, viral) 480.9
  gram-negative bacteria NEC 482.83
    anaerobic 482.81
  grippal 487.0
  Hemophilus influenzae (bronchial) (lobar) 482.2
  hypostatic (broncho-) (lobar) 514
  in
    actinomycosis 039.1
    anthrax 022.1 *[484.5]*
    aspergillosis 117.3 *[484.6]*
    candidiasis 112.4
    coccidioidomycosis 114.0
    cytomegalic inclusion disease 078.5 *[484.1]*
    histoplasmosis (*see also* Histoplasmosis)
      115.95
    infectious disease NEC 136.9 *[484.8]*
    measles 055.1
    mycosis, systemic NEC 117.9 *[484.7]*
    nocardiasis, nocardiosis 039.1
    ornithosis 073.0
    pneumocystosis 136.3
    psittacosis 073.0
    Q fever 083.0 *[484.8]*
    salmonellosis 003.22
    toxoplasmosis 130.4
    tularemia 021.2
    typhoid (fever) 002.0 *[484.8]*
    varicella 052.1
    whooping cough (*see also* Whooping cough)
      033.9 *[484.3]*
  infective, acquired prenatally 770.0
  influenzal (broncho) (lobar) (virus) 487.0
  inhalation (*see also* Pneumonia, aspiration)
    507.0
    fumes or vapors (chemical) 506.0
  interstitial 516.8
    with influenzal 487.0
    acute 136.3
    chronic (*see also* Fibrosis, lung) 515
    desquamative 516.8
    hypostatic 514
    lipoid 507.1
    lymphoid 516.8
    plasma cell 136.3
    pseudomonas 482.1
  intrauterine (infective) 770.0
    aspiration 770.1
  Klebsiella pneumoniae 482.0
  Legionnaires' 482.84
  lipid, lipoid (exogenous) (interstitial) 507.1
    endogenous 516.8
  lobar (diplococcal) (disseminated) (double)
    (interstitial) (pneumococcal, any type) 481
    with influenza 487.0
    bacterial 482.9
      specified type NEC 482.89

Pneumonia—*continued*
  chronic (*see also* Fibrosis, lung) 515
  Escherichia coli (E. coli) 482.82
  Friedländer's bacillus 482.0
  Hemophilus influenzae (H. influenzae) 482.2
  hypostatic 514
  influenzal 487.0
  Klebsiella 482.0
  ornithosis 073.0
  Proteus 482.83
  pseudomonas 482.1
  psittacosis 073.0
  specified organism NEC 483.8
    bacterial NEC 482.89
  staphylococcal 482.40
    aureus 482.41
    specified type NEC 482.49
  streptococcal—*see* Pneumonia, streptococcal
  viral, virus (*see also* Pneumonia, viral) 480.9
  lobular (confluent)—*see* Pneumonia, broncho-
  Löffler's 518.3
  massive—*see* Pneumonia, lobar
  meconium 770.1
  metastatic NEC 038.8 *[484.8]*
  Mycoplasma (pneumoniae) 483.0
  necrotic 513.0
  nitrogen dioxide 506.9
  orthostatic 514
  parainfluenza virus 480.2
  parenchymatous (*see also* Fibrosis, lung) 515
  passive 514
  patchy—*see* Pneumonia, broncho
  Peptococcus 482.81
  Peptostreptococcus 482.81
  plasma cell 136.3
  pleurolobar—*see* Pneumonia, lobar
  pleuropneumonia-like organism (PPLO) 483.0
  pneumococcal (broncho) (lobar) 481
  Pneumocystis (carinii) 136.3
  postinfectional NEC 136.9 *[484.8]*
  postmeasles 055.1
  postoperative 997.3
  primary atypical 486
  Proprionibacterium 482.81
  Proteus 482.83
  pseudomonas 482.1
  psittacosis 073.0
  radiation 508.0
  respiratory syncytial virus 480.1
  resulting from a procedure 997.3
  rheumatic 390 *[517.1]*
  Salmonella 003.22
  segmented, segmental—*see* Pneumonia,
    broncho-
  Serratia (marcescens) 482.83
  specified
    bacteria NEC 482.89
    organism NEC 483.8
    virus NEC 480.8
  spirochetal 104.8 *[484.8]*
  staphylococcal (broncho) (lobar) 482.40
    aureus 482.41
    specified type NEC 482.49
  static, stasis 514
  streptococcal (broncho) (lobar) NEC 482.30
    Group
      A 482.31
      B 482.32
      specified NEC 482.39
    pneumoniae 481
    specified type NEC 482.39

Pneumonia—*continued*
　Streptococcus pneumoniae 481
　traumatic (complication) (early) (secondary)
　　958.8
　tuberculous (any) (*see also* Tuberculosis) 011.6
　tularemic 021.2
　TWAR agent 483.1
　varicella 052.1
　Veillonella 482.81
　viral, virus (broncho) (interstitial) (lobar) 480.9
　　with influenza, flu, or grippe 487.0
　　adenoviral 480.0
　　parainfluenza 480.2
　　respiratory syncytial 480.1
　　specified type NEC 480.8
　white (congenital) 090.0
Pneumonic —*see* condition
Pneumonitis (acute) (primary) (*see also*
　　Pneumonia) 486
　allergic 495.9
　　specified type NEC 495.8
　aspiration 507.0
　　due to fumes or gases 506.0
　　newborn 770.1
　　obstetric 668.0
　chemical 506.0
　　due to fumes or gases 506.0
　cholesterol 516.8
　chronic (*see also* Fibrosis, lung) 515
　congenital rubella 771.0
　due to
　　fumes or vapors 506.0
　　inhalation
　　　food (regurgitated), milk, vomitus 507.0
　　　oils, essences 507.1
　　　saliva 507.0
　　　solids, liquids NEC 507.8
　　toxoplasmosis (acquired) 130.4
　　　congenital (active) 771.2 *[484.8]*
　eosinophilic 518.3
　fetal aspiration 770.1
　hypersensitivity 495.9
　interstitial (chronic) (*see also* Fibrosis, lung) 515
　　lymphoid 516.8
　lymphoid, interstitial 516.8
　meconium 770.1
　postanesthetic
　　correct substance properly administered 507.0
　　obstetric 668.0
　　overdose or wrong substance given 968.4
　　　specified anesthetic—*see* Table of drugs
　　　　and chemicals
　postoperative 997.3
　　obstetric 668.0
　radiation 508.0
　rubella, congenital 771.0
　"ventilation" 495.7
　wood-dust 495.8
Pneumonoconiosis —*see* Pneumoconiosis
Pneumoparotid 527.8
Pneumopathy NEC 518.89
　alveolar 516.9
　　specified NEC 516.8
　due to dust NEC 504
　parietoalveolar 516.9
　　specified condition NEC 516.8
Pneumopericarditis (*see also* Pericarditis) 423.9
　acute 420.90

Pneumopericardium —*see also* Pericarditis
　congenital 770.2
　fetus or newborn 770.2
　traumatic (post) (*see also* Pneumothorax,
　　traumatic) 860.0
　　with open wound into thorax 860.1
Pneumoperitoneum 568.89
　fetus or newborn 770.2
Pneumophagia (psychogenic) 306.4
Pneumopleurisy, pneumopleuritis (*see also*
　　Pneumonia) 486
Pneumopyopericardium 420.99
Pneumopyothorax (*see also* Pyopneumothorax)
　　510.9
　with fistula 510.0
Pneumorrhagia 786.3
　newborn 770.3
　tuberculous (*see also* Tuberculosis, pulmonary)
　　011.9
Pneumosiderosis (occupational) 503
Pneumothorax (acute) (chronic) 512.8
　congenital 770.2
　due to operative injury of chest wall or lung
　　512.1
　　accidental puncture or laceration 512.1
　fetus or newborn 770.2
　iatrogenic 512.1
　postoperative 512.1
　spontaneous 512.8
　　fetus or newborn 770.2
　　tension 512.0
　sucking 512.8
　　iatrogenic 512.1
　　postoperative 512.1
　tense valvular, infectional 512.0
　tension 512.0
　　iatrogenic 512.1
　　postoperative 512.1
　　spontaneous 512.0
　traumatic 860.0
　　with
　　　hemothorax 860.4
　　　　with open wound into thorax 860.5
　　　open wound into thorax 860.1
　tuberculous (*see also* Tuberculosis) 011.7
Pocket (s)
　endocardial (*see also* Endocarditis) 424.90
　periodontal 523.8
Podagra 274.9
Podencephalus 759.89
Poikilocytosis 790.09
Poikiloderma 709.09
　Civatte's 709.09
　congenital 757.33
　vasculare atrophicans 696.2
Poikilodermatomyositis 710.3
Pointed ear 744.29
Poise imperfect 729.9
Poisoned —*see* Poisoning
Poisoning (acute)—*see also* Table of drugs and
　　chemicals
　Bacillus, B.
　　aertrycke (*see also* Infection, Salmonella)
　　　003.9
　　botulinus 005.1
　　cholerae (suis) (*see also* Infection,
　　　Salmonella) 003.9
　　paratyphosus (*see also* Infection, Salmonella)
　　　003.9
　　suipestifer (*see also* Infection, Salmonella)
　　　003.9

Pollitzer's disease (hidradenitis suppurativa)
705.83
Polyadenitis (*see also* Adenitis) 289.3
malignant 020.0
Polyalgia 729.9
Polyangiitis (essential) 446.0
Polyarteritis (nodosa) (renal) 446.0
Polyarthralgia 719.49
psychogenic 306.0
Polyarthritis, polyarthropathy NEC 716.59
due to or associated with other specified
conditions—*see* Arthritis, due to or
associated with
endemic (*see also* Disease, Kaschin-Beck) 716.0
inflammatory 714.9
specified type NEC 714.89
juvenile (chronic) 714.30
acute 714.31
migratory—*see* Fever, rheumatic
rheumatic 714.0
fever (acute)—*see* Fever, rheumatic
Polycarential syndrome of infancy 260
Polychondritis (atrophic) (chronic) (relapsing)
733.99
Polycoria 743.46
Polycystic (congenital) (disease) 759.89
degeneration, kidney—*see* Polycystic, kidney
kidney (congenital) 753.12
adult type (APKD) 753.13
autosomal dominant 753.13
autosomal recessive 753.14
childhood type (CPKD) 753.14
infantile type 753.14
liver 751.62
lung 518.89
congenital 748.4
ovary, ovaries 256.4
spleen 759.0
Polycythemia (primary) (rubra) (vera)
(M9950/1) 238.4
acquired 289.0
benign 289.0
familial 289.6
due to
donor twin 776.4
fall in plasma volume 289.0
high altitude 289.0
maternal-fetal transfusion 776.4
stress 289.0
emotional 289.0
erythropoietin 289.0
familial (benign) 289.6
Gaisböck's (hypertonica) 289.0
high altitude 289.0
hypertonica 289.0
hypoxemic 289.0
neonatorum 776.4
nephrogenous 289.0
relative 289.0
secondary 289.0
spurious 289.0
stress 289.0
Polycytosis cryptogenica 289.0
Polydactylism, polydactyly 755.00
fingers 755.01
toes 755.02
Polydipsia 783.5
Polydystrophic oligophrenia 277.5
Polyembryoma (M9072/3)—*see* Neoplasm, by
site, malignant
Polygalactia 676.6

Polyglandular
deficiency 258.9
dyscrasia 258.9
dysfunction 258.9
syndrome 258.8
Polyhydramnios (*see also* Hydramnios) 657
Polymastia 757.6
Polymenorrhea 626.2
Polymicrogyria 742.2
Polymyalgia 725
arteritica 446.5
rheumatica 725
Polymyositis (acute) (chronic) (hemorrhagic)
710.4
with involvement of
lung 710.4 *[517.8]*
skin 710.3
ossificans (generalisata) (progressiva) 728.19
Wagner's (dermatomyositis) 710.3
Polyneuritis, polyneuritic (*see also*
Polyneuropathy) 356.9
alcoholic 357.5
with psychosis 291.1
cranialis 352.6
demyelinating, chronic inflammatory 357.81
diabetic 250.6 *[357.2]*
due to lack of vitamin NEC 269.2 *[357.4]*
endemic 265.0 *[357.4]*
erythredema 985.0
febrile 357.0
hereditary ataxic 356.3
idiopathic, acute 357.0
infective (acute) 357.0
nutritional 269.9 *[357.4]*
postinfectious 357.0
Polyneuropathy (peripheral) 356.9
alcoholic 357.5
amyloid 277.3 *[357.4]*
arsenical 357.7
critical illness 357.82
diabetic 250.6 *[357.2]*
due to
antitetanus serum 357.6
arsenic 357.7
drug or medicinal substance 357.6
correct substance properly administered
357.6
overdose or wrong substance given or taken
977.9
specified drug—*see* Table of drugs and
chemicals
lack of vitamin NEC 269.2 *[357.4]*
lead 357.7
organophosphate compounds 357.7
pellagra 265.2 *[357.4]*
porphyria 277.1 *[357.4]*
serum 357.6
toxic agent NEC 357.7
hereditary 356.0
idiopathic 356.9
progressive 356.4
in
amyloidosis 277.3 *[357.4]*
avitaminosis 269.2 *[357.4]*
specified NEC 269.1 *[357.4]*
beriberi 265.0 *[357.4]*
collagen vascular disease NEC 710.9 *[357.1]*
deficiency
B-complex NEC 266.2 *[357.4]*
vitamin B 266.9 *[357.4]*
vitamin B6 266.1 *[357.4]*

Polyneuropathy—*continued*
  diabetes 250.6 *[357.2]*
  diphtheria (*see also* Diphtheria) 032.89
    [357.4]
  disseminated lupus erythematosus 710.0
    [357.1]
  herpes zoster 053.13
  hypoglycemia 251.2 *[357.4]*
  malignant neoplasm (M8000/3) NEC 199.1
    [357.3]
  mumps 072.72
  pellagra 265.2 *[357.4]*
  polyarteritis nodosa 446.0 *[357.1]*
  porphyria 277.1 *[357.4]*
  rheumatoid arthritis 714.0 *[357.1]*
  sarcoidosis 135 *[357.4]*
  uremia 585 *[357.4]*
  lead 357.7
  nutritional 269.9 *[357.4]*
    specified NEC 269.8 *[357.4]*
  postherpetic 053.13
  progressive 356.4
  sensory (hereditary) 356.2
Polyonychia 757.5
Polyopia 368.2
  refractive 368.15
Polyorchism, polyorchidism (three testes) 752.8
Polyorrhymenitis (peritoneal) (*see also*
    Polyserositis) 568.82
  pericardial 423.2
Polyostotic fibrous dysplasia 756.54
Polyotia 744.1
Polyp, polypus

> *Note—Polyps of organs or sites that do not*
> *appear in the list below should be coded to the*
> *residual category for diseases of the organ or*
> *site concerned.*

  accessory sinus 471.8
  adenoid tissue 471.0
  adenomatous (M8210/0)—*see also* Neoplasm,
    by site, benign
    adenocarcinoma in (M8210/3)—*see*
      Neoplasm, by site, malignant
    carcinoma in (M8210/3)—*see* Neoplasm, by
      site, malignant
    multiple (M8221/0)—*see* Neoplasm, by site,
      benign
  antrum 471.8
  anus, anal (canal) (nonadenomatous) 569.0
    adenomatous 211.4
  Bartholin's gland 624.6
  bladder (M8120/1) 236.7
  broad ligament 620.8—
  cervix (uteri) 622.7
    adenomatous 219.0
    in pregnancy or childbirth 654.6
      affecting fetus or newborn 763.89
      causing obstructed labor 660.2
    mucous 622.7
    nonneoplastic 622.7
  choanal 471.0
  cholesterol 575.6
  clitoris 624.6
  colon (M8210/0) (*see also* Polyp, adenomatous)
    211.3
  corpus uteri 621.0
  dental 522.0
  ear (middle) 385.30
  endometrium 621.0
  ethmoidal (sinus) 471.8

Polyp, polypus—*continued*
  fallopian tube 620.8
  female genital organs NEC 624.8
  frontal (sinus) 471.8
  gallbladder 575.6
  gingiva 523.8
  gum 523.8
  labia 624.6
  larynx (mucous) 478.4
  malignant (M8000/3)—*see* Neoplasm, by site,
    malignant
  maxillary (sinus) 471.8
  middle ear 385.30
  myometrium 621.0
  nares
    anterior 471.9
    posterior 471.0
  nasal (mucous) 471.9
    cavity 471.0
    septum 471.9
  nasopharyngeal 471.0
  neoplastic (M8210/0)—*see* Neoplasm, by site,
    benign
  nose (mucous) 471.9
  oviduct 620.8
  paratubal 620.8
  pharynx 478.29
    congenital 750.29
  placenta, placental 674.4
  prostate 600.2
  pudenda 624.6
  pulp (dental) 522.0
  rectosigmoid 211.4
  rectum (nonadenomatous) 569.0
    adenomatous 211.4
  septum (nasal) 471.9
  sinus (accessory) (ethmoidal) (frontal)
    (maxillary) (sphenoidal) 471.8
  sphenoidal (sinus) 471.8
  stomach (M8210/0) 211.1
  tube, fallopian 620.8
  turbinate, mucous membrane 471.8
  ureter 593.89
  urethra 599.3
  uterine
    ligament 620.8
    tube 620.8
  uterus (body) (corpus) (mucous) 621.0
    in pregnancy or childbirth 654.1
      affecting fetus or newborn 763.89
      causing obstructed labor 660.2
  vagina 623.7—
  vocal cord (mucous) 478.4
  vulva 624.6
Polyphagia 783.6
Polypoid —*see* condition
Polyposis —*see also* Polyp
  coli (adenomatous) (M8220/0) 211.3
    adenocarcinoma in (M8220/3) 153.9
    carcinoma in (M8220/3) 153.9
  familial (M8220/0) 211.3
  intestinal (adenomatous) (M8220/0) 211.3
  multiple (M8221/0)—*see* Neoplasm, by site,
    benign
Polyradiculitis (acute) 357.0
Polyradiculoneuropathy (acute) (segmentally
    demyelinating) 357.0
Polysarcia 278.00
Polyserositis (peritoneal) 568.82
  due to pericarditis 423.2
  paroxysmal (familial) 277.3

Polyserositis—*continued*
  pericardial 423.2
  periodic 277.3
  pleural—*see* Pleurisy
  recurrent 277.3
  tuberculous (*see also* Tuberculosis,
      polyserositis) 018.9
Polysialia 527.7
Polysplenia syndrome 759.0
Polythelia 757.6
Polytrichia (*see also* Hypertrichosis) 704.1
Polyunguia (congenital) 757.5
  acquired 703.8
Polyuria 788.42
Pompe's disease (glycogenosis II) 271.0
Pompholyx 705.81
Poncet's disease (tuberculous rheumatism) (*see
      also* Tuberculosis) 015.9
Pond fracture —*see* Fracture, skull, vault
Ponos 085.0
Pons, pontine —*see* condition
Poor
  contractions, labor 661.2
    affecting fetus or newborn 763.7
  fetal growth NEC 764.9
    affecting management of pregnancy 656.5
  incorporation
    artificial skin graft 996.55
    decellularized allodermis graft 996.55
  obstetrical history V13.49
    affecting management of current pregnancy
        V23.49
      pre-term labor V23.41
      pre-term labor V13.41
  sucking reflex (newborn) 796.1
  vision NEC 369.9
Poradenitis, nostras 099.1
Porencephaly (congenital) (development) (true)
      742.4
  acquired 348.0
  nondevelopmental 348.0
  traumatic (post) 310.2
Porocephaliasis 134.1
Porokeratosis 757.39
  disseminated superficial actinic (DSAP) 692.75
Poroma, eccrine (M8402/0)—*see* Neoplasm,
      skin, benign
Porphyria (acute) (congenital) (constitutional)
      (erythropoietic) (familial) (hepatica)
      (idiopathic) (idiosyncratic) (intermittent)
      (latent) (mixed hepatic) (photosensitive)
      (South African genetic) (Swedish) 277.1
  acquired 277.1
  cutaneatarda
    hereditaria 277.1
    symptomatica 277.1
  due to drugs
    correct substance properly administered 277.1
    overdose or wrong substance given or taken
        977.9
      specified drug—*see* Table of drugs and
          chemicals
  secondary 277.1
  toxic NEC 277.1
  variegata 277.1
Porphyrinuria (acquired) (congenital)
      (secondary) 277.1
Porphyruria (acquired) (congenital) 277.1
Portal —*see* condition
Port wine nevus or mark 757.32
Posadas-Wernicke disease 114.9

Position
  fetus, abnormal (*see also* Presentation, fetal)
      652.9
  teeth, faulty 524.3
Positive
  culture (nonspecific) 795.39
    AIDS virus V08
    blood 790.7
    HIV V08
    human immunodeficiency virus V08
    nose 795.39
    skin lesion NEC 795.39
    spinal fluid 792.0
    sputum 795.39
    stool 792.1
    throat 795.39
    urine 791.9
    wound 795.39
  findings, anthrax 795.31
  HIV V08
  human immunodeficiency virus (HIV) V08
  PPD 795.5
  serology
    AIDS virus V08
      inconclusive 795.71
    HIV V08
      inconclusive 795.71
    human immunodeficiency virus V08
      inconclusive 795.71
    syphilis 097.1
      with signs or symptoms—*see* Syphilis, by
          site and stage
      false 795.6
  skin test 795.7
    tuberculin (without active tuberculosis) 795.5
  VDRL 097.1
    with signs or symptoms—*see* Syphilis, by site
        and stage
    false 795.6
  Wassermann reaction 097.1
    false 795.6
Postcardiotomy syndrome 429.4
Postcaval ureter 753.4
Postcholecystectomy syndrome 576.0
Postclimacteric bleeding 627.1
Postcommissurotomy syndrome 429.4
Postconcussional syndrome 310.2
Postcontusional syndrome 310.2
Postcricoid region —*see* condition
Post-dates (pregnancy) —*see* Pregnancy
Postencephalitic —*see also* condition syndrome
      310.8
Posterior —*see* condition
Posterolateral sclerosis (spinal cord)—*see*
      Degeneration, combined
Postexanthematous —*see* condition
Postfebrile —*see* condition
Postgastrectomy dumping syndrome 564.2
Posthemiplegic chorea 344.89
Posthemorrhagic anemia (chronic) 280.0
  acute 285.1
  newborn 776.5
Posthepatitis syndrome 780.79
Postherpetic neuralgia (intercostal) (syndrome)
      (zoster) 053.19
  geniculate ganglion 053.11
  ophthalmica 053.19
  trigeminal 053.12
Posthitis 607.1
Postimmunization complication or reaction
      —*see* Complications, vaccination
Postinfectious —*see* condition

Pregnancy (single) (uterine) (without sickness) V22.2

> *Note—Use the following fifth-digit subclassification with categories 640-648, 651-676:*
>
> 0 *unspecified as to episode of care*
> 1 *delivered, with or without mention of antepartum condition*
> 2 *delivered, with mention of postpartum complication*
> 3 *antepartum condition or complication*
> 4 *postpartum condition or complication*

abdominal (ectopic) 633.00
  affecting fetus or newborn 761.4
  with intrauterine pregnancy 633.01
abnormal NEC 646.9
ampullar—*see* Pregnancy, tubal
broad ligament—*see* Pregnancy, cornual
cervical—*see* Pregnancy, cornual
combined (extrauterine and intrauterine)—*see* Pregnancy, cornual
complicated (by) 646.9
  abnormal, abnormality NEC 646.9
    cervix 654.6
    cord (umbilical) 663.9
    glucose tolerance (conditions classifiable to 790.2) 648.8
    pelvic organs or tissues NEC 654.9
    pelvis (bony) 653.0
    perineum or vulva 654.8
    placenta, placental (vessel) 656.7
    position
      cervix 654.4
      placenta 641.1
        without hemorrhage 641.0
      uterus 654.4
    size, fetus 653.5
    uterus (congenital) 654.0
  abscess or cellulitis
    bladder 646.6
    genitourinary tract (conditions classifiable to 590, 595, 597, 599.0, 614-616) 646.6
    kidney 646.6
    urinary tract NEC 646.6
  air embolism 673.0
  albuminuria 646.2
    with hypertension—*see* Toxemia, of pregnancy
  amnionitis 658.4
  amniotic fluid embolism 673.1
  anemia (conditions classifiable to 280-285) 648.2
  atrophy, yellow (acute) (liver) (subacute) 646.7
  bacilluria, asymptomatic 646.5
  bacteriuria, asymptomatic 646.5
  bicornis or bicornuate uterus 654.0
  bone and joint disorders (conditions classifiable to 720-724 or conditions affecting lower limbs classifiable to 711-719, 725-738) 648.7
  breech presentation 652.2
    with successful version 652.1
  cardiovascular disease (conditions classifiable to 390-398, 410-429) 648.6
    congenital (conditions classifiable to 745-747) 648.5
  cerebrovascular disorders conditions (classifiable to 430-434, 436-437) 674.0

Pregnancy—*continued*
  cervicitis (conditions classifiable to 616.0) 646.6
  chloasma (gravidarum) 646.8
  cholelithiasis 646.8
  chorea (gravidarum)—*see* Eclampsia, pregnancy
  contraction, pelvis (general) 653.1
    inlet 653.2
    outlet 653.3
  convulsions (eclamptic) (uremic) 642.6
    with pre-existing hypertension 642.7
  current disease or condition (nonobstetric)
    abnormal glucose tolerance 648.8
    anemia 648.2
    bone and joint (lower limb) 648.7
    cardiovascular 648.6
      congenital 648.5
    cerebrovascular 674.0
    diabetic 648.0
    drug dependence 648.3
    genital organ or tract 646.6
    gonorrheal 647.1
    hypertensive 642.2
      renal 642.1
    infectious 647.9
      specified type NEC 647.8
    liver 646.7
    malarial 647.4
    nutritional deficiency 648.9
    parasitic NEC 647.8
    renal 646.2
      hypertensive 642.1
    rubella 647.5
    specified condition NEC 648.9
    syphilitic 647.0
    thyroid 648.1
    tuberculous 647.3
    urinary 646.6
    venereal 647.2
    viral NEC 647.6
  cystitis 646.6
  cystocele 654.4
  death of fetus (near term) 656.4
    early pregnancy (before 22 completed weeks gestation) 632
  deciduitis 646.6
  decreased fetal movements 655.7
  diabetes (mellitus) (conditions classifiable to 250) 648.0
  disorders of liver 646.7
  displacement, uterus NEC 654.4
  disproportion—*see* Disproportion
  double uterus 654.0
  drug dependence (conditions classifiable to 304) 648.3
  dysplasia, cervix 654.6
  early onset of delivery (spontaneous) 644.2
  eclampsia, eclamptic (coma) (convulsions) (delirium) (nephritis) (uremia) 642.6
    with pre-existing hypertension 642.7
  edema 646.1
    with hypertension—*see* Toxemia, of pregnancy
  effusion, amniotic fluid 658.1
    delayed delivery following 658.2
  embolism
    air 673.0
    amniotic fluid 673.1
    blood-clot 673.2
    cerebral 674.0

Pregnancy—*continued*
 false 300.11
  labor (pains) 644.1
 fatigue 646.8
 illegitimate V61.6
 incidental finding V22.2
 in double uterus 654.0
 interstitial—*see* Pregnancy, cornual
 intraligamentous—*see* Pregnancy, cornual
 intramural—*see* Pregnancy, cornual
 intraperitoneal—*see* Pregnancy, abdominal
 isthmian—*see* Pregnancy, tubal
 management affected by
  abnormal, abnormality
   fetus (suspected) 655.9
    specified NEC 655.8
   placenta 656.7
  advanced maternal age NEC 659.6
   multigravida 659.6
   primigravida 659.5
  antibodies (maternal)
   anti-c 656.1
   anti-d 656.1
   anti-e 656.1
   blood group (ABO) 656.2
    Rh(esus) 656.1
  elderly multigravida 659.6
  elderly primigravida 659.5
  fetal (suspected)
   abnormality 655.9
    acid-base balance 656.8
    heart rate or rhythm 659.7
    specified NEC 655.8
   acidemia 656.3
   anencephaly 655.0
   bradycardia 659.7
   central nervous system malformation 655.0
   chromosomal abnormalities (conditions
     classifiable to 758.0-758.9) 655.1
   damage from
    drugs 655.5
     obstetric, anesthetic, or sedative 655.5
    environmental toxins 655.8
    intrauterine contraceptive device 655.8
    maternal
     alcohol addiction 655.4
     disease NEC 655.4
     drug use 655.5
     listeriosis 655.4
     rubella 655.3
     toxoplasmosis 655.4
     viral infection 655.3
    radiation 655.6
   death (near term) 656.4
    early (before 22 completed weeks
      gestation) 632
   distress 656.8
   excessive growth 656.6
   growth retardation 656.5
   hereditary disease 655.2
   hydrocephalus 655.0
   intrauterine death 656.4
   poor growth 656.5
   spina bifida (with myelomeningocele) 655.0
  fetal-maternal hemorrhage 656.0
  hereditary disease in family (possibly)
    affecting fetus 655.2
  incompatibility, blood groups (ABO) 656.2
   rh(esus) 656.1
  insufficient prenatal care V23.7
  intrauterine death 656.4

Pregnancy—*continued*
  isoimmunization (ABO) 656.2
   rh(esus) 656.1
  large-for-dates fetus 656.6
  light-for-dates fetus 656.5
  meconium in liquor 656.8
  mental disorder (conditions classifiable to
    290-303, 305-316, 317-319) 648.4
  multiparity (grand) 659.4
  poor obstetric history V23.49
   pre-term labor V23.41
  postmaturity
   post term 645.1
   prolonged 645.2
  post term pregnancy 645.1
  previous
   abortion V23.2
    habitual 646.3
   cesarean delivery 654.2
   difficult delivery V23.49
   forceps delivery V23.49
   habitual abortions 646.3
   hemorrhage, antepartum or postpartum
     V23.49
   hydatidiform mole V23.1
   infertility V23.0
   malignancy NEC V23.8
   nonobstetrical conditions V23.8
   premature delivery V23.41
   trophoblastic disease (conditions in 630)
     V23.1
   vesicular mole V23.1
  prolonged pregnancy 645.2
  small-for-dates fetus 656.5
  young maternal age 659.8
 maternal death NEC 646.9
 mesometric (mural)—*see* Pregnancy, cornual
 molar 631
  hydatidiform (*see also* Hydatidiform mole)
    630
   previous, affecting management of
     pregnancy V23.1
  previous, affecting management of pregnancy
    V23.49
 multiple NEC 651.9
  with fetal loss and retention of one or more
    fetus(es) 651.6
  affecting fetus or newborn 761.5
  specified type NEC 651.8
   with fetal loss and retention of one or more
     fetus(es) 651.6
 mural—*see* Pregnancy, cornual
 observation NEC V22.1
  first pregnancy V22.0
  high-risk V23.9
   specified problem NEC V23.8
 ovarian 633.20
  affecting fetus or newborn 761.4
  with intrauterine pregnancy 633.21
 postmature
  post term 645.1
  prolonged 645.2
 post term 645.1
 prenatal care only V22.1
  first pregnancy V22.0
  high-risk V23.9
   specified problem NEC V23.8
 prolonged 645.2
 quadruplet NEC 651.2
  with fetal loss and retention of one or more
    fetus(es) 651.5

Presentation—*continued*
    affecting fetus or newborn, any, except
      breech 763.1
  in multiple gestation (one or more) 652.6
  specified NEC 652.8
  arm 652.7
    causing obstructed labor 660.0
  breech (buttocks) (complete) (frank) 652.2
    with successful version 652.1
      before labor, affecting fetus or newborn
        761.7
      before labor, affecting fetus or newborn 761.7
  brow 652.4
    causing obstructed labor 660.0
  buttocks 652.2
  chin 652.4
  complete 652.2
  compound 652.8
  cord 663.0
  extended head 652.4
  face 652.4
    to pubes 652.8
  footling 652.8
  frank 652.2
  hand, leg, or foot NEC 652.8
  incomplete 652.8
  mentum 652.4
  multiple gestation (one fetus or more) 652.6
  oblique 652.3
    with successful version 652.1
  shoulder 652.8
    affecting fetus or newborn 763.1
  transverse 652.3
    with successful version 652.1
  umbilical cord 663.0
  unstable 652.0
Prespondylolisthesis (congenital) (lumbosacral)
  756.11
Pressure
  area, skin ulcer (*see also* Decubitus) 707.0
  atrophy, spine 733.99
  birth, fetus or newborn NEC 767.9
  brachial plexus 353.0
  brain 348.4
    injury at birth 767.0
  cerebral—*see* Pressure, brain
  chest 786.59
  cone, tentorial 348.4
    injury at birth 767.0
  funis—*see* Compression, umbilical cord
  hyposystolic (*see also* Hypotension) 458.9
  increased
    intracranial 781.99
      due to
        benign intracranial hypertension 348.2
        hydrocephalus—*see* hydrocephalus
        injury at birth 767.8
    intraocular 365.00
  lumbosacral plexus 353.1
  mediastinum 519.3
  necrosis (chronic) (skin) (*see also* Decubitus)
    707.0
  nerve—*see* Compression, nerve
  paralysis (*see also* Neuropathy, entrapment)
    355.9
  sore (chronic) (*see also* Decubitus) 707.0
  spinal cord 336.9
  ulcer (chronic) (*see also* Decubitus) 707.0
  umbilical cord—*see* Compression, umbilical
    cord
  venous, increased 459.89
Pre-syncope 780.2

Preterm infant NEC 765.1
  extreme 765.0
Priapism (penis) 607.3
Prickling sensation (*see also* Disturbance,
  sensation) 782.0
Prickly heat 705.1
Primary —*see* condition
Primigravida, elderly
  affecting
    fetus or newborn 763.89
    management of pregnancy, labor, and delivery
      659.5
Primipara, old
  affecting
    fetus or newborn 763.89
    management of pregnancy, labor, and delivery
      659.5
Primula dermatitis 692.6
Primus varus (bilateral) (metatarsus) 754.52
P.R.I.N.D. 436
Pringle's disease (tuberous sclerosis) 759.5
Prinzmetal's angina 413.1
Prinzmetal-Massumi syndrome (anterior chest
  wall) 786.52
Prizefighter ear 738.7
Problem (with) V49.9
  academic V62.3
  acculturation V62.4
  adopted child V61.29
  aged
    in-law V61.3
    parent V61.3
    person NEC V61.8
  alcoholism in family V61.41
  anger reaction (*see also* Disturbance, conduct)
    312.0
  behavior, child 312.9
  behavioral V40.9
    specified NEC V40.3
  betting V69.3
  cardiorespiratory NEC V47.2
  care of sick or handicapped person in family or
    household V61.49
  career choice V62.2
  communication V40.1
  conscience regarding medical care V62.6
  delinquency (juvenile) 312.9
  diet, inappropriate V69.1
  digestive NEC V47.3
  ear NEC V41.3
  eating habits, inappropriate V69.1
  economic V60.2
    affecting care V60.9
      specified type NEC V60.8
  educational V62.3
  enuresis, child 307.6
  exercise, lack of V69.0
  eye NEC V41.1
  family V61.9
    specified circumstance NEC V61.8
  fear reaction, child 313.0
  feeding (elderly) (infant) 783.3
    newborn 779.3
    nonorganic 307.50
  fetal, affecting management of pregnancy 656.9
    specified type NEC 656.8
  financial V60.2
  foster child V61.29
    specified NEC V41.8
  functional V41.9
    specified type NEC V41.8

Problem—*continued*
  gambling V69.3
  genital NEC V47.5
  head V48.9
    deficiency V48.0
    disfigurement V48.6
    mechanical V48.2
    motor V48.2
    movement of V48.2
    sensory V48.4
    specified condition NEC V48.8
  hearing V41.2
  high-risk sexual behavior V69.2
  influencing health status NEC V49.89
  internal organ NEC V47.9
    deficiency V47.0
    mechanical or motor V47.1
  interpersonal NEC V62.81
  jealousy, child 313.3
  learning V40.0
  legal V62.5
  life circumstance NEC V62.89
  lifestyle V69.9
    specified NEC V69.8
  limb V49.9
    deficiency V49.0
    disfigurement V49.4
    mechanical V49.1
    motor V49.2
    movement, involving
      musculoskeletal system V49.1
      nervous system V49.2
    sensory V49.3
    specified condition NEC V49.5
  litigation V62.5
  living alone V60.3
  loneliness NEC V62.89
  marital V61.10
    involving
      divorce V61.0
      estrangement V61.0
      psychosexual disorder 302.9
      sexual function V41.7
  mastication V41.6
  medical care, within family V61.49
  mental V40.9
    specified NEC V40.2
  mental hygiene, adult V40.9
  multiparity V61.5
  nail biting, child 307.9
  neck V48.9
    deficiency V48.1
    disfigurement V48.7
    mechanical V48.3
    motor V48.3
    movement V48.3
    sensory V48.5
    specified condition NEC V48.8
  neurological NEC 781.99
  none (feared complaint unfounded) V65.5
  occupational V62.2
  parent-child V61.20
  partner V61.10
  personal NEC V62.89
    interpersonal conflict NEC V62.81
  personality (*see also* Disorder, personality)
    301.9
  phase of life V62.89
  placenta, affecting management of pregnancy
    656.9
    specified type NEC 656.8

Problem—*continued*
  poverty V60.2
  presence of sick or handicapped person in
    family or household V61.49
  psychiatric 300.9
  psychosocial V62.9
    specified type NEC V62.89
  relational NEC V62.81
  relationship, childhood 313.3
  religious or spiritual belief
    other than medical care V62.89
    regarding medical care V62.6
  self-damaging behavior V69.8
  sexual
    behavior, high-risk V69.2
    function NEC V41.7
  sibling, relational V61.8
  sight V41.0
  sleep disorder, child 307.40
  smell V41.5
  speech V40.1
  spite reaction, child (*see also* Disturbance,
    conduct) 312.0
  spoiled child reaction (*see also* Disturbance,
    conduct) 312.1
  swallowing V41.6
  tantrum, child (*see also* Disturbance, conduct)
    312.1
  taste V41.5
  thumb sucking, child 307.9
  tic, child 307.21
  trunk V48.9
    deficiency V48.1
    disfigurement V48.7
    mechanical V48.3
    motor V48.3
    movement V48.3
    sensory V48.5
    specified condition NEC V48.8
  unemployment V62.0
  urinary NEC V47.4
  voice production V41.4
Procedure (surgical) not done NEC V64.3
  because of
    contraindication V64.1
    patient's decision V64.2
      for reasons of conscience or religion V62.6
    specified reason NEC V64.3
Procidentia
  anus (sphincter) 569.1
  rectum (sphincter) 569.1
  stomach 537.89
  uteri 618.1
Proctalgia 569.42
  fugax 564.6
  spasmodic 564.6
    psychogenic 307.89
Proctitis 569.49
  amebic 006.8
  chlamydial 099.52
  gonococcal 098.7
  granulomatous 555.1
  idiopathic 556.2
    with ulcerative sigmoiditis 556.3
  tuberculous (*see also* Tuberculosis) 014.8
  ulcerative (chronic) (nonspecific) 556.2
    with ulcerative sigmoiditis 556.3
Proctocele
  female (without uterine prolapse) 618.0
    with uterine prolapse 618.4
      complete 618.3

Prominence
  auricle (ear) (congenital) 744.29
    acquired 380.32
  ischial spine or sacral promontory
    with disproportion (fetopelvic) 653.3
      affecting fetus or newborn 763.1
      causing obstructed labor 660.1
        affecting fetus or newborn 763.1
  nose (congenital) 748.1
    acquired 738.0
Pronation
  ankle 736.79
  foot 736.79
    congenital 755.67
Prophylactic
  administration of
    antibiotics V07.39
    antitoxin, any V07.2
    antivenin V07.2
    chemotherapeutic agent NEC V07.39
      fluoride V07.31
    diphtheria antitoxin V07.2
    gamma globulin V07.2
    immune sera (gamma globulin) V07.2
    RhoGAM V07.2
    tetanus antitoxin V07.2
  chemotherapy NEC V07.39
    fluoride V07.31
  immunotherapy V07.2
  measure V07.9
    specified type NEC V07.8
  postmenopausal hormone replacement V07.4
  sterilization V25.2
Proptosis (ocular) (*see also* Exophthalmos)
  376.30
  thyroid 242.0
Propulsion
  eyeball 360.81
Prosecution, anxiety concerning V62.5
Prostate, prostatic —*see* condition
Prostatism 600.9
Prostatitis (congestive) (suppurative) 601.9
  acute 601.0
  cavitary 601.8
  chlamydial 099.54
  chronic 601.1
  diverticular 601.8
  due to Trichomonas (vaginalis) 131.03
  fibrous 600.9
  gonococcal (acute) 098.12
    chronic or duration of 2 months or over 098.32
  granulomatous 601.8
  hypertrophic 600.0
  specified type NEC 601.8
  subacute 601.1
  trichomonal 131.03
  tuberculous (*see also* Tuberculosis) 016.5
    [601.4]
Prostatocystitis 601.3
Prostatorrhea 602.8
Prostatoseminovesiculitis, trichomonal 131.03
Prostration 780.79
  heat 992.5
    anhydrotic 992.3
    due to
      salt (and water) depletion 992.4
      water depletion 992.3
  nervous 300.5
  newborn 779.89
  senile 797
Protanomaly 368.51

Protanopia (anomalous trichromat) (complete)
  (incomplete) 368.51
Protein
  deficiency 260
  malnutrition 260
  sickness (prophylactic) (therapeutic) 999.5
Proteinemia 790.99
Proteinosis
  alveolar, lung or pulmonary 516.0
  lipid 272.8
Proteinosis
  lipoid (of Urbach) 272.8
Proteinuria (*see also* Albuminuria) 791.0
  Bence-Jones NEC 791.0
  gestational 646.2
    with hypertension—*see* Toxemia, of
      pregnancy
  orthostatic 593.6
  postural 593.6
Proteolysis, pathologic 286.6
Protocoproporphyria 277.1
Protoporphyria (erythrohepatic) (erythropoietic)
  277.1
Protrusio acetabuli 718.65
Protrusion
  acetabulum (into pelvis) 718.65
  device, implant, or graft—*see* Complications,
    mechanical
  ear, congenital 744.29
  intervertebral disc—*see* Displacement,
    intervertebral disc
  nucleus pulposus—*see* Displacement,
    intervertebral disc
Proud flesh 701.5
Prune belly (syndrome) 756.71
Prurigo (ferox) (gravis) (Hebra's) (hebrae)
  (mitis) (simplex) 698.2
  agria 698.3
  asthma syndrome 691.8
  Besnier's (atopic dermatitis) (infantile eczema)
    691.8
  eczematodes allergicum 691.8
  estivalis (Hutchinson's) 692.72
  Hutchinson's 692.72
  nodularis 698.3
  psychogenic 306.3
Pruritus, pruritic 698.9
  ani 698.0
    psychogenic 306.3
  conditions NEC 698.9
    psychogenic 306.3
  due to Onchocerca volvulus 125.3
  ear 698.9
  essential 698.9
  genital organ(s) 698.1
    psychogenic 306.3
  gravidarum 646.8
  hiemalis 698.8
  neurogenic (any site) 306.3
  perianal 698.0
  psychogenic (any site) 306.3
  scrotum 698.1
    psychogenic 306.3
  senile, senilis 698.8
  Trichomonas 131.9
  vulva, vulvae 698.1
    psychogenic 306.3
Psammocarcinoma (M8140/3)—*see* Neoplasm,
  by site, malignant
Pseudarthrosis, pseudoarthrosis (bone) 733.82
  joint following fusion V45.4

Pseudoacanthosis
 nigricans 701.8
Pseudoaneurysm —*see* Aneurysm
Pseudoangina (pectoris)—*see* Angina
Pseudoangioma 452
Pseudo-Argyll-Robertson pupil 379.45
Pseudoarteriosus 747.89
Pseudoarthrosis —*see* Pseudarthrosis
Pseudoataxia 799.8
Pseudobursa 727.89
Pseudocholera 025
Pseudochromidrosis 705.89
Pseudocirrhosis, liver, pericardial 423.2
Pseudocoarctation 747.21
Pseudocowpox 051.1
Pseudocoxalgia 732.1
Pseudocroup 478.75
Pseudocyesis 300.11
Pseudocyst
 lung 518.89
 pancreas 577.2
 retina 361.19
Pseudodementia 300.16
Pseudoelephantiasis neuroarthritica 757.0
Pseudoemphysema 518.89
Pseudoencephalitis
 superior (acute) hemorrhagic 265.1
Pseudoerosion cervix, congenital 752.49
Pseudoexfoliation, lens capsule 366.11
Pseudofracture (idiopathic) (multiple)
  (spontaneous) (symmetrical) 268.2
Pseudoglanders 025
Pseudoglioma 360.44
Pseudogout —*see* Chondrocalcinosis
Pseudohallucination 780.1
Pseudohemianesthesia 782.0
Pseudohemophilia (Bernuth's) (hereditary) (type
  B) 286.4
 type A 287.8
 vascular 287.8
Pseudohermaphroditism 752.7
 with chromosomal anomaly—*see* Anomaly,
  chromosomal
 adrenal 255.2
 female (without adrenocortical disorder) 752.7
  with adrenocortical disorder 255.2
  adrenal 255.2
 male (without gonadal disorder) 752.7
  with
   adrenocortical disorder 255.2
   cleft scrotum 752.7
   feminizing testis 257.8
   gonadal disorder 257.9
  adrenal 255.2
Pseudohole, macula 362.54
Pseudo-Hurler's disease (mucolipidosis III)
  272.7
Pseudohydrocephalus 348.2
Pseudohypertrophic muscular dystrophy
  (Erb's) 359.1
Pseudohypertrophy, muscle 359.1
Pseudohypoparathyroidism 275.49
Psuedopseudohypoparathyroidism 275.49
Pseudoinfluenza 487.1
Pseudoinsomnia 307.49
Pseudoleukemia 288.8
 infantile 285.8
Pseudomembranous —*see* condition
Pseudomeningocele (cerebral) (infective)
  (surgical) 349.2
 spinal 349.2
Pseudomenstruation 626.8

Pseudomucinous
 cyst (ovary) (M8470/0) 220
 peritoneum 568.89
Pseudomyeloma 273.1
Pseudomyxoma peritonei (M8480/6) 197.6
Pseudoneuritis optic (nerve) 377.24
 papilla 377.24
  congenital 743.57
Pseudoneuroma —*see* Injury, nerve, by site
Pseudo-obstruction
 intestine 564.89
Pseudopapilledema 377.24
Pseudoparalysis
 arm or leg 781.4
 atonic, congenital 358.8
Pseudopelade 704.09
Pseudophakia V43.1
Pseudopolycythemia 289.0
Pseudopolyposis, colon 556.4
Pseudoporencephaly 348.0
Pseudopseudohypoparathyroidism 275.49
Pseudopsychosis 300.16
Pseudopterygium 372.52
Pseudoptosis (eyelid) 374.34
Pseudorabies 078.89
Pseudoretinitis, pigmentosa 362.65
Pseudorickets 588.0
 senile (Pozzi's) 731.0
Pseudorubella 057.8
Pseudoscarlatina 057.8
Pseudosclerema 778.1
Pseudosclerosis (brain)
 Jakob's 046.1
 of Westphal (-Strümpell) (hepatolenticular
  degeneration) 275.1
 spastic 046.1
  with dementia
   with behavioral disturbance 046.1 *[294.11]*
   without behavioral disturbance 046.1
    [294.10]
Pseudoseizure 780.39
 non-psychiatric 780.39
 psychiatric 300.11
Pseudotabes 799.8
 diabetic 250.6 *[337.1]*
Pseudotetanus (*see also* Convulsions) 780.39
Pseudotetany 781.7
 hysterical 300.11
Pseudothalassemia 285.0
Pseudotrichinosis 710.3
Pseudotruncus arteriosus 747.29
Pseudotuberculosis, pasteurella (infection)
  027.2
Pseudotumor
 cerebri 348.2
 orbit (inflammatory) 376.11
Pseudo-Turner's syndrome 759.89
Pseudoxanthoma elasticum 757.39
Psilosis (sprue) (tropical) 579.1
 Monilia 112.89
 nontropical 579.0
 not sprue 704.00
Psittacosis 073.9
Psoitis 728.89
Psora NEC 696.1
Psoriasis 696.1
 any type, except arthropathic 696.1
 arthritic, arthropathic 696.0
 buccal 528.6
 flexural 696.1
 follicularis 696.1

Psychosis—*continued*
  of childhood (*see also* Psychosis, childhood)
    299.8
    prepubertal 299.8
  brief reactive 298.8
  childhood, with origin specific to 299.9

> *Note—Use the following fifth-digit*
> *subclassification with category 299:*
>
> *0 current or active state*
> *1 residual state*

    atypical 299.8
    specified type NEC 299.8
  circular (*see also* Psychosis, manic-depressive,
    circular) 296.7
  climacteric (*see also* Psychosis, involutional)
    298.8
  confusional 298.9
    acute 293.0
    reactive 298.2
    subacute 293.1
  depressive (*see also* Psychosis, affective) 296.2
    atypical 296.82
    involutional 296.2
      recurrent episode 296.3
      single episode 296.2
    psychogenic 298.0
    reactive (emotional stress) (psychological
      trauma) 298.0
    recurrent episode 296.3
      with hypomania (bipolar II) 296.89
    single episode 296.2
  disintegrative (childhood) (*see also* Psychosis,
    childhood) 299.1
  drug 292.9
    with
      affective syndrome 292.84
      amnestic syndrome 292.83
      anxiety 292.89
      delirium 292.81
        withdrawal 292.0
      delusional syndrome 292.11
      dementia 292.82
      depressive state 292.84
      hallucinosis 292.12
      mood disturbance 292.84
      organic personality syndrome NEC 292.89
      sexual dysfunction 292.89
      sleep disturbance 292.89
      withdrawal syndrome (and delirium) 292.0
    affective syndrome 292.84
    delusional state 292.11
    hallucinatory state 292.12
    hallucinosis 292.12
    paranoid state 292.11
    specified type NEC 292.89
    withdrawal syndrome (and delirium) 292.0
  due to or associated with physical condition (*see*
    also Psychosis, organic) 293.9
  epileptic NEC 294.8
  excitation (psychogenic) (reactive) 298.1
  exhaustive (*see also* Reaction, stress, acute)
    308.9
  hypomanic (*see also* Psychosis, affective) 296.0
    recurrent episode 296.1
    single episode 296.0
  hysterical 298.8
    acute 298.1
  incipient 298.8
    schizophrenic (*see also* Schizophrenia) 295.5

Psychosis—*continued*
  induced 297.3
  infantile (*see also* Psychosis, childhood) 299.0
  infective 293.9
    acute 293.0
    subacute 293.1
  in pregnancy, childbirth, or puerperium 648.4
  interactional (childhood) (*see also* Psychosis,
    childhood) 299.1
  involutional 298.8
    depressive (*see also* Psychosis, affective)
      296.2
      recurrent episode 296.3
      single episode 296.2
    melancholic 296.2
      recurrent episode 296.3
      single episode 296.2
    paranoid state 297.2
    paraphrenia 297.2
  Korsakoff's, Korakov's, Korsakow's
    (nonalcoholic) 294.0
    alcoholic 291.1
  mania (phase) (*see also* Psychosis, affective)
    296.0
    recurrent episode 296.1
    single episode 296.0
  manic (*see also* Psychosis, affective) 296.0
    atypical 296.81
    recurrent episode 296.1
    single episode 296.0
  manic-depressive 296.80
    circular 296.7
      currently
        depressed 296.5
        manic 296.4
      mixed 296.6
    depressive 296.2
      recurrent episode 296.3
        with hypomania (bipolar II) 296.89
      single episode 296.2
    hypomanic 296.0
      recurrent episode 296.1
      single episode 296.0
    manic 296.0
      atypical 296.81
      recurrent episode 296.1
      single episode 296.0
    mixed NEC 296.89
    perplexed 296.89
    stuporous 296.89
  menopausal (*see also* Psychosis, involutional)
    298.8
  mixed schizophrenic and affective (*see also*
    Schizophrenia) 295.7
  multi-infarct (cerebrovascular) (*see also*
    Psychosis, arteriosclerotic) 290.40
  organic NEC 294.9
    due to or associated with
      addiction
        alcohol (*see also* Psychosis, alcoholic)
          291.9
        drug (*see also* Psychosis, drug) 292.9
      alcohol intoxication, acute (*see also*
        Psychosis, alcoholic) 291.9
      alcoholism (*see also* Psychosis, alcoholic)
        291.9
      arteriosclerosis (cerebral) (*see also*
        Psychosis, arteriosclerotic) 290.40
      cerebrovascular disease
        acute (psychosis) 293.0

Puerperal—*continued*
   vaginorectal 646.6
   vulvovaginal gland 646.6
  accident 674.9
  adnexitis 670
  afibrinogenemia, or other coagulation defect
    666.3
  albuminuria (acute) (subacute) 646.2
   pre-eclamptic 642.4
  anemia (conditions classifiable to 280-285)
    648.2
  anuria 669.3
  apoplexy 674.0
  asymptomatic bacteriuria 646.5
  atrophy, breast 676.3
  blood dyscrasia 666.3
  caked breast 676.2
  cardiomyopathy 674.8
  cellulitis—*see* Puerperal, abscess
  cerebrovascular disorder (conditions classifiable
    to 430-434, 436-437) 674.0
  cervicitis (conditions classifiable to 616.0) 646.6
  coagulopathy (any) 666.3
  complications 674.9
   specified type NEC 674.8
  convulsions (eclamptic) (uremic) 642.6
   with pre-existing hypertension 642.7
  cracked nipple 676.1
  cystitis 646.6
  cystopyelitis 646.6
  deciduitis (acute) 670
  delirium NEC 293.9
  diabetes (mellitus) (conditions classifiable to
    250) 648.0
  disease 674.9
   breast NEC 676.3
   cerebrovascular (acute) 674.0
   nonobstetric NEC (*see also* Pregnancy,
     complicated, current disease or condition)
     648.9
   pelvis inflammatory 670
   renal NEC 646.2
   tubo-ovarian 670
   Valsuani's (progressive pernicious anemia)
     648.2
  disorder
   lactation 676.9
    specified type NEC 676.8
   nonobstetric NEC (*see also* Pregnancy,
     complicated, current disease or condition)
     648.9
  disruption
   cesarean wound 674.1
   episiotomy wound 674.2
   perineal laceration wound 674.2
  drug dependence (conditions classifiable to 304)
    648.3
  eclampsia 642.6
   with pre-existing hypertension 642.7
  embolism (pulmonary) 673.2
   air 673.0
   amniotic fluid 673.1
   blood-clot 673.2
   brain or cerebral 674.0
   cardiac 674.8
   fat 673.8
   intracranial sinus (venous) 671.5
   pyemic 673.3
   septic 673.3
   spinal cord 671.5

Puerperal—*continued*
  endometritis (conditions classifiable to
    615.0-615.9) 670
  endophlebitis—*see* Puerperal, phlebitis
  endotrachelitis 646.6
  engorgement, breasts 676.2
  erysipelas 670
  failure
   lactation 676.4
   renal, acute 669.3
  fever 670
   meaning pyrexia (of unknown origin) 672
   meaning sepsis 670
  fissure, nipple 676.1
  fistula
   breast 675.1
   mammary gland 675.1
   nipple 675.0
  galactophoritis 675.2
  galactorrhea 676.6
  gangrene
   gas 670
   uterus 670
  gonorrhea (conditions classifiable to 098) 647.1
  hematoma, subdural 674.0
  hematosalpinx, infectional 670
  hemiplegia, cerebral 674.0
  hemorrhage 666.1
   brain 674.0
   bulbar 674.0
   cerebellar 674.0
   cerebral 674.0
   cortical 674.0
   delayed (after 24 hours) (uterine) 666.2
   extradural 674.0
   internal capsule 674.0
   intracranial 674.0
   intrapontine 674.0
   meningeal 674.0
   pontine 674.0
   subarachnoid 674.0
   subcortical 674.0
   subdural 674.0
   uterine, delayed 666.2
   ventricular 674.0
  hemorrhoids 671.8
  hepatorenal syndrome 674.8
  hypertrophy
   breast 676.3
   mammary gland 676.3
  induration breast (fibrous) 676.3
  infarction
   lung—*see* Puerperal, embolism
   pulmonary—*see* Puerperal, embolism
  infection
   Bartholin's gland 646.6
   breast 675.2
    with nipple 675.9
     specified type NEC 675.8
   cervix 646.6
   endocervix 646.6
   fallopian tube 670
   generalized 670
   genital tract (major) 670
    minor or localized 646.6
   kidney (bacillus coli) 646.6
   mammary gland 675.2
    with nipple 675.9
     specified type NEC 675.8
   nipple 675.0
    with breast 675.9

Puerperal—*continued*
  sudden death (cause unknown) 674.9
  suppuration—*see* Puerperal, abscess
  syphilis (conditions classifiable to 090-097) 647.0
  tetanus 670
  thelitis 675.0
  thrombocytopenia 666.3
  thrombophlebitis (superficial) 671.2
    deep 671.4
    pelvic 671.4
    specified site NEC 671.5
  thrombosis (venous)—*see* Thrombosis, puerperal
  thyroid dysfunction (conditions classifiable to 240-246) 648.1
  toxemia (*see also* Toxemia, of pregnancy) 642.4
    eclamptic 642.6
      with pre-existing hypertension 642.7
    pre-eclamptic (mild) 642.4
      with
        convulsions 642.6
        pre-existing hypertension 642.7
      severe 642.5
  tuberculosis (conditions classifiable to 010-018) 647.3
  uremia 669.3
  vaginitis (conditions classifiable to 616.1) 646.6
  varicose veins (legs) 671.0
    vulva or perineum 671.1
  vulvitis (conditions classifiable to 616.1) 646.6
  vulvovaginitis (conditions classifiable to 616.1) 646.6
  white leg 671.4
Pulled muscle —*see* Sprain, by site
Pulmolithiasis 518.89
Pulmonary —*see* condition
Pulmonitis (unknown etiology) 486
Pulpitis (acute) (anachoretic) (chronic) (hyperplastic) (putrescent) (suppurative) (ulcerative) 522.0
Pulpless tooth 522.9
Pulse
  alternating 427.89
    psychogenic 306.2
  bigeminal 427.89
  fast 785.0
  feeble, rapid, due to shock following injury 958.4
  rapid 785.0
  slow 427.89
  strong 785.9
  trigeminal 427.89
  water-hammer (*see also* Insufficiency, aortic) 424.1
  weak 785.9
Pulseless disease 446.7
Pulsus
  alternans or trigeminy 427.89
    psychogenic 306.2
Punch drunk 310.2
Puncta lacrimalia occlusion 375.52
Punctiform hymen 752.49
Puncture (traumatic)—*see also* Wound, open, by site
  accidental, complicating surgery 998.2
  bladder, nontraumatic 596.6
  by
    device, implant, or graft—*see* Complications, mechanical

Puncture—*continued*
  foreign body
    internal organs—*see also* Injury, internal, by site
      by ingested object—*see* Foreign body
    left accidentally in operation wound 998.4
  instrument (any) during a procedure, accidental 998.2
  internal organs, abdomen, chest, or pelvis—*see* Injury, internal, by site
  kidney, nontraumatic 593.89
Pupil —*see* condition
Pupillary membrane 364.74
  persistent 743.46
Pupillotonia 379.46
  pseudotabetic 379.46
Purpura 287.2
  abdominal 287.0
  allergic 287.0
  anaphylactoid 287.0
  annularis telangiectodes 709.1
  arthritic 287.0
  autoerythrocyte sensitization 287.2
  autoimmune 287.0
  bacterial 287.0
  Bateman's (senile) 287.2
  capillary fragility (hereditary) (idiopathic) 287.8
  cryoglobulinemic 273.2
  devil's pinches 287.2
  fibrinolytic (*see also* Fibrinolysis) 286.6
  fulminans, fulminous 286.6
  gangrenous 287.0
  hemorrhagic (*see also* Purpura, thrombocytopenic) 287.3
    nodular 272.7
    nonthrombocytopenic 287.0
    thrombocytopenic 287.3
  Henoch's (purpura nervosa) 287.0
  Henoch-Schönlein (allergic) 287.0
  hypergammaglobulinemic (benign primary) (Waldenström's) 273.0
  idiopathic 287.3
    nonthrombocytopenic 287.0
    thrombocytopenic 287.3
  infectious 287.0
  malignant 287.0
  neonatorum 772.6
  nervosa 287.0
  newborn NEC 772.6
  nonthrombocytopenic 287.2
    hemorrhagic 287.0
    idiopathic 287.0
  nonthrombopenic 287.2
  peliosis rheumatica 287.0
  pigmentaria, progressiva 709.09
  posttransfusion 287.4
  primary 287.0
  primitive 287.0
  red cell membrane sensitivity 287.2
  rheumatica 287.0
  Schönlein (-Henoch) (allergic) 287.0
  scorbutic 267
  senile 287.2
  simplex 287.2
  symptomatica 287.0
  telangiectasia annularis 709.1
  thrombocytopenic (congenital) (essential) (hereditary) (idiopathic) (primary) (*see also* Thrombocytopenia) 287.3

Purpura—*continued*
  neonatal, transitory (*see also*
    Thrombocytopenia, neonatal transitory)
    776.1
    puerperal, postpartum 666.3
    thrombotic 446.6
  thrombohemolytic (*see also* Fibrinolysis) 286.6
  thrombopenic (congenital) (essential) (*see also*
    Thrombocytopenia) 287.3
  thrombotic 446.6
    thrombocytic 446.6
    thrombocytopenic 446.6
  toxic 287.0
  variolosa 050.0
  vascular 287.0
  visceral symptoms 287.0
  Werlhof's (*see also* Purpura, thrombocytopenic)
    287.3
Purpuric spots 782.7
Purulent —*see* condition
Pus
  absorption, general—*see* Septicemia
  in
    stool 792.1
    urine 791.9
  tube (rupture) (*see also* Salpingo-oophoritis)
    614.2
Pustular rash 782.1
Pustule 686.9
  malignant 022.0
  nonmalignant 686.9
Putnam's disease (subacute combined sclerosis
  with pernicious anemia) 281.0 *[336.2]*
Putnam-Dana syndrome (subacute combined
  sclerosis with pernicious anemia) 281.0
  [336.2]
Putrefaction, intestinal 569.89
Putrescent pulp (dental) 522.1
Pyarthritis —*see* Pyarthrosis
Pyarthrosis (*see also* Arthritis, pyogenic) 711.0
  tuberculous—*see* Tuberculosis, joint
Pycnoepilepsy, pycnolepsy (idiopathic) (*see also*
  Epilepsy) 345.0
Pyelectasia 593.89
Pyelectasis 593.89
Pyelitis (congenital) (uremic) 590.80
  with
    abortion—*see* Abortion, by type, with
      specified complication NEC
    contracted kidney 590.00
    ectopic pregnancy (*see also* categories
      633.0-633.9) 639.8
    molar pregnancy (*see also* categories
      630-632) 639.8
  acute 590.10
    with renal medullary necrosis 590.11
  chronic 590.00
    with
      renal medullary necrosis 590.01
  complicating pregnancy, childbirth, or
    puerperium 646.6
    affecting fetus or newborn 760.1
  cystica 590.3
  following
    abortion 639.8
    ectopic or molar pregnancy 639.8
  gonococcal 098.19
    chronic or duration of 2 months or over 098.39
  tuberculous (*see also* Tuberculosis) 016.0
    [590.81]
Pyelocaliectasis 593.89
Pyelocystitis (*see also* Pyelitis) 590.80

Pyelohydronephrosis 591
Pyelonephritis (*see also* Pyelitis) 590.80
  acute 590.10
    with renal medullary necrosis 590.11
  chronic 590.00
  syphilitic (late) 095.4
  tuberculous (*see also* Tuberculosis) 016.0
    [590.81]
Pyelonephrosis (*see also* Pyelitis) 590.80
  chronic 590.00
Pyelophlebitis 451.89
Pyelo-ureteritis cystica 590.3
Pyemia, pyemic (purulent) (*see also* Septicemia)
  038.9
  abscess—*see* Abscess
  arthritis (*see also* Arthritis, pyogenic) 711.0
  Bacillus coli 038.42
  embolism—*see* Embolism, pyemic
  fever 038.9
  infection 038.9
  joint (*see also* Arthritis, pyogenic) 711.0
  liver 572.1
  meningococcal 036.2
  newborn 771.81
  phlebitis—*see* Phlebitis
  pneumococcal 038.2
  portal 572.1
  postvaccinal 999.3
  specified organism NEC 038.8
  staphylococcal 038.10
    aureus 038.11
    specified organism NEC 038.19
  streptococcal 038.0
  tuberculous—*see* Tuberculosis, miliary
Pygopagus 759.4
Pykno-epilepsy, pyknolepsy (idiopathic) (*see
  also* Epilepsy) 345.0
Pyle (-Cohn) disease (craniometaphyseal
  dysplasia) 756.89
Pylephlebitis (suppurative) 572.1
Pylethrombophlebitis 572.1
Pylethrombosis 572.1
Pyloritis (*see also* Gastritis) 535.5
Pylorospasm (reflex) 537.81
  congenital or infantile 750.5
  neurotic 306.4
  newborn 750.5
  psychogenic 306.4
Pylorus, pyloric —*see* condition
Pyoarthrosis —*see* Pyarthrosis
Pyocele
  mastoid 383.00
  sinus (accessory) (nasal) (*see also* Sinusitis)
    473.9
  turbinate (bone) 473.9
  urethra (*see also* Urethritis) 597.0
Pyococcal dermatitis 686.00
Pyococcide, skin 686.00
Pyocolpos (*see also* Vaginitis) 616.10
Pyocyaneus dermatitis 686.09
Pyocystitis (*see also* Cystitis) 595.9
Pyoderma, pyodermia NEC 686.00
  gangrenosum 686.01
  specified type NEC 686.09
  vegetans 686.8
Pyodermatitis 686.00
  vegetans 686.8
Pyogenic —*see* condition
Pyohemia —*see* Septicemia
Pyohydronephrosis (*see also* Pyelitis) 590.80
Pyometra 615.9
Pyometritis (*see also* Endometritis) 615.9

Q

Q fever 083.0
　with pneumonia 083.0 *[484.8]*
Quadricuspid aortic valve 746.89
Quadrilateral fever 083.0
Quadriparesis —*see* Quadriplegia
Quadriplegia 344.00
　with fracture, vertebra (process)—*see* Fracture,
　　　vertebra, cervical, with spinal cord injury
　brain (current episode) 437.8
　cerebral (current episode) 437.8
　C1-C4
　　complete 344.01
　　incomplete 344.02
　C5-C7
　　complete 344.03
　　incomplete 344.04
　congenital or infantile (cerebral) (spastic)
　　　(spinal) 343.2
　cortical 437.8
　embolic (current episode) (*see also* Embolism,
　　　brain) 434.1
　infantile (cerebral) (spastic) (spinal) 343.2
　newborn NEC 767.0
　specified NEC 344.09
　thrombotic (current episode) (*see also*
　　　Thrombosis, brain) 434.0
　traumatic—*see* Injury, spinal, cervical
Quadruplet
　affected by maternal complications of
　　　pregnancy 761.5
　healthy liveborn—*see* Newborn, multiple
　pregnancy (complicating delivery) NEC 651.8
　　with fetal loss and retention of one or more
　　　　fetus(es) 651.5
Quarrelsomeness 301.3
Quartan
　fever 084.2
　malaria (fever) 084.2
Queensland fever 083.0
　coastal 083.0
　seven-day 100.89
Quervain's disease 727.04
　thyroid (subacute granulomatous thyroiditis)
　　　245.1
Queyrat's erythroplasia (M8080/2)
　specified site—*see* Neoplasm, skin, in situ
　unspecified site 233.5
Quincke's disease or edema —*see* Edema,
　　angioneurotic
Quinquaud's disease (acne decalvans) 704.09
Quinsy (gangrenous) 475
Quintan fever 083.1
Quintuplet
　affected by maternal complications of
　　　pregnancy 761.5
　healthy liveborn—*see* Newborn, multiple
　pregnancy (complicating delivery) NEC 651.2
　　with fetal loss and retention of one or more
　　　　fetus(es) 651.6
Quotidian
　fever 084.0
　malaria (fever) 084.0

R

Rabbia 071
Rabbit fever (*see also* Tularemia) 021.9
Rabies 071
　contact V01.5
　exposure to V01.5
　inoculation V04.5
　　reaction—*see* Complications, vaccination
　vaccination, prophylactic (against) V04.5
Rachischisis (*see also* Spina bifida) 741.9
Rachitic —*see also* condition
　deformities of spine 268.1
　pelvis 268.1
　　with disproportion (fetopelvic) 653.2
　　　affecting fetus or newborn 763.1
　　　causing obstructed labor 660.1
　　　　affecting fetus or newborn 763.1
Rachitis, rachitism —*see also* Rickets
　acute 268.0
　fetalis 756.4
　renalis 588.0
　tarda 268.0
Racket nail 757.5
Radial nerve —*see* condition
Radiation effects or sickness —*see also* Effect,
　　adverse, radiation
　cataract 366.46
　dermatitis 692.82
　　sunburn (*see also* Sunburn) 692.71
Radiculitis (pressure) (vertebrogenic) 729.2
　accessory nerve 723.4
　anterior crural 724.4
　arm 723.4
　brachial 723.4
　cervical NEC 723.4
　due to displacement of intervertebral disc—*see*
　　　Neuritis, due to, displacement intervertebral
　　　disc
　leg 724.4
　lumbar NEC 724.4
　lumbosacral 724.4
　rheumatic 729.2
　syphilitic 094.89
　thoracic (with visceral pain) 724.4
Radiculomyelitis 357.0
　toxic, due to
　　Clostridium tetani 037
　　Corynebacterium diphtheriae 032.89
Radiculopathy (*see also* Radiculitis) 729.2
Radioactive substances, adverse effect —*see*
　　Effect, adverse, radioactive substance
Radiodermal burns (acute) (chronic)
　　(occupational)—*see* Burn, by site
Radiodermatitis 692.82
Radionecrosis —*see* Effect, adverse, radiation
Radiotherapy session V58.0
Radium, adverse effect —*see* Effect, adverse,
　　radioactive substance
Raeder-Harbitz syndrome (pulseless disease)
　　446.7
Rage (*see also* Disturbance, conduct) 312.0
　meaning rabies 071
Rag sorters' disease 022.1
Raillietiniasis 123.8
Railroad neurosis 300.16
Railway spine 300.16
Raised —*see* Elevation
Raiva 071
Rake teeth, tooth 524.3

Removal (of)—*continued*
   vascular V58.81
   cerebral ventricle (communicating) shunt
      V53.01
   device—*see also* Fitting (of)
    contraceptive V25.42
    fixation
      external V54.89
      internal V54.0
    traction V54.89
   dressing V58.3
   ileostomy V55.2
   Kirschner wire V54.89
   non-vascular catheter V58.82
   pin V54.0
   plaster cast V54.89
   plate (fracture) V54.0
   rod V54.0
   screw V54.0
   splint, external V54.89
   subdermal implantable contraceptive V25.43
   suture V58.3
   traction device, external V54.89
   vascular catheter V58.81
Ren
   arcuatus 753.3
   mobile, mobilis (*see also* Disease, renal) 593.0
    congenital 753.3
   unguliformis 753.3
Renal —*see also* condition
   glomerulohyalinosis-diabetic syndrome 250.4
    [581.81]
Rendu-Osler-Weber disease or syndrome
   (familial hemorrhagic telangiectasia) 448.0
Reninoma (M8361/1) 236.91
Rénon-Delille syndrome 253.8
Repair
   pelvic floor, previous, in pregnancy or
      childbirth 654.4
    affecting fetus or newborn 763.89
   scarred tissue V51
Replacement by artificial or mechanical device
   or prosthesis of (*see also* Fitting (of))
   artificial skin V43.83
   bladder V43.5
   blood vessel V43.4
   breast V43.82
   eye globe V43.0
   heart V43.2
    valve V43.3
   intestine V43.89
   joint V43.60
    ankle 43.66
    elbow V43.62
    finger V43.69
    hip (partial) (total) V43.64
    knee V43.65
    shoulder V43.61
    specified NEC V43.69
    wrist V43.63
   kidney V43.89
   larynx V43.81
   lens V43.1
   limb(s) V43.7
   liver V43.89
   lung V43.89
   organ NEC V43.89
   pancreas V43.89
   skin (artificial) V43.83
   tissue NEC V43.89
Reprogramming
   cardiac pacemaker V53.31

Request for expert evidence V68.2
Reserve, decreased or low
   cardiac—*see* Disease, heart
   kidney (*see also* Disease, renal) 593.9
Residual —*see also* condition
   bladder 596.8
   foreign body—*see* Retention, foreign body
   state, schizophrenic (*see also* Schizophrenia)
    295.6
   urine 788.69
Resistance, resistant (to)

> *Note—Use the following subclassification for
> categories V09.5, V09.7, V09.8, V09.9.:*
>
> *0 without mention of resistance to multiple
>   drugs*
> *1 with resistance to multiple drugs*
>
> *V09.5   quinolones and fluoroquinolones*
> *V09.7   antimycobacterial agents*
> *V09.8   specified drugs NEC*
> *V09.9   unspecified drugs*
>
> *9 multiple sites*

   drugs by microorganisms V09.90
    Amikacin V09.4
    aminoglycosides V09.4
    Amodiaquine V09.5
    Amoxicillin V09.0
    Ampicillin V09.0
    antimycobacterial agents V09.7
    Azithromycin V09.2
    Azlocillin V09.0
    Aztreonam V09.1
    B-lactam antibiotics V09.1
    Bacampicillin V09.0
    Bacitracin V09.8
    Benznidazole V09.8
    Capreomycin V09.7
    Carbenicillin V09.0
    Cefaclor V09.1
    Cefadroxil V09.1
    Cefamandole V09.1
    Cefatetan V09.1
    Cefazolin V09.1
    Cefixime V09.1
    Cefonicid V09.1
    Cefoperazone V09.1
    Ceforanide V09.1
    Cefotaxime V09.1
    Cefoxitin V09.1
    Ceftazidine V09.1
    Ceftizoxime V09.1
    Ceftriaxone V09.1
    Cefuroxime V09.1
    Cephalexin V09.1
    Cephaloglycin V09.1
    Cephaloridine V09.1
    cephalosporins V09.1
    Cephalothin V09.1
    Cephapirin V09.1
    Cephradine V09.1
    Chloramphenicol V09.8
    Chloraquine V09.5
    Chlorguanide V09.8
    Chlorproguanil V09.8
    Chlortetracycline V09.3
    Cinoxacin V09.5
    Ciprofloxacin V09.5
    Clarithromycin V09.2

Rest, rests
  mesonephric duct 752.8
    fallopian tube 752.11
  ovarian, in fallopian tubes 752.19
  wolffian duct 752.8
Restless leg (syndrome) 333.99
Restlessness 799.2
**Restoration of organ continuity from previous
    sterilization** (tuboplasty) (vasoplasty) V26.0
Restriction of housing space V60.1
Restzustand, schizophrenic (*see also*
    Schizophrenia) 295.6
Retained —*see* Retention
Retardation
  development, developmental, specific (*see also*
      Disorder, development, specific) 315.9
    learning, specific 315.2
      arithmetical 315.1
      language (skills) 315.31
        expressive 315.31
        mixed receptive-expressive 315.32
      mathematics 315.1
      reading 315.00
        phonological 315.39
      written expression 315.2
    motor 315.4
  endochondral bone growth 733.91
  growth (physical) in childhood 783.43
    due to malnutrition 263.2
    fetal (intrauterine) 764.9
      affecting management of pregnancy 656.5
  intrauterine growth 764.9
    affecting management of pregnancy 656.5
  mental 319
    borderline V62.89
    mild, IQ 50-70 317
    moderate, IQ 35-49 318.0
    profound, IQ under 20 318.2
    severe, IQ 20-34 318.1
  motor, specific 315.4
  physical 783.43
    child 783.43
    due to malnutrition 263.2
    fetus (intrauterine) 764.9
      affecting management of pregnancy 656.5
  psychomotor NEC 307.9
  reading 315.00
Retching —*see* Vomiting
Retention, retained
  bladder NEC (*see also* Retention, urine) 788.20
    psychogenic 306.53
  carbon dioxide 276.2
  cyst—*see* Cyst
  dead
    fetus (after 22 completed weeks gestation)
        656.4
      early fetal death (before 22 completed
          weeks gestation) 632
    ovum 631
  decidua (following delivery) (fragments) (with
      hemorrhage) 666.2
    without hemorrhage 667.1
  deciduous tooth 520.6
  dental root 525.3
  fecal (*see also* Constipation) 564.00
  fluid 276.6
  foreign body—*see also* Foreign body, retained
    bone 733.99
    current trauma—*see* Foreign body, by site or
        type
    middle ear 385.83

Retention, retained—*continued*
    muscle 729.6
    soft tissue NEC 729.6
  gastric 536.8
  membranes (following delivery) (with
      hemorrhage) 666.2
    with abortion—*see* Abortion, by type
    without hemorrhage 667.1
  menses 626.8
  milk (puerperal) 676.2
  nitrogen, extrarenal 788.9
  placenta (total) (with hemorrhage) 666.0
    with abortion—*see* Abortion, by type
    portions or fragments 666.2
      without hemorrhage 667.1
    without hemorrhage 667.0
  products of conception
    early pregnancy (fetal death before 22
        completed weeks gestation) 632
    following
      abortion—*see* Abortion, by type
      delivery 666.2
        with hemorrhage 666.2
        without hemorrhage 667.1
  secundines (following delivery) (with
      hemorrhage) 666.2
    with abortion—*see* Abortion, by type
    complicating puerperium (delayed
        hemorrhage) 666.2
    without hemorrhage 667.1
  smegma, clitoris 624.8
  urine NEC 788.20
    bladder, incomplete emptying 788.21
    psychogenic 306.53
    specified NEC 788.29
  water (in tissue) (*see also* Edema) 782.3
Reticulation, dust (occupational) 504
Reticulocytosis NEC 790.99
Reticuloendotheliosis
  acute infantile (M9722/3) 202.5
  leukemic (M9940/3) 202.4
  malignant (M9720/3) 202.3
  nonlipid (M9722/3) 202.5
Reticulohistiocytoma (giant cell) 277.8
Reticulohistiocytosis, multicentric 272.8
Reticulolymphosarcoma (diffuse) (M9613/3)
    200.8
  follicular (M9691/3) 202.0
  nodular (M9691/3) 202.0
Reticulosarcoma (M9640/3) 200.0
  odular (M9642/3) 200.0
  pleomorphic cell type (M9641/3) 200.0
Reticulosis (skin)
  acute of infancy (M9722/3) 202.5
  histiocytic medullary (M9721/3) 202.3
  lipomelanotic 695.89
  malignant (M9720/3) 202.3
  Sézary's (M9701/3) 202.2
Retina, retinal —*see* condition
Retinitis (*see also* Chorioretinitis) 363.20
  albuminurica 585 *[363.10]*
  arteriosclerotic 440.8 *[362.13]*
  central angiospastic 362.41
  Coat's 362.12
  diabetic 250.5 *[362.01]*
  disciformis 362.52
  disseminated 363.10
    metastatic 363.14
    neurosyphilitic 094.83
    pigment epitheliopathy 363.15
  exudative 362.12

Retinitis—*continued*
  focal 363.00
    in histoplasmosis 115.92
      capsulatum 115.02
      duboisii 115.12
    juxtapapillary 363.05
    macular 363.06
    paramacular 363.06
    peripheral 363.08
    posterior pole NEC 363.07
  gravidarum 646.8
  hemorrhagica externa 362.12
  juxtapapillary (Jensen's) 363.05
  luetic—*see* Retinitis, syphilitic
  metastatic 363.14
  pigmentosa 362.74
  proliferans 362.29
  proliferating 362.29
  punctata albescens 362.76
  renal 585 *[363.13]*
  syphilitic (secondary) 091.51
    congenital 090.0 *[363.13]*
    early 091.51
    late 095.8 *[363.13]*
  syphilitica, central, recurrent 095.8 *[363.13]*
  tuberculous (*see also* Tuberculous) 017.3
    [363.13]
Retinoblastoma (M9510/3) 190.5
  differentiated type (M9511/3) 190.5
  undifferentiated type (M9512/3) 190.5
Retinochoroiditis (*see also* Chorioretinitis)
  363.20
  central angiospastic 362.41
  disseminated 363.10
    metastatic 363.14
    neurosyphilitic 094.83
    pigment epitheliopathy 363.15
    syphilitic 094.83
  due to toxoplasmosis (acquired) (focal) 130.2
  focal 363.00
    in histoplasmosis 115.92
      capsulatum 115.02
      duboisii 115.12
    juxtapapillary (Jensen's) 363.05
    macular 363.06
    paramacular 363.06
    peripheral 363.08
    posterior pole NEC 363.07
  juxtapapillaris 363.05
  syphilitic (disseminated) 094.83
Retinopathy (background) 362.10
  arteriosclerotic 440.8 *[362.13]*
  atherosclerotic 440.8 *[362.13]*
  central serous 362.41
  circinate 362.10
  Coat's 362.12
  diabetic 250.5 *[362.01]*
    proliferative 250.5 *[362.02]*
  exudative 362.12
  hypertensive 362.11
  of prematurity 362.21
  pigmentary, congenital 362.74
  proliferative 362.29
    diabetic 250.5 *[362.02]*
    sickle-cell 282.60 *[362.29]*
  solar 363.31
Retinoschisis 361.10
  bullous 361.12
  congenital 743.56
  flat 361.11
  juvenile 362.73
Retractile testis 752.52

Retraction
  cervix (*see also* Retroversion, uterus) 621.6
  drum (membrane) 384.82
  eyelid 374.41
  finger 736.29
  head 781.0
  lid 374.41
  lung 518.89
  mediastinum 519.3
  nipple 611.79
    congenital 757.6
    puerperal, postpartum 676.0
  palmar fascia 728.6
  pleura (*see also* Pleurisy) 511.0
  ring, uterus (Bandl's) (pathological) 661.4
    affecting fetus or newborn 763.7
  sternum (congenital) 756.3
    acquired 738.3
    during respiration 786.9
  substernal 738.3
  supraclavicular 738.8
  syndrome (Duane's) 378.71
  uterus (*see also* Retroversion, uterus) 621.6
  valve (heart)—*see* Endocarditis
Retrobulbar —*see* condition
Retrocaval ureter 753.4
Retrocecal —*see also* condition
  appendix (congenital) 751.5
Retrocession —*see* Retroversion
Retrodisplacement —*see* Retroversion
Retroflection, retroflexion —*see* Retroversion
Retrognathia, retrognathism (mandibular)
  (maxillary) 524.06
Retrograde
  ejaculation 608.87
  menstruation 626.8
Retroiliac ureter 753.4
Retroperineal —*see* condition
Retroperitoneal —*see* condition
Retroperitonitis (*see also* Peritonitis) 567.9
Retropharyngeal —*see* condition
Retroplacental —*see* condition
Retroposition —*see* Retroversion
Retrosternal thyroid (congenital) 759.2
Retroversion, retroverted
  cervix (*see also* Retroversion, uterus) 621.6
  female NEC (*see also* Retroversion, uterus)
    621.6
  iris 364.70
  testis (congenital) 752.51
  uterus, uterine (acquired) (acute) (adherent)
    (any degree) (asymptomatic) (cervix)
    (postinfectional) (postpartal, old) 621.6
    congenital 752.3
    in pregnancy or childbirth 654.3
      affecting fetus or newborn 763.89
      causing obstructed labor 660.2
        affecting fetus or newborn 763.1
Retrusion, premaxilla (developmental) 524.04
Rett's syndrome 330.8
Reverse, reversed
  peristalsis 787.4
Reye's syndrome 331.81
Reye-Sheehan syndrome (postpartum pituitary
  necrosis) 253.2
Rh (factor)
  hemolytic disease 773.0
  incompatibility, immunization, or sensitization
    affecting management of pregnancy 656.1
    fetus or newborn 773.0
    transfusion reaction 999.7

Rhinitis—*continued*
  infective 460
  obstructive 472.0
  pneumococcal 460
  syphilitic 095.8
    congenital 090.0
  tuberculous (*see also* Tuberculosis) 012.8
  vasomotor (*see also* Fever, hay) 477.9
Rhinoantritis (chronic) 473.0
  acute 461.0
Rhinodacryolith 375.57
Rhinolalia (aperta) (clausa) (open) 784.49
Rhinolith 478.1
  nasal sinus (*see also* Sinusitis) 473.9
Rhinomegaly 478.1
Rhinopharyngitis (acute) (subacute) (*see also*
    Nasopharyngitis) 460
  chronic 472.2
  destructive ulcerating 102.5
  mutilans 102.5
Rhinophyma 695.3
Rhinorrhea 478.1
  cerebrospinal (fluid) 349.81
  paroxysmal (*see also* Fever, hay) 477.9
  spasmodic (*see also* Fever, hay) 477.9
Rhinosalpingitis 381.50
  acute 381.51
  chronic 381.52
Rhinoscleroma 040.1
Rhinosporidiosis 117.0
Rhinovirus infection 079.3
Rhizomelique, pseudopolyarthritic 446.5
Rhoads and Bomford anemia (refractory) 284.9
Rhus
  diversiloba dermatitis 692.6
  radicans dermatitis 692.6
  toxicodendron dermatitis 692.6
  venenata dermatitis 692.6
  verniciflua dermatitis 692.6
Rhythm
  atrioventricular nodal 427.89
  disorder 427.9
    coronary sinus 427.89
    ectopic 427.89
    nodal 427.89
  escape 427.89
  heart, abnormal 427.9
    fetus or newborn—*see* Abnormal, heart rate
  idioventricular 426.89
    accelerated 427.89
  nodal 427.89
  sleep, inversion 780.55
    nonorganic origin 307.45
Rhytidosis facialis 701.8
Rib —*see also* condition
  cervical 756.2
Riboflavin deficiency 266.0
Rice bodies (*see also* Loose, body, joint) 718.1
  knee 717.6
Richter's hernia —*see* Hernia, Richter's
Ricinism 988.2
Rickets (active) (acute) (adolescent) (adult)
    (chest wall) (congenital) (current) (infantile)
    (intestinal) 268.0
  celiac 579.0
  fetal 756.4
  hemorrhagic 267
  hypophosphatemic with nephrotic-glycosuric
    dwarfism 270.0
  kidney 588.0
  late effect 268.1

Rickets—*continued*
  renal 588.0
  scurvy 267
  vitamin D-resistant 275.3
Rickettsial disease 083.9
  specified type NEC 083.8
Rickettsialpox 083.2
Rickettsiosis NEC 083.9
  specified type NEC 083.8
  tick-borne 082.9
    specified type NEC 082.8
  vesicular 083.2
Ricord's chancre 091.0
Riddoch's syndrome (visual disorientation)
    368.16
Rider's
  bone 733.99
  chancre 091.0
Ridge, alveolus —*see also* condition
  flabby 525.2
Ridged ear 744.29
Riedel's
  disease (ligneous thyroiditis) 245.3
  lobe, liver 751.69
  struma (ligneous thyroiditis) 245.3
  thyroiditis (ligneous) 245.3
Rieger's anomaly or syndrome (mesodermal
    dysgenesis, anterior ocular segment) 743.44
Riehl's melanosis 709.09
Rietti-Greppi-Micheli anemia or syndrome
    282.4
Rieux's hernia —*see* Hernia, Rieux's
Rift Valley fever 066.3
Riga's disease (cachectic aphthae) 529.0
Riga-Fede disease (cachectic aphthae) 529.0
Riggs' disease (compound periodontitis) 523.4
Right middle lobe syndrome 518.0
Rigid, rigidity —*see also* condition
  abdominal 789.4
  articular, multiple congenital 754.89
  back 724.8
  cervix uteri
    in pregnancy or childbirth 654.6
      affecting fetus or newborn 763.89
      causing obstructed labor 660.2
        affecting fetus or newborn 763.1
  hymen (acquired) (congenital) 623.3
  nuchal 781.6
  pelvic floor
    in pregnancy or childbirth 654.4
      affecting fetus or newborn 763.89
      causing obstructed labor 660.2
        affecting fetus or newborn 763.1
  perineum or vulva
    in pregnancy or childbirth 654.8
      affecting fetus or newborn 763.89
      causing obstructed labor 660.2
        affecting fetus or newborn 763.1
  spine 724.8
  vagina
    in pregnancy or childbirth 654.7
      affecting fetus or newborn 763.89
      causing obstructed labor 660.2
        affecting fetus or newborn 763.1
Rigors 780.99
Riley-Day syndrome (familial dysautonomia)
    742.8
Ring(s)
  aorta 747.21
  Bandl's, complicating delivery 661.4
    affecting fetus or newborn 763.7

Ring(s)—*continued*
  contraction, complicating delivery 661.4
    affecting fetus or newborn 763.7
  esophageal (congenital) 750.3
  Fleischer (-Kayser) (cornea) 275.1 *[371.14]*
  hymenal, tight (acquired) (congenital) 623.3
  Kayser-Fleischer (cornea) 275.1 *[371.14]*
  retraction, uterus, pathological 661.4
    affecting fetus or newborn 763.7
  Schatzki's (esophagus) (congenital) (lower) 750.3
    acquired 530.3
  Soemmering's 366.51
  trachea, abnormal 748.3
  vascular (congenital) 747.21
  Vossius' 921.3
    late effect 366.21
Ringed hair (congenital) 757.4
Ringing in the ear (*see also* Tinnitus) 388.30
Ringworm 110.9
  beard 110.0
  body 110.5
  Burmese 110.9
  corporeal 110.5
  foot 110.4
  groin 110.3
  hand 110.2
  honeycomb 110.0
  nails 110.1
  perianal (area) 110.3
  scalp 110.0
  specified site NEC 110.8
  Tokelau 110.5
Rise, venous pressure 459.89
Risk
  factor —*see* Problem
  suicidal 300.9
Ritter's disease (dermatitis exfoliativa neonatorum) 695.81
Rivalry, sibling 313.3
Rivalta's disease (cervicofacial actinomycosis) 039.3
River blindness 125.3 *[360.13]*
Robert's pelvis 755.69
  with disproportion (fetopelvic) 653.0
    affecting fetus or newborn 763.1
    causing obstructed labor 660.1
      affecting fetus or newborn 763.1
Robin's syndrome 756.0
Robinson's (hidrotic) ectodermal dysplasia 757.31
Robles' disease (onchocerciasis) 125.3 *[360.13]*
Rochalimea —*see* Rickettsial disease
Rocky Mountain fever (spotted) 082.0
Rodent ulcer (M8090/3)—*see also* Neoplasm, skin, malignant
  cornea 370.07
Roentgen ray, adverse effect —*see* Effect, adverse, x-ray
Roetheln 056.9
Roger's disease (congenital interventricular septal defect) 745.4
Rokitansky's
  disease (*see also* Necrosis, liver) 570
  tumor 620.2
Rokitansky-Aschoff sinuses (mucosal outpouching of gallbladder) (*see also* Disease, gallbladder) 575.8
Rokitansky-Kuster-Hauser syndrome (congenital absence vagina) 752.49
Rollet's chancre (syphilitic) 091.0
Rolling of head 781.0

Romano-Ward syndrome (prolonged Q-T interval) 794.31
Romanus lesion 720.1
Romberg's disease or syndrome 349.89
Roof, mouth —*see* condition
Rosacea 695.3
  acne 695.3
  keratitis 695.3 *[370.49]*
Rosary, rachitic 268.0
Rose
  cold 477.0
  fever 477.0
  rash 782.1
    epidemic 056.9
    of infants 057.8
Rosen-Castleman-Liebow syndrome (pulmonary proteinosis) 516.0
Rosenbach's erysipelatoid or erysipeloid 027.1
Rosenthal's disease (factor XI deficiency) 286.2
Roseola 057.8
  infantum, infantilis 057.8
Rossbach's disease (hyperchlorhydria) 536.8
  psychogenic 306.4
Rössle-Urbach-Wiethe lipoproteinosis 272.8
Ross river fever 066.3
Rostan's asthma (cardiac) (*see also* Failure, ventricular, left) 428.1
Rot
  Barcoo (*see also* Ulcer, skin) 707.9
  knife-grinders' (*see also* Tuberculosis) 011.4
Rot-Bernhardt disease 355.1
Rotation
  anomalous, incomplete or insufficient—*see* Malrotation
  cecum (congenital) 751.4
  colon (congenital) 751.4
  manual, affecting fetus or newborn 763.89
  spine, incomplete or insufficient 737.8
  tooth, teeth 524.3
  vertebra, incomplete or insufficient 737.8
Röteln 056.9
Roth's disease or meralgia 355.1
Roth-Bernhardt disease or syndrome 355.1
Rothmund (-Thomson) syndrome 757.33
Rotor's disease or syndrome (idiopathic hyperbilirubinemia) 277.4
Rotundum ulcus —*see* Ulcer, stomach
Round
  back (with wedging of vertebrae) 737.10
    late effect of rickets 268.1
  hole, retina 361.31
    with detachment 361.01
  ulcer (stomach)—*see* Ulcer, stomach
  worms (infestation) (large) NEC 127.0
Roussy-Lévy syndrome 334.3
Routine postpartum follow-up V24.2
Roy (-Jutras) syndrome (acropachyderma) 757.39
Rubella (German measles) 056.9
  complicating pregnancy, childbirth, or puerperium 647.5
  complication 056.8
    neurological 056.00
      encephalomyelitis 056.01
      specified type NEC 056.09
    specified type NEC 056.79
  congenital 771.0
  contact V01.4
  exposure to V01.4
  maternal
    with suspected fetal damage affecting management of pregnancy 655.3

Rupture, ruptured—*continued*
  tricuspid (heart) (valve)—*see* Endocarditis,
      tricuspid
  tube, tubal 620.8
    abscess (*see also* Salpingo-oophoritis) 614.2
    due to pregnancy—*see* Pregnancy, tubal
  tympanum, tympanic (membrane) (*see also*
      Perforation, tympanum) 384.20
    with otitis media—*see* Otitis media
    traumatic—*see* Wound, open, ear, drum
  umbilical cord 663.8
    fetus or newborn 772.0
  ureter (traumatic) (*see also* Injury, internal,
      ureter) 867.2
    nontraumatic 593.89
  urethra 599.84
    with
      abortion—*see* Abortion, by type, with
          damage to pelvic organs
      ectopic pregnancy (*see also* categories
          633.0-633.9) 639.2
      molar pregnancy (*see also* categories
          630-632) 639.2
    following
      abortion 639.2
      ectopic or molar pregnancy 639.2
    obstetrical trauma 665.5
    traumatic—*see* Injury, internal urethra
  uterosacral ligament 620.8
  uterus (traumatic)—*see also* Injury, internal
      uterus
    affecting fetus or newborn 763.89
    during labor 665.1
    nonpuerperal, nontraumatic 621.8
    nontraumatic 621.8
    pregnant (during labor) 665.1
      before labor 665.0
  vaginal 878.6
    complicated 878.7
    complicating delivery—*see* Laceration,
        vagina, complicating delivery
  valve, valvular (heart)—*see* Endocarditis
  varicose vein—*see* Varicose, vein
  varix—*see* Varix
  vena cava 459.0
  ventricle (free wall) (left) (*see also* Infarct,
      myocardium) 410.9
  vesical (urinary) 596.6
    traumatic—*see* Injury, internal, bladder
  vessel (blood) 459.0
    pulmonary 417.8
  viscus 799.8
  vulva 878.4
    complicated 878.5
    complicating delivery 664.0
Russell's dwarf (uterine dwarfism and
  craniofacial dysostosis) 759.89
Russell's dysentery 004.8
Russell (-Silver) syndrome (congenital
  hemihypertrophy and short stature) 759.89
Russian spring-summer type encephalitis 063.0
Rust's disease (tuberculous spondylitis) 015.0
  [720.81]
Rustitskii's disease (multiple myeloma)
  (M9730/3) 203.0
Ruysch's disease (Hirschsprung's disease) 751.3
Rytand-Lipsitch syndrome (complete
  atrioventricular block) 426.0

S

Saber
shin 090.5
tibia 090.5
Sac, lacrimal —*see* condition
Saccharomyces infection (*see also* Candidiasis)
112.9
Saccharopinuria 270.7
Saccular —*see* condition
Sacculation
aorta (nonsyphilitic) (*see also* Aneurysm, aorta)
441.9
ruptured 441.5
syphilitic 093.0
bladder 596.3
colon 569.89
intralaryngeal (congenital) (ventricular) 748.3
larynx (congenital) (ventricular) 748.3
organ or site, congenital—*see* Distortion
pregnant uterus, complicating delivery 654.4
affecting fetus or newborn 763.1
causing obstructed labor 660.2
affecting fetus or newborn 763.1
rectosigmoid 569.89
sigmoid 569.89
ureter 593.89
urethra 599.2
vesical 596.3
Sachs (-Tay) disease (amaurotic familial idiocy)
330.1
Sacks-Libman disease 710.0 *[424.91]*
Sacralgia 724.6
Sacralization
fifth lumbar vertebra 756.15
incomplete (vertebra) 756.15
Sacrodynia 724.6
Sacroiliac joint —*see* condition
Sacroiliitis NEC 720.2
Sacrum —*see* condition
Saddle
back 737.8
embolus, aorta 444.0
nose 738.0
congenital 754.0
due to syphilis 090.5
Sadism (sexual) 302.84
Saemisch's ulcer 370.04
Saenger's syndrome 379.46
Sago spleen 277.3
Sailors' skin 692.74
Saint
Anthony's fire (*see also* Erysipelas) 035
Guy's dance—*see* Chorea
Louis-type encephalitis 062.3
triad (*see also* Hernia, diaphragm) 553.3
Vitus' dance—*see* Chorea
Salicylism
correct substance properly administered 535.4
overdose or wrong substance given or taken
965.1
Salivary duct or gland —*see also* condition
virus disease 078.5
Salivation (excessive) (*see also* Ptyalism) 527.7
Salmonella (aertrycke) (choleraesuis)
(enteritidis) (gallinarum) (suipestifer)
(typhimurium) (*see also* Infection,
Salmonella) 003.9
arthritis 003.23
carrier (suspected) of V02.3

Salmonella—*continued*
meningitis 003.21
osteomyelitis 003.24
pneumonia 003.22
septicemia 003.1
typhosa 002.0
carrier (suspected) of V02.1
Salmonellosis 003.0
with pneumonia 003.22
Salpingitis (catarrhal) (fallopian tube) (nodular)
(pseudofollicular) (purulent) (septic) (*see also*
Salpingo-oophoritis) 614.2
ear 381.50
acute 381.51
chronic 381.52
Eustachian (tube) 381.50
acute 381.51
chronic 381.52
follicularis 614.1
gonococcal (chronic) 098.37
acute 098.17
interstitial, chronic 614.1
isthmica nodosa 614.1
old—*see* Salpingo-oophoritis, chronic
puerperal, postpartum, childbirth 670
specific (chronic) 098.37
acute 098.17
tuberculous (acute) (chronic) (*see also*
Tuberculosis) 016.6
venereal (chronic) 098.37
acute 098.17
Salpingocele 620.4
Salpingo-oophoritis (catarrhal) (purulent)
(ruptured) (septic) (suppurative) 614.2
acute 614.0
with
abortion—*see* Abortion, by type, with sepsis
ectopic pregnancy (*see also* categories
633.0-633.9) 639.0
molar pregnancy (*see also* categories
630-632) 639.0
following
abortion 639.0
ectopic or molar pregnancy 639.0
gonococcal 098.17
puerperal, postpartum, childbirth 670
tuberculous (*see also* Tuberculosis) 016.6
chronic 614.1
gonococcal 098.37
tuberculous (*see also* Tuberculosis) 016.6
complicating pregnancy 646.6
affecting fetus or newborn 760.8
gonococcal (chronic) 098.37
acute 098.17
old—*see* Salpingo-oophoritis, chronic
puerperal 670
specific—*see* Salpingo-oophoritis, gonococcal
subacute (*see also* Salpingo-oophoritis, acute)
614.0
tuberculous (acute) (chronic) (*see also*
Tuberculosis) 016.6
venereal—*see* Salpingo-oophoritis, gonococcal
Salpingo-ovaritis (*see also* Salpingo-oophoritis)
614.2
Salpingoperitonitis (*see also*
Salpingo-oophoritis) 614.2

Schizoid personality 301.20
  introverted 301.21
  schizotypal 301.22
Schizophrenia, schizophrenic (reaction) 295.9

> *Note—Use the following fifth-digit*
> *subclassification with category 295:*
>
> *0 unspecified*
> *1 subchronic*
> *2 chronic*
> *3 subchronic with acute exacerbation*
> *4 chronic with acute exacerbation*
> *5 in remission*

  acute (attack) NEC 295.8
    episode 295.4
  atypical form 295.8
  borderline 295.5
  catalepsy 295.2
  catatonic (type) (acute) (excited) (withdrawn)
    295.2
  childhood (type) (*see also* Psychosis,
    childhood) 299.9
  chronic NEC 295.6
  coenesthesiopathic 295.8
  cyclic (type) 295.7
  disorganized (type) 295.1
  flexibilitas cerea 295.2
  hebephrenic (type) (acute) 295.1
  incipient 295.5
  latent 295.5
  paranoid (type) (acute) 295.3
  paraphrenic (acute) 295.3
  prepsychotic 295.5
  primary (acute) 295.0
  prodromal 295.5
  pseudoneurotic 295.5
  pseudopsychopathic 295.5
  reaction 295.9
  residual (state) (type) 295.6
  restzustand 295.6
  schizo-affective (type) (depressed) (excited)
    295.7
  schizophreniform type 295.4
  simple (type) (acute) 295.0
  simplex (acute) 295.0
  specified type NEC 295.8
  syndrome of childhood NEC (*see also*
    Psychosis, childhood) 299.9
  undifferentiated 295.9
    acute 295.8
    chronic 295.6
Schizothymia 301.20
  introverted 301.21
  schizotypal 301.22
Schlafkrankheit 086.5
Schlatter's tibia (osteochondrosis) 732.4
Schlatter-Osgood disease (osteochondrosis,
  tibial tubercle) 732.4
Schloffer's tumor (*see also* Peritonitis) 567.2
Schmidt's syndrome
  sphallo-pharyngo-laryngeal hemiplegia 352.6
  thyroid-adrenocortical insufficiency 258.1
  vagoaccessory 352.6
Schmincke
  carcinoma (M8082/3)—*see* Neoplasm,
    nasopharynx, malignant
  tumor (M8082/3)—*see* Neoplasm,
    nasopharynx, malignant
Schmitz (-Stutzer) dysentery 004.0

Schmorl's disease or nodes 722.30
  lumbar, lumbosacral 722.32
  specified region NEC 722.39
  thoracic, thoracolumbar 722.31
Schneider's syndrome 047.9
Schneiderian
  carcinoma (M8121/3)
    specified site—*see* Neoplasm, by site,
      malignant
    unspecified site 160.0
  papilloma (M8121/0)
    specified site—*see* Neoplasm, by site, benign
    unspecified site 212.0
Schoffer's tumor (*see also* Peritonitis) 567.2
Scholte's syndrome (malignant carcinoid) 259.2
Scholz's disease 330.0
Scholz (-Bielschowsky-Henneberg) syndrome
  330.0
Schönlein (-Henoch) disease (primary) (purpura)
  (rheumatic) 287.0
School examination V70.3
Schottmüller's disease (*see also* Fever,
  paratyphoid) 002.9
Schroeder's syndrome (endocrine-hypertensive)
  255.3
Schüller-Christian disease or syndrome
  (chronic histiocytosis X) 277.8
Schultz's disease or syndrome (agranulocytosis)
  288.0
Schultze's acroparesthesia, simple 443.89
Schwalbe-Ziehen-Oppenheimer disease 333.6
Schwannoma (M9560/0)—*see also* Neoplasm,
  connective tissue, benign
  malignant (M9560/3)—*see* Neoplasm,
    connective tissue, malignant
Schwartz (-Jampel) syndrome 756.89
Schwartz-Bartter syndrome (inappropriate
  secretion of antidiuretic hormone) 253.6
Schweninger-Buzzi disease (macular atrophy)
  701.3
Sciatic —*see* condition
Sciatica (infectional) 724.3
  due to
    displacement of intervertebral disc 722.10
    herniation, nucleus pulposus 722.10
Scimitar syndrome (anomalous venous
  drainage, right lung to inferior vena cava)
  747.49
Sclera —*see* condition
Sclerectasia 379.11
Scleredema
  adultorum 710.1
  Buschke's 710.1
  newborn 778.1
Sclerema
  adiposum (newborn) 778.1
  adultorum 710.1
  edematosum (newborn) 778.1
  neonatorum 778.1
  newborn 778.1
Scleriasis —*see* Scleroderma
Scleritis 379.00
  with corneal involvement 379.05
  anterior (annular) (localized) 379.03
  brawny 379.06
  granulomatous 379.09
  posterior 379.07
  specified NEC 379.09
  suppurative 379.09
  syphilitic 095.0
  tuberculous (nodular) (*see also* Tuberculosis)
    017.3 *[379.09]*

Sclerochoroiditis (*see also* Scleritis) 379.00
Scleroconjunctivitis (*see also* Scleritis) 379.00
Sclerocystic ovary (syndrome) 256.4
Sclerodactylia 701.0
Scleroderma, sclerodermia (acrosclerotic)
 (diffuse) (generalized) (progressive)
 (pulmonary) 710.1
 circumscribed 701.0
 linear 701.0
 localized (linear) 701.0
 newborn 778.1
Sclerokeratitis 379.05
 meaning sclerosing keratitis 370.54
 tuberculous (*see also* Tuberculosis) 017.3
  [379.09]
Scleroma, trachea 040.1
Scleromalacia
 multiple 731.0
 perforans 379.04
Scleromyxedema 701.8
Scleroperikeratitis 379.05
Sclerose en plaques 340
Sclerosis, sclerotic
 adrenal (gland) 255.8
 Alzheimer's 331.0
  with dementia—*see* Alzheimer's, demential
 amyotrophic (lateral) 335.20
 annularis fibrosi
  aortic 424.1
  mitral 424.0
 aorta, aortic 440.0
  valve (*see also* Endocarditis, aortic) 424.1
 artery, arterial, arteriolar, arteriovascular—*see*
  Arteriosclerosis
 ascending multiple 340
 Baló's (concentric) 341.1
 basilar—*see* Sclerosis, brain
 bone (localized) NEC 733.99
 brain (general) (lobular) 341.9
  Alzheimer's—*see* Alzheimer's dementia
  artery, arterial 437.0
  atrophic lobar 331.0
   with dementia
    with behavioral disturbance 331.0 *[294.11]*
    without behavioral disturbance 331.0
     [294.10]
  diffuse 341.1
   familial (chronic) (infantile) 330.0
   infantile (chronic) (familial) 330.0
   Pelizaeus-Merzbacher type 330.0
  disseminated 340
  hereditary 334.2
  infantile, (degenerative) (diffuse) 330.0
  insular 340
  Krabbe's 330.0
  miliary 340
  multiple 340
  Pelizaeus-Merzbacher 330.0
  progressive familial 330.0
  senile 437.0
  tuberous 759.5
 bulbar, progressive 340
 bundle of His 426.50
  left 426.3
  right 426.4
 cardiac —*see* Arteriosclerosis, coronary
 cardiorenal (*see also* Hypertension, cardiorenal)
  404.90
 cardiovascular (*see also* Disease,
  cardiovascular) 429.2

Sclerosis, sclerotic—*continued*
 renal (*see also* Hypertension, cardiorenal)
  404.90
 centrolobar, familial 330.0
 cerebellar—*see* Sclerosis, brain
 cerebral—*see* Sclerosis, brain
 cerebrospinal 340
  disseminated 340
  multiple 340
 cerebrovascular 437.0
 choroid 363.40
  diffuse 363.56
 combined (spinal cord)—*see also* Degeneration,
  combined
  multiple 340
 concentric, Baló's 341.1
 cornea 370.54
 coronary (artery) —*see* Arteriosclerosis,
  coronary
 corpus cavernosum
  female 624.8
  male 607.89
 Dewitzky's
  aortic 424.1
  mitral 424.0
 diffuse NEC 341.1
 disease, heart —*see* Arteriosclerosis, coronary
 disseminated 340
 dorsal 340
 dorsolateral (spinal cord)—*see* Degeneration,
  combined
 endometrium 621.8
 extrapyramidal 333.90
 eye, nuclear (senile) 366.16
 Friedreich's (spinal cord) 334.0
 funicular (spermatic cord) 608.89
 gastritis 535.4
 general (vascular)—*see* Arteriosclerosis
 gland (lymphatic) 457.8
 hepatic 571.9
 hereditary
  cerebellar 334.2
  spinal 334.0
 idiopathic cortical (Garré's) (*see also*
  Osteomyelitis) 730.1
 ilium, piriform 733.5
 insular 340
  pancreas 251.8
 Islands of Langerhans 251.8
 kidney—*see* Sclerosis, renal
 larynx 478.79
 lateral 335.24
  amyotrophic 335.20
  descending 335.24
  primary 335.24
  spinal 335.24
 liver 571.9
 lobar, atrophic (of brain) 331.0
  with dementia
   with behavioral disturbance 331.0 *[294.11]*
   without behavioral disturbance 331.0
    [294.10]
 lung (*see also* Fibrosis, lung) 515
 mastoid 383.1
 mitral—*see* Endocarditis, mitral
 Mönckeberg's (medial) (*see also*
  Arteriosclerosis, extremities) 440.20
 multiple (brain stem) (cerebral) (generalized)
  (spinal cord) 340
 myocardium, myocardial —*see*
  Arteriosclerosis, coronary

Sclerosis, sclerotic—*continued*
  nuclear (senile), eye 366.16
  ovary 620.8
  pancreas 577.8
  penis 607.89
  peripheral arteries NEC (*see also*
    Arteriosclerosis, extremities) 440.20
  plaques 340
  pluriglandular 258.8
  polyglandular 258.8
  posterior (spinal cord) (syphilitic) 094.0
  posterolateral (spinal cord)—*see* Degeneration,
    combined
  prepuce 607.89
  primary lateral 335.24
  progressive systemic 710.1
  pulmonary (*see also* Fibrosis, lung) 515
    artery 416.0
    valve (heart) (*see also* Endocarditis,
      pulmonary) 424.3
  renal 587
    with
      cystine storage disease 270.0
      hypertension (*see also* Hypertension,
        kidney) 403.90
      hypertensive heart disease (conditions
        classifiable to 402) (*see also*
        Hypertension, cardiorenal) 404.90
      arteriolar (hyaline) (*see also* Hypertension,
        kidney) 403.90
      hyperplastic (*see also* Hypertension, kidney)
        403.90
  retina (senile) (vascular) 362.17
  rheumatic
    aortic valve 395.9
    mitral valve 394.9
  Schilder's 341.1
  senile—*see* Arteriosclerosis
  spinal (cord) (general) (progressive)
    (transverse) 336.8
    ascending 357.0
    combined—*see also* Degeneration, combined
      multiple 340
      syphilitic 094.89
    disseminated 340
    dorsolateral—*see* Degeneration, combined
    hereditary (Friedreich's) (mixed form) 334.0
    lateral (amyotrophic) 335.24
    multiple 340
    posterior (syphilitic) 094.0
  stomach 537.89
  subendocardial, congenital 425.3
  systemic (progressive) 710.1
    with lung involvement 710.1 *[517.2]*
  tricuspid (heart) (valve)—*see* Endocarditis,
    tricuspid
  tuberous (brain) 759.5
  tympanic membrane (*see also*
    Tympanosclerosis) 385.00
  valve, valvular (heart)—*see* Endocarditis
  vascular—*see* Arteriosclerosis
  vein 459.89
Sclerotenonitis 379.07
Sclerotitis (*see also* Scleritis) 379.00
  syphilitic 095.0
  tuberculous (*see also* Tuberculosis) 017.3
    [379.09]
Scoliosis (acquired) (postural) 737.30
  congenital 754.2
  due to or associated with
    Charcot-Marie-Tooth disease 356.1 *[737.43]*

Scoliosis—*continued*
    mucopolysaccharidosis 277.5 *[737.43]*
    neurofibromatosis 237.71 *[737.43]*
    osteitis
      deformans 731.0 *[737.43]*
      fibrosa cystica 252.0 *[737.43]*
    osteoporosis (*see also* Osteoporosis) 733.00
      [737.43]
    poliomyelitis 138 *[737.43]*
    radiation 737.33
    tuberculosis (*see also* Tuberculosis) 015.0
      [737.43]
  idiopathic 737.30
    infantile
      progressive 737.32
      resolving 737.31
  paralytic 737.39
  rachitic 268.1
  sciatic 724.3
  specified NEC 737.39
  thoracogenic 737.34
  tuberculous (*see also* Tuberculosis) 015.0
    [737.43]
Scoliotic pelvis 738.6
  with disproportion (fetopelvic) 653.0
    affecting fetus or newborn 763.1
    causing obstructed labor 660.1
      affecting fetus or newborn 763.1
Scorbutus, scorbutic 267
  anemia 281.8
Scotoma (ring) 368.44
  arcuate 368.43
  Bjerrum 368.43
  blind spot area 368.42
  central 368.41
  centrocecal 368.41
  paracecal 368.42
  paracentral 368.41
  scintillating 368.12
  Seidel 368.43
Scratch —*see* Injury, superficial, by site
Screening (for) V82.9
  alcoholism V79.1
  anemia, deficiency NEC V78.1
    iron V78.0
  anomaly, congenital V82.89
  antenatal V28.9
    alphafetoprotein levels, raised V28.1
    based on amniocentesis V28.2
      chromosomal anomalies V28.0
      raised alphafetoprotein levels V28.1
    fetal growth retardation using ultrasonics
      V28.4
    isoimmunization V28.5
    malformations using ultrasonics V28.3
    raised alphafetoprotein levels V28.1
    specified condition NEC V28.8
    Streptococcus B V28.6
  arterial hypertension V81.1
  arthropod-borne viral disease NEC V73.5
  asymptomatic bacteriuria V81.5
  bacterial
    conjunctivitis V74.4
    disease V74.9
      specified condition NEC V74.8
  bacteriuria, asymptomatic V81.5
  blood disorder NEC V78.9
    specified type NEC V78.8
  bronchitis, chronic V81.3
  brucellosis V74.8
  cancer—*see* Screening, malignant neoplasm

Secretion—*continued*
  by
    carcinoid tumor 259.2
      pheochromocytoma 255.6
    ectopic NEC 259.3
  urinary
    excessive 788.42
    suppression 788.5
Section
  cesarean
    affecting fetus or newborn 763.4
    post mortem, affecting fetus or newborn 761.6
    previous, in pregnancy or childbirth 654.2
      affecting fetus or newborn 763.89
  nerve, traumatic—*see* Injury, nerve, by site
Seeligmann's syndrome (ichthyosis congenita)
  757.1
Segmentation, incomplete (congenital)—*see*
  also Fusion
  bone NEC 756.9
  lumbosacral (joint) 756.15
  vertebra 756.15
    lumbosacral 756.15
Seizure 780.39
  akinetic (idiopathic) (*see also* Epilepsy) 345.0
    psychomotor 345.4
  apoplexy, apoplectic (*see also* Disease,
    cerebrovascular, acute) 436
  atonic (*see also* Epilepsy) 345.0
  autonomic 300.11
  brain or cerebral (*see also* Disease,
    cerebrovascular, acute) 436
  convulsive (*see also* Convulsions) 780.39
  cortical (focal) (motor) (*see also* Epilepsy) 345.5
  epilepsy, epileptic (cryptogenic) (*see also*
    Epilepsy) 345.9
  epileptiform, epileptoid 780.39
    focal (*see also* Epilepsy) 345.5
  febrile 780.31
  heart—*see* Disease, heart
  hysterical 300.11
  Jacksonian (focal) (*see also* Epilepsy) 345.5
    motor type 345.5
    sensory type 345.5
  newborn 779.0
  paralysis (*see also* Disease, cerebrovascular,
    acute) 436
  recurrent 780.39
    epileptic—*see* Epilepsy
  repetitive 780.39
    epileptic—*see* Epilepsy
  salaam (*see also* Epilepsy) 345.6
  uncinate (*see also* Epilepsy) 345.4
Self-mutilation 300.9
Semicoma 780.09
Semiconsciousness 780.09
Seminal
  vesicle—*see* condition
  vesiculitis (*see also* Vesiculitis) 608.0
Seminoma (M9061/3)
  anaplastic type (M9062/3)
    specified site—*see* Neoplasm, by site,
      malignant
    unspecified site 186.9
  specified site—*see* Neoplasm, by site, malignant
  spermatocytic (M9063/3)
    specified site—*see* Neoplasm, by site,
      malignant
    unspecified site 186.9
  unspecified site 186.9
Semliki Forest encephalitis 062.8

Senear-Usher disease or syndrome (pemphigus
  erythematosus) 694.4
Senecio jacobae dermatitis 692.6
Senectus 797
Senescence 797
Senile (*see also* condition) 797
  cervix (atrophic) 622.8
  degenerative atrophy, skin 701.3
  endometrium (atrophic) 621.8
  fallopian tube (atrophic) 620.3
  heart (failure) 797
  lung 492.8
  ovary (atrophic) 620.3
  syndrome 259.8
  vagina, vaginitis (atrophic) 627.3
  wart 702.0
Senility 797
  with
    acute confusional state 290.3
    delirium 290.3
    mental changes 290.9
    psychosis NEC (*see also* Psychosis, senile)
      290.20
  premature (syndrome) 259.8
Sensation
  burning (*see also* Disturbance, sensation) 782.0
    tongue 529.6
  choking 784.9
  loss of (*see also* Disturbance, sensation) 782.0
  prickling (*see also* Disturbance, sensation) 782.0
  tingling (*see also* Disturbance, sensation) 782.0
Sense loss (touch) (*see also* Disturbance,
  sensation) 782.0
  smell 781.1
  taste 781.1
Sensibility disturbance NEC (cortical) (deep)
  (vibratory) (*see also* Disturbance, sensation)
  782.0
Sensitive dentine 521.8
Sensitiver Beziehungswahn 297.8
Sensitivity, sensitization —*see also* Allergy
  autoerythrocyte 287.2
  carotid sinus 337.0
  child (excessive) 313.21
  cold, autoimmune 283.0
  methemoglobin 289.7
  suxamethonium 289.8
  tuberculin, without clinical or radiological
    symptoms 795.5
Sensory
  extinction 781.8
  neglect 781.8
Separation
  acromioclavicular—*see* Dislocation, shoulder
  anxiety, abnormal 309.21
  apophysis, traumatic—*see* Fracture, by site
  choroid 363.70
    hemorrhagic 363.72
    serous 363.71
  costochondral (simple) (traumatic)—*see*
    Dislocation, costochondral
  epiphysis, epiphyseal
    nontraumatic 732.9
      upper femoral 732.2
    traumatic—*see* Fracture, by site
  fracture—*see* Fracture, by site
  infundibulum cardiac from right ventricle by a
    partition 746.83
  joint (current) (traumatic)—*see* Dislocation, by
    site

Separation—*continued*
  placenta (normally implanted)—*see* Placenta,
    separation
  pubic bone, obstetrical trauma 665.6
  retina, retinal (*see also* Detachment, retina)
    361.9
    layers 362.40
      sensory (*see also* Retinoschisis) 361.10
      pigment epithelium (exudative) 362.42
        hemorrhagic 362.43
  sternoclavicular (traumatic)—*see* Dislocation,
    sternoclavicular
  symphysis pubis, obstetrical trauma 665.6
  tracheal ring, incomplete (congenital) 748.3
Sepsis (generalized) (*see also* Septicemia) 038.9
  with
    abortion—*see* Abortion, by type, with sepsis
    ectopic pregnancy (*see also* categories
      633.0-633.9) 639.0
    molar pregnancy (*see also* categories
      630-632) 639.0
  buccal 528.3
  complicating labor 659.3
  dental (pulpal origin) 522.4
  female genital organ NEC 614.9
  fetus (intrauterine) 771.81
  following
    abortion 639.0
    ectopic or molar pregnancy 639.0
    infusion, perfusion, or transfusion 999.3
  Friedländer's 038.49
  intraocular 360.00
  localized
    in operation wound 998.59
    skin (*see also* Abscess) 682.9
  malleus 024
  nadir 038.9
  newborn (umbilical) (organism unspecified)
    NEC 771.81
  oral 528.3
  puerperal, postpartum, childbirth (pelvic) 670
  resulting from infusion, injection, transfusion,
    or vaccination 999.3
  severe 995.92
  skin, localized (*see also* Abscess) 682.9
  umbilical (newborn) (organism unspecified)
    771.89
    tetanus 771.3
  urinary 599.0
Septate —*see also* Septum
Septic —*see also* condition
  adenoids 474.01
    and tonsils 474.02
  arm (with lymphangitis) 682.3
  embolus—*see* Embolism
  finger (with lymphangitis) 681.00
  foot (with lymphangitis) 682.7
  gallbladder (*see also* Cholecystitis) 575.8
  hand (with lymphangitis) 682.4
  joint (*see also* Arthritis, septic) 711.0
  kidney (*see also* Infection, kidney) 590.9
  leg (with lymphangitis) 682.6
  mouth 528.3
  nail 681.9
    finger 681.02
    toe 681.11
  shock (endotoxic) 785.59
  sore (*see also* Abscess) 682.9
    throat 034.0
      milk-borne 034.0
      streptococcal 034.0

Septic—*continued*
  spleen (acute) 289.59
  teeth (pulpal origin) 522.4
  throat 034.0
  thrombus—*see* Thrombosis
  toe (with lymphangitis) 681.10
  tonsils 474.00
    and adenoids 474.02
  umbilical cord (newborn) (organism
    unspecified) 771.89
  uterus (*see also* Endometritis) 615.9
Septicemia, septicemic (generalized)
  (suppurative) 038.9
  with
    abortion—*see* Abortion, by type, with sepsis
    ectopic pregnancy (*see also* categories
      633.0-633.9) 639.0
    molar pregnancy (*see also* categories
      630-632) 639.0
  Aerobacter aerogenes 038.49
  anaerobic 038.3
  anthrax 022.3
  Bacillus coli 038.42
  Bacteroides 038.3
  Clostridium 038.3
  complicating labor 659.3
  cryptogenic 038.9
  enteric gram-negative bacilli 038.40
  Enterobacter aerogenes 038.49
  Erysipelothrix (insidiosa) (rhusiopathiae) 027.1
  Escherichia coli 038.42
  following
    abortion 639.0
    ectopic or molar pregnancy 639.0
    infusion, injection, transfusion, or vaccination
      999.3
  Friedländer's (bacillus) 038.49
  gangrenous 038.9
  gonococcal 098.89
  gram-negative (organism) 038.40
    anaerobic 038.3
  Hemophilus influenzae 038.41
  herpes (simplex) 054.5
  herpetic 054.5
  Listeria monocytogenes 027.0
  meningeal—*see* Meningitis
  meningococcal (chronic) (fulminating) 036.2
  navel, newborn (organism unspecified) 771.89
  newborn (umbilical) (organism unspecified)
    771.81
  plague 020.2
  pneumococcal 038.2
  postabortal 639.0
  postoperative 998.59
  Proteus vulgaris 038.49
  Pseudomonas (aeruginosa) 038.43
  puerperal, postpartum 670
  Salmonella (aertrycke) (callinarum)
    (choleraesuis) (enteritidis) (suipestifer) 003.1
  Serratia 038.44
  Shigella (*see also* Dysentery, bacillary) 004.9
  specified organism NEC 038.8
  staphylococcal 038.10
    aureus 038.11
    specified organism NEC 038.19
  streptococcal (anaerobic) 038.0
  suipestifer 003.1
  umbilicus, newborn (organism unspecified)
    771.89
  viral 079.99
  Yersinia enterocolitica 038.49

Septum, septate (congenital)—*see also*
Anomaly, specified type NEC
anal 751.2
aqueduct of Sylvius 742.3
with spina bifida (*see also* Spina bifida) 741.0
hymen 752.49
uterus (*see also* Double, uterus) 752.2
vagina 752.49
in pregnancy or childbirth 654.7
affecting fetus or newborn 763.89
causing obstructed labor 660.2
affecting fetus or newborn 763.1
Sequestration
lung (congenital) (extralobar) (intralobar) 748.5
orbit 376.10
pulmonary artery (congenital) 747.3
Sequestrum
bone (*see also* Osteomyelitis) 730.1
jaw 526.4
dental 525.8
jaw bone 526.4
sinus (accessory) (nasal) (*see also* Sinusitis)
473.9
maxillary 473.0
Sequoiosis asthma 495.8
Serology for syphilis
doubtful
with signs or symptoms—*see* Syphilis, by site
and stage
follow-up of latent syphilis—*see* Syphilis,
latent
false positive 795.6
negative, with signs or symptoms—*see*
Syphilis, by site and stage
positive 097.1
with signs or symptoms—*see* Syphilis, by site
and stage
false 795.6
follow-up of latent syphilis—*see* Syphilis,
latent
only finding—*see* Syphilis, latent
reactivated 097.1
Seroma (postoperative) (non-infected) 998.13
infected 998.51
Seropurulent —*see* condition
Serositis, multiple 569.89
pericardial 423.2
peritoneal 568.82
pleural—*see* Pleurisy
Serotonin syndrome 333.99
Serous —*see* condition
Sertoli cell
adenoma (M8640/0)
specified site—*see* Neoplasm, by site, benign
unspecified site
female 220
male 222.0
carcinoma (M8640/3)
specified site—*see* Neoplasm, by site,
malignant
unspecified site 186.9
syndrome (germinal aplasia) 606.0
tumor (M8640/0)
with lipid storage (M8641/0)
specified site—*see* Neoplasm, by site,
benign
unspecified site
female 220
male 222.0
specified site—*see* Neoplasm, by site, benign

Sertoli cell—*continued*
unspecified site
female 220
male 222.0
Sertoli-Leydig cell tumor (M8631/0)
specified site—*see* Neoplasm, by site, benign
unspecified site
female 220
male 222.0
Serum
allergy, allergic reaction 999.5
shock 999.4
arthritis 999.5 *[713.6]*
complication or reaction NEC 999.5
disease NEC 999.5
hepatitis 070.3
intoxication 999.5
jaundice (homologous) *see* Hepatitis, viral
neuritis 999.5
poisoning NEC 999.5
rash NEC 999.5
reaction NEC 999.5
sickness NEC 999.5
Sesamoiditis 733.99
Seven-day fever 061
of
Japan 100.89
Queensland 100.89
Sever's disease or osteochondrosis (calcaneum)
732.5
Sex chromosome mosaics 758.81
Sextuplet
affected by maternal complications of
pregnancy 761.5
healthy liveborn—*see* Newborn, multiple
pregnancy (complicating delivery) NEC 651.8
with fetal loss and retention of one or more
fetus(es) 651.6
Sexual
anesthesia 302.72
deviation (*see also* Deviation, sexual) 302.9
disorder (*see also* Deviation, sexual) 302.9
frigidity (female) 302.72
function, disorder of (psychogenic) 302.70
specified type NEC 302.79
immaturity (female) (male) 259.0
impotence (psychogenic) 302.72
organic origin NEC 607.84
precocity (constitutional) (cryptogenic) (female)
(idiopathic) (male) NEC 259.1
with adrenal hyperplasia 255.2
sadism 302.84
Sexuality, pathological (*see also* Deviation,
sexual) 302.9
Sézary's disease, reticulosis, or syndrome
(M9701/3) 202.2
Shadow, lung 793.1
Shaken infant syndrome 995.55
Shaking
head (tremor) 781.0
palsy or paralysis (*see also* Parkinsonism) 332.0
Shallowness, acetabulum 736.39
Shaver's disease or syndrome (bauxite
pneumoconiosis) 503
Shearing
artificial skin graft 996.55
decellularized allodermis graft 996.55
Sheath (tendon)—*see* condition
Shedding
nail 703.8
teeth, premature, primary (deciduous) 520.6

Shock—*continued*
    ectopic pregnancy (*see also* categories 633.0-633.9) 639.5
    molar pregnancy (*see also* categories 630-632) 639.5
   due to
    surgical procedure 998.0
    transfusion NEC 999.8
     bone marrow 996.85
   following
    abortion 639.5
    ectopic or molar pregnancy 639.5
    surgical procedure 998.0
    transfusion NEC 999.8
     bone marrow 996.85
  spinal—*see also* Injury, spinal, by site
   with spinal bone injury—*see* Fracture, vertebra, by site, with spinal cord injury
  surgical 998.0
  therapeutic misadventure NEC (*see also* Complications) 998.89
  thyroxin 962.7
  toxic 040.82
  transfusion—*see* Complications, transfusion
  traumatic (immediate) (delayed) 958.4
Shoemakers' chest 738.3
Short, shortening, shortness
  Achilles tendon (acquired) 727.81
  arm 736.89
   congenital 755.20
  back 737.9
  bowel syndrome 579.3
  breath 786.05
  common bile duct, congenital 751.69
  cord (umbilical) 663.4
   affecting fetus or newborn 762.6
  cystic duct, congenital 751.69
  esophagus (congenital) 750.4
  femur (acquired) 736.81
   congenital 755.34
  frenulum linguae 750.0
  frenum, lingual 750.0
  hamstrings 727.81
  hip (acquired) 736.39
   congenital 755.63
  leg (acquired) 736.81
   congenital 755.30
  metatarsus (congenital) 754.79
   acquired 736.79
  organ or site, congenital NEC—*see* Distortion
  palate (congenital) 750.26
  P-R interval syndrome 426.81
  radius (acquired) 736.09
   congenital 755.26
  round ligament 629.8
  sleeper 307.49
  stature, constitutional (hereditary) 783.43
  tendon 727.81
   Achilles (acquired) 727.81
    congenital 754.79
   congenital 756.89
  thigh (acquired) 736.81
   congenital 755.34
  tibialis anticus 727.81
  umbilical cord 663.4
   affecting fetus or newborn 762.6
  urethra 599.84
  uvula (congenital) 750.26
  vagina 623.8
Shortsightedness 367.1
Shoshin (acute fulminating beriberi) 265.0
Shoulder —*see* condition

Shovel-shaped incisors 520.2
Shower, thromboembolic —*see* Embolism
Shunt (status)
  aortocoronary bypass V45.81
  arterial-venous (dialysis) V45.1
  arteriovenous, pulmonary (acquired) 417.0
   congenital 747.3
   traumatic (complication) 901.40
  cerebral ventricle (communicating) in situ V45.2
  coronary artery bypass V45.81
  surgical, prosthetic, with complications—*see* Complications, shunt
  vascular NEC V45.89
Shutdown
  renal 586
   with
    abortion—*see* Abortion, by type, with renal failure
    ectopic pregnancy (*see also* categories 633.0-633.9) 639.3
    molar pregnancy (*see also* categories 630-632) 639.3
   complicating
    abortion 639.3
    ectopic or molar pregnancy 639.3
   following labor and delivery 669.3
Shwachman's syndrome 288.0
Shy-Drager syndrome (orthostatic hypotension with multisystem degeneration) 333.0
Sialadenitis (any gland) (chronic) (suppurative) 527.2
  epidemic—*see* Mumps
Sialadenosis, periodic 527.2
Sialaporia 527.7
Sialectasia 527.8
Sialitis 527.2
Sialoadenitis (*see also* Sialadenitis) 527.2
Sialoangitis 527.2
Sialodochitis (fibrinosa) 527.2
Sialodocholithiasis 527.5
Sialolithiasis 527.5
Sialorrhea (*see also* Ptyalism) 527.7
  periodic 527.2
Sialosis 527.8
  rheumatic 710.2
Siamese twin 759.4
Sicard's syndrome 352.6
Sicca syndrome (keratoconjunctivitis) 710.2
Sick 799.9
  cilia syndrome 759.89
  or handicapped person in family V61.49
Sickle-cell
  anemia (*see also* Disease, sickle-cell) 282.60
  disease (*see also* Disease, sickle-cell) 282.60
  hemoglobin
   C disease 282.63
   D disease 282.69
   E disease 282.69
  thalassemia 282.4
  trait 282.5
Sicklemia (*see also* Disease, sickle-cell) 282.60
  trait 282.5
Sickness
  air (travel) 994.6
  airplane 994.6
  alpine 993.2
  altitude 993.2
  Andes 993.2
  aviators' 993.2
  balloon 993.2
  car 994.6

Sirenomelia 759.89
Siriasis 992.0
Sirkari's disease 085.0
SIRS (systemic inflammatory response
        syndrome) 995.90
    due to
        infectious disease 995.91
            with organ dysfunction 995.92
        non-infectious process 995.93
            with organ dysfunction 995.94
Siti 104.0
Sitophobia 300.29
Situation, psychiatric 300.9
Situational
    disturbance (transient) (*see also* Reaction,
        adjustment) 309.9
        acute 308.3
    maladjustment, acute (*see also* Reaction,
        adjustment) 309.9
    reaction (*see also* Reaction, adjustment) 309.9
        acute 308.3
Situs inversus or transversus 759.3
    abdominalis 759.3
    thoracis 759.3
Sixth disease 057.8
Sjögren (-Gougerot) syndrome or disease
        (keratoconjunctivitis sicca) 710.2
    with lung involvement 710.2 *[517.8]*
Sjögren-Larsson syndrome (ichthyosis
        congenita) 757.1
Skeletal —*see* condition
Skene's gland —*see* condition
Skenitis (*see also* Urethritis) 597.89
    gonorrheal (acute) 098.0
        chronic or duration of 2 months or over 098.2
Skerljevo 104.0
Skevas-Zerfus disease 989.5
Skin —*see also* condition
    donor V59.1
    hidebound 710.9
SLAP lesion (superior glenoid labrum) 840.7
Slate-dressers' lung 502
Slate-miners' lung 502
Sleep
    disorder 780.50
        with apnea—*see* Apnea, sleep
        child 307.40
        nonorganic origin 307.40
            specified type NEC 307.49
    disturbance 780.50
        with apnea—*see* Apnea, sleep
        nonorganic origin 307.40
            specified type NEC 307.49
    drunkenness 307.47
    paroxysmal 347
    rhythm inversion 780.55
        nonorganic origin 307.45
    walking 307.46
        hysterical 300.13
Sleeping sickness 086.5
    late effect 139.8
Sleeplessness (*see also* Insomnia) 780.52
    menopausal 627.2
    nonorganic origin 307.41
Slipped, slipping
    epiphysis (postinfectional) 732.9
        traumatic (old) 732.9
            current—*see* Fracture, by site
        upper femoral (nontraumatic) 732.2
    intervertebral disc—*see* Displacement,
        intervertebral disc

Slipped, slipping—*continued*
    ligature, umbilical 772.3
    patella 717.89
    rib 733.99
    sacroiliac joint 724.6
    tendon 727.9
    ulnar nerve, nontraumatic 354.2
    vertebra NEC (*see also* Spondylolisthesis)
        756.12
Slocumb's syndrome 255.3
Sloughing (multiple) (skin) 686.9
    abscess—*see* Abscess, by site
    appendix 543.9
    bladder 596.8
    fascia 728.9
    graft—*see* Complications, graft
    phagedena (*see also* Gangrene) 785.4
    reattached extremity (*see also* Complications,
        reattached extremity) 996.90
    rectum 569.49
    scrotum 608.89
    tendon 727.9
    transplanted organ (*see also* Rejection,
        transplant, organ, by site) 996.80
    ulcer (*see also* Ulcer, skin) 707.9
Slow
    feeding newborn 779.3
    fetal, growth NEC 764.9
        affecting management of pregnancy 656.5
Slowing
    heart 427.89
    urinary stream 788.62
Sluder's neuralgia or syndrome 337.0
Slurred, slurring, speech 784.5
Small, smallness
    cardiac reserve—*see* Disease, heart
    for dates
        fetus or newborn 764.0
            with malnutrition 764.1
            affecting management of pregnancy 656.5
    infant, term 764.0
        with malnutrition 764.1
        affecting management of pregnancy 656.5
    introitus, vagina 623.3
    kidney, unknown cause 589.9
        bilateral 589.1
        unilateral 589.0
    ovary 620.8
    pelvis
        with disproportion (fetopelvic) 653.1
            affecting fetus or newborn 763.1
        causing obstructed labor 660.1
            affecting fetus or newborn 763.1
    placenta—*see* Placenta, insufficiency
    uterus 621.8
    white kidney 582.9
Small-for-dates (*see also* Light-for-dates) 764.0
    affecting management of pregnancy 656.5
Smallpox 050.9
    contact V01.3
    exposure to V01.3
    hemorrhagic (pustular) 050.0
    malignant 050.0
    modified 050.2
    vaccination
        complications—*see* Complications,
            vaccination
        prophylactic (against) V04.1
Smith's fracture (separation) (closed) 813.41
    open 813.51
Smith-Lemli-Opitz syndrome
        (cerebrohepatorenal syndrome) 759.89

Spasm, spastic, spasticity—*continued*
  retinal (*see also* Occlusion, retinal, artery)
    362.30
    vertebral 435.1
    vertebrobasilar 435.3
  Bell's 351.0
  bladder (sphincter, external or internal) 596.8
  bowel 564.9
    psychogenic 306.4
  bronchus, bronchiole 519.1
  cardia 530.0
  cardiac—*see* Angina
  carpopedal (*see also* Tetany) 781.7
  cecum 564.9
    psychogenic 306.4
  cerebral (arteries) (vascular) 435.9
    specified artery NEC 435.8
  cerebrovascular 435.9
  cervix, complicating delivery 661.4
    affecting fetus or newborn 763.7
  ciliary body (of accommodation) 367.53
  colon 564.1
    psychogenic 306.4
  common duct (*see also* Disease, biliary) 576.8
  compulsive 307.22
  conjugate 378.82
  convergence 378.84
  coronary (artery)—*see* Angina
  diaphragm (reflex) 786.8
    psychogenic 306.1
  duodenum, duodenal (bulb) 564.89
  esophagus (diffuse) 530.5
    psychogenic 306.4
  facial 351.8
  fallopian tube 620.8
  gait 781.2
  gastrointestinal (tract) 536.8
    psychogenic 306.4
  glottis 478.75
    hysterical 300.11
    psychogenic 306.1
      specified as conversion reaction 300.11
    reflex through recurrent laryngeal nerve
      478.75
  habit 307.20
    chronic 307.22
    transient of childhood 307.21
  heart—*see* Angina
  hourglass—*see* Contraction, hourglass
  hysterical 300.11
  infantile (*see also* Epilepsy) 345.6
  internal oblique, eye 378.51
  intestinal 564.9
    psychogenic 306.4
  larynx, laryngeal 478.75
    hysterical 300.11
    psychogenic 306.1
      specified as conversion reaction 300.11
  levator palpebrae superioris 333.81
  lightning (*see also* Epilepsy) 345.6
  mobile 781.0
  muscle 728.85
    back 724.8
    psychogenic 306.0
  nerve, trigeminal 350.1
  nervous 306.0
  nodding 307.3
    infantile (*see also* Epilepsy) 345.6
  occupational 300.89
  oculogyric 378.87
  ophthalmic artery 362.30

Spasm, spastic, spasticity—*continued*
  orbicularis 781.0
  perineal 625.8
  peroneo-extensor (*see also* Flat, foot) 734
  pharynx (reflex) 478.29
    hysterical 300.11
    psychogenic 306.1
      specified as conversion reaction 300.11
  pregnant uterus, complicating delivery 661.4
  psychogenic 306.0
  pylorus 537.81
    adult hypertrophic 537.0
    congenital or infantile 750.5
    psychogenic 306.4
  rectum (sphincter) 564.6
    psychogenic 306.4
  retinal artery NEC (*see also* Occlusion, retina,
    artery) 362.30
  sacroiliac 724.6
  salaam (infantile) (*see also* Epilepsy) 345.6
  saltatory 781.0
  sigmoid 564.9
    psychogenic 306.4
  sphincter of Oddi (*see also* Disease,
    gallbladder) 576.5
  stomach 536.8
    neurotic 306.4
  throat 478.29
    hysterical 300.11
    psychogenic 306.1
      specified as conversion reaction 300.11
  tic 307.20
    chronic 307.22
    transient of childhood 307.21
  tongue 529.8
  torsion 333.6
  trigeminal nerve 350.1
    postherpetic 053.12
  ureter 593.89
  urethra (sphincter) 599.84
  uterus 625.8
    complicating labor 661.4
      affecting fetus or newborn 763.7
  vagina 625.1
    psychogenic 306.51
  vascular NEC 443.9
  vasomotor NEC 443.9
  vein NEC 459.89
  vesical (sphincter, external or internal) 596.8
  viscera 789.0
Spasmodic —*see* condition
Spasmophilia (*see also* Tetany) 781.7
Spasmus nutans 307.3
Spastic —*see also* Spasm
  child 343.9
Spasticity —*see also* Spasm
  cerebral, child 343.9
Speakers' throat 784.49
Specific, specified —*see* condition
Speech
  defect, disorder, disturbance, impediment NEC
    784.5
    psychogenic 307.9
  therapy V57.3
Spells 780.39
  breath-holding 786.9
Spencer's disease (epidemic vomiting) 078.82
Spens' syndrome (syncope with heart block)
  426.9
Spermatic cord —*see* condition
Spermatocele 608.1
  congenital 752.8

Spermatocystitis 608.4
Spermatocytoma (M9063/3)
  specified site—*see* Neoplasm, by site, malignant
  unspecified site 186.9
Spermatorrhea 608.89
Sperm counts
  fertility testing V26.21
  following sterilization reversal V26.22
  postvasectomy V25.8
Sphacelus (*see also* Gangrene) 785.4
Sphenoidal —*see* condition
Sphenoiditis (chronic) (*see also* Sinusitis,
    sphenoidal) 473.3
Sphenopalatine ganglion neuralgia 337.0
Sphericity, increased, lens 743.36
Spherocytosis (congenital) (familial) (hereditary)
    282.0
  hemoglobin disease 287.7
  sickle-cell (disease) 282.60
Spherophakia 743.36
Sphincter —*see* condition
Sphincteritis, sphincter of Oddi (*see also*
    Cholecystitis) 576.8
Sphingolipidosis 272.7
Sphingolipodystrophy 272.7
Sphingomyelinosis 272.7
Spicule tooth 520.2
Spider
  finger 755.59
  nevus 448.1
  vascular 448.1
Spiegler-Fendt sarcoid 686.8
Spielmeyer-Stock disease 330.1
Spielmeyer-Vogt disease 330.1
Spina bifida (aperta) 741.9

---

*Note—Use the following fifth-digit
subclassification with category 741:*

0 unspecified region
1 cervical region
2 dorsal [thoracic] region
3 lumbar region

---

  with hydrocephalus 741.0
  fetal (suspected), affecting management of
    pregnancy 655.0
  occulta 756.17
Spindle, Krukenberg's 371.13
Spine, spinal —*see* condition
Spiradenoma (eccrine) (M8403/0)—*see*
    Neoplasm, skin, benign
Spirillosis NEC (*see also* Fever, relapsing) 087.9
Spirillum minus 026.0
Spirillum obermeieri infection 087.0
Spirochetal —*see* condition
Spirochetosis 104.9
  arthritic, arthritica 104.9 *[711.8]*
  bronchopulmonary 104.8
  icterohemorrhagica 100.0
  lung 104.8
Spitting blood (*see also* Hemoptysis) 786.3
Splanchnomegaly 569.89
Splanchnoptosis 569.89
Spleen, splenic —*see also* condition
  agenesis 759.0
  flexure syndrome 569.89
  neutropenia syndrome 288.0
  sequestration syndrome 282.60
Splenectasis (*see also* Splenomegaly) 789.2

Splenitis (interstitial) (malignant) (nonspecific)
    289.59
  malarial (*see also* Malaria) 084.6
  tuberculous (*see also* Tuberculosis) 017.7
Splenocele 289.59
Splenomegalia —*see* Splenomegaly
Splenomegalic —*see* condition
Splenomegaly 789.2
  Bengal 789.2
  cirrhotic 289.51
  congenital 759.0
  congestive, chronic 289.51
  cryptogenic 789.2
  Egyptian 120.1
  Gaucher's (cerebroside lipidosis) 272.7
  idiopathic 789.2
  malarial (*see also* Malaria) 084.6
  neutropenic 288.0
  Niemann-Pick (lipid histiocytosis) 272.7
  siderotic 289.51
  syphilitic 095.8
    congenital 090.0
  tropical (Bengal) (idiopathic) 789.2
Splenopathy 289.50
Splenopneumonia —*see* Pneumonia
Splenoptosis 289.59
Splinter —*see* Injury, superficial, by site
Split, splitting
  heart sounds 427.89
  lip, congenital (*see also* Cleft, lip) 749.10
  nails 703.8
  urinary stream 788.61
Spoiled child reaction (*see also* Disturbance,
    conduct) 312.1
Spondylarthritis (*see also* Spondylosis) 721.90
Spondylarthrosis (*see also* Spondylosis) 721.90
Spondylitis 720.9
  ankylopoietica 720.0
  ankylosing (chronic) 720.0
  atrophic 720.9
    ligamentous 720.9
  chronic (traumatic) (*see also* Spondylosis)
    721.90
  deformans (chronic) (*see also* Spondylosis)
    721.90
  gonococcal 098.53
  gouty 274.0
  hypertrophic (*see also* Spondylosis) 721.90
  infectious NEC 720.9
  juvenile (adolescent) 720.0
  Kümmell's 721.7
  Marie-Strümpell (ankylosing) 720.0
  muscularis 720.9
  ossificans ligamentosa 721.6
  osteoarthritica (*see also* Spondylosis) 721.90
  posttraumatic 721.7
  proliferative 720.0
  rheumatoid 720.0
  rhizomelica 720.0
  sacroiliac NEC 720.2
  senescent (*see also* Spondylosis) 721.90
  senile (*see also* Spondylosis) 721.90
  static (*see also* Spondylosis) 721.90
  traumatic (chronic) (*see also* Spondylosis)
    721.90
  tuberculous (*see also* Tuberculosis) 015.0
    [720.81]
  typhosa 002.0 *[720.81]*
Spondyloarthrosis (*see also* Spondylosis) 721.90

Staphylococcemia 038.10
  aureus 038.11
  specified organism NEC 038.19
Staphylococcus, staphylococcal —*see* condition
Staphyloderma (skin) 686.00
Staphyloma 379.11
  anterior, localized 379.14
  ciliary 379.11
  cornea 371.73
  equatorial 379.13
  posterior 379.12
  posticum 379.12
  ring 379.15
  sclera NEC 379.11
Starch eating 307.52
Stargardt's disease 362.75
Starvation (inanition) (due to lack of food) 994.2
  edema 262
  voluntary NEC 307.1
Stasis
  bile (duct) (*see also* Disease, biliary) 576.8
  bronchus (*see also* Bronchitis) 490
  cardiac (*see also* Failure, heart) 428.0
  cecum 564.89
  colon 564.89
  dermatitis (*see also* Varix, with stasis
    dermatitis) 454.1
  duodenal 536.8
  eczema (*see also* Varix, with stasis dermatitis)
    454.1
  edema (*see also* Hypertension, venous) 459.30
  foot 991.4
  gastric 536.3
  ileocecal coil 564.89
  ileum 564.89
  intestinal 564.89
  jejunum 564.89
  kidney 586
  liver 571.9
    cirrhotic—*see* Cirrhosis, liver
  lymphatic 457.8
  pneumonia 514
  portal 571.9
  pulmonary 514
  rectal 564.89
  renal 586
    tubular 584.5
  stomach 536.3
  ulcer
    with varicose veins 454.0
    without varicose veins 459.81
  urine NEC (*see also* Retention, urine) 788.20
  venous 459.81
State
  affective and paranoid, mixed, organic
    psychotic 294.8
  agitated 307.9
    acute reaction to stress 308.2
  anxiety (neurotic) (*see also* Anxiety) 300.00
    specified type NEC 300.09
  apprehension (*see also* Anxiety) 300.00
    specified type NEC 300.09
  climacteric, female 627.2
    following induced menopause 627.4
  clouded
    epileptic (*see also* Epilepsy) 345.9
    paroxysmal (idiopathic) (*see also* Epilepsy)
      345.9
  compulsive (mixed) (with obsession) 300.3
  confusional 298.9

State—*continued*
  acute 293.0
    with
      arteriosclerotic dementia 290.41
      presenile brain disease 290.11
      senility 290.3
    alcoholic 291.0
    drug-induced 292.81
    epileptic 293.0
    postoperative 293.9
    reactive (emotional stress) (psychological
      trauma) 298.2
    subacute 293.1
  constitutional psychopathic 301.9
  convulsive (*see also* Convulsions) 780.39
  depressive NEC 311
    induced by drug 292.84
    neurotic 300.4
  dissociative 300.15
  hallucinatory 780.1
    induced by drug 292.12
  hyperdynamic beta-adrenergic circulatory
    429.82
  locked-in 344.81
  menopausal 627.2
    artificial 627.4
    following induced menopause 627.4
  neurotic NEC 300.9
    with depersonalization episode 300.6
  obsessional 300.3
  oneiroid (*see also* Schizophrenia) 295.4
  panic 300.01
  paranoid 297.9
    alcohol-induced 291.5
    arteriosclerotic 290.42
    climacteric 297.2
    drug-induced 292.11
    in
      presenile brain disease 290.12
      senile brain disease 290.20
    involutional 297.2
    menopausal 297.2
    senile 290.20
    simple 297.0
  postleukotomy 310.0
  pregnant (*see also* Pregnancy) V22.2
  psychogenic, twilight 298.2
  psychotic, organic (*see also* Psychosis, organic)
    294.9
    mixed paranoid and affective 294.8
    senile or presenile NEC 290.9
    transient NEC 293.9
      with
        anxiety 293.84
        delusions 293.81
        depression 293.83
        hallucinations 293.82
  residual schizophrenic (*see also* Schizophrenia)
    295.6
  tension (*see also* Anxiety) 300.9
  transient organic psychotic 293.9
    anxiety type 293.84
    depressive type 293.83
    hallucinatory type 293.83
    paranoid type 293.81
    specified type NEC 293.89
  twilight
    epileptic 293.0
    psychogenic 298.2
  vegetative (persistent) 780.03

Status (post)
  absence
    epileptic (*see also* Epilepsy) 345.2
    of organ, acquired (postsurgical)—*see*
      Absence, by site, acquired
  anastomosis of intestine (for bypass) V45.3
  angioplasty, percutaneous transluminal coronary
    V45.82
  anginosus 413.9
  ankle prosthesis V43.66
  aortocoronary bypass or shunt V45.81
  arthrodesis V45.4
  artificially induced condition NEC V45.89
  artificial opening (of) V44.9
    gastrointestinal tract NEC V44.4
    specified site NEC V44.8
    urinary tract NEC V44.6
    vagina V44.7
  aspirator V46.0
  asthmaticus (*see also* Asthma) 493.9
  breast implant removal V45.83
  cardiac
    device (in situ) V45.00
      defibrillator, automatic implantable V45.02
      pacemaker V45.01
        fitting or adjustment V53.3
      carotid sinus V45.09
        fitting or adjustment V53.3
  carotid sinus stimulator V45.09
  cataract extraction V45.61
  chemotherapy V66.2
    current V58.69
  colostomy V44.3
  contraceptive device V45.59
    intrauterine V45.51
    subdermal V45.52
  convulsivus idiopathicus (*see also* Epilepsy)
    345.3
  coronary artery bypass or shunt V45.81
  cystostomy V44.50
    appendico-vesicostomy V44.52
    cutaneous-vesicostomy V44.51
    specified type NEC V44.59
  defibrillator, automatic implantable cardiac
    V45.02
  dental crowns V45.84
  dental fillings V45.84
  dental restoration V45.84
  dental sealant V49.82
  dialysis V45.1
  donor V59.9
  drug therapy or regimen V67.59
    high-risk medication NEC V67.51
  elbow prosthesis V43.62
  enterostomy V44.4
  epileptic, epilepticus (absence) (grand mal) (*see*
    also Epilepsy) 345.3
    focal motor 345.7
    partial 345.7
    petit mal 345.2
    psychomotor 345.7
    temporal lobe 345.7
  eye (adnexa) surgery V45.69
  filtering bleb (eye) (postglaucoma) V45.69
    with rupture or complication 997.99
    postcataract extraction (complication) 997.99
  finger joint prosthesis V43.69
  gastrostomy V44.1
  grand mal 345.3
  heart valve prosthesis V43.3
  hip prosthesis (joint) (partial) (total) V43.64

Status (post)—*continued*
  ileostomy V44.2
  intestinal bypass V45.3
  intrauterine contraceptive device V45.51
  jejunostomy V44.4
  knee joint prosthesis V43.65
  lacunaris 437.8
  lacunosis 437.8
  low birth weight V21.30
    less than 500 grams V21.31
    500-999 grams V21.32
    1000-1499 grams V21.33
    1500-1999 grams V21.34
    2000-2500 grams V21.35
  lymphaticus 254.8
  malignant neoplasm, ablated or excised—*see*
    History, malignant neoplasm
  marmoratus 333.7
  nephrostomy V44.6
  neuropacemaker NEC V45.89
    brain V45.89
    carotid sinus V45.09
    neurologic NEC V45.89
  organ replacement
    by artificial or mechanical device or
      prosthesis of
      artery V43.4
      artificial skin V43.83
      bladder V43.5
      blood vessel V43.4
      breast V43.82
      eye globe V43.0
      heart V43.2
        valve V43.3
      intestine V43.89
      joint V43.60
        ankle V43.66
        elbow V43.62
        finger V43.69
        hip (partial) (total) V43.64
        knee V43.65
        shoulder V43.61
        specified NEC 43.69
        wrist V43.63
      kidney V43.89
      larynx V43.81
      lens V43.1
      limb(s) V43.7
      liver V43.89
      lung V43.89
      organ NEC V43.89
      pancreas V43.89
      skin (artificial) V43.83
      tissue NEC V43.89
      vein V43.4
    by organ transplant (heterologous)
      (homologous)—*see* Status, transplant
  pacemaker
    brain V45.89
    cardiac V45.01
    carotid sinus V45.09
    neurologic NEC V45.89
    specified site NEC V45.89
  percutaneous transluminal coronary angioplasty
    V45.82
  petit mal 345.2
  postcommotio cerebri 310.2
  postmenopausal (age related) (natural) V49.81
  postoperative NEC V45.89
  postpartum NEC V24.2
    care immediately following delivery V24.0

Stricture—*continued*
  digestive organs NEC, congenital 751.8
  duodenum 537.3
    congenital 751.1
  ear canal (external) (congenital) 744.02
    acquired 380.50
      secondary to
        inflammation 380.53
        surgery 380.52
        trauma 380.51
  ejaculatory duct 608.85
  enterostomy 569.62
  esophagus (corrosive) (peptic) 530.3
    congenital 750.3
    syphilitic 095.8
      congenital 090.5
  Eustachian tube (*see also* Obstruction,
      Eustachian tube) 381.60
    congenital 744.24
  fallopian tube 628.2
    gonococcal (chronic) 098.37
      acute 098.17
    tuberculous (*see also* Tuberculosis) 016.6
  gallbladder (*see also* Obstruction, gallbladder)
      575.2
    congenital 751.69
  glottis 478.74
  heart—*see also* Disease, heart
    congenital NEC 746.89
    valve—*see also* Endocarditis
      congenital NEC 746.89
        aortic 746.3
        mitral 746.5
        pulmonary 746.02
        tricuspid 746.1
  hepatic duct (*see also* Obstruction, biliary) 576.2
  hourglass, of stomach 537.6
  hymen 623.3
  hypopharynx 478.29
  intestine (*see also* Obstruction, intestine) 560.9
    congenital (small) 751.1
      large 751.2
    ischemic 557.1
  lacrimal
    canaliculi 375.53
      congenital 743.65
    punctum 375.52
      congenital 743.65
    sac 375.54
      congenital 743.65
  lacrimonasal duct 375.56
    congenital 743.65
    neonatal 375.55
  larynx 478.79
    congenital 748.3
    syphilitic 095.8
      congenital 090.5
  lung 518.89
  meatus
    ear (congenital) 744.02
      acquired (*see also* Stricture, ear canal,
          acquired) 380.50
      osseous (congenital) (ear) 744.03
        acquired (*see also* Stricture, ear canal,
            acquired) 380.50
    urinarius (*see also* Stricture, urethra) 598.9
      congenital 753.6
  mitral (valve) (*see also* Stenosis, mitral) 394.0
    congenital 746.5
    specified cause, except rheumatic 424.0

Stricture—*continued*
  myocardium, myocardial (*see also*
      Degeneration, myocardial) 429.1
    hypertrophic subaortic (idiopathic) 425.1
  nares (anterior) (posterior) 478.1
    congenital 748.0
  nasal duct 375.56
    congenital 743.65
    neonatal 375.55
  nasolacrimal duct 375.56
    congenital 743.65
    neonatal 375.55
  nasopharynx 478.29
    syphilitic 095.8
  nephrostomy 997.5
  nose 478.1
    congenital 748.0
  nostril (anterior) (posterior) 478.1
    congenital 748.0
  organ or site, congenital NEC—*see* Atresia
  osseous meatus (congenital) (ear) 744.03
    acquired (*see also* Stricture, ear canal,
        acquired) 380.50
  os uteri (*see also* Stricture, cervix) 622.4
  oviduct—*see* Stricture, fallopian tube
  pelviureteric junction 593.3
  pharynx (dilation) 478.29
  prostate 602.8
  pulmonary, pulmonic
    artery (congenital) 747.3
      acquired 417.8
      noncongenital 417.8
    infundibulum (congenital) 746.83
    valve (*see also* Endocarditis, pulmonary) 424.3
      congenital 746.02
    vein (congenital) 747.49
      acquired 417.8
    vessel NEC 417.8
  punctum lacrimale 375.52
    congenital 743.65
  pylorus (hypertrophic) 537.0
    adult 537.0
    congenital 750.5
    infantile 750.5
  rectosigmoid 569.89
  rectum (sphincter) 569.2
    congenital 751.2
    due to
      chemical burn 947.3
      irradiation 569.2
      lymphogranuloma venereum 099.1
    gonococcal 098.7
    inflammatory 099.1
    syphilitic 095.8
    tuberculous (*see also* Tuberculosis) 014.8
  renal artery 440.1
  salivary duct or gland (any) 527.8
  sigmoid (flexure) (*see also* Obstruction,
      intestine) 560.9
  spermatic cord 608.85
  stoma (following) (of)
    colostomy 569.62
    cystostomy 997.5
    enterostomy 569.62
    gastrostomy 536.42
    ileostomy 569.62
    nephrostomy 997.5
    tracheostomy 519.02
    ureterostomy 997.5
  stomach 537.89
    congenital 750.7

Suppuration, suppurative—*continued*
  salivary duct or gland (any) 527.2
  sinus (nasal) (*see also* Sinusitis) 473.9
  sphenoidal (sinus) (chronic) (*see also* Sinusitis,
      sphenoidal) 473.3
  thymus (gland) 254.1
  thyroid (gland) 245.0
  tonsil 474.8
  uterus (*see also* Endometritis) 615.9
  vagina 616.10
  wound—*see also* Wound, open, by site,
      complicated
    dislocation—*see* Dislocation, by site,
        compound
    fracture—*see* Fracture, by site, open
    scratch or other superficial injury—*see* Injury,
        superficial, by site
Supraglottitis 464.50
  with obstruction 464.51
Suprapubic drainage 596.8
Suprarenal (gland)—*see* condition
Suprascapular nerve —*see* condition
Suprasellar —*see* condition
Supraspinatus syndrome 726.10
Surfer knots 919.8
  infected 919.9
Surgery
  cosmetic NEC V50.1
    following healed injury or operation V51
    hair transplant V50.0
  elective V50.9
    breast augmentation reduction V50.1
    circumcision, ritual or routine (in absence of
        medical indication) V50.2
    cosmetic NEC V50.1
    ear piercing V50.3
    face-lift V50.1
    following healed injury or operation V51
    hair transplant V50.0
  not done because of
    contraindication V64.1
    patient's decision V64.2
    specified reason NEC V64.3
  plastic
    breast augmentation or reduction V50.1
    cosmetic V50.1
    face-lift V50.1
    following healed injury or operation V51
    repair of scarred tissue (following healed
        injury or operation) V51
    specified type NEC V50.8
  previous, in pregnancy or childbirth
    cervix 654.6
      affecting fetus or newborn 763.89
      causing obstructed labor 660.2
        affecting fetus or newborn 763.1
    pelvic soft tissues NEC 654.9
      affecting fetus or newborn 763.89
      causing obstructed labor 660.2
        affecting fetus or newborn 763.1
    perineum or vulva 654.8
    uterus NEC 654.9
      affecting fetus or newborn 763.89
      causing obstructed labor 660.2
        affecting fetus or newborn 763.1
      due to previous cesarean delivery 654.2
    vagina 654.7

Surgical
  abortion—*see* Abortion, legal
  emphysema 998.81
  kidney (*see also* Pyelitis) 590.80
  operation NEC 799.9
  procedures, complication or misadventure—*see*
      Complications, surgical procedure
  shock 998.0
Suspected condition, ruled out (*see also*
      Observation, suspected) V71.9
  specified condition NEC V71.89
Suspended uterus, in pregnancy or childbirth
      654.4
  affecting fetus or newborn 763.89
  causing obstructed labor 660.2
    affecting fetus or newborn 763.1
Sutton's disease 709.09
Sutton and Gull's disease (arteriolar
      nephrosclerosis) (*see also* Hypertension,
      kidney) 403.90
Suture
  burst (in external operation wound) 998.32
    internal 998.31
  inadvertently left in operation wound 998.4
  removal V58.3
  Shirodkar, in pregnancy (with or without
      cervical incompetence) 654.5
Swab inadvertently left in operation wound
      998.4
Swallowed, swallowing
  difficulty (*see also* Dysphagia) 787.2
  foreign body NEC (*see also* Foreign body) 938
Swamp fever 100.89
Swan neck hand (intrinsic) 736.09
Sweat (s), sweating
  disease or sickness 078.2
  excessive 780.8
  fetid 705.89
  fever 078.2
  gland disease 705.9
    specified type NEC 705.89
  miliary 078.2
  night 780.8
Sweeley-Klionsky disease (angiokeratoma
      corporis diffusum) 272.7
Sweet's syndrome (acute febrile neutrophilic
      dermatosis) 695.89
Swelling
  abdominal (not referable to specific organ) 789.3
  adrenal gland, cloudy 255.8
  ankle 719.07
  anus 787.99
  arm 729.81
  breast 611.72
  Calabar 125.2
  cervical gland 785.6
  cheek 784.2
  chest 786.6
  ear 388.8
  epigastric 789.3
  extremity (lower) (upper) 729.81
  eye 379.92
  female genital organ 625.8
  finger 729.81
  foot 729.81
  glands 785.6
  gum 784.2
  hand 729.81
  head 784.2
  inflammatory—*see* Inflammation

Syncope (near) (pre-) 780.2
  anginosa 413.9
  bradycardia 427.89
  cardiac 780.2
  carotid sinus 337.0
  complicating delivery 669.2
  due to lumbar puncture 349.0
  fatal 798.1
  heart 780.2
  heat 992.1
  laryngeal 786.2
  tussive 786.2
  vasoconstriction 780.2
  vasodepressor 780.2
  vasomotor 780.2
  vasovagal 780.2
Syncytial infarct —*see* Placenta, abnormal
Syndactylism, syndactyly (multiple sites) 755.10
  fingers (without fusion of bone) 755.11
    with fusion of bone 755.12
  toes (without fusion of bone) 755.13
    with fusion of bone 755.14
Syndrome —*see also* Disease
  abdominal
    acute 789.0
    migraine 346.2
    muscle deficiency 756.79
  Abercrombie's (amyloid degeneration) 277.3
  abnormal innervation 374.43
  abstinence
    alcohol 291.81
    drug 292.0
  Abt-Letterer-Siwe (acute histiocytosis X)
      (M9722/3) 202.5
  Achard-Thiers (adrenogenital) 255.2
  acid pulmonary aspiration 997.3
    obstetric (Mendelson's) 668.0
  acquired immune deficiency 042
  acquired immunodeficiency 042
  acrocephalosyndactylism 755.55
  acute abdominal 789.0
  acute chest 282.62
  acute coronary 411.1
  Adair-Dighton (brittle bones and blue sclera,
      deafness) 756.51
  Adams-Stokes (-Morgagni) (syncope with heart
      block) 426.9
  addisonian 255.4
  Adie (-Holmes) (pupil) 379.46
  adiposogenital 253.8
  adrenal
    hemorrhage 036.3
    meningococcic 036.3
  adrenocortical 255.3
  adrenogenital (acquired) (congenital) 255.2
    feminizing 255.2
    iatrogenic 760.79
    virilism (acquired) (congenital) 255.2
  affective organic NEC 293.89
    drug-induced 292.84
  afferent loop NEC 537.89
  African macroglobulinemia 273.3
  Ahumada-Del Castillo (nonpuerperal
      galactorrhea and amenorrhea) 253.1
  air blast concussion—*see* Injury, internal, by site
  Albright (-Martin) (pseudohypoparathyroidism)
      275.49
  Albright-McCune-Sternberg (osteitis fibrosa
      disseminata) 756.59
  alcohol withdrawal 291.81
  Alder's (leukocyte granulation anomaly) 288.2

Syndrome—*continued*
  Aldrich (-Wiskott) (eczema-thrombocytopenia)
      279.12
  Alibert-Bazin (mycosis, fungoides) (M9700/3)
      202.1
  Alice in Wonderland 293.89
  Allen-Masters 620.6
  Alligator baby (ichthyosis congenita) 757.1
  Alport's (hereditary hematuria-nephropathy-
      deafness) 759.89
  Alvarez (transient cerebral ischemia) 435.9
  alveolar capillary block 516.3
  Alzheimer's 331.0
    with dementia—*see* Alzheimer's, dementia
  amnestic (confabulatory) 294.0
    alcoholic 291.1
    drug-induced 292.83
    posttraumatic 294.0
  amotivational 292.89
  amyostatic 275.1
  amyotrophic lateral sclerosis 335.20
  angina (*see also* Angina) 413.9
  ankyloglossia superior 750.0
  anterior
    chest wall 786.52
    compartment (tibial) 958.8
    spinal artery 433.8
      compression 721.1
    tibial (compartment) 958.8
  antibody deficiency 279.00
    agammaglobulinemic 279.00
    congenital 279.04
    hypogammaglobulinemic 279.00
  anticardiolipin antibody 795.79
  antimongolism 758.3
  antiphospholipid antibody 795.79
  Anton (-Babinski) (hemiasomatognosia) 307.9
  anxiety (*see also* Anxiety) 300.00
    organic 293.84
  aortic
    arch 446.7
    bifurcation (occlusion) 444.0
    ring 747.21
  Apert's (acrocephalosyndactyly) 755.55
  Apert-Gallais (adrenogenital) 255.2
  aphasia-apraxia-alexia 784.69
  "approximate answers" 300.16
  arcuate ligament (-celiac axis) 447.4
  arcus aortae 446.7
  arc-welders' 370.24
  argentaffin, argintaffinoma 259.2
  Argonz-Del Castillo (nonpuerperal galactorrhea
      and amenorrhea) 253.1
  Argyll Robertson's (syphilitic) 094.89
    nonsyphilitic 379.45
  arm-shoulder (*see also* Neuropathy, peripheral,
      autonomic) 337.9
  Arnold-Chiari (*see also* Spina bifida) 741.0
    type I 348.4
    type II 741.0
    type III 742.0
    type IV 742.2
  Arrillaga-Ayerza (pulmonary artery sclerosis
      with pulmonary hypertension) 416.0
  arteriomesenteric duodenum occlusion 537.89
  arteriovenous steal 996.73
  arteritis, young female (obliterative
      brachiocephalic) 446.7
  aseptic meningitis—*see* Meningitis, aseptic
  Asherman's 621.5
  asphyctic (*see also* Anxiety) 300.00

Syndrome—*continued*
  mesenteric
    artery, superior 557.1
    vascular insufficiency (with gangrene) 557.1
  metastatic carcinoid 259.2
  Meyenburg-Altherr-Uehlinger 733.99
  Meyer-Schwickerath and Weyers (dysplasia
    oculodentodigitalis) 759.89
  Micheli-Rietti (thalassemia minor) 282.4
  Michotte's 721.5
  micrognathia-glossoptosis 756.0
  microphthalmos (congenital) 759.89
  midbrain 348.8
  middle
    lobe (lung) (right) 518.0
    radicular 353.0
  Miescher's
    familial acanthosis nigricans 701.2
    granulomatosis disciformis 709.3
  Mieten's 759.89
  migraine 346.0
  Mikity-Wilson (pulmonary dysmaturity) 770.7
  Mikulicz's (dryness of mouth, absent or
    decreased lacrimation) 527.1
  milk alkali (milk drinkers') 999.9
  Milkman (-Looser) (osteomalacia with
    pseudofractures) 268.2
  Millard-Gubler 344.89
  Miller Fisher's 357.0
  Milles' (encephalocutaneous angiomatosis)
    759.6
  Minkowski-Chauffard (*see also* Spherocytosis)
    282.0
  Mirizzi's (hepatic duct stenosis) 576.2
    with calculus, cholelithiasis, or stones—*see*
      Choledocholithiasis
  mitral
    click (-murmur) 785.2
    valve prolapse 424.0
  Möbius'
    congenital oculofacial paralysis 352.6
    ophthalmoplegic migraine 346.8
  Mohr's (Types I and II) 759.89
  monofixation 378.34
  Moore's (*see also* Epilepsy) 345.5
  Morel-Moore (hyperostosis frontalis interna)
    733.3
  Morel-Morgagni (hyperostosis frontalis interna)
    733.3
  Morgagni (-Stewart-Morel) (hyperostosis
    frontalis interna) 733.3
  Morgagni-Adams-Stokes (syncope with heart
    block) 426.9
  Morquio (-Brailsford) (-Ullrich)
    (mucopolysaccharidosis IV) 277.5
  Morris (testicular feminization) 257.8
  Morton's (foot) (metatarsalgia) (metatarsal
    neuralgia) (neuralgia) (neuroma) (toe) 355.6
  Moschcowitz (-Singer-Symmers) (thrombotic
    thrombocytopenic purpura) 446.6
  Mounier-Kuhn 494.0
    with acute exacerbation 494.1
  Mucha-Haberman (acute parapsoriasis
    varioliformis) 696.2
  mucocutaneous lymph node (acute) (febrile)
    (infantile) (MCLS) 446.1
  multiple
    deficiency 260
    operations 301.51
  Munchausen's 301.51
  Münchmeyer's (exostosis luxurians) 728.11

Syndrome—*continued*
  Murchison-Sanderson—*see* Disease, Hodgkin's
  myasthenic—*see* Myasthenia, syndrome
  myelodysplastic 238.7
  myeloproliferative (chronic) (M9960/1) 238.7
  myofascial pain NEC 729.1
  Naffziger's 353.0
  Nager-de Reynier (dysostosis mandibularis)
    756.0
  nail-patella (hereditary osteo-onychodysplasia)
    756.89
  Nebécourt's 253.3
  Neill-Dingwall (microencephaly and dwarfism)
    759.89
  nephrotic (*see also* Nephrosis) 581.9
    diabetic 250.4 *[581.81]*
  Netherton's (ichthyosiform erythroderma) 757.1
  neurocutaneous 759.6
  neuroleptic malignant 333.92
  Nezelof's (pure alymphocytosis) 279.13
  Niemann-Pick (lipid histiocytosis) 272.7
  Nonne-Milroy-Meige (chronic hereditary
    edema) 757.0
  nonsense 300.16
  Noonan's 759.89
  Nothnagel's
    ophthalmoplegia-cerebellar ataxia 378.52
    vasomotor acroparesthesia 443.89
  nucleus ambiguous-hypoglossal 352.6
  OAV (oculoauriculovertebral dysplasia) 756.0
  obsessional 300.3
  oculocutaneous 364.24
  oculomotor 378.81
  oculourethroarticular 099.3
  Ogilvie's (sympathicotonic colon obstruction)
    560.89
  ophthalmoplegia-cerebellar ataxia 378.52
  Oppenheim-Urbach (necrobiosis lipoidica
    diabeticorum) 250.8 *[709.3]*
  oral-facial-digital 759.89
  organic
    affective NEC 293.83
      drug-induced 292.84
    anxiety 293.84
    delusional 293.81
      alcohol-induced 291.5
      drug-induced 292.11
      due to or associated with
        arteriosclerosis 290.42
        presenile brain disease 290.12
        senility 290.20
    depressive 293.83
      drug-induced 292.84
      due to or associated with
        arteriosclerosis 290.43
        presenile brain disease 290.13
        senile brain disease 290.21
    hallucinosis 293.82
      drug-induced 292.84
  organic affective 293.83
    induced by drug 292.84
  organic personality 310.1
    induced by drug 292.89
  Ormond's 593.4
  orodigitofacial 759.89
  orthostatic hypotensive-dysautonomic-
    dyskinetic 333.0
  Osler-Weber-Rendu (familial hemorrhagic
    telangiectasia) 448.0
  osteodermopathic hyperostosis 757.39
  osteoporosis-osteomalacia 268.2

Syndrome—*continued*
 blind loop 579.2
 postpartum panhypopituitary 253.2
 postperfusion NEC 999.8
  bone marrow 996.85
 postpericardiotomy 429.4
 postphlebitic (asymptomatic) 459.10
  with
   complications NEC 459.19
   inflammatin 459.12
    and ulcer 459.13
   stasis dermatitis 459.12
    with ulcer 459.13
   ulcer 459.11
    with inflammation 459.13
 postpolio (myelitis) 138
 postvagotomy 564.2
 postvalvulotomy 429.4
 postviral (asthenia) NEC 780.79
 Potain's (gastrectasis with dyspepsia) 536.1
 potassium intoxication 276.7
 Potter's 753.0
 Prader (-Labhart) -Willi (-Fanconi) 759.81
 preinfarction 411.1
 preleukemic 238.7
 premature senility 259.8
 premenstrual 625.4
 premenstrual tension 625.4
 pre ulcer 536.9
 Prinzmetal-Massumi (anterior chest wall
  syndrome) 786.52
 Profichet's 729.9
 progeria 259.8
 progressive pallidal degeneration 333.0
 prolonged gestation 766.2
 Proteus (dermal hypoplasia) 757.39
 prune belly 756.71
 prurigo-asthma 691.8
 pseudocarpal tunnel (sublimis) 354.0
 pseudohermaphroditism-virilism-hirsutism 255.2
 pseudoparalytica 358.0
 pseudo-Turner's 759.89
 psycho-organic 293.9
  acute 293.0
  anxiety type 293.84
  depressive type 293.83
  hallucinatory type 293.82
  nonpsychotic severity 310.1
   specified focal (partial) NEC 310.8
  paranoid type 293.81
  specified type NEC 293.89
  subacute 293.1
 pterygolymphangiectasia 758.6
 ptosis-epicanthus 270.2
 pulmonary
  arteriosclerosis 416.0
  hypoperfusion (idiopathic) 769
  renal (hemorrhagic) 446.21
 pulseless 446.7
 Putnam-Dana (subacute combined sclerosis
  with pernicious anemia) 281.0 *[336.2]*
 pyloroduodenal 537.89
 pyramidopallidonigral 332.0
 pyriformis 355.0
 Q-T interval prolongation 794.31
 radicular NEC 729.2
  lower limbs 724.4
  upper limbs 723.4
   newborn 767.4
 Raeder-Harbitz (pulseless disease) 446.7

Syndrome—*continued*
 Ramsay Hunt's
  dyssynergia cerebellaris myoclonica 334.2
  herpetic geniculate ganglionitis 053.11
 rapid time-zone change 307.45
 Raymond (-Céstan) 433.8
 Raynaud's (paroxysmal digital cyanosis) 443.0
 RDS (respiratory distress syndrome, newborn)
  769
 Refsum's (heredopathia atactica
  polyneuritiformis) 356.3
 Reichmann's (gastrosuccorrhea) 536.8
 Reifenstein's (hereditary familial
  hypogonadism, male) 257.2
 Reilly's (*see also* Neuropathy, peripheral,
  autonomic) 337.9
 Reiter's 099.3
 renal glomerulohyalinosis-diabetic 250.4
  [581.81]
 Rendu-Osler-Weber (familial hemorrhagic
  telangiectasia) 448.0
 renofacial (congenital biliary fibroangiomatosis)
  753.0
 Rénon-Delille 253.8
 respiratory distress (idiopathic) (newborn) 769
  adult (following shock, surgery, or trauma)
   518.5
   specified NEC 518.82
 restless leg 333.99
 retraction (Duane's) 378.71
 retroperitoneal fibrosis 593.4
 Rett's 330.8
 Reye's 331.81
 Reye-Sheehan (postpartum pituitary necrosis)
  253.2
 Riddoch's (visual disorientation) 368.16
 Ridley's (*see also* Failure, ventricular, left)
  428.1
 Rieger's (mesodermal dysgenesis, anterior
  ocular segment) 743.44
 Rietti-Greppi-Micheli (thalassemia minor) 282.4
 right ventricular obstruction—*see* Failure heart
 Riley-Day (familial dysautonomia) 742.8
 Robin's 756.0
 Rokitansky-Kuster-Hauser (congenital absence,
  vagina) 752.49
 Romano-Ward (prolonged Q-T interval) 794.31
 Romberg's 349.89
 Rosen-Castleman-Liebow (pulmonary
  proteinosis) 516.0
 rotator cuff, shoulder 726.10
 Roth's 355.1
 Rothmund's (congenital poikiloderma) 757.33
 Rotor's (idiopathic hyperbilirubinemia) 277.4
 Roussy-Lévy 334.3
 Roy (-Jutras) (acropachyderma) 757.39
 rubella (congenital) 771.0
 Rubinstein-Taybi's (brachydactylia, short
  stature, and mental retardation) 759.89
 Rud's (mental deficiency, epilepsy, and
  infantilism) 759.89
 Ruiter-Pompen (-Wyers) (angiokeratoma
  corporis diffusum) 272.7
 Runge's (postmaturity) 766.2
 Russell (-Silver) (congenital hemihypertrophy
  and short stature) 759.89
 Rytand-Lipsitch (complete atrioventricular
  block) 426.0
 sacralization-scoliosis-sciatica 756.15
 sacroiliac 724.6
 Saenger's 379.46

Syphilis, syphilitic—*continued*
  uterus 095.8
  uveal tract (secondary) 091.50
    late 095.8 *[363.13]*
  uveitis (secondary) 091.50
    late 095.8 *[363.13]*
  uvula (late) 095.8
    perforated 095.8
  vagina 091.0
    late 095.8
  valvulitis NEC 093.20
  vascular 093.89
    brain or cerebral 094.89
  vein 093.89
    cerebral 094.89
  ventriculi 095.8
  vesicae urinariae 095.8
  viscera (abdominal) 095.2
    secondary 091.69
  vitreous (hemorrhage) (opacities) 095.8
  vulva 091.0
    late 095.8
    secondary 091.3
Syphiloma 095.9
  cardiovascular system 093.9
  central nervous system 094.9
  circulatory system 093.9
  congenital 090.5
Syphilophobia 300.29
Syringadenoma (M8400/0)—*see also*
    Neoplasm, skin, benign
  papillary (M8406/0)—*see* Neoplasm, skin,
    benign
Syringobulbia 336.0
Syringocarcinoma (M8400/3)—*see* Neoplasm,
  skin, malignant
Syringocystadenoma (M8400/0)—*see also*
    Neoplasm, skin, benign
  papillary (M8406/0)—*see* Neoplasm, skin,
    benign
Syringocystoma (M8407/0)—*see* Neoplasm,
  skin, benign
Syringoma (M8407/0)—*see also* Neoplasm,
  skin, benign
  chondroid (M8940/0)—*see* Neoplasm, by site,
    benign
Syringomyelia 336.0
Syringomyelitis 323.9
  late effect—*see* category 326
Syringomyelocele (*see also* Spina bifida) 741.9
Syringopontia 336.0
System, systemic —*see also* condition
  disease, combined—*see* Degeneration,
    combined
  fibrosclerosing syndrome 710.8
  inflammatory response syndrome (SIRS) 995.90
    due to
      infectious process 995.91
        with organ dysfunction 995.92
      non-infectious process 995.93
        with organ dysfunction 995.94
  lupus erythematosus 710.0
    inhibitor 286.5

T

Tab —*see* Tag
Tabacism 989.8
Tabacosis 989.8
Tabardillo 080
  flea-borne 081.0
  louse-borne 080
Tabes, tabetic
  with
    central nervous system syphilis 094.0
    Charcot's joint 094.0 *[713.5]*
    cord bladder 094.0
    crisis, viscera (any) 094.0
    paralysis, general 094.1
    paresis (general) 094.1
    perforating ulcer 094.0
  arthropathy 094.0 *[713.5]*
  bladder 094.0
  bone 094.0
  cerebrospinal 094.0
  congenital 090.40
  conjugal 094.0
  dorsalis 094.0
    neurosyphilis 094.0
  early 094.0
  juvenile 090.40
  latent 094.0
  mesenterica (*see also* Tuberculosis) 014.8
  paralysis insane, general 094.1
  peripheral (nonsyphilitic) 799.8
  spasmodic 094.0
    not dorsal or dorsalis 343.9
  syphilis (cerebrospinal) 094.0
Taboparalysis 094.1
Taboparesis (remission) 094.1
  with
    Charcot's joint 094.1 *[713.5]*
    cord bladder 094.1
    perforating ulcer 094.1
  juvenile 090.40
Tachyalimentation 579.3
Tachyarrhythmia, tachyrhythmia —*see also*
  Tachycardia
  paroxysmal with sinus bradycardia 427.81
Tachycardia 785.0
  atrial 427.89
  auricular 427.89
  newborn 779.82
  nodal 427.89
    nonparoxysmal atrioventricular 426.89
  nonparoxysmal atrioventricular (nodal) 426.89
  paroxysmal 427.2
    with sinus bradycardia 427.81
    atrial (PAT) 427.0
      psychogenic 316 *[427.0]*
    atrioventricular (AV) 427.0
      psychogenic 316 *[427.0]*
    essential 427.2
    junctional 427.0
    nodal 427.0
    psychogenic 316 *[427.2]*
      atrial 316 *[427.0]*
      supraventricular 316 *[427.0]*
      ventricular 316 *[427.1]*
    supraventricular 427.0
      psychogenic 316 *[427.0]*
    ventricular 427.1
      psychogenic 316 *[427.1]*
  postoperative 997.1

Tachycardia—*continued*
  psychogenic 306.2
  sick sinus 427.81
  sinoauricular 427.89
  sinus 427.89
  supraventricular 427.89
  ventricular (paroxysmal) 427.1
    psychogenic 316 *[427.1]*
Tachypnea 786.06
  hysterical 300.11
  newborn (idiopathic) (transitory) 770.6
  psychogenic 306.1
  transitory, of newborn 770.6
Taenia (infection) (infestation) (*see also*
  Infestation, taenia) 123.3
  diminuta 123.6
  echinococcal infestation (*see also*
    Echinococcus) 122.9
  nana 123.6
  saginata infestation 123.2
  solium (intestinal form) 123.0
    larval form 123.1
Taeniasis (intestine) (*see also* Infestation,
  Taenia) 123.3
  saginata 123.2
  solium 123.0
Taenzer's disease 757.4
Tag (hypertrophied skin) (infected) 701.9
  adenoid 474.8
  anus 455.9
  endocardial (*see also* Endocarditis) 424.90
  hemorrhoidal 455.9
  hymen 623.8
  perineal 624.8
  preauricular 744.1
  rectum 455.9
  sentinel 455.9
  skin 701.9
    accessory 757.39
    anus 455.9
    congenital 757.39
    preauricular 744.1
    rectum 455.9
  tonsil 474.8
  urethra, urethral 599.84
  vulva 624.8
Tahyna fever 062.5
Takayasu (-Onishi) disease or syndrome
  (pulseless disease) 446.7
Talc granuloma 728.82
Talcosis 502
Talipes (congenital) 754.70
  acquired NEC 736.79
    planus 734
  asymmetric 754.79
    acquired 736.79
  calcaneovalgus 754.62
    acquired 736.76
  calcaneovarus 754.59
    acquired 736.76
  calcaneus 754.79
    acquired 736.76
  cavovarus 754.59
    acquired 736.75
  cavus 754.71
    acquired 736.73
  equinovalgus 754.69
    acquired 736.72

Test(s)—*continued*
  bacterial disease NEC (*see also* Screening, by
    name of disease) V74.9
  basal metabolic rate V72.6
  blood-alcohol V70.4
  blood-drug V70.4
    for therapeutic drug monitoring V58.83
  developmental, infant or child V20.2
  Dick V74.8
  fertility V26.21
  genetic V26.3
  hearing V72.1
  HIV V72.6
  human immunodeficiency virus V72.6
  Kveim V82.89
  laboratory V72.6
    for medicolegal reason V70.4
  Mantoux (for tuberculosis) V74.1
  mycotic organism V75.4
  parasitic agent NEC V75.8
  paternity V70.4
  peritoneal equilibration V56.32
  pregnancy
    positive V22.1
      first pregnancy V22.0
    unconfirmed V72.4
  preoperative V72.84
    cardiovascular V72.81
    respiratory V72.82
    specified NEC V72.83
  procreative management NEC V26.29
  sarcoidosis V82.89
  Schick V74.3
  Schultz-Charlton V74.8
  skin, diagnostic
    allergy V72.7
    bacterial agent NEC (*see also* Screening, by
      name of disease) V74.9
    Dick V74.8
    hypersensitivity V72.7
    Kveim V82.89
    Mantoux V74.1
    mycotic organism V75.4
    parasitic agent NEC V75.8
    sarcoidosis V82.89
    Schick V74.3
    Schultz-Charlton V74.8
    tuberculin V74.1
  specified type NEC V72.85
  tuberculin V74.1
  vision V72.0
  Wassermann
    positive (*see also* Serology for syphilis,
      positive) 097.1
    false 795.6
Testicle, testicular, testis —*see also* condition
  feminization (syndrome) 257.8
Tetanus, tetanic (cephalic) (convulsions) 037
  with
    abortion—*see* Abortion, by type, with sepsis
    ectopic pregnancy (*see also* categories
      633.0-633.9) 639.0
    molar pregnancy (*see* categories 630-632)
      639.0
  following
    abortion 639.0
    ectopic or molar pregnancy 639.0
  inoculation V03.7
    reaction (due to serum)—*see* Complications,
      vaccination
  neonatorum 771.3
  puerperal, postpartum, childbirth 670

Tetany, tetanic 781.7
  alkalosis 276.3
  associated with rickets 268.0
  convulsions 781.7
    hysterical 300.11
  functional (hysterical) 300.11
  hyperkinetic 781.7
    hysterical 300.11
  hyperpnea 786.01
    hysterical 300.11
    psychogenic 306.1
  hyperventilation 786.01
    hysterical 300.11
    psychogenic 306.1
  hypocalcemic, neonatal 775.4
  hysterical 300.11
  neonatal 775.4
  parathyroid (gland) 252.1
  parathyroprival 252.1
  postoperative 252.1
  postthyroidectomy 252.1
  pseudotetany 781.7
    hysterical 300.11
  psychogenic 306.1
    specified as conversion reaction 300.11
Tetralogy of Fallot 745.2
Tetraplegia —*see* Quadriplegia
Thailand hemorrhagic fever 065.4
Thalassanemia 282.4
Thalassemia (alpha) (beta) (disease) (Hb-C)
  (Hb-D) (Hb-E) (Hb-H) (Hb-I) (Hb-S) (high
  fetal gene) (high fetal hemoglobin)
  (intermedia) (major) (minima) (minor)
  (mixed) (sickle-cell) (trait) (with other
  hemoglobinopathy) 282.4
Thalassemic variants 282.4
Thaysen-Gee disease (nontropical sprue) 579.0
Thecoma (M8600/0) 220
  malignant (M8600/3) 183.0
Thelarche, precocious 259.1
Thelitis 611.0
  puerperal, postpartum 675.0
Therapeutic —*see* condition
Therapy V57.9
  blood transfusion, without reported diagnosis
    V58.2
  breathing V57.0
  chemotherapy V58.1
    fluoride V07.31
    prophylactic NEC V07.39
  dialysis (intermittent) (treatment)
    extracorporeal V56.0
    peritoneal V56.8
    renal V56.0
    specified type NEC V56.8
  exercise NEC V57.1
    breathing V57.0
  extracorporeal dialysis (renal) V56.0
  fluoride prophylaxis V07.31
  hemodialysis V56.0
  long term oxygen therapy V46.2
  occupational V57.21
  orthoptic V57.4
  orthotic V57.81
  peritoneal dialysis V56.8
  physical NEC V57.1
  postmenopausal hormone replacement V07.4
  radiation V58.0
  speech V57.3
  vocational V57.22
Thermalgesia 782.0
Thermalgia 782.0

Thrombophlebitis—*continued*
  cavernous (venous) sinus—*see*
      Thrombophlebitis, intracranial venous sinus
  cephalic vein 451.82
  cerebral (sinus) (vein) 325
    late effect—*see* category 326
    nonpyogenic 437.6
      in pregnancy or puerperium 671.5
      late effect—*see* Late effect(s) (of)
          cerebrovascular disease
  due to implanted device—*see* Complications,
      due to (presence of) any device, implant, or
      graft classified to 996.0-996.5 NEC
  during or resulting from a procedure NEC 997.2
  femoral 451.11
  femoropopliteal 451.19
  following infusion, perfusion, or transfusion
      999.2
  hepatic (vein) 451.89
  idiopathic, recurrent 453.1
  iliac vein 451.81
  iliofemoral 451.11
  intracranial venous sinus (any) 325
    late effect—*see* category 326
    nonpyogenic 437.6
      in pregnancy or puerperium 671.5
      late effect—*see* Late effect(s) (of)
          cerebrovascular disease
  jugular vein 451.89
  lateral (venous) sinus—*see* Thrombophlebitis,
      intracranial venous sinus
  leg 451.2
    deep (vessels) 451.19
      femoral vein 451.11
      specified vessel NEC 451.19
    superficial (vessels) 451.0
      femoral vein 451.11
  longitudinal (venous) sinus—*see*
      Thrombophlebitis, intracranial venous sinus
  lower extremity 451.2
    deep (vessels) 451.19
      femoral vein 451.11
      specified vessel NEC 451.19
    superficial (vessels) 451.0
  migrans, migrating 453.1
  pelvic
    with
      abortion—*see* Abortion, by type, with sepsis
      ectopic pregnancy (*see also* categories
          633.0-633.9) 639.0
      molar pregnancy (*see also* categories
          630-632) 639.0
    following
      abortion 639.0
      ectopic or molar pregnancy 639.0
    puerperal 671.4
  popliteal vein 451.19
  portal (vein) 572.1
  postoperative 997.2
  pregnancy (superficial) 671.2
    affecting fetus or newborn 760.3
    deep 671.3
  puerperal, postpartum, childbirth (extremities)
      (superficial) 671.2
    deep 671.4
    pelvic 671.4
    specified site NEC 671.5
  radial vein 451.83
  saphenous (greater) (lesser) 451.0
  sinus (intracranial)—*see* Thrombophlebitis,
      intracranial venous sinus

Thrombophlebitis—*continued*
  specified site NEC 451.89
  tibial vein 451.19
Thrombosis, thrombotic (marantic) (multiple)
    (progressive) (septic) (vein) (vessel) 453.9
  with childbirth or during the puerperium—*see*
      Thrombosis, puerperal, postpartum
  antepartum—*see* Thrombosis, pregnancy
  aorta, aortic 444.1
    abdominal 444.0
    bifurcation 444.0
    saddle 444.0
    terminal 444.0
    thoracic 444.1
    valve—*see* Endocarditis, aortic
  apoplexy (*see also* Thrombosis, brain) 434.0
    late effect—*see* Late effect(s) (of)
        cerebrovascular disease
  appendix, septic—*see* Appendicitis, acute
  arteriolar-capillary platelet, disseminated 446.6
  artery, arteries (postinfectional) 444.9
    auditory, internal 433.8
    basilar (*see also* Occlusion, artery, basilar)
        433.0
    carotid (common) (internal) (*see also*
        Occlusion, artery, carotid) 433.1
      with other precerebral artery 433.3
    cerebellar (anterior inferior) (posterior
        inferior) (superior) 433.8
    cerebral (*see also* Thrombosis, brain) 434.0
    choroidal (anterior) 433.8
    communicating posterior 433.8
    coronary (*see also* Infarct, myocardium) 410.9
      due to syphilis 093.89
      healed or specified as old 412
      without myocardial infarction 411.81
    extremities 444.22
      lower 444.22
      upper 444.21
    femoral 444.22
    hepatic 444.89
    hypophyseal 433.8
    meningeal, anterior or posterior 433.8
    mesenteric (with gangrene) 557.0
    ophthalmic (*see also* Occlusion, retina) 362.30
    pontine 433.8
    popliteal 444.22
    precerebral—*see* Occlusion, artery,
        precerebral NEC
    pulmonary 415.19
      iatrogenic 415.11
      postoperative 415.11
    renal 593.81
    retinal (*see also* Occlusion, retina) 362.30
    specified site NEC 444.89
    spinal, anterior or posterior 433.8
    traumatic (complication) (early) (*see also*
        Injury, blood vessel, by site) 904.9
    vertebral (*see also* Occlusion, artery,
        vertebral) 433.2
      with other precerebral artery 433.3
  atrial (endocardial) 424.90
    due to syphilis 093.89
  auricular (*see also* Infarct, myocardium) 410.9
  axillary (vein) 453.8
  basilar (artery) (*see also* Occlusion, artery,
      basilar) 433.0
  bland NEC 453.9
  brain (artery) (stem) 434.0
    due to syphilis 094.89
    iatrogenic 997.02

Thrombosis, thrombotic—*continued*
   resulting from presence of shunt or other
      internal prosthetic device—*see*
      Complications, due to (presence of) any
      device, implant, or graft classified to
      996.0-996.5 NEC
   retina, retinal (artery) 362.30
    arterial branch 362.32
    central 362.31
    partial 362.33
    vein
      central 362.35
      tributary (branch) 362.36
   scrotum 608.83
   seminal vesicle 608.83
   sigmoid (venous) sinus (*see* Thrombosis,
    intracranial venous sinus) 325
   silent NEC 453.9
   sinus, intracranial (venous) (any) (*see also*
    Thrombosis, intracranial venous sinus) 325
   softening, brain (*see also* Thrombosis, brain)
    434.0
   specified site NEC 453.8
   spermatic cord 608.83
   spinal cord 336.1
    due to syphilis 094.89
    in pregnancy or puerperium 671.5
    pyogenic origin 324.1
     late effect—*see* category 326
   spleen, splenic 289.59
    artery 444.89
   testis 608.83
   traumatic (complication) (early) (*see also*
    Injury, blood vessel, by site) 904.9
   tricuspid—*see* Endocarditis, tricuspid
   tunica vaginalis 608.83
   umbilical cord (vessels) 663.6
    affecting fetus or newborn 762.6
   vas deferens 608.83
   vena cava (inferior) (superior) 453.2
Thrombus —*see* Thrombosis
Thrush 112.0
   newborn 771.7
Thumb —*see also* condition
   gamekeeper's 842.12
   sucking (child problem) 307.9
Thygeson's superficial punctate keratitis
   370.21
Thymergasia (*see also* Psychosis, affective)
   296.80
Thymitis 254.8
Thymoma (benign) (M8580/0) 212.6
   malignant (M8580/3) 164.0
Thymus, thymic (gland)—*see* condition
Thyrocele (*see also* Goiter) 240.9
Thyroglossal —*see also* condition
   cyst 759.2
   duct, persistent 759.2
Thyroid (body) (gland)—*see also* condition
   lingual 759.2
Thyroiditis 245.9
   acute (pyogenic) (suppurative) 245.0
    nonsuppurative 245.0
   autoimmune 245.2
   chronic (nonspecific) (sclerosing) 245.8
    fibrous 245.3
    lymphadenoid 245.2
    lymphocytic 245.2
    lymphoid 245.2
   complicating pregnancy, childbirth, or
    puerperium 648.1

Thyroiditis—*continued*
   de Quervain's (subacute granulomatous) 245.1
   fibrous (chronic) 245.3
   giant (cell) (follicular) 245.1
   granulomatous (de Quervain's) (subacute) 245.1
   Hashimoto's (struma lymphomatosa) 245.2
   iatrogenic 245.4
   invasive (fibrous) 245.3
   ligneous 245.3
   lymphocytic (chronic) 245.2
   lymphoid 245.2
   lymphomatous 245.2
   pseudotuberculous 245.1
   pyogenic 245.0
   radiation 245.4
   Riedel's (ligneous) 245.3
   subacute 245.1
   suppurative 245.0
   tuberculous (*see also* Tuberculosis) 017.5
   viral 245.1
   woody 245.3
Thyrolingual duct, persistent 759.2
Thyromegaly 240.9
Thyrotoxic
   crisis or storm (*see also* Thyrotoxicosis) 242.9
   heart failure (*see also* Thyrotoxicosis) 242.9
    [425.7]
Thyrotoxicosis 242.9

> *Note—Use the following fifth-digit*
> *subclassification with category 242:*
>
> 0 *without mention of thyrotoxic crisis or storm*
> 1 *with mention of thyrotoxic crisis or storm*

   with
    goiter (diffuse) 242.0
     adenomatous 242.3
      multinodular 242.2
      uninodular 242.1
     nodular 242.3
      multinodular 242.2
      uninodular 242.1
    infiltrative
     dermopathy 242.0
     ophthalmopathy 242.0
    thyroid acropachy 242.0
   complicating pregnancy, childbirth, or
    puerperium 648.1
   due to
    ectopic thyroid nodule 242.4
    ingestion of (excessive) thyroid material 242.8
    specified cause NEC 242.8
   factitia 242.8
   heart 242.9 *[425.7]*
   neonatal (transient) 775.3
TIA (transient ischemic attack) 435.9
   with transient neurologic deficit 435.9
   late effect—*see* Late effect(s) (of)
    cerebrovascular disease
Tibia vara 732.4
Tic 307.20
   breathing 307.20
   child problem 307.21
   compulsive 307.22
   convulsive 307.20
   degenerative (generalized) (localized) 333.3
    facial 351.8
   douloureux (*see also* Neuralgia, trigeminal)
    350.1
    atypical 350.2

Tornwaldt's bursitis (disease) (pharyngeal
bursitis) 478.29
cyst 478.26
Torpid liver 573.9
Torsion
accessory tube 620.5
adnexa (female) 620.5
aorta (congenital) 747.29
acquired 447.1
appendix epididymis 608.2
bile duct 576.8
with calculus, choledocholithiasis or
stones—*see* Choledocholithiasis
congenital 751.69
bowel, colon, or intestine 560.2
cervix (*see also* Malposition, uterus) 621.6
duodenum 537.3
dystonia—*see* Dystonia, torsion
epididymis 608.2
appendix 608.2
fallopian tube 620.5
gallbladder (*see also* Disease, gallbladder) 575.8
congenital 751.69
gastric 537.89
hydatid of Morgagni (female) 620.5
kidney (pedicle) 593.89
Meckel's diverticulum (congenital) 751.0
mesentery 560.2
omentum 560.2
organ or site, congenital NEC—*see* Anomaly,
specified type NEC
ovary (pedicle) 620.5
congenital 752.0
oviduct 620.5
penis 607.89
congenital 752.69
renal 593.89
spasm—*see* Dystonia, torsion
spermatic cord 608.2
spleen 289.59
testicle, testis 608.2
tibia 736.89
umbilical cord—*see* Compression, umbilical
cord
uterus (*see also* Malposition, uterus) 621.6
Torticollis (intermittent) (spastic) 723.5
congenital 754.1
sternomastoid 754.1
due to birth injury 767.8
hysterical 300.11
ocular 781.93
psychogenic 306.0
specified as conversion reaction 300.11
rheumatic 723.5
rheumatoid 714.0
spasmodic 333.83
traumatic, current NEC 847.0
Tortuous
artery 447.1
fallopian tube 752.19
organ or site, congenital NEC—*see* Distortion
renal vessel, congenital 747.62
retina vessel (congenital) 743.58
acquired 362.17
ureter 593.4
urethra 599.84
vein—*see* Varicose, vein
Torula, torular (infection) 117.5
histolytica 117.5
lung 117.5
Torulosis 117.5

Torus
fracture
fibula 823.41
with tibia 823.42
radius 813.45
tibia 823.40
with fibula 823.42
mandibularis 526.81
palatinus 526.81
Touch, vitreous 997.99
Touraine's syndrome (hereditary
osteo-onychodysplasia) 756.89
Touraine-Solente-Golé syndrome
(acropachyderma) 757.39
Tourette's disease (motor-verbal tic) 307.23
Tower skull 756.0
with exophthalmos 756.0
Toxemia 799.8
with
abortion—*see* Abortion, by type, with toxemia
bacterial—*see* Septicemia
biliary (*see also* Disease, biliary) 576.8
burn—*see* Burn, by site
congenital NEC 779.89
eclamptic 642.6
with pre-existing hypertension 642.7
erysipelatous (*see also* Erysipelas) 035
fatigue 799.8
fetus or newborn NEC 779.89
food (*see also* Poisoning, food) 005.9
gastric 537.89
gastrointestinal 558.2
intestinal 558.2
kidney (*see also* Disease, renal) 593.9
lung 518.89
malarial NEC (*see also* Malaria) 084.6
maternal (of pregnancy), affecting fetus or
newborn 760.0
myocardial—*see* Myocarditis, toxic
of pregnancy (mild) (pre-eclamptic) 642.4
with
convulsions 642.6
pre-existing hypertension 642.7
affecting fetus or newborn 760.0
severe 642.5
pre-eclamptic—*see* Toxemia, of pregnancy
puerperal, postpartum—*see* Toxemia, of
pregnancy
pulmonary 518.89
renal (*see also* Disease, renal) 593.9
septic (*see also* Septicemia) 038.9
small intestine 558.2
staphylococcal 038.10
aureus 038.11
due to food 005.0
specified organism NEC 038.19
stasis 799.8
stomach 537.89
uremic (*see also* Uremia) 586
urinary 586
Toxemica cerebropathia psychica
(nonalcoholic) 294.0
alcoholic 291.1
Toxic (poisoning)—*see also* condition
from drug or poison—*see* Table of drugs and
chemicals
oil syndrome 710.5
shock syndrome 040.82
thyroid (gland) (*see also* Thyrotoxicosis) 242.9
Toxicemia —*see* Toxemia

Triplet—*continued*
  healthy liveborn—*see* Newborn, multiple
  pregnancy (complicating delivery) NEC 651.1
    with fetal loss and retention of one or more
      fetus(es) 651.4
Triplex placenta —*see* Placenta, abnormal
Triplication —*see* Accessory
Trismus 781.0
  neonatorum 771.3
  newborn 771.3
Trisomy (syndrome) NEC 758.5
  13 (partial) 758.1
  16-18 758.2
  18 (partial) 758.2
  21 (partial) 758.0
  22 758.0
  autosomes NEC 758.5
  D_1 758.1
  E_3 758.2
  G (group) 758.0
  group D_1 758.1
  group E 758.2
  group G 758.0
Tritanomaly 368.53
Tritanopia 368.53
Troisier-Hanot-Chauffard syndrome (bronze
    diabetes) 275.0
Trombidiosis 133.8
Trophedema (hereditary) 757.0
  congenital 757.0
Trophoblastic disease (*see also* Hydatidiform
    mole) 630
  previous, affecting management of pregnancy
    V23.1
Tropholymphedema 757.0
Trophoneurosis NEC 356.9
  arm NEC 354.9
  disseminated 710.1
  facial 349.89
  leg NEC 355.8
  lower extremity NEC 355.8
  upper extremity NEC 354.9
Tropical —*see also* condition
  maceration feet (syndrome) 991.4
  wet foot (syndrome) 991.4
Trouble —*see also* Disease
  bowel 569.9
  heart—*see* Disease, heart
  intestine 569.9
  kidney (*see also* Disease, renal) 593.9
  nervous 799.2
  sinus (*see also* Sinusitis) 473.9
Trousseau's syndrome (thrombophlebitis
    migrans) 453.1
Truancy, childhood —*see also* Disturbance,
    conduct
  socialized 312.2
  undersocialized, unsocialized 312.1
Truncus
  arteriosus (persistent) 745.0
  common 745.0
  communis 745.0
Trunk —*see* condition
Trychophytide —*see* Dermatophytosis
Trypanosoma infestation —*see*
  Trypanosomiasis
Trypanosomiasis 086.9
  with meningoencephalitis 086.9 *[323.2]*
  African 086.5
    due to Trypanosoma 086.5
      gambiense 086.3

Trypanosomiasis—*continued*
    rhodesiense 086.4
  American 086.2
    with
      heart involvement 086.0
      other organ involvement 086.1
    without mention of organ involvement 086.2
  Brazilian—*see* Trypanosomiasis, American
  Chagas'—*see* Trypanosomiasis, American
  due to Trypanosoma
    cruzi—*see* Trypanosomiasis, American
    gambiense 086.3
    rhodesiense 086.4
  gambiensis, Gambian 086.3
  North American—*see* Trypanosomiasis,
    American
  rhodesiensis, Rhodesian 086.4
  South American—*see* Trypanosomiasis,
    American
T-shaped incisors 520.2
Tsutsugamushi fever 081.2
Tube, tubal, tubular —*see also* condition
  ligation, admission for V25.2
Tubercle —*see also* Tuberculosis
  brain, solitary 013.2
  Darwin's 744.29
  epithelioid noncaseating 135
  Ghon, primary infection 010.0
Tuberculid, tuberculide (indurating) (lichenoid)
    (miliary) (papulonecrotic) (primary) (skin)
    (subcutaneous) (*see also* Tuberculosis) 017.0
Tuberculoma —*see also* Tuberculosis
  brain (any part) 013.2
  meninges (cerebral) (spinal) 013.1
  spinal cord 013.4
Tuberculosis, tubercular, tuberculous
    (calcification) (calcified) (caseous)
    (chromogenic acid-fast bacilli) (congenital)
    (degeneration) (disease) (fibrocaseous)
    (fistula) (gangrene) (interstitial) (isolated
    circumscribed lesions) (necrosis)
    (parenchymatous) (ulcerative) 011.9

---

*Note—Use the following fifth-digit
subclassification with categories 010-018:*

0 unspecified
*1 bacteriological or histological examination
   not done*
*2 bacteriological or histological examination
   unknown (at present)*
*3 tubercle bacilli found (in sputum) by
   microscopy*
*4 tubercle bacilli not found (in sputum) by
   microscopy, but found by bacterial culture*
*5 tubercle bacilli not found by bacteriological
   examination, but tuberculosis confirmed
   histologically*
*6 tubercle bacilli not found by bacteriological or
   histological examination, but tuberculosis
   confirmed by other methods [inoculation of
   animals]*

*For tuberculous conditions specified as late
effects or sequelae, see category 137.*

---

  abdomen 014.8
    lymph gland 014.8
  abscess 011.9
    arm 017.9
    bone (*see also* Osteomyelitis, due to,
      tuberculosis) 015.9 *[730.8]*

Tuberculosis, tubercular, tuberculous—*cont.*
  caries (*see also* Tuberculosis, bone) 015.9
    [730.8]
  cartilage (*see also* Tuberculosis, bone) 015.9
    [730.8]
    intervertebral 015.0 *[730.88]*
  catarrhal (*see also* Tuberculosis, pulmonary)
    011.9
  cecum 014.8
  cellular tissue (primary) 017.0
  cellulitis (primary) 017.0
  central nervous system 013.9
    specified site NEC 013.8
  cerebellum (current) 013.2
  cerebral (current) 013.2
    meninges 013.0
  cerebrospinal 013.6
    meninges 013.0
  cerebrum (current) 013.2
  cervical 017.2
    gland 017.2
    lymph nodes 017.2
  cervicitis (uteri) 016.7
  cervix 016.7
  chest (*see also* Tuberculosis, pulmonary) 011.9
  childhood type or first infection 010.0
  choroid 017.3 *[363.13]*
  choroiditis 017.3 *[363.13]*
  ciliary body 017.3 *[364.11]*
  colitis 014.8
  colliers' 011.4
  colliquativa (primary) 017.0
  colon 014.8
    ulceration 014.8
  complex, primary 010.0
  complicating pregnancy, childbirth, or
    puerperium 647.3
    affecting fetus or newborn 760.2
  congenital 771.2
  conjunctiva 017.3 *[370.31]*
  connective tissue 017.9
    bone—*see* Tuberculosis, bone
  contact V01.1
  converter (tuberculin skin test) (without disease)
    795.5
  cornea (ulcer) 017.3 *[370.31]*
  Cowper's gland 016.5
  coxae 015.1 *[730.85]*
  coxalgia 015.1 *[730.85]*
  cul-de-sac of Douglas 014.8
  curvature, spine 015.0 *[737.40]*
  cutis (colliquativa) (primary) 017.0
  cyst, ovary 016.6
  cystitis 016.1
  dacryocystitis 017.3 *[375.32]*
  dactylitis 015.5
  diarrhea 014.8
  diffuse (*see also* Tuberculosis, miliary) 018.9
    lung—*see* Tuberculosis, pulmonary
    meninges 013.0
  digestive tract 014.8
  disseminated (*see also* Tuberculosis, miliary)
    018.9
    meninges 013.0
  duodenum 014.8
  dura (mater) 013.9
    abscess 013.8
      cerebral 013.3
      spinal 013.5
  dysentery 014.8
  ear (inner) (middle) 017.4

Tuberculosis, tubercular, tuberculous—*cont.*
  bone 015.6
    external (primary) 017.0
    skin (primary) 017.0
  elbow 015.8
  emphysema—*see* Tuberculosis, pulmonary
  empyema 012.0
  encephalitis 013.6
  endarteritis 017.9
  endocarditis (any valve) 017.9 *[424.91]*
  endocardium (any valve) 017.9 *[424.91]*
  endocrine glands NEC 017.9
  endometrium 016.7
  enteric, enterica 014.8
  enteritis 014.8
  enterocolitis 014.8
  epididymis 016.4
  epididymitis 016.4
  epidural abscess 013.8
    brain 013.3
    spinal cord 013.5
  epiglottis 012.3
  episcleritis 017.3 *[379.00]*
  erythema (induratum) (nodosum) (primary)
    017.1
  esophagus 017.8
  Eustachian tube 017.4
  exposure to V01.1
  exudative 012.0
    primary, progressive 010.1
  eye 017.3
    glaucoma 017.3 *[365.62]*
  eyelid (primary) 017.0
    lupus 017.0 *[373.4]*
  fallopian tube 016.6
  fascia 017.9
  fauces 012.8
  finger 017.9
  first infection 010.0
  fistula, perirectal 014.8
  Florida 011.6
  foot 017.9
  funnel pelvis 137.3
  gallbladder 017.9
  galloping (*see also* Tuberculosis, pulmonary)
    011.9
  ganglionic 015.9
  gastritis 017.9
  gastrocolic fistula 014.8
  gastroenteritis 014.8
  gastrointestinal tract 014.8
  general, generalized 018.9
    acute 018.0
    chronic 018.8
  genital organs NEC 016.9
    female 016.7
    male 016.5
  genitourinary NEC 016.9
  genu 015.2
  glandulae suprarenalis 017.6
  glandular, general 017.2
  glottis 012.3
  grinders' 011.4
  groin 017.2
  gum 017.9
  hand 017.9
  heart 017.9 *[425.8]*
  hematogenous—*see* Tuberculosis, miliary
  hemoptysis (*see also* Tuberculosis, pulmonary)
    011.9

Tuberculosis, tubercular, tuberculous—*cont.*
  sternoclavicular joint 015.8
  stomach 017.9
  stonemasons' 011.4
  struma 017.2
  subcutaneous tissue (cellular) (primary) 017.0
  subcutis (primary) 017.0
  subdeltoid bursa 017.9
  submaxillary 017.9
    region 017.9
  supraclavicular gland 017.2
  suprarenal (capsule) (gland) 017.6
  swelling, joint (*see also* Tuberculosis, joint)
    015.9
  symphysis pubis 015.7 *[730.88]*
  synovitis 015.9 *[727.01]*
    hip 015.1 *[727.01]*
    knee 015.2 *[727.01]*
    specified site NEC 015.8 *[727.01]*
    spine or vertebra 015.0 *[727.01]*
  systemic—*see* Tuberculosis, miliary
  tarsitis (eyelid) 017.0 *[373.4]*
    ankle (bone) 015.5 *[730.87]*
  tendon (sheath)—*see* Tuberculosis,
    tenosynovitis
  tenosynovitis 015.9 *[727.01]*
    hip 015.1 *[727.01]*
    knee 015.2 *[727.01]*
    specified site NEC 015.8 *[727.01]*
    spine or vertebra 015.0 *[727.01]*
  testis 016.5 *[608.81]*
  throat 012.8
  thymus gland 017.9
  thyroid gland 017.5
  toe 017.9
  tongue 017.9
  tonsil (lingual) 012.8
  tonsillitis 012.8
  trachea, tracheal 012.8
    gland 012.1
      primary, progressive 010.8
    isolated 012.2
  tracheobronchial 011.3
    glandular 012.1
      primary, progressive 010.8
    isolated 012.2
    lymph gland or node 012.1
      primary, progressive 010.8
  tubal 016.6
  tunica vaginalis 016.5
  typhlitis 014.8
  ulcer (primary) (skin) 017.0
    bowel or intestine 014.8
    specified site NEC—*see* Tuberculosis, by site
  unspecified site—*see* Tuberculosis, pulmonary
  ureter 016.2
  urethra, urethral 016.3
  urinary organ or tract 016.3
    kidney 016.0
  uterus 016.7
  uveal tract 017.3 *[363.13]*
  uvula 017.9
  vaccination, prophylactic (against) V03.2
  vagina 016.7
  vas deferens 016.5
  vein 017.9
  verruca (primary) 017.0
  verrucosa (cutis) (primary) 017.0
  vertebra (column) 015.0 *[730.88]*
  vesiculitis 016.5 *[608.81]*
  viscera NEC 014.8

Tuberculosis, tubercular, tuberculous—*cont.*
  vulva 016.7 *[616.51]*
  wrist (joint) 015.8
    bone 015.5 *[730.83]*
Tuberculum
  auriculae 744.29
  occlusal 520.2
  paramolare 520.2
Tuberous sclerosis (brain) 759.5
Tubo-ovarian —*see* condition
Tuboplasty, after previous sterilization V26.0
Tubotympanitis 381.10
Tularemia 021.9
  with
    conjunctivitis 021.3
    pneumonia 021.2
  bronchopneumonic 021.2
  conjunctivitis 021.3
  cryptogenic 021.1
  disseminated 021.8
  enteric 021.1
  generalized 021.8
  glandular 021.8
  intestinal 021.1
  oculoglandular 021.3
  ophthalmic 021.3
  pneumonia 021.2
  pulmonary 021.2
  specified NEC 021.8
  typhoidal 021.1
  ulceroglandular 021.0
  vaccination, prophylactic (against) V03.4
Tularensis conjunctivitis 021.3
Tumefaction —*see also* Swelling
  liver (*see also* Hypertrophy, liver) 789.1
Tumor (M8000/1)—*see also* Neoplasm, by site,
  unspecified nature
  Abrikossov's (M9580/0)—*see also* Neoplasm,
    connective tissue, benign
    malignant (M9580/3)—*see* Neoplasm,
      connective tissue, malignant
  acinar cell (M8550/1)—*see* Neoplasm, by site,
    uncertain behavior
  acinic cell (M8550/1)—*see* Neoplasm, by site,
    uncertain behavior
  adenomatoid (M9054/0)—*see also* Neoplasm,
    by site, benign
    odontogenic (M9300/0) 213.1
      upper jaw (bone) 213.0
  adnexal (skin) (M8390/0)—*see* Neoplasm, skin,
    benign
  adrenal
    cortical (benign) (M8370/0) 227.0
      malignant (M8370/3) 194.0
    rest (M8671/0)—*see* Neoplasm, by site,
      benign
  alpha cell (M8152/0)
    malignant (M8152/3)
      pancreas 157.4
      specified site NEC—*see* Neoplasm, by site,
        malignant
      unspecified site 157.4
    pancreas 211.7
    specified site NEC—*see* Neoplasm, by site,
      benign
    unspecified site 211.7
  aneurysmal (*see also* Aneurysm) 442.9
  aortic body (M8691/1) 237.3
    malignant (M8691/3) 194.6
  argentaffin (M8241/1)—*see* Neoplasm, by site,
    uncertain behavior

Tumor—*continued*
  basal cell (M8090/1)—*see also* Neoplasm, skin,
    uncertain behavior
  benign (M8000/0)—*see* Neoplasm, by site,
    benign
  beta cell (M8151/0)
    malignant (M8151/3)
      pancreas 157.4
      specified site—*see* Neoplasm, by site,
        malignant
      unspecified site 157.4
    pancreas 211.7
    specified site NEC—*see* Neoplasm, by site,
      benign
    unspecified site 211.7
  blood—*see* Hematoma
  brenner (M9000/0) 220
    borderline malignancy (M9000/1) 236.2
    malignant (M9000/3) 183.0
    proliferating (M9000/1) 236.2
  Brooke's (M8100/0)—*see* Neoplasm, skin,
    benign
  brown fat (M8880/0)—*see* Lipoma, by site
  Burkitt's (M9750/3) 200.2
  calcifying epithelial odontogenic (M9340/0)
    213.1
    upper jaw (bone) 213.0
  carcinoid (M8240/1)—*see* Carcinoid
  carotid body (M8692/1) 237.3
    malignant (M8692/3) 194.5
  Castleman's (mediastinal lymph node
    hyperplasia) 785.6
  cells (M8001/1)—*see also* Neoplasm, by site,
    unspecified nature
    benign (M8001/0)—*see* Neoplasm, by site,
      benign
    malignant (M8001/3)—*see* Neoplasm, by site,
      malignant
    uncertain whether benign or malignant
      (M8001/1)—*see* Neoplasm, by site,
      uncertain nature
  cervix
    in pregnancy or childbirth 654.6
      affecting fetus or newborn 763.89
      causing obstructed labor 660.2
        affecting fetus or newborn 763.1
  chondromatous giant cell (M9230/0)—*see*
    Neoplasm, bone, benign
  chromaffin (M8700/0)—*see also* Neoplasm, by
    site, benign
    malignant (M8700/3)—*see* Neoplasm, by site,
      malignant
  Cock's peculiar 706.2
  Codman's (benign chondroblastoma)
    (M9230/0)—*see* Neoplasm, bone, benign
  dentigerous, mixed (M9282/0) 213.1
    upper jaw (bone) 213.0
  dermoid (M9084/0)—*see* Neoplasm, by site,
    benign
    with malignant transformation (M9084/3)
      183.0
  desmoid (extra-abdominal) (M8821/1)—*see*
    also Neoplasm, connective tissue, uncertain
    behavior
    abdominal (M8822/1)—*see* Neoplasm,
      connective tissue, uncertain behavior
  embryonal (mixed) (M9080/1)—*see also*
    Neoplasm, by site, uncertain behavior
    liver (M9080/3) 155.0
  endodermal sinus (M9071/3)

Tumor—*continued*
    specified site—*see* Neoplasm, by site,
      malignant
    unspecified site
      female 183.0
      male 186.9
  epithelial
    benign (M8010/0)—*see* Neoplasm, by site,
      benign
    malignant (M8010/3)—*see* Neoplasm, by site,
      malignant
  Ewing's (M9260/3)—*see* Neoplasm, bone,
    malignant
  fatty—*see* Lipoma
  fetal, causing disproportion 653.7
    causing obstructed labor 660.1
  fibroid (M8890/0)—*see* Leiomyoma
  G cell (M8153/1)
    malignant (M8153/3)
      pancreas 157.4
      specified site NEC—*see* Neoplasm, by site,
        malignant
      unspecified site 157.4
    specified site—*see* Neoplasm, by site,
      uncertain behavior
    unspecified site 235.5
  giant cell (type) (M8003/1)—*see also*
    Neoplasm, by site, unspecified nature
    bone (M9250/1) 238.0
      malignant (M9250/3)—*see* Neoplasm, bone,
        malignant
    chondromatous (M9230/0)—*see* Neoplasm,
      bone, benign
    malignant (M8003/3)—*see* Neoplasm, by site,
      malignant
    peripheral (gingiva) 523.8
    soft parts (M9251/1)—*see also* Neoplasm,
      connective tissue, uncertain behavior
      malignant (M9251/3)—*see* Neoplasm,
        connective tissue, malignant
    tendon sheath 727.02
  glomus (M8711/0)—*see also* Hemangioma, by
    site
    jugulare (M8690/1) 237.3
      malignant (M8690/3) 194.6
  gonadal stromal (M8590/1)—*see* Neoplasm, by
    site, uncertain behavior
  granular cell (M9580/0)—*see also* Neoplasm,
    connective tissue, benign
    malignant (M9580/3)—*see* Neoplasm,
      connective tissue, malignant
  granulosa cell (M8620/1) 236.2
    malignant (M8620/3) 183.0
  granulosa cell-theca cell (M8621/1) 236.2
    malignant (M8621/3) 183.0
  Grawitz's (hypernephroma) (M8312/3) 189.0
  hazard-crile (M8350/3) 193
  hemorrhoidal—*see* Hemorrhoids
  hilar cell (M8660/0) 220
  hurthle cell (benign) (M8290/0) 226
    malignant (M8290/3) 193
  hydatid (*see also* Echinococcus) 122.9
  hypernephroid (M8311/1)—*see also* Neoplasm,
    by site, uncertain behavior
  interstitial cell (M8650/1)—*see also* Neoplasm,
    by site, uncertain behavior
    benign (M8650/0)—*see* Neoplasm, by site,
      benign
    malignant (M8650/3)—*see* Neoplasm, by site,
      malignant
  islet cell (M8150/0)

Tumor—*continued*
  with lipid storage (M8641/0)
    specified site—*see* Neoplasm, by site,
      benign
    unspecified site
      female 220
      male 222.0
  specified site—*see* Neoplasm, by site, benign
  unspecified site
    female 220
    male 222.0
  Sertoli-Leydig cell (M8631/0)
    specified site—*see* Neoplasm, by site, benign
    unspecified site
      female 220
      male 222.0
  sex cord (-stromal) (M8590/1)—*see* Neoplasm,
    by site, uncertain behavior
  skin appendage (M8390/0)—*see* Neoplasm,
    skin, benign
  soft tissue
    benign (M8800/0)—*see* Neoplasm,
      connective tissue, benign
    malignant (M8800/3)—*see* Neoplasm,
      connective tissue, malignant
  sternomastoid 754.1
  superior sulcus (lung) (pulmonary) (syndrome)
    (M8010/3) 162.3
  suprasulcus (M8010/3) 162.3
  sweat gland (M8400/1)—*see also* Neoplasm,
    skin, uncertain behavior
    benign (M8400/0)—*see* Neoplasm, skin,
      benign
    malignant (M8400/3)—*see* Neoplasm, skin,
      malignant
  syphilitic brain 094.89
    congenital 090.49
  testicular stromal (M8590/1) 236.4
  theca cell (M8600/0) 220
  theca cell-granulosa cell (M8621/1) 236.2
  theca-lutein (M8610/0) 220
  turban (M8200/0) 216.4
  uterus
    in pregnancy or childbirth 654.1
      affecting fetus or newborn 763.89
      causing obstructed labor 660.2
        affecting fetus or newborn 763.1
  vagina
    in pregnancy or childbirth 654.7
      affecting fetus or newborn 763.89
      causing obstructed labor 660.2
        affecting fetus or newborn 763.1
  varicose (*see also* Varicose, vein) 454.9
  von Recklinghausen's (M9540/1) 237.71
  vulva
    in pregnancy or childbirth 654.8
      affecting fetus or newborn 763.89
      causing obstructed labor 660.2
        affecting fetus or newborn 763.1
  Warthin's (salivary gland) (M8561/0) 210.2
  white—*see also* Tuberculosis, arthritis
  White-Darier 757.39
  Wilms' (nephroblastoma) (M8960/3) 189.0
  yolk sac (M9071/3)
    specified site—*see* Neoplasm, by site,
      malignant
    unspecified site
      female 183.0
      male 186.9
Tumorlet (M8040/1)—*see* Neoplasm, by site,
  uncertain behavior
Tungiasis 134.1

Tunica vasculosa lentis 743.39
Tunnel vision 368.45
Turban tumor (M8200/0) 216.4
Türck's trachoma (chronic catarrhal laryngitis)
  476.0
Türk's syndrome (ocular retraction syndrome)
  378.71
Turner's
  hypoplasia (tooth) 520.4
  syndrome 758.6
  tooth 520.4
Turner-Kieser syndrome (hereditary
  osteo-onychodysplasia) 756.89
Turner-Varny syndrome 758.6
Turricephaly 756.0
Tussis convulsiva (*see also* Whooping cough)
  033.9
Twin
  affected by maternal complications of
    pregnancy 761.5
  conjoined 759.4
  healthy liveborn—*see* Newborn, twin
  pregnancy (complicating delivery) NEC 651.0
    with fetal loss and retention of one fetus 651.3
Twinning, teeth 520.2
Twist, twisted
  bowel, colon, or intestine 560.2
  hair (congenital) 757.4
  mesentery 560.2
  omentum 560.2
  organ or site, congenital NEC—*see* Anomaly,
    specified type NEC
  ovarian pedicle 620.5
    congenital 752.0
  umbilical cord—*see* Compression, umbilical
    cord
Twitch 781.0
Tylosis 700
  buccalis 528.6
  gingiva 523.8
  linguae 528.6
  palmaris et plantaris 757.39
Tympanism 787.3
Tympanites (abdominal) (intestine) 787.3
Tympanitis —*see* Myringitis
Tympanosclerosis 385.00
  involving
    combined sites NEC 385.09
      with tympanic membrane 385.03
    tympanic membrane 385.01
      with ossicles 385.02
        and middle ear 385.03
Tympanum —*see* condition
Tympany
  abdomen 787.3
  chest 786.7
Typhlitis (*see also* Appendicitis) 541
Typhoenteritis 002.0
Typhogastric fever 002.0
Typhoid (abortive) (ambulant) (any site) (fever)
  (hemorrhagic) (infection) (intermittent)
  (malignant) (rheumatic) 002.0
  with pneumonia 002.0 *[484.8]*
  abdominal 002.0
  carrier (suspected) of V02.1
  cholecystitis (current) 002.0
  clinical (Widal and blood test negative) 002.0
  endocarditis 002.0 *[421.1]*
  inoculation reaction—*see* Complications,
    vaccination
  meningitis 002.0 *[320.7]*

Typhoid—*continued*
  mesenteric lymph nodes 002.0
  myocarditis 002.0 *[422.0]*
  osteomyelitis (*see also* Osteomyelitis, due to,
    typhoid) 002.0 *[730.8]*
  perichondritis, larynx 002.0 *[478.71]*
  pneumonia 002.0 *[484.8]*
  spine 002.0 *[720.81]*
  ulcer (perforating) 002.0
  vaccination, prophylactic (against) V03.1
  Widal negative 002.0
Typhomalaria (fever) (*see also* Malaria) 084.6
Typhomania 002.0
Typhoperitonitis 002.0
Typhus (fever) 081.9
  abdominal, abdominalis 002.0
  African tick 082.1
  amarillic (*see also* Fever, Yellow) 060.9
  brain 081.9
  cerebral 081.9
  classical 080
  endemic (flea-borne) 081.0
  epidemic (louse-borne) 080
  exanthematic NEC 080
  exanthematicus SAI 080
    brillii SAI 081.1
    Mexicanus SAI 081.0
    pediculo vestimenti causa 080
    typhus murinus 081.0
  flea-borne 081.0
  Indian tick 082.1
  Kenya tick 082.1
  louse-borne 080
  Mexican 081.0
    flea-borne 081.0
    louse-borne 080
    tabardillo 080
  mite-borne 081.2
  murine 081.0
  North Asian tick-borne 082.2
  petechial 081.9
  Queensland tick 082.3
  rat 081.0
  recrudescent 081.1
  recurrent (*see also* Fever, relapsing) 087.9
  São Paulo 082.0
  scrub (China) (India) (Malaya) (New Guinea)
    081.2
  shop (of Malaya) 081.0
  Siberian tick 082.2
  tick-borne NEC 082.9
  tropical 081.2
  vaccination, prophylactic (against) V05.8
Tyrosinemia 270.2
  neonatal 775.8
Tyrosinosis (Medes) (Sakai) 270.2
Tyrosinuria 270.2
Tyrosyluria 270.2

U

Uehlinger's syndrome (acropachyderma) 757.39
Uhl's anomaly or disease (hypoplasia of
    myocardium, right ventricle) 746.84
**Ulcer, ulcerated, ulcerating, ulceration, ulcera-
    tive** 707.9
  with gangrene 707.9 *[785.4]*
  abdomen (wall) (*see also* Ulcer, skin) 707.8
  ala, nose 478.1
  alveolar process 526.5
  amebic (intestine) 006.9
    skin 006.6
  anastomotic—*see* Ulcer, gastrojejunal
  anorectal 569.41
  antral—*see* Ulcer, stomach
  anus (sphincter) (solitary) 569.41
    varicose—*see* Varicose, ulcer, anus
  aphthous (oral) (recurrent) 528.2
    genital organ(s)
      female 616.8
      male 608.89
    mouth 528.2
  arm (*see also* Ulcer, skin) 707.8
  arteriosclerotic plaque—*see* Arteriosclerosis, by
    site
  artery NEC 447.2
    without rupture 447.8
  atrophic NEC—*see* Ulcer, skin
  Barrett's (chronic peptic ulcer of esophagus)
    530.2
  bile duct 576.8
  bladder (solitary) (sphincter) 596.8
    bilharzial (*see also* Schistosomiasis) 120.9
      [595.4]
    submucosal (*see also* Cystitis) 595.1
    tuberculous (*see also* Tuberculosis) 016.1
  bleeding NEC—*see* Ulcer, peptic, with
    hemorrhage
  bone 730.9
  bowel (*see also* Ulcer, intestine) 569.82
  breast 611.0
  bronchitis 491.8
  bronchus 519.1
  buccal (cavity) (traumatic) 528.9
  burn (acute)—*see* Ulcer, duodenum
  Buruli 031.1
  buttock (*see also* Ulcer, skin) 707.8
    decubitus (*see also* Ulcer, decubitus) 707.0
  cancerous (M8000/3)—*see* Neoplasm, by site,
    malignant
  cardia—*see* Ulcer, stomach
  cardio-esophageal (peptic) 530.2
  cecum (*see also* Ulcer, intestine) 569.82
  cervix (uteri) (trophic) 622.0
    with mention of cervicitis 616.0
  chancroidal 099.0
  chest (wall) (*see also* Ulcer, skin) 707.8
  Chiclero 085.4
  chin (pyogenic) (*see also* Ulcer, skin) 707.8
  chronic (cause unknown)—*see also* Ulcer, skin
    penis 607.89
  Cochin-China 085.1
  colitis —*see* Colitis, ulcerative
  colon (*see also* Ulcer, intestine) 569.82
  conjunctiva (acute) (postinfectional) 372.00

Ulcer, ulcerated, ulcerating—*continued*
  cornea (infectional) 370.00
    with perforation 370.06
    annular 370.02
    catarrhal 370.01
    central 370.03
    dendritic 054.42
    marginal 370.01
    mycotic 370.05
    phlyctenular, tuberculous (*see also*
      Tuberculosis) 017.3 *[370.31]*
    ring 370.02
    rodent 370.07
    serpent, serpiginous 370.04
    superficial marginal 370.01
    tuberculous (*see also* Tuberculosis) 017.3
      [370.31]
  corpus cavernosum (chronic) 607.89
  crural—*see* Ulcer, lower extremity
  Curling's—*see* Ulcer, duodenum
  Cushing's—*see* Ulcer, peptic
  cystitis (interstitial) 595.1
  decubitus (any site) 707.0
    with gangrene 707.0 *[785.4]*
  dendritic 054.42
  diabetes, diabetic (mellitus) 250.8 *[707.9]*
    lower limb 250.8 *[707.10]*
      ankle 250.8 *[707.13]*
      calf 250.8 *[707.12]*
      foot 250.8 *[707.15]*
      heel 250.8 *[707.14]*
      knee 250.8 *[707.19]*
      specified site NEC 250.8 *[707.19]*
      thigh 250.8 *[707.11]*
      toes 250.8 *[707.15]*
    specified site NEC 250.8 *[707.8]*
  Dieulafoy's—*see* Lesion, Dieulafoy
  due to
    infection NEC—*see* Ulcer, skin
    radiation, radium—*see* Ulcer, by site
    trophic disturbance (any region)—*see* Ulcer,
      skin
    x-ray—*see* Ulcer, by site
  duodenum, duodenal (eroded) (peptic) 532.9

> *Note—Use the following fifth-digit
> subclassification with categories 531-534:*
>
> *0 without mention of obstruction*
> *1 with obstruction*

    with
      hemorrhage (chronic) 532.4
        and perforation 532.6
      perforation (chronic) 532.5
        and hemorrhage 532.6
    acute 532.3
      with
        hemorrhage 532.0
          and perforation 532.2
        perforation 532.1
          and hemorrhage 532.2
    bleeding (recurrent)—*see* Ulcer, duodenum,
      with hemorrhage
    chronic 532.7
      with
        hemorrhage 532.4
          and perforation 532.6

> *Note—Use the following fifth-digit*
> *subclassification with categories 531-534:*
>
> *0 without mention of obstruction*
> *1 with obstruction*

Ulcer, ulcerated, ulcerating—*continued*
  lower extremity (atrophic) (chronic)
    (neurogenic) (perforating) (pyogenic)
    (trophic) (tropical) 707.10
    with gangrene (*see also* Ulcer, lower
      extremity) 707.10 *[785.4]*
      arteriosclerotic 440.24
    ankle 707.13
    arteriosclerotic 440.23
      with gangrene 440.24
    calf 707.12
    decubitus 707.0
      with gangrene 707.0 *[785.4]*
    foot 707.15
    heel 707.14
    knee 707.19
    specified site NEC 707.19
    thigh 707.11
    toes 707.15
    varicose 454.0
      inflamed or infected 454.2
  luetic—*see* Ulcer, syphilitic
  lung 518.89
    tuberculous (*see also* Tuberculosis) 011.2
  malignant (M8000/3)—*see* Neoplasm, by site,
    malignant
  marginal NEC—*see* Ulcer, gastrojejunal
  meatus (urinarius) 597.89
  Meckel's diverticulum 751.0
  Meleney's (chronic undermining) 686.09
  Mooren's (cornea) 370.07
  mouth (traumatic) 528.9
  mycobacterial (skin) 031.1
  nasopharynx 478.29
  navel cord (newborn) 771.4
  neck (*see also* Ulcer, skin) 707.8
    uterus 622.0
  neurogenic NEC—*see* Ulcer, skin
  nose, nasal (infectional) (passage) 478.1
    septum 478.1
      varicose 456.8
    skin—*see* Ulcer, skin
    spirochetal NEC 104.8
  oral mucosa (traumatic) 528.9
  palate (soft) 528.9
  penetrating NEC—*see* Ulcer, peptic, with
    perforation
  penis (chronic) 607.89
  peptic (site unspecified) 533.9

> *Note—Use the following fifth-digit*
> *subclassification with categories 531-534:*
>
> *0 without mention of obstruction*
> *1 with obstruction*

    with
      hemorrhage 533.4
        and perforation 533.6
      perforation (chronic) 533.5
        and hemorrhage 533.6
    acute 533.3
      with
        hemorrhage 533.0
          and perforation 533.2
        perforation 533.1
          and hemorrhage 533.2
    bleeding (recurrent)—*see* Ulcer, peptic, with
      hemorrhage

Ulcer, ulcerated, ulcerating—*continued*
  chronic 533.7
    with
      hemorrhage 533.4
        and perforation 533.6
      perforation 533.5
        and hemorrhage 533.6
  penetrating—*see* Ulcer, peptic, with
    perforation
  perforating NEC (*see also* Ulcer, peptic, with
    perforation) 533.5
    skin 707.9
  perineum (*see also* Ulcer, skin) 707.8
  peritonsillar 474.8
  phagedenic (tropical) NEC—*see* Ulcer, skin
  pharynx 478.29
  phlebitis—*see* Phlebitis
  plaster (*see also* Ulcer, decubitus) 707.0
  popliteal space—*see* Ulcer, lower extremity
  postpyloric—*see* Ulcer, duodenum
  prepuce 607.89
  prepyloric—*see* Ulcer, stomach
  pressure (*see also* Ulcer, decubitus) 707.0
  primary of intestine 569.82
    with perforation 569.83
  proctitis 556.2
    with ulcerative sigmoiditis 556.3
  prostate 601.8
  pseudopeptic—*see* Ulcer, peptic
  pyloric—*see* Ulcer, stomach
  rectosigmoid 569.82
    with perforation 569.83
  rectum (sphincter) (solitary) 569.41
    stercoraceous, stercoral 569.41
    varicose—*see* Varicose, ulcer, anus
  retina (*see also* Chorioretinitis) 363.20
  rodent (M8090/3)—*see also* Neoplasm, skin,
    malignant
    cornea 370.07
  round—*see* Ulcer, stomach
  sacrum (region) (*see also* Ulcer, skin) 707.8
  Saemisch's 370.04
  scalp (*see also* Ulcer, skin) 707.8
  sclera 379.09
  scrofulous (*see also* Tuberculosis) 017.2
  scrotum 608.89
    tuberculous (*see also* Tuberculosis) 016.5
    varicose 456.4
  seminal vesicle 608.89
  sigmoid 569.82
    with perforation 569.83
  skin (atrophic) (chronic) (neurogenic)
    (non-healing) (perforating) (pyogenic)
    (trophic) 707.9
    with gangrene 707.9 *[785.4]*
    amebic 006.6
    decubitus 707.0
      with gangrene 707.0 *[785.4]*
    in granulocytopenia 288.0
    lower extremity (*see also* Ulcer, lower
      extremity) 707.10
      with gangrene 707.10 *[785.4]*
        arteriosclerotic 440.24
      ankle 707.13
      arteriosclerotic 440.23
        with gangrene 440.24
      calf 707.12
      foot 707.15
      heel 707.14
      knee 707.19
      specified site NEC 707.19

Ulcer, ulcerated, ulcerating—*continued*
  thigh 707.11
  toes 707.15
  mycobacterial 031.1
  syphilitic (early) (secondary) 091.3
  tuberculous (primary) (*see also* Tuberculosis)
    017.0
  varicose—*see* Ulcer, varicose
 sloughing NEC—*see* Ulcer, skin
 soft palate 528.9
 solitary, anus or rectum (sphincter) 569.41
 sore throat 462
  streptococcal 034.0
 spermatic cord 608.89
 spine (tuberculous) 015.0 *[730.88]*
 stasis (leg) (venous) 454.0
  inflamed or infected 454.2
  without varicose veins 459.81
 stercoral, stercoraceous 569.82
  with perforation 569.83
  anus or rectum 569.41
 stoma, stomal—*see* Ulcer, gastrojejunal
 stomach (eroded) (peptic) (round) 531.9

> *Note—Use the following fifth-digit*
> *subclassification with categories 531-534:*
>
> *0 without mention of obstruction*
> *1 with obstruction*

  with
    hemorrhage 531.4
      and perforation 531.6
    perforation (chronic) 531.5
      and hemorrhage 531.6
  acute 531.3
    with
      hemorrhage 531.0
        and perforation 531.2
      perforation 531.1
        and hemorrhage 531.2
  bleeding (recurrent)—*see* Ulcer, stomach,
    with hemorrhage
  chronic 531.7
    with
      hemorrhage 531.4
        and perforation 531.6
      perforation 531.5
        and hemorrhage 531.6
  penetrating—*see* Ulcer, stomach, with
    perforation
  perforating—*see* Ulcer, stomach, with
    perforation
 stomatitis 528.0
 stress—*see* Ulcer, peptic
 strumous (tuberculous) (*see also* Tuberculosis)
   017.2
 submental (*see also* Ulcer, skin) 707.8
 submucosal, bladder 595.1
 syphilitic (any site) (early) (secondary) 091.3
  late 095.9
    perforating 095.9
      foot 094.0
 testis 608.89
 thigh—*see* Ulcer, lower extremity
 throat 478.29
  diphtheritic 032.0
 toe—*see* Ulcer, lower extremity
 tongue (traumatic) 529.0
 tonsil 474.8
  diphtheritic 032.0
 trachea 519.1

Ulcer, ulcerated, ulcerating—*continued*
  trophic—*see* Ulcer, skin
  tropical NEC (*see also* Ulcer, skin) 707.9
  tuberculous—*see* Tuberculosis, ulcer
  tunica vaginalis 608.89
  turbinate 730.9
  typhoid (fever) 002.0
    perforating 002.0
  umbilicus (newborn) 771.4
  unspecified site NEC—*see* Ulcer, skin
  urethra (meatus) (*see also* Urethritis) 597.89
  uterus 621.8
    cervix 622.0
      with mention of cervicitis 616.0
    neck 622.0
      with mention of cervicitis 616.0
  vagina 616.8
  valve, heart 421.0
  varicose (lower extremity, any part) 454.0
    anus—*see* Varicose, ulcer, anus
    broad ligament 456.5
    esophagus (*see also* Varix, esophagus) 456.1
      bleeding (*see also* Varix, esophagus,
        bleeding) 456.0
    inflamed or infected 454.2
    nasal septum 456.8
    perineum 456.6
    rectum—*see* Varicose, ulcer, anus
    scrotum 456.4
    specified site NEC 456.8
    sublingual 456.3
    vulva 456.6
  vas deferens 608.89
  vesical (*see also* Ulcer, bladder) 596.8
  vulva (acute) (infectional) 616.50
    Behçet's syndrome 136.1 *[616.51]*
    herpetic 054.12
    tuberculous 016.7 *[616.51]*
  vulvobuccal, recurring 616.50
  x-ray—*see* Ulcer, by site
  yaws 102.4
Ulcerosa scarlatina 034.1
Ulcus —*see also* Ulcer
  cutis tuberculosum (*see also* Tuberculosis) 017.0
  duodeni—*see* Ulcer, duodenum
  durum 091.0
    extragenital 091.2
  gastrojejunale—*see* Ulcer, gastrojejunal
  hypostaticum—*see* Ulcer, varicose
  molle (cutis) (skin) 099.0
  serpens cornea (pneumococcal) 370.04
  ventriculi—*see* Ulcer, stomach
Ulegyria 742.4
Ulerythema
  acneiforma 701.8
  centrifugum 695.4
  ophryogenes 757.4
Ullrich (-Bonnevie) (-Turner) syndrome 758.6
Ullrich-Feichtiger syndrome 759.89
Ulnar —*see* condition
Ulorrhagia 523.8
Ulorrhea 523.8
Umbilicus, umbilical —*see also* condition
  cord necrosis, affecting fetus or newborn 762.6
Unavailability of medical facilities (at) V63.9
  due to
    investigation by social service agency V63.8
    lack of services at home V63.1
    remoteness from facility V63.0
    waiting list V63.2
  home V63.1

Unavailability of medical facilities— *continued*
  outpatient clinic V63.0
  specified reason NEC V63.8
Uncinaria americana infestation 126.1
Uncinariasis (*see also* Ancylostomiasis) 126.9
Unconscious, unconsciousness 780.09
Underdevelopment —*see also* Undeveloped
  sexual 259.0
Undernourishment 269.9
Undernutrition 269.9
Under observation —*see* Observation
Underweight 783.22
  for gestational age—*see* Light-for-dates
Underwood's disease (sclerema neonatorum)
  778.1
Undescended —*see also* Malposition, congenital
  cecum 751.4
  colon 751.4
  testis 752.51
Undetermined diagnosis or cause 799.9
Undeveloped, undevelopment —*see also*
    Hypoplasia
  brain (congenital) 742.1
  cerebral (congenital) 742.1
  fetus or newborn 764.9
  heart 746.89
  lung 748.5
  testis 257.2
  uterus 259.0
Undiagnosed (disease) 799.9
Undulant fever (*see also* Brucellosis) 023.9
Unemployment, anxiety concerning V62.0
Unequal leg (acquired) (length) 736.81
  congenital 755.30
Unerupted teeth, tooth 520.6
Unextracted dental root 525.3
Unguis incarnatus 703.0
Unicornis uterus 752.3
Unicorporeus uterus 752.3
Uniformis uterus 752.3
Unilateral —*see also* condition
  development, breast 611.8
  organ or site, congenital NEC—*see* Agenesis
  vagina 752.49
Unilateralis uterus 752.3
Unilocular heart 745.8
Uninhibited (neurogenic) bladder 596.54
  with cauda equina syndrome 344.61
  neurogenic—*see* Neurogenic, bladder 596.54
Union, abnormal —*see also* Fusion
  divided tendon 727.89
  larynx and trachea 748.3
Universal
  joint, cervix 620.6
  mesentery 751.4
Unknown
  cause of death 799.9
  diagnosis 799.9
Unna's disease (seborrheic dermatitis) 690.10
Unresponsiveness, adrenocorticotropin
  (ACTH) 255.4
Unsoundness of mind (*see also* Psychosis) 298.9
Unspecified cause of death 799.9
Unstable
  back NEC 724.9
  colon 569.89
  joint—*see* Instability, joint
  lie 652.0
    affecting fetus or newborn (before labor) 761.7
    causing obstructed labor 660.0
      affecting fetus or newborn 763.1

Unstable—*continued*
  lumbosacral joint (congenital) 756.19
    acquired 724.6
  sacroiliac 724.6
  spine NEC 724.9
Untruthfulness, child problem (*see also*
  Disturbance, conduct) 312.0
Unverricht (-Lundborg) disease, syndrome, or
  epilepsy 333.2
Unverricht-Wagner syndrome
  (dermatomyositis) 710.3
Upper respiratory —*see* condition
Upset
  gastric 536.8
    psychogenic 306.4
  gastrointestinal 536.8
    psychogenic 306.4
    virus (*see also* Enteritis, viral) 008.8
  intestinal (large) (small) 564.9
    psychogenic 306.4
  menstruation 626.9
  mental 300.9
  stomach 536.8
    psychogenic 306.4
Urachus —*see also* condition
  patent 753.7
  persistent 753.7
Uratic arthritis 274.0
Urbach's lipoid proteinosis 272.8
Urbach-Oppenheim disease or syndrome
  (necrobiosis lipoidica diabeticorum) 250.8
  [709.3]
Urbach-Wiethe disease or syndrome (lipoid
  proteinosis) 272.8
Urban yellow fever 060.1
Urea, blood, high —*see* Uremia
Uremia, uremic (absorption) (amaurosis)
  (amblyopia) (aphasia) (apoplexy) (coma)
  (delirium) (dementia) (dropsy) (dyspnea)
  (fever) (intoxication) (mania) (paralysis)
  (poisoning) (toxemia) (vomiting) 586
  with
    abortion—*see* Abortion, by type, with renal
      failure
    ectopic pregnancy (*see also* categories
      633.0-633.9) 639.3
    hypertension (*see also* Hypertension, kidney)
      403.91
    molar pregnancy (*see also* categories
      630-632) 639.3
  chronic 585
  complicating
    abortion 639.3
    ectopic or molar pregnancy 639.3
    hypertension (*see also* Hypertension, kidney)
      403.91
    labor and delivery 669.3
  congenital 779.89
  extrarenal 788.9
  hypertensive (chronic) (*see also* Hypertension,
    kidney) 403.91
  maternal NEC, affecting fetus or newborn 760.1
  neuropathy 585 *[357.4]*
  pericarditis 585 *[420.0]*
  prerenal 788.9
  pyelitic (*see also* Pyelitis) 590.80
Ureter, ureteral —*see* condition
Ureteralgia 788.0
Ureterectasis 593.89

V

Vaccination
complication or reaction—*see* Complications, vaccination
not done (contraindicated) V64.0
  because of patient's decision V64.2
prophylactic (against) V05.9
  arthropod-borne viral
    disease NEC V05.1
    encephalitis V05.0
  chickenpox V05.4
  cholera (alone) V03.0
    with typhoid-paratyphoid (cholera + TAB) V06.0
  common cold V04.7
  diphtheria (alone) V03.5
    with
      poliomyelitis (DTP + polio) V06.3
      tetanus V06.5
        -pertussis combined [DTP] V06.1
      typhoid-paratyphoid (DTP + TAB) V06.2
  disease (single) NEC V05.9
    bacterial NEC V03.9
      specified type NEC V03.89
    combinations NEC V06.9
      specified type NEC V06.8
    specified type NEC V05.8
  encephalitis, viral, arthropod-borne V05.0
  Hemophilus influenzae, type B [Hib] V03.81
  hepatitis, viral V05.3
  influenza V04.8
    with
      Streptococcus pneumoniae [pneumococcus] V06.6
  lileishmaniasis V05.2
  measles (alone) V04.2
    with mumps-rubella (MMR) V06.4
  mumps (alone) V04.6
    with measles and rubella (MMR) V06.4
  pertussis alone V03.6
  plague V03.3
  poliomyelitis V04.0
    with diphtheria-tetanus-pertussis (DTP + polio) V06.3
  rabies V04.5
  rubella (alone) V04.3
    with measles and mumps (MMR) V06.4
  smallpox V04.1
  Streptococcus pneumoniae [pneumococcus] V03.82
    with
      influenza V06.6
  tetanus toxoid (alone) V03.7
    with diphtheria [Td] V06.5
      with
        pertussis (DTP) V06.1
          with poliomyelitis (DTP + polio) V06.3
  tuberculosis (BCG) V03.2
  tularemia V03.4
  typhoid-paratyphoid (TAB) (alone) V03.1
    with diphtheria-tetanus-pertussis (TAB + DTP) V06.2
  varicella V05.4
  viral
    encephalitis, arthropod-borne V05.0
    hepatitis V05.3
  yellow fever V04.4

Vaccinia (generalized) 999.0
congenital 771.2
conjunctiva 999.3
eyelids 999.0 *[373.5]*
localized 999.3
nose 999.3
not from vaccination 051.0
  eyelid 051.0 *[373.5]*
sine vaccinatione 051.0
without vaccination 051.0
Vacuum
extraction of fetus or newborn 763.3
in sinus (accessory) (nasal) (*see also* Sinusitis) 473.9
Vagabond V60.0
Vagabondage V60.0
Vagabonds' disease 132.1
Vagina, vaginal —*see* condition
Vaginalitis (tunica) 608.4
Vaginismus (reflex) 625.1
functional 306.51
hysterical 300.11
psychogenic 306.51
Vaginitis (acute) (chronic) (circumscribed) (diffuse) (emphysematous) (Hemophilus vaginalis) (nonspecific) (nonvenereal) (ulcerative) 616.10
with
  abortion—*see* Abortion, by type, with sepsis
  ectopic pregnancy (*see also* categories 633.0-633.9) 639.0
  molar pregnancy (*see also* categories 630-632) 639.0
adhesive, congenital 752.49
atrophic, postmenopausal 627.3
bacterial 616.10
blennorrhagic (acute) 098.0
  chronic or duration of 2 months or over 098.2
candidal 112.1
chlamydial 099.53
complicating pregnancy or puerperium 646.6
  affecting fetus or newborn 760.8
congenital (adhesive) 752.49
due to
  C. albicans 112.1
  Trichomonas (vaginalis) 131.01
following
  abortion 639.0
  ectopic or molar pregnancy 639.0
gonococcal (acute) 098.0
  chronic or duration of 2 months or over 098.2
granuloma 099.2
Monilia 112.1
mycotic 112.1
pinworm 127.4 *[616.11]*
postirradiation 616.10
postmenopausal atrophic 627.3
senile (atrophic) 627.3
syphilitic (early) 091.0
  late 095.8
trichomonal 131.01
tuberculous (*see also* Tuberculosis) 016.7
venereal NEC 099.8
Vaginosis —*see* Vaginitis
Vagotonia 352.3
Vagrancy V60.0
Vallecula —*see* condition
Valley fever 114.0

Valsuani's disease (progressive pernicious anemia, puerperal) 648.2
Valve, valvular (formation)—*see also* condition
  cerebral ventricle (communicating) in situ V45.2
  cervix, internal os 752.49
  colon 751.5
  congenital NEC—*see* Atresia
  formation, congenital NEC—*see* Atresia
  heart defect—*see* Anomaly, heart, valve
  ureter 753.29
    pelvic junction 753.21
    vesical orifice 753.22
  urethra 753.6
Valvulitis (chronic) (*see also* Endocarditis) 424.90
  rheumatic (chronic) (inactive) (with chorea) 397.9
    active or acute (aortic) (mitral) (pulmonary) (tricuspid) 391.1
  syphilitic NEC 093.20
    aortic 093.22
    mitral 093.21
    pulmonary 093.24
    tricuspid 093.23
Valvulopathy —*see* Endocarditis
van Bogaert's leukoencephalitis (sclerosing) (subacute) 046.2
van Bogaert-Nijssen (-Peiffer) disease 330.0
van Buchem's syndrome (hyperostosis corticalis) 733.3
van Creveld-von Gierke disease (glycogenosis I) 271.0
van den Bergh's disease (enterogenous cyanosis) 289.7
van der Hoeve's syndrome (brittle bones and blue sclera, deafness) 756.51
van der Hoeve-Halbertsma-Waardenburg syndrome (ptosis-epicanthus) 270.2
van der Hoeve-Waardenburg-Gualdi syndrome (ptosis epicanthus) 270.2
Vanillism 692.89
Vanishing lung 492.0
Vanishing twin 651.33
van Neck (-Odelberg) disease or syndrome (juvenile osteochondrosis) 732.1
Vapor asphyxia or suffocation NEC 987.9
  specified agent—*see* Table of drugs and chemicals
Vaquez's disease (M9950/1) 238.4
Vaquez-Osler disease (polycythemia vera) (M9950/1) 238.4
Variance, lethal ball, prosthetic heart valve 996.02
Variants, thalassemic 282.4
Variations in hair color 704.3
Varicella 052.9
  with
    complication 052.8
      specified NEC 052.7
    pneumonia 052.1
  vaccination and inoculation (prophylactic) V05.4
Varices —*see* Varix
Varicocele (scrotum) (thrombosed) 456.4
  ovary 456.5
  perineum 456.6
  spermatic cord (ulcerated) 456.4

Varicose
  aneurysm (ruptured) (*see also* Aneurysm) 442.9
  dermatitis (lower extremity)—*see* Varicose, vein, inflamed or infected
  eczema—*see* Varicose, vein
  phlebitis—*see* Varicose, vein, inflamed or infected
  placental vessel—*see* Placenta, abnormal
  tumor—*see* Varicose, vein
  ulcer (lower extremity, any part) 454.0
    anus 455.8
      external 455.5
      internal 455.2
    esophagus (*see also* Varix, esophagus) 456.1
      bleeding (*see also* Varix, esophagus, bleeding) 456.0
    inflamed or infected 454.2
    nasal septum 456.8
    perineum 456.6
    rectum—*see* Varicose, ulcer, anus
    scrotum 456.4
    specified site NEC 456.8
  vein (lower extremity) (ruptured) (*see also* Varix) 454.9
    with
      complications NEC 454.8
      edema 454.8
      inflammation or infection 454.1
        ulcerated 454.2
      pain 454.8
      stasis dermatitis 454.1
        with ulcer 454.2
      swelling 454.8
      ulcer 454.0
        inflamed or infected 454.2
    anus—*see* Hemorrhoids
    broad ligament 456.5
    congenital (peripheral) NEC 747.60
      gastrointestinal 747.61
      lower limb 747.64
      renal 747.62
      specified NEC 747.69
      upper limb 747.63
    esophagus (ulcerated) (*see also* Varix, esophagus) 456.1
      bleeding (*see also* Varix, esophagus, bleeding) 456.0
    inflamed or infected 454.1
      with ulcer 454.2
    in pregnancy or puerperium 671.0
      vulva or perineum 671.1
    nasal septum (with ulcer) 456.8
    pelvis 456.5
    perineum 456.6
      in pregnancy, childbirth, or puerperium 671.1
    rectum—*see* Hemorrhoids
    scrotum (ulcerated) 456.4
    specified site NEC 456.8
    sublingual 456.3
    ulcerated 454.0
      inflamed or infected 454.2
    umbilical cord, affecting fetus or newborn 762.6
    urethra 456.8
    vulva 456.6
      in pregnancy, childbirth, or puerperium 671.1
  vessel—*see also* Varix
    placenta—*see* Placenta, abnormal

Varicosis, varicosities, varicosity (*see also* Varix) 454.9
Variola 050.9
  hemorrhagic (pustular) 050.0
  major 050.0
  minor 050.1
  modified 050.2
Varioloid 050.2
Variolosa, purpura 050.0
Varix (lower extremity) (ruptured) 454.9
  with
    complications NEC 454.8
    edema 454.8
    inflammation or infection 454.1
      with ulcer 454.2
    pain 454.8
    stasis dermatitis 454.1
      with ulcer 454.2
    swelling 454.8
    ulcer 454.0
      with inflammation or infection 454.2
  aneurysmal (*see also* Aneurysm) 442.9
  anus—*see* Hemorrhoids
  arteriovenous (congenital) (peripheral) NEC
    747.60
    gastrointestinal 747.61
    lower limb 747.64
    renal 747.62
    specified NEC 747.69
    spinal 747.82
    upper limb 747.63
  bladder 456.5
  broad ligament 456.5
  congenital (peripheral) NEC 747.60
  esophagus (ulcerated) 456.1
    bleeding 456.0
      in
        cirrhosis of liver 571.5 *[456.20]*
        portal hypertension 572.3 *[456.20]*
    congenital 747.69
    in
      cirrhosis of liver 571.5 *[456.21]*
        with bleeding 571.5 *[456.20]*
      portal hypertension 572.3 *[456.21]*
        with bleeding 572.3 *[456.20]*
  gastric 456.8
  inflamed or infected 454.1
    ulcerated 454.2
  in pregnancy or puerperium 671.0
    perineum 671.1
    vulva 671.1
  labia (majora) 456.6
  orbit 456.8
    congenital 747.69
  ovary 456.5
  papillary 448.1
  pelvis 456.5
  perineum 456.6
    in pregnancy or puerperium 671.1
  pharynx 456.8
  placenta—*see* Placenta, abnormal
  prostate 456.8
  rectum—*see* Hemorrhoids
  renal papilla 456.8
  retina 362.17
  scrotum (ulcerated) 456.4
  sigmoid colon 456.8
  specified site NEC 456.8
  spinal (cord) (vessels) 456.8
  spleen, splenic (vein) (with phlebolith) 456.8
  sublingual 456.3

Varix—*continued*
  ulcerated 454.0
    inflamed or infected 454.2
  umbilical cord, affecting fetus or newborn 762.6
  uterine ligament 456.5
  vocal cord 456.8
  vulva 456.6
    in pregnancy, childbirth, or puerperium 671.1
Vasa previa 663.5
  affecting fetus or newborn 762.6
  hemorrhage from, affecting fetus or newborn
    772.0
Vascular —*see also* condition
  loop on papilla (optic) 743.57
  sheathing, retina 362.13
  spasm 443.9
  spider 448.1
Vascularity, pulmonary, congenital 747.3
Vascularization
  choroid 362.16
  cornea 370.60
    deep 370.63
    localized 370.61
  retina 362.16
  subretinal 362.16
Vasculitis 447.6
  allergic 287.0
  cryoglobulinemic 273.2
  disseminated 447.6
  kidney 447.8
  leukocytoclastic 446.29
  nodular 695.2
  retinal 362.18
  rheumatic—*see* Fever, rheumatic
Vas deferens —*see* condition
Vas deferentitis 608.4
Vasectomy, admission for V25.2
Vasitis 608.4
  nodosa 608.4
  scrotum 608.4
  spermatic cord 608.4
  testis 608.4
  tuberculous (*see also* Tuberculosis) 016.5
  tunica vaginalis 608.4
  vas deferens 608.4
Vasodilation 443.9
Vasomotor —*see* condition
Vasoplasty, after previous sterilization V26.0
Vasoplegia, splanchnic (*see also* Neuropathy,
  peripheral, autonomic) 337.9
Vasospasm 443.9
  cerebral (artery) 435.9
    with transient neurologic deficit 435.9
  nerve
    arm NEC 354.9
    autonomic 337.9
    brachial plexus 353.0
    cervical plexus 353.2
    leg NEC 355.8
    lower extremity NEC 355.8
    peripheral NEC 355.9
    spinal NEC 355.9
    sympathetic 337.9
    upper extremity NEC 354.9
  peripheral NEC 443.9
  retina (artery) (*see also* Occlusion, retinal,
    artery) 362.30
Vasospastic —*see* condition
Vasovagal attack (paroxysmal) 780.2
  psychogenic 306.2
Vater's ampulla —*see* condition
VATER syndrome 759.89

Vegetation, vegetative
  adenoid (nasal fossa) 474.2
  consciousness (persistent) 780.03
  endocarditis (acute) (any valve) (chronic)
      (subacute) 421.0
  heart (mycotic) (valve) 421.0
  state (persistent) 780.03
Veil
  Jackson's 751.4
  over face (causing asphyxia) 768.9
Vein, venous *—see* condition
Veldt sore (*see also* Ulcer, skin) 707.9
Velpeau's hernia *—see* Hernia, femoral
Venereal
  balanitis NEC 099.8
  bubo 099.1
  disease 099.9
    specified nature or type NEC 099.8
  granuloma inguinale 099.2
  lymphogranuloma (Durand-Nicolas-Favre), any
      site 099.1
  salpingitis 098.37
  urethritis (*see also* Urethritis, nongonococcal)
      099.40
  vaginitis NEC 099.8
  warts 078.19
Vengefulness, in child (*see also* Disturbance,
    conduct) 312.0
Venofibrosis 459.89
Venom, venomous
  bite or sting (animal or insect) 989.5
  poisoning 989.5
Venous *—see* condition
Ventouse delivery NEC 669.5
  affecting fetus or newborn 763.3
Ventral *—see* condition
Ventricle, ventricular *—see also* condition
  escape 427.69
  standstill (*see also* Arrest, cardiac) 427.5
Ventriculitis, cerebral (*see also* Meningitis)
    322.9
Ventriculostomy status V45.2
Verbiest's syndrome (claudicatio intermittens
    spinalis) 435.1
Vernet's syndrome 352.6
Verneuil's disease (syphilitic bursitis) 095.7
Verruca (filiformis) 078.10
  acuminata (any site) 078.11
  necrogenica (primary) (*see also* Tuberculosis)
      017.0
  peruana 088.0
  peruviana 088.0
  plana (juvenilis) 078.19
  plantaris 078.19
  seborrheica 702.19
    inflamed 702.11
  senilis 702.0
  tuberculosa (primary) (*see also* Tuberculosis)
      017.0
  venereal 078.19
  viral NEC 078.10
Verrucosities (*see also* Verruca) 078.10
Verrucous endocarditis (acute) (any valve)
    (chronic) (subacute) 710.0 *[424.91]*
  nonbacterial 710.0 *[424.91]*
Verruga
  peruana 088.0
  peruviana 088.0
Verse's disease (calcinosis intervertebralis)
    275.49 *[722.90]*

Version
  before labor, affecting fetus or newborn 761.7
  cephalic (correcting previous malposition) 652.1
    affecting fetus or newborn 763.1
  cervix (*see also* Malposition, uterus) 621.6
  uterus (postinfectional) (postpartal, old) (*see
      also* Malposition, uterus) 621.6
    forward—*see* Anteversion, uterus
    lateral—*see* Lateroversion, uterus
Vertebra, vertebral *—see* condition
Vertigo 780.4
  auditory 386.19
  aural 386.19
  benign paroxysmal positional 386.11
  central origin 386.2
  cerebral 386.2
  Dix and Hallpike (epidemic) 386.12
  endemic paralytic 078.81
  epidemic 078.81
    Dix and Hallpike 386.12
    Gerlier's 078.81
    Pedersen's 386.12
    vestibular neuronitis 386.12
  epileptic—*see* Epilepsy
  Gerlier's (epidemic) 078.81
  hysterical 300.11
  labyrinthine 386.10
  laryngeal 786.2
  malignant positional 386.2
  Ménière's (*see also* Disease, Ménière's) 386.00
  menopausal 627.2
  otogenic 386.19
  paralytic 078.81
  paroxysmal positional, benign 386.11
  Pedersen's (epidemic) 386.12
  peripheral 386.10
    specified type NEC 386.19
  positional
    benign paroxysmal 386.11
    malignant 386.2
Verumontanitis (chronic) (*see also* Urethritis)
    597.89
Vesania (*see also* Psychosis) 298.9
Vesical *—see* condition
Vesicle
  cutaneous 709.8
  seminal—*see* condition
  skin 709.8
Vesicocolic *—see* condition
Vesicoperineal *—see* condition
Vesicorectal *—see* condition
Vesicourethrorectal *—see* condition
Vesicovaginal *—see* condition
Vesicular *—see* condition
Vesiculitis (seminal) 608.0
  amebic 006.8
  gonorrheal (acute) 098.14
    chronic or duration of 2 months or over 098.34
  trichomonal 131.09
  tuberculous (*see also* Tuberculosis) 016.5
    [608.81]
Vestibulitis (ear) (*see also* Labyrinthitis) 386.30
  nose (external) 478.1
  vulvar 616.10
Vestibulopathy, acute peripheral (recurrent)
    386.12
Vestige, vestigial *—see also* Persistence
  branchial 744.41
  structures in vitreous 743.51
Vibriosis NEC 027.9
Vidal's disease (lichen simplex chronicus) 698.3
Video display tube syndrome 723.8

W

Waardenburg's syndrome 756.89
  meaning ptosis-epicanthus 270.2
Waardenburg-Klein syndrome
    (ptosis-epicanthus) 270.2
Wagner's disease (colloid milium) 709.3
Wagner (-Unverricht) syndrome
    (dermatomyositis) 710.3
Waiting list, person on V63.2
  undergoing social agency investigation V63.8
Wakefulness disorder (*see also* Hypersomnia)
    780.54
  nonorganic origin 307.43
Waldenström's
  disease (osteochondrosis, capital femoral) 732.1
  hepatitis (lupoid hepatitis) 571.49
  hypergammaglobulinemia 273.0
  macroglobulinemia 273.3
  purpura, hypergammaglobulinemic 273.0
  syndrome (macroglobulinemia) 273.3
Waldenström-Kjellberg syndrome (sideropenic
    dysphagia) 280.8
Walking
  difficulty 719.7
    psychogenic 307.9
  sleep 307.46
    hysterical 300.13
Wall, abdominal —*see* condition
Wallenberg's syndrome (posterior inferior
    cerebellar artery) (*see also* Disease,
    cerebrovascular, acute) 436
Wallgren's
  disease (obstruction of splenic vein with
      collateral circulation) 459.89
  meningitis (*see also* Meningitis, aseptic) 047.9
Wandering
  acetabulum 736.39
  gallbladder 751.69
  kidney, congenital 753.3
  organ or site, congenital NEC—*see*
      Malposition, congenital
  pacemaker (atrial) (heart) 427.89
  spleen 289.59
Wardrop's disease (with lymphangitis) 681.9
  finger 681.02
  toe 681.11
War neurosis 300.16
Wart (common) (digitate) (filiform) (infectious)
    (juvenile) (plantar) (viral) 078.10
  external genital organs (venereal) 078.19
  fig 078.19
  Hassall-Henle's (of cornea) 371.41
  Henle's (of cornea) 371.41
  juvenile 078.19
  moist 078.10
  Peruvian 088.0
  plantar 078.19
  prosector (*see also* Tuberculosis) 017.0
  seborrheic 702.19
    inflamed 702.11
  senile 702.0
  specified NEC 078.19
  syphilitic 091.3
  tuberculous (*see also* Tuberculosis) 017.0
  venereal (female) (male) 078.19
Warthin's tumor (salivary gland) (M8561/0)
    210.2
Washerwoman's itch 692.4

Wassilieff's disease (leptospiral jaundice) 100.0
Wasting
  disease 799.4
    due to malnutrition 261
  extreme (due to malnutrition) 261
  muscular NEC 728.2
  palsy, paralysis 335.21
Water
  clefts 366.12
  deprivation of 994.3
  in joint (*see also* Effusion, joint) 719.0
  intoxication 276.6
  itch 120.3
  lack of 994.3
  loading 276.6
  on
    brain—*see* Hydrocephalus
    chest 511.8
  poisoning 276.6
Waterbrash 787.1
Water-hammer pulse (*see also* Insufficiency,
    aortic) 424.1
Waterhouse (-Friderichsen) disease or syndrome
    036.3
Water-losing nephritis 588.8
Wax in ear 380.4
Waxy
  degeneration, any site 277.3
  disease 277.3
  kidney 277.3 [583.81]
  liver (large) 277.3
  spleen 277.3
Weak, weakness (generalized) 780.79
  arches (acquired) 734
    congenital 754.61
  bladder sphincter 596.59
  congenital 779.89
  eye muscle—*see* Strabismus
  foot (double)—*see* Weak, arches
  heart, cardiac (*see also* Failure, heart) 428.9
    congenital 746.9
  mind 317
  muscle 728.9
  myocardium (*see also* Failure, heart) 428.9
  newborn 779.89
  pelvic fundus 618.8
  pulse 785.9
  senile 797
  valvular—*see* Endocarditis
Wear, worn, tooth, teeth (approximal) (hard
    tissues) (interproximal) (occlusal) 521.1
Weather, weathered
  effects of
    cold NEC 991.9
      specified effect NEC 991.8
    hot (*see also* Heat) 992.9
  skin 692.74
Web, webbed (congenital)—*see also* Anomaly,
    specified type NEC
  canthus 743.63
  digits (*see also* Syndactylism) 755.10
  esophagus 750.3
  fingers (*see also* Syndactylism, fingers) 755.11
  larynx (glottic) (subglottic) 748.2
  neck (pterygium colli) 744.5
  Paterson-Kelly (sideropenic dysphagia) 280.8
  popliteal syndrome 756.89
  toes (*see also* Syndactylism, toes) 755.13

Note—For fracture with open wound, see Fracture. For laceration, traumatic rupture, tear or penetrating wound of internal organs, such as heart, lung, liver, kidney, pelvic organs, etc., whether or not accompanied by open wound or fracture in the same region, see Injury, internal. For contused wound, see Contusion. For crush injury, see Crush. For abrasion, insect bite (nonvenomous), blister, or scratch, see Injury, superficial.

Complicated includes wounds with:
delayed healing
delayed treatment
foreign body
primary infection

For late effect of open wound, see Late, effect, wound, open, by site.

Wound, open—*continued*
  intracranial—*see* Injury, intracranial, with open
    intracranial wound
  intraocular 871.9
    with
      partial loss (of intraocular tissue) 871.2
      prolapse or exposure (of intraocular tissue)
        871.1
    laceration (*see also* Laceration, eyeball) 871.4
    penetrating 871.7
      with foreign body (nonmagnetic) 871.6
        magnetic 871.5
    without prolapse (of intraocular tissue) 871.0
  iris (*see also* Wound, open, eyeball) 871.9
  jaw (fracture not involved) 873.44
    with fracture—*see* Fracture, jaw
    complicated 873.54
  knee 891.0
    with tendon involvement 891.2
    complicated 891.1
  labium (majus) (minus) 878.4
    complicated 878.5
  lacrimal apparatus, gland, or sac 870.8
    with laceration of eyelid 870.2
  larynx 874.01
    with trachea 874.00
      complicated 874.10
    complicated 874.11
  leg (multiple) 891.0
    with tendon involvement 891.2
    complicated 891.1
    lower 891.0
      with tendon involvement 891.2
      complicated 891.1
    thigh 890.0
      with tendon involvement 890.2
      complicated 890.1
    upper 890.0
      with tendon involvement 890.2
      complicated 890.1
  lens (eye) (alone) (*see also* Cataract, traumatic)
    366.20
    with involvement of other eye structures—*see*
      Wound, open, eyeball
  limb
    lower (multiple) NEC 894.0
      with tendon involvement 894.2
      complicated 894.1
    upper (multiple) NEC 884.0
      with tendon involvement 884.2
      complicated 884.1
  lip 873.43
    complicated 873.53
  loin 876.0
    complicated 876.1
  lumbar region 876.0
    complicated 876.1
  malar region 873.41
    complicated 873.51
  mastoid region 873.49
    complicated 873.59
  mediastinum—*see* Injury, internal, mediastinum
  midthoracic region 875.0
    complicated 875.1
  mouth 873.60
    complicated 873.70
    floor 873.64
      complicated 873.74
    multiple sites 873.69
      complicated 873.79

Wound, open—*continued*
  specified site NEC 873.69
    complicated 873.79
  multiple, unspecified site(s) 879.8

> *Note—Multiple open wounds of sites classifiable to the same four-digit category should be classified to that category unless they are in different limbs.*
>
> *Multiple open wounds of sites classifiable to different four-digit categories, or to different limbs, should be coded separately.*

    complicated 879.9
    lower limb(s) (one or both) (sites classifiable
      to more than one three-digit category in
      890 to 893) 894.0
      with tendon involvement 894.2
      complicated 894.1
    upper limb(s) (one or both) (sites classifiable
      to more than one three-digit category in
      880 to 883) 884.0
      with tendon involvement 884.2
      complicated 884.1
  muscle—*see* Sprain, by site
  nail
    finger(s) 883.0
      complicated 883.1
    thumb 883.0
      complicated 883.1
    toe(s) 893.0
      complicated 893.1
  nape (neck) 874.8
    complicated 874.9
    specified part NEC 874.8
      complicated 874.9
  nasal—*see also* Wound, open, nose
    cavity 873.22
      complicated 873.32
    septum 873.21
      complicated 873.31
    sinuses 873.23
      complicated 873.33
  nasopharynx 873.22
    complicated 873.32
  neck 874.8
    complicated 874.9
    nape 874.8
      complicated 874.9
    specified part NEC 874.8
      complicated 874.9
  nerve—*see* Injury, nerve, by site
  non-healing surgical 998.83
  nose 873.20
    complicated 873.30
    multiple sites 873.29
      complicated 873.39
    septum 873.21
      complicated 873.31
    sinuses 873.23
      complicated 873.33
  occipital region—*see* Wound, open, scalp
  ocular NEC 871.9
    adnexa 870.9
      specified region NEC 870.8
    laceration (*see also* Laceration, ocular) 871.4
    muscle (extraocular) 870.3
      with foreign body 870.4
      eyelid 870.1
    intraocular—*see* Wound, open, eyeball

X

Y

Yawning 786.09
  psychogenic 306.1
Yaws 102.9
  bone or joint lesions 102.6
  butter 102.1
  chancre 102.0
  cutaneous, less than five years after infection
      102.2
  early (cutaneous) (macular) (maculopapular)
      (micropapular) (papular) 102.2
    frambeside 102.2
    skin lesions NEC 102.2
  eyelid 102.9 [373.4]
  ganglion 102.6
  gangosis, gangosa 102.5
  gumma, gummata 102.4
    bone 102.6
  gummatous
    frambeside 102.4
    osteitis 102.6
    periostitis 102.6
  hydrarthrosis 102.6
  hyperkeratosis (early) (late) (palmar) (plantar)
      102.3
  initial lesions 102.0
  joint lesions 102.6
  juxta-articular nodules 102.7
  late nodular (ulcerated) 102.4
  latent (without clinical manifestations) (with
      positive serology) 102.8
  mother 102.0
  mucosal 102.7
  multiple papillomata 102.1
  nodular, late (ulcerated) 102.4
  osteitis 102.6
  papilloma, papillomata (palmar) (plantar) 102.1
  periostitis (hypertrophic) 102.6
  ulcers 102.4
  wet crab 102.1
Yeast infection (*see also* Candidiasis) 112.9
Yellow
  atrophy (liver) 570
    chronic 571.8
    resulting from administration of blood,
        plasma, serum, or other biological
        substance (within 8 months of
        administration)—*see* Hepatitis, viral
  fever—*see* Fever, yellow
  jack (*see also* Fever, yellow) 060.9
  jaundice (*see also* Jaundice) 782.4
Yersinia septica 027.8

Z

Zagari's disease (xerostomia) 527.7
Zahorsky's disease (exanthema subitum) 057.8
  syndrome (herpangina) 074.0
Zenker's diverticulum (esophagus) 530.6
Ziehen-Oppenheim disease 333.6
Zieve's syndrome (jaundice, hyperlipemia, and
    hemolytic anemia) 571.1
Zika fever 066.3
Zollinger-Ellison syndrome (gastric
    hypersecretion with pancreatic islet cell
    tumor) 251.5
Zona (*see also* Herpes, zoster) 053.9
Zoophilia (erotica) 302.1
Zoophobia 300.29
Zoster (herpes) (*see also* Herpes, zoster) 053.9
Zuelzer (-Ogden) anemia or syndrome
    (nutritional megaloblastic anemia) 281.2
Zygodactyly (*see also* Syndactylism) 755.10
Zygomycosis 117.7
Zymotic —*see* condition

SECTION 2

ALPHABETIC INDEX TO POISONING AND EXTERNAL CAUSES OF ADVERSE EFFECTS OF DRUGS AND OTHER CHEMICAL SUBSTANCES

TABLE OF DRUGS AND CHEMICALS

This table contains a classification of drugs and other chemical substances to identify poisoning states and external causes of adverse effects.

Each of the listed substances in the table is assigned a code according to the poisoning classification (960–989). These codes are used when there is a statement of poisoning, overdose, wrong substance given or taken, or intoxication.

The table also contains a listing of external causes of adverse effects. An adverse effect is a pathologic manifestation due to ingestion or exposure to drugs or other chemical substances (e.g., dermatitis, hypersensitivity reaction, aspirin gastritis). The adverse effect is to be identified by the appropriate code found in Section 1, Index to Diseases and Injuries. An external cause code can then be used to identify the circumstances involved. The table headings pertaining to external causes are defined below:

> **Accidental poisoning (E850–E869)**—accidental overdose of drug, wrong substance given or taken, drug taken inadvertently, accidents in the usage of drugs and biologicals in medical and surgical procedures, and to show external causes of poisonings classifiable to 980–989.

> **Therapeutic use (E930–E949)**—a correct substance properly administered in therapeutic or prophylactic dosage as the external cause of adverse effects.

> **Suicide attempt (E950–E952)**—instances in which self–inflicted injuries or poisonings are involved.

> **Assault (E961–E962)**—injury or poisoning inflicted by another person with the intent to injure or kill.

> **Undetermined (E980–E982)**—to be used when the intent of the poisoning or injury cannot be determined whether it was intentional or accidental.

The American Hospital Formulary Service list numbers are included in the table to help classify new drugs not identified in the table by name. The AHFS list numbers are keyed to the continually revised American Hospital Formulary Service (AHFS).* These listings are found in the table under the main term **Drug**.

Excluded from the table are radium and other radioactive substances. The classification of adverse effects and complications pertaining to these substances will be found in Section 1, Index to Diseases and Injuries, and Section 3, Index to External Causes of Injuries.

Although certain substances are indexed with one or more subentries, the majority are listed according to one use or state. It is recognized that many substances may be used in various ways, in medicine and in industry, and may cause adverse effects whatever the state of the agent (solid, liquid, or fumes arising from a liquid). In cases in which the reported data indicates a use or state not in the table, or which is clearly different from the one listed, an attempt should be made to classify the substance in the form which most nearly expresses the reported facts.

---

*American Hospital Formulary Service, 2 vol. (Washington, DC: American Society of Hospital Pharmacists, 1959-)

Substance	Poisoning	External Cause (E-Code)				
		Accident	Therapeutic Use	Suicide Attempt	Assault	Undetermined
1–propanol	980.3	E860.4	—	E950.9	E962.1	E980.9
2–propanol	980.2	E860.3	—	E950.9	E962.1	E980.9
2, 4–D (dichlorophenoxyacetic acid)	989.4	E863.5	—	E950.6	E962.1	E980.7
2, 4–toluene diisocyanate	983.0	E864.0	—	E950.7	E962.1	E980.6
2, 4, 5–T (trichlorophenoxyacetic acid)	989.2	E863.5	—	E950.6	E962.1	E980.7
14–hydroxydihydromorphinone	965.09	E850.2	E935.2	E950.0	E962.0	E980.0
ABOB	961.7	E857	E931.7	E950.4	E962.0	E980.4
Abrus (seed)	988.2	E865.3	—	E950.9	E962.1	E980.9
Absinthe	980.0	E860.1	—	E950.9	E962.1	E980.9
beverage	980.0	E860.0	—	E950.9	E962.1	E980.9
Acenocoumarin, acenocoumarol	964.2	E858.2	E934.2	E950.4	E962.0	E980.4
Acepromazine	969.1	E853.0	E939.1	E950.3	E962.0	E980.3
Acetal	982.8	E862.4	—	E950.9	E962.1	E980.9
Acetaldehyde (vapor)	987.8	E869.8	—	E952.8	E962.2	E982.8
liquid	989.89	E866.8	—	E950.9	E962.1	E980.9
Acetaminophen	965.4	E850.4	E935.4	E950.0	E962.0	E980.0
Acetaminosalol	965.1	E850.3	E935.3	E950.0	E962.0	E980.0
Acetanilid(e)	965.4	E850.4	E935.4	E950.0	E962.0	E980.0
Acetarsol, acetarsone	961.1	E857	E931.1	E950.4	E962.0	E980.4
Acetazolamide	974.2	E858.5	E944.2	E950.4	E962.0	E980.4
Acetic						
acid	983.1	E864.1	—	E950.7	E962.1	E980.6
with sodium acetate (ointment)	976.3	E858.7	E946.3	E950.4	E962.0	E980.4
irrigating solution	974.5	E858.5	E944.5	E950.4	E962.0	E980.4
lotion	976.2	E858.7	E946.2	E950.4	E962.0	E980.4
anhydride	983.1	E864.1	—	E950.7	E962.1	E980.6
ether (vapor)	982.8	E862.4	—	E950.9	E962.1	E980.9
Acetohexamide	962.3	E858.0	E932.3	E950.4	E962.0	E980.4
Acetomenaphthone	964.3	E858.2	E934.3	E950.4	E962.0	E980.4
Acetomorphine	965.01	E850.0	E935.0	E950.0	E962.0	E980.0
Acetone (oils) (vapor)	982.8	E862.4	—	E950.9	E962.1	E980.9
Acetophenazine (maleate)	969.1	E853.0	E939.1	E950.3	E962.0	E980.3
Acetophenetidin	965.4	E850.4	E935.4	E950.0	E962.0	E980.0
Acetophenone	982.0	E862.4	—	E950.9	E962.1	E980.9
Acetorphine	965.09	E850.2	E935.2	E950.0	E962.0	E980.0
Acetosulfone (sodium)	961.8	E857	E931.8	E950.4	E962.0	E980.4
Acetrizoate (sodium)	977.8	E858.8	E947.8	E950.4	E962.0	E980.4
Acetylcarbromal	967.3	E852.2	E937.3	E950.2	E962.0	E980.2
Acetylcholine (chloride)	971.0	E855.3	E941.0	E950.4	E962.0	E980.4
Acetylcysteine	975.5	E858.6	E945.5	E950.4	E962.0	E980.4
Acetyldigitoxin	972.1	E858.3	E942.1	E950.4	E962.0	E980.4
Acetyldihydrocodeine	965.09	E850.2	E935.2	E950.0	E962.0	E980.0
Acetyldihydrocodeinone	965.09	E850.2	E935.2	E950.0	E962.0	E980.0
Acetylene (gas) (industrial)	987.1	E868.1	—	E951.8	E962.2	E981.8
incomplete combustion of — *see* Carbon monoxide, fuel, utility						
tetrachloride (vapor)	982.3	E862.4	—	E950.9	E962.1	E980.9
Acetyliodosalicylic acid	965.1	E850.3	E935.3	E950.0	E962.0	E980.0
Acetylphenylhydrazine	965.8	E850.8	E935.8	E950.0	E962.0	E980.0
Acetylsalicylic acid	965.1	E850.3	E935.3	E950.0	E962.0	E980.0
Achromycin	960.4	E856	E930.4	E950.4	E962.0	E980.4
ophthalmic preparation	976.5	E858.7	E946.5	E950.4	E962.0	E980.4
topical NEC	976.0	E858.7	E946.0	E950.4	E962.0	E980.4
Acidifying agents	963.2	E858.1	E933.2	E950.4	E962.0	E980.4
Acids (corrosive) NEC	983.1	E864.1	—	E950.7	E962.1	E980.6
Aconite (wild)	988.2	E865.4	—	E950.9	E962.1	E980.9
Aconitine (liniment)	976.8	E858.7	E946.8	E950.4	E962.0	E980.4

Substance	Poisoning	External Cause (E-Code)				
		Accident	Therapeutic Use	Suicide Attempt	Assault	Undetermined
Aconitum ferox	988.2	E865.4	—	E950.9	E962.1	E980.9
Acridine	983.0	E864.0	—	E950.7	E962.1	E980.6
vapor	987.8	E869.8	—	E952.8	E962.2	E982.8
Acriflavine	961.9	E857	E931.9	E950.4	E962.0	E980.4
Acrisorcin	976.0	E858.7	E946.0	E950.4	E962.0	E980.4
Acrolein (gas)	987.8	E869.8	—	E952.8	E962.2	E982.8
liquid	989.89	E866.8	—	E950.9	E962.1	E980.9
Actaea spicata	988.2	E865.4	—	E950.9	E962.1	E980.9
Acterol	961.5	E857	E931.5	E950.4	E962.0	E980.4
ACTH	962.4	E858.0	E932.4	E950.4	E962.0	E980.4
Acthar	962.4	E858.0	E932.4	E950.4	E962.0	E980.4
Actinomycin (C) (D)	960.7	E856	E930.7	E950.4	E962.0	E980.4
Adalin (acetyl)	967.3	E852.2	E937.3	E950.2	E962.0	E980.2
Adenosine (phosphate)	977.8	E858.8	E947.8	E950.4	E962.0	E980.4
Adhesives	989.89	E866.6	—	E950.9	E962.1	E980.9
ADH	962.5	E858.0	E932.5	E950.4	E962.0	E980.4
Adicillin	960.0	E856	E930.0	E950.4	E962.0	E980.4
Adiphenine	975.1	E855.6	E945.1	E950.4	E962.0	E980.4
Adjunct, pharmaceutical	977.4	E858.8	E947.4	E950.4	E962.0	E980.4
Adrenal (extract, cortex or medulla) (glucocorticoids) (hormones) (mineralocorticoids)	962.0	E858.0	E932.0	E950.4	E962.0	E980.4
ENT agent	976.6	E858.7	E946.6	E950.4	E962.0	E980.4
ophthalmic preparation	976.5	E858.7	E946.5	E950.4	E962.0	E980.4
topical NEC	976.0	E858.7	E946.0	E950.4	E962.0	E980.4
Adrenalin	971.2	E855.5	E941.2	E950.4	E962.0	E980.4
Adrenergic blocking agents	971.3	E855.6	E941.3	E950.4	E962.0	E980.4
Adrenergics	971.2	E855.5	E941.2	E950.4	E962.0	E980.4
Adrenochrome (derivatives)	972.8	E858.3	E942.8	E950.4	E962.0	E980.4
Adrenocorticotropic hormone	962.4	E858.0	E932.4	E950.4	E962.0	E980.4
Adrenocorticotropin	962.4	E858.0	E932.4	E950.4	E962.0	E980.4
Adriamycin	960.7	E856	E930.7	E950.4	E962.0	E980.4
Aerosol spray — *see* Sprays						
Aerosporin	960.8	E856	E930.8	E950.4	E962.0	E980.4
ENT agent	976.6	E858.7	E946.6	E950.4	E962.0	E980.4
ophthalmic preparation	976.5	E858.7	E946.5	E950.4	E962.0	E980.4
topical NEC	976.0	E858.7	E946.0	E950.4	E962.0	E980.4
Aethusa cynapium	988.2	E865.4	—	E950.9	E962.1	E980.9
Afghanistan black	969.6	E854.1	E939.6	E950.3	E962.0	E980.3
Aflatoxin	989.7	E865.9	—	E950.9	E962.1	E980.9
African boxwood	988.2	E865.4	—	E950.9	E962.1	E980.9
Agar (–agar)	973.3	E858.4	E943.3	E950.4	E962.0	E980.4
Agricultural agent NEC	989.89	E863.9	—	E950.6	E962.1	E980.7
Agrypnal	967.0	E851	E937.0	E950.1	E962.0	E980.1
Air contaminant(s), source or type not specified	987.9	E869.9	—	E952.9	E962.2	E982.9
specified type — *see* specific substance						
Akee	988.2	E865.4	—	E950.9	E962.1	E980.9
Akrinol	976.0	E858.7	E946.0	E950.4	E962.0	E980.4
Alantolactone	961.6	E857	E931.6	E950.4	E962.0	E980.4
Albamycin	960.8	E856	E930.8	E950.4	E962.0	E980.4
Albumin (normal human serum)	964.7	E858.2	E934.7	E950.4	E962.0	E980.4
Albuterol	975.7	E858.6	E945.7	E950.4	E962.0	E980.4
Alcohol	980.9	E860.9	—	E950.9	E962.1	E980.9
absolute	980.0	E860.1	—	E950.9	E962.1	E980.9
beverage	980.0	E860.0	E947.8	E950.9	E962.1	E980.9
amyl	980.3	E860.4	—	E950.9	E962.1	E980.9

Substance	Poisoning	External Cause (E-Code)				
		Accident	Therapeutic Use	Suicide Attempt	Assault	Undetermined
antifreeze	980.1	E860.2	—	E950.9	E962.1	E980.9
butyl	980.3	E860.4	—	E950.9	E962.1	E980.9
dehydrated	980.0	E860.1	—	E950.9	E862.1	E980.9
beverage	980.0	E860.0	E947.8	E950.9	E962.1	E980.9
denatured	980.0	E860.1	—	E950.9	E962.1	E980.9
deterrents	977.3	E858.8	E947.3	E950.4	E962.0	E980.4
diagnostic (gastric function)	977.8	E858.8	E947.8	E950.4	E962.0	E980.4
ethyl	980.0	E860.1	—	E950.9	E962.1	E980.9
beverage	980.0	E860.0	E947.8	E950.9	E962.1	E980.9
grain	980.0	E860.1	—	E950.9	E962.1	E980.9
beverage	980.0	E860.0	E947.8	E950.9	E962.1	E980.9
industrial	980.9	E860.9	—	E950.9	E962.1	E980.9
isopropyl	980.2	E860.3	—	E950.9	E962.1	E980.9
methyl	980.1	E860.2	—	E950.9	E962.1	E980.9
preparation for consumption	980.0	E860.0	E947.8	E950.9	E962.1	E980.9
propyl	980.3	E860.4	—	E950.9	E962.1	E980.9
secondary	980.2	E860.3	—	E950.9	E962.1	E980.9
radiator	980.1	E860.2	—	E950.9	E962.1	E980.9
rubbing	980.2	E860.3	—	E950.9	E962.1	E980.9
specified type NEC	980.8	E860.8	—	E950.9	E962.1	E980.9
surgical	980.9	E860.9	—	E950.9	E962.1	E980.9
vapor (from any type of alcohol)	987.8	E869.8	—	E952.8	E962.2	E982.8
wood	980.1	E860.2	—	E950.9	E962.1	E980.9
Alcuronium chloride	975.2	E858.6	E945.2	E950.4	E962.0	E980.4
Aldactone	974.4	E858.5	E944.4	E950.4	E962.0	E980.4
Aldicarb	989.3	E863.2	—	E950.6	E962.1	E980.7
Aldomet	972.6	E858.3	E942.6	E950.4	E962.0	E980.4
Aldosterone	962.0	E858.0	E932.0	E950.4	E962.0	E980.4
Aldrin (dust)	989.2	E863.0	—	E950.6	E962.1	E980.7
Algeldrate	973.0	E858.4	E943.0	E950.4	E962.0	E980.4
Alidase	963.4	E858.1	E933.4	E950.4	E962.0	E980.4
Aliphatic thiocyanates	989.0	E866.8	—	E950.9	E962.1	E980.9
Alkaline antiseptic solution (aromatic)	976.6	E858.7	E946.6	E950.4	E962.0	E980.4
Alkalinizing agents (medicinal)	963.3	E858.1	E933.3	E950.4	E962.0	E980.4
Alkalis, caustic	983.2	E864.2	—	E950.7	E962.1	E980.6
Alkalizing agents (medicinal)	963.3	E858.1	E933.3	E950.4	E962.0	E980.4
Alka–seltzer	965.1	E850.3	E935.3	E950.0	E962.0	E980.0
Alkavervir	972.6	E858.3	E942.6	E950.4	E962.0	E980.4
Allegron	969.0	E854.0	E939.0	E950.3	E962.0	E980.3
Alleve *see* Naproxen						
Allobarbital, allobarbitone	967.0	E851	E937.0	E950.1	E962.0	E980.1
Allopurinol	974.7	E858.5	E944.7	E950.4	E962.0	E980.4
Allylestrenol	962.2	E858.0	E932.2	E950.4	E962.0	E980.4
Allylisopropylacetylurea	967.8	E852.8	E937.8	E950.2	E962.0	E980.2
Allylisopropylmalonylurea	967.0	E851	E937.0	E950.1	E962.0	E980.1
Allyltribromide	967.3	E852.2	E937.3	E950.2	E962.0	E980.2
Aloe, aloes, aloin	973.1	E858.4	E943.1	E950.4	E962.0	E980.4
Alosetron	973.8	E858.4	E943.8	E950.4	E962.0	E980.4
Aloxidone	966.0	E855.0	E936.0	E950.4	E962.0	E980.4
Aloxiprin	965.1	E850.3	E935.3	E950.0	E962.0	E980.0
Alpha amylase	963.4	E858.1	E933.4	E950.4	E962.0	E980.4
Alphaprodine (hydrochloride)	965.09	E850.2	E935.2	E950.0	E962.0	E980.0
Alpha tocopherol	963.5	E858.1	E933.5	E950.4	E962.0	E980.4
Alseroxylon	972.6	E858.3	E942.6	E950.4	E962.0	E980.4
Alum (ammonium) (potassium)	983.2	E864.2	—	E950.7	E962.1	E980.6
medicinal (astringent) NEC	976.2	E858.7	E946.2	E950.4	E962.0	E980.4
Aluminium, aluminum (gel) (hydroxide)	973.0	E858.4	E943.0	E950.4	E962.0	E980.4

Substance	Poisoning	External Cause (E-Code)				
		Accident	Therapeutic Use	Suicide Attempt	Assault	Undetermined
acetate solution	976.2	E858.7	E946.2	E950.4	E962.0	E980.4
aspirin	965.1	E850.3	E935.3	E950.0	E962.0	E980.0
carbonate	973.0	E858.4	E943.0	E950.4	E962.0	E980.4
glycinate	973.0	E858.4	E943.0	E950.4	E962.0	E980.4
nicotinate	972.2	E858.3	E942.2	E950.4	E962.0	E980.4
ointment (surgical) (topical)	976.3	E858.7	E946.3	E950.4	E962.0	E980.4
phosphate	973.0	E858.4	E943.0	E950.4	E962.0	E980.4
subacetate	976.2	E858.7	E946.2	E950.4	E962.0	E980.4
topical NEC	976.3	E858.7	E946.3	E950.4	E962.0	E980.4
Alurate	967.0	E851	E937.0	E950.1	E962.0	E980.1
Alverine (citrate)	975.1	E858.6	E945.1	E950.4	E962.0	E980.4
Alvodine	965.09	E850.2	E935.2	E950.0	E962.0	E980.0
Amanita phalloides	988.1	E865.5	—	E950.9	E962.1	E980.9
Amantadine (hydrochloride)	966.4	E855.0	E936.4	E950.4	E962.0	E980.4
Ambazone	961.9	E857	E931.9	E950.4	E962.0	E980.4
Ambenonium	971.0	E855.3	E941.0	E950.4	E962.0	E980.4
Ambutonium bromide	971.1	E855.4	E941.1	E950.4	E962.0	E980.4
Ametazole	977.8	E858.8	E947.8	E950.4	E962.0	E980.4
Amethocaine (infiltration) (topical)	968.5	E855.2	E938.5	E950.4	E962.0	E980.4
nerve block (peripheral) (plexus)	968.6	E855.2	E938.6	E950.4	E962.0	E980.4
spinal	968.7	E855.2	E938.7	E950.4	E962.0	E980.4
Amethopterin	963.1	E858.1	E933.1	E950.4	E962.0	E980.4
Amfepramone	977.0	E858.8	E947.0	E950.4	E962.0	E980.4
Amidon	965.02	E850.1	E935.1	E950.0	E962.0	E980.0
Amidopyrine	965.5	E850.5	E935.5	E950.0	E962.0	E980.0
Aminacrine	976.0	E858.7	E946.0	E950.4	E962.0	E980.4
Aminitrozole	961.5	E857	E931.5	E950.4	E962.0	E980.4
Aminoacetic acid	974.5	E858.5	E944.5	E950.4	E962.0	E980.4
Amino acids	974.5	E858.5	E944.5	E950.4	E962.0	E980.4
Aminocaproic acid	964.4	E858.2	E934.4	E950.4	E962.0	E980.4
Aminoethylisothiourium	963.8	E858.1	E933.8	E950.4	E962.0	E980.4
Aminoglutethimide	966.3	E855.0	E936.3	E950.4	E962.0	E980.4
Aminometradine	974.3	E858.5	E944.3	E950.4	E962.0	E980.4
Aminopentamide	971.1	E855.4	E941.1	E950.4	E962.0	E980.4
Aminophenazone	965.5	E850.5	E935.5	E950.0	E962.0	E980.0
Aminophenol	983.0	E864.0	—	E950.7	E962.1	E980.6
Aminophenylpyridone	969.5	E853.8	E939.5	E950.3	E962.0	E980.3
Aminophyllin	975.7	E858.6	E945.7	E950.4	E962.0	E980.4
Aminopterin	963.1	E858.1	E933.1	E950.4	E962.0	E980.4
Aminopyrine	965.5	E850.5	E935.5	E950.0	E962.0	E980.0
Aminosalicylic acid	961.8	E857	E931.8	E950.4	E962.0	E980.4
Amiphenazole	970.1	E854.3	E940.1	E950.4	E962.0	E980.4
Amiquinsin	972.6	E858.3	E942.6	E950.4	E962.0	E980.4
Amisometradine	974.3	E858.5	E944.3	E950.4	E962.0	E980.4
Amitriptyline	969.0	E854.0	E939.0	E950.3	E962.0	E980.3
Ammonia (fumes) (gas) (vapor)	987.8	E869.8	—	E952.8	E962.2	E982.8
liquid (household) NEC	983.2	E861.4	—	E950.7	E962.1	E980.6
spirit, aromatic	970.8	E854.3	E940.8	E950.4	E962.0	E980.4
Ammoniated mercury	976.0	E858.7	E946.0	E950.4	E962.0	E980.4
Ammonium						
carbonate	983.2	E864.2	—	E950.7	E962.1	E980.6
chloride (acidifying agent)	963.2	E858.1	E933.2	E950.4	E962.0	E980.4
expectorant	975.5	E858.6	E945.5	E950.4	E962.0	E980.4
compounds (household) NEC	983.2	E861.4	—	E950.7	E962.1	E980.6
fumes (any usage)	987.8	E869.8	—	E952.8	E962.2	E982.8
industrial	983.2	E864.2	—	E950.7	E962.1	E980.6
ichthyosulfonate	976.4	E858.7	E946.4	E950.4	E962.0	E980.4

Substance	Poisoning	External Cause (E-Code)				
		Accident	Therapeutic Use	Suicide Attempt	Assault	Undetermined
mandelate	961.9	E857	E931.9	E950.4	E962.0	E980.4
Amobarbital	967.0	E851	E937.0	E950.1	E962.0	E980.1
Amodiaquin(e)	961.4	E857	E931.4	E950.4	E962.0	E980.4
Amopyroquin(e)	961.4	E857	E931.4	E950.4	E962.0	E980.4
Amphenidone	969.5	E853.8	E939.5	E950.3	E962.0	E980.3
Amphetamine	969.7	E854.2	E939.7	E950.3	E962.0	E980.3
Amphomycin	960.8	E856	E930.8	E950.4	E962.0	E980.4
Amphotericin B	960.1	E856	E930.1	E950.4	E962.0	E980.4
topical	976.0	E858.7	E946.0	E950.4	E962.0	E980.4
Ampicillin	960.0	E856	E930.0	E950.4	E962.0	E980.4
Amprotropine	971.1	E855.4	E941.1	E950.4	E962.0	E980.4
Amygdalin	977.8	E858.8	E947.8	E950.4	E962.0	E980.4
Amyl						
acetate (vapor)	982.8	E862.4	—	E950.9	E962.1	E980.9
alcohol	980.3	E860.4	—	E950.9	E962.1	E980.9
nitrite (medicinal)	972.4	E858.3	E942.4	E950.4	E962.0	E980.4
Amylase (alpha)	963.4	E858.1	E933.4	E950.4	E962.0	E980.4
Amylene hydrate	980.8	E860.8	—	E950.9	E962.1	E980.9
Amylobarbitone	967.0	E851	E937.0	E950.1	E962.0	E980.1
Amylocaine	968.9	E855.2	E938.9	E950.4	E962.0	E980.4
infiltration (subcutaneous)	968.5	E855.2	E938.5	E950.4	E962.0	E980.4
nerve block (peripheral) (plexus)	968.6	E855.2	E938.6	E950.4	E962.0	E980.4
spinal	968.7	E855.2	E938.7	E950.4	E962.0	E980.4
topical (surface)	968.5	E855.2	E938.5	E950.4	E962.0	E980.4
Amytal (sodium)	967.0	E851	E937.0	E950.1	E962.0	E980.1
Analeptics	970.0	E854.3	E940.0	E950.4	E962.0	E980.4
Analgesics	965.9	E850.9	E935.9	E950.0	E962.0	E980.0
aromatic NEC	965.4	E850.4	E935.4	E950.0	E962.0	E980.0
non–narcotic NEC	965.7	E850.7	E935.7	E950.0	E962.0	E980.0
specified NEC	965.8	E850.8	E935.8	E950.0	E962.0	E980.0
Anamirta cocculus	988.2	E865.3	—	E950.9	E962.1	E980.9
Ancillin	960.0	E856	E930.0	E950.4	E962.0	E980.4
Androgens (anabolic congeners)	962.1	E858.0	E932.1	E950.4	E962.0	E980.4
Androstalone	962.1	E858.0	E932.1	E950.4	E962.0	E980.4
Androsterone	962.1	E858.0	E932.1	E950.4	E962.0	E980.4
Anemone pulsatilla	988.2	E865.4	—	E950.9	E962.1	E980.9
Anesthesia, anesthetic (general) NEC	968.4	E855.1	E938.4	E950.4	E962.0	E980.4
block (nerve) (plexus)	968.6	E855.2	E938.6	E950.4	E962.0	E980.4
gaseous NEC	968.2	E855.1	E938.2	E950.4	E962.0	E980.4
halogenated hydrocarbon derivatives NEC	968.2	E855.1	E938.2	E950.4	E962.0	E980.4
infiltration (intradermal) (subcutaneous) (submucosal)	968.5	E855.2	E938.5	E950.4	E962.0	E980.4
intravenous	968.3	E855.1	E938.3	E950.4	E962.0	E980.4
local NEC	968.9	E855.2	E938.9	E950.4	E962.0	E980.4
nerve blocking (peripheral) (plexus)	968.6	E855.2	E938.6	E950.4	E962.0	E980.4
rectal NEC	968.3	E855.1	E938.3	E950.4	E962.0	E980.4
spinal	968.7	E855.2	E938.7	E950.4	E962.0	E980.4
surface	968.5	E855.2	E938.5	E950.4	E962.0	E980.4
topical	968.5	E855.2	E938.5	E950.4	E962.0	E980.4
Aneurine	963.5	E858.1	E933.5	E950.4	E962.0	E980.4
Angio–Conray	977.8	E858.8	E947.8	E950.4	E962.0	E980.4
Angininesee Glyceryl trinitrate						
Angiotensin	971.2	E855.5	E941.2	E950.4	E962.0	E980.4
Anhydrohydroxyprogesterone	962.2	E858.0	E932.2	E950.4	E962.0	E980.4
Anhydron	974.3	E858.5	E944.3	E950.4	E962.0	E980.4
Anileridine	965.09	E850.2	E935.2	E950.0	E962.0	E980.0

Substance	Poisoning	External Cause (E-Code)				
		Accident	Therapeutic Use	Suicide Attempt	Assault	Undetermined
Aniline (dye) (liquid)	983.0	E864.0	—	E950.7	E962.1	E980.6
analgesic	965.4	E850.4	E935.4	E950.0	E962.0	E980.0
derivatives, therapeutic NEC	965.4	E850.4	E935.4	E950.0	E962.0	E980.0
vapor	987.8	E869.8	—	E952.8	E962.2	E982.8
Anisindione	964.2	E858.2	E934.2	E950.4	E962.0	E980.4
Anisotropine	971.1	E855.4	E941.1	E950.4	E962.0	E980.4
Anorexic agents	977.0	E858.8	E947.0	E950.4	E962.0	E980.4
Ant (bite) (sting)	989.5	E905.5	—	E950.9	E962.1	E980.9
Antabuse	977.3	E858.8	E947.3	E950.4	E962.0	E980.4
Antacids	973.0	E858.4	E943.0	E950.4	E962.0	E980.4
Antazoline	963.0	E858.1	E933.0	E950.4	E962.0	E980.4
Anthelmintics	961.6	E857	E931.6	E950.4	E962.0	E980.4
Anthralin	976.4	E858.7	E946.4	E950.4	E962.0	E980.4
Anthramycin	960.7	E856	E930.7	E950.4	E962.0	E980.4
Antiadrenergics	971.3	E855.6	E941.3	E950.4	E962.0	E980.4
Antiallergic agents	963.0	E858.1	E933.0	E950.4	E962.0	E980.4
Antianemic agents NEC	964.1	E858.2	E934.1	E950.4	E962.0	E980.4
Antiaris toxicaria	988.2	E865.4	—	E950.9	E962.1	E980.9
Antiarteriosclerotic agents	972.2	E858.3	E942.2	E950.4	E962.0	E980.4
Antiasthmatics	975.7	E858.6	E945.7	E950.4	E962.0	E980.4
Antibiotics	960.9	E856	E930.9	E950.4	E962.0	E980.4
antifungal	960.1	E856	E930.1	E950.4	E962.0	E980.4
antimycobacterial	960.6	E856	E930.6	E950.4	E962.0	E980.4
antineoplastic	960.7	E856	E930.7	E950.4	E962.0	E980.4
cephalosporin (group)	960.5	E856	E930.5	E950.4	E962.0	E980.4
chloramphenicol (group)	960.2	E856	E930.2	E950.4	E962.0	E980.4
macrolides	960.3	E856	E930.3	E950.4	E962.0	E980.4
specified NEC	960.8	E856	E930.8	E950.4	E962.0	E980.4
tetracycline (group)	960.4	E856	E930.4	E950.4	E962.0	E980.4
Anticancer agents NEC	963.1	E858.1	E933.1	E950.4	E962.0	E980.4
antibiotics	960.7	E856	E930.7	E950.4	E962.0	E980.4
Anticholinergics	971.1	E855.4	E941.1	E950.4	E962.0	E980.4
Anticholinesterase (organophosphorus) (reversible)	971.0	E855.3	E941.0	E950.4	E962.0	E980.4
Anticoagulants	964.2	E858.2	E934.2	E950.4	E962.0	E980.4
antagonists	964.5	E858.2	E934.5	E950.4	E962.0	E980.4
Anti–common cold agents NEC	975.6	E858.6	E945.6	E950.4	E962.0	E980.4
Anticonvulsants NEC	966.3	E855.0	E936.3	E950.4	E962.0	E980.4
Antidepressants	969.0	E854.0	E939.0	E950.3	E962.0	E980.3
Antidiabetic agents	962.3	E858.0	E932.3	E950.4	E962.0	E980.4
Antidiarrheal agents	973.5	E858.4	E943.5	E950.4	E962.0	E980.4
Antidiuretic hormone	962.5	E858.0	E932.5	E950.4	E962.0	E980.4
Antidotes NEC	977.2	E858.8	E947.2	E950.4	E962.0	E980.4
Antiemetic agents	963.0	E858.1	E933.0	E950.4	E962.0	E980.4
Antiepilepsy agent NEC	966.3	E855.0	E936.3	E950.4	E962.0	E980.4
Antifertility pills	962.2	E858.0	E932.2	E950.4	E962.0	E980.4
Antiflatulents	973.8	E858.4	E943.8	E950.4	E962.0	E980.4
Antifreeze	989.89	E866.8	—	E950.9	E962.1	E980.9
alcohol	980.1	E860.2	—	E950.9	E962.1	E980.9
ethylene glycol	982.8	E862.4	—	E950.9	E962.1	E980.9
Antifungals (nonmedicinal) (sprays)	989.4	E863.6	—	E950.6	E962.1	E980.7
medicinal NEC	961.9	E857	E931.9	E950.4	E962.0	E980.4
antibiotic	960.1	E856	E930.1	E950.4	E962.0	E980.4
topical	976.0	E858.7	E946.0	E950.4	E962.0	E980.4
Antigastric secretion agents	973.0	E858.4	E943.0	E950.4	E962.0	E980.4
Antihelmintics	961.6	E857	E931.6	E950.4	E962.0	E980.4
Antihemophilic factor (human)	964.7	E858.2	E934.7	E950.4	E962.0	E980.4

Substance	Poisoning	External Cause (E-Code)				
		Accident	Therapeutic Use	Suicide Attempt	Assault	Undetermined
Antihistamine	963.0	E858.1	E933.0	E950.4	E962.0	E980.4
Antihypertensive agents NEC	972.6	E858.3	E942.6	E950.4	E962.0	E980.4
Anti–infectives NEC	961.9	E857	E931.9	E950.4	E962.0	E980.4
antibiotics	960.9	E856	E930.9	E950.4	E962.0	E980.4
specified NEC	960.8	E856	E930.8	E950.4	E962.0	E980.4
antihelmintic	961.6	E857	E931.6	E950.4	E962.0	E980.4
antimalarial	961.4	E857	E931.4	E950.4	E962.0	E980.4
antimycobacterial NEC	961.8	E857	E931.8	E950.4	E962.0	E980.4
antibiotics	960.6	E856	E930.6	E950.4	E962.0	E980.4
antiprotozoal NEC	961.5	E857	E931.5	E950.4	E962.0	E980.4
blood	961.4	E857	E931.4	E950.4	E962.0	E980.4
antiviral	961.7	E857	E931.7	E950.4	E962.0	E980.4
arsenical	961.1	E857	E931.1	E950.4	E962.0	E980.4
ENT agents	976.6	E858.7	E946.6	E950.4	E962.0	E980.4
heavy metals NEC	961.2	E857	E931.2	E950.4	E962.0	E980.4
local	976.0	E858.7	E946.0	E950.4	E962.0	E980.4
ophthalmic preparation	976.5	E858.7	E946.5	E950.4	E962.0	E980.4
topical NEC	976.0	E858.7	E946.0	E950.4	E962.0	E980.4
Anti–inflammatory agents (topical)	976.0	E858.7	E946.0	E950.4	E962.0	E980.4
Antiknock (tetraethyl lead)	984.1	E862.1	—	E950.9	E962.1	E980.9
Antilipemics	972.2	E858.3	E942.2	E950.4	E962.0	E980.4
Antimalarials	961.4	E857	E931.4	E950.4	E962.0	E980.4
Antimony (compounds) (vapor) NEC	985.4	E866.2	—	E950.9	E962.1	E980.9
anti–infectives	961.2	E857	E931.2	E950.4	E962.0	E980.4
pesticides (vapor)	985.4	E863.4	—	E950.6	E962.2	E980.7
potassium tartrate	961.2	E857	E931.2	E950.4	E962.0	E980.4
tartrated	961.2	E857	E931.2	E950.4	E962.0	E980.4
Antimuscarinic agents	971.1	E855.4	E941.1	E950.4	E962.0	E980.4
Antimycobacterials NEC	961.8	E857	E931.8	E950.4	E962.0	E980.4
antibiotics	960.6	E856	E930.6	E950.4	E962.0	E980.4
Antineoplastic agents	963.1	E858.1	E933.1	E950.4	E962.0	E980.4
antibiotics	960.7	E856	E930.7	E950.4	E962.0	E980.4
Anti–Parkinsonism agents	966.4	E855.0	E936.4	E950.4	E962.0	E980.4
Antiphlogistics	965.69	E850.6	E935.6	E950.0	E962.0	E980.0
Antiprotozoals NEC	961.5	E857	E931.5	E950.4	E962.0	E980.4
blood	961.4	E857	E931.4	E950.4	E962.0	E980.4
Antipruritics (local)	976.1	E858.7	E946.1	E950.4	E962.0	E980.4
Antipsychotic agents NEC	969.3	E853.8	E939.3	E950.3	E962.0	E980.3
Antipyretics	965.9	E850.9	E935.9	E950.0	E962.0	E980.0
specified NEC	965.8	E850.8	E935.8	E950.0	E962.0	E980.0
Antipyrine	965.5	E850.5	E935.5	E950.0	E962.0	E980.0
Antirabies serum (equine)	979.9	E858.8	E949.9	E950.4	E962.0	E980.4
Antirheumatics	965.69	E850.6	E935.6	E950.0	E962.0	E980.0
Antiseborrheics	976.4	E858.7	E946.4	E950.4	E962.0	E980.4
Antiseptics (external) (medicinal)	976.0	E858.7	E946.0	E950.4	E962.0	E980.4
Antistine	963.0	E858.1	E933.0	E950.4	E962.0	E980.4
Antithyroid agents	962.8	E858.0	E932.8	E950.4	E962.0	E980.4
Antitoxin, any	979.9	E858.8	E949.9	E950.4	E962.0	E980.4
Antituberculars	961.8	E857	E931.8	E950.4	E962.0	E980.4
antibiotics	960.6	E856	E930.6	E950.4	E962.0	E980.4
Antitussives	975.4	E858.6	E945.5	E950.4	E962.0	E980.4
Antivaricose agents (sclerosing)	972.7	E858.3	E942.7	E950.4	E962.0	E980.4
Antivenin (crotaline) (spider–bite)	979.9	E858.8	E949.9	E950.4	E962.0	E980.4
Antivert	963.0	E858.1	E933.0	E950.4	E962.0	E980.4
Antivirals NEC	961.7	E857	E931.7	E950.4	E962.0	E980.4
Ant poisons — *see* Pesticides						
Antrol	989.4	E863.4	—	E950.6	E962.1	E980.7

Substance	Poisoning	Accident	Therapeutic Use	Suicide Attempt	Assault	Undetermined
fungicide	989.4	E863.6	—	E950.6	E962.1	E980.7
Apomorphine hydrochloride (emetic)	973.6	E858.4	E943.6	E950.4	E962.0	E980.4
Appetite depressants, central	977.0	E858.8	E947.0	E950.4	E962.0	E980.4
Apresoline	972.6	E858.3	E942.6	E950.4	E962.0	E980.4
Aprobarbital, aprobarbitone	967.0	E851	E937.0	E950.1	E962.0	E980.1
Apronalide	967.8	E852.8	E937.8	E950.2	E962.0	E980.2
Aqua fortis	983.1	E864.1	—	E950.7	E962.1	E980.6
Arachis oil (topical)	976.3	E858.7	E946.3	E950.4	E962.0	E980.4
cathartic	973.2	E858.4	E943.2	E950.4	E962.0	E980.4
Aralen	961.4	E857	E931.4	E950.4	E962.0	E980.4
Arginine salts	974.5	E858.5	E944.5	E950.4	E962.0	E980.4
Argyrol	976.0	E858.7	E946.0	E950.4	E962.0	E980.4
ENT agent	976.6	E858.7	E946.6	E950.4	E962.0	E980.4
ophthalmic preparation	976.5	E858.7	E946.5	E950.4	E962.0	E980.4
Aristocort	962.0	E858.0	E932.0	E950.4	E962.0	E980.4
ENT agent	976.6	E858.7	E946.6	E950.4	E962.0	E980.4
ophthalmic preparation	976.5	E858.7	E946.5	E950.4	E962.0	E980.4
topical NEC	976.0	E858.7	E946.0	E950.4	E962.0	E980.4
Aromatics, corrosive	983.0	E864.0	—	E950.7	E962.1	E980.6
disinfectants	983.0	E861.4	—	E950.7	E962.1	E980.6
Arsenate of lead (insecticide)	985.1	E863.4	—	E950.8	E962.1	E980.8
herbicide	985.1	E863.5	—	E950.8	E962.1	E980.8
Arsenic, arsenicals (compounds) (dust) (fumes) (vapor) NEC	985.1	E866.3	—	E950.8	E962.1	E980.8
anti–infectives	961.1	E857	E931.1	E950.4	E962.0	E980.4
pesticide (dust) (fumes)	985.1	E863.4	—	E950.8	E962.1	E980.8
Arsine (gas)	985.1	E866.3	—	E950.8	E962.1	E980.8
Arsphenamine (silver)	961.1	E857	E931.1	E950.4	E962.0	E980.4
Arsthinol	961.1	E857	E931.1	E950.4	E962.0	E980.4
Artane	971.1	E855.4	E941.1	E950.4	E962.0	E980.4
Arthropod (venomous) NEC	989.5	E905.5	—	E950.9	E962.1	E980.9
Asbestos	989.81	E866.8	—	E950.9	E962.1	E980.9
Ascaridole	961.6	E857	E931.6	E950.4	E962.0	E980.4
Ascorbic acid	963.5	E858.1	E933.5	E950.4	E962.0	E980.4
Asiaticoside	976.0	E858.7	E946.0	E950.4	E962.0	E980.4
Aspidium (oleoresin)	961.6	E857	E931.6	E950.4	E962.0	E980.4
Aspirin	965.1	E850.3	E935.3	E950.0	E962.0	E980.0
Astringents (local)	976.2	E858.7	E946.2	E950.4	E962.0	E980.4
Atabrine	961.3	E857	E931.3	E950.4	E962.0	E980.4
Ataractics	969.5	E853.8	E939.5	E950.3	E962.0	E980.3
Atonia drug, intestinal	973.3	E858.4	E943.3	E950.4	E962.0	E980.4
Atophan	974.7	E858.5	E944.7	E950.4	E962.0	E980.4
Atropine	971.1	E855.4	E941.1	E950.4	E962.0	E980.4
Attapulgite	973.5	E858.4	E943.5	E950.4	E962.0	E980.4
Attenuvax	979.4	E858.8	E949.4	E950.4	E962.0	E980.4
Aureomycin	960.4	E856	E930.4	E950.4	E962.0	E980.4
ophthalmic preparation	976.5	E858.7	E946.5	E950.4	E962.0	E980.4
topical NEC	976.0	E858.7	E946.0	E950.4	E962.0	E980.4
Aurothioglucose	965.69	E850.6	E935.6	E950.0	E962.0	E980.0
Aurothioglycanide	965.69	E850.6	E935.6	E950.0	E962.0	E980.0
Aurothiomalate	965.69	E850.6	E935.6	E950.0	E962.0	E980.0
Automobile fuel	981	E862.1	—	E950.9	E962.1	E980.9
Autonomic nervous system agents NEC	971.9	E855.9	E941.9	E950.4	E962.0	E980.4
Avlosulfon	961.8	E857	E931.8	E950.4	E962.0	E980.4
Avomine	967.8	E852.8	E937.8	E950.2	E962.0	E980.2
Azacyclonol	969.5	E853.8	E939.5	E950.3	E962.0	E980.3
Azapetine	971.3	E855.6	E941.3	E950.4	E962.0	E980.4

Substance	Poisoning	External Cause (E-Code)				
		Accident	Therapeutic Use	Suicide Attempt	Assault	Undetermined
Azaribine	963.1	E858.1	E933.1	E950.4	E962.0	E980.4
Azaserine	960.7	E856	E930.7	E950.4	E962.0	E980.4
Azathioprine	963.1	E858.1	E933.1	E950.4	E962.0	E980.4
Azosulfamide	961.0	E857	E931.0	E950.4	E962.0	E980.4
Azulfidine	961.0	E857	E931.0	E950.4	E962.0	E980.4
Azuresin	977.8	E858.8	E947.8	E950.4	E962.0	E980.4
Bacimycin	976.0	E858.7	E946.0	E950.4	E962.0	E980.4
ophthalmic preparation	976.5	E858.7	E946.5	E950.4	E962.0	E980.4
Bacitracin	960.8	E856	E930.8	E950.4	E962.0	E980.4
ENT agent	976.6	E858.7	E946.6	E950.4	E962.0	E980.4
ophthalmic preparation	976.5	E858.7	E946.5	E950.4	E962.0	E980.4
topical NEC	976.0	E858.7	E946.0	E950.4	E962.0	E980.4
Baking soda	963.3	E858.1	E933.3	E950.4	E962.0	E980.4
BAL	963.8	E858.1	E933.8	E950.4	E962.0	E980.4
Bamethan (sulfate)	972.5	E858.3	E942.5	E950.4	E962.0	E980.4
Bamipine	963.0	E858.1	E933.0	E950.4	E962.0	E980.4
Baneberry	988.2	E865.4	—	E950.9	E962.1	E980.9
Banewort	988.2	E865.4	—	E950.9	E962.1	E980.9
Barbenyl	967.0	E851	E937.0	E950.1	E962.0	E980.1
Barbital, barbitone	967.0	E851	E937.0	E950.1	E962.0	E980.1
Barbiturates, barbituric acid	967.0	E851	E937.0	E950.1	E962.0	E980.1
anesthetic (intravenous)	968.3	E855.1	E938.3	E950.4	E962.0	E980.4
Barium (carbonate) (chloride) (sulfate)	985.8	E866.4	—	E950.9	E962.1	E980.9
diagnostic agent	977.8	E858.8	E947.8	E950.4	E962.0	E980.4
pesticide	985.8	E863.4	—	E950.6	E962.1	E980.7
rodenticide	985.8	E863.7	—	E950.6	E962.1	E980.7
Barrier cream	976.3	E858.7	E946.3	E950.4	E962.0	E980.4
Battery acid or fluid	983.1	E864.1	—	E950.7	E962.1	E980.6
Bay rum	980.8	E860.8	—	E950.9	E962.1	E980.9
BCG vaccine	978.0	E858.8	E948.0	E950.4	E962.0	E980.4
Bearsfoot	988.2	E865.4	—	E950.9	E962.1	E980.9
Beclamide	966.3	E855.0	E936.3	E950.4	E962.0	E980.4
Bee (sting) (venom)	989.5	E905.3	—	E950.9	E962.1	E980.9
Belladonna (alkaloids)	971.1	E855.4	E941.1	E950.4	E962.0	E980.4
Bemegride	970.0	E854.3	E940.0	E950.4	E962.0	E980.4
Benactyzine	969.8	E855.8	E939.8	E950.3	E962.0	E980.3
Benadryl	963.0	E858.1	E933.0	E950.4	E962.0	E980.4
Bendrofluazide	974.3	E858.5	E944.3	E950.4	E962.0	E980.4
Bendroflumethiazide	974.3	E858.5	E944.3	E950.4	E962.0	E980.4
Benemid	974.7	E858.5	E944.7	E950.4	E962.0	E980.4
Benethamine penicillin G	960.0	E856	E930.0	E950.4	E962.0	E980.4
Benisone	976.0	E858.7	E946.0	E950.4	E962.0	E980.4
Benoquin	976.8	E858.7	E946.8	E950.4	E962.0	E980.4
Benoxinate	968.5	E855.2	E938.5	E950.4	E962.0	E980.4
Bentonite	976.3	E858.7	E946.3	E950.4	E962.0	E980.4
Benzalkonium (chloride)	976.0	E858.7	E946.0	E950.4	E962.0	E980.4
ophthalmic preparation	976.5	E858.7	E946.5	E950.4	E962.0	E980.4
Benzamidosalicylate (calcium)	961.8	E857	E931.8	E950.4	E962.0	E980.4
Benzathine penicillin	960.0	E856	E930.0	E950.4	E962.0	E980.4
Benzcarbimine	963.1	E858.1	E933.1	E950.4	E962.0	E980.4
Benzedrex	971.2	E855.5	E941.2	E950.4	E962.0	E980.4
Benzedrine (amphetamine)	969.7	E854.2	E939.7	E950.3	E962.0	E980.3
Benzene (acetyl) (dimethyl) (methyl) (solvent) (vapor)	982.0	E862.4	—	E950.9	E962.1	E980.9
hexachloride (gamma) (insecticide) (vapor)	989.2	E863.0	—	E950.6	E962.1	E980.7
Benzethonium	976.0	E858.7	E946.0	E950.4	E962.0	E980.4

Substance	Poisoning	External Cause (E-Code)				
		Accident	Therapeutic Use	Suicide Attempt	Assault	Undetermined
Benzhexol (chloride)	966.4	E855.0	E936.4	E950.4	E962.0	E980.4
Benzilonium	971.1	E855.4	E941.1	E950.4	E962.0	E980.4
Benzin(e) — *see* Ligroin						
Benziodarone	972.4	E858.3	E942.4	E950.4	E962.0	E980.4
Benzocaine	968.5	E855.2	E938.5	E950.4	E962.0	E980.4
Benzodiapin	969.4	E853.2	E939.4	E950.3	E962.0	E980.3
Benzodiazepines (tranquilizers) NEC	969.4	E853.2	E939.4	E950.3	E962.0	E980.3
Benzoic acid (with salicylic acid) (anti–infective)	976.0	E858.7	E946.0	E950.4	E962.0	E980.4
Benzoin	976.3	E858.7	E946.3	E950.4	E962.0	E980.4
Benzol (vapor)	982.0	E862.4	—	E950.9	E962.1	E980.9
Benzomorphan	965.09	E850.2	E935.2	E950.0	E962.0	E980.0
Benzonatate	975.4	E858.6	E945.4	E950.4	E962.0	E980.4
Benzothiadiazides	974.3	E858.5	E944.3	E950.4	E962.0	E980.4
Benzoylpas	961.8	E857	E931.8	E950.4	E962.0	E980.4
Benzperidol	969.5	E853.8	E939.5	E950.3	E962.0	E980.3
Benzphetamine	977.0	E858.8	E947.0	E950.4	E962.0	E980.4
Benzpyrinium	971.0	E855.3	E941.0	E950.4	E962.0	E980.4
Benzquinamide	963.0	E858.1	E933.0	E950.4	E962.0	E980.4
Benzthiazide	974.3	E858.5	E944.3	E950.4	E962.0	E980.4
Benztropine	971.1	E855.4	E941.1	E950.4	E962.0	E980.4
Benzyl						
acetate	982.8	E862.4	—	E950.9	E962.1	E980.9
benzoate (anti–infective)	976.0	E858.7	E946.0	E950.4	E962.0	E980.4
morphine	965.09	E850.2	E935.2	E950.0	E962.0	E980.0
penicillin	960.0	E856	E930.0	E950.4	E962.0	E980.4
Bephenium hydroxynapthoate	961.6	E857	E931.6	E950.4	E962.0	E980.4
Bergamot oil	989.89	E866.8	—	E950.9	E962.1	E980.9
Berries, poisonous	988.2	E865.3	—	E950.9	E962.1	E980.9
Beryllium (compounds) (fumes)	985.3	E866.4	—	E950.9	E962.1	E980.9
Beta–carotene	976.3	E858.7	E946.3	E950.4	E962.0	E980.4
Beta–Chlor	967.1	E852.0	E937.1	E950.2	E962.0	E980.2
Betamethasone	962.0	E858.0	E932.0	E950.4	E962.0	E980.4
topical	976.0	E858.7	E946.0	E950.4	E962.0	E980.4
Betazole	977.8	E858.8	E947.8	E950.4	E962.0	E980.4
Bethanechol	971.0	E855.3	E941.0	E950.4	E962.0	E980.4
Bethanidine	972.6	E858.3	E942.6	E950.4	E962.0	E980.4
Betula oil	976.3	E858.7	E946.3	E950.4	E962.0	E980.4
Bhang	969.6	E854.1	E939.6	E950.3	E962.0	E980.3
Bialamicol	961.5	E857	E931.5	E950.4	E962.0	E980.4
Bichloride of mercury — *see* Mercury, chloride						
Bichromates (calcium) (crystals) (potassium) (sodium)	983.9	E864.3	—	E950.7	E962.1	E980.6
fumes	987.8	E869.8		E952.8	E962.2	E982.8
Biguanide derivatives, oral	962.3	E858.0	E932.3	E950.4	E962.0	E980.4
Biligrafin	977.8	E858.8	E947.8	E950.4	E962.0	E980.4
Bilopaque	977.8	E858.8	E947.8	E950.4	E962.0	E980.4
Bioflavonoids	972.8	E858.3	E942.8	E950.4	E962.0	E980.4
Biological substance NEC	979.9	E858.8	E949.9	E950.4	E962.0	E980.4
Biperiden	966.4	E855.0	E936.4	E950.4	E962.0	E980.4
Bisacodyl	973.1	E858.4	E943.1	E950.4	E962.0	E980.4
Bishydroxycoumarin	964.2	E858.2	E934.2	E950.4	E962.0	E980.4
Bismarsen	961.1	E857	E931.1	E950.4	E962.0	E980.4
Bismuth (compounds) NEC	985.8	E866.4	—	E950.9	E962.1	E980.9
anti–infectives	961.2	E857	E931.2	E950.4	E962.0	E980.4
subcarbonate	973.5	E858.4	E943.5	E950.4	E962.0	E980.4

Substance	Poisoning	Accident	Therapeutic Use	Suicide Attempt	Assault	Undetermined
				External Cause (E-Code)		
sulfarsphenamine	961.1	E857	E931.1	E950.4	E962.0	E980.4
Bithionol	961.6	E857	E931.6	E950.4	E962.0	E980.4
Bitter almond oil	989.0	E866.8	—	E950.9	E962.1	E980.9
Bittersweet	988.2	E865.4	—	E950.9	E962.1	E980.9
Black						
flag	989.4	E863.4	—	E950.6	E962.1	E980.7
henbane	988.2	E865.4	—	E950.9	E962.1	E980.9
leaf (40)	989.4	E863.4	—	E950.6	E962.1	E980.7
widow spider (bite)	989.5	E905.1	—	E950.9	E962.1	E980.9
antivenin	979.9	E858.8	E949.9	E950.4	E962.0	E980.4
Blast furnace gas (carbon monoxide from)	986	E868.8	—	E952.1	E962.2	E982.1
Bleach NEC	983.9	E864.3	—	E950.7	E962.1	E980.6
Bleaching solutions	983.9	E864.3	—	E950.7	E962.1	E980.6
Bleomycin (sulfate)	960.7	E856	E930.7	E950.4	E962.0	E980.4
Blockain	968.9	E855.2	E938.9	E950.4	E962.0	E980.4
infiltration (subcutaneous)	968.5	E855.2	E938.5	E950.4	E962.0	E980.4
nerve block (peripheral) (plexus)	968.6	E855.2	E938.6	E950.4	E962.0	E980.4
topical (surface)	968.5	E855.2	E938.5	E950.4	E962.0	E980.4
Blood (derivatives) (natural) (plasma)						
(whole)	964.7	E858.2	E934.7	E950.4	E962.0	E980.4
affecting agent	964.9	E858.2	E934.9	E950.4	E962.0	E980.4
specified NEC	964.8	E858.2	E934.8	E950.4	E962.0	E980.4
substitute (macromolecular)	964.8	E858.2	E934.8	E950.4	E962.0	E980.4
Blue velvet	965.09	E850.2	E935.2	E950.0	E962.0	E980.0
Bone meal	989.89	E866.5	—	E950.9	E962.1	E980.9
Bonine	963.0	E858.1	E933.0	E950.4	E962.0	E980.4
Boracic acid	976.0	E858.7	E946.0	E950.4	E962.0	E980.4
ENT agent	976.6	E858.7	E946.6	E950.4	E962.0	E980.4
ophthalmic preparation	976.5	E858.7	E946.5	E950.4	E962.0	E980.4
Borate (cleanser) (sodium)	989.6	E861.3	—	E950.9	E962.1	E980.9
Borax (cleanser)	989.6	E861.3	—	E950.9	E962.1	E980.9
Boric acid	976.0	E858.7	E946.0	E950.4	E962.0	E980.4
ENT agent	976.6	E858.7	E946.6	E950.4	E962.0	E980.4
ophthalmic preparation	976.5	E858.7	E946.5	E950.4	E962.0	E980.4
Boron hydride NEC	989.89	E866.8	—	E950.9	E962.1	E980.9
fumes or gas	987.8	E869.8	—	E952.8	E962.2	E982.8
Brake fluid vapor	987.8	E869.8	—	E952.8	E962.2	E982.8
Brass (compounds) (fumes)	985.8	E866.4	—	E950.9	E962.1	E980.9
Brasso	981	E861.3	—	E950.9	E962.1	E980.9
Bretylium (tosylate)	972.6	E858.3	E942.6	E950.4	E962.0	E980.4
Brevital (sodium)	968.3	E855.1	E938.3	E950.4	E962.0	E980.4
British antilewisite	963.8	E858.1	E933.8	E950.4	E962.0	E980.4
Bromal (hydrate)	967.3	E852.2	E937.3	E950.2	E962.0	E980.2
Bromelains	963.4	E858.1	E933.4	E950.4	E962.0	E980.4
Bromides NEC	967.3	E852.2	E937.3	E950.2	E962.0	E980.2
Bromine (vapor)	987.8	E869.8	—	E952.8	E962.2	E982.8
compounds (medicinal)	967.3	E852.2	E937.3	E950.2	E962.0	E980.2
Bromisovalum	967.3	E852.2	E937.3	E950.2	E962.0	E980.2
Bromobenzyl cyanide	987.5	E869.3	—	E952.8	E962.2	E982.8
Bromodiphenhydramine	963.0	E858.1	E933.0	E950.4	E962.0	E980.4
Bromoform	967.3	E852.2	E937.3	E950.2	E962.0	E980.2
Bromophenol blue reagent	977.8	E858.8	E947.8	E950.4	E962.0	E980.4
Bromosalicylhydroxamic acid	961.8	E857	E931.8	E950.4	E962.0	E980.4
Bromo–seltzer	965.4	E850.4	E935.4	E950.0	E962.0	E980.0
Brompheniramine	963.0	E858.1	E933.0	E950.4	E962.0	E980.4
Bromural	967.3	E852.2	E937.3	E950.2	E962.0	E980.2
Brown spider (bite) (venom)	989.5	E905.1	—	E950.9	E962.1	E980.9

Substance	Poisoning	External Cause (E-Code)				
		Accident	Therapeutic Use	Suicide Attempt	Assault	Undetermined
Brucia	988.2	E865.3	—	E950.9	E962.1	E980.9
Brucine	989.1	E863.7	—	E950.6	E962.1	E980.7
Brunswick green — *see* Copper						
Bruten — *see* Ibuperofen						
Bryonia (alba) (dioica)	988.2	E865.4	—	E950.9	E962.1	E980.9
Buclizine	969.5	E853.8	E939.5	E950.3	E962.0	E980.3
Bufferin	965.1	E850.3	E935.3	E950.0	E962.0	E980.0
Bufotenine	969.6	E854.1	E939.6	E950.3	E962.0	E980.3
Buphenine	971.2	E855.5	E941.2	E950.4	E962.0	E980.4
Bupivacaine	968.9	E855.2	E938.9	E950.4	E962.0	E980.4
infiltration (subcutaneous)	968.5	E855.2	E938.5	E950.4	E962.0	E980.4
nerve block (peripheral) (plexus)	968.6	E855.2	E938.6	E950.4	E962.0	E980.4
Busulfan	963.1	E858.1	E933.1	E950.4	E962.0	E980.4
Butabarbital (sodium)	967.0	E851	E937.0	E950.1	E962.0	E980.1
Butabarbitone	967.0	E851	E937.0	E950.1	E962.0	E980.1
Butabarpal	967.0	E851	E937.0	E950.1	E962.0	E980.1
Butacaine	968.5	E855.2	E938.5	E950.4	E962.0	E980.4
Butallylonal	967.0	E851	E937.0	E950.1	E962.0	E980.1
Butane (distributed in mobile container)	987.0	E868.0	—	E951.1	E962.2	E981.1
distributed through pipes	987.0	E867	—	E951.0	E962.2	E981.0
incomplete combustion of — *see*						
Carbon monoxide, butane						
Butanol	980.3	E860.4	—	E950.9	E962.1	E980.9
Butanone	982.8	E862.4	—	E950.9	E962.1	E980.9
Butaperazine	969.1	E853.0	E939.1	E950.3	E962.0	E980.3
Butazolidin	965.5	E850.5	E935.5	E950.0	E962.0	E980.0
Butethal	967.0	E851	E937.0	E950.1	E962.0	E980.1
Butethamate	971.1	E855.4	E941.1	E950.4	E962.0	E980.4
Buthalitone (sodium)	968.3	E855.1	E938.3	E950.4	E962.0	E980.4
Butisol (sodium)	967.0	E851	E937.0	E950.1	E962.0	E980.1
Butobarbital, butobarbitone	967.0	E851	E937.0	E950.1	E962.0	E980.1
Butriptyline	969.0	E854.0	E939.0	E950.3	E962.0	E980.3
Buttercups	988.2	E865.4	—	E950.9	E962.1	E980.9
Butter of antimony — *see* Antimony						
Butyl						
acetate (secondary)	982.8	E862.4	—	E950.9	E962.1	E980.9
alcohol	980.3	E860.4	—	E950.9	E962.1	E980.9
carbinol	980.8	E860.8	—	E950.9	E962.1	E980.9
carbitol	982.8	E862.4	—	E950.9	E962.1	E980.9
cellosolve	982.8	E862.4	—	E950.9	E962.1	E980.9
chloral (hydrate)	967.1	E852.0	E937.1	E950.2	E962.0	E980.2
formate	982.8	E862.4	—	E950.9	E962.1	E980.9
scopolammonium bromide	971.1	E855.4	E941.1	E950.4	E962.0	E980.4
Butyn	968.5	E855.2	E938.5	E950.4	E962.0	E980.4
Butyrophenone (–based tranquilizers)	969.2	E853.1	E939.2	E950.3	E962.0	E980.3
Cacodyl, cacodylic acid — *see* Arsenic						
Cactinomycin	960.7	E856	E930.7	E950.4	E962.0	E980.4
Cade oil	976.4	E858.7	E946.4	E950.4	E962.0	E980.4
Cadmium (chloride) (compounds) (dust)						
(fumes) (oxide)	985.5	E866.4	—	E950.9	E962.1	E980.9
sulfide (medicinal) NEC	976.4	E858.7	E946.4	E950.4	E962.0	E980.4
Caffeine	969.7	E854.2	E939.7	E950.3	E962.0	E980.3
Calabar bean	988.2	E865.4	—	E950.9	E962.1	E980.9
Caladium seguinium	988.2	E865.4	—	E950.9	E962.1	E980.9
Calamine (liniment) (lotion)	976.3	E858.7	E946.3	E950.4	E962.0	E980.4
Calciferol	963.5	E858.1	E933.5	E950.4	E962.0	E980.4
Calcium (salts) NEC	974.5	E858.5	E944.5	E950.4	E962.0	E980.4

Substance	Poisoning	Accident	Therapeutic Use	Suicide Attempt	Assault	Undetermined
acetylsalicylate	965.1	E850.3	E935.3	E950.0	E962.0	E980.0
benzamidosalicylate	961.8	E857	E931.8	E950.4	E962.0	E980.4
carbaspirin	965.1	E850.3	E935.3	E950.0	E962.0	E980.0
carbamide (citrated)	977.3	E858.8	E947.3	E950.4	E962.0	E980.4
carbonate (antacid)	973.0	E858.4	E943.0	E950.4	E962.0	E980.4
cyanide (citrated)	977.3	E858.8	E947.3	E950.4	E962.0	E980.4
dioctyl sulfosuccinate	973.2	E858.4	E943.2	E950.4	E962.0	E980.4
disodium edathamil	963.8	E858.1	E933.8	E950.4	E962.0	E980.4
disodium edetate	963.8	E858.1	E933.8	E950.4	E962.0	E980.4
EDTA	963.8	E858.1	E933.8	E950.4	E962.0	E980.4
hydrate, hydroxide	983.2	E864.2	—	E950.7	E962.1	E980.6
mandelate	961.9	E857	E931.9	E950.4	E962.0	E980.4
oxide	983.2	E864.2	—	E950.7	E962.1	E980.6
Calomel — *see* Mercury, chloride						
Caloric agents NEC	974.5	E858.5	E944.5	E950.4	E962.0	E980.4
Calusterone	963.1	E858.1	E933.1	E950.4	E962.0	E980.4
Camoquin	961.4	E857	E931.4	E950.4	E962.0	E980.4
Camphor (oil)	976.1	E858.7	E946.1	E950.4	E962.0	E980.4
Candeptin	976.0	E858.7	E946.0	E950.4	E962.0	E980.4
Candicidin	976.0	E858.7	E946.0	E950.4	E962.0	E980.4
Cannabinols	969.6	E854.1	E939.6	E950.3	E962.0	E980.3
Cannabis (derivatives) (indica) (sativa)	969.6	E854.1	E939.6	E950.3	E962.0	E980.3
Canned heat	980.1	E860.2	—	E950.9	E962.1	E980.9
Cantharides, cantharidin, cantharis	976.8	E858.7	E946.8	E950.4	E962.0	E980.4
Capillary agents	972.8	E858.3	E942.8	E950.4	E962.0	E980.4
Capreomycin	960.6	E856	E930.6	E950.4	E962.0	E980.4
Captodiame, captodiamine	969.5	E853.8	E939.5	E950.3	E962.0	E980.3
Caramiphen (hydrochloride)	971.1	E855.4	E941.1	E950.4	E962.0	E980.4
Carbachol	971.0	E855.3	E941.0	E950.4	E962.0	E980.4
Carbacrylamine resins	974.5	E858.5	E944.5	E950.4	E962.0	E980.4
Carbamate (sedative)	967.8	E852.8	E937.8	E950.2	E962.0	E980.2
herbicide	989.3	E863.5	—	E950.6	E962.1	E980.7
insecticide	989.3	E863.2	—	E950.6	E962.1	E980.7
Carbamazepine	966.3	E855.0	E936.3	E950.4	E962.0	E980.4
Carbamic esters	967.8	E852.8	E937.8	E950.2	E962.0	E980.2
Carbamide	974.4	E858.5	E944.4	E950.4	E962.0	E980.4
topical	976.8	E858.7	E946.8	E950.4	E962.0	E980.4
Carbamylcholine chloride	971.0	E855.3	E941.0	E950.4	E962.0	E980.4
Carbarsone	961.1	E857	E931.1	E950.4	E962.0	E980.4
Carbaryl	989.3	E863.2	—	E950.6	E962.1	E980.7
Carbaspirin	965.1	E850.3	E935.3	E950.0	E962.0	E980.0
Carbazochrome	972.8	E858.3	E942.8	E950.4	E962.0	E980.4
Carbenicillin	960.0	E856	E930.0	E950.4	E962.0	E980.4
Carbenoxolone	973.8	E858.4	E943.8	E950.4	E962.0	E980.4
Carbetapentane	975.4	E858.6	E945.4	E950.4	E962.0	E980.4
Carbimazole	962.8	E858.0	E932.8	E950.4	E962.0	E980.4
Carbinol	980.1	E860.2	—	E950.9	E962.1	E980.9
Carbinoxamine	963.0	E858.1	E933.0	E950.4	E962.0	E980.4
Carbitol	982.8	E862.4	—	E950.9	E962.1	E980.9
Carbocaine	968.9	E855.2	E938.9	E950.4	E962.0	E980.4
infiltration (subcutaneous)	968.5	E855.2	E938.5	E950.4	E962.0	E980.4
nerve block (peripheral) (plexus)	968.6	E855.2	E938.6	E950.4	E962.0	E980.4
topical (surface)	968.5	E855.2	E938.5	E950.4	E962.0	E980.4
Carbol–fuchsin solution	976.0	E858.7	E946.0	E950.4	E962.0	E980.4
Carbolic acid (*see also* Phenol)	983.0	E864.0	—	E950.7	E962.1	E980.6
Carbomycin	960.8	E856	E930.8	E950.4	E962.0	E980.4
Carbon						

Substance	Poisoning	Accident	Therapeutic Use	Suicide Attempt	Assault	Undetermined
bisulfide (liquid) (vapor)	982.2	E862.4	—	E950.9	E962.1	E980.9
dioxide (gas)	987.8	E869.8	—	E952.8	E962.2	E982.8
disulfide (liquid) (vapor)	982.2	E862.4	—	E950.9	E962.1	E980.9
monoxide (from incomplete combustion of) (in) NEC	986	E868.9	—	E952.1	E962.2	E982.1
blast furnace gas	986	E868.8	—	E952.1	E962.2	E982.1
butane (distributed in mobile container)	986	E868.0	—	E951.1	E962.2	E981.1
distributed through pipes	986	E867	—	E951.0	E962.2	E981.0
charcoal fumes	986	E868.3	—	E952.1	E962.2	E982.1
coal						
gas (piped)	986	E867	—	E951.0	E962.2	E981.0
solid (in domestic stoves, fireplaces)	986	E868.3	—	E952.1	E962.2	E982.1
coke (in domestic stoves, fireplaces)	986	E868.3	—	E952.1	E962.2	E982.1
exhaust gas (motor) not in transit	986	E868.2	—	E952.0	E962.2	E982.0
combustion engine, any not in watercraft	986	E868.2	—	E952.0	E962.2	E982.0
farm tractor, not in transit	986	E868.2	—	E952.0	E962.2	E982.0
gas engine	986	E868.2	—	E952.0	E962.2	E982.0
motor pump	986	E868.2	—	E952.0	E962.2	E982.0
motor vehicle, not in transit	986	E868.2	—	E952.0	E962.2	E982.0
fuel (in domestic use)	986	E868.3	—	E952.1	E962.2	E982.1
gas (piped)	986	E867	—	E951.0	E962.2	E981.0
in mobile container	986	E868.0	—	E951.1	E962.2	E981.1
utility	986	E868.1	—	E951.8	E962.2	E981.1
in mobile container	986	E868.0	—	E951.1	E962.2	E981.1
piped (natural)	986	E867	—	E951.0	E962.2	E981.0
illuminating gas	986	E868.1	—	E951.8	E962.2	E981.8
industrial fuels or gases, any	986	E868.8	—	E952.1	E962.2	E982.1
kerosene (in domestic stoves, fireplaces)	986	E868.3	—	E952.1	E962.2	E982.1
kiln gas or vapor	986	E868.8	—	E952.1	E962.2	E982.1
motor exhaust gas, not in transit	986	E868.2	—	E952.0	E962.2	E982.0
piped gas (manufactured) (natural)	986	E867	—	E951.0	E962.2	E981.0
producer gas	986	E868.8	—	E952.1	E962.2	E982.1
propane (distributed in mobile container)	986	E868.0	—	E951.1	E962.2	E981.1
distributed through pipes	986	E867	—	E951.0	E962.2	E981.0
specified source NEC	986	E868.8	—	E952.1	E962.2	E982.1
stove gas	986	E868.1	—	E951.8	E962.2	E981.8
piped	986	E867	—	E951.0	E962.2	E981.0
utility gas	986	E868.1	—	E951.8	E962.2	E981.8
piped	986	E867	—	E951.0	E962.2	E981.0
water gas	986	E868.1		E951.8	E962.2	E981.8
wood (in domestic stoves, fireplaces)	986	E868.3	—	E952.1	E962.2	E982.1
tetrachloride (vapor) NEC	987.8	E869.8	—	E952.8	E962.2	E982.8
liquid (cleansing agent) NEC	982.1	E861.3	—	E950.9	E962.1	E980.9
solvent	982.1	E862.4	—	E950.9	E962.1	E980.9
Carbonic acid (gas)	987.8	E869.8	—	E952.8	E962.2	E982.8
anhydrase inhibitors	974.2	E858.5	E944.2	E950.4	E962.0	E980.4
Carbowax	976.3	E858.7	E946.3	E950.4	E962.0	E980.4
Carbrital	967.0	E851	E937.0	E950.1	E962.0	E980.1
Carbromal (derivatives)	967.3	E852.2	E937.3	E950.2	E962.0	E980.2
Cardiac						
depressants	972.0	E858.3	E942.0	E950.4	E962.0	E980.4
rhythm regulators	972.0	E858.3	E942.0	E950.4	E962.0	E980.4

Substance	Poisoning	External Cause (E-Code)				
		Accident	Therapeutic Use	Suicide Attempt	Assault	Undetermined
Cardiografin	977.8	E858.8	E947.8	E950.4	E962.0	E980.4
Cardio–green	977.8	E858.8	E947.8	E950.4	E962.0	E980.4
Cardiotonic glycosides	972.1	E858.3	E942.1	E950.4	E962.0	E980.4
Cardiovascular agents NEC	972.9	E858.3	E942.9	E950.4	E962.0	E980.4
Cardrase	974.2	E858.5	E944.2	E950.4	E962.0	E980.4
Carfusin	976.0	E858.7	E946.0	E950.4	E962.0	E980.4
Carisoprodol	968.0	E855.1	E938.0	E950.4	E962.0	E980.4
Carmustine	963.1	E858.1	E933.1	E950.4	E962.0	E980.4
Carotene	963.5	E858.1	E933.5	E950.4	E962.0	E980.4
Carphenazine (maleate)	969.1	E853.0	E939.1	E950.3	E962.0	E980.3
Carter's Little Pills	973.1	E858.4	E943.1	E950.4	E962.0	E980.4
Cascara (sagrada)	973.1	E858.4	E943.1	E950.4	E962.0	E980.4
Cassava	988.2	E865.4	—	E950.9	E962.1	E980.9
Castellani's paint	976.0	E858.7	E946.0	E950.4	E962.0	E980.4
Castor						
bean	988.2	E865.3	—	E950.9	E962.1	E980.9
oil	973.1	E858.4	E943.1	E950.4	E962.0	E980.4
Caterpillar (sting)	989.5	E905.5	—	E950.9	E962.1	E980.9
Catha (edulis)	970.8	E854.3	E940.8	E950.4	E962.0	E980.4
Cathartics NEC	973.3	E858.4	E943.3	E950.4	E962.0	E980.4
contact	973.1	E858.4	E943.1	E950.4	E962.0	E980.4
emollient	973.2	E858.4	E943.2	E950.4	E962.0	E980.4
intestinal irritants	973.1	E858.4	E943.1	E950.4	E962.0	E980.4
saline	973.3	E858.4	E943.3	E950.4	E962.0	E980.4
Cathomycin	960.8	E856	E930.8	E950.4	E962.0	E980.4
Caustic(s)	983.9	E864.4	—	E950.7	E962.1	E980.6
alkali	983.2	E864.2	—	E950.7	E962.1	E980.6
hydroxide	983.2	E864.2	—	E950.7	E962.1	E980.6
potash	983.2	E864.2	—	E950.7	E962.1	E980.6
soda	983.2	E864.2	—	E950.7	E962.1	E980.6
specified NEC	983.9	E864.3	—	E950.7	E962.1	E980.6
Ceepryn	976.0	E858.7	E946.0	E950.4	E962.0	E980.4
ENT agent	976.6	E858.7	E946.6	E950.4	E962.0	E980.4
lozenges	976.6	E858.7	E946.6	E950.4	E962.0	E980.4
Celestone	962.0	E858.0	E932.0	E950.4	E962.0	E980.4
topical	976.0	E858.7	E946.0	E950.4	E962.0	E980.4
Cellosolve	982.8	E862.4	—	E950.9	E962.1	E980.9
Cell stimulants and proliferants	976.8	E858.7	E946.8	E950.4	E962.0	E980.4
Cellulose derivatives, cathartic	973.3	E858.4	E943.3	E950.4	E962.0	E980.4
nitrates (topical)	976.3	E858.7	E946.3	E950.4	E962.0	E980.4
Centipede (bite)	989.5	E905.4	—	E950.9	E962.1	E980.9
Central nervous system						
depressants	968.4	E855.1	E938.4	E950.4	E962.0	E980.4
anesthetic (general) NEC	968.4	E855.1	E938.4	E950.4	E962.0	E980.4
gases NEC	968.2	E855.1	E938.2	E950.4	E962.0	E980.4
intravenous	968.3	E855.1	E938.3	E950.4	E962.0	E980.4
barbiturates	967.0	E851	E937.0	E950.1	E962.0	E980.1
bromides	967.3	E852.2	E937.3	E950.2	E962.0	E980.2
cannabis sativa	969.6	E854.1	E939.6	E950.3	E962.0	E980.3
chloral hydrate	967.1	E852.0	E937.1	E950.2	E962.0	E980.2
hallucinogenics	969.6	E854.1	E939.6	E950.3	E962.0	E980.3
hypnotics	967.9	E852.9	E937.9	E950.2	E962.0	E980.2
specified NEC	967.8	E852.8	E937.8	E950.2	E962.0	E980.2
muscle relaxants	968.0	E855.1	E938.0	E950.4	E962.0	E980.4
paraldehyde	967.2	E852.1	E937.2	E950.2	E962.0	E980.2
sedatives	967.9	E852.9	E937.9	E950.2	E962.0	E980.2
mixed NEC	967.6	E852.5	E937.6	E950.2	E962.0	E980.2

Substance	Poisoning	Accident	Therapeutic Use	Suicide Attempt	Assault	Undetermined
specified NEC	967.8	E852.8	E937.8	E950.2	E962.0	E980.2
muscle–tone depressants	968.0	E855.1	E938.0	E950.4	E962.0	E980.4
stimulants	970.9	E854.3	E940.9	E950.4	E962.0	E980.4
amphetamines	969.7	E854.2	E939.7	E950.3	E962.0	E980.3
analeptics	970.0	E854.3	E940.0	E950.4	E962.0	E980.4
antidepressants	969.0	E854.0	E939.0	E950.3	E962.0	E980.3
opiate antagonists	970.1	E854.3	E940.0	E950.4	E962.0	E980.4
specified NEC	970.8	E854.3	E940.8	E950.4	E962.0	E980.4
Cephalexin	960.5	E856	E930.5	E950.4	E962.0	E980.4
Cephaloglycin	960.5	E856	E930.5	E950.4	E962.0	E980.4
Cephaloridine	960.5	E856	E930.5	E950.4	E962.0	E980.4
Cephalosporins NEC	960.5	E856	E930.5	E950.4	E962.0	E980.4
N (adicillin)	960.0	E856	E930.0	E950.4	E962.0	E980.4
Cephalothin (sodium)	960.5	E856	E930.5	E950.4	E962.0	E980.4
Cerbera (odallam)	988.2	E865.4	—	E950.9	E962.1	E980.9
Cerberin	972.1	E858.3	E942.1	E950.4	E962.0	E980.4
Cerebral stimulants	970.9	E854.3	E940.9	E950.4	E962.0	E980.4
psychotherapeutic	969.7	E854.2	E939.7	E950.3	E962.0	E980.3
specified NEC	970.8	E854.3	E940.8	E950.4	E962.0	E980.4
Cetalkonium (chloride)	976.0	E858.7	E946.0	E950.4	E962.0	E980.4
Cetoxime	963.0	E858.1	E933.0	E950.4	E962.0	E980.4
Cetrimide	976.2	E858.7	E946.2	E950.4	E962.0	E980.4
Cetylpyridinium	976.0	E858.7	E946.0	E950.4	E962.0	E980.4
ENT agent	976.6	E858.7	E946.6	E950.4	E962.0	E980.4
lozenges	976.6	E858.7	E946.6	E950.4	E962.0	E980.4
Cevadilla — *see* Sabadilla						
Cevitamic acid	963.5	E858.1	E933.5	E950.4	E962.0	E980.4
Chalk, precipitated	973.0	E858.4	E943.0	E950.4	E962.0	E980.4
Charcoal						
fumes (carbon monoxide)	986	E868.3	—	E952.1	E962.2	E982.1
industrial	986	E868.8	—	E952.1	E962.2	E982.1
medicinal (activated)	973.0	E858.4	E943.0	E950.4	E962.0	E980.4
Chelating agents NEC	977.2	E858.8	E947.2	E950.4	E962.0	E980.4
Chelidonium majus	988.2	E865.4	—	E950.9	E962.1	E980.9
Chemical substance	989.9	E866.9	—	E950.9	E962.1	E980.9
specified NEC	989.89	E866.8	—	E950.9	E962.1	E980.9
Chemotherapy, antineoplastic	963.1	E858.1	E933.1	E950.4	E962.0	E980.4
Chenopodium (oil)	961.6	E857	E931.6	E950.4	E962.0	E980.4
Cherry laurel	988.2	E865.4	—	E950.9	E962.1	E980.9
Chiniofon	961.3	E857	E931.3	E950.4	E962.0	E980.4
Chlophedianol	975.4	E858.6	E945.4	E950.4	E962.0	E980.4
Chloral (betaine) (formamide) (hydrate)	967.1	E852.0	E937.1	E950.2	E962.0	E980.2
Chloralamide	967.1	E852.0	E937.1	E950.2	E962.0	E980.2
Chlorambucil	963.1	E858.1	E933.1	E950.4	E962.0	E980.4
Chloramphenicol	960.2	E856	E930.2	E950.4	E962.0	E980.4
ENT agent	976.6	E858.7	E946.6	E950.4	E962.0	E980.4
ophthalmic preparation	976.5	E858.7	E946.5	E950.4	E962.0	E980.4
topical NEC	976.0	E858.7	E946.0	E950.4	E962.0	E980.4
Chlorate(s) (potassium) (sodium) NEC	983.9	E864.3	—	E950.7	E962.1	E980.6
herbicides	989.4	E863.5	—	E950.6	E962.1	E980.7
Chlorcyclizine	963.0	E858.1	E933.0	E950.4	E962.0	E980.4
Chlordan(e) (dust)	989.2	E863.0	—	E950.6	E962.1	E980.7
Chlordantoin	976.0	E858.7	E946.0	E950.4	E962.0	E980.4
Chlordiazepoxide	969.4	E853.2	E939.4	E950.3	E962.0	E980.3
Chloresium	976.8	E858.7	E946.8	E950.4	E962.0	E980.4
Chlorethiazol	967.1	E852.0	E937.1	E950.2	E962.0	E980.2
Chlorethyl — *see* Ethyl, chloride						

Substance	Poisoning	External Cause (E-Code)				
		Accident	Therapeutic Use	Suicide Attempt	Assault	Undetermined
Chloretone	967.1	E852.0	E937.1	E950.2	E962.0	E980.2
Chlorex	982.3	E862.4	—	E950.9	E962.1	E980.9
Chlorhexadol	967.1	E852.0	E937.1	E950.2	E962.0	E980.2
Chlorhexidine (hydrochloride)	976.0	E858.7	E946.0	E950.4	E962.0	E980.4
Chlorhydroxyquinolin	976.0	E858.7	E946.0	E950.4	E962.0	E980.4
Chloride of lime (bleach)	983.9	E864.3	—	E950.7	E962.1	E980.6
Chlorinated						
camphene	989.2	E863.0	—	E950.6	E962.1	E980.7
diphenyl	989.89	E866.8	—	E950.9	E962.1	E980.9
hydrocarbons NEC	989.2	E863.0	—	E950.6	E962.1	E980.7
solvent	982.3	E862.4	—	E950.9	E962.1	E980.9
lime (bleach)	983.9	E864.3	—	E950.7	E962.1	E980.6
naphthalene — *see* Naphthalene						
pesticides NEC	989.2	E863.0	—	E950.6	E962.1	E980.7
soda — *see* Sodium, hypochlorite						
Chlorine (fumes) (gas)	987.6	E869.8	—	E952.8	E962.2	E982.8
bleach	983.9	E864.3	—	E950.7	E962.1	E980.6
compounds NEC	983.9	E864.3	—	E950.7	E962.1	E980.6
disinfectant	983.9	E861.4	—	E950.7	E962.1	E980.6
releasing agents NEC	983.9	E864.3	—	E950.7	E962.1	E980.6
Chlorisondamine	972.3	E858.3	E942.3	E950.4	E962.0	E980.4
Chlormadinone	962.2	E858.0	E932.2	E950.4	E962.0	E980.4
Chlormerodrin	974.0	E858.5	E944.0	E950.4	E962.0	E980.4
Chlormethiazole	967.1	E852.0	E937.1	E950.2	E962.0	E980.2
Chlormethylenecycline	960.4	E856	E930.4	E950.4	E962.0	E980.4
Chlormezanone	969.5	E853.8	E939.5	E950.3	E962.0	E980.3
Chloroacetophenone	987.5	E869.3	—	E952.8	E962.2	E982.8
Chloroaniline	983.0	E864.0	—	E950.7	E962.1	E980.6
Chlorobenzene, chlorobenzol	982.0	E862.4	—	E950.9	E962.1	E980.9
Chlorobutanol	967.1	E852.0	E937.1	E950.2	E962.0	E980.2
Chlorodinitrobenzene	983.0	E864.0	—	E950.7	E962.1	E980.6
dust or vapor	987.8	E869.8	—	E952.8	E962.2	E982.8
Chloroethane — *see* Ethyl, chloride						
Chloroform (fumes) (vapor)	987.8	E869.8	—	E952.8	E962.2	E982.8
anesthetic (gas)	968.2	E855.1	E938.2	E950.4	E962.0	E980.4
liquid NEC	968.4	E855.1	E938.4	E950.4	E962.0	E980.4
solvent	982.3	E862.4	—	E950.9	E962.1	E980.9
Chloroguanide	961.4	E857	E931.4	E950.4	E962.0	E980.4
Chloromycetin	960.2	E856	E930.2	E950.4	E962.0	E980.4
ENT agent	976.6	E858.7	E946.6	E950.4	E962.0	E980.4
ophthalmic preparation	976.5	E858.7	E946.5	E950.4	E962.0	E980.4
otic solution	976.6	E858.7	E946.6	E950.4	E962.0	E980.4
topical NEC	976.0	E858.7	E946.0	E950.4	E962.0	E980.4
Chloronitrobenzene	983.0	E864.0	—	E950.7	E962.1	E980.6
dust or vapor	987.8	E869.8	—	E952.8	E962.2	E982.8
Chlorophenol	983.0	E864.0	—	E950.7	E962.1	E980.6
Chlorophenothane	989.2	E863.0	—	E950.6	E962.1	E980.7
Chlorophyll (derivatives)	976.8	E858.7	E946.8	E950.4	E962.0	E980.4
Chloropicrin (fumes)	987.8	E869.8	—	E952.8	E962.2	E982.8
fumigant	989.4	E863.8	—	E950.6	E962.1	E980.7
fungicide	989.4	E863.6	—	E950.6	E962.1	E980.7
pesticide (fumes)	989.4	E863.4	—	E950.6	E962.1	E980.7
Chloroprocaine	968.9	E855.2	E938.9	E950.4	E962.0	E980.4
infiltration (subcutaneous)	968.5	E855.2	E938.5	E950.4	E962.0	E980.4
nerve block (peripheral) (plexus)	968.6	E855.2	E938.6	E950.4	E962.0	E980.4
Chloroptic	976.5	E858.7	E946.5	E950.4	E962.0	E980.4
Chloropurine	963.1	E858.1	E933.1	E950.4	E962.0	E980.4

Substance	Poisoning	Accident	Therapeutic Use	Suicide Attempt	Assault	Undetermined
Chloroquine (hydrochloride) (phosphate)	961.4	E857	E931.4	E950.4	E962.0	E980.4
Chlorothen	963.0	E858.1	E933.0	E950.4	E962.0	E980.4
Chlorothiazide	974.3	E858.5	E944.3	E950.4	E962.0	E980.4
Chlorotrianisene	962.2	E858.0	E932.2	E950.4	E962.0	E980.4
Chlorovinyldichloroarsine	985.1	E866.3	—	E950.8	E962.1	E980.8
Chloroxylenol	976.0	E858.7	E946.0	E950.4	E962.0	E980.4
Chlorphenesin (carbamate)	968.0	E855.1	E938.0	E950.4	E962.0	E980.4
topical (antifungal)	976.0	E858.7	E946.0	E950.4	E962.0	E980.4
Chlorpheniramine	963.0	E858.1	E933.0	E950.4	E962.0	E980.4
Chlorophenoxamine	966.4	E855.0	E936.4	E950.4	E962.0	E980.4
Chlorophentermine	977.0	E858.8	E947.0	E950.4	E962.0	E980.4
Chlorproguanil	961.4	E857	E931.4	E950.4	E962.0	E980.4
Chlorpromazine	969.1	E853.0	E939.1	E950.3	E962.0	E980.3
Chlorpropamide	962.3	E858.0	E932.3	E950.4	E962.0	E980.4
Chlorprothixene	969.3	E853.8	E939.3	E950.3	E962.0	E980.3
Chlorquinaldol	976.0	E858.7	E946.0	E950.4	E962.0	E980.4
Chlortetracycline	960.4	E856	E930.4	E950.4	E962.0	E980.4
Chlorthalidone	974.4	E858.5	E944.4	E950.4	E962.0	E980.4
Chlortrianisene	962.2	E858.0	E932.2	E950.4	E962.0	E980.4
Chlor–Trimeton	963.0	E858.1	E933.0	E950.4	E962.0	E980.4
Chlorzoxazone	968.0	E855.1	E938.0	E950.4	E962.0	E980.4
Choke damp	987.8	E869.8	—	E952.8	E962.2	E982.8
Cholebrine	977.8	E858.8	E947.8	E950.4	E962.0	E980.4
Cholera vaccine	978.2	E858.8	E948.2	E950.4	E962.0	E980.4
Cholesterol–lowering agents	972.2	E858.3	E942.2	E950.4	E962.0	E980.4
Cholestyramine (resin)	972.2	E858.3	E942.2	E950.4	E962.0	E980.4
Cholic acid	973.4	E858.4	E943.4	E950.4	E962.0	E980.4
Choline						
dihydrogen citrate	977.1	E858.8	E947.1	E950.4	E962.0	E980.4
salicylate	965.1	E850.3	E935.3	E950.0	E962.0	E980.0
theophyllinate	974.1	E858.5	E944.1	E950.4	E962.0	E980.4
Cholinergics	971.0	E855.3	E941.0	E950.4	E962.0	E980.4
Cholografin	977.8	E858.8	E947.8	E950.4	E962.0	E980.4
Chorionic gonadotropin	962.4	E858.0	E932.4	E950.4	E962.0	E980.4
Chromates	983.9	E864.3	—	E950.7	E962.1	E980.6
dust or mist	987.8	E869.8	—	E952.8	E962.2	E982.8
lead	984.0	E866.0	—	E950.9	E962.1	E980.9
paint	984.0	E861.5	—	E950.9	E962.1	E980.9
Chromic acid	983.9	E864.3	—	E950.7	E962.1	E980.6
dust or mist	987.8	E869.8	—	E952.8	E962.2	E982.8
Chromium	985.6	E866.4	—	E950.9	E962.1	E980.9
compounds — *see* Chromates						
Chromonar	972.4	E858.3	E942.4	E950.4	E962.0	E980.4
Chromyl chloride	983.9	E864.3	—	E950.7	E962.1	E980.6
Chrysarobin (ointment)	976.4	E858.7	E946.4	E950.4	E962.0	E980.4
Chrysazin	973.1	E858.4	E943.1	E950.4	E962.0	E980.4
Chymar	963.4	E858.1	E933.4	E950.4	E962.0	E980.4
ophthalmic preparation	976.5	E858.7	E946.5	E950.4	E962.0	E980.4
Chymotrypsin	963.4	E858.1	E933.4	E950.4	E962.0	E980.4
ophthalmic preparation	976.5	E858.7	E946.5	E950.4	E962.0	E980.4
Cicuta maculata or virosa	988.2	E865.4	—	E950.9	E962.1	E980.9
Cigarette lighter fluid	981	E862.1	—	E950.9	E962.1	E980.9
Cinchocaine (spinal)	968.7	E855.2	E938.7	E950.4	E962.0	E980.4
topical (surface)	968.5	E855.2	E938.5	E950.4	E962.0	E980.4
Cinchona	961.4	E857	E931.4	E950.4	E962.0	E980.4
Cinchonine alkaloids	961.4	E857	E931.4	E950.4	E962.0	E980.4
Cinchophen	974.7	E858.5	E944.7	E950.4	E962.0	E980.4

Substance	Poisoning	Accident	Therapeutic Use	Suicide Attempt	Assault	Undetermined
		External Cause (E-Code)				
Cinnarizine	963.0	E858.1	E933.0	E950.4	E962.0	E980.4
Citanest	968.9	E855.2	E938.9	E950.4	E962.0	E980.4
infiltration (subcutaneous)	968.5	E855.2	E938.5	E950.4	E962.0	E980.4
nerve block (peripheral) (plexus)	968.6	E855.2	E938.6	E950.4	E962.0	E980.4
Citric acid	989.89	E866.8	—	E950.9	E962.1	E980.9
Citrovorum factor	964.1	E858.2	E934.1	E950.4	E962.0	E980.4
Claviceps purpurea	988.2	E865.4	—	E950.9	E962.1	E980.9
Cleaner, cleansing agent NEC	989.89	E861.3	—	E950.9	E962.1	E980.9
of paint or varnish	982.8	E862.9	—	E950.9	E962.1	E980.9
Clematis vitalba	988.2	E865.4	—	E950.9	E962.1	E980.9
Clemizole	963.0	E858.1	E933.0	E950.4	E962.0	E980.4
penicillin	960.0	E856	E930.0	E950.4	E962.0	E980.4
Clidinium	971.1	E855.4	E941.1	E950.4	E962.0	E980.4
Clindamycin	960.8	E856	E930.8	E950.4	E962.0	E980.4
Cliradon	965.09	E850.2	E935.2	E950.0	E962.0	E980.0
Clocortolone	962.0	E858.0	E932.0	E950.4	E962.0	E980.4
Clofedanol	975.4	E858.6	E945.4	E950.4	E962.0	E980.4
Clofibrate	972.2	E858.3	E942.2	E950.4	E962.0	E980.4
Clomethiazole	967.1	E852.0	E937.1	E950.2	E962.0	E980.2
Clomiphene	977.8	E858.8	E947.8	E950.4	E962.0	E980.4
Clonazepam	969.4	E853.2	E939.4	E950.3	E962.0	E980.3
Clonidine	972.6	E858.3	E942.6	E950.4	E962.0	E980.4
Clopamide	974.3	E858.5	E944.3	E950.4	E962.0	E980.4
Clorazepate	969.4	E853.2	E939.4	E950.3	E962.0	E980.3
Clorexolone	974.4	E858.5	E944.4	E950.4	E962.0	E980.4
Clorox (bleach)	983.9	E864.3	—	E950.7	E962.1	E980.6
Clortermine	977.0	E858.8	E947.0	E950.4	E962.0	E980.4
Clotrimazole	976.0	E858.7	E946.0	E950.4	E962.0	E980.4
Cloxacillin	960.0	E856	E930.0	E950.4	E962.0	E980.4
Coagulants NEC	964.5	E858.2	E934.5	E950.4	E962.0	E980.4
Coal (carbon monoxide from) — *see also* Carbon, monoxide, coal						
oil — *see* Kerosene						
tar NEC	983.0	E864.0	—	E950.7	E962.1	E980.6
fumes	987.8	E869.8	—	E952.8	E962.2	E982.8
medicinal (ointment)	976.4	E858.7	E946.4	E950.4	E962.0	E980.4
analgesics NEC	965.5	E850.5	E935.5	E950.0	E962.0	E980.0
naphtha (solvent)	981	E862.0	—	E950.9	E962.1	E980.9
Cobalt (fumes) (industrial)	985.8	E866.4	—	E950.9	E962.1	E980.9
Cobra (venom)	989.5	E905.0	—	E950.9	E962.1	E980.9
Coca (leaf)	970.8	E854.3	E940.8	E950.4	E962.0	E980.4
Cocaine (hydrochloride) (salt)	970.8	E854.3	E940.8	E950.4	E962.0	E980.4
topical anesthetic	968.5	E855.2	E938.5	E950.4	E962.0	E980.4
Coccidioidin	977.8	E858.8	E947.8	E950.4	E962.0	E980.4
Cocculus indicus	988.2	E865.3	—	E950.9	E962.1	E980.9
Cochineal	989.89	E866.8	—	E950.9	E962.1	E980.9
medicinal products	977.4	E858.8	E947.4	E950.4	E962.0	E980.4
Codeine	965.09	E850.2	E935.2	E950.0	E962.0	E980.0
Coffee	989.89	E866.8	—	E950.9	E962.1	E980.9
Cogentin	971.1	E855.4	E941.1	E950.4	E962.0	E980.4
Coke fumes or gas (carbon monoxide)	986	E868.3	—	E952.1	E962.2	E982.1
industrial use	986	E868.8	—	E952.1	E962.2	E982.1
Colace	973.2	E858.4	E943.2	E950.4	E962.0	E980.4
Colchicine	974.7	E858.5	E944.7	E950.4	E962.0	E980.4
Colchicum	988.2	E865.3	—	E950.9	E962.1	E980.9
Cold cream	976.3	E858.7	E946.3	E950.4	E962.0	E980.4
Colestipol	972.2	E858.3	E942.2	E950.4	E962.0	E980.4

Substance	Poisoning	External Cause (E-Code)				
		Accident	Therapeutic Use	Suicide Attempt	Assault	Undetermined
Colistimethate	960.8	E856	E930.8	E950.4	E962.0	E980.4
Colistin	960.8	E856	E930.8	E950.4	E962.0	E980.4
Collagen	977.8	E866.8	E947.8	E950.9	E962.1	E980.9
Collagenase	976.8	E858.7	E946.8	E950.4	E962.0	E980.4
Collodion (flexible)	976.3	E858.7	E946.3	E950.4	E962.0	E980.4
Colocynth	973.1	E858.4	E943.1	E950.4	E962.0	E980.4
Coloring matter — *see* Dye(s)						
Combustion gas — *see* Carbon, monoxide						
Compazine	969.1	E853.0	E939.1	E950.3	E962.0	E980.3
Compound						
42 (warfarin)	989.4	E863.7	—	E950.6	E962.1	E980.7
269 (endrin)	989.2	E863.0	—	E950.6	E962.1	E980.7
497 (dieldrin)	989.2	E863.0	—	E950.6	E962.1	E980.7
1080 (sodium fluoroacetate)	989.4	E863.7	—	E950.6	E962.1	E980.7
3422 (parathion)	989.3	E863.1	—	E950.6	E962.1	E980.7
3911 (phorate)	989.3	E863.1	—	E950.6	E962.1	E980.7
3956 (toxaphene)	989.2	E863.0	—	E950.6	E962.1	E980.7
4049 (malathion)	989.3	E863.1	—	E950.6	E962.1	E980.7
4124 (dicapthon)	989.4	E863.4	—	E950.6	E962.1	E980.7
E (cortisone)	962.0	E858.0	E932.0	E950.4	E962.0	E980.4
F (hydrocortisone)	962.0	E858.0	E932.0	E950.4	E962.0	E980.4
Congo red	977.8	E858.8	E947.8	E950.4	E962.0	E980.4
Coniine, conine	965.7	E850.7	E935.7	E950.0	E962.0	E980.0
Conium (maculatum)	988.2	E865.4	—	E950.9	E962.1	E980.9
Conjugated estrogens (equine)	962.2	E858.0	E932.2	E950.4	E962.0	E980.4
Contac	975.6	E858.6	E945.6	E950.4	E962.0	E980.4
Contact lens solution	976.5	E858.7	E946.5	E950.4	E962.0	E980.4
Contraceptives (oral)	962.2	E858.0	E932.2	E950.4	E962.0	E980.4
vaginal	976.8	E858.7	E946.8	E950.4	E962.0	E980.4
Contrast media (roentgenographic)	977.8	E858.8	E947.8	E950.4	E962.0	E980.4
Convallaria majalis	988.2	E865.4	—	E950.9	E962.1	E980.9
Copper (dust) (fumes) (salts) NEC	985.8	E866.4	—	E950.9	E962.1	E980.9
arsenate, arsenite	985.1	E866.3	—	E950.8	E962.1	E980.8
insecticide	985.1	E863.4	—	E950.8	E962.1	E980.8
emetic	973.6	E858.4	E943.6	E950.4	E962.0	E980.4
fungicide	985.8	E863.6	—	E950.6	E962.1	E980.7
insecticide	985.8	E863.4	—	E950.6	E962.1	E980.7
oleate	976.0	E858.7	E946.0	E950.4	E962.0	E980.4
sulfate	983.9	E864.3	—	E950.7	E962.1	E980.6
fungicide	983.9	E863.6	—	E950.7	E962.1	E980.6
cupric	973.6	E858.4	E943.6	E950.4	E962.0	E980.4
cuprous	983.9	E864.3	—	E950.7	E962.1	E980.6
Copperhead snake (bite) (venom)	989.5	E905.0	—	E950.9	E962.1	E980.9
Coral (sting)	989.5	E905.6	—	E950.9	E962.1	E980.9
snake (bite) (venom)	989.5	E905.0	—	E950.9	E962.1	E980.9
Cordran	976.0	E858.7	E946.0	E950.4	E962.0	E980.4
Corn cures	976.4	E858.7	E946.4	E950.4	E962.0	E980.4
Cornhusker's lotion	976.3	E858.7	E946.3	E950.4	E962.0	E980.4
Corn starch	976.3	E858.7	E946.3	E950.4	E962.0	E980.4
Corrosive	983.9	E864.4	—	E950.7	E962.1	E980.6
acids NEC	983.1	E864.1	—	E950.7	E962.1	E980.6
aromatics	983.0	E864.0	—	E950.7	E962.1	E980.6
disinfectant	983.0	E861.4	—	E950.7	E962.1	E980.6
fumes NEC	987.9	E869.9	—	E952.9	E962.2	E982.9
specified NEC	983.9	E864.3	—	E950.7	E962.1	E980.6
sublimate — *see* Mercury, chloride						
Cortate	962.0	E858.0	E932.0	E950.4	E962.0	E980.4

Substance	Poisoning	External Cause (E-Code)				
		Accident	Therapeutic Use	Suicide Attempt	Assault	Undetermined
Cort–Dome	962.0	E858.0	E932.0	E950.4	E962.0	E980.4
ENT agent	976.6	E858.7	E946.6	E950.4	E962.0	E980.4
ophthalmic preparation	976.5	E858.7	E946.5	E950.4	E962.0	E980.4
topical NEC	976.0	E858.7	E946.0	E950.4	E962.0	E980.4
Cortef	962.0	E858.0	E932.0	E950.4	E962.0	E980.4
ENT agent	976.6	E858.7	E946.6	E950.4	E962.0	E980.4
ophthalmic preparation	976.5	E858.7	E946.5	E950.4	E962.0	E980.4
topical NEC	976.0	E858.7	E946.0	E950.4	E962.0	E980.4
Corticosteroids (fluorinated)	962.0	E858.0	E932.0	E950.4	E962.0	E980.4
ENT agent	976.6	E858.7	E946.6	E950.4	E962.0	E980.4
ophthalmic preparation	976.5	E858.7	E946.5	E950.4	E962.0	E980.4
topical NEC	976.0	E858.7	E946.0	E950.4	E962.0	E980.4
Corticotropin	962.4	E858.0	E932.4	E950.4	E962.0	E980.4
Cortisol	962.0	E858.0	E932.0	E950.4	E962.0	E980.4
ENT agent	976.6	E858.7	E946.6	E950.4	E962.0	E980.4
ophthalmic preparation	976.5	E858.7	E946.5	E950.4	E962.0	E980.4
topical NEC	976.0	E858.7	E946.0	E950.4	E962.0	E980.4
Cortisone derivatives (acetate)	962.0	E858.0	E932.0	E950.4	E962.0	E980.4
ENT agent	976.6	E858.7	E946.6	E950.4	E962.0	E980.4
ophthalmic preparation	976.5	E858.7	E946.5	E950.4	E962.0	E980.4
topical NEC	976.0	E858.7	E946.0	E950.4	E962.0	E980.4
Cortogen	962.0	E858.0	E932.0	E950.4	E962.0	E980.4
ENT agent	976.6	E858.7	E946.6	E950.4	E962.0	E980.4
ophthalmic preparation	976.5	E858.7	E946.5	E950.4	E962.0	E980.4
Cortone	962.0	E858.0	E932.0	E950.4	E962.0	E980.4
ENT agent	976.6	E858.7	E946.6	E950.4	E962.0	E980.4
ophthalmic preparation	976.5	E858.7	E946.5	E950.4	E962.0	E980.4
Cortril	962.0	E858.0	E932.0	E950.4	E962.0	E980.4
ENT agent	976.6	E858.7	E946.6	E950.4	E962.0	E980.4
ophthalmic preparation	976.5	E858.7	E946.5	E950.4	E962.0	E980.4
topical NEC	976.0	E858.7	E946.0	E950.4	E962.0	E980.4
Cosmetics	989.89	E866.7	—	E950.9	E962.1	E980.9
Cosyntropin	977.8	E858.8	E947.8	E950.4	E962.0	E980.4
Cotarnine	964.5	E858.2	E934.5	E950.4	E962.0	E980.4
Cottonseed oil	976.3	E858.7	E946.3	E950.4	E962.0	E980.4
Cough mixtures (antitussives)	975.4	E858.6	E945.4	E950.4	E962.0	E980.4
containing opiates	965.09	E850.2	E935.2	E950.0	E962.0	E980.0
expectorants	975.5	E858.6	E945.5	E950.4	E962.0	E980.4
Coumadin	964.2	E858.2	E934.2	E950.4	E962.0	E980.4
rodenticide	989.4	E863.7	—	E950.6	E962.1	E980.7
Coumarin	964.2	E858.2	E934.2	E950.4	E962.0	E980.4
Coumetarol	964.2	E858.2	E934.2	E950.4	E962.0	E980.4
Cowbane	988.2	E865.4	—	E950.9	E962.1	E980.9
Cozyme	963.5	E858.1	E933.5	E950.4	E962.0	E980.4
Crack	970.8	E854.3	E940.8	E950.4	E962.0	E980.4
Creolin	983.0	E864.0	—	E950.7	E962.1	E980.6
disinfectant	983.0	E861.4	—	E950.7	E962.1	E980.6
Creosol (compound)	983.0	E864.0	—	E950.7	E962.1	E980.6
Creosote (beechwood) (coal tar)	983.0	E864.0	—	E950.7	E962.1	E980.6
medicinal (expectorant)	975.5	E858.6	E945.5	E950.4	E962.0	E980.4
syrup	975.5	E858.6	E945.5	E950.4	E962.0	E980.4
Cresol	983.0	E864.0	—	E950.7	E962.1	E980.6
disinfectant	983.0	E861.4	—	E950.7	E962.1	E980.6
Cresylic acid	983.0	E864.0	—	E950.7	E962.1	E980.6
Cropropamide	965.7	E850.7	E935.7	E950.0	E962.0	E980.0
with crotethamide	970.0	E854.3	E940.0	E950.4	E962.0	E980.4
Crotamiton	976.0	E858.7	E946.0	E950.4	E962.0	E980.4

Substance	Poisoning	External Cause (E-Code)				
		Accident	Therapeutic Use	Suicide Attempt	Assault	Undetermined
Crotethamide	965.7	E850.7	E935.7	E950.0	E962.0	E980.0
with cropropamide	970.0	E854.3	E940.0	E950.4	E962.0	E980.4
Croton (oil)	973.1	E858.4	E943.1	E950.4	E962.0	E980.4
chloral	967.1	E852.0	E937.1	E950.2	E962.0	E980.2
Crude oil	981	E862.1	—	E950.9	E962.1	E980.9
Cryogenine	965.8	E850.8	E935.8	E950.0	E962.0	E980.0
Cryolite (pesticide)	989.4	E863.4	—	E950.6	E962.1	E980.7
Cryptenamine	972.6	E858.3	E942.6	E950.4	E962.0	E980.4
Crystal violet	976.0	E858.7	E946.0	E950.4	E962.0	E980.4
Cuckoopint	988.2	E865.4	—	E950.9	E962.1	E980.9
Cumetharol	964.2	E858.2	E934.2	E950.4	E962.0	E980.4
Cupric sulfate	973.6	E858.4	E943.6	E950.4	E962.0	E980.4
Cuprous sulfate	983.9	E864.3	—	E950.7	E962.1	E980.6
Curare, curarine	975.2	E858.6	E945.2	E950.4	E962.0	E980.4
Cyanic acid — *see* Cyanide(s)						
Cyanide(s) (compounds) (hydrogen) (potassium) (sodium) NEC	989.0	E866.8	—	E950.9	E962.1	E980.9
dust or gas (inhalation) NEC	987.7	E869.8	—	E952.8	E962.2	E982.8
fumigant	989.0	E863.8	—	E950.6	E962.1	E980.7
mercuric — *see* Mercury						
pesticide (dust) (fumes)	989.0	E863.4	—	E950.6	E962.1	E980.7
Cyanocobalamin	964.1	E858.2	E934.1	E950.4	E962.0	E980.4
Cyanogen (chloride) (gas) NEC	987.8	E869.8	—	E952.8	E962.2	E982.8
Cyclaine	968.5	E855.2	E938.5	E950.4	E962.0	E980.4
Cyclamen europaeum	988.2	E865.4	—	E950.9	E962.1	E980.9
Cyclandelate	972.5	E858.3	E942.5	E950.4	E962.0	E980.4
Cyclazocine	965.09	E850.2	E935.2	E950.0	E962.0	E980.0
Cyclizine	963.0	E858.1	E933.0	E950.4	E962.0	E980.4
Cyclobarbital, cyclobarbitone	967.0	E851	E937.0	E950.1	E962.0	E980.1
Cycloguanil	961.4	E857	E931.4	E950.4	E962.0	E980.4
Cyclohexane	982.0	E862.4	—	E950.9	E962.1	E980.9
Cyclohexanol	980.8	E860.8	—	E950.9	E962.1	E980.9
Cyclohexanone	982.8	E862.4	—	E950.9	E962.1	E980.9
Cyclomethycaine	968.5	E855.2	E938.5	E950.4	E962.0	E980.4
Cyclopentamine	971.2	E855.5	E941.2	E950.4	E962.0	E980.4
Cyclopenthiazide	974.3	E858.5	E944.3	E950.4	E962.0	E980.4
Cyclopentolate	971.1	E855.4	E941.1	E950.4	E962.0	E980.4
Cyclophosphamide	963.1	E858.1	E933.1	E950.4	E962.0	E980.4
Cyclopropane	968.2	E855.1	E938.2	E950.4	E962.0	E980.4
Cycloserine	960.6	E856	E930.6	E950.4	E962.0	E980.4
Cyclothiazide	974.3	E858.5	E944.3	E950.4	E962.0	E980.4
Cycrimine	966.4	E855.0	E936.4	E950.4	E962.0	E980.4
Cymarin	972.1	E858.3	E942.1	E950.4	E962.0	E980.4
Cyproheptadine	963.0	E858.1	E933.0	E950.4	E962.0	E980.4
Cyprolidol	969.0	E854.0	E939.0	E950.3	E962.0	E980.3
Cytarabine	963.1	E858.1	E933.1	E950.4	E962.0	E980.4
Cytisus						
laburnum	988.2	E865.4	—	E950.9	E962.1	E980.9
scoparius	988.2	E865.4	—	E950.9	E962.1	E980.9
Cytomel	962.7	E858.0	E932.7	E950.4	E962.0	E980.4
Cytosine (antineoplastic)	963.1	E858.1	E933.1	E950.4	E962.0	E980.4
Cytoxan	963.1	E858.1	E933.1	E950.4	E962.0	E980.4
Dacarbazine	963.1	E858.1	E933.1	E950.4	E962.0	E980.4
Dactinomycin	960.7	E856	E930.7	E950.4	E962.0	E980.4
DADPS	961.8	E857	E931.8	E950.4	E962.0	E980.4
Dakin's solution (external)	976.0	E858.7	E946.0	E950.4	E962.0	E980.4
Dalmane	969.4	E853.2	E939.4	E950.3	E962.0	E980.3

Substance	Poisoning	External Cause (E-Code)				
		Accident	Therapeutic Use	Suicide Attempt	Assault	Undetermined
DAM	977.2	E858.8	E947.2	E950.4	E962.0	E980.4
Danilone	964.2	E858.2	E934.2	E950.4	E962.0	E980.4
Danthron	973.1	E858.4	E943.1	E950.4	E962.0	E980.4
Dantrolene	975.2	E858.6	E945.2	E950.4	E962.0	E980.4
Daphne (gnidium) (mezereum)	988.2	E865.4	—	E950.9	E962.1	E980.9
berry	988.2	E865.3	—	E950.9	E962.1	E980.9
Dapsone	961.8	E857	E931.8	E950.4	E962.0	E980.4
Daraprim	961.4	E857	E931.4	E950.4	E962.0	E980.4
Darnel	988.2	E865.3	—	E950.9	E962.1	E980.9
Darvon	965.8	E850.8	E935.8	E950.0	E962.0	E980.0
Daunorubicin	960.7	E856	E930.7	E950.4	E962.0	E980.4
DBI	962.3	E858.0	E932.3	E950.4	E962.0	E980.4
D–Con (rodenticide)	989.4	E863.7	—	E950.6	E962.1	E980.7
DDS	961.8	E857	E931.8	E950.4	E962.0	E980.4
DDT	989.2	E863.0	—	E950.6	E962.1	E980.7
Deadly nightshade	988.2	E865.4	—	E950.9	E962.1	E980.9
berry	988.2	E865.3	—	E950.9	E962.1	E980.9
Deanol	969.7	E854.2	E939.7	E950.3	E962.0	E980.3
Debrisoquine	972.6	E858.3	E942.6	E950.4	E962.0	E980.4
Decaborane	989.89	E866.8	—	E950.9	E962.1	E980.9
fumes	987.8	E869.8	—	E952.8	E962.2	E982.8
Decadron	962.0	E858.0	E932.0	E950.4	E962.0	E980.4
ENT agent	976.6	E858.7	E946.6	E950.4	E962.0	E980.4
ophthalmic preparation	976.5	E858.7	E946.5	E950.4	E962.0	E980.4
topical NEC	976.0	E858.7	E946.0	E950.4	E962.0	E980.4
Decahydronaphthalene	982.0	E862.4	—	E950.9	E962.1	E980.9
Decalin	982.0	E862.4	—	E950.9	E962.1	E980.9
Decamethonium	975.2	E858.6	E945.2	E950.4	E962.0	E980.4
Decholin	973.4	E858.4	E943.4	E950.4	E962.0	E980.4
sodium (diagnostic)	977.8	E858.8	E947.8	E950.4	E962.0	E980.4
Declomycin	960.4	E856	E930.4	E950.4	E962.0	E980.4
Deferoxamine	963.8	E858.1	E933.8	E950.4	E962.0	E980.4
Dehydrocholic acid	973.4	E858.4	E943.4	E950.4	E962.0	E980.4
DeKalin	982.0	E862.4	—	E950.9	E962.1	E980.9
Delalutin	962.2	E858.0	E932.2	E950.4	E962.0	E980.4
Delphinium	988.2	E865.3	—	E950.9	E962.1	E980.9
Deltasone	962.0	E858.0	E932.0	E950.4	E962.0	E980.4
Deltra	962.0	E858.0	E932.0	E950.4	E962.0	E980.4
Delvinal	967.0	E851	E937.0	E950.1	E962.0	E980.1
Demecarium (bromide)	971.0	E855.3	E941.0	E950.4	E962.0	E980.4
Demeclocycline	960.4	E856	E930.4	E950.4	E962.0	E980.4
Demecolcine	963.1	E858.1	E933.1	E950.4	E962.0	E980.4
Demelanizing agents	976.8	E858.7	E946.8	E950.4	E962.0	E980.4
Demerol	965.09	E850.2	E935.2	E950.0	E962.0	E980.0
Demethylchlortetracycline	960.4	E856	E930.4	E950.4	E962.0	E980.4
Demethyltetracycline	960.4	E856	E930.4	E950.4	E962.0	E980.4
Demeton	989.3	E863.1	—	E950.6	E962.1	E980.7
Demulcents	976.3	E858.7	E946.3	E950.4	E962.0	E980.4
Demulen	962.2	E858.0	E932.2	E950.4	E962.0	E980.4
Denatured alcohol	980.0	E860.1	—	E950.9	E962.1	E980.9
Dendrid	976.5	E858.7	E946.5	E950.4	E962.0	E980.4
Dental agents, topical	976.7	E858.7	E946.7	E950.4	E962.0	E980.4
Deodorant spray (feminine hygiene)	976.8	E858.7	E946.8	E950.4	E962.0	E980.4
Deoxyribonuclease	963.4	E858.1	E933.4	E950.4	E962.0	E980.4
Depressants						
appetite, central	977.0	E858.8	E947.0	E950.4	E962.0	E980.4
cardiac	972.0	E858.3	E942.0	E950.4	E962.0	E980.4

Substance	Poisoning	Accident	Therapeutic Use	Suicide Attempt	Assault	Undetermined
central nervous system (anesthetic)	968.4	E855.1	E938.4	E950.4	E962.0	E980.4
psychotherapeutic	969.5	E853.9	E939.5	E950.3	E962.0	E980.3
Dequalinium	976.0	E858.7	E946.0	E950.4	E962.0	E980.4
Dermolate	976.2	E858.7	E946.2	E950.4	E962.0	E980.4
DES	962.2	E858.0	E932.2	E950.4	E962.0	E980.4
Desenex	976.0	E858.7	E946.0	E950.4	E962.0	E980.4
Deserpidine	972.6	E858.3	E942.6	E950.4	E962.0	E980.4
Desipramine	969.0	E854.0	E939.0	E950.3	E962.0	E980.3
Deslanoside	972.1	E858.3	E942.1	E950.4	E962.0	E980.4
Desocodeine	965.09	E850.2	E935.2	E950.0	E962.0	E980.0
Desomorphine	965.09	E850.2	E935.2	E950.0	E962.0	E980.0
Desonide	976.0	E858.7	E946.0	E950.4	E962.0	E980.4
Desoxycorticosterone derivatives	962.0	E858.0	E932.0	E950.4	E962.0	E980.4
Desoxyephedrine	969.7	E854.2	E939.7	E950.3	E962.0	E980.3
DET	969.6	E854.1	E939.6	E950.3	E962.0	E980.3
Detergents (ingested) (synthetic)	989.6	E861.0	—	E950.9	E962.1	E980.9
external medication	976.2	E858.7	E946.2	E950.4	E962.0	E980.4
Deterrent, alcohol	977.3	E858.8	E947.3	E950.4	E962.0	E980.4
Detrothyronine	962.7	E858.0	E932.7	E950.4	E962.0	E980.4
Dettol (external medication)	976.0	E858.7	E946.0	E950.4	E962.0	E980.4
Dexamethasone	962.0	E858.0	E932.0	E950.4	E962.0	E980.4
ENT agent	976.6	E858.7	E946.6	E950.4	E962.0	E980.4
ophthalmic preparation	976.5	E858.7	E946.5	E950.4	E962.0	E980.4
topical NEC	976.0	E858.7	E946.0	E950.4	E962.0	E980.4
Dexamphetamine	969.7	E854.2	E939.7	E950.3	E962.0	E980.3
Dexedrine	969.7	E854.2	E939.7	E950.3	E962.0	E980.3
Dexpanthenol	963.5	E858.1	E933.5	E950.4	E962.0	E980.4
Dextran	964.8	E858.2	E934.8	E950.4	E962.0	E980.4
Dextriferron	964.0	E858.2	E934.0	E950.4	E962.0	E980.4
Dextroamphetamine	969.7	E854.2	E939.7	E950.3	E962.0	E980.3
Dextro calcium pantothenate	963.5	E858.1	E933.5	E950.4	E962.0	E980.4
Dextromethorphan	975.4	E858.6	E945.4	E950.4	E962.0	E980.4
Dextromoramide	965.09	E850.2	E935.2	E950.0	E962.0	E980.0
Dextro pantothenyl alcohol	963.5	E858.1	E933.5	E950.4	E962.0	E980.4
topical	976.8	E858.7	E946.8	E950.4	E962.0	E980.4
Dextropropoxyphene (hydrochloride)	965.8	E850.8	E935.8	E950.0	E962.0	E980.0
Dextrorphan	965.09	E850.2	E935.2	E950.0	E962.0	E980.0
Dextrose NEC	974.5	E858.5	E944.5	E950.4	E962.0	E980.4
Dextrothyroxin	962.7	E858.0	E932.7	E950.4	E962.0	E980.4
DFP	971.0	E855.3	E941.0	E950.4	E962.0	E980.4
DHE–45	972.9	E858.3	E942.9	E950.4	E962.0	E980.4
Diabinese	962.3	E858.0	E932.3	E950.4	E962.0	E980.4
Diacetyl monoxime	977.2	E858.8	E947.2	E950.4	E962.0	E980.4
Diacetylmorphine	965.01	E850.0	E935.0	E950.0	E962.0	E980.0
Diagnostic agents	977.8	E858.8	E947.8	E950.4	E962.0	E980.4
Dial (soap)	976.2	E858.7	E946.2	E950.4	E962.0	E980.4
sedative	967.0	E851	E937.0	E950.1	E962.0	E980.1
Diallylbarbituric acid	967.0	E851	E937.0	E950.1	E962.0	E980.1
Diaminodiphenylsulfone	961.8	E857	E931.8	E950.4	E962.0	E980.4
Diamorphine	965.01	E850.0	E935.0	E950.0	E962.0	E980.0
Diamox	974.2	E858.5	E944.2	E950.4	E962.0	E980.4
Diamthazole	976.0	E858.7	E946.0	E950.4	E962.0	E980.4
Diaphenylsulfone	961.8	E857	E931.8	E950.4	E962.0	E980.4
Diasone (sodium)	961.8	E857	E931.8	E950.4	E962.0	E980.4
Diazepam	969.4	E853.2	E939.4	E950.3	E962.0	E980.3
Diazinon	989.3	E863.1	—	E950.6	E962.1	E980.7
Diazomethane (gas)	987.8	E869.8	—	E952.8	E962.2	E982.8

Substance	Poisoning	External Cause (E-Code)				
		Accident	Therapeutic Use	Suicide Attempt	Assault	Undetermined
Diazoxide	972.5	E858.3	E942.5	E950.4	E962.0	E980.4
Dibenamine	971.3	E855.6	E941.3	E950.4	E962.0	E980.4
Dibenzheptropine	963.0	E858.1	E933.0	E950.4	E962.0	E980.4
Dibenzyline	971.3	E855.6	E941.3	E950.4	E962.0	E980.4
Diborane (gas)	987.8	E869.8	—	E952.8	E962.2	E982.8
Dibromomannitol	963.1	E858.1	E933.1	E950.4	E962.0	E980.4
Dibucaine (spinal)	968.7	E855.2	E938.7	E950.4	E962.0	E980.4
topical (surface)	968.5	E855.2	E938.5	E950.4	E962.0	E980.4
Dibunate sodium	975.4	E858.6	E945.4	E950.4	E962.0	E980.4
Dibutoline	971.1	E855.4	E941.1	E950.4	E962.0	E980.4
Dicapthon	989.4	E863.4	—	E950.6	E962.1	E980.7
Dichloralphenazone	967.1	E852.0	E937.1	E950.2	E962.0	E980.2
Dichlorodifluoromethane	987.4	E869.2	—	E952.8	E962.2	E982.8
Dichloroethane	982.3	E862.4	—	E950.9	E962.1	E980.9
Dichloroethylene	982.3	E862.4	—	E950.9	E962.1	E980.9
Dichloroethyl sulfide	987.8	E869.8	—	E952.8	E962.2	E982.8
Dichlorohydrin	982.3	E862.4	—	E950.9	E962.1	E980.9
Dichloromethane (solvent) (vapor)	982.3	E862.4	—	E950.9	E962.1	E980.9
Dichlorophen(e)	961.6	E857	E931.6	E950.4	E962.0	E980.4
Dichlorphenamide	974.2	E858.5	E944.2	E950.4	E962.0	E980.4
Dichlorvos	989.3	E863.1	—	E950.6	E962.1	E980.7
Diclofenac sodium	965.69	E850.6	E935.6	E950.0	E962.0	E980.0
Dicoumarin, dicumarol	964.2	E858.2	E934.2	E950.4	E962.0	E980.4
Dicyanogen (gas)	987.8	E869.8	—	E952.8	E962.2	E982.8
Dicyclomine	971.1	E855.4	E941.1	E950.4	E962.0	E980.4
Dieldrin (vapor)	989.2	E863.0	—	E950.6	E962.1	E980.7
Dienestrol	962.2	E858.0	E932.2	E950.4	E962.0	E980.4
Dietetics	977.0	E858.8	E947.0	E950.4	E962.0	E980.4
Diethazine	966.4	E855.0	E936.4	E950.4	E962.0	E980.4
Diethyl						
barbituric acid	967.0	E851	E937.0	E950.1	E962.0	E980.1
carbamazine	961.6	E857	E931.6	E950.4	E962.0	E980.4
carbinol	980.8	E860.8	—	E950.9	E962.1	E980.9
carbonate	982.8	E862.4	—	E950.9	E962.1	E980.9
ether (vapor) — *see* Ether(s)						
propion	977.0	E858.8	E947.0	E950.4	E962.0	E980.4
stilbestrol	962.2	E858.0	E932.2	E950.4	E962.0	E980.4
Diethylene						
dioxide	982.8	E862.4	—	E950.9	E962.1	E980.9
glycol (monoacetate) (monoethyl ether)	982.8	E862.4	—	E950.9	E962.1	E980.9
Diethylsulfone–diethylmethane	967.8	E852.8	E937.8	E950.2	E962.0	E980.2
Difencloxazine	965.09	E850.2	E935.2	E950.0	E962.0	E980.0
Diffusin	963.4	E858.1	E933.4	E950.4	E962.0	E980.4
Diflos	971.0	E855.3	E941.0	E950.4	E962.0	E980.4
Digestants	973.4	E858.4	E943.4	E950.4	E962.0	E980.4
Digitalin(e)	972.1	E858.3	E942.1	E950.4	E962.0	E980.4
Digitalis glycosides	972.1	E858.3	E942.1	E950.4	E962.0	E980.4
Digitoxin	972.1	E858.3	E942.1	E950.4	E962.0	E980.4
Digoxin	972.1	E858.3	E942.1	E950.4	E962.0	E980.4
Dihydrocodeine	965.09	E850.2	E935.2	E950.0	E962.0	E980.0
Dihydrocodeinone	965.09	E850.2	E935.2	E950.0	E962.0	E980.0
Dihydroergocristine	972.9	E858.3	E942.9	E950.4	E962.0	E980.4
Dihydroergotamine	972.9	E858.3	E942.9	E950.4	E962.0	E980.4
Dihydroergotoxine	972.9	E858.3	E942.9	E950.4	E962.0	E980.4
Dihydrohydroxycodeinone	965.09	E850.2	E935.2	E950.0	E962.0	E980.0
Dihydrohydroxymorphinone	965.09	E850.2	E935.2	E950.0	E962.0	E980.0
Dihydroisocodeine	965.09	E850.2	E935.2	E950.0	E962.0	E980.0

Substance	Poisoning	External Cause (E-Code)				
		Accident	Therapeutic Use	Suicide Attempt	Assault	Undetermined
Dihydromorphine	965.09	E850.2	E935.2	E950.0	E962.0	E980.0
Dihydromorphinone	965.09	E850.2	E935.2	E950.0	E962.0	E980.0
Dihydrostreptomycin	960.6	E856	E930.6	E950.4	E962.0	E980.4
Dihydrotachysterol	962.6	E858.0	E932.6	E950.4	E962.0	E980.4
Dihydroxyanthraquinone	973.1	E858.4	E943.1	E950.4	E962.0	E980.4
Dihydroxycodeinone	965.09	E850.2	E935.2	E950.0	E962.0	E980.0
Diiodohydroxyquin	961.3	E857	E931.3	E950.4	E962.0	E980.4
topical	976.0	E858.7	E946.0	E950.4	E962.0	E980.4
Diiodohydroxyquinoline	961.3	E857	E931.3	E950.4	E962.0	E980.4
Dilantin	966.1	E855.0	E936.1	E950.4	E962.0	E980.4
Dilaudid	965.09	E850.2	E935.2	E950.0	E962.0	E980.0
Diloxanide	961.5	E857	E931.5	E950.4	E962.0	E980.4
Dimefline	970.0	E854.3	E940.0	E950.4	E962.0	E980.4
Dimenhydrinate	963.0	E858.1	E933.0	E950.4	E962.0	E980.4
Dimercaprol	963.8	E858.1	E933.8	E950.4	E962.0	E980.4
Dimercaptopropanol	963.8	E858.1	E933.8	E950.4	E962.0	E980.4
Dimetane	963.0	E858.1	E933.0	E950.4	E962.0	E980.4
Dimethicone	976.3	E858.7	E946.3	E950.4	E962.0	E980.4
Dimethindene	963.0	E858.1	E933.0	E950.4	E962.0	E980.4
Dimethisoquin	968.5	E855.2	E938.5	E950.4	E962.0	E980.4
Dimethisterone	962.2	E858.0	E932.2	E950.4	E962.0	E980.4
Dimethoxanate	975.4	E858.6	E945.4	E950.4	E962.0	E980.4
Dimethyl						
arsine, arsinic acid — *see* Arsenic						
carbinol	980.2	E860.3	—	E950.9	E962.1	E980.9
diguanide	962.3	E858.0	E932.3	E950.4	E962.0	E980.4
ketone	982.8	E862.4	—	E950.9	E962.1	E980.9
vapor	987.8	E869.8	—	E952.8	E962.2	E982.8
meperidine	965.09	E850.2	E935.2	E950.0	E962.0	E980.0
parathion	989.3	E863.1	—	E950.6	E962.1	E980.7
polysiloxane	973.8	E858.4	E943.8	E950.4	E962.0	E980.4
sulfate (fumes)	987.8	E869.8	—	E952.8	E962.2	E982.8
liquid	983.9	E864.3	—	E950.7	E962.1	E980.6
sulfoxide NEC	982.8	E862.4	—	E950.9	E962.1	E980.9
medicinal	976.4	E858.7	E946.4	E950.4	E962.0	E980.4
triptamine	969.6	E854.1	E939.6	E950.3	E962.0	E980.3
tubocurarine	975.2	E858.6	E945.2	E950.4	E962.0	E980.4
Dindevan	964.2	E858.2	E934.2	E950.4	E962.0	E980.4
Dinitro (–ortho–) cresol (herbicide) (spray)	989.4	E863.5	—	E950.6	E962.1	E980.7
insecticide	989.4	E863.4	—	E950.6	E962.1	E980.7
Dinitrobenzene	983.0	E864.0	—	E950.7	E962.1	E980.6
vapor	987.8	E869.8	—	E952.8	E962.2	E982.8
Dinitro–orthocresol (herbicide)	989.4	E863.5	—	E950.6	E962.1	E980.7
insecticide	989.4	E863.4	—	E950.6	E962.1	E980.7
Dinitrophenol (herbicide) (spray)	989.4	E863.5	—	E950.6	E962.1	E980.7
insecticide	989.4	E863.4	—	E950.6	E962.1	E980.7
Dinoprost	975.0	E858.6	E945.0	E950.4	E962.0	E980.4
Dioctyl sulfosuccinate (calcium) (sodium)	973.2	E858.4	E943.2	E950.4	E962.0	E980.4
Diodoquin	961.3	E857	E931.3	E950.4	E962.0	E980.4
Dione derivatives NEC	966.3	E855.0	E936.3	E950.4	E962.0	E980.4
Dionin	965.09	E850.2	E935.2	E950.0	E962.0	E980.0
Dioxane	982.8	E862.4	—	E950.9	E962.1	E980.9
Dioxin — *see* herbicide						
Dioxyline	972.5	E858.3	E942.5	E950.4	E962.0	E980.4
Dipentene	982.8	E862.4	—	E950.9	E962.1	E980.9
Diphemanil	971.1	E855.4	E941.1	E950.4	E962.0	E980.4
Diphenadione	964.2	E858.2	E934.2	E950.4	E962.0	E980.4

Substance	Poisoning	External Cause (E-Code)				
		Accident	Therapeutic Use	Suicide Attempt	Assault	Undetermined
Diphenhydramine	963.0	E858.1	E933.0	E950.4	E962.0	E980.4
Diphenidol	963.0	E858.1	E933.0	E950.4	E962.0	E980.4
Diphenoxylate	973.5	E858.4	E943.5	E950.4	E962.0	E980.4
Diphenylchloroarsine	985.1	E866.3	—	E950.8	E962.1	E980.8
Diphenylhydantoin (sodium)	966.1	E855.0	E936.1	E950.4	E962.0	E980.4
Diphenylpyraline	963.0	E858.1	E933.0	E950.4	E962.0	E980.4
Diphtheria						
antitoxin	979.9	E858.8	E949.9	E950.4	E962.0	E980.4
toxoid	978.5	E858.8	E948.5	E950.4	E962.0	E980.4
with tetanus toxoid	978.9	E858.8	E948.9	E950.4	E962.0	E980.4
with pertussis component	978.6	E858.8	E948.6	E950.4	E962.0	E980.4
vaccine	978.5	E858.8	E948.5	E950.4	E962.0	E980.4
Dipipanone	965.09	E850.2	E935.2	E950.0	E962.0	E980.0
Diplovax	979.5	E858.8	E949.5	E950.4	E962.0	E980.4
Diprophylline	975.1	E858.6	E945.1	E950.4	E962.0	E980.4
Dipyridamole	972.4	E858.3	E942.4	E950.4	E962.0	E980.4
Dipyrone	965.5	E850.5	E935.5	E950.0	E962.0	E980.0
Diquat	989.4	E863.5	—	E950.6	E962.1	E980.7
Disinfectant NEC	983.9	E861.4	—	E950.7	E962.1	E980.6
alkaline	983.2	E861.4	—	E950.7	E962.1	E980.6
aromatic	983.0	E861.4	—	E950.7	E962.1	E980.6
Disipal	966.4	E855.0	E936.4	E950.4	E962.0	E980.4
Disodium edetate	963.8	E858.1	E933.8	E950.4	E962.0	E980.4
Disulfamide	974.4	E858.5	E944.4	E950.4	E962.0	E980.4
Disulfanilamide	961.0	E857	E931.0	E950.4	E962.0	E980.4
Disulfiram	977.3	E858.8	E947.3	E950.4	E962.0	E980.4
Dithiazanine	961.6	E857	E931.6	E950.4	E962.0	E980.4
Dithioglycerol	963.8	E858.1	E933.8	E950.4	E962.0	E980.4
Dithranol	976.4	E858.7	E946.4	E950.4	E962.0	E980.4
Diucardin	974.3	E858.5	E944.3	E950.4	E962.0	E980.4
Diupres	974.3	E858.5	E944.3	E950.4	E962.0	E980.4
Diuretics NEC	974.4	E858.5	E944.4	E950.4	E962.0	E980.4
carbonic acid anhydrase inhibitors	974.2	E858.5	E944.2	E950.4	E962.0	E980.4
mercurial	974.0	E858.5	E944.0	E950.4	E962.0	E980.4
osmotic	974.4	E858.5	E944.4	E950.4	E962.0	E980.4
purine derivatives	974.1	E858.5	E944.1	E950.4	E962.0	E980.4
saluretic	974.3	E858.5	E944.3	E950.4	E962.0	E980.4
Diuril	974.3	E858.5	E944.3	E950.4	E962.0	E980.4
Divinyl ether	968.2	E855.1	E938.2	E950.4	E962.0	E980.4
D–lysergic acid diethylamide	969.6	E854.1	E939.6	E950.3	E962.0	E980.3
DMCT	960.4	E856	E930.4	E950.4	E962.0	E980.4
DMSO	982.8	E862.4	—	E950.9	E962.1	E980.9
DMT	969.6	E854.1	E939.6	E950.3	E962.0	E980.3
DNOC	989.4	E863.5	—	E950.6	E962.1	E980.7
DOCA	962.0	E858.0	E932.0	E950.4	E962.0	E980.4
Dolophine	965.02	E850.1	E935.1	E950.0	E962.0	E980.0
Doloxene	965.8	E850.8	E935.8	E950.0	E962.0	E980.0
DOM	969.6	E854.1	E939.6	E950.3	E962.0	E980.3
Domestic gas — *see* Gas, utility						
Domiphen (bromide) (lozenges)	976.6	E858.7	E946.6	E950.4	E962.0	E980.4
Dopa (levo)	966.4	E855.0	E936.4	E950.4	E962.0	E980.4
Dopamine	971.2	E855.5	E941.2	E950.4	E962.0	E980.4
Doriden	967.5	E852.4	E937.5	E950.2	E962.0	E980.2
Dormiral	967.0	E851	E937.0	E950.1	E962.0	E980.1
Dormison	967.8	E852.8	E937.8	E950.2	E962.0	E980.2
Dornase	963.4	E858.1	E933.4	E950.4	E962.0	E980.4
Dorsacaine	968.5	E855.2	E938.5	E950.4	E962.0	E980.4

Substance	Poisoning	External Cause (E-Code)				
		Accident	Therapeutic Use	Suicide Attempt	Assault	Undetermined
Dothiepin hydrochloride	969.0	E854.0	E939.0	E950.3	E962.0	E980.3
Doxapram	970.0	E854.3	E940.0	E950.4	E962.0	E980.4
Doxepin	969.0	E854.0	E939.0	E950.3	E962.0	E980.3
Doxorubicin	960.7	E856	E930.7	E950.4	E962.0	E980.4
Doxycycline	960.4	E856	E930.4	E950.4	E962.0	E980.4
Doxylamine	963.0	E858.1	E933.0	E950.4	E962.0	E980.4
Dramamine	963.0	E858.1	E933.0	E950.4	E962.0	E980.4
Drano (drain cleaner)	983.2	E864.2	—	E950.7	E962.1	E980.6
Dromoran	965.09	E850.2	E935.2	E950.0	E962.0	E980.0
Dromostanolone	962.1	E858.0	E932.1	E950.4	E962.0	E980.4
Droperidol	969.2	E853.1	E939.2	E950.3	E962.0	E980.3
Drug	977.9	E858.9	E947.9	E950.5	E962.0	E980.5
specified NEC	977.8	E858.8	E947.8	E950.4	E962.0	E980.4
AHFS List						
4:00 antihistamine drugs	963.0	E858.1	E933.0	E950.4	E962.0	E980.4
8:04 amebacides	961.5	E857	E931.5	E950.4	E962.0	E980.4
arsenical anti–infectives	961.1	E857	E931.1	E950.4	E962.0	E980.4
quinoline derivatives	961.3	E857	E931.3	E950.4	E962.0	E980.4
8:08 anthelmintics	961.6	E857	E931.6	E950.4	E962.0	E980.4
quinoline derivatives	961.3	E857	E931.3	E950.4	E962.0	E980.4
8:12.04 antifungal antibiotics	960.1	E856	E930.1	E950.4	E962.0	E980.4
8:12.06 cephalosporins	960.5	E856	E930.5	E950.4	E962.0	E980.4
8:12.08 chloramphenicol	960.2	E856	E930.2	E950.4	E962.0	E980.4
8:12.12 erythromycins	960.3	E856	E930.3	E950.4	E962.0	E980.4
8:12.16 penicillins	960.0	E856	E930.0	E950.4	E962.0	E980.4
8:12.20 streptomycins	960.6	E856	E930.6	E950.4	E962.0	E980.4
8:12.24 tetracyclines	960.4	E856	E930.4	E950.4	E962.0	E980.4
8:12.28 other antibiotics	960.8	E856	E930.8	E950.4	E962.0	E980.4
antimycobacterial	960.6	E856	E930.6	E950.4	E962.0	E980.4
macrolides	960.3	E856	E930.3	E950.4	E962.0	E980.4
8:16 antituberculars	961.8	E857	E931.8	E950.4	E962.0	E980.4
antibiotics	960.6	E856	E930.6	E950.4	E962.0	E980.4
8:18 antivirals	961.7	E857	E931.7	E950.4	E962.0	E980.4
8:20 plasmodicides (antimalarials)	961.4	E857	E931.4	E950.4	E962.0	E980.4
8:24 sulfonamides	961.0	E857	E931.0	E950.4	E962.0	E980.4
8:26 sulfones	961.8	E857	E931.8	E950.4	E962.0	E980.4
8:28 treponemicides	961.2	E857	E931.2	E950.4	E962.0	E980.4
8:32 trichomonacides	961.5	E857	E931.5	E950.4	E962.0	E980.4
quinoline derivatives	961.3	E857	E931.3	E950.4	E962.0	E980.4
nitrofuran derivatives	961.9	E857	E931.9	E950.4	E962.0	E980.4
8:36 urinary germicides	961.9	E857	E931.9	E950.4	E962.0	E980.4
quinoline derivatives	961.3	E857	E931.3	E950.4	E962.0	E980.4
8:40 other anti–infectives	961.9	E857	E931.9	E950.4	E962.0	E980.4
10·00 antineoplastic agents	963.1	E858.1	E933.1	E950.4	E962.0	E980.4
antibiotics	960.7	E856	E930.7	E950.4	E962.0	E980.4
progestogens	962.2	E858.0	E932.2	E950.4	E962.0	E980.4
12:04 parasympathomimetic (cholinergic) agents	971.0	E855.3	E941.0	E950.4	E962.0	E980.4
12:08 parasympatholytic (cholinergic –blocking) agents	971.1	E855.4	E941.1	E950.4	E962.0	E980.4
12:12 Sympathomimetic (adrenergic) agents	971.2	E855.5	E941.2	E950.4	E962.0	E980.4
12:16 sympatholytic (adrenergic– blocking) agents	971.3	E855.6	E941.3	E950.4	E962.0	E980.4
12:20 skeletal muscle relaxants central nervous system muscle-tone depressants	968.0	E855.1	E938.0	E950.4	E962.0	E980.4

Substance	Poisoning	Accident	Therapeutic Use	Suicide Attempt	Assault	Undetermined
myoneural blocking agents	975.2	E858.6	E945.2	E950.4	E962.0	E980.4
16:00 blood derivatives	964.7	E858.2	E934.7	E950.4	E962.0	E980.4
20:04 antianemia drugs	964.1	E858.2	E934.1	E950.4	E962.0	E980.4
20:04.04 iron preparations	964.0	E858.2	E934.0	E950.4	E962.0	E980.4
20:04.08 liver and stomach preparations	964.1	E858.2	E934.1	E950.4	E962.0	E980.4
20:12.04 anticoagulants	964.2	E858.2	E934.2	E950.4	E962.0	E980.4
20:12.08 antiheparin agents	964.5	E858.2	E934.5	E950.4	E962.0	E980.4
20:12.12 coagulants	964.5	E858.2	E934.5	E950.4	E962.0	E980.4
20:12.16 hemostatics NEC	964.5	E858.2	E934.5	E950.4	E962.0	E980.4
capillary active drugs	972.8	E858.3	E942.8	E950.4	E962.0	E980.4
24:04 cardiac drugs	972.9	E858.3	E942.9	E950.4	E962.0	E980.4
cardiotonic agents	972.1	E858.3	E942.1	E950.4	E962.0	E980.4
rhythm regulators	972.0	E858.3	E942.0	E950.4	E962.0	E980.4
24:06 antilipemic agents	972.2	E858.3	E942.2	E950.4	E962.0	E980.4
thyroid derivatives	962.7	E858.0	E932.7	E950.4	E962.0	E980.4
24:08 hypotensive agents	972.6	E858.3	E942.6	E950.4	E962.0	E980.4
adrenergic blocking agents	971.3	E855.6	E941.3	E950.4	E962.0	E980.4
ganglion blocking agents	972.3	E858.3	E942.3	E950.4	E962.0	E980.4
vasodilators	972.5	E858.3	E942.5	E950.4	E962.0	E980.4
24:12 vasodilating agents NEC	972.5	E858.3	E942.5	E950.4	E962.0	E980.4
coronary	972.4	E858.3	E942.4	E950.4	E962.0	E980.4
nicotinic acid derivatives	972.2	E858.3	E942.2	E950.4	E962.0	E980.4
24:16 sclerosing agents	972.7	E858.3	E942.7	E950.4	E962.0	E980.4
28:04 general anesthetics	968.4	E855.1	E938.4	E950.4	E962.0	E980.4
gaseous anesthetics	968.2	E855.1	E938.2	E950.4	E962.0	E980.4
halothane	968.1	E855.1	E938.1	E950.4	E962.0	E980.4
intravenous anesthetics	968.3	E855.1	E938.3	E950.4	E962.0	E980.4
28:08 analgesics and antipyretics	965.9	E850.9	E935.9	E950.0	E962.0	E980.0
antirheumatics	965.69	E850.6	E935.6	E950.0	E962.0	E980.0
aromatic analgesics	965.4	E850.4	E935.4	E950.0	E962.0	E980.0
non–narcotic NEC	965.7	E850.7	E935.7	E950.0	E962.0	E980.0
opium alkaloids	965.00	E850.2	E935.2	E950.0	E962.0	E980.0
heroin	965.01	E850.0	E935.0	E950.0	E962.0	E980.0
methadone	965.02	E850.1	E935.1	E950.0	E962.0	E980.0
specified type NEC	965.09	E850.2	E935.2	E950.0	E962.0	E980.0
pyrazole derivatives	965.5	E850.5	E935.5	E950.0	E962.0	E980.0
salicylates	965.1	E850.3	E935.3	E950.0	E962.0	E980.0
specified NEC	965.8	E850.8	E935.8	E950.0	E962.0	E980.0
28:10 narcotic antagonists	970.1	E854.3	E940.1	E950.4	E962.0	E980.4
28:12 anticonvulsants	966.3	E855.0	E936.3	E950.4	E962.0	E980.4
barbiturates	967.0	E851	E937.0	E950.1	E962.0	E980.1
benzodiazepine–based tranquilizers	969.4	E853.2	E939.4	E950.3	E962.0	E980.3
bromides	967.3	E852.2	E937.3	E950.2	E962.0	E980.2
hydantoin derivatives	966.1	E855.0	E936.1	E950.4	E962.0	E980.4
oxazolidine (derivatives)	966.0	E855.0	E936.0	E950.4	E962.0	E980.4
succinimides	966.2	E855.0	E936.2	E950.4	E962.0	E980.4
28:16.04 antidepressants	969.0	E854.0	E939.0	E950.3	E962.0	E980.3
28:16.08 tranquilizers	969.5	E853.9	E939.5	E950.3	E962.0	E980.3
benzodiazepine–based	969.4	E853.2	E939.4	E950.3	E962.0	E980.3
butyrophenone–based	969.2	E853.1	E939.2	E950.3	E962.0	E980.3
major NEC	969.3	E853.8	E939.3	E950.3	E962.0	E980.3
phenothiazine–based	969.1	E853.0	E939.1	E950.3	E962.0	E980.3
28:16.12 other psychotherapeutic agents	969.8	E855.8	E939.8	E950.3	E962.0	E980.3
28:20 respiratory and cerebral stimulants	970.9	E854.3	E940.9	E950.4	E962.0	E980.4
analeptics	970.0	E854.3	E940.0	E950.4	E962.0	E980.4
anorexigenic agents	977.0	E858.8	E947.0	E950.4	E962.0	E980.4

Substance	Poisoning	External Cause (E-Code)				
		Accident (Therapeutic Use)	Therapeutic Use	Suicide Attempt	Assault	Undetermined
psychostimulants	969.7	E854.2	E939.7	E950.3	E962.0	E980.3
specified NEC	970.8	E854.3	E940.8	E950.4	E962.0	E980.4
28:24 sedatives and hypnotics	967.9	E852.9	E937.9	E950.2	E962.0	E980.2
barbiturates	967.0	E851	E937.0	E950.1	E962.0	E980.1
benzodiazepine–based tranquilizers	969.4	E853.2	E939.4	E950.3	E962.0	E980.3
chloral hydrate (group)	967.1	E852.0	E937.1	E950.2	E962.0	E980.2
glutethamide group	967.5	E852.4	E937.5	E950.2	E962.0	E980.2
intravenous anesthetics	968.3	E855.1	E938.3	E950.4	E962.0	E980.4
methaqualone (compounds)	967.4	E852.3	E937.4	E950.2	E962.0	E980.2
paraldehyde	967.2	E852.1	E937.2	E950.2	E962.0	E980.2
phenothiazine–based tranquilizers	969.1	E853.0	E939.1	E950.3	E962.0	E980.3
specified NEC	967.8	E852.8	E937.8	E950.2	E962.0	E980.2
thiobarbiturates	968.3	E855.1	E938.3	E950.4	E962.0	E980.4
tranquilizer NEC	969.5	E853.9	E939.5	E950.3	E962.0	E980.3
36:04 to 36:88 diagnostic agents	977.8	E858.8	E947.8	E950.4	E962.0	E980.4
40:00 electrolyte, caloric, and water balance agents NEC	974.5	E858.5	E944.5	E950.4	E962.0	E980.4
40:04 acidifying agents	963.2	E858.1	E933.2	E950.4	E962.0	E980.4
40:08 alkalinizing agents	963.3	E858.1	E933.3	E950.4	E962.0	E980.4
40:10 ammonia detoxicants	974.5	E858.5	E944.5	E950.4	E962.0	E980.4
40:12 replacement solutions	974.5	E858.5	E944.5	E950.4	E962.0	E980.4
plasma expanders	964.8	E858.2	E934.8	E950.4	E962.0	E980.4
40:16 sodium–removing resins	974.5	E858.5	E944.5	E950.4	E962.0	E980.4
40:18 potassium–removing resins	974.5	E858.5	E944.5	E950.4	E962.0	E980.4
40:20 caloric agents	974.5	E858.5	E944.5	E950.4	E962.0	E980.4
40:24 salt and sugar substitutes	974.5	E858.5	E944.5	E950.4	E962.0	E980.4
40:28 diuretics NEC	974.4	E858.5	E944.4	E950.4	E962.0	E980.4
carbonic acid anhydrase inhibitors	974.2	E858.5	E944.2	E950.4	E962.0	E980.4
mercurials	974.0	E858.5	E944.0	E950.4	E962.0	E980.4
purine derivatives	974.1	E858.5	E944.1	E950.4	E962.0	E980.4
saluretics	974.3	E858.5	E944.3	E950.4	E962.0	E980.4
thiazides	974.3	E858.5	E944.3	E950.4	E962.1	E980.4
40:36 irrigating solutions	974.5	E858.5	E944.5	E950.4	E962.0	E980.4
40:40 uricosuric agents	974.7	E858.5	E944.7	E950.4	E962.0	E980.4
44:00 enzymes	963.4	E858.1	E933.4	E950.4	E962.0	E980.4
fibrinolysis–affecting agents	964.4	E858.2	E934.4	E950.4	E962.0	E980.4
gastric agents	973.4	E858.4	E943.4	E950.4	E962.0	E980.4
48:00 expectorants and cough preparations						
antihistamine agents	963.0	E858.1	E933.0	E950.4	E962.0	E980.4
antitussives	975.4	E858.6	E945.4	E950.4	E962.0	E980.4
codeine derivatives	965.09	E850.2	E935.2	E950.0	E962.0	E980.0
expectorants	975.5	E858.6	E945.5	E950.4	E962.0	E980.4
narcotic agents NEC	965.09	E850.2	E935.2	E950.0	E962.0	E980.0
52:04 anti–infectives (EENT)						
ENT agent	976.6	E858.7	E946.6	E950.4	E962.0	E980.4
ophthalmic preparation	976.5	E858.7	E946.5	E950.4	E962.0	E980.4
52:04.04 antibiotics (EENT)						
ENT agent	976.6	E858.7	E946.6	E950.4	E962.0	E980.4
ophthalmic preparation	976.5	E858.7	E946.5	E950.4	E962.0	E980.4
52:04.06 antivirals (EENT)						
ENT agent	976.6	E858.7	E946.6	E950.4	E962.0	E980.4
ophthalmic preparation	976.5	E858.7	E946.5	E950.4	E962.0	E980.4
52:04.08 sulfonamides (EENT)						
ENT agent	976.6	E858.7	E946.6	E950.4	E962.0	E980.4
ophthalmic preparation	976.5	E858.7	E946.5	E950.4	E962.0	E980.4
52:04.12 miscellaneous anti–infectives (EENT)						
ENT agent	976.6	E858.7	E946.6	E950.4	E962.0	E980.4

Substance	Poisoning	External Cause (E-Code)				
		Accident	Therapeutic Use	Suicide Attempt	Assault	Undetermined
ophthalmic preparation	976.5	E858.7	E946.5	E950.4	E962.0	E980.4
52:08 anti–inflammatory agents (EENT)						
ENT agent	976.6	E858.7	E946.6	E950.4	E962.0	E980.4
ophthalmic preparation	976.5	E858.7	E946.5	E950.4	E962.0	E980.4
52:10 carbonic anhydrase inhibitors	974.2	E858.5	E944.2	E950.4	E962.0	E980.4
52:12 contact lens solutions	976.5	E858.7	E946.5	E950.4	E962.0	E980.4
52:16 local anesthetics (EENT)	968.5	E855.2	E938.5	E950.4	E962.0	E980.4
52:20 miotics	971.0	E855.3	E941.0	E950.4	E962.0	E980.4
52:24 mydriatics						
adrenergics	971.2	E855.5	E941.2	E950.4	E962.0	E980.4
anticholinergics	971.1	E855.4	E941.1	E950.4	E962.0	E980.4
antimuscarinics	971.1	E855.4	E941.1	E950.4	E962.0	E980.4
parasympatholytics	971.1	E855.4	E941.1	E950.4	E962.0	E980.4
spasmolytics	971.1	E855.4	E941.1	E950.4	E962.0	E980.4
sympathomimetics	971.2	E855.5	E941.2	E950.4	E962.0	E980.4
52:28 mouth washes and gargles	976.6	E858.7	E946.6	E950.4	E962.0	E980.4
52:32 vasoconstrictors (EENT)	971.2	E855.5	E941.2	E950.4	E962.0	E980.4
52:36 unclassified agents (EENT)						
ENT agent	976.6	E858.7	E946.6	E950.4	E962.0	E980.4
ophthalmic preparation	976.5	E858.7	E946.5	E950.4	E962.0	E980.4
56:04 antacids and adsorbents	973.0	E858.4	E943.0	E950.4	E962.0	E980.4
56:08 Antidiarrhea agents	973.5	E858.4	E943.5	E950.4	E962.0	E980.4
56:10 antiflatulents	973.8	E858.4	E943.8	E950.4	E962.0	E980.4
56:12 cathartics NEC	973.3	E858.4	E943.3	E950.4	E962.0	E980.4
emollients	973.2	E858.4	E943.2	E950.4	E962.0	E980.4
irritants	973.1	E858.4	E943.1	E950.4	E962.0	E980.4
56:16 digestants	973.4	E858.4	E943.4	E950.4	E962.0	E980.4
56:20 emetics and antiemetics						
antiemetics	963.0	E858.1	E933.0	E950.4	E962.0	E980.4
emetics	973.6	E858.4	E943.6	E950.4	E962.0	E980.4
56:24 lipotropic agents	977.1	E858.8	E947.1	E950.4	E962.0	E980.4
56:40 miscellaneous G.I. drugs	973.8	E858.4	E943.8	E950.4	E962.0	E980.4
60:00 gold compounds	965.69	E850.6	E935.6	E950.0	E962.0	E980.0
64:00 heavy metal antagonists	963.8	E858.1	E933.8	E950.4	E962.0	E980.4
68:04 adrenals	962.0	E858.0	E932.0	E950.4	E962.0	E980.4
68:08 androgens	962.1	E858.0	E932.1	E950.4	E962.0	E980.4
68:12 contraceptives, oral	962.2	E858.0	E932.2	E950.4	E962.0	E980.4
68:16 estrogens	962.2	E858.0	E932.2	E950.4	E962.0	E980.4
68:18 gonadotropins	962.4	E858.0	E932.4	E950.4	E962.0	E980.4
68:20 insulins and antidiabetic agents	962.3	E858.0	E932.3	E950.4	E962.0	E980.4
68:20.08 insulins	962.3	E858.0	E932.3	E950.4	E962.0	E980.4
68:24 parathyroid	962.6	E858.0	E932.6	E950.4	E962.0	E980.4
68:28 pituitary (posterior)	962.5	E858.0	E932.5	E950.4	E962.0	E980.4
anterior	962.4	E858.0	E932.4	E950.4	E962.0	E980.4
68:32 progestogens	962.2	E858.0	E932.2	E950.4	E962.0	E980.4
68:34 other corpus luteum hormones NEC	962.2	E858.0	E932.2	E950.4	E962.0	E980.4
68:36 thyroid and antithyroid						
antithyroid	962.8	E858.0	E932.8	E950.4	E962.0	E980.4
thyroid (derivatives)	962.7	E858.0	E932.7	E950.4	E962.0	E980.4
72:00 local anesthetics NEC	968.9	E855.2	E938.9	E950.4	E962.0	E980.4
topical (surface)	968.5	E855.2	E938.5	E950.4	E962.0	E980.4
infiltration (intradermal) (subcutaneous) (submucosal)	968.5	E855.2	E938.5	E950.4	E962.0	E980.4
nerve blocking (peripheral) (plexus) (regional)	968.6	E855.2	E938.6	E950.4	E962.0	E980.4
spinal	968.7	E855.2	E938.7	E950.4	E962.0	E980.4

Substance	Poisoning	External Cause (E-Code)				
		Accident	Therapeutic Use	Suicide Attempt	Assault	Undetermined
76:00 oxytocics	975.0	E858.6	E945.0	E950.4	E962.0	E980.4
78:00 radioactive agents	990	—	—	—	—	—
80:04 serums NEC	979.9	E858.8	E949.9	E950.4	E962.0	E980.4
immune gamma globulin (human)	964.6	E858.2	E934.6	E950.4	E962.0	E980.4
80:08 toxoids NEC	978.8	E858.8	E948.8	E950.4	E962.0	E980.4
diphtheria	978.5	E858.8	E948.5	E950.4	E962.0	E980.4
and tetanus	978.9	E858.8	E948.9	E950.4	E962.0	E980.4
with pertussis component	978.6	E858.8	E948.6	E950.4	E962.0	E980.4
tetanus	978.4	E858.8	E948.4	E950.4	E962.0	E980.4
and diphtheria	978.9	E858.8	E948.9	E950.4	E962.0	E980.4
with pertussis component	978.6	E858.8	E948.6	E950.4	E962.0	E980.4
80:12 vaccines	979.9	E858.8	E949.9	E950.4	E962.0	E980.4
bacterial NEC	978.8	E858.8	E948.8	E950.4	E962.0	E980.4
with						
other bacterial components	978.9	E858.8	E948.9	E950.4	E962.0	E980.4
pertussis component	978.6	E858.8	E948.6	E950.4	E962.0	E980.4
viral and rickettsial components	979.7	E858.8	E949.7	E950.4	E962.0	E980.4
rickettsial NEC	979.6	E858.8	E949.6	E950.4	E962.0	E980.4
with						
bacterial component	979.7	E858.8	E949.7	E950.4	E962.0	E980.4
pertussis component	978.6	E858.8	E948.6	E950.4	E962.0	E980.4
viral component	979.7	E858.8	E949.7	E950.4	E962.0	E980.4
viral NEC	979.6	E858.8	E949.6	E950.4	E962.0	E980.4
with						
bacterial component	979.7	E858.8	E949.7	E950.4	E962.0	E980.4
pertussis component	978.6	E858.8	E948.6	E950.4	E962.0	E980.4
rickettsial component	979.7	E858.8	E949.7	E950.4	E962.0	E980.4
84:04.04 antibiotics (skin and mucous membrane)	976.0	E858.7	E946.0	E950.4	E962.0	E980.4
84:04.08 fungicides (skin and mucous membrane)	976.0	E858.7	E946.0	E950.4	E962.0	E980.4
84:04.12 scabicides and pediculicides (skin and mucous membrane)	976.0	E858.7	E946.0	E950.4	E962.0	E980.4
84:04.16 miscellaneous local anti–infectives (skin and mucous membrane)	976.0	E858.7	E946.0	E950.4	E962.0	E980.4
84:06 anti–inflammatory agents (skin and mucous membrane)	976.0	E858.7	E946.0	E950.4	E962.0	E980.4
84:08 antipruritics and local anesthetics						
antipruritics	976.1	E858.7	E946.1	E950.4	E962.0	E980.4
local anesthetics	968.5	E855.2	E938.5	E950.4	E962.0	E980.4
84:12 astringents	976.2	E858.7	E946.2	E950.4	E962.0	E980.4
84:16 cell stimulants and proliferants	976.8	E858.7	E946.8	E950.4	E962.0	E980.4
84:20 detergents	976.2	E858.7	E946.2	E950.4	E962.0	E980.4
84:24 emollients, demulcents, and protectants	976.3	E858.7	E946.3	E950.4	E962.0	E980.4
84:28 keratolytic agents	976.4	E858.7	E946.4	E950.4	E962.0	E980.4
84:32 keratoplastic agents	976.4	E858.7	E946.4	E950.4	E962.0	E980.4
84:36 miscellaneous agents (skin and mucous membrane)	976.8	E858.7	E946.8	E950.4	E962.0	E980.4
86:00 spasmolytic agents	975.1	E858.6	E945.1	E950.4	E962.0	E980.4
antiasthmatics	975.7	E858.6	E945.7	E950.4	E962.0	E980.4
papaverine	972.5	E858.3	E942.5	E950.4	E962.0	E980.4
theophylline	974.1	E858.5	E944.1	E950.4	E962.0	E980.4
88:04 vitamin A	963.5	E858.1	E933.5	E950.4	E962.0	E980.4
88:08 vitamin B complex	963.5	E858.1	E933.5	E950.4	E962.0	E980.4

Substance	Poisoning	External Cause (E-Code)				
		Accident	Therapeutic Use	Suicide Attempt	Assault	Undetermined
hematopoietic vitamin	964.1	E858.2	E934.1	E950.4	E962.0	E980.4
nicotinic acid derivatives	972.2	E858.3	E942.2	E950.4	E962.0	E980.4
88:12 vitamin C	963.5	E858.1	E933.5	E950.4	E962.0	E980.4
88:16 vitamin D	963.5	E858.1	E933.5	E950.4	E962.0	E980.4
88:20 vitamin E	963.5	E858.1	E933.5	E950.4	E962.0	E980.4
88:24 vitamin K activity	964.3	E858.2	E934.3	E950.4	E962.0	E980.4
88:28 multivitamin preparations	963.5	E858.1	E933.5	E950.4	E962.0	E980.4
92:00 unclassified therapeutic agents	977.8	E858.8	E947.8	E950.4	E962.0	E980.4
Duboisine	971.1	E855.4	E941.1	E950.4	E962.0	E980.4
Dulcolax	973.1	E858.4	E943.1	E950.4	E962.0	E980.4
Duponol (C) (EP)	976.2	E858.7	E946.2	E950.4	E962.0	E980.4
Durabolin	962.1	E858.0	E932.1	E950.4	E962.0	E980.4
Dyclone	968.5	E855.2	E938.5	E950.4	E962.0	E980.4
Dyclonine	968.5	E855.2	E938.5	E950.4	E962.0	E980.4
Dydrogesterone	962.2	E858.0	E932.2	E950.4	E962.0	E980.4
Dyes NEC	989.89	E866.8	—	E950.9	E962.1	E980.9
diagnostic agents	977.8	E858.8	E947.8	E950.4	E962.0	E980.4
pharmaceutical NEC	977.4	E858.8	E947.4	E950.4	E962.0	E980.4
Dyfols	971.0	E855.3	E941.0	E950.4	E962.0	E980.4
Dymelor	962.3	E858.0	E932.3	E950.4	E962.0	E980.4
Dynamite	989.89	E866.8	—	E950.9	E962.1	E980.9
fumes	987.8	E869.8	—	E952.8	E962.2	E982.8
Dyphylline	975.1	E858.6	E945.1	E950.4	E962.0	E980.4
Ear preparations	976.6	E858.7	E946.6	E950.4	E962.0	E980.4
Echothiopate, ecothiopate	971.0	E855.3	E941.0	E950.4	E962.0	E980.4
Ectylurea	967.8	E852.8	E937.8	E950.2	E962.0	E980.2
Edathamil disodium	963.8	E858.1	E933.8	E950.4	E962.0	E980.4
Edecrin	974.4	E858.5	E944.4	E950.4	E962.0	E980.4
Edetate, disodium (calcium)	963.8	E858.1	E933.8	E950.4	E962.0	E980.4
Edrophonium	971.0	E855.3	E941.0	E950.4	E962.0	E980.4
Elase	976.8	E858.7	E946.8	E950.4	E962.0	E980.4
Elaterium	973.1	E858.4	E943.1	E950.4	E962.0	E980.4
Elder	988.2	E865.4	—	E950.9	E962.1	E980.9
berry (unripe)	988.2	E865.3	—	E950.9	E962.1	E980.9
Electrolytes NEC	974.5	E858.5	E944.5	E950.4	E962.0	E980.4
Electrolytic agent NEC	974.5	E858.5	E944.5	E950.4	E962.0	E980.4
Embramine	963.0	E858.1	E933.0	E950.4	E962.0	E980.4
Emetics	973.6	E858.4	E943.6	E950.4	E962.0	E980.4
Emetine (hydrochloride)	961.5	E857	E931.5	E950.4	E962.0	E980.4
Emollients	976.3	E858.7	E946.3	E950.4	E962.0	E980.4
Emylcamate	969.5	E853.8	E939.5	E950.3	E962.0	E980.3
Encyprate	969.0	E854.0	E939.0	E950.3	E962.0	E980.3
Endocaine	968.5	E855.2	E938.5	E950.4	E962.0	E980.4
Endrin	989.2	E863.0	—	E950.6	E962.1	E980.7
Enflurane	968.2	E855.1	E938.2	E950.4	E962.0	E980.4
Enovid	962.2	E858.0	E932.2	E950.4	E962.0	E980.4
ENT preparations (anti–infectives)	976.6	E858.7	E946.6	E950.4	E962.0	E980.4
Enzodase	963.4	E858.1	E933.4	E950.4	E962.0	E980.4
Enzymes NEC	963.4	E858.1	E933.4	E950.4	E962.0	E980.4
Epanutin	966.1	E855.0	E936.1	E950.4	E962.0	E980.4
Ephedra (tincture)	971.2	E855.5	E941.2	E950.4	E962.0	E980.4
Ephedrine	971.2	E855.5	E941.2	E950.4	E962.0	E980.4
Epiestriol	962.2	E858.0	E932.2	E950.4	E962.0	E980.4
Epilim — *see* Sodium valproate						
Epinephrine	971.2	E855.5	E941.2	E950.4	E962.0	E980.4
Epsom salt	973.3	E858.4	E943.3	E950.4	E962.0	E980.4
Equanil	969.5	E853.8	E939.5	E950.3	E962.0	E980.3

Substance	Poisoning	External Cause (E-Code)				
		Accident	Therapeutic Use	Suicide Attempt	Assault	Undetermined
Equisetum (diuretic)	974.4	E858.5	E944.4	E950.4	E962.0	E980.4
Ergometrine	975.0	E858.6	E945.0	E950.4	E962.0	E980.4
Ergonovine	975.0	E858.6	E945.0	E950.4	E962.0	E980.4
Ergot NEC	988.2	E865.4	—	E950.9	E962.1	E980.9
medicinal (alkaloids)	975.0	E858.6	E945.0	E950.4	E962.0	E980.4
Ergotamine (tartrate) (for migraine) NEC	972.9	E858.3	E942.9	E950.4	E962.0	E980.4
Ergotrate	975.0	E858.6	E945.0	E950.4	E962.0	E980.4
Erythrityl tetranitrate	972.4	E858.3	E942.4	E950.4	E962.0	E980.4
Erythrol tetranitrate	972.4	E858.3	E942.4	E950.4	E962.0	E980.4
Erythromycin	960.3	E856	E930.3	E950.4	E962.0	E980.4
ophthalmic preparation	976.5	E858.7	E946.5	E950.4	E962.0	E980.4
topical NEC	976.0	E858.7	E946.0	E950.4	E962.0	E980.4
Eserine	971.0	E855.3	E941.0	E950.4	E962.0	E980.4
Eskabarb	967.0	E851	E937.0	E950.1	E962.0	E980.1
Eskalith	969.8	E855.8	E939.8	E950.3	E962.0	E980.3
Estradiol (cypionate) (dipropionate) (valerate)	962.2	E858.0	E932.2	E950.4	E962.0	E980.4
Estriol	962.2	E858.0	E932.2	E950.4	E962.0	E980.4
Estrogens (with progestogens)	962.2	E858.0	E932.2	E950.4	E962.0	E980.4
Estrone	962.2	E858.0	E932.2	E950.4	E962.0	E980.4
Etafedrine	971.2	E855.5	E941.2	E950.4	E962.0	E980.4
Ethacrynate sodium	974.4	E858.5	E944.4	E950.4	E962.0	E980.4
Ethacrynic acid	974.4	E858.5	E944.4	E950.4	E962.0	E980.4
Ethambutol	961.8	E857	E931.8	E950.4	E962.0	E980.4
Ethamide	974.2	E858.5	E944.2	E950.4	E962.0	E980.4
Ethamivan	970.0	E854.3	E940.0	E950.4	E962.0	E980.4
Ethamsylate	964.5	E858.2	E934.5	E950.4	E962.0	E980.4
Ethanol	980.0	E860.1	—	E950.9	E962.1	E980.9
beverage	980.0	E860.0	—	E950.9	E962.1	E980.9
Ethchlorvynol	967.8	E852.8	E937.8	E950.2	E962.0	E980.2
Ethebenecid	974.7	E858.5	E944.7	E950.4	E962.0	E980.4
Ether(s) (diethyl) (ethyl) (vapor)	987.8	E869.8	—	E952.8	E962.2	E982.8
anesthetic	968.2	E855.1	E938.2	E950.4	E962.0	E980.4
petroleum — *see* Ligroin						
solvent	982.8	E862.4	—	E950.9	E962.1	E980.9
Ethidine chloride (vapor)	987.8	E869.8	—	E952.8	E962.2	E982.8
liquid (solvent)	982.3	E862.4	—	E950.9	E962.1	E980.9
Ethinamate	967.8	E852.8	E937.8	E950.2	E962.0	E980.2
Ethinylestradiol	962.2	E858.0	E932.2	E950.4	E962.0	E980.4
Ethionamide	961.8	E857	E931.8	E950.4	E962.0	E980.4
Ethisterone	962.2	E858.0	E932.2	E950.4	E962.0	E980.4
Ethobral	967.0	E851	E937.0	E950.1	E962.0	E980.1
Ethocaine (infiltration) (topical)	968.5	E855.2	E938.5	E950.4	E962.0	E980.4
nerve block (peripheral) (plexus)	968.6	E855.2	E938.6	E950.4	E962.0	E980.4
spinal	968.7	E855.2	E938.7	E950.4	E962.0	E980.4
Ethoheptazine (citrate)	965.7	E850.7	E935.7	E950.0	E962.0	E980.0
Ethopropazine	966.4	E855.0	E936.4	E950.4	E962.0	E980.4
Ethosuximide	966.2	E855.0	E936.2	E950.4	E962.0	E980.4
Ethotoin	966.1	E855.0	E936.1	E950.4	E962.0	E980.4
Ethoxazene	961.9	E857	E931.9	E950.4	E962.0	E980.4
Ethoxzolamide	974.2	E858.5	E944.2	E950.4	E962.0	E980.4
Ethyl						
acetate (vapor)	982.8	E862.4	—	E950.9	E962.1	E980.9
alcohol	980.0	E860.1	—	E950.9	E962.1	E980.9
beverage	980.0	E860.0	—	E950.9	E962.1	E980.9
aldehyde (vapor)	987.8	E869.8	—	E952.8	E962.2	E982.8
liquid	989.89	E866.8	—	E950.9	E962.1	E980.9

Substance	Poisoning	External Cause (E-Code)				
		Accident	Therapeutic Use	Suicide Attempt	Assault	Undetermined
aminobenzoate	968.5	E855.2	E938.5	E950.4	E962.0	E980.4
biscoumacetate	964.2	E858.2	E934.2	E950.4	E962.0	E980.4
bromide (anesthetic)	968.2	E855.1	E938.2	E950.4	E962.0	E980.4
carbamate (antineoplastic)	963.1	E858.1	E933.1	E950.4	E962.0	E980.4
carbinol	980.3	E860.4	—	E950.9	E962.1	E980.9
chaulmoograte	961.8	E857	E931.8	E950.4	E962.0	E980.4
chloride (vapor)	987.8	E869.8	—	E952.8	E962.2	E982.8
anesthetic (local)	968.5	E855.2	E938.5	E950.4	E962.0	E980.4
inhaled	968.2	E855.1	E938.2	E950.4	E962.0	E980.4
solvent	982.3	E862.4	—	E950.9	E962.1	E980.9
estranol	962.1	E858.0	E932.1	E950.4	E962.0	E980.4
ether — *see* Ether(s)						
formate (solvent) NEC	982.8	E862.4	—	E950.9	E962.1	E980.9
iodoacetate	987.5	E869.3	—	E952.8	E962.2	E982.8
lactate (solvent) NEC	982.8	E862.4	—	E950.9	E962.1	E980.9
methylcarbinol	980.8	E860.8	—	E950.9	E962.1	E980.9
morphine	965.09	E850.2	E935.2	E950.0	E962.0	E980.0
Ethylene (gas)	987.1	E869.8	—	E952.8	E962.2	E982.8
anesthetic (general)	968.2	E855.1	E938.2	E950.4	E962.0	E980.4
chlorohydrin (vapor)	982.3	E862.4	—	E950.9	E962.1	E980.9
dichloride (vapor)	982.3	E862.4	—	E950.9	E962.1	E980.9
glycol(s) (any) (vapor)	982.8	E862.4	—	E950.9	E962.1	E980.9
Ethylidene						
chloride NEC	982.3	E862.4	—	E950.9	E962.1	E980.9
diethyl ether	982.8	E862.4	—	E950.9	E962.1	E980.9
Ethynodiol	962.2	E858.0	E932.2	E950.4	E962.0	E980.4
Etidocaine	968.9	E855.2	E938.9	E950.4	E962.0	E980.4
infiltration (subcutaneous)	968.5	E855.2	E938.5	E950.4	E962.0	E980.4
nerve (peripheral) (plexus)	968.6	E855.2	E938.6	E950.4	E962.0	E980.4
Etilfen	967.0	E851	E937.0	E950.1	E962.0	E980.1
Etomide	965.7	E850.7	E935.7	E950.0	E962.0	E980.0
Etorphine	965.09	E850.2	E935.2	E950.0	E962.0	E980.0
Etoval	967.0	E851	E937.0	E950.1	E962.0	E980.1
Etryptamine	969.0	E854.0	E939.0	E950.3	E962.0	E980.3
Eucaine	968.5	E855.2	E938.5	E950.4	E962.0	E980.4
Eucalyptus (oil) NEC	975.5	E858.6	E945.5	E950.4	E962.0	E980.4
Eucatropine	971.1	E855.4	E941.1	E950.4	E962.0	E980.4
Eucodal	965.09	E850.2	E935.2	E950.0	E962.0	E980.0
Euneryl	967.0	E851	E937.0	E950.1	E962.0	E980.1
Euphthalmine	971.1	E855.4	E941.1	E950.4	E962.0	E980.4
Eurax	976.0	E858.7	E946.0	E950.4	E962.0	E980.4
Euresol	976.4	E858.7	E946.4	E950.4	E962.0	E980.4
Euthroid	962.7	E858.0	E932.7	E950.4	E962.0	E980.4
Evans blue	977.8	E858.8	E947.8	E950.4	E962.0	E980.4
Evipal	967.0	E851	E937.0	E950.1	E962.0	E980.1
sodium	968.3	E855.1	E938.3	E950.4	E962.0	E980.4
Evipan	967.0	E851	E937.0	E950.1	E962.0	E980.1
sodium	968.3	E855.1	E938.3	E950.4	E962.0	E980.4
Exalgin	965.4	E850.4	E935.4	E950.0	E962.0	E980.0
Excipients, pharmaceutical	977.4	E858.8	E947.4	E950.4	E962.0	E980.4
Exhaust gas — *see* Carbon, monoxide						
Ex–Lax (phenolphthalein)	973.1	E858.4	E943.1	E950.4	E962.0	E980.4
Expectorants	975.5	E858.6	E945.5	E950.4	E962.0	E980.4
External medications (skin) (mucous membrane)	976.9	E858.7	E946.9	E950.4	E962.0	E980.4
dental agent	976.7	E858.7	E946.7	E950.4	E962.0	E980.4
ENT agent	976.6	E858.7	E946.6	E950.4	E962.0	E980.4

Substance	Poisoning	Accident	Therapeutic Use	Suicide Attempt	Assault	Undetermined
			External Cause (E-Code)			
ophthalmic preparation	976.5	E858.7	E946.5	E950.4	E962.0	E980.4
specified NEC	976.8	E858.7	E946.8	E950.4	E962.0	E980.4
Eye agents (anti–infective)	976.5	E858.7	E946.5	E950.4	E962.0	E980.4
Factor IX complex (human)	964.5	E858.2	E934.5	E950.4	E962.0	E980.4
Fecal softeners	973.2	E858.4	E943.2	E950.4	E962.0	E980.4
Fenbutrazate	977.0	E858.8	E947.0	E950.4	E962.0	E980.4
Fencamfamin	970.8	E854.3	E940.8	E950.4	E962.0	E980.4
Fenfluramine	977.0	E858.8	E947.0	E950.4	E962.0	E980.4
Fenoprofen	965.61	E850.6	E935.6	E950.0	E962.0	E980.0
Fentanyl	965.09	E850.2	E935.2	E950.0	E962.0	E980.0
Fentazin	969.1	E853.0	E939.1	E950.3	E962.0	E980.3
Fenticlor, fentichlor	976.0	E858.7	E946.0	E950.4	E962.0	E980.4
Fer de lance (bite) (venom)	989.5	E905.0	—	E950.9	E962.1	E980.9
Ferric — *see* Iron						
Ferrocholinate	964.0	E858.2	E934.0	E950.4	E962.0	E980.4
Ferrous fumarate, gluconate, lactate, salt						
NEC, sulfate (medicinal)	964.0	E858.2	E934.0	E950.4	E962.0	E980.4
Ferrum — *see* Iron						
Fertilizers NEC	989.89	E866.5	—	E950.9	E962.1	E980.4
with herbicide mixture	989.4	E863.5	—	E950.6	E962.1	E980.7
Fibrinogen (human)	964.7	E858.2	E934.7	E950.4	E962.0	E980.4
Fibrinolysin	964.4	E858.2	E934.4	E950.4	E962.0	E980.4
Fibrinolysis–affecting agents	964.4	E858.2	E934.4	E950.4	E962.0	E980.4
Filix mas	961.6	E857	E931.6	E950.4	E962.0	E980.4
Fiorinal	965.1	E850.3	E935.3	E950.0	E962.0	E980.0
Fire damp	987.1	E869.8	—	E952.8	E962.2	E982.8
Fish, nonbacterial or noxious	988.0	E865.2	—	E950.9	E962.1	E980.9
shell	988.0	E865.1	—	E950.9	E962.1	E980.9
Flagyl	961.5	E857	E931.5	E950.4	E962.0	E980.4
Flavoxate	975.1	E858.6	E945.1	E950.4	E962.0	E980.4
Flaxedil	975.2	E858.6	E945.2	E950.4	E962.0	E980.4
Flaxseed (medicinal)	976.3	E858.7	E946.3	E950.4	E962.0	E980.4
Florantyrone	973.4	E858.4	E943.4	E950.4	E962.0	E980.4
Floraquin	961.3	E857	E931.3	E950.4	E962.0	E980.4
Florinef	962.0	E858.0	E932.0	E950.4	E962.0	E980.4
ENT agent	976.6	E858.7	E946.6	E950.4	E962.0	E980.4
ophthalmic preparation	976.5	E858.7	E946.5	E950.4	E962.0	E980.4
topical NEC	976.0	E858.7	E946.0	E950.4	E962.0	E980.4
Flowers of sulfur	976.4	E858.7	E946.4	E950.4	E962.0	E980.4
Floxuridine	963.1	E858.1	E933.1	E950.4	E962.0	E980.4
Flucytosine	961.9	E857	E931.9	E950.4	E962.0	E980.4
Fludrocortisone	962.0	E858.0	E932.0	E950.4	E962.0	E980.4
ENT agent	976.6	E858.7	E946.6	E950.4	E962.0	E980.4
ophthalmic preparation	976.5	E858.7	E946.5	E950.4	E962.0	E980.4
topical NEC	976.0	E858.7	E946.0	E950.4	E962.0	E980.4
Flumethasone	976.0	E858.7	E946.0	E950.4	E962.0	E980.4
Flumethiazide	974.3	E858.5	E944.3	E950.4	E962.0	E980.4
Flumidin	961.7	E857	E931.7	E950.4	E962.0	E980.4
Flunitrazepam	969.4	E853.2	E939.4	E950.3	E962.0	E980.3
Fluocinolone	976.0	E858.7	E946.0	E950.4	E962.0	E980.4
Fluocortolone	962.0	E858.0	E932.0	E950.4	E962.0	E980.4
Fluohydrocortisone	962.0	E858.0	E932.0	E950.4	E962.0	E980.4
ENT agent	976.6	E858.7	E946.6	E950.4	E962.0	E980.4
ophthalmic preparation	976.5	E858.7	E946.5	E950.4	E962.0	E980.4
topical NEC	976.0	E858.7	E946.0	E950.4	E962.0	E980.4
Fluonid	976.0	E858.7	E946.0	E950.4	E962.0	E980.4
Fluopromazine	969.1	E853.0	E939.1	E950.3	E962.0	E980.3

Substance	Poisoning	External Cause (E-Code)				
		Accident	Therapeutic Use	Suicide Attempt	Assault	Undetermined
Fluoracetate	989.4	E863.7	—	E950.6	E962.1	E980.7
Fluorescein (sodium)	977.8	E858.8	E947.8	E950.4	E962.0	E980.4
Fluoride(s) (pesticides) (sodium) NEC	989.4	E863.4	—	E950.6	E962.1	E980.7
hydrogen — *see* Hydrofluoric acid						
medicinal	976.7	E858.7	E946.7	E950.4	E962.0	E980.4
not pesticide NEC	983.9	E864.4	—	E950.7	E962.1	E980.6
stannous	976.7	E858.7	E946.7	E950.4	E962.0	E980.4
Fluorinated corticosteroids	962.0	E858.0	E932.0	E950.4	E962.0	E980.4
Fluorine (compounds) (gas)	987.8	E869.8	—	E952.8	E962.2	E982.8
salt — *see* Fluoride(s)						
Fluoristan	976.7	E858.7	E946.7	E950.4	E962.0	E980.4
Fluoroacetate	989.4	E863.7	—	E950.6	E962.1	E980.7
Fluorodeoxyuridine	963.1	E858.1	E933.1	E950.4	E962.0	E980.4
Fluorometholone (topical) NEC	976.0	E858.7	E946.0	E950.4	E962.0	E980.4
ophthalmic preparation	976.5	E858.7	E946.5	E950.4	E962.0	E980.4
Fluorouracil	963.1	E858.1	E933.1	E950.4	E962.0	E980.4
Fluothane	968.1	E855.1	E938.1	E950.4	E962.0	E980.4
Fluoxetine hydrochloride	969.0	E854.0	E939.0	E950.3	E962.0	E980.3
Fluoxymesterone	962.1	E858.0	E932.1	E950.4	E962.0	E980.4
Fluphenazine	969.1	E853.0	E939.1	E950.3	E962.0	E980.3
Fluprednisolone	962.0	E858.0	E932.0	E950.4	E962.0	E980.4
Flurandrenolide	976.0	E858.7	E946.0	E950.4	E962.0	E980.4
Flurazepam (hydrochloride)	969.4	E853.2	E939.4	E950.3	E962.0	E980.3
Flurbiprofen	965.61	E850.6	E935.6	E950.0	E962.0	E980.0
Flurobate	976.0	E858.7	E946.0	E950.4	E962.0	E980.4
Flurothyl	969.8	E855.8	E939.8	E950.3	E962.0	E980.3
Fluroxene	968.2	E855.1	E938.2	E950.4	E962.0	E980.4
Folacin	964.1	E858.2	E934.1	E950.4	E962.0	E980.4
Folic acid	964.1	E858.2	E934.1	E950.4	E962.0	E980.4
Follicle stimulating hormone	962.4	E858.0	E932.4	E950.4	E962.0	E980.4
Food, foodstuffs, nonbacterial or noxious	988.9	E865.9	—	E950.9	E962.1	E980.9
berries, seeds	988.2	E865.3	—	E950.9	E962.1	E980.9
fish	988.0	E865.2	—	E950.9	E962.1	E980.9
mushrooms	988.1	E865.5	—	E950.9	E962.1	E980.9
plants	988.2	E865.9	—	E950.9	E962.1	E980.9
specified type NEC	988.2	E865.4	—	E950.9	E962.1	E980.9
shellfish	988.0	E865.1	—	E950.9	E962.1	E980.9
specified NEC	988.8	E865.8	—	E950.9	E962.1	E980.9
Fool's parsley	988.2	E865.4	—	E950.9	E962.1	E980.9
Formaldehyde (solution)	989.89	E861.4	—	E950.9	E962.1	E980.9
fungicide	989.4	E863.6	—	E950.6	E962.1	E980.7
gas or vapor	987.8	E869.8	—	E952.8	E962.2	E982.8
Formalin	989.89	E861.4	—	E950.9	E962.1	E980.9
fungicide	989.4	E863.6	—	E950.6	E962.1	E980.7
vapor	987.8	E869.8	—	E952.8	E962.2	E982.8
Formic acid	983.1	E864.1	—	E950.7	E962.1	E980.6
vapor	987.8	E869.8	—	E952.8	E962.2	E982.8
Fowler's solution	985.1	E866.3	—	E950.8	E962.1	E980.8
Foxglove	988.2	E865.4	—	E950.9	E962.1	E980.9
Fox green	977.8	E858.8	E947.8	E950.4	E962.0	E980.4
Framycetin	960.8	E856	E930.8	E950.4	E962.0	E980.4
Frangula (extract)	973.1	E858.4	E943.1	E950.4	E962.0	E980.4
Frei antigen	977.8	E858.8	E947.8	E950.4	E962.0	E980.4
Freons	987.4	E869.2	—	E952.8	E962.2	E982.8
Fructose	974.5	E858.5	E944.5	E950.4	E962.0	E980.4
Frusemide	974.4	E858.5	E944.4	E950.4	E962.0	E980.4
FSH	962.4	E858.0	E932.4	E950.4	E962.0	E980.4

Substance	Poisoning	Accident	Therapeutic Use	Suicide Attempt	Assault	Undetermined
Fuel						
automobile	981	E862.1	—	E950.9	E962.1	E980.9
exhaust gas, not in transit	986	E868.2	—	E952.0	E962.2	E982.0
vapor NEC	987.1	E869.8	—	E952.8	E962.2	E982.8
gas (domestic use) — *see also* Carbon, monoxide, fuel						
utility	987.1	E868.1	—	E951.8	E962.2	E981.8
incomplete combustion of — *see* Carbon, monoxide, fuel, utility						
in mobile container	987.0	E868.0	—	E951.1	E962.2	E981.1
piped (natural)	987.1	E867	—	E951.0	E962.2	E981.0
industrial, incomplete combustion	986	E868.3	—	E952.1	E962.2	E982.1
Fugillin	960.8	E856	E930.8	E950.4	E962.0	E980.4
Fulminate of mercury	985.0	E866.1	—	E950.9	E961.1	E980.9
Fulvicin	960.1	E856	E930.1	E950.4	E962.0	E980.4
Fumadil	960.8	E856	E930.8	E950.4	E962.0	E980.4
Fumagillin	960.8	E856	E930.8	E950.4	E962.0	E980.4
Fumes (from)	987.9	E869.9	—	E952.9	E962.2	E982.9
carbon monoxide — *see* Carbon, monoxide						
charcoal (domestic use)	986	E868.3	—	E952.1	E962.2	E982.1
chloroform — *see* Chloroform						
coke (in domestic stoves, fireplaces)	986	E868.3	—	E952.1	E962.2	E982.1
corrosive NEC	987.8	E869.8	—	E952.8	E962.2	E982.8
ether — *see* Ether(s)						
freons	987.4	E869.2	—	E952.8	E962.2	E982.8
hydrocarbons	987.1	E869.8	—	E952.8	E962.2	E982.8
petroleum (liquefied)	987.0	E868.0	—	E951.1	E962.2	E981.1
distributed through pipes (pure or mixed with air)	987.0	E867	—	E951.0	E962.2	E981.0
lead — *see* Lead						
metals — *see* specified metal						
nitrogen dioxide	987.2	E869.0	—	E952.8	E962.2	E982.8
pesticides — *see* Pesticides						
petroleum (liquefied)	987.0	E868.0	—	E951.1	E962.2	E981.1
distributed through pipes (pure or mixed with air)	987.0	E867	—	E951.0	E962.2	E981.0
polyester	987.8	E869.8	—	E952.8	E962.2	E982.8
specified source, other (see also substance specified)	987.8	E869.8	—	E952.8	E962.2	E982.8
sulfur dioxide	987.3	E869.1	—	E952.8	E962.2	E982.8
Fumigants	989.4	E863.8	—	E950.6	E962.1	E980.7
Fungi, noxious, used as food	988.1	E865.5	—	E950.9	E962.1	E980.9
Fungicides (*see also* Antifungals)	989.4	E863.6	—	E950.6	E962.1	E980.7
Fungizone	960.1	E856	E930.1	E950.4	E962.0	E980.4
topical	976.0	E858.7	E946.0	E950.4	E962.0	E980.4
Furacin	976.0	E858.7	E946.0	E950.4	E962.0	E980.4
Furadantin	961.9	E857	E931.9	E950.4	E962.0	E980.4
Furazolidone	961.9	E857	E931.9	E950.4	E962.0	E980.4
Furnace (coal burning) (domestic), gas from	986	E868.3	—	E952.1	E962.2	E982.1
industrial	986	E868.8	—	E952.1	E962.2	E982.1
Furniture polish	989.89	E861.2	—	E950.9	E962.1	E980.9
Furosemide	974.4	E858.5	E944.4	E950.4	E962.0	E980.4
Furoxone	961.9	E857	E931.9	E950.4	E962.0	E980.4
Fusel oil (amyl) (butyl) (propyl)	980.3	E860.4	—	E950.9	E962.1	E980.9
Fusidic acid	960.8	E856	E930.8	E950.4	E962.0	E980.4
Gallamine	975.2	E858.6	E945.2	E950.4	E962.0	E980.4

Substance	External Cause (E-Code)					
	Poisoning	Accident	Therapeutic Use	Suicide Attempt	Assault	Undetermined
Gallotannic acid	976.2	E858.7	E946.2	E950.4	E962.0	E980.4
Gamboge	973.1	E858.4	E943.1	E950.4	E962.0	E980.4
Gamimune	964.6	E858.2	E934.6	E950.4	E962.0	E980.4
Gamma–benzene hexachloride (vapor)	989.2	E863.0	—	E950.6	E962.1	E980.7
Gamma globulin	964.6	E858.2	E934.6	E950.4	E962.0	E980.4
Gamma Hydroxy Butyrate (GHB)	968.4	E855.1	E938.4	E950.4	E962.0	E980.4
Gamulin	964.6	E858.2	E934.6	E950.4	E962.0	E980.4
Ganglionic blocking agents	972.3	E858.3	E942.3	E950.4	E962.0	E980.4
Ganja	969.6	E854.1	E939.6	E950.3	E962.0	E980.3
Garamycin	960.8	E856	E930.8	E950.4	E962.0	E980.4
ophthalmic preparation	976.5	E858.7	E946.5	E950.4	E962.0	E980.4
topical NEC	976.0	E858.7	E946.0	E950.4	E962.0	E980.4
Gardenal	967.0	E851	E937.0	E950.1	E962.0	E980.1
Gardepanyl	967.0	E851	E937.0	E950.1	E962.0	E980.1
Gas	987.9	E869.9	—	E952.9	E962.2	E982.9
acetylene	987.1	E868.1	—	E951.8	E962.2	E981.8
incomplete combustion of — *see* Carbon, monoxide, fuel, utility						
air contaminants, source or type not specified	987.9	E869.9	—	E952.9	E962.2	E982.9
anesthetic (general) NEC	968.2	E855.1	E938.2	E950.4	E962.0	E980.4
blast furnace	986	E868.8	—	E952.1	E962.2	E982.1
butane — *see* Butane						
carbon monoxide — *see* Carbon, monoxide						
chlorine	987.6	E869.8	—	E952.8	E962.2	E982.8
coal — *see* Carbon, monoxide, coal						
cyanide	987.7	E869.8	—	E952.8	E962.2	E982.8
dicyanogen	987.8	E869.8	—	E952.8	E962.2	E982.8
domestic — *see* Gas, utility						
exhaust — *see* Carbon, monoxide, exhaust gas						
from wood– or coal–burning stove or fireplace	986	E868.3	—	E952.1	E962.2	E982.1
fuel (domestic use) — *see also* Carbon, monoxide, fuel						
industrial use	986	E868.8	—	E952.1	E962.2	E982.1
utility	987.1	E868.1	—	E951.8	E962.2	E981.8
incomplete combustion of — *see* Carbon, monoxide, fuel, utility						
in mobile container	987.0	E868.0	—	E951.1	E962.2	E981.1
piped (natural)	987.1	E867	—	E951.0	E962.2	E981.0
garage	986	E868.2	—	E952.0	E962.2	E982.0
hydrocarbon NEC	987.1	E869.8	—	E952.8	E962.2	E982.8
incomplete combustion of — *see* Carbon, monoxide, fuel, utility						
liquefied (mobile container)	987.0	E868.0	—	E951.1	E962.2	E981.1
piped	987.0	E867	—	E951.0	E962.2	E981.0
hydrocyanic acid	987.7	E869.8	—	E952.8	E962.2	E982.8
illuminating — *see* Gas, utility						
incomplete combustion, any — *see* Carbon, monoxide						
kiln	986	E868.8	—	E952.1	E962.2	E982.1
lacrimogenic	987.5	E869.3	—	E952.8	E962.2	E982.8
marsh	987.1	E869.8	—	E952.8	E962.2	E982.8
motor exhaust, not in transit	986	E868.8	—	E952.1	E962.2	E982.1
mustard — *see* Mustard, gas						
natural	987.1	E867	—	E951.0	E962.2	E981.0
nerve (war)	987.9	E869.9	—	E952.9	E962.2	E982.9

Substance	Poisoning	External Cause (E-Code)				
		Accident	Therapeutic Use	Suicide Attempt	Assault	Undetermined
oils	981	E862.1	—	E950.9	E962.1	E980.9
petroleum (liquefied) (distributed in mobile containers)	987.0	E868.0	—	E951.1	E962.2	E981.1
piped (pure or mixed with air)	987.0	E867	—	E951.1	E962.2	E981.1
piped (manufactured) (natural) NEC	987.1	E867	—	E951.0	E962.2	E981.0
producer	986	E868.8	—	E952.1	E962.2	E982.1
propane — *see* Propane						
refrigerant (freon)	987.4	E869.2	—	E952.8	E962.2	E982.8
not freon	987.9	E869.9	—	E952.9	E962.2	E982.9
sewer	987.8	E869.8	—	E952.8	E962.2	E982.8
specified source NEC (*see also* substance specified)	987.8	E869.8	—	E952.8	E962.2	E982.8
stove — *see* Gas, utility						
tear	987.5	E869.3	—	E952.8	E962.2	E982.8
utility (for cooking, heating, or lighting) (piped) NEC	987.1	E868.1	—	E951.8	E962.2	E981.8
incomplete combustion of — *see* Carbon, monoxide, fuel, utility						
in mobile container	987.0	E868.0	—	E951.1	E962.2	E981.1
piped (natural)	987.1	E867	—	E951.0	E962.2	E981.0
water	987.1	E868.1	—	E951.8	E962.2	E981.8
incomplete combustion of — *see* Carbon, monoxide, fuel, utility						
Gaseous substance — *see* Gas						
Gasoline, gasolene	981	E862.1	—	E950.9	E962.1	E980.9
vapor	987.1	E869.8	—	E952.8	E962.2	E982.8
Gastric enzymes	973.4	E858.4	E943.4	E950.4	E962.0	E980.4
Gastrografin	977.8	E858.8	E947.8	E950.4	E962.0	E980.4
Gastrointestinal agents	973.9	E858.4	E943.9	E950.4	E962.0	E980.4
specified NEC	973.8	E858.4	E943.8	E950.4	E962.0	E980.4
Gaultheria procumbens	988.2	E865.4	—	E950.9	E962.1	E980.9
Gelatin (intravenous)	964.8	E858.2	E934.8	E950.4	E962.0	E980.4
absorbable (sponge)	964.5	E858.2	E934.5	E950.4	E962.0	E980.4
Gelfilm	976.8	E858.7	E946.8	E950.4	E962.0	E980.4
Gelfoam	964.5	E858.2	E934.5	E950.4	E962.0	E980.4
Gelsemine	970.8	E854.3	E940.8	E950.4	E962.0	E980.4
Gelsemium (sempervirens)	988.2	E865.4	—	E950.9	E962.1	E980.9
Gemonil	967.0	E851	E937.0	E950.1	E962.0	E980.1
Gentamicin	960.8	E856	E930.8	E950.4	E962.0	E980.4
ophthalmic preparation	976.5	E858.7	E946.5	E950.4	E962.0	E980.4
topical NEC	976.0	E858.7	E946.0	E950.4	E962.0	E980.4
Gentian violet	976.0	E858.7	E946.0	E950.4	E962.0	E980.4
Gexane	976.0	E858.7	E946.0	E950.4	E962.0	E980.4
Gila monster (venom)	989.5	E905.0	—	E950.9	E962.1	E980.9
Ginger, Jamaica	989.89	E866.8		E950.9	E962.1	E980.9
Gitalin	972.1	E858.3	E942.1	E950.4	E962.0	E980.4
Gitoxin	972.1	E858.3	E942.1	E950.4	E962.0	E980.4
Glandular extract (medicinal) NEC	977.9	E858.9	E947.9	E950.5	E962.0	E980.5
Glaucarubin	961.5	E857	E931.5	E950.4	E962.0	E980.4
Globin zinc insulin	962.3	E858.0	E932.3	E950.4	E962.0	E980.4
Glucagon	962.3	E858.0	E932.3	E950.4	E962.0	E980.4
Glucochloral	967.1	E852.0	E937.1	E950.2	E962.0	E980.2
Glucocorticoids	962.0	E858.0	E932.0	E950.4	E962.0	E980.4
Glucose	974.5	E858.5	E944.5	E950.4	E962.0	E980.4
oxidase reagent	977.8	E858.8	E947.8	E950.4	E962.0	E980.4
Glucosulfone sodium	961.8	E857	E931.8	E950.4	E962.0	E980.4
Glue(s)	989.89	E866.6	—	E950.9	E962.1	E980.9

Substance	Poisoning	External Cause (E-Code)				
		Accident	Therapeutic Use	Suicide Attempt	Assault	Undetermined
Glutamic acid (hydrochloride)	973.4	E858.4	E943.4	E950.4	E962.0	E980.4
Glutathione	963.8	E858.1	E933.8	E950.4	E962.0	E980.4
Glutethimide (group)	967.5	E852.4	E937.5	E950.2	E962.0	E980.2
Glycerin (lotion)	976.3	E858.7	E946.3	E950.4	E962.0	E980.4
Glycerol (topical)	976.3	E858.7	E946.3	E950.4	E962.0	E980.4
Glyceryl						
guaiacolate	975.5	E858.6	E945.5	E950.4	E962.0	E980.4
triacetate (topical)	976.0	E858.7	E946.0	E950.4	E962.0	E980.4
trinitrate	972.4	E858.3	E942.4	E950.4	E962.0	E980.4
Glycine	974.5	E858.5	E944.5	E950.4	E962.0	E980.4
Glycobiarsol	961.1	E857	E931.1	E950.4	E962.0	E980.4
Glycols (ether)	982.8	E862.4	—	E950.9	E962.1	E980.9
Glycopyrrolate	971.1	E855.4	E941.1	E950.4	E962.0	E980.4
Glymidine	962.3	E858.0	E932.3	E950.4	E962.0	E980.4
Gold (compounds) (salts)	965.69	E850.6	E935.6	E950.0	E962.0	E980.0
Golden sulfide of antimony	985.4	E866.2	—	E950.9	E962.1	E980.9
Goldylocks	988.2	E865.4	—	E950.9	E962.1	E980.9
Gonadal tissue extract	962.9	E858.0	E932.9	E950.4	E962.0	E980.4
female	962.2	E858.0	E932.2	E950.4	E962.0	E980.4
male	962.1	E858.0	E932.1	E950.4	E962.0	E980.4
Gonadotropin	962.4	E858.0	E932.4	E950.4	E962.0	E980.4
Grain alcohol	980.0	E860.1	—	E950.9	E962.1	E980.9
beverage	980.0	E860.0	—	E950.9	E962.1	E980.9
Gramicidin	960.8	E856	E930.8	E950.4	E962.0	E980.4
Gratiola officinalis	988.2	E865.4	—	E950.9	E962.1	E980.9
Grease	989.89	E866.8	—	E950.9	E962.1	E980.9
Green hellebore	988.2	E865.4	—	E950.9	E962.1	E980.9
Green soap	976.2	E858.7	E946.2	E950.4	E962.0	E980.4
Grifulvin	960.1	E856	E930.1	E950.4	E962.0	E980.4
Griseofulvin	960.1	E856	E930.1	E950.4	E962.0	E980.4
Growth hormone	962.4	E858.0	E932.4	E950.4	E962.0	E980.4
Guaiacol	975.5	E858.6	E945.5	E950.4	E962.0	E980.4
Guaiac reagent	977.8	E858.8	E947.8	E950.4	E962.0	E980.4
Guaifenesin	975.5	E858.6	E945.5	E950.4	E962.0	E980.4
Guaiphenesin	975.5	E858.6	E945.5	E950.4	E962.0	E980.4
Guanatol	961.4	E857	E931.4	E950.4	E962.0	E980.4
Guanethidine	972.6	E858.3	E942.6	E950.4	E962.0	E980.4
Guano	989.89	E866.5	—	E950.9	E962.1	E980.9
Guanochlor	972.6	E858.3	E942.6	E950.4	E962.0	E980.4
Guanoctine	972.6	E858.3	E942.6	E950.4	E962.0	E980.4
Guanoxan	972.6	E858.3	E942.6	E950.4	E962.0	E980.4
Hair treatment agent NEC	976.4	E858.7	E946.4	E950.4	E962.0	E980.4
Halcinonide	976.0	E858.7	E946.0	E950.4	E962.0	E980.4
Halethazole	976.0	E858.7	E946.0	E950.4	E962.0	E980.4
Hallucinogens	969.6	E854.1	E939.6	E950.3	E962.0	E980.3
Haloperidol	969.2	E853.1	E939.2	E950.3	E962.0	E980.3
Haloprogin	976.0	E858.7	E946.0	E950.4	E962.0	E980.4
Halotex	976.0	E858.7	E946.0	E950.4	E962.0	E980.4
Halothane	968.1	E855.1	E938.1	E950.4	E962.0	E980.4
Halquinols	976.0	E858.7	E946.0	E950.4	E962.0	E980.4
Harmonyl	972.6	E858.3	E942.6	E950.4	E962.0	E980.4
Hartmann's solution	974.5	E858.5	E944.5	E950.4	E962.0	E980.4
Hashish	969.6	E854.1	E939.6	E950.3	E962.0	E980.3
Hawaiian wood rose seeds	969.6	E854.1	E939.6	E950.3	E962.0	E980.3
Headache cures, drugs, powders NEC	977.9	E858.9	E947.9	E950.5	E962.0	E980.9
Heavenly Blue (morning glory)	969.6	E854.1	E939.6	E950.3	E962.0	E980.3
Heavy metal						

Substance	Poisoning	External Cause (E-Code)				
		Accident	Therapeutic Use	Suicide Attempt	Assault	Undetermined
antagonists	963.8	E858.1	E933.8	E950.4	E962.0	E980.4
anti–infectives	961.2	E857	E931.2	E950.4	E962.0	E980.4
Hedaquinium	976.0	E858.7	E946.0	E950.4	E962.0	E980.4
Hedge hyssop	988.2	E865.4	—	E950.9	E962.1	E980.9
Heet	976.8	E858.7	E946.8	E950.4	E962.0	E980.4
Helenin	961.6	E857	E931.6	E950.4	E962.0	E980.4
Hellebore (black) (green) (white)	988.2	E865.4	—	E950.9	E962.1	E980.9
Hemlock	988.2	E865.4	—	E950.9	E962.1	E980.9
Hemostatics	964.5	E858.2	E934.5	E950.4	E962.0	E980.4
capillary active drugs	972.8	E858.3	E942.8	E950.4	E962.0	E980.4
Henbane	988.2	E865.4	—	E950.9	E962.1	E980.9
Heparin (sodium)	964.2	E858.2	E934.2	E950.4	E962.0	E980.4
Heptabarbital, heptabarbitone	967.0	E851	E937.0	E950.1	E962.0	E980.1
Heptachlor	989.2	E863.0	—	E950.6	E962.1	E980.7
Heptalgin	965.09	E850.2	E935.2	E950.0	E962.0	E980.0
Herbicides	989.4	E863.5	—	E950.6	E962.1	E980.7
Heroin	965.01	E850.0	E935.0	E950.0	E962.0	E980.0
Herplex	976.5	E858.7	E946.5	E950.4	E962.0	E980.4
HES	964.8	E858.2	E934.8	E950.4	E962.0	E980.4
Hetastarch	964.8	E858.2	E934.8	E950.4	E962.0	E980.4
Hexachlorocyclohexane	989.2	E863.0	—	E950.6	E962.1	E980.7
Hexachlorophene	976.2	E858.7	E946.2	E950.4	E962.0	E980.4
Hexadimethrine (bromide)	964.5	E858.2	E934.5	E950.4	E962.0	E980.4
Hexafluorenium	975.2	E858.6	E945.2	E950.4	E962.0	E980.4
Hexa–germ	976.2	E858.7	E946.2	E950.4	E962.0	E980.4
Hexahydrophenol	980.8	E860.8	—	E950.9	E962.1	E980.9
Hexalin	980.8	E860.8	—	E950.9	E962.1	E980.9
Hexamethonium	972.3	E858.3	E942.3	E950.4	E962.0	E980.4
Hexamethyleneamine	961.9	E857	E931.9	E950.4	E962.0	E980.4
Hexamine	961.9	E857	E931.9	E950.4	E962.0	E980.4
Hexanone	982.8	E862.4	—	E950.9	E962.1	E980.9
Hexapropymate	967.8	E852.8	E937.8	E950.2	E962.0	E980.2
Hexestrol	962.2	E858.0	E932.2	E950.4	E962.0	E980.4
Hexethal (sodium)	967.0	E851	E937.0	E950.1	E962.0	E980.1
Hexetidine	976.0	E858.7	E946.0	E950.4	E962.0	E980.4
Hexobarbital, hexobarbitone	967.0	E851	E937.0	E950.1	E962.0	E980.1
sodium (anesthetic)	968.3	E855.1	E938.3	E950.4	E962.0	E980.4
soluble	968.3	E855.1	E938.3	E950.4	E962.0	E980.4
Hexocyclium	971.1	E855.4	E941.1	E950.4	E962.0	E980.4
Hexoestrol	962.2	E858.0	E932.2	E950.4	E962.0	E980.4
Hexone	982.8	E862.4	—	E950.9	E962.1	E980.9
Hexylcaine	968.5	E855.2	E938.5	E950.4	E962.0	E980.4
Hexylresorcinol	961.6	E857	E931.6	E950.4	E962.0	E980.4
Hinkle's pills	973.1	E858.4	E943.1	E950.4	E962.0	E980.4
Histalog	977.8	E858.8	E947.8	E950.4	E962.0	E980.4
Histamine (phosphate)	972.5	E858.3	E942.5	E950.4	E962.0	E980.4
Histoplasmin	977.8	E858.8	E947.8	E950.4	E962.0	E980.4
Holly berries	988.2	E865.3	—	E950.9	E962.1	E980.9
Homatropine	971.1	E855.4	E941.1	E950.4	E962.0	E980.4
Homo–tet	964.6	E858.2	E934.6	E950.4	E962.0	E980.4
Hormones (synthetic substitute) NEC	962.9	E858.0	E932.9	E950.4	E962.0	E980.4
adrenal cortical steroids	962.0	E858.0	E932.0	E950.4	E962.0	E980.4
antidiabetic agents	962.3	E858.0	E932.3	E950.4	E962.0	E980.4
follicle stimulating	962.4	E858.0	E932.4	E950.4	E962.0	E980.4
gonadotropic	962.4	E858.0	E932.4	E950.4	E962.0	E980.4
growth	962.4	E858.0	E932.4	E950.4	E962.0	E980.4
ovarian (substitutes)	962.2	E858.0	E932.2	E950.4	E962.0	E980.4

Substance	Poisoning	Accident	Therapeutic Use	Suicide Attempt	Assault	Undetermined
parathyroid (derivatives)	962.6	E858.0	E932.6	E950.4	E962.0	E980.4
pituitary (posterior)	962.5	E858.0	E932.5	E950.4	E962.0	E980.4
anterior	962.4	E858.0	E932.4	E950.4	E962.0	E980.4
thyroid (derivative)	962.7	E858.0	E932.7	E950.4	E962.0	E980.4
Hornet (sting)	989.5	E905.3	—	E950.9	E962.1	E980.9
Horticulture agent NEC	989.4	E863.9	—	E950.6	E962.1	E980.7
Hyaluronidase	963.4	E858.1	E933.4	E950.4	E962.0	E980.4
Hyazyme	963.4	E858.1	E933.4	E950.4	E962.0	E980.4
Hycodan	965.09	E850.2	E935.2	E950.0	E962.0	E980.0
Hydantoin derivatives	966.1	E855.0	E936.1	E950.4	E962.0	E980.4
Hydeltra	962.0	E858.0	E932.0	E950.4	E962.0	E980.4
Hydergine	971.3	E855.6	E941.3	E950.4	E962.0	E980.4
Hydrabamine penicillin	960.0	E856	E930.0	E950.4	E962.0	E980.4
Hydralazine, hydrallazine	972.6	E858.3	E942.6	E950.4	E962.0	E980.4
Hydrargaphen	976.0	E858.7	E946.0	E950.4	E962.0	E980.4
Hydrazine	983.9	E864.3	—	E950.7	E962.1	E980.6
Hydriodic acid	975.5	E858.6	E945.5	E950.4	E962.0	E980.4
Hydrocarbon gas	987.1	E869.8	—	E952.8	E962.2	E982.8
incomplete combustion of — *see* Carbon, monoxide, fuel, utility						
liquefied (mobile container)	987.0	E868.0	—	E951.1	E962.2	E981.1
piped (natural)	987.0	E867	—	E951.0	E962.2	E981.0
Hydrochloric acid (liquid)	983.1	E864.1	—	E950.7	E962.1	E980.6
medicinal	973.4	E858.4	E943.4	E950.4	E962.0	E980.4
vapor	987.8	E869.8	—	E952.8	E962.2	E982.8
Hydrochlorothiazide	974.3	E858.5	E944.3	E950.4	E962.0	E980.4
Hydrocodone	965.09	E850.2	E935.2	E950.0	E962.0	E980.0
Hydrocortisone	962.0	E858.0	E932.0	E950.4	E962.0	E980.4
ENT agent	976.6	E858.7	E946.6	E950.4	E962.0	E980.4
ophthalmic preparation	976.5	E858.7	E946.5	E950.4	E962.0	E980.4
topical NEC	976.0	E858.7	E946.0	E950.4	E962.0	E980.4
Hydrocortone	962.0	E858.0	E932.0	E950.4	E962.0	E980.4
ENT agent	976.6	E858.7	E946.6	E950.4	E962.0	E980.4
ophthalmic preparation	976.5	E858.7	E946.5	E950.4	E962.0	E980.4
topical NEC	976.0	E858.7	E946.0	E950.4	E962.0	E980.4
Hydrocyanic acid — *see* Cyanide(s)						
Hydroflumethiazide	974.3	E858.5	E944.3	E950.4	E962.0	E980.4
Hydrofluoric acid (liquid)	983.1	E864.1	—	E950.7	E962.1	E980.6
vapor	987.8	E869.8	—	E952.8	E962.2	E982.8
Hydrogen	987.8	E869.8	—	E952.8	E962.2	E982.8
arsenide	985.1	E866.3	—	E950.8	E962.1	E980.8
arseniureted	985.1	E866.3	—	E950.8	E962.1	E980.8
cyanide (salts)	989.0	E866.8	—	E950.9	E962.1	E980.9
gas	987.7	E869.8	—	E952.8	E962.2	E982.8
fluoride (liquid)	983.1	E864.1	—	E950.7	E962.1	E980.6
vapor	987.8	E869.8	—	E952.8	E962.2	E982.8
peroxide (solution)	976.6	E858.7	E946.6	E950.4	E962.0	E980.4
phosphureted	987.8	E869.8	—	E952.8	E962.2	E982.8
sulfide (gas)	987.8	E869.8	—	E952.8	E962.2	E982.8
arseniureted	985.1	E866.3	—	E950.8	E962.1	E980.8
sulfureted	987.8	E869.8	—	E952.8	E962.2	E982.8
Hydromorphinol	965.09	E850.2	E935.2	E950.0	E962.0	E980.0
Hydromorphinone	965.09	E850.2	E935.2	E950.0	E962.0	E980.0
Hydromorphone	965.09	E850.2	E935.2	E950.0	E962.0	E980.0
Hydromox	974.3	E858.5	E944.3	E950.4	E962.0	E980.4
Hydrophilic lotion	976.3	E858.7	E946.3	E950.4	E962.0	E980.4
Hydroquinone	983.0	E864.0	—	E950.7	E962.1	E980.6

Substance	Poisoning	Accident	Therapeutic Use	Suicide Attempt	Assault	Undetermined
			External Cause (E-Code)			
vapor	987.8	E869.8	—	E952.8	E962.2	E982.8
Hydrosulfuric acid (gas)	987.8	E869.8	—	E952.8	E962.2	E982.8
Hydrous wool fat (lotion)	976.3	E858.7	E946.3	E950.4	E962.0	E980.4
Hydroxide, caustic	983.2	E864.2	—	E950.7	E962.1	E980.6
Hydroxocobalamin	964.1	E858.2	E934.1	E950.4	E962.0	E980.4
Hydroxyamphetamine	971.2	E855.5	E941.2	E950.4	E962.0	E980.4
Hydroxychloroquine	961.4	E857	E931.4	E950.4	E962.0	E980.4
Hydroxydihydrocodeinone	965.09	E850.2	E935.2	E950.0	E962.0	E980.0
Hydroxyethyl starch	964.8	E858.2	E934.8	E950.4	E962.0	E980.4
Hydroxyphenamate	969.5	E853.8	E939.5	E950.3	E962.0	E980.3
Hydroxyphenylbutazone	965.5	E850.5	E935.5	E950.0	E962.0	E980.0
Hydroxyprogesterone	962.2	E858.0	E932.2	E950.4	E962.0	E980.4
Hydroxyquinoline derivatives	961.3	E857	E931.3	E950.4	E962.0	E980.4
Hydroxystilbamidine	961.5	E857	E931.5	E950.4	E962.0	E980.4
Hydroxyurea	963.1	E858.1	E933.1	E950.4	E962.0	E980.4
Hydroxyzine	969.5	E853.8	E939.5	E950.3	E962.0	E980.3
Hyoscine (hydrobromide)	971.1	E855.4	E941.1	E950.4	E962.0	E980.4
Hyoscyamine	971.1	E855.4	E941.1	E950.4	E962.0	E980.4
Hyoscyamus (albus) (niger)	988.2	E865.4	—	E950.9	E962.1	E980.9
Hypaque	977.8	E858.8	E947.8	E950.4	E962.0	E980.4
Hypertussis	964.6	E858.2	E934.6	E950.4	E962.0	E980.4
Hypnotics NEC	967.9	E852.9	E937.9	E950.2	E962.0	E980.2
Hypochlorites — *see* Sodium, hypochlorite						
Hypotensive agents NEC	972.6	E858.3	E942.6	E950.4	E962.0	E980.4
Ibufenac	965.69	E850.6	E935.6	E950.0	E962.0	E980.0
Ibuprofen	965.61	E850.6	E935.6	E950.0	E962.0	E980.0
ICG	977.8	E858.8	E947.8	E950.4	E962.0	E980.4
Ichthammol	976.4	E858.7	E946.4	E950.4	E962.0	E980.4
Ichthyol	976.4	E858.7	E946.4	E950.4	E962.0	E980.4
Idoxuridine	976.5	E858.7	E946.5	E950.4	E962.0	E980.4
IDU	976.5	E858.7	E946.5	E950.4	E962.0	E980.4
Iletin	962.3	E858.0	E932.3	E950.4	E962.0	E980.4
Ilex	988.2	E865.4	—	E950.9	E962.1	E980.9
Illuminating gas — *see* Gas, utility						
Ilopan	963.5	E858.1	E933.5	E950.4	E962.0	E980.4
Ilotycin	960.3	E856	E930.3	E950.4	E962.0	E980.4
ophthalmic preparation	976.5	E858.7	E946.5	E950.4	E962.0	E980.4
topical NEC	976.0	E858.7	E946.0	E950.4	E962.0	E980.4
Imipramine	969.0	E854.0	E939.0	E950.3	E962.0	E980.3
Immu–G	964.6	E858.2	E934.6	E950.4	E962.0	E980.4
Immuglobin	964.6	E858.2	E934.6	E950.4	E962.0	E980.4
Immune serum globulin	964.6	E858.2	E934.6	E950.4	E962.0	E980.4
Immunosuppressive agents	963.1	E858.1	E933.1	E950.4	E962.0	E980.4
Immu–tetanus	964.6	E858.2	E934.6	E950.4	E962.0	E980.4
Indandione (derivatives)	964.2	E858.2	E934.2	E950.4	E962.0	E980.4
Inderal	972.0	E858.3	E942.0	E950.4	E962.0	E980.4
Indian						
hemp	969.6	E854.1	E939.6	E950.3	E962.0	E980.3
tobacco	988.2	E865.4	—	E950.9	E962.1	E980.9
Indigo carmine	977.8	E858.8	E947.8	E950.4	E962.0	E980.4
Indocin	965.69	E850.6	E935.6	E950.0	E962.0	E980.0
Indocyanine green	977.8	E858.8	E947.8	E950.4	E962.0	E980.4
Indomethacin	965.69	E850.6	E935.6	E950.0	E962.0	E980.0
Industrial						
alcohol	980.9	E860.9	—	E950.9	E962.1	E980.9
fumes	987.8	E869.8	—	E952.8	E962.2	E982.8
solvents (fumes) (vapors)	982.8	E862.9	—	E950.9	E962.1	E980.9

Substance	Poisoning	Accident	Therapeutic Use	Suicide Attempt	Assault	Undetermined
			External Cause (E-Code)			
Influenza vaccine	979.6	E858.8	E949.6	E950.4	E962.0	E982.8
Ingested substances NEC	989.9	E866.9	—	E950.9	E962.1	E980.9
INH (isoniazid)	961.8	E857	E931.8	E950.4	E962.0	E980.4
Inhalation, gas (noxious) — *see* Gas						
Ink	989.89	E866.8	—	E950.9	E962.1	E980.9
Innovar	967.6	E852.5	E937.6	E950.2	E962.0	E980.2
Inositol niacinate	972.2	E858.3	E942.2	E950.4	E962.0	E980.4
Inproquone	963.1	E858.1	E933.1	E950.4	E962.0	E980.4
Insect (sting), venomous	989.5	E905.5	—	E950.9	E962.1	E980.9
Insecticides (*see also* Pesticides)	989.4	E863.4	—	E950.6	E962.1	E980.7
chlorinated	989.2	E863.0	—	E950.6	E962.1	E980.7
mixtures	989.4	E863.3	—	E950.6	E962.1	E980.7
organochlorine (compounds)	989.2	E863.0	—	E950.6	E962.1	E980.7
organophosphorus (compounds)	989.3	E863.1	—	E950.6	E962.1	E980.7
Insular tissue extract	962.3	E858.0	E932.3	E950.4	E962.0	E980.4
Insulin (amorphous) (globin) (isophane) (Lente) (NPH) (protamine) (Semilente) (Ultralente) (zinc)	962.3	E858.0	E932.3	E950.4	E962.0	E980.4
Intranarcon	968.3	E855.1	E938.3	E950.4	E962.0	E980.4
Inulin	977.8	E858.8	E947.8	E950.4	E962.0	E980.4
Invert sugar	974.5	E858.5	E944.5	E950.4	E962.0	E980.4
Inza—*see* Naproxen						
Iodide NEC (*see also* Iodine)	976.0	E858.7	E946.0	E950.4	E962.0	E980.4
mercury (ointment)	976.0	E858.7	E946.0	E950.4	E962.0	E980.4
methylate	976.0	E858.7	E946.0	E950.4	E962.0	E980.4
potassium (expectorant) NEC	975.5	E858.6	E945.5	E950.4	E962.0	E980.4
Iodinated glycerol	975.5	E858.6	E945.5	E950.4	E962.0	E980.4
Iodine (antiseptic, external) (tincture) NEC	976.0	E858.7	E946.0	E950.4	E962.0	E980.4
diagnostic	977.8	E858.8	E947.8	E950.4	E962.0	E980.4
for thyroid conditions (antithyroid)	962.8	E858.0	E932.8	E950.4	E962.0	E980.4
vapor	987.8	E869.8	—	E952.8	E962.2	E982.8
Iodized oil	977.8	E858.8	E947.8	E950.4	E962.0	E980.4
Iodobismitol	961.2	E857	E931.2	E950.4	E962.0	E980.4
Iodochlorhydroxyquin	961.3	E857	E931.3	E950.4	E962.0	E980.4
topical	976.0	E858.7	E946.0	E950.4	E962.0	E980.4
Iodoform	976.0	E858.7	E946.0	E950.4	E962.0	E980.4
Iodopanoic acid	977.8	E858.8	E947.8	E950.4	E962.0	E980.4
Iodophthalein	977.8	E858.8	E947.8	E950.4	E962.0	E980.4
Ion exchange resins	974.5	E858.5	E944.5	E950.4	E962.0	E980.4
Iopanoic acid	977.8	E858.8	E947.8	E950.4	E962.0	E980.4
Iophendylate	977.8	E858.8	E947.8	E950.4	E962.0	E980.4
Iothiouracil	962.8	E858.0	E932.8	E950.4	E962.0	E980.4
Ipecac	973.6	E858.4	E943.6	E950.4	E962.0	E980.4
Ipecacuanha	973.6	E858.4	E943.6	E950.4	E962.0	E980.4
Ipodate	977.8	E858.8	E947.8	E950.4	E962.0	E980.4
Ipral	967.0	E851	E937.0	E950.1	E962.0	E980.1
Ipratropium	975.1	E858.6	E945.1	E950.4	E962.0	E980.4
Iproniazid	969.0	E854.0	E939.0	E950.3	E962.0	E980.3
Iron (compounds) (medicinal) (preparations)	964.0	E858.2	E934.0	E950.4	E962.0	E980.4
dextran	964.0	E858.2	E934.0	E950.4	E962.0	E980.4
nonmedicinal (dust) (fumes) NEC	985.8	E866.4	—	E950.9	E962.1	E980.9
Irritant drug	977.9	E858.9	E947.9	E950.5	E962.0	E980.5
Ismelin	972.6	E858.3	E942.6	E950.4	E962.0	E980.4
Isoamyl nitrite	972.4	E858.3	E942.4	E950.4	E962.0	E980.4
Isobutyl acetate	982.8	E862.4	—	E950.9	E962.1	E980.9

Substance	Poisoning	External Cause (E-Code)				
		Accident	Therapeutic Use	Suicide Attempt	Assault	Undetermined
Isocarboxazid	969.0	E854.0	E939.0	E950.3	E962.0	E980.3
Isoephedrine	971.2	E855.5	E941.2	E950.4	E962.0	E980.4
Isoetharine	971.2	E855.5	E941.2	E950.4	E962.0	E980.4
Isofluorophate	971.0	E855.3	E941.0	E950.4	E962.0	E980.4
Isoniazid (INH)	961.8	E857	E931.8	E950.4	E962.0	E980.4
Isopentaquine	961.4	E857	E931.4	E950.4	E962.0	E980.4
Isophane insulin	962.3	E858.0	E932.3	E950.4	E962.0	E980.4
Isopregnenone	962.2	E858.0	E932.2	E950.4	E962.0	E980.4
Isoprenaline	971.2	E855.5	E941.2	E950.4	E962.0	E980.4
Isopropamide	971.1	E855.4	E941.1	E950.4	E962.0	E980.4
Isopropanol	980.2	E860.3	—	E950.9	E962.1	E980.9
topical (germicide)	976.0	E858.7	E946.0	E950.4	E962.0	E980.4
Isopropyl						
acetate	982.8	E862.4	—	E950.9	E962.1	E980.9
alcohol	980.2	E860.3	—	E950.9	E962.1	E980.9
topical (germicide)	976.0	E858.7	E946.0	E950.4	E962.0	E980.4
ether	982.8	E862.4	—	E950.9	E962.1	E980.9
Isoproterenol	971.2	E855.5	E941.2	E950.4	E962.0	E980.4
Isosorbide dinitrate	972.4	E858.3	E942.4	E950.4	E962.0	E980.4
Isothipendyl	963.0	E858.1	E933.0	E950.4	E962.0	E980.4
Isoxazolyl penicillin	960.0	E856	E930.0	E950.4	E962.0	E980.4
Isoxsuprine hydrochloride	972.5	E858.3	E942.5	E950.4	E962.0	E980.4
I–thyroxine sodium	962.7	E858.0	E932.7	E950.4	E962.0	E980.4
Jaborandi (pilocarpus) (extract)	971.0	E855.3	E941.0	E950.4	E962.0	E980.4
Jalap	973.1	E858.4	E943.1	E950.4	E962.0	E980.4
Jamaica						
dogwood (bark)	965.7	E850.7	E935.7	E950.0	E962.0	E980.0
ginger	989.89	E866.8	—	E950.9	E962.1	E980.9
Jatropha	988.2	E865.4	—	E950.9	E962.1	E980.9
curcas	988.2	E865.3	—	E950.9	E962.1	E980.9
Jectofer	964.0	E858.2	E934.0	E950.4	E962.0	E980.4
Jellyfish (sting)	989.5	E905.6	—	E950.9	E962.1	E980.9
Jequirity (bean)	988.2	E865.3	—	E950.9	E962.1	E980.9
Jimson weed	988.2	E865.4	—	E950.9	E962.1	E980.9
seeds	988.2	E865.3	—	E950.9	E962.1	E980.9
Juniper tar (oil) (ointment)	976.4	E858.7	E946.4	E950.4	E962.0	E980.4
Kallikrein	972.5	E858.3	E942.5	E950.4	E962.0	E980.4
Kanamycin	960.6	E856	E930.6	E950.4	E962.0	E980.4
Kantrex	960.6	E856	E930.6	E950.4	E962.0	E980.4
Kaolin	973.5	E858.4	E943.5	E950.4	E962.0	E980.4
Karaya (gum)	973.3	E858.4	E943.3	E950.4	E962.0	E980.4
Kemithal	968.3	E855.1	E938.3	E950.4	E962.0	E980.4
Kenacort	962.0	E858.0	E932.0	E950.4	E962.0	E980.4
Keratolytics	976.4	E858.7	E946.4	E950.4	E962.0	E980.4
Keratoplastics	976.4	E858.7	E946.4	E950.4	E962.0	E980.4
Kerosene, kerosine (fuel) (solvent) NEC	981	E862.1	—	E950.9	E962.1	E980.9
insecticide	981	E863.4	—	E950.6	E962.1	E980.7
vapor	987.1	E869.8	—	E952.8	E962.2	E982.8
Ketamine	968.3	E855.1	E938.3	E950.4	E962.0	E980.4
Ketobemidone	965.09	E850.2	E935.2	E950.0	E962.0	E980.0
Ketols	982.8	E862.4	—	E950.9	E962.1	E980.9
Ketone oils	982.8	E862.4	—	E950.9	E962.1	E980.9
Ketoprofen	965.61	E850.6	E935.6	E950.0	E962.0	E980.0
Kiln gas or vapor (carbon monoxide)	986	E868.8	—	E952.1	E962.2	E982.1
Konsyl	973.3	E858.4	E943.3	E950.4	E962.0	E980.4
Kosam seed	988.2	E865.3	—	E950.9	E962.1	E980.9
Krait (venom)	989.5	E905.0	—	E950.9	E962.1	E980.9

Substance	Poisoning	External Cause (E-Code)				
		Accident	Therapeutic Use	Suicide Attempt	Assault	Undetermined
Kwell (insecticide)	989.2	E863.0	—	E950.6	E962.1	E980.7
anti–infective (topical)	976.0	E858.7	E946.0	E950.4	E962.0	E980.4
Laburnum (flowers) (seeds)	988.2	E865.3	—	E950.9	E962.1	E980.9
leaves	988.2	E865.4	—	E950.9	E962.1	E980.9
Lacquers	989.89	E861.6	—	E950.9	E962.1	E980.9
Lacrimogenic gas	987.5	E869.3	—	E952.8	E962.2	E982.8
Lactic acid	983.1	E864.1	—	E950.7	E962.1	E980.6
Lactobacillus acidophilus	973.5	E858.4	E943.5	E950.4	E962.0	E980.4
Lactoflavin	963.5	E858.1	E933.5	E950.4	E962.0	E980.4
Lactuca (virosa) (extract)	967.8	E852.8	E937.8	E950.2	E962.0	E980.2
Lactucarium	967.8	E852.8	E937.8	E950.2	E962.0	E980.2
Laevulose	974.5	E858.5	E944.5	E950.4	E962.0	E980.4
Lanatoside(C)	972.1	E858.3	E942.1	E950.4	E962.0	E980.4
Lanolin (lotion)	976.3	E858.7	E946.3	E950.4	E962.0	E980.4
Largactil	969.1	E853.0	E939.1	E950.3	E962.0	E980.3
Larkspur	988.2	E865.3	—	E950.9	E962.1	E980.9
Laroxyl	969.0	E854.0	E939.0	E950.3	E962.0	E980.3
Lasix	974.4	E858.5	E944.4	E950.4	E962.0	E980.4
Latex	989.82	E866.8	—	E950.9	E962.1	E980.9
Lathyrus (seed)	988.2	E865.3	—	E950.9	E962.1	E980.9
Laudanum	965.09	E850.2	E935.2	E950.0	E962.0	E980.0
Laudexium	975.2	E858.6	E945.2	E950.4	E962.0	E980.4
Laurel, black or cherry	988.2	E865.4	—	E950.9	E962.1	E980.9
Laurolinium	976.0	E858.7	E946.0	E950.4	E962.0	E980.4
Lauryl sulfoacetate	976.2	E858.7	E946.2	E950.4	E962.0	E980.4
Laxatives NEC	973.3	E858.4	E943.3	E950.4	E962.0	E980.4
emollient	973.2	E858.4	E943.2	E950.4	E962.0	E980.4
L–dopa	966.4	E855.0	E936.4	E950.4	E962.0	E980.4
L Tryptophan—*see* amino acid						
Lead (dust) (fumes) (vapor) NEC	984.9	E866.0	—	E950.9	E962.1	E980.9
acetate (dust)	984.1	E866.0	—	E950.9	E962.1	E980.9
anti–infectives	961.2	E857	E931.2	E950.4	E962.0	E980.4
antiknock compound (tetraethyl)	984.1	E862.1	—	E950.9	E962.1	E980.9
arsenate, arsenite (dust) (insecticide) (vapor)	985.1	E863.4	—	E950.8	E962.1	E980.8
herbicide	985.1	E863.5	—	E950.8	E962.1	E980.8
carbonate	984.0	E866.0	—	E950.9	E962.1	E980.9
paint	984.0	E861.5	—	E950.9	E962.1	E980.9
chromate	984.0	E866.0	—	E950.9	E962.1	E980.9
paint	984.0	E861.5	—	E950.9	E962.1	E980.9
dioxide	984.0	E866.0	—	E950.9	E962.1	E980.9
inorganic (compound)	984.0	E866.0	—	E950.9	E962.1	E980.9
paint	984.0	E861.5	—	E950.9	E962.1	E980.9
iodine	984.0	E866.0	—	E950.9	E962.1	E980.9
pigment (paint)	984.0	E861.5	—	E950.9	E962.1	E980.9
monoxide (dust)	984.0	E866.0	—	E950.9	E962.1	E980.9
paint	984.0	E861.5	—	E950.9	E962.1	E980.9
organic	984.1	E866.0	—	E950.9	E962.1	E980.9
oxide	984.0	E866.0	—	E950.9	E962.1	E980.9
paint	984.0	E861.5	—	E950.9	E962.1	E980.9
paint	984.0	E861.5	—	E950.9	E962.1	E980.9
salts	984.0	E866.0	—	E950.9	E962.1	E980.9
specified compound NEC	984.8	E866.0	—	E950.9	E962.1	E980.9
tetra–ethyl	984.1	E862.1	—	E950.9	E962.1	E980.9
Lebanese red	969.6	E854.1	E939.6	E950.3	E962.0	E980.3
Lente Iletin (insulin)	962.3	E858.0	E932.3	E950.4	E962.0	E980.4
Leptazol	970.0	E854.3	E940.0	E950.4	E962.0	E980.4

Substance	Poisoning	External Cause (E-Code)				
		Accident	Therapeutic Use	Suicide Attempt	Assault	Undetermined
Leritine	965.09	E850.2	E935.2	E950.0	E962.0	E980.0
Letter	962.7	E858.0	E932.7	E950.4	E962.0	E980.4
Lettuce opium	967.8	E852.8	E937.8	E950.2	E962.0	E980.2
Leucovorin (factor)	964.1	E858.2	E934.1	E950.4	E962.0	E980.4
Leukeran	963.1	E858.1	E933.1	E950.4	E962.0	E980.4
Levalbuterol	975.7	E858.6	E945.7	E950.4	E962.0	E980.4
Levallorphan	970.1	E854.3	E940.1	E950.4	E962.0	E980.4
Levanil	967.8	E852.8	E937.8	E950.2	E962.0	E980.2
Levarterenol	971.2	E855.5	E941.2	E950.4	E962.0	E980.4
Levodopa	966.4	E855.0	E936.4	E950.4	E962.0	E980.4
Levo–dromoran	965.09	E850.2	E935.2	E950.0	E962.0	E980.0
Levoid	962.7	E858.0	E932.7	E950.4	E962.0	E980.4
Levo–iso–methadone	965.02	E850.1	E935.1	E950.0	E962.0	E980.0
Levomepromazine	967.8	E852.8	E937.8	E950.2	E962.0	E980.2
Levoprome	967.8	E852.8	E937.8	E950.2	E962.0	E980.2
Levopropoxyphene	975.4	E858.6	E945.4	E950.4	E962.0	E980.4
Levorphan, levophanol	965.09	E850.2	E935.2	E950.0	E962.0	E980.0
Levothyroxine (sodium)	962.7	E858.0	E932.7	E950.4	E962.0	E980.4
Levsin	971.1	E855.4	E941.1	E950.4	E962.0	E980.4
Levulose	974.5	E858.5	E944.5	E950.4	E962.0	E980.4
Lewisite (gas)	985.1	E866.3	—	E950.8	E962.1	E980.8
Librium	969.4	E853.2	E939.4	E950.3	E962.0	E980.3
Lidex	976.0	E858.7	E946.0	E950.4	E962.0	E980.4
Lidocaine (infiltration) (topical)	968.5	E855.2	E938.5	E950.4	E962.0	E980.4
nerve block (peripheral) (plexus)	968.6	E855.2	E938.6	E950.4	E962.0	E980.4
spinal	968.7	E855.2	E938.7	E950.4	E962.0	E980.4
Lighter fluid	981	E862.1	—	E950.9	E962.1	E980.9
Lignocaine (infiltration) (topical)	968.5	E855.2	E938.5	E950.4	E962.0	E980.4
nerve block (peripheral) (plexus)	968.6	E855.2	E938.6	E950.4	E962.0	E980.4
spinal	968.7	E855.2	E938.7	E950.4	E962.0	E980.4
Ligroin(e) (solvent)	981	E862.0	—	E950.9	E962.1	E980.9
vapor	987.1	E869.8	—	E952.8	E962.2	E982.8
Ligustrum vulgare	988.2	E865.3	—	E950.9	E962.1	E980.9
Lily of the valley	988.2	E865.4	—	E950.9	E962.1	E980.9
Lime (chloride)	983.2	E864.2	—	E950.7	E962.1	E980.6
solution, sulferated	976.4	E858.7	E946.4	E950.4	E962.0	E980.4
Limonene	982.8	E862.4	—	E950.9	E962.1	E980.9
Lincomycin	960.8	E856	E930.8	E950.4	E962.0	E980.4
Lindane (insecticide) (vapor)	989.2	E863.0	—	E950.6	E962.1	E980.7
anti–infective (topical)	976.0	E858.7	E946.0	E950.4	E962.0	E980.4
Liniments NEC	976.9	E858.7	E946.9	E950.4	E962.0	E980.4
Linoleic acid	972.2	E858.3	E942.2	E950.4	E962.0	E980.4
Liothyronine	962.7	E858.0	E932.7	E950.4	E962.0	E980.4
Liotrix	962.7	E858.0	E932.7	E950.4	E962.0	E980.4
Lipancreatin	973.4	E858.4	E943.4	E950.4	E962.0	E980.4
Lipo–Lutin	962.2	E858.0	E932.2	E950.4	E962.0	E980.4
Lipotropic agents	977.1	E858.8	E947.1	E950.4	E962.0	E980.4
Liquefied petroleum gases	987.0	E868.0	—	E951.1	E962.2	E981.1
piped (pure or mixed with air)	987.0	E867	—	E951.0	E962.2	E981.0
Liquid petrolatum	973.2	E858.4	E943.2	E950.4	E962.0	E980.4
substance	989.9	E866.9	—	E950.9	E962.1	E980.9
specified NEC	989.89	E866.8	—	E950.9	E962.1	E980.9
Lirugen	979.4	E858.8	E949.4	E950.4	E962.0	E980.4
Lithane	969.8	E855.8	E939.8	E950.3	E962.0	E980.3
Lithium	985.8	E866.4	—	E950.9	E962.1	E980.9
carbonate	969.8	E855.8	E939.8	E950.3	E962.0	E980.3
Lithonate	969.8	E855.8	E939.8	E950.3	E962.0	E980.3

Substance	Poisoning	Accident	Therapeutic Use	Suicide Attempt	Assault	Undetermined
Liver (extract) (injection) (preparations)	964.1	E858.2	E934.1	E950.4	E962.0	E980.4
Lizard (bite) (venom)	989.5	E905.0	—	E950.9	E962.1	E980.9
LMD	964.8	E858.2	E934.8	E950.4	E962.0	E980.4
Lobelia	988.2	E865.4	—	E950.9	E962.1	E980.9
Lobeline	970.0	E854.3	E940.0	E950.4	E962.0	E980.4
Locorten	976.0	E858.7	E946.0	E950.4	E962.0	E980.4
Lolium temulentum	988.2	E865.3	—	E950.9	E962.1	E980.9
Lomotil	973.5	E858.4	E943.5	E950.4	E962.0	E980.4
Lomustine	963.1	E858.1	E933.1	E950.4	E962.0	E980.4
Lophophora williamsii	969.6	E854.1	E939.6	E950.3	E962.0	E980.3
Lorazepam	969.4	E853.2	E939.4	E950.3	E962.0	E980.3
Lotions NEC	976.9	E858.7	E946.9	E950.4	E962.0	E980.4
Lotronex	973.8	E858.4	E943.8	E950.4	E962.0	E980.4
Lotusate	967.0	E851	E937.0	E950.1	E962.0	E980.1
Lowila	976.2	E858.7	E946.2	E950.4	E962.0	E980.4
Loxapine	969.3	E853.8	E939.3	E950.3	E962.0	E980.3
Lozenges (throat)	976.6	E858.7	E946.6	E950.4	E962.0	E980.4
LSD (25)	969.6	E854.1	E939.6	E950.3	E962.0	E980.3
Lubricating oil NEC	981	E862.2	—	E950.9	E962.1	E980.9
Lucanthone	961.6	E857	E931.6	E950.4	E962.0	E980.4
Luminal	967.0	E851	E937.0	E950.1	E962.0	E980.1
Lung irritant (gas) NEC	987.9	E869.9	—	E952.9	E962.2	E982.9
Lutocylol	962.2	E858.0	E932.2	E950.4	E962.0	E980.4
Lutromone	962.2	E858.0	E932.2	E950.4	E962.0	E980.4
Lututrin	975.0	E858.6	E945.0	E950.4	E962.0	E980.4
Lye (concentrated)	983.2	E864.2	—	E950.7	E962.1	E980.6
Lygranum (skin test)	977.8	E858.8	E947.8	E950.4	E962.0	E980.4
Lymecycline	960.4	E856	E930.4	E950.4	E962.0	E980.4
Lymphogranuloma venereum antigen	977.8	E858.8	E947.8	E950.4	E962.0	E980.4
Lynestrenol	962.2	E858.0	E932.2	E950.4	E962.0	E980.4
Lyovac Sodium Edecrin	974.4	E858.5	E944.4	E950.4	E962.0	E980.4
Lypressin	962.5	E858.0	E932.5	E950.4	E962.0	E980.4
Lysergic acid (amide) (diethylamide)	969.6	E854.1	E939.6	E950.3	E962.0	E980.3
Lysergide	969.6	E854.1	E939.6	E950.3	E962.0	E980.3
Lysine vasopressin	962.5	E858.0	E932.5	E950.4	E962.0	E980.4
Lysol	983.0	E864.0	—	E950.7	E962.1	E980.6
Lytta (vitatta)	976.8	E858.7	E946.8	E950.4	E962.0	E980.4
Mace	987.5	E869.3	—	E952.8	E962.2	E982.8
Macrolides (antibiotics)	960.3	E856	E930.3	E950.4	E962.0	E980.4
Mafenide	976.0	E858.7	E946.0	E950.4	E962.0	E980.4
Magaldrate	973.0	E858.4	E943.0	E950.4	E962.0	E980.4
Magic mushroom	969.6	E854.1	E939.6	E950.3	E962.0	E980.3
Magnamycin	960.8	E856	E930.8	E950.4	E962.0	E980.4
Magnesia magma	973.0	E858.4	E943.0	E950.4	E962.0	E980.4
Magnesium (compounds) (fumes) NEC	985.8	E866.4	—	E950.9	E962.1	E980.9
antacid	973.0	E858.4	E943.0	E950.4	E962.0	E980.4
carbonate	973.0	E858.4	E943.0	E950.4	E962.0	E980.4
cathartic	973.3	E858.4	E943.3	E950.4	E962.0	E980.4
citrate	973.3	E858.4	E943.3	E950.4	E962.0	E980.4
hydroxide	973.0	E858.4	E943.0	E950.4	E962.0	E980.4
oxide	973.0	E858.4	E943.0	E950.4	E962.0	E980.4
sulfate (oral)	973.3	E858.4	E943.3	E950.4	E962.0	E980.4
intravenous	966.3	E855.0	E936.3	E950.4	E962.0	E980.4
trisilicate	973.0	E858.4	E943.0	E950.4	E962.0	E980.4
Malathion (insecticide)	989.3	E863.1	—	E950.6	E962.1	E980.7
Male fern (oleoresin)	961.6	E857	E931.6	E950.4	E962.0	E980.4
Mandelic acid	961.9	E857	E931.9	E950.4	E962.0	E980.4

Substance	Poisoning	External Cause (E-Code)				
		Accident	Therapeutic Use	Suicide Attempt	Assault	Undetermined
Manganese compounds (fumes) NEC	985.2	E866.4	—	E950.9	E962.1	E980.9
Mannitol (diuretic) (medicinal) NEC	974.4	E858.5	E944.4	E950.4	E962.0	E980.4
hexanitrate	972.4	E858.3	E942.4	E950.4	E962.0	E980.4
mustard	963.1	E858.1	E933.1	E950.4	E962.0	E980.4
Mannomustine	963.1	E858.1	E933.1	E950.4	E962.0	E980.4
MAO inhibitors	969.0	E854.0	E939.0	E950.3	E962.0	E980.3
Mapharsen	961.1	E857	E931.1	E950.4	E962.0	E980.4
Marcaine	968.9	E855.2	E938.9	E950.4	E962.0	E980.4
infiltration (subcutaneous)	968.5	E855.2	E938.5	E950.4	E962.0	E980.4
nerve block (peripheral) (plexus)	968.6	E855.2	E938.6	E950.4	E962.0	E980.4
Marezine	963.0	E858.1	E933.0	E950.4	E962.0	E980.4
Marihuana, marijuana (derivatives)	969.6	E854.1	E939.6	E950.3	E962.0	E980.3
Marine animals or plants (sting)	989.5	E905.6	—	E950.9	E962.1	E980.9
Marplan	969.0	E854.0	E939.0	E950.3	E962.0	E980.3
Marsh gas	987.1	E869.8	—	E952.8	E962.2	E982.8
Marsilid	969.0	E854.0	E939.0	E950.3	E962.0	E980.3
Matulane	963.1	E858.1	E933.1	E950.4	E962.0	E980.4
Mazindol	977.0	E858.8	E947.0	E950.4	E962.0	E980.4
Meadow saffron	988.2	E865.3	—	E950.9	E962.1	E980.9
Measles vaccine	979.4	E858.8	E949.4	E950.4	E962.0	E980.4
Meat, noxious or nonbacterial	988.8	E865.0	—	E950.9	E962.1	E980.9
Mebanazine	969.0	E854.0	E939.0	E950.3	E962.0	E980.3
Mebaral	967.0	E851	E937.0	E950.1	E962.0	E980.1
Mebendazole	961.6	E857	E931.6	E950.4	E962.0	E980.4
Mebeverine	975.1	E858.6	E945.1	E950.4	E962.0	E980.4
Mebhydroline	963.0	E858.1	E933.0	E950.4	E962.0	E980.4
Mebrophenhydramine	963.0	E858.1	E933.0	E950.4	E962.0	E980.4
Mebutamate	969.5	E853.8	E939.5	E950.3	E962.0	E980.3
Mecamylamine (chloride)	972.3	E858.3	E942.3	E950.4	E962.0	E980.4
Mechlorethamine hydrochloride	963.1	E858.1	E933.1	E950.4	E962.0	E980.4
Meclizene (hydrochloride)	963.0	E858.1	E933.0	E950.4	E962.0	E980.4
Meclofenoxate	970.0	E854.3	E940.0	E950.4	E962.0	E980.4
Meclozine (hydrochloride)	963.0	E858.1	E933.0	E950.4	E962.0	E980.4
Medazepam	969.4	E853.2	E939.4	E950.3	E962.0	E980.3
Medicine, medicinal substance	977.9	E858.9	E947.9	E950.5	E962.0	E980.5
specified NEC	977.8	E858.8	E947.8	E950.4	E962.0	E980.4
Medinal	967.0	E851	E937.0	E950.1	E962.0	E980.1
Medomin	967.0	E851	E937.0	E950.1	E962.0	E980.1
Medroxyprogesterone	962.2	E858.0	E932.2	E950.4	E962.0	E980.4
Medrysone	976.5	E858.7	E946.5	E950.4	E962.0	E980.4
Mefenamic acid	965.7	E850.7	E935.7	E950.0	E962.0	E980.0
Megahallucinogen	969.6	E854.1	E939.6	E950.3	E962.0	E980.3
Megestrol	962.2	E858.0	E932.2	E950.4	E962.0	E980.4
Meglumine	977.8	E858.8	E947.8	E950.4	E962.0	E980.4
Meladinin	976.3	E858.7	E946.3	E950.4	E962.0	E980.4
Melanizing agents	976.3	E858.7	E946.3	E950.4	E962.0	E980.4
Melarsoprol	961.1	E857	E931.1	E950.4	E962.0	E980.4
Melia azedarach	988.2	E865.3	—	E950.9	E962.1	E980.9
Mellaril	969.1	E853.0	E939.1	E950.3	E962.0	E980.3
Meloxine	976.3	E858.7	E946.3	E950.4	E962.0	E980.4
Melphalan	963.1	E858.1	E933.1	E950.4	E962.0	E980.4
Menadiol sodium diphosphate	964.3	E858.2	E934.3	E950.4	E962.0	E980.4
Menadione (sodium bisulfate)	964.3	E858.2	E934.3	E950.4	E962.0	E980.4
Menaphthone	964.3	E858.2	E934.3	E950.4	E962.0	E980.4
Meningococcal vaccine	978.8	E858.8	E948.8	E950.4	E962.0	E980.4
Menningovax–C	978.8	E858.8	E948.8	E950.4	E962.0	E980.4
Menotropins	962.4	E858.0	E932.4	E950.4	E962.0	E980.4

Substance	Poisoning	External Cause (E-Code)				
		Accident	Therapeutic Use	Suicide Attempt	Assault	Undetermined
Menthol NEC	976.1	E858.7	E946.1	E950.4	E962.0	E980.4
Mepacrine	961.3	E857	E931.3	E950.4	E962.0	E980.4
Meparfynol	967.8	E852.8	E937.8	E950.2	E962.0	E980.2
Mepazine	969.1	E853.0	E939.1	E950.3	E962.0	E980.3
Mepenzolate	971.1	E855.4	E941.1	E950.4	E962.0	E980.4
Meperidine	965.09	E850.2	E935.2	E950.0	E962.0	E980.0
Mephenamin(e)	966.4	E855.0	E936.4	E950.4	E962.0	E980.4
Mephenesin (carbamate)	968.0	E855.1	E938.0	E950.4	E962.0	E980.4
Mephenoxalone	969.5	E853.8	E939.5	E950.3	E962.0	E980.3
Mephentermine	971.2	E855.5	E941.2	E950.4	E962.0	E980.4
Mephenytoin	966.1	E855.0	E936.1	E950.4	E962.0	E980.4
Mephobarbital	967.0	E851	E937.0	E950.1	E962.0	E980.1
Mepiperphenidol	971.1	E855.4	E941.1	E950.4	E962.0	E980.4
Mepivacaine	968.9	E855.2	E938.9	E950.4	E962.0	E980.4
infiltration (subcutaneous)	968.5	E855.2	E938.5	E950.4	E962.0	E980.4
nerve block (peripheral) (plexus)	968.6	E855.2	E938.6	E950.4	E962.0	E980.4
topical (surface)	968.5	E855.2	E938.5	E950.4	E962.0	E980.4
Meprednisone	962.0	E858.0	E932.0	E950.4	E962.0	E980.4
Meprobam	969.5	E853.8	E939.5	E950.3	E962.0	E980.3
Meprobamate	969.5	E853.8	E939.5	E950.3	E962.0	E980.3
Mepyramine (maleate)	963.0	E858.1	E933.0	E950.4	E962.0	E980.4
Meralluride	974.0	E858.5	E944.0	E950.4	E962.0	E980.4
Merbaphen	974.0	E858.5	E944.0	E950.4	E962.0	E980.4
Merbromin	976.0	E858.7	E946.0	E950.4	E962.0	E980.4
Mercaptomerin	974.0	E858.5	E944.0	E950.4	E962.0	E980.4
Mercaptopurine	963.1	E858.1	E933.1	E950.4	E962.0	E980.4
Mercumatilin	974.0	E858.5	E944.0	E950.4	E962.0	E980.4
Mercuramide	974.0	E858.5	E944.0	E950.4	E962.0	E980.4
Mercuranin	976.0	E858.7	E946.0	E950.4	E962.0	E980.4
Mercurochrome	976.0	E858.7	E946.0	E950.4	E962.0	E980.4
Mercury, mercuric, mercurous (compounds) (cyanide) (fumes) (nonmedicinal) (vapor) NEC	985.0	E866.1	—	E950.9	E962.1	E980.9
ammoniated	976.0	E858.7	E946.0	E950.4	E962.0	E980.4
anti–infective	961.2	E857	E931.2	E950.4	E962.0	E980.4
topical	976.0	E858.7	E946.0	E950.4	E962.0	E980.4
chloride (antiseptic) NEC	976.0	E858.7	E946.0	E950.4	E962.0	E980.4
fungicide	985.0	E863.6	—	E950.6	E962.1	E980.7
diuretic compounds	974.0	E858.5	E944.0	E950.4	E962.0	E980.4
fungicide	985.0	E863.6	—	E950.6	E962.1	E980.7
organic (fungicide)	985.0	E863.6	—	E950.6	E962.1	E980.7
Merethoxylline	974.0	E858.5	E944.0	E950.4	E962.0	E980.4
Mersalyl	974.0	E858.5	E944.0	E950.4	E962.0	E980.4
Merthiolate (topical)	976.0	E858.7	E946.0	E950.4	E962.0	E980.4
ophthalmic preparation	976.5	E858.7	E946.5	E950.4	E962.0	E980.4
Meruvax	979.4	E858.8	E949.4	E950.4	E962.0	E980.4
Mescal buttons	969.6	E854.1	E939.6	E950.3	E962.0	E980.3
Mescaline (salts)	969.6	E854.1	E939.6	E950.3	E962.0	E980.3
Mesoridazine besylate	969.1	E853.0	E939.1	E950.3	E962.0	E980.3
Mestanolone	962.1	E858.0	E932.1	E950.4	E962.0	E980.4
Mestranol	962.2	E858.0	E932.2	E950.4	E962.0	E980.4
Metacresylacetate	976.0	E858.7	E946.0	E950.4	E962.0	E980.4
Metaldehyde (snail killer) NEC	989.4	E863.4	—	E950.6	E962.1	E980.7
Metals (heavy) (nonmedicinal) NEC	985.9	E866.4	—	E950.9	E962.1	E980.9
dust, fumes, or vapor NEC	985.9	E866.4	—	E950.9	E962.1	E980.9
light NEC	985.9	E866.4	—	E950.9	E962.1	E980.9
dust, fumes, or vapor NEC	985.9	E866.4	—	E950.9	E962.1	E980.9

Substance	Poisoning	External Cause (E-Code)				
		Accident	Therapeutic Use	Suicide Attempt	Assault	Undetermined
pesticides (dust) (vapor)	985.9	E863.4	—	E950.6	E962.1	E980.7
Metamucil	973.3	E858.4	E943.3	E950.4	E962.0	E980.4
Metaphen	976.0	E858.7	E946.0	E950.4	E962.0	E980.4
Metaproterenol	975.1	E858.6	E945.1	E950.4	E962.0	E980.4
Metaraminol	972.8	E858.3	E942.8	E950.4	E962.0	E980.4
Metaxalone	968.0	E855.1	E938.0	E950.4	E962.0	E980.4
Metformin	962.3	E858.0	E932.3	E950.4	E962.0	E980.4
Methacycline	960.4	E856	E930.4	E950.4	E962.0	E980.4
Methadone	965.02	E850.1	E935.1	E950.0	E962.0	E980.0
Methallenestril	962.2	E858.0	E932.2	E950.4	E962.0	E980.4
Methamphetamine	969.7	E854.2	E939.7	E950.3	E962.0	E980.3
Methandienone	962.1	E858.0	E932.1	E950.4	E962.0	E980.4
Methandriol	962.1	E858.0	E932.1	E950.4	E962.0	E980.4
Methandrostenolone	962.1	E858.0	E932.1	E950.4	E962.0	E980.4
Methane gas	987.1	E869.8	—	E952.8	E962.2	E982.8
Methanol	980.1	E860.2	—	E950.9	E962.1	E980.9
vapor	987.8	E869.8	—	E952.8	E962.2	E982.8
Methantheline	971.1	E855.4	E941.1	E950.4	E962.0	E980.4
Methaphenilene	963.0	E858.1	E933.0	E950.4	E962.0	E980.4
Methapyrilene	963.0	E858.1	E933.0	E950.4	E962.0	E980.4
Methaqualone (compounds)	967.4	E852.3	E937.4	E950.2	E962.0	E980.2
Metharbital, metharbitone	967.0	E851	E937.0	E950.1	E962.0	E980.1
Methazolamide	974.2	E858.5	E944.2	E950.4	E962.0	E980.4
Methdilazine	963.0	E858.1	E933.0	E950.4	E962.0	E980.4
Methedrine	969.7	E854.2	E939.7	E950.3	E962.0	E980.3
Methenamine (mandelate)	961.9	E857	E931.9	E950.4	E962.0	E980.4
Methenolone	962.1	E858.0	E932.1	E950.4	E962.0	E980.4
Methergine	975.0	E858.6	E945.0	E950.4	E962.0	E980.4
Methiacil	962.8	E858.0	E932.8	E950.4	E962.0	E980.4
Methicillin (sodium)	960.0	E856	E930.0	E950.4	E962.0	E980.4
Methimazole	962.8	E858.0	E932.8	E950.4	E962.0	E980.4
Methionine	977.1	E858.8	E947.1	E950.4	E962.0	E980.4
Methisazone	961.7	E857	E931.7	E950.4	E962.0	E980.4
Methitural	967.0	E851	E937.0	E950.1	E962.0	E980.1
Methixene	971.1	E855.4	E941.1	E950.4	E962.0	E980.4
Methobarbital, methobarbitone	967.0	E851	E937.0	E950.1	E962.0	E980.1
Methocarbamol	968.0	E855.1	E938.0	E950.4	E962.0	E980.4
Methohexital, methohexitone (sodium)	968.3	E855.1	E938.3	E950.4	E962.0	E980.4
Methoin	966.1	E855.0	E936.1	E950.4	E962.0	E980.4
Methopholine	965.7	E850.7	E935.7	E950.0	E962.0	E980.0
Methorate	975.4	E858.6	E945.4	E950.4	E962.0	E980.4
Methoserpidine	972.6	E858.3	E942.6	E950.4	E962.0	E980.4
Methotrexate	963.1	E858.1	E933.1	E950.4	E962.0	E980.4
Methotrimeprazine	967.8	E852.8	E937.8	E950.2	E962.0	E980.2
Methoxa–Dome	976.3	E858.7	E946.3	E950.4	E962.0	E980.4
Methoxamine	971.2	E855.5	E941.2	E950.4	E962.0	E980.4
Methoxsalen	976.3	E858.7	E946.3	E950.4	E962.0	E980.4
Methoxybenzyl penicillin	960.0	E856	E930.0	E950.4	E962.0	E980.4
Methoxychlor	989.2	E863.0	—	E950.6	E962.1	E980.7
Methoxyflurane	968.2	E855.1	E938.2	E950.4	E962.0	E980.4
Methoxyphenamine	971.2	E855.5	E941.2	E950.4	E962.0	E980.4
Methoxypromazine	969.1	E853.0	E939.1	E950.3	E962.0	E980.3
Methoxypsoralen	976.3	E858.7	E946.3	E950.4	E962.0	E980.4
Methscopolamine (bromide)	971.1	E855.4	E941.1	E950.4	E962.0	E980.4
Methsuximide	966.2	E855.0	E936.2	E950.4	E962.0	E980.4
Methyclothiazide	974.3	E858.5	E944.3	E950.4	E962.0	E980.4
Methyl						

Substance	Poisoning	External Cause (E-Code)				
		Accident	Therapeutic Use	Suicide Attempt	Assault	Undetermined
acetate	982.8	E862.4	—	E950.9	E962.1	E980.9
acetone	982.8	E862.4	—	E950.9	E962.1	E980.9
alcohol	980.1	E860.2	—	E950.9	E962.1	E980.9
amphetamine	969.7	E854.2	E939.7	E950.3	E962.0	E980.3
androstanolone	962.1	E858.0	E932.1	E950.4	E962.0	E980.4
atropine	971.1	E855.4	E941.1	E950.4	E962.0	E980.4
benzene	982.0	E862.4	—	E950.9	E962.1	E980.9
bromide (gas)	987.8	E869.8	—	E952.8	E962.2	E982.8
fumigant	987.8	E863.8	—	E950.6	E962.2	E980.7
butanol	980.8	E860.8	—	E950.9	E962.1	E980.9
carbinol	980.1	E860.2	—	E950.9	E962.1	E980.9
cellosolve	982.8	E862.4	—	E950.9	E962.1	E980.9
cellulose	973.3	E858.4	E943.3	E950.4	E962.0	E980.4
chloride (gas)	987.8	E869.8	—	E952.8	E962.2	E982.8
cyclohexane	982.8	E862.4	—	E950.9	E962.1	E980.9
cyclohexanone	982.8	E862.4	—	E950.9	E962.1	E980.9
dihydromorphinone	965.09	E850.2	E935.2	E950.0	E962.0	E980.0
ergometrine	975.0	E858.6	E945.0	E950.4	E962.0	E980.4
ergonovine	975.0	E858.6	E945.0	E950.4	E962.0	E980.4
ethyl ketone	982.8	E862.4	—	E950.9	E962.1	E980.9
hydrazine	983.9	E864.3	—	E950.7	E961.1	E980.6
isobutyl ketone	982.8	E862.4	—	E950.9	E962.1	E980.9
morphine NEC	965.09	E850.2	E935.2	E950.0	E962.0	E980.0
parafynol	967.8	E852.8	E937.8	E950.2	E962.0	E980.2
parathion	989.3	E863.1	—	E950.6	E961.1	E980.7
pentynol NEC	967.8	E852.8	E937.8	E950.2	E962.0	E980.2
peridol	969.2	E853.1	E939.2	E950.3	E962.0	E980.3
phenidate	969.7	E854.2	E939.7	E950.3	E962.0	E980.3
prednisolone	962.0	E858.0	E932.0	E950.4	E962.0	E980.4
ENT agent	976.6	E858.7	E946.6	E950.4	E962.0	E980.4
ophthalmic preparation	976.5	E858.7	E946.5	E950.4	E962.0	E980.4
topical NEC	976.0	E858.7	E946.0	E950.4	E962.0	E980.4
propylcarbinol	980.8	E860.8	—	E950.9	E962.1	E980.9
rosaniline NEC	976.0	E858.7	E946.0	E950.4	E962.0	E980.4
salicylate NEC	976.3	E858.7	E946.3	E950.4	E962.0	E980.4
sulfate (fumes)	987.8	E869.8	—	E952.8	E962.2	E982.8
liquid	983.9	E864.3	—	E950.7	E961.1	E980.6
sulfonal	967.8	E852.8	E937.8	E950.2	E962.0	E980.2
testosterone	962.1	E858.0	E932.1	E950.4	E962.0	E980.4
thiouracil	962.8	E858.0	E932.8	E950.4	E962.0	E980.4
Methylated spirit	980.0	E860.1	—	E950.9	E962.1	E980.9
Methyldopa	972.6	E858.3	E942.6	E950.4	E962.0	E980.4
Methylene						
blue	961.9	E857	E931.9	E950.4	E962.0	E980.4
chloride or dichloride (solvent) NEC	982.3	E862.4	—	E950.9	E962.1	E980.9
Methylhexabital	967.0	E851	E937.0	E950.1	E962.0	E980.1
Methylparaben (ophthalmic)	976.5	E858.7	E946.5	E950.4	E962.0	E980.4
Methyprylon	967.5	E852.4	E937.5	E950.2	E962.0	E980.2
Methysergide	971.3	E855.6	E941.3	E950.4	E962.0	E980.4
Metoclopramide	963.0	E858.1	E933.0	E950.4	E962.0	E980.4
Metofoline	965.7	E850.7	E935.7	E950.0	E962.0	E980.0
Metopon	965.09	E850.2	E935.2	E950.0	E962.0	E980.0
Metronidazole	961.5	E857	E931.5	E950.4	E962.0	E980.4
Metycaine	968.9	E855.2	E938.9	E950.4	E962.0	E980.4
infiltration (subcutaneous)	968.5	E855.2	E938.5	E950.4	E962.0	E980.4
nerve block (peripheral) (plexus)	968.6	E855.2	E938.6	E950.4	E962.0	E980.4
topical (surface)	968.5	E855.2	E938.5	E950.4	E962.0	E980.4

Substance	Poisoning	Accident	External Cause (E-Code) Therapeutic Use	Suicide Attempt	Assault	Undetermined
Metyrapone	977.8	E858.8	E947.8	E950.4	E962.0	E980.4
Mevinphos	989.3	E863.1	—	E950.6	E962.1	E980.7
Mezereon (berries)	988.2	E865.3	—	E950.9	E962.1	E980.9
Micatin	976.0	E858.7	E946.0	E950.4	E962.0	E980.4
Miconazole	976.0	E858.7	E946.0	E950.4	E962.0	E980.4
Midol	965.1	E850.3	E935.3	E950.0	E962.0	E980.0
Mifepristone	962.9	E858.0	E932.9	E950.4	E962.0	E980.4
Milk of magnesia	973.0	E858.4	E943.0	E950.4	E962.0	E980.4
Millipede (tropical) (venomous)	989.5	E905.4	—	E950.9	E962.1	E980.9
Miltown	969.5	E853.8	E939.5	E950.3	E962.0	E980.3
Mineral						
oil (medicinal)	973.2	E858.4	E943.2	E950.4	E962.0	E980.4
nonmedicinal	981	E862.1	—	E950.9	E962.1	E980.9
topical	976.3	E858.7	E946.3	E950.4	E962.0	E980.4
salts NEC	974.6	E858.5	E944.6	E950.4	E962.0	E980.4
spirits	981	E862.0	—	E950.9	E962.1	E980.9
Minocycline	960.4	E856	E930.4	E950.4	E962.0	E980.4
Mithramycin (antineoplastic)	960.7	E856	E930.7	E950.4	E962.0	E980.4
Mitobronitol	963.1	E858.1	E933.1	E950.4	E962.0	E980.4
Mitomycin (antineoplastic)	960.7	E856	E930.7	E950.4	E962.0	E980.4
Mitotane	963.1	E858.1	E933.1	E950.4	E962.0	E980.4
Moderil	972.6	E858.3	E942.6	E950.4	E962.0	E980.4
Mogadon—*see* Nitrazepam						
Molindone	969.3	E853.8	E939.3	E950.3	E962.0	E980.3
Monistat	976.0	E858.7	E946.0	E950.4	E962.0	E980.4
Monkshood	988.2	E865.4	—	E950.9	E962.1	E980.9
Monoamine oxidase inhibitors	969.0	E854.0	E939.0	E950.3	E962.0	E980.3
Monochlorobenzene	982.0	E862.4	—	E950.9	E962.1	E980.9
Monosodium glutamate	989.89	E866.8	—	E950.9	E962.1	E980.9
Monoxide, carbon — *see* Carbon, monoxide						
Moperone	969.2	E853.1	E939.2	E950.3	E962.0	E980.3
Morning glory seeds	969.6	E854.1	E939.6	E950.3	E962.0	E980.3
Moroxydine (hydrochloride)	961.7	E857	E931.7	E950.4	E962.0	E980.4
Morphazinamide	961.8	E857	E931.8	E950.4	E962.0	E980.4
Morphinans	965.09	E850.2	E935.2	E950.0	E962.0	E980.0
Morphine NEC	965.09	E850.2	E935.2	E950.0	E962.0	E980.0
antagonists	970.1	E854.3	E940.1	E950.4	E962.0	E980.4
Morpholinylethylmorphine	965.09	E850.2	E935.2	E950.0	E962.0	E980.0
Morrhuate sodium	972.7	E858.3	E942.7	E950.4	E962.0	E980.4
Moth balls (*see also* Pesticides)	989.4	E863.4	—	E950.6	E962.1	E980.7
naphthalene	983.0	E863.4	—	E950.7	E962.1	E980.6
Motor exhaust gas — *see* Carbon, monoxide, exhaust gas						
Mouth wash	976.6	E858.7	E946.6	E950.4	E962.0	E980.4
Mucolytic agent	975.5	E858.6	E945.5	E950.4	E962.0	E980.4
Mucomyst	975.5	E858.6	E945.5	E950.4	E962.0	E980.4
Mucous membrane agents (external)	976.9	E858.7	E946.9	E950.4	E962.0	E980.4
specified NEC	976.8	E858.7	E946.8	E950.4	E962.0	E980.4
Mumps						
immune globulin (human)	964.6	E858.2	E934.6	E950.4	E962.0	E980.4
skin test antigen	977.8	E858.8	E947.8	E950.4	E962.0	E980.4
vaccine	979.6	E858.8	E949.6	E950.4	E962.0	E980.4
Mumpsvax	979.6	E858.8	E949.6	E950.4	E962.0	E980.4
Muriatic acid — *see* Hydrochloric acid						
Muscarine	971.0	E855.3	E941.0	E950.4	E962.0	E980.4
Muscle affecting agents NEC	975.3	E858.6	E945.3	E950.4	E962.0	E980.4
oxytocic	975.0	E858.6	E945.0	E950.4	E962.0	E980.4

Substance	Poisoning	External Cause (E-Code)				
		Accident	Therapeutic Use	Suicide Attempt	Assault	Undetermined
relaxants	975.3	E858.6	E945.3	E950.4	E962.0	E980.4
central nervous system	968.0	E855.1	E938.0	E950.4	E962.0	E980.4
skeletal	975.2	E858.6	E945.2	E950.4	E962.0	E980.4
smooth	975.1	E858.6	E945.1	E950.4	E962.0	E980.4
Mushrooms, noxious	988.1	E865.5	—	E950.9	E962.1	E980.9
Mussel, noxious	988.0	E865.1	—	E950.9	E962.1	E980.9
Mustard (emetic)	973.6	E858.4	E943.6	E950.4	E962.0	E980.4
gas	987.8	E869.8	—	E952.8	E962.2	E982.8
nitrogen	963.1	E858.1	E933.1	E950.4	E962.0	E980.4
Mustine	963.1	E858.1	E933.1	E950.4	E962.0	E980.4
M–vac	979.4	E858.8	E949.4	E950.4	E962.0	E980.4
Mycifradin	960.8	E856	E930.8	E950.4	E962.0	E980.4
topical	976.0	E858.7	E946.0	E950.4	E962.0	E980.4
Mycitracin	960.8	E856	E930.8	E950.4	E962.0	E980.4
ophthalmic preparation	976.5	E858.7	E946.5	E950.4	E962.0	E980.4
Mycostatin	960.1	E856	E930.1	E950.4	E962.0	E980.4
topical	976.0	E858.7	E946.0	E950.4	E962.0	E980.4
Mydriacyl	971.1	E855.4	E941.1	E950.4	E962.0	E980.4
Myelobromal	963.1	E858.1	E933.1	E950.4	E962.0	E980.4
Myleran	963.1	E858.1	E933.1	E950.4	E962.0	E980.4
Myochrysin(e)	965.69	E850.6	E935.6	E950.0	E962.0	E980.0
Myoneural blocking agents	975.2	E858.6	E945.2	E950.4	E962.0	E980.4
Myristica fragrans	988.2	E865.3	—	E950.9	E962.1	E980.9
Myristicin	988.2	E865.3	—	E950.9	E962.1	E980.9
Mysoline	966.3	E855.0	E936.3	E950.4	E962.0	E980.4
Nafcillin (sodium)	960.0	E856	E930.0	E950.4	E962.0	E980.4
Nail polish remover	982.8	E862.4	—	E950.9	E962.1	E980.9
Nalidixic acid	961.9	E857	E931.9	E950.4	E962.0	E980.4
Nalorphine	970.1	E854.3	E940.1	E950.4	E962.0	E980.4
Naloxone	970.1	E854.3	E940.1	E950.4	E962.0	E980.4
Nandrolone (decanoate) (phenproprioate)	962.1	E858.0	E932.1	E950.4	E962.0	E980.4
Naphazoline	971.2	E855.5	E941.2	E950.4	E962.0	E980.4
Naphtha (painter's) (petroleum)	981	E862.0	—	E950.9	E962.1	E980.9
solvent	981	E862.0	—	E950.9	E962.1	E980.9
vapor	987.1	E869.8	—	E952.8	E962.2	E982.8
Naphthalene (chlorinated)	983.0	E864.0	—	E950.7	E962.1	E980.6
insecticide or moth repellent	983.0	E863.4	—	E950.7	E962.1	E980.6
vapor	987.8	E869.8	—	E952.8	E962.2	E982.8
Naphthol	983.0	E864.0	—	E950.7	E962.1	E980.6
Naphthylamine	983.0	E864.0	—	E950.7	E962.1	E980.6
Naprosyn—*see* Naproxen						
Naproxen	965.61	E850.6	E935.6	E950.0	E962.0	E980.0
Narcotic (drug)	967.9	E852.9	E937.9	E950.2	E962.0	E980.2
analgesic NEC	965.8	E850.8	E935.8	E950.0	E962.0	E980.0
antagonist	970.1	E854.3	E940.1	E950.4	E962.0	E980.4
specified NEC	967.8	E852.8	E937.8	E950.2	E962.0	E980.2
Narcotine	975.4	E858.6	E945.4	E950.4	E962.0	E980.4
Nardil	969.0	E854.0	E939.0	E950.3	E962.0	E980.3
Natrium cyanide — *see* Cyanide(s)						
Natural						
blood (product)	964.7	E858.2	E934.7	E950.4	E962.0	E980.4
gas (piped)	987.1	E867	—	E951.0	E962.2	E981.0
incomplete combustion	986	E867	—	E951.0	E962.2	E981.0
Nealbarbital, nealbarbitone	967.0	E851	E937.0	E950.1	E962.0	E980.1
Nectadon	975.4	E858.6	E945.4	E950.4	E962.0	E980.4
Nematocyst (sting)	989.5	E905.6	—	E950.9	E962.1	E980.9
Nembutal	967.0	E851	E937.0	E950.1	E962.0	E980.1

Substance	Poisoning	External Cause (E-Code)				
		Accident	Therapeutic Use	Suicide Attempt	Assault	Undetermined
Neoarsphenamine	961.1	E857	E931.1	E950.4	E962.0	E980.4
Neocinchophen	974.7	E858.5	E944.7	E950.4	E962.0	E980.4
Neomycin	960.8	E856	E930.8	E950.4	E962.0	E980.4
ENT agent	976.6	E858.7	E946.6	E950.4	E962.0	E980.4
ophthalmic preparation	976.5	E858.7	E946.5	E950.4	E962.0	E980.4
topical NEC	976.0	E858.7	E946.0	E950.4	E962.0	E980.4
Neonal	967.0	E851	E937.0	E950.1	E962.0	E980.1
Neoprontosil	961.0	E857	E931.0	E950.4	E962.0	E980.4
Neosalvarsan	961.1	E857	E931.1	E950.4	E962.0	E980.4
Neosilversalvarsan	961.1	E857	E931.1	E950.4	E962.0	E980.4
Neosporin	960.8	E856	E930.8	E950.4	E962.0	E980.4
ENT agent	976.6	E858.7	E946.6	E950.4	E962.0	E980.4
ophthalmic preparation	976.5	E858.7	E946.5	E950.4	E962.0	E980.4
topical NEC	976.0	E858.7	E946.0	E950.4	E962.0	E980.4
Neostigmine	971.0	E855.3	E941.0	E950.4	E962.0	E980.4
Neraval	967.0	E851	E937.0	E950.1	E962.0	E980.1
Neravan	967.0	E851	E937.0	E950.1	E962.0	E980.1
Nerium oleander	988.2	E865.4	—	E950.9	E962.1	E980.9
Nerve gases (war)	987.9	E869.9	—	E952.9	E962.2	E982.9
Nesacaine	968.9	E855.2	E938.9	E950.4	E962.0	E980.4
infiltration (subcutaneous)	968.5	E855.2	E938.5	E950.4	E962.0	E980.4
nerve block (peripheral) (plexus)	968.6	E855.2	E938.6	E950.4	E962.0	E980.4
Neurobarb	967.0	E851	E937.0	E950.1	E962.0	E980.1
Neuroleptics NEC	969.3	E853.8	E939.3	E950.3	E962.0	E980.3
Neuroprotective agent	977.8	E858.8	E947.8	E950.4	E962.0	E980.4
Neutral spirits	980.0	E860.1	—	E950.9	E962.1	E980.9
beverage	980.0	E860.0	—	E950.9	E962.1	E980.9
Niacin, niacinamide	972.2	E858.3	E942.2	E950.4	E962.0	E980.4
Nialamide	969.0	E854.0	E939.0	E950.3	E962.0	E980.3
Nickle (carbonyl) (compounds) (fumes) (tetracarbonyl) (vapor)	985.8	E866.4	—	E950.9	E962.1	E980.9
Niclosamide	961.6	E857	E931.6	E950.4	E962.0	E980.4
Nicomorphine	965.09	E850.2	E935.2	E950.0	E962.0	E980.0
Nicotinamide	972.2	E858.3	E942.2	E950.4	E962.0	E980.4
Nicotine (insecticide) (spray) (sulfate) NEC	989.4	E863.4	—	E950.6	E962.1	E980.7
not insecticide	989.89	E866.8	—	E950.9	E962.1	E980.9
Nicotinic acid (derivatives)	972.2	E858.3	E942.2	E950.4	E962.0	E980.4
Nicotinyl alcohol	972.2	E858.3	E942.2	E950.4	E962.0	E980.4
Nicoumalone	964.2	E858.2	E934.2	E950.4	E962.0	E980.4
Nifenazone	965.5	E850.5	E935.5	E950.0	E962.0	E980.0
Nifuraldezone	961.9	E857	E931.9	E950.4	E962.0	E980.4
Nightshade (deadly)	988.2	E865.4	—	E950.9	E962.1	E980.9
Nikethamide	970.0	E854.3	E940.0	E950.4	E962.0	E980.4
Nilstat	960.1	E856	E930.1	E950.4	E962.0	E980.4
topical	976.0	E858.7	E946.0	E950.4	E962.0	E980.4
Nimodipine	977.8	E858.8	E947.8	E950.4	E962.0	E980.4
Niridazole	961.6	E857	E931.6	E950.4	E962.0	E980.4
Nisentil	965.09	E850.2	E935.2	E950.0	E962.0	E980.0
Nitrates	972.4	E858.3	E942.4	E950.4	E962.0	E980.4
Nitrazepam	969.4	E853.2	E939.4	E950.3	E962.0	E980.3
Nitric						
acid (liquid)	983.1	E864.1	—	E950.7	E962.1	E980.6
vapor	987.8	E869.8	—	E952.8	E962.2	E982.8
oxide (gas)	987.2	E869.0	—	E952.8	E962.2	E982.8
Nitrite, amyl (medicinal) (vapor)	972.4	E858.3	E942.4	E950.4	E962.0	E980.4
Nitroaniline	983.0	E864.0	—	E950.7	E962.1	E980.6
vapor	987.8	E869.8	—	E952.8	E962.2	E982.8

Substance	Poisoning	External Cause (E-Code)				
		Accident	Therapeutic Use	Suicide Attempt	Assault	Undetermined
Nitrobenzene, nitrobenzol	983.0	E864.0	—	E950.7	E962.1	E980.6
vapor	987.8	E869.8	—	E952.8	E962.2	E982.8
Nitrocellulose	976.3	E858.7	E946.3	E950.4	E962.0	E980.4
Nitrofuran derivatives	961.9	E857	E931.9	E950.4	E962.0	E980.4
Nitrofurantoin	961.9	E857	E931.9	E950.4	E962.0	E980.4
Nitrofurazone	976.0	E858.7	E946.0	E950.4	E962.0	E980.4
Nitrogen (dioxide) (gas) (oxide)	987.2	E869.0	—	E952.8	E962.2	E982.8
mustard (antineoplastic)	963.1	E858.1	E933.1	E950.4	E962.0	E980.4
Nitroglycerin, nitroglycerol (medicinal)	972.4	E858.3	E942.4	E950.4	E962.0	E980.4
nonmedicinal	989.89	E866.8	—	E950.9	E962.1	E980.9
fumes	987.8	E869.8	—	E952.8	E962.2	E982.8
Nitrohydrochloric acid	983.1	E864.1	—	E950.7	E962.1	E980.6
Nitromersol	976.0	E858.7	E946.0	E950.4	E962.0	E980.4
Nitronaphthalene	983.0	E864.0	—	E950.7	E962.2	E980.6
Nitrophenol	983.0	E864.0	—	E950.7	E962.2	E980.6
Nitrothiazol	961.6	E857	E931.6	E950.4	E962.0	E980.4
Nitrotoluene, nitrotoluol	983.0	E864.0	—	E950.7	E962.1	E980.6
vapor	987.8	E869.8	—	E952.8	E962.2	E982.8
Nitrous	968.2	E855.1	E938.2	E950.4	E962.0	E980.4
acid (liquid)	983.1	E864.1	—	E950.7	E962.1	E980.6
fumes	987.2	E869.0	—	E952.8	E962.2	E982.8
oxide (anesthetic) NEC	968.2	E855.1	E938.2	E950.4	E962.0	E980.4
Nitrozone	976.0	E858.7	E946.0	E950.4	E962.0	E980.4
Noctec	967.1	E852.0	E937.1	E950.2	E962.0	E980.2
Noludar	967.5	E852.4	E937.5	E950.2	E962.0	E980.2
Noptil	967.0	E851	E937.0	E950.1	E962.0	E980.1
Noradrenalin	971.2	E855.5	E941.2	E950.4	E962.0	E980.4
Noramidopyrine	965.5	E850.5	E935.5	E950.0	E962.0	E980.0
Norepinephrine	971.2	E855.5	E941.2	E950.4	E962.0	E980.4
Norethandrolone	962.1	E858.0	E932.1	E950.4	E962.0	E980.4
Norethindrone	962.2	E858.0	E932.2	E950.4	E962.0	E980.4
Norethisterone	962.2	E858.0	E932.2	E950.4	E962.0	E980.4
Norethynodrel	962.2	E858.0	E932.2	E950.4	E962.0	E980.4
Norlestrin	962.2	E858.0	E932.2	E950.4	E962.0	E980.4
Norlutin	962.2	E858.0	E932.2	E950.4	E962.0	E980.4
Normison—*see* Benzodiazepines						
Normorphine	965.09	E850.2	E935.2	E950.0	E962.0	E980.0
Nortriptyline	969.0	E854.0	E939.0	E950.3	E962.0	E980.3
Noscapine	975.4	E858.6	E945.4	E950.4	E962.0	E980.4
Nose preparations	976.6	E858.7	E946.6	E950.4	E962.0	E980.4
Novobiocin	960.8	E856	E930.8	E950.4	E962.0	E980.4
Novocain (infiltration) (topical)	968.5	E855.2	E938.5	E950.4	E962.0	E980.4
nerve block (peripheral) (plexus)	968.6	E855.2	E938.6	E950.4	E962.0	E980.4
spinal	968.7	E855.2	E938.7	E950.4	E962.0	E980.4
Noxythiolin	961.9	E857	E931.9	E950.4	E962.0	E980.4
NPH Iletin (insulin)	962.3	E858.0	E932.3	E950.4	E962.0	E980.4
Numorphan	965.09	E850.2	E935.2	E950.0	E962.0	E980.0
Nunol	967.0	E851	E937.0	E950.1	E962.0	E980.1
Nupercaine (spinal anesthetic)	968.7	E855.2	E938.7	E950.4	E962.0	E980.4
topical (surface)	968.5	E855.2	E938.5	E950.4	E962.0	E980.4
Nutmeg oil (liniment)	976.3	E858.7	E946.3	E950.4	E962.0	E980.4
Nux vomica	989.1	E863.7	—	E950.6	E962.1	E980.7
Nydrazid	961.8	E857	E931.8	E950.4	E962.0	E980.4
Nylidrin	971.2	E855.5	E941.2	E950.4	E962.0	E980.4
Nystatin	960.1	E856	E930.1	E950.4	E962.0	E980.4
topical	976.0	E858.7	E946.0	E950.4	E962.0	E980.4
Nytol	963.0	E858.1	E933.0	E950.4	E962.0	E980.4

Substance	Poisoning	External Cause (E-Code)				
		Accident	Therapeutic Use	Suicide Attempt	Assault	Undetermined
Oblivion	967.8	E852.8	E937.8	E950.2	E962.0	E980.2
Octyl nitrite	972.4	E858.3	E942.4	E950.4	E962.0	E980.4
Oestradiol (cypionate) (dipropionate) (valerate)	962.2	E858.0	E932.2	E950.4	E962.0	E980.4
Oestriol	962.2	E858.0	E932.2	E950.4	E962.0	E980.4
Oestrone	962.2	E858.0	E932.2	E950.4	E962.0	E980.4
Oil (of) NEC	989.89	E866.8	—	E950.9	E962.1	E980.9
bitter almond	989.0	E866.8	—	E950.9	E962.1	E980.9
camphor	976.1	E858.7	E946.1	E950.4	E962.0	E980.4
colors	989.89	E861.6	—	E950.9	E962.1	E980.9
fumes	987.8	E869.8	—	E952.8	E962.2	E982.8
lubricating	981	E862.2	—	E950.9	E962.1	E980.9
specified source, other — *see* substance specified						
vitriol (liquid)	983.1	E864.1	—	E950.7	E962.1	E980.6
fumes	987.8	E869.8	—	E952.8	E962.2	E982.8
wintergreen (bitter) NEC	976.3	E858.7	E946.3	E950.4	E962.0	E980.4
Ointments NEC	976.9	E858.7	E946.9	E950.4	E962.0	E980.4
Oleander	988.2	E865.4	—	E950.9	E962.1	E980.9
Oleandomycin	960.3	E856	E930.3	E950.4	E962.0	E980.4
Oleovitamin A	963.5	E858.1	E933.5	E950.4	E962.0	E980.4
Oleum ricini	973.1	E858.4	E943.1	E950.4	E962.0	E980.4
Olive oil (medicinal) NEC	973.2	E858.4	E943.2	E950.4	E962.0	E980.4
OMPA	989.3	E863.1	—	E950.6	E962.1	E980.7
Oncovin	963.1	E858.1	E933.1	E950.4	E962.0	E980.4
Ophthaine	968.5	E855.2	E938.5	E950.4	E962.0	E980.4
Ophthetic	968.5	E855.2	E938.5	E950.4	E962.0	E980.4
Opiates, opioids, opium NEC	965.00	E850.2	E935.2	E950.0	E962.0	E980.0
antagonists	970.1	E854.3	E940.1	E950.4	E962.0	E980.4
Oracon	962.2	E858.0	E932.2	E950.4	E962.0	E980.4
Oragrafin	977.8	E858.8	E947.8	E950.4	E962.0	E980.4
Oral contraceptives	962.2	E858.0	E932.2	E950.4	E962.0	E980.4
Orciprenaline	975.1	E858.6	E945.1	E950.4	E962.0	E980.4
Organidin	975.5	E858.6	E945.5	E950.4	E962.0	E980.4
Organophosphates	989.3	E863.1	—	E950.6	E962.1	E980.7
Orimune	979.5	E858.8	E949.5	E950.4	E962.0	E980.4
Orinase	962.3	E858.0	E932.3	E950.4	E962.0	E980.4
Orphenadrine	966.4	E855.0	E936.4	E950.4	E962.0	E980.4
Ortal (sodium)	967.0	E851	E937.0	E950.1	E962.0	E980.1
Orthoboric acid	976.0	E858.7	E946.0	E950.4	E962.0	E980.4
ENT agent	976.6	E858.7	E946.6	E950.4	E962.0	E980.4
ophthalmic preparation	976.5	E858.7	E946.5	E950.4	E962.0	E980.4
Orthocaine	968.5	E855.2	E938.5	E950.4	E962.0	E980.4
Ortho–Novum	962.2	E858.0	E932.2	E950.4	E962.0	E980.4
Orthotolidine (reagent)	977.8	E858.8	E947.8	E950.4	E962.0	E980.4
Osmic acid (liquid)	983.1	E864.1	—	E950.7	E962.1	E980.6
fumes	987.8	E869.8	—	E952.8	E962.2	E982.8
Osmotic diuretics	974.4	E858.5	E944.4	E950.4	E962.0	E980.4
Ouabain	972.1	E858.3	E942.1	E950.4	E962.0	E980.4
Ovarian hormones (synthetic substitutes)	962.2	E858.0	E932.2	E950.4	E962.0	E980.4
Ovral	962.2	E858.0	E932.2	E950.4	E962.0	E980.4
Ovulation suppressants	962.2	E858.0	E932.2	E950.4	E962.0	E980.4
Ovulen	962.2	E858.0	E932.2	E950.4	E962.0	E980.4
Oxacillin (sodium)	960.0	E856	E930.0	E950.4	E962.0	E980.4
Oxalic acid	983.1	E864.1	—	E950.7	E962.1	E980.6
Oxanamide	969.5	E853.8	E939.5	E950.3	E962.0	E980.3
Oxandrolone	962.1	E858.0	E932.1	E950.4	E962.0	E980.4

Substance	Poisoning	External Cause (E-Code)				
		Accident	Therapeutic Use	Suicide Attempt	Assault	Undetermined
Oxaprozin	965.61	E850.6	E935.6	E950.0	E962.0	E980.0
Oxazepam	969.4	E853.2	E939.4	E950.3	E962.0	E980.3
Oxazolidine derivatives	966.0	E855.0	E936.0	E950.4	E962.0	E980.4
Ox bile extract	973.4	E858.4	E943.4	E950.4	E962.0	E980.4
Oxedrine	971.2	E855.5	E941.2	E950.4	E962.0	E980.4
Oxeladin	975.4	E858.6	E945.4	E950.4	E962.0	E980.4
Oxethazaine NEC	968.5	E855.2	E938.5	E950.4	E962.0	E980.4
Oxidizing agents NEC	983.9	E864.3	—	E950.7	E962.1	E980.6
Oxolinic acid	961.3	E857	E931.3	E950.4	E962.0	E980.4
Oxophenarsine	961.1	E857	E931.1	E950.4	E962.0	E980.4
Oxsoralen	976.3	E858.7	E946.3	E950.4	E962.0	E980.4
Oxtriphylline	975.7	E858.6	E945.7	E950.4	E962.0	E980.4
Oxybuprocaine	968.5	E855.2	E938.5	E950.4	E962.0	E980.4
Oxybutynin	975.1	E858.6	E945.1	E950.4	E962.0	E980.4
Oxycodone	965.09	E850.2	E935.2	E950.0	E962.0	E980.0
Oxygen	987.8	E869.8	—	E952.8	E962.2	E982.8
Oxylone	976.0	E858.7	E946.0	E950.4	E962.0	E980.4
ophthalmic preparation	976.5	E858.7	E946.5	E950.4	E962.0	E980.4
Oxymesterone	962.1	E858.0	E932.1	E950.4	E962.0	E980.4
Oxymetazoline	971.2	E855.5	E941.2	E950.4	E962.0	E980.4
Oxymetholone	962.1	E858.0	E932.1	E950.4	E962.0	E980.4
Oxymorphone	965.09	E850.2	E935.2	E950.0	E962.0	E980.0
Oxypertine	969.0	E854.0	E939.0	E950.3	E962.0	E980.3
Oxyphenbutazone	965.5	E850.5	E935.5	E950.0	E962.0	E980.0
Oxyphencyclimine	971.1	E855.4	E941.1	E950.4	E962.0	E980.4
Oxyphenisatin	973.1	E858.4	E943.1	E950.4	E962.0	E980.4
Oxyphenonium	971.1	E855.4	E941.1	E950.4	E962.0	E980.4
Oxyquinoline	961.3	E857	E931.3	E950.4	E962.0	E980.4
Oxytetracycline	960.4	E856	E930.4	E950.4	E962.0	E980.4
Oxytocics	975.0	E858.6	E945.0	E950.4	E962.0	E980.4
Oxytocin	975.0	E858.6	E945.0	E950.4	E962.0	E980.4
Ozone	987.8	E869.8	—	E952.8	E962.2	E982.8
PABA	976.3	E858.7	E946.3	E950.4	E962.0	E980.4
Packed red cells	964.7	E858.2	E934.7	E950.4	E962.0	E980.4
Paint NEC	989.89	E861.6	—	E950.9	E962.1	E980.9
cleaner	982.8	E862.9	—	E950.9	E962.1	E980.9
fumes NEC	987.8	E869.8	—	E952.8	E962.1	E982.8
lead (fumes)	984.0	E861.5	—	E950.9	E962.1	E980.9
solvent NEC	982.8	E862.9	—	E950.9	E962.1	E980.9
stripper	982.8	E862.9	—	E950.9	E962.1	E980.9
Palfium	965.09	E850.2	E935.2	E950.0	E962.0	E980.0
Palivizumab	979.9	E858.8	E949.6	E950.4	E962.0	E980.4
Paludrine	961.4	E857	E931.4	E950.4	E962.0	E980.4
PAM	977.2	E855.8	E947.2	E950.4	E962.0	E980.4
Pamaquine (naphthoate)	961.4	E857	E931.4	E950.4	E962.0	E980.4
Pamprin	965.1	E850.3	E935.3	E950.0	E962.0	E980.0
Panadol	965.4	E850.4	E935.4	E950.0	E962.0	E980.0
Pancreatic dornase (mucolytic)	963.4	E858.1	E933.4	E950.4	E962.0	E980.4
Pancreatin	973.4	E858.4	E943.4	E950.4	E962.0	E980.4
Pancrelipase	973.4	E858.4	E943.4	E950.4	E962.0	E980.4
Pangamic acid	963.5	E858.1	E933.5	E950.4	E962.0	E980.4
Panthenol	963.5	E858.1	E933.5	E950.4	E962.0	E980.4
topical	976.8	E858.7	E946.8	E950.4	E962.0	E980.4
Pantopaque	977.8	E858.8	E947.8	E950.4	E962.0	E980.4
Pantopon	965.00	E850.2	E935.2	E950.0	E962.0	E980.0
Pantothenic acid	963.5	E858.1	E933.5	E950.4	E962.0	E980.4
Panwarfin	964.2	E858.2	E934.2	E950.4	E962.0	E980.4

Substance	Poisoning	External Cause (E-Code)				
		Accident	Therapeutic Use	Suicide Attempt	Assault	Undetermined
Papain	973.4	E858.4	E943.4	E950.4	E962.0	E980.4
Papaverine	972.5	E858.3	E942.5	E950.4	E962.0	E980.4
Para–aminobenzoic acid	976.3	E858.7	E946.3	E950.4	E962.0	E980.4
Para–aminophenol derivatives	965.4	E850.4	E935.4	E950.0	E962.0	E980.0
Para–aminosalicylic acid (derivatives)	961.8	E857	E931.8	E950.4	E962.0	E980.4
Paracetaldehyde (medicinal)	967.2	E852.1	E937.2	E950.2	E962.0	E980.2
Paracetamol	965.4	E850.4	E935.4	E950.0	E962.0	E980.0
Paracodin	965.09	E850.2	E935.2	E950.0	E962.0	E980.0
Paradione	966.0	E855.0	E936.0	E950.4	E962.0	E980.4
Paraffin(s) (wax)	981	E862.3	—	E950.9	E962.1	E980.9
liquid (medicinal)	973.2	E858.4	E943.2	E950.4	E962.0	E980.4
nonmedicinal (oil)	981	E962.1	—	E950.9	E962.1	E980.9
Paraldehyde (medicinal)	967.2	E852.1	E937.2	E950.2	E962.0	E980.2
Paramethadione	966.0	E855.0	E936.0	E950.4	E962.0	E980.4
Paramethasone	962.0	E858.0	E932.0	E950.4	E962.0	E980.4
Paraquat	989.4	E863.5	—	E950.6	E962.1	E980.7
Parasympatholytics	971.1	E855.4	E941.1	E950.4	E962.0	E980.4
Parasympathomimetics	971.0	E855.3	E941.0	E950.4	E962.0	E980.4
Parathion	989.3	E863.1	—	E950.6	E962.1	E980.7
Parathormone	962.6	E858.0	E932.6	E950.4	E962.0	E980.4
Parathyroid (derivatives)	962.6	E858.0	E932.6	E950.4	E962.0	E980.4
Paratyphoid vaccine	978.1	E858.8	E948.1	E950.4	E962.0	E980.4
Paredrine	971.2	E855.5	E941.2	E950.4	E962.0	E980.4
Paregoric	965.00	E850.2	E935.2	E950.0	E962.0	E980.0
Pargyline	972.3	E858.3	E942.3	E950.4	E962.0	E980.4
Paris green	985.1	E866.3	—	E950.8	E962.1	E980.8
insecticide	985.1	E863.4	—	E950.8	E962.1	E980.8
Parnate	969.0	E854.0	E939.0	E950.3	E962.0	E980.3
Paromomycin	960.8	E856	E930.8	E950.4	E962.0	E980.4
Paroxypropione	963.1	E858.1	E933.1	E950.4	E962.0	E980.4
Parzone	965.09	E850.2	E935.2	E950.0	E962.0	E980.0
PAS	961.8	E857	E931.8	E950.4	E962.0	E980.4
PCBs	981	E862.3	—	E950.9	E962.1	E980.9
PCP (pentachlorophenol)	989.4	E863.6	—	E950.6	E962.1	E980.7
herbicide	989.4	E863.5	—	E950.6	E962.1	E980.7
insecticide	989.4	E863.4	—	E950.6	E962.1	E980.7
phencyclidine	968.3	E855.1	E938.3	E950.4	E962.0	E980.4
Peach kernel oil (emulsion)	973.2	E858.4	E943.2	E950.4	E962.0	E980.4
Peanut oil (emulsion) NEC	973.2	E858.4	E943.2	E950.4	E962.0	E980.4
topical	976.3	E858.7	E946.3	E950.4	E962.0	E980.4
Pearly Gates (morning glory seeds)	969.6	E854.1	E939.6	E950.3	E962.0	E980.3
Pecazine	969.1	E853.0	E939.1	E950.3	E962.0	E980.3
Pecilocin	960.1	E856	E930.1	E950.4	E962.0	E980.4
Pectin (with kaolin) NEC	973.5	E858.4	E943.5	E950.4	E962.0	E980.4
Pelletierine tannate	961.6	E857	E931.6	E950.4	E962.0	E980.4
Pemoline	969.7	E854.2	E939.7	E950.3	E962.0	E980.3
Pempidine	972.3	E858.3	E942.3	E950.4	E962.0	E980.4
Penamecillin	960.0	E856	E930.0	E950.4	E962.0	E980.4
Penethamate hydriodide	960.0	E856	E930.0	E950.4	E962.0	E980.4
Penicillamine	963.8	E858.1	E933.8	E950.4	E962.0	E980.4
Penicillin (any type)	960.0	E856	E930.0	E950.4	E962.0	E980.4
Penicillinase	963.4	E858.1	E933.4	E950.4	E962.0	E980.4
Pentachlorophenol (fungicide)	989.4	E863.6	—	E950.6	E962.1	E980.7
herbicide	989.4	E863.5	—	E950.6	E962.1	E980.7
insecticide	989.4	E863.4	—	E950.6	E962.1	E980.7
Pentaerythritol	972.4	E858.3	E942.4	E950.4	E962.0	E980.4
chloral	967.1	E852.0	E937.1	E950.2	E962.0	E980.2

Substance	Poisoning	External Cause (E-Code)				
		Accident	Therapeutic Use	Suicide Attempt	Assault	Undetermined
tetranitrate NEC	972.4	E858.3	E942.4	E950.4	E962.0	E980.4
Pentagastrin	977.8	E858.8	E947.8	E950.4	E962.0	E980.4
Pentalin	982.3	E862.4	—	E950.9	E962.1	E980.9
Pentamethonium (bromide)	972.3	E858.3	E942.3	E950.4	E962.0	E980.4
Pentamidine	961.5	E857	E931.5	E950.4	E962.0	E980.4
Pentanol	980.8	E860.8	—	E950.9	E962.1	E980.9
Pentaquine	961.4	E857	E931.4	E950.4	E962.0	E980.4
Pentazocine	965.8	E850.8	E935.8	E950.0	E962.0	E980.0
Penthienate	971.1	E855.4	E941.1	E950.4	E962.0	E980.4
Pentobarbital, pentobarbitone (sodium)	967.0	E851	E937.0	E950.1	E962.0	E980.1
Pentolinium (tartrate)	972.3	E858.3	E942.3	E950.4	E962.0	E980.4
Pentothal	968.3	E855.1	E938.3	E950.4	E962.0	E980.4
Pentylenetetrazol	970.0	E854.3	E940.0	E950.4	E962.0	E980.4
Pentylsalicylamide	961.8	E857	E931.8	E950.4	E962.0	E980.4
Pepsin	973.4	E858.4	E943.4	E950.4	E962.0	E980.4
Peptavlon	977.8	E858.8	E947.8	E950.4	E962.0	E980.4
Percaine (spinal)	968.7	E855.2	E938.7	E950.4	E962.0	E980.4
topical (surface)	968.5	E855.2	E938.5	E950.4	E962.0	E980.4
Perchloroethylene (vapor)	982.3	E862.4	—	E950.9	E962.1	E980.9
medicinal	961.6	E857	E931.6	E950.4	E962.0	E980.4
Percodan	965.09	E850.2	E935.2	E950.0	E962.0	E980.0
Percogesic	965.09	E850.2	E935.2	E950.0	E962.0	E980.0
Percorten	962.0	E858.0	E932.0	E950.4	E962.0	E980.4
Pergonal	962.4	E858.0	E932.4	E950.4	E962.0	E980.4
Perhexiline	972.4	E858.3	E942.4	E950.4	E962.0	E980.4
Periactin	963.0	E858.1	E933.0	E950.4	E962.0	E980.4
Periclor	967.1	E852.0	E937.1	E950.2	E962.0	E980.2
Pericyazine	969.1	E853.0	E939.1	E950.3	E962.0	E980.3
Peritrate	972.4	E858.3	E942.4	E950.4	E962.0	E980.4
Permanganates NEC	983.9	E864.3	—	E950.7	E962.1	E980.6
potassium (topical)	976.0	E858.7	E946.0	E950.4	E962.0	E980.4
Pernocton	967.0	E851	E937.0	E950.1	E962.0	E980.1
Pernoston	967.0	E851	E937.0	E950.1	E962.0	E980.1
Peronin(e)	965.09	E850.2	E935.2	E950.0	E962.0	E980.0
Perphenazine	969.1	E853.0	E939.1	E950.3	E962.0	E980.3
Pertofrane	969.0	E854	E939.0	E950.3	E962.0	E980.3
Pertussis						
immune serum (human)	964.6	E858.2	E934.6	E950.4	E962.0	E980.4
vaccine (with diphtheria toxoid) (with tetanus toxoid)	978.6	E858.8	E948.6	E950.4	E962.0	E980.4
Peruvian balsam	976.8	E858.7	E946.8	E950.4	E962.0	E980.4
Pesticides (dust) (fumes) (vapor)	989.4	E863.4	—	E950.6	E962.1	E980.7
arsenic	985.1	E863.4	—	E950.8	E962.1	E980.8
chlorinated	989.2	E863.0	—	E950.6	E962.1	E980.7
cyanide	989.0	E863.4	—	E950.6	E962.1	E980.7
kerosene	981	E863.4	—	E950.6	E962.1	E980.7
mixture (of compounds)	989.4	E863.3	—	E950.6	E962.1	E980.7
naphthalene	983.0	E863.4	—	E950.7	E962.1	E980.6
organochlorine (compounds)	989.2	E863.0	—	E950.6	E962.1	E980.7
petroleum (distillate) (products) NEC	981	E863.4	—	E950.6	E962.1	E980.7
specified ingredient NEC	989.4	E863.4	—	E950.6	E962.1	E980.7
strychnine	989.1	E863.4	—	E950.6	E962.1	E980.7
thallium	985.8	E863.7	—	E950.6	E962.1	E980.7
Pethidine (hydrochloride)	965.09	E850.2	E935.2	E950.0	E962.0	E980.0
Petrichloral	967.1	E852.0	E937.1	E950.2	E962.0	E980.2
Petrol	981	E862.1	—	E950.9	E962.1	E980.9

Substance	Poisoning	External Cause (E-Code)				
		Accident	Therapeutic Use	Suicide Attempt	Assault	Undetermined
vapor	987.1	E869.8	—	E952.8	E962.2	E982.8
Petrolatum (jelly) (ointment)	976.3	E858.7	E946.3	E950.4	E962.0	E980.4
hydrophilic	976.3	E858.7	E946.3	E950.4	E962.0	E980.4
liquid	973.2	E858.4	E943.2	E950.4	E962.0	E980.4
topical	976.3	E858.7	E946.3	E950.4	E962.0	E980.4
nonmedicinal	981	E862.1	—	E950.9	E962.1	E980.9
Petroleum (cleaners) (fuels) (products) NEC	981	E862.1	—	E950.9	E962.1	E980.9
benzin(e) — *see* Ligroin						
ether — *see* Ligroin						
jelly — *see* Petrolatum						
naphtha — *see* Ligroin						
pesticide	981	E863.4	—	E950.6	E962.1	E980.7
solids	981	E862.3	—	E950.9	E962.1	E980.9
solvents	981	E862.0	—	E950.9	E962.1	E980.9
vapor	987.1	E869.8	—	E952.8	E962.2	E982.8
Peyote	969.6	E854.1	E939.6	E950.3	E962.0	E980.3
Phanodorm, phanodorn	967.0	E851	E937.0	E950.1	E962.0	E980.1
Phanquinone, phanquone	961.5	E857	E931.5	E950.4	E962.0	E980.4
Pharmaceutical excipient or adjunct	977.4	E858.8	E947.4	E950.4	E962.0	E980.4
Phenacemide	966.3	E855.0	E936.3	E950.4	E962.0	E980.4
Phenacetin	965.4	E850.4	E935.4	E950.0	E962.0	E980.0
Phenadoxone	965.09	E850.2	E935.2	E950.0	E962.0	E980.0
Phenaglycodol	969.5	E853.8	E939.5	E950.3	E962.0	E980.3
Phenantoin	966.1	E855.0	E936.1	E950.4	E962.0	E980.4
Phenaphthazine reagent	977.8	E858.8	E947.8	E950.4	E962.0	E980.4
Phenazocine	965.09	E850.2	E935.2	E950.0	E962.0	E980.0
Phenazone	965.5	E850.5	E935.5	E950.0	E962.0	E980.0
Phenazopyridine	976.1	E858.7	E946.1	E950.4	E962.0	E980.4
Phenbenicillin	960.0	E856	E930.0	E950.4	E962.0	E980.4
Phenbutrazate	977.0	E858.8	E947.0	E950.4	E962.0	E980.4
Phencyclidine	968.3	E855.1	E938.3	E950.4	E962.0	E980.4
Phendimetrazine	977.0	E858.8	E947.0	E950.4	E962.0	E980.4
Phenelzine	969.0	E854.0	E939.0	E950.3	E962.0	E980.3
Phenergan	967.8	E852.8	E937.8	E950.2	E962.0	E980.2
Phenethicillin (potassium)	960.0	E856	E930.0	E950.4	E962.0	E980.4
Phenetsal	965.1	E850.3	E935.3	E950.0	E962.0	E980.0
Pheneturide	966.3	E855.0	E936.3	E950.4	E962.0	E980.4
Phenformin	962.3	E858.0	E932.3	E950.4	E962.0	E980.4
Phenglutarimide	971.1	E855.4	E941.1	E950.4	E962.0	E980.4
Phenicarbazide	965.8	E850.8	E935.8	E950.0	E962.0	E980.0
Phenindamine (tartrate)	963.0	E858.1	E933.0	E950.4	E962.0	E980.4
Phenindione	964.2	E858.2	E934.2	E950.4	E962.0	E980.4
Pheniprazine	969.0	E854.0	E939.0	E950.3	E962.0	E980.3
Pheniramine (maleate)	963.0	E858.1	E933.0	E950.4	E962.0	E980.4
Phenmetrazine	977.0	E858.8	E947.0	E950.4	E962.0	E980.4
Phenobal	967.0	E851	E937.0	E950.1	E962.0	E980.1
Phenobarbital	967.0	E851	E937.0	E950.1	E962.0	E980.1
Phenobarbitone	967.0	E851	E937.0	E950.1	E962.0	E980.1
Phenoctide	976.0	E858.7	E946.0	E950.4	E962.0	E980.4
Phenol (derivatives) NEC	983.0	E864.0	—	E950.7	E962.1	E980.6
disinfectant	983.0	E864.0	—	E950.7	E962.1	E980.6
pesticide	989.4	E863.4	—	E950.6	E962.1	E980.7
red	977.8	E858.8	E947.8	E950.4	E962.0	E980.4
Phenolphthalein	973.1	E858.4	E943.1	E950.4	E962.0	E980.4
Phenolsulfonphthalein	977.8	E858.8	E947.8	E950.4	E962.0	E980.4
Phenomorphan	965.09	E850.2	E935.2	E950.0	E962.0	E980.0

Substance	Poisoning	External Cause (E-Code)				
		Accident	Therapeutic Use	Suicide Attempt	Assault	Undetermined
Phenonyl	967.0	E851	E937.0	E950.1	E962.0	E980.1
Phenoperidine	965.09	E850.2	E935.2	E950.0	E962.0	E980.0
Phenoquin	974.7	E858.5	E944.7	E950.4	E962.0	E980.4
Phenothiazines (tranquilizers) NEC	969.1	E853.0	E939.1	E950.3	E962.0	E980.3
insecticide	989.3	E863.4	—	E950.6	E962.1	E980.7
Phenoxybenzamine	971.3	E855.6	E941.3	E950.4	E962.0	E980.4
Phenoxymethyl penicillin	960.0	E856	E930.0	E950.4	E962.0	E980.4
Phenprocoumon	964.2	E858.2	E934.2	E950.4	E962.0	E980.4
Phensuximide	966.2	E855.0	E936.2	E950.4	E962.0	E980.4
Phentermine	977.0	E858.8	E947.0	E950.4	E962.0	E980.4
Phentolamine	971.3	E855.6	E941.3	E950.4	E962.0	E980.4
Phenyl						
butazone	965.5	E850.5	E935.5	E950.0	E962.0	E980.0
enediamine	983.0	E864.0	—	E950.7	E962.1	E980.6
hydrazine	983.0	E864.0	—	E950.7	E962.1	E980.6
antineoplastic	963.1	E858.1	E933.1	E950.4	E962.0	E980.4
mercuric compounds — *see* Mercury						
salicylate	976.3	E858.7	E946.3	E950.4	E962.0	E980.4
Phenylephrin	971.2	E855.5	E941.2	E950.4	E962.0	E980.4
Phenylethybiguanide	962.3	E858.0	E932.3	E950.4	E962.0	E980.4
Phenylpropanolamine	971.2	E855.5	E941.2	E950.4	E962.0	E980.4
Phenylsulfthion	989.3	E863.1	—	E950.6	E962.1	E980.7
Phenyramidol, phenyramidon	965.7	E850.7	E935.7	E950.0	E962.0	E980.0
Phenytoin	966.1	E855.0	E936.1	E950.4	E962.0	E980.4
pHisoHex	976.2	E858.7	E946.2	E950.4	E962.0	E980.4
Pholcodine	965.09	E850.2	E935.2	E950.0	E962.0	E980.0
Phorate	989.3	E863.1	—	E950.6	E962.1	E980.7
Phosdrin	989.3	E863.1	—	E950.6	E962.1	E980.7
Phosgene (gas)	987.8	E869.8	—	E952.8	E962.2	E982.8
Phosphate (tricresyl)	989.89	E866.8	—	E950.9	E962.1	E980.9
organic	989.3	E863.1	—	E950.6	E962.1	E980.7
solvent	982.8	E862.4	—	E950.9	E926.1	E980.9
Phosphine	987.8	E869.8	—	E952.8	E962.2	E982.8
fumigant	987.8	E863.8	—	E950.6	E962.2	E980.7
Phospholine	971.0	E855.3	E941.0	E950.4	E962.0	E980.4
Phosphoric acid	983.1	E864.1	—	E950.7	E962.1	E980.6
Phosphorus (compounds) NEC	983.9	E864.3	—	E950.7	E962.1	E980.6
rodenticide	983.9	E863.7	—	E950.7	E962.1	E980.6
Phthalimidogluarimide	967.8	E852.8	E937.8	E950.2	E962.0	E980.2
Phthalylsulfathiazole	961.0	E857	E931.0	E950.4	E962.0	E980.4
Phylloquinone	964.3	E858.2	E934.3	E950.4	E962.0	E980.4
Physeptone	965.02	E850.1	E935.1	E950.0	E962.0	E980.0
Physostigma venenosum	988.2	E865.4	—	E950.9	E962.1	E980.9
Physostigmine	971.0	E855.3	E941.0	E950.4	E962.0	E980.4
Phytolacca decandra	988.2	E865.4	—	E950.9	E962.1	E980.9
Phytomenadione	964.3	E858.2	E934.3	E950.4	E962.0	E980.4
Phytonadione	964.3	E858.2	E934.3	E950.4	E962.0	E980.4
Picric (acid)	983.0	E864.0	—	E950.7	E962.1	E980.6
Picrotoxin	970.0	E854.3	E940.0	E950.4	E962.0	E980.4
Pilocarpine	971.0	E855.3	E941.0	E950.4	E962.0	E980.4
Pilocarpus (jaborandi) extract	971.0	E855.3	E941.0	E950.4	E962.0	E980.4
Pimaricin	960.1	E856	E930.1	E950.4	E962.0	E980.4
Piminodine	965.09	E850.2	E935.2	E950.0	E962.0	E980.0
Pine oil, pinesol (disinfectant)	983.9	E861.4	—	E950.7	E962.1	E980.6
Pinkroot	961.6	E857	E931.6	E950.4	E962.0	E980.4
Pipadone	965.09	E850.2	E935.2	E950.0	E962.0	E980.0
Pipamazine	963.0	E858.1	E933.0	E950.4	E962.0	E980.4

Substance	Poisoning	Accident	Therapeutic Use	Suicide Attempt	Assault	Undetermined
			External Cause (E-Code)			
Pipazethate	975.4	E858.6	E945.4	E950.4	E962.0	E980.4
Pipenzolate	971.1	E855.4	E941.1	E950.4	E962.0	E980.4
Piperacetazine	969.1	E853.0	E939.1	E950.3	E962.0	E980.3
Piperazine NEC	961.6	E857	E931.6	E950.4	E962.0	E980.4
estrone sulfate	962.2	E858.0	E932.2	E950.4	E962.0	E980.4
Piper cubeba	988.2	E865.4	—	E950.9	E962.1	E980.9
Piperidione	975.4	E858.6	E945.4	E950.4	E962.0	E980.4
Piperidolate	971.1	E855.4	E941.1	E950.4	E962.0	E980.4
Piperocaine	968.9	E855.2	E938.9	E950.4	E962.0	E980.4
infiltration (subcutaneous)	968.5	E855.2	E938.5	E950.4	E962.0	E980.4
nerve block (peripheral) (plexus)	968.6	E855.2	E938.6	E950.4	E962.0	E980.4
topical (surface)	968.5	E855.2	E938.5	E950.4	E962.0	E980.4
Pipobroman	963.1	E858.1	E933.1	E950.4	E962.0	E980.4
Pipradrol	970.8	E854.3	E940.8	E950.4	E962.0	E980.4
Piscidia (bark) (erythrina)	965.7	E850.7	E935.7	E950.0	E962.0	E980.0
Pitch	983.0	E864.0	—	E950.7	E962.1	E980.6
Pitkin's solution	968.7	E855.2	E938.7	E950.4	E962.0	E980.4
Pitocin	975.0	E858.6	E945.0	E950.4	E962.0	E980.4
Pitressin (tannate)	962.5	E858.0	E932.5	E950.4	E962.0	E980.4
Pituitary extracts (posterior)	962.5	E858.0	E932.5	E950.4	E962.0	E980.4
anterior	962.4	E858.0	E932.4	E950.4	E962.0	E980.4
Pituitrin	962.5	E858.0	E932.5	E950.4	E962.0	E980.4
Placental extract	962.9	E858.0	E932.9	E950.4	E962.0	E980.4
Placidyl	967.8	E852.8	E937.8	E950.2	E962.0	E980.2
Plague vaccine	978.3	E858.8	E948.3	E950.4	E962.0	E980.4
Plant foods or fertilizers NEC	989.89	E866.5	—	E950.9	E962.1	E980.9
mixed with herbicides	989.4	E863.5	—	E950.6	E962.1	E980.7
Plants, noxious, used as food	988.2	E865.9	—	E950.9	E962.1	E980.9
berries and seeds	988.2	E865.3	—	E950.9	E962.1	E980.9
specified type NEC	988.2	E865.4	—	E950.9	E962.1	E980.9
Plasma (blood)	964.7	E858.2	E934.7	E950.4	E962.0	E980.4
expanders	964.8	E858.2	E934.8	E950.4	E962.0	E980.4
Plasmanate	964.7	E858.2	E934.7	E950.4	E962.0	E980.4
Plegicil	969.1	E853.0	E939.1	E950.3	E962.0	E980.3
Podophyllin	976.4	E858.7	E946.4	E950.4	E962.0	E980.4
Podophyllum resin	976.4	E858.7	E946.4	E950.4	E962.0	E980.4
Poison NEC	989.9	E866.9	—	E950.9	E962.1	E980.9
Poisonous berries	988.2	E865.3	—	E950.9	E962.1	E980.9
Pokeweed (any part)	988.2	E865.4	—	E950.9	E962.1	E980.9
Poldine	971.1	E855.4	E941.1	E950.4	E962.0	E980.4
Poliomyelitis vaccine	979.5	E858.8	E949.5	E950.4	E962.0	E980.4
Poliovirus vaccine	979.5	E858.8	E949.5	E950.4	E962.0	E980.4
Polish (car) (floor) (furniture) (metal) (silver)	989.89	E861.2	—	E950.9	E962.1	E980.9
abrasive	989.89	E861.3	—	E950.9	E962.1	E980.9
porcelain	989.89	E861.3	—	E950.9	E962.1	E980.9
Poloxalkol	973.2	E858.4	E943.2	E950.4	E962.0	E980.4
Polyaminostyrene resins	974.5	E858.5	E944.5	E950.4	E962.0	E980.4
Polychlorinated biphenyl—*see* PCBs						
Polycycline	960.4	E856	E930.4	E950.4	E962.0	E980.4
Polyester resin hardener	982.8	E862.4	—	E950.9	E962.1	E980.9
fumes	987.8	E869.8	—	E952.8	E962.2	E982.8
Polyestradiol (phosphate)	962.2	E858.0	E932.2	E950.4	E962.0	E980.4
Polyethanolamine alkyl sulfate	976.2	E858.7	E946.2	E950.4	E962.0	E980.4
Polyethylene glycol	976.3	E858.7	E946.3	E950.4	E962.0	E980.4
Polyferose	964.0	E858.2	E934.0	E950.4	E962.0	E980.4
Polymyxin B	960.8	E856	E930.8	E950.4	E962.0	E980.4

Substance	Poisoning	External Cause (E-Code) Accident	Therapeutic Use	Suicide Attempt	Assault	Undetermined
ENT agent	976.6	E858.7	E946.6	E950.4	E962.0	E980.4
ophthalmic preparation	976.5	E858.7	E946.5	E950.4	E962.0	E980.4
topical NEC	976.0	E858.7	E946.0	E950.4	E962.0	E980.4
Polynoxylin(e)	976.0	E858.7	E946.0	E950.4	E962.0	E980.4
Polyoxymethyleneurea	976.0	E858.7	E946.0	E950.4	E962.0	E980.4
Polytetrafluoroethylene (inhaled)	987.8	E869.8	—	E952.8	E962.2	E982.8
Polythiazide	974.3	E858.5	E944.3	E950.4	E962.0	E980.4
Polyvinylpyrrolidone	964.8	E858.2	E934.8	E950.4	E962.0	E980.4
Pontocaine (hydrochloride) (infiltration) (topical)	968.5	E855.2	E938.5	E950.4	E962.0	E980.4
nerve block (peripheral) (plexus)	968.6	E855.2	E938.6	E950.4	E962.0	E980.4
spinal	968.7	E855.2	E938.7	E950.4	E962.0	E980.4
Pot	969.6	E854.1	E939.6	E950.3	E962.0	E980.3
Potash (caustic)	983.2	E864.2	—	E950.7	E962.1	E980.6
Potassic saline injection (lactated)	974.5	E858.5	E944.5	E950.4	E962.0	E980.4
Potassium (salts) NEC	974.5	E858.5	E944.5	E950.4	E962.0	E980.4
aminosalicylate	961.8	E857	E931.8	E950.4	E962.0	E980.4
arsenite (solution)	985.1	E866.3	—	E950.8	E962.1	E980.8
bichromate	983.9	E864.3	—	E950.7	E962.1	E980.6
bisulfate	983.9	E864.3	—	E950.7	E962.1	E980.6
bromide (medicinal) NEC	967.3	E852.2	E937.3	E950.2	E962.0	E980.2
carbonate	983.2	E864.2	—	E950.7	E962.1	E980.6
chlorate NEC	983.9	E864.3	—	E950.7	E962.1	E980.6
cyanide — *see* Cyanide						
hydroxide	983.2	E864.2	—	E950.7	E962.1	E980.6
iodide (expectorant) NEC	975.5	E858.6	E945.5	E950.4	E962.0	E980.4
nitrate	989.89	E866.8	—	E950.9	E962.1	E980.9
oxalate	983.9	E864.3	—	E950.7	E962.1	E980.6
perchlorate NEC	977.8	E858.8	E947.8	E950.4	E962.0	E980.4
antithyroid	962.8	E858.0	E932.8	E950.4	E962.0	E980.4
permanganate	976.0	E858.7	E946.0	E950.4	E962.0	E980.4
nonmedicinal	983.9	E864.3	—	E950.7	E962.1	E980.6
Povidone–iodine (anti–infective) NEC	976.0	E858.7	E946.0	E950.4	E962.0	E980.4
Practolol	972.0	E858.3	E942.0	E950.4	E962.0	E980.4
Pralidoxime (chloride)	977.2	E858.8	E947.2	E950.4	E962.0	E980.4
Pramoxine	968.5	E855.2	E938.5	E950.4	E962.0	E980.4
Prazosin	972.6	E858.3	E942.6	E950.4	E962.0	E980.4
Prednisolone	962.0	E858.0	E932.0	E950.4	E962.0	E980.4
ENT agent	976.6	E858.7	E946.6	E950.4	E962.0	E980.4
ophthalmic preparation	976.5	E858.7	E946.5	E950.4	E962.0	E980.4
topical NEC	976.0	E858.7	E946.0	E950.4	E962.0	E980.4
Prednisone	962.0	E858.0	E932.0	E950.4	E962.0	E980.4
Pregnanediol	962.2	E858.0	E932.2	E950.4	E962.0	E980.4
Pregneninolone	962.2	E858.0	E932.2	E950.4	E962.0	E980.4
Preludin	977.0	E858.8	E947.0	E950.4	E962.0	E980.4
Premarin	962.2	E858.0	E932.2	E950.4	E962.0	E980.4
Prenylamine	972.4	E858.3	E942.4	E950.4	E962.0	E980.4
Preparation H	976.8	E858.7	E946.8	E950.4	E962.0	E980.4
Preservatives	989.89	E866.8	—	E950.9	E962.1	E980.9
Pride of China	988.2	E865.3	—	E950.9	E962.1	E980.9
Prilocaine	968.9	E855.2	E938.9	E950.4	E962.0	E980.4
infiltration (subcutaneous)	968.5	E855.2	E938.5	E950.4	E962.0	E980.4
nerve block (peripheral) (plexus)	968.6	E855.2	E938.6	E950.4	E962.0	E980.4
Primaquine	961.4	E857	E931.4	E950.4	E962.0	E980.4
Primidone	966.3	E855.0	E936.3	E950.4	E962.0	E980.4
Primula (veris)	988.2	E865.4	—	E950.9	E962.1	E980.9
Prinadol	965.09	E850.2	E935.2	E950.0	E962.0	E980.0

Substance	Poisoning	External Cause (E-Code)				
		Accident	Therapeutic Use	Suicide Attempt	Assault	Undetermined
Priscol, Priscoline	971.3	E855.6	E941.3	E950.4	E962.0	E980.4
Privet	988.2	E865.4	—	E950.9	E962.1	E980.9
Privine	971.2	E855.5	E941.2	E950.4	E962.0	E980.4
Pro–Banthine	971.1	E855.4	E941.1	E950.4	E962.0	E980.4
Probarbital	967.0	E851	E937.0	E950.1	E962.0	E980.1
Probenecid	974.7	E858.5	E944.7	E950.4	E962.0	E980.4
Procainamide (hydrochloride)	972.0	E858.3	E942.0	E950.4	E962.0	E980.4
Procaine (hydrochloride) (infiltration) (topical)	968.5	E855.2	E938.5	E950.4	E962.0	E980.4
nerve block (peripheral) (plexus)	968.6	E855.2	E938.6	E950.4	E962.0	E980.4
penicillin G	960.0	E856	E930.0	E950.4	E962.0	E980.4
spinal	968.7	E855.2	E938.7	E950.4	E962.0	E980.4
Procalmidol	969.5	E853.8	E939.5	E950.3	E962.0	E980.3
Procarbazine	963.1	E858.1	E933.1	E950.4	E962.0	E980.4
Prochlorperazine	969.1	E853.0	E939.1	E950.3	E962.0	E980.3
Procyclidine	966.4	E855.0	E936.4	E950.4	E962.0	E980.4
Producer gas	986	E868.8	—	E952.1	E962.2	E982.1
Profenamine	966.4	E855.0	E936.4	E950.4	E962.0	E980.4
Profenil	975.1	E858.6	E945.1	E950.4	E962.0	E980.4
Progesterones	962.2	E858.0	E932.2	E950.4	E962.0	E980.4
Progestin	962.2	E858.0	E932.2	E950.4	E962.0	E980.4
Progestogens (with estrogens)	962.2	E858.0	E932.2	E950.4	E962.0	E980.4
Progestone	962.2	E858.0	E932.2	E950.4	E962.0	E980.4
Proguanil	961.4	E857	E931.4	E950.4	E962.0	E980.4
Prolactin	962.4	E858.0	E932.4	E950.4	E962.0	E980.4
Proloid	962.7	E858.0	E932.7	E950.4	E962.0	E980.4
Proluton	962.2	E858.0	E932.2	E950.4	E962.0	E980.4
Promacetin	961.8	E857	E931.8	E950.4	E962.0	E980.4
Promazine	969.1	E853.0	E939.1	E950.3	E962.0	E980.3
Promedol	965.09	E850.2	E935.2	E950.0	E962.0	E980.0
Promethazine	967.8	E852.8	E937.8	E950.2	E962.0	E980.2
Promin	961.8	E857	E931.8	E950.4	E962.0	E980.4
Pronestyl (hydrochloride)	972.0	E858.3	E942.0	E950.4	E962.0	E980.4
Pronetalol, pronethalol	972.0	E858.3	E942.0	E950.4	E962.0	E980.4
Prontosil	961.0	E857	E931.0	E950.4	E962.0	E980.4
Propamidine isethionate	961.5	E857	E931.5	E950.4	E962.0	E980.4
Propanal (medicinal)	967.8	E852.8	E937.8	E950.2	E962.0	E980.2
Propane (gas) (distributed in mobile container)	987.0	E868.0	—	E951.1	E962.2	E981.1
distributed through pipes	987.0	E867	—	E951.0	E962.2	E981.0
incomplete combustion of – *see* Carbon monoxide, Propane						
Propanidid	968.3	E855.1	E938.3	E950.4	E962.0	E980.4
Propanol	980.3	E860.4	—	E950.9	E962.1	E980.9
Propantheline	971.1	E855.4	E941.1	E950.4	E962.0	E980.4
Proparacaine	968.5	E855.2	E938.5	E950.4	E962.0	E980.4
Propatyl nitrate	972.4	E858.3	E942.4	E950.4	E962.0	E980.4
Propicillin	960.0	E856	E930.0	E950.4	E962.0	E980.4
Propiolactone (vapor)	987.8	E869.8	—	E952.8	E962.2	E982.8
Propiomazine	967.8	E852.8	E937.8	E950.2	E962.0	E980.2
Propionaldehyde (medicinal)	967.8	E852.8	E937.8	E950.2	E962.0	E980.2
Propionate compound	976.0	E858.7	E946.0	E950.4	E962.0	E980.4
Propion gel	976.0	E858.7	E946.0	E950.4	E962.0	E980.4
Propitocaine	968.9	E855.2	E938.9	E950.4	E962.0	E980.4
infiltration (subcutaneous)	968.5	E855.2	E938.5	E950.4	E962.0	E980.4
nerve block (peripheral) (plexus)	968.6	E855.2	E938.6	E950.4	E962.0	E980.4
Propoxur	989.3	E863.2	—	E950.6	E962.1	E980.7

Substance	Poisoning	External Cause (E-Code)				
		Accident	Therapeutic Use	Suicide Attempt	Assault	Undetermined
Propoxycaine	968.9	E855.2	E938.9	E950.4	E962.0	E980.4
infiltration (subcutaneous)	968.5	E855.2	E938.5	E950.4	E962.0	E980.4
nerve block (peripheral) (plexus)	968.6	E855.2	E938.6	E950.4	E962.0	E980.4
topical (surface)	968.5	E855.2	E938.5	E950.4	E962.0	E980.4
Propoxyphene (hydrochloride)	965.8	E850.8	E935.8	E950.0	E962.0	E980.0
Propranolol	972.0	E858.3	E942.0	E950.4	E962.0	E980.4
Propyl						
alcohol	980.3	E860.4	—	E950.9	E962.1	E980.9
carbinol	980.3	E860.4	—	E950.9	E962.1	E980.9
hexadrine	971.2	E855.5	E941.2	E950.4	E962.0	E980.4
iodone	977.8	E858.8	E947.8	E950.4	E962.0	E980.4
thiouracil	962.8	E858.0	E932.8	E950.4	E962.0	E980.4
Propylene	987.1	E869.8	—	E952.8	E962.2	E982.8
Propylparaben (ophthalmic)	976.5	E858.7	E946.5	E950.4	E962.0	E980.4
Proscillaridin	972.1	E858.3	E942.1	E950.4	E962.0	E980.4
Prostaglandins	975.0	E858.6	E945.0	E950.4	E962.0	E980.4
Prostigmin	971.0	E855.3	E941.0	E950.4	E962.0	E980.4
Protamine (sulfate)	964.5	E858.2	E934.5	E950.4	E962.0	E980.4
zinc insulin	962.3	E858.0	E932.3	E950.4	E962.0	E980.4
Protectants (topical)	976.3	E858.7	E946.3	E950.4	E962.0	E980.4
Protein hydrolysate	974.5	E858.5	E944.5	E950.4	E962.0	E980.4
Prothiaden—*see* Dothiepin hydrochloride						
Prothionamide	961.8	E857	E931.8	E950.4	E962.0	E980.4
Prothipendyl	969.5	E853.8	E939.5	E950.3	E962.0	E980.3
Protokylol	971.2	E855.5	E941.2	E950.4	E962.0	E980.4
Protopam	977.2	E858.8	E947.2	E950.4	E962.0	E980.4
Protoveratrine(s) (A) (B)	972.6	E858.3	E942.6	E950.4	E962.0	E980.4
Protriptyline	969.0	E854.0	E939.0	E950.3	E962.0	E980.3
Provera	962.2	E858.0	E932.2	E950.4	E962.0	E980.4
Provitamin A	963.5	E858.1	E933.5	E950.4	E962.0	E980.4
Proxymetacaine	968.5	E855.2	E938.5	E950.4	E962.0	E980.4
Proxyphylline	975.1	E858.6	E945.1	E950.4	E962.0	E980.4
Prozac—*see* Fluoxetine hydrochloride						
Prunus						
laurocerasus	988.2	E865.4	—	E950.9	E962.1	E980.9
virginiana	988.2	E865.4	—	E950.9	E962.1	E980.9
Prussic acid	989.0	E866.8	—	E950.9	E962.1	E980.9
vapor	987.7	E869.8	—	E952.8	E962.2	E982.8
Pseudoephedrine	971.2	E855.5	E941.2	E950.4	E962.0	E980.4
Psilocin	969.6	E854.1	E939.6	E950.3	E962.0	E980.3
Psilocybin	969.6	E854.1	E939.6	E950.3	E962.0	E980.3
PSP	977.8	E858.8	E947.8	E950.4	E962.0	E980.4
Psychedelic agents	969.6	E854.1	E939.6	E950.3	E962.0	E980.3
Psychodysleptics	969.6	E854.1	E939.6	E950.3	E962.0	E980.3
Psychostimulants	969.7	E854.2	E939.7	E950.3	E962.0	E980.3
Psychotherapeutic agents	969.9	E855.9	E939.9	E950.3	E962.0	E980.3
antidepressants	969.0	E854.0	E939.0	E950.3	E962.0	E980.3
specified NEC	969.8	E855.8	E939.8	E950.3	E962.0	E980.3
tranquilizers NEC	969.5	E853.9	E939.5	E950.3	E962.0	E980.3
Psychotomimetic agents	969.6	E854.1	E939.6	E950.3	E962.0	E980.3
Psychotropic agents	969.9	E854.8	E939.9	E950.3	E962.0	E980.3
specified NEC	969.8	E854.8	E939.8	E950.3	E962.0	E980.3
Psyllium	973.3	E858.4	E943.3	E950.4	E962.0	E980.4
Pteroylglutamic acid	964.1	E858.2	E934.1	E950.4	E962.0	E980.4
Pteroyltriglutamate	963.1	E858.1	E933.1	E950.4	E962.0	E980.4
PTFE	987.8	E869.8	—	E952.8	E962.2	E982.8
Pulsatilla	988.2	E865.4	—	E950.9	E962.1	E980.9

Substance	Poisoning	External Cause (E-Code)				
		Accident	Therapeutic Use	Suicide Attempt	Assault	Undetermined
Purex (bleach)	983.9	E864.3	—	E950.7	E962.1	E980.6
Purine diuretics	974.1	E858.5	E944.1	E950.4	E962.0	E980.4
Purinethol	963.1	E858.1	E933.1	E950.4	E962.0	E980.4
PVP	964.8	E858.2	E934.8	E950.4	E962.0	E980.4
Pyrabital	965.7	E850.7	E935.7	E950.0	E962.0	E980.0
Pyramidon	965.5	E850.5	E935.5	E950.0	E962.0	E980.0
Pyrantel (pamoate)	961.6	E857	E931.6	E950.4	E962.0	E980.4
Pyrathiazine	963.0	E858.1	E933.0	E950.4	E962.0	E980.4
Pyrazinamide	961.8	E857	E931.8	E950.4	E962.0	E980.4
Pyrazinoic acid (amide)	961.8	E857	E931.8	E950.4	E962.0	E980.4
Pyrazole (derivatives)	965.5	E850.5	E935.5	E950.0	E962.0	E980.0
Pyrazolone (analgesics)	965.5	E850.5	E935.5	E950.0	E962.0	E980.0
Pyrethrins, pyrethrum	989.4	E863.4	—	E950.6	E962.1	E980.7
Pyribenzamine	963.0	E858.1	E933.0	E950.4	E962.0	E980.4
Pyridine (liquid) (vapor)	982.0	E862.4	—	E950.9	E962.1	E980.9
aldoxime chloride	977.2	E858.8	E947.2	E950.4	E962.0	E980.4
Pyridium	976.1	E858.7	E946.1	E950.4	E962.0	E980.4
Pyridostigmine	971.0	E855.3	E941.0	E950.4	E962.0	E980.4
Pyridoxine	963.5	E858.1	E933.5	E950.4	E962.0	E980.4
Pyrilamine	963.0	E858.1	E933.0	E950.4	E962.0	E980.4
Pyrimethamine	961.4	E857	E931.4	E950.4	E962.0	E980.4
Pyrogallic acid	983.0	E864.0	—	E950.7	E962.1	E980.6
Pyroxylin	976.3	E858.7	E946.3	E950.4	E962.0	E980.4
Pyrrobutamine	963.0	E858.1	E933.0	E950.4	E962.0	E980.4
Pyrrocaine	968.5	E855.2	E938.5	E950.4	E962.0	E980.4
Pyrvinium (pamoate)	961.6	E857	E931.6	E950.4	E962.0	E980.4
PZI	962.3	E858.0	E932.3	E950.4	E962.0	E980.4
Quaalude	967.4	E852.3	E937.4	E950.2	E962.0	E980.2
Quaternary ammonium derivatives	971.1	E855.4	E941.1	E950.4	E962.0	E980.4
Quicklime	983.2	E864.2	—	E950.7	E962.1	E980.6
Quinacrine	961.3	E857	E931.3	E950.4	E962.0	E980.4
Quinaglute	972.0	E858.3	E942.0	E950.4	E962.0	E980.4
Quinalbarbitone	967.0	E851	E937.0	E950.1	E962.0	E980.1
Quinestradiol	962.2	E858.0	E932.2	E950.4	E962.0	E980.4
Quinethazone	974.3	E858.5	E944.3	E950.4	E962.0	E980.4
Quinidine (gluconate) (polygalacturonate) (salts) (sulfate)	972.0	E858.3	E942.0	E950.4	E962.0	E980.4
Quinine	961.4	E857	E931.4	E950.4	E962.0	E980.4
Quiniobine	961.3	E857	E931.3	E950.4	E962.0	E980.4
Quinolines	961.3	E857	E931.3	E950.4	E962.0	E980.4
Quotane	968.5	E855.2	E938.5	E950.4	E962.0	E980.4
Rabies						
immune globulin (human)	964.6	E858.2	E934.6	E950.4	E962.0	E980.4
vaccine	979.1	E858.8	E949.1	E950.4	E962.0	E980.4
Racemoramide	965.09	E850.2	E935.2	E950.0	E962.0	E980.0
Racemorphan	965.09	E850.2	E935.2	E950.0	E962.0	E980.0
Radiator alcohol	980.1	E860.2	—	E950.9	E962.1	E980.9
Radio–opaque (drugs) (materials)	977.8	E858.8	E947.8	E950.4	E962.0	E980.4
Ranunculus	988.2	E865.4	—	E950.9	E962.1	E980.9
Rat poison	989.4	E863.7	—	E950.6	E962.1	E980.7
Rattlesnake (venom)	989.5	E905.0	—	E950.9	E962.1	E980.9
Raudixin	972.6	E858.3	E942.6	E950.4	E962.0	E980.4
Rautensin	972.6	E858.3	E942.6	E950.4	E962.0	E980.4
Rautina	972.6	E858.3	E942.6	E950.4	E962.0	E980.4
Rautotal	972.6	E858.3	E942.6	E950.4	E962.0	E980.4
Rauwiloid	972.6	E858.3	E942.6	E950.4	E962.0	E980.4
Rauwoldin	972.6	E858.3	E942.6	E950.4	E962.0	E980.4

Substance	Poisoning	External Cause (E-Code)				
		Accident	Therapeutic Use	Suicide Attempt	Assault	Undetermined
Rauwolfia (alkaloids)	972.6	E858.3	E942.6	E950.4	E962.0	E980.4
Realgar	985.1	E866.3	—	E950.8	E962.1	E980.8
Red cells, packed	964.7	E858.2	E934.7	E950.4	E962.0	E980.4
Reducing agents, industrial NEC	983.9	E864.3	—	E950.7	E962.1	E980.6
Refrigerant gas (freon)	987.4	E869.2	—	E952.8	E962.2	E982.8
not freon	987.9	E869.9	—	E952.9	E962.2	E982.9
Regroton	974.4	E858.5	E944.4	E950.4	E962.0	E980.4
Rela	968.0	E855.1	E938.0	E950.4	E962.0	E980.4
Relaxants, skeletal muscle (autonomic)	975.2	E858.6	E945.2	E950.4	E962.0	E980.4
central nervous system	968.0	E855.1	E938.0	E950.4	E962.0	E980.4
Renese	974.3	E858.5	E944.3	E950.4	E962.0	E980.4
Renografin	977.8	E858.8	E947.8	E950.4	E962.0	E980.4
Replacement solutions	974.5	E858.5	E944.5	E950.4	E962.0	E980.4
Rescinnamine	972.6	E858.3	E942.6	E950.4	E962.0	E980.4
Reserpine	972.6	E858.3	E942.6	E950.4	E962.0	E980.4
Resorcin, resorcinol	976.4	E858.7	E946.4	E950.4	E962.0	E980.4
Respaire	975.5	E858.6	E945.5	E950.4	E962.0	E980.4
Respiratory agents NEC	975.8	E858.6	E945.8	E950.4	E962.0	E980.4
Retinoic acid	976.8	E858.7	E946.8	E950.4	E962.0	E980.4
Retinol	963.5	E858.1	E933.5	E950.4	E962.0	E980.4
Rh$_0$ (D) immune globulin (human)	964.6	E858.2	E934.6	E950.4	E962.0	E980.4
Rhodine	965.1	E850.3	E935.3	E950.0	E962.0	E980.0
RhoGAM	964.6	E858.2	E934.6	E950.4	E962.0	E980.4
Riboflavin	963.5	E858.1	E933.5	E950.4	E962.0	E980.4
Ricin	989.89	E866.8	—	E950.9	E962.1	E980.9
Ricinus communis	988.2	E865.3	—	E950.9	E962.1	E980.9
Rickettsial vaccine NEC	979.6	E858.8	E949.6	E950.4	E962.0	E980.4
with viral and bacterial vaccine	979.7	E858.8	E949.7	E950.4	E962.0	E980.4
Rifampin	960.6	E856	E930.6	E950.4	E962.0	E980.4
Rimifon	961.8	E857	E931.8	E950.4	E962.0	E980.4
Ringer's injection (lactated)	974.5	E858.5	E944.5	E950.4	E962.0	E980.4
Ristocetin	960.8	E856	E930.8	E950.4	E962.0	E980.4
Ritalin	969.7	E854.2	E939.7	E950.3	E962.0	E980.3
Roach killers — *see* Pesticides						
Rocky Mountain spotted fever vaccine	979.6	E858.8	E949.6	E950.4	E962.0	E980.4
Rodenticides	989.4	E863.7	—	E950.6	E962.1	E980.7
Rohypnol	969.4	E853.2	E939.4	E950.3	E962.0	E980.3
Rolaids	973.0	E858.4	E943.0	E950.4	E962.0	E980.4
Rolitetracycline	960.4	E856	E930.4	E950.4	E962.0	E980.4
Romilar	975.4	E858.6	E945.4	E950.4	E962.0	E980.4
Rose water ointment	976.3	E858.7	E946.3	E950.4	E962.0	E980.4
Rotenone	989.4	E863.7	—	E950.6	E962.1	E980.7
Rotoxamine	963.0	E858.1	E933.0	E950.4	E962.0	E980.4
Rough–on–rats	989.4	E863.7	—	E950.6	E962.1	E980.7
Rubbing alcohol	980.2	E860.3	—	E950.9	E962.1	E980.9
Rubella virus vaccine	979.4	E858.8	E949.4	E950.4	E962.0	E980.4
Rubelogen	979.4	E858.8	E949.4	E950.4	E962.0	E980.4
Rubeovax	979.4	E858.8	E949.4	E950.4	E962.0	E980.4
Rubidomycin	960.7	E856	E930.7	E950.4	E962.0	E980.4
Rue	988.2	E865.4	—	E950.9	E962.1	E980.9
RU486	962.9	E858.0	E932.9	E950.4	E962.0	E980.4
Ruta	988.2	E865.4	—	E950.9	E962.1	E980.9
Sabadilla (medicinal)	976.0	E858.7	E946.0	E950.4	E962.0	E980.4
pesticide	989.4	E863.4	—	E950.6	E962.1	E980.7
Sabin oral vaccine	979.5	E858.8	E949.5	E950.4	E962.0	E980.4
Saccharated iron oxide	964.0	E858.2	E934.0	E950.4	E962.0	E980.4
Saccharin	974.5	E858.5	E944.5	E950.4	E962.0	E980.4

Substance	Poisoning	External Cause (E-Code)				
		Accident	Therapeutic Use	Suicide Attempt	Assault	Undetermined
Safflower oil	972.2	E858.3	E942.2	E950.4	E962.0	E980.4
Salbutamol sulfate	975.7	E858.6	E945.7	E950.4	E962.0	E980.4
Salicylamide	965.1	E850.3	E935.3	E950.0	E962.0	E980.0
Salicylate(s)	965.1	E850.3	E935.3	E950.0	E962.0	E980.0
methyl	976.3	E858.7	E946.3	E950.4	E962.0	E980.4
theobromine calcium	974.1	E858.5	E944.1	E950.4	E962.0	E980.4
Salicylazosulfapyridine	961.0	E857	E931.0	E950.4	E962.0	E980.4
Salicylhydroxamic acid	976.0	E858.7	E946.0	E950.4	E962.0	E980.4
Salicylic acid (keratolytic) NEC	976.4	E858.7	E946.4	E950.4	E962.0	E980.4
congeners	965.1	E850.3	E935.3	E950.0	E962.0	E980.0
salts	965.1	E850.3	E935.3	E950.0	E962.0	E980.0
Saliniazid	961.8	E857	E931.8	E950.4	E962.0	E980.4
Salol	976.3	E858.7	E946.3	E950.4	E962.0	E980.4
Salt (substitute) NEC	974.5	E858.5	E944.5	E950.4	E962.0	E980.4
Saluretics	974.3	E858.5	E944.3	E950.4	E962.0	E980.4
Saluron	974.3	E858.5	E944.3	E950.4	E962.0	E980.4
Salvarsan 606 (neosilver) (silver)	961.1	E857	E931.1	E950.4	E962.0	E980.4
Sambucus canadensis	988.2	E865.4	—	E950.9	E962.1	E980.9
berry	988.2	E865.3	—	E950.9	E962.1	E980.9
Sandril	972.6	E858.3	E942.6	E950.4	E962.0	E980.4
Sanguinaria canadensis	988.2	E865.4	—	E950.9	E962.1	E980.9
Saniflush (cleaner)	983.9	E861.3	—	E950.7	E962.1	E980.6
Santonin	961.6	E857	E931.6	E950.4	E962.0	E980.4
Santyl	976.8	E858.7	E946.8	E950.4	E962.0	E980.4
Sarkomycin	960.7	E856	E930.7	E950.4	E962.0	E980.4
Saroten	969.0	E854.0	E939.0	E950.3	E962.0	E980.3
Saturnine – *see* Lead						
Savin (oil)	976.4	E858.7	E946.4	E950.4	E962.0	E980.4
Scammony	973.1	E858.4	E943.1	E950.4	E962.0	E980.4
Scarlet red	976.8	E858.7	E946.8	E950.4	E962.0	E980.4
Scheele's green	985.1	E866.3	—	E950.8	E962.1	E980.8
insecticide	985.1	E863.4	—	E950.8	E962.1	E980.8
Schradan	989.3	E863.1	—	E950.6	E962.1	E980.7
Schweinfurt (h) green	985.1	E866.3	—	E950.8	E962.1	E980.8
insecticide	985.1	E863.4	—	E950.8	E962.1	E980.8
Scilla — *see* Squill						
Sclerosing agents	972.7	E858.3	E942.7	E950.4	E962.0	E980.4
Scopolamine	971.1	E855.4	E941.1	E950.4	E962.0	E980.4
Scouring powder	989.89	E861.3	—	E950.9	E962.1	E980.9
Sea						
anemone (sting)	989.5	E905.6	—	E950.9	E962.1	E980.9
cucumber (sting)	989.5	E905.6	—	E950.9	E962.1	E980.9
snake (bite) (venom)	989.5	E905.0	—	E950.9	E962.1	E980.9
urchin spine (puncture)	989.5	E905.6	—	E950.9	E962.1	E980.9
Secbutabarbital	967.0	E851	E937.0	E950.1	E962.0	E980.1
Secbutabaritone	967.0	E851	E937.0	E950.1	E962.0	E980.1
Secobarbital	967.0	E851	E937.0	E950.1	E962.0	E980.1
Seconal	967.0	E851	E937.0	E950.1	E962.0	E980.1
Secretin	977.8	E858.8	E947.8	E950.4	E962.0	E980.4
Sedatives, nonbarbiturate	967.9	E852.9	E937.9	E950.2	E962.0	E980.2
specified NEC	967.8	E852.8	E937.8	E950.2	E962.0	E980.2
Sedormid	967.8	E852.8	E937.8	E950.2	E962.0	E980.2
Seed (plant)	988.2	E865.3	—	E950.9	E962.1	E980.9
disinfectant or dressing	989.89	E866.5	—	E950.9	E962.1	E980.9
Selenium (fumes) NEC	985.8	E866.4	—	E950.9	E962.1	E980.9
disulfide or sulfide	976.4	E858.7	E946.4	E950.4	E962.0	E980.4
Selsun	976.4	E858.7	E946.4	E950.4	E962.0	E980.4

Substance	Poisoning	External Cause (E-Code)				
		Accident	Therapeutic Use	Suicide Attempt	Assault	Undetermined
Senna	973.1	E858.4	E943.1	E950.4	E962.0	E980.4
Septisol	976.2	E858.7	E946.2	E950.4	E962.0	E980.4
Serax	969.4	E853.2	E939.4	E950.3	E962.0	E980.3
Serenesil	967.8	E852.8	E937.8	E950.2	E962.0	E980.2
Serenium (hydrochloride)	961.9	E857	E931.9	E950.4	E962.0	E980.4
Serepax—*see* Oxazepam						
Sernyl	968.3	E855.1	E938.3	E950.4	E962.0	E980.4
Serotonin	977.8	E858.8	E947.8	E950.4	E962.0	E980.4
Serpasil	972.6	E858.3	E942.6	E950.4	E962.0	E980.4
Sewer gas	987.8	E869.8	—	E952.8	E962.2	E982.8
Shampoo	989.6	E861.0	—	E950.9	E962.1	E980.9
Shellfish, nonbacterial or noxious	988.0	E865.1	—	E950.9	E962.1	E980.9
Silicones NEC	989.83	E866.8	E947.8	E950.9	E962.1	E980.9
Silvadene	976.0	E858.7	E946.0	E950.4	E962.0	E980.4
Silver (compound) (medicinal) NEC	976.0	E858.7	E946.0	E950.4	E962.0	E980.4
anti–infectives	976.0	E858.7	E946.0	E950.4	E962.0	E980.4
arsphenamine	961.1	E857	E931.1	E950.4	E962.0	E980.4
nitrate	976.0	E858.7	E946.0	E950.4	E962.0	E980.4
ophthalmic preparation	976.5	E858.7	E946.5	E950.4	E962.0	E980.4
toughened (keratolytic)	976.4	E858.7	E946.4	E950.4	E962.0	E980.4
nonmedicinal (dust)	985.8	E866.4	—	E950.9	E962.1	E980.9
protein (mild) (strong)	976.0	E858.7	E946.0	E950.4	E962.0	E980.4
salvarsan	961.1	E857	E931.1	E950.4	E962.0	E980.4
Simethicone	973.8	E858.4	E943.8	E950.4	E962.0	E980.4
Sinequan	969.0	E854.0	E939.0	E950.3	E962.0	E980.3
Singoserp	972.6	E858.3	E942.6	E950.4	E962.0	E980.4
Sintrom	964.2	E858.2	E934.2	E950.4	E962.0	E980.4
Sitosterols	972.2	E858.3	E942.2	E950.4	E962.0	E980.4
Skeletal muscle relaxants	975.2	E858.6	E945.2	E950.4	E962.0	E980.4
Skin						
agents (external)	976.9	E858.7	E946.9	E950.4	E962.0	E980.4
specified NEC	976.8	E858.7	E946.8	E950.4	E962.0	E980.4
test antigen	977.8	E858.8	E947.8	E950.4	E962.0	E980.4
Sleep–eze	963.0	E858.1	E933.0	E950.4	E962.0	E980.4
Sleeping draught (drug) (pill) (tablet)	967.9	E852.9	E937.9	E950.2	E962.0	E980.2
Smallpox vaccine	979.0	E858.8	E949.0	E950.4	E962.0	E980.4
Smelter fumes NEC	985.9	E866.4	—	E950.9	E962.1	E980.9
Smog	987.3	E869.1	—	E952.8	E962.2	E982.8
Smoke NEC	987.9	E869.9	—	E952.9	E962.2	E982.9
Smooth muscle relaxant	975.1	E858.6	E945.1	E950.4	E962.0	E980.4
Snail killer	989.4	E863.4	—	E950.6	E962.1	E980.7
Snake (bite) (venom)	989.5	E905.0	—	E950.9	E962.1	E980.9
Snuff	989.89	E866.8	—	E950.9	E962.1	E980.9
Soap (powder) (product)	989.6	E861.1	—	E950.9	E962.1	E980.9
medicinal, soft	976.2	E858.7	E946.2	E950.4	E962.0	E980.4
Soda (caustic)	983.2	E864.2	—	E950.7	E962.1	E980.6
bicarb	963.3	E858.1	E933.3	E950.4	E962.0	E980.4
chlorinated — *see* Sodium, hypochlorite						
Sodium						
acetosulfone	961.8	E857	E931.8	E950.4	E962.0	E980.4
acetrizoate	977.8	E858.8	E947.8	E950.4	E962.0	E980.4
amytal	967.0	E851	E937.0	E950.1	E962.0	E980.1
arsenate — *see* Arsenic						
bicarbonate	963.3	E858.1	E933.3	E950.4	E962.0	E980.4
bichromate	983.9	E864.3	—	E950.7	E962.1	E980.6
biphosphate	963.2	E858.1	E933.2	E950.4	E962.0	E980.4
bisulfate	983.9	E864.3	—	E950.7	E962.1	E980.6

Substance	Poisoning	External Cause (E-Code)				
		Accident	Therapeutic Use	Suicide Attempt	Assault	Undetermined
borate (cleanser)	989.6	E861.3	—	E950.9	E962.1	E980.9
bromide NEC	967.3	E852.2	E937.3	E950.2	E962.0	E980.2
cacodylate (nonmedicinal) NEC	978.8	E858.8	E948.8	E950.4	E962.0	E980.4
anti–infective	961.1	E857	E931.1	E950.4	E962.0	E980.4
herbicide	989.4	E863.5	—	E950.6	E962.1	E980.7
calcium edetate	963.8	E858.1	E933.8	E950.4	E962.0	E980.4
carbonate NEC	983.2	E864.2	—	E950.7	E962.1	E980.6
chlorate NEC	983.9	E864.3	—	E950.7	E962.1	E980.6
herbicide	983.9	E863.5	—	E950.7	E962.1	E980.6
chloride NEC	974.5	E858.5	E944.5	E950.4	E962.0	E980.4
chromate	983.9	E864.3	—	E950.7	E962.1	E980.6
citrate	963.3	E858.1	E933.3	E950.4	E962.0	E980.4
cyanide — *see* Cyanide(s)						
cyclamate	974.5	E858.5	E944.5	E950.4	E962.0	E980.4
diatrizoate	977.8	E858.8	E947.8	E950.4	E962.0	E980.4
dibunate	975.4	E858.6	E945.4	E950.4	E962.0	E980.4
dioctyl sulfosuccinate	973.2	E858.4	E943.2	E950.4	E962.0	E980.4
edetate	963.8	E858.1	E933.8	E950.4	E962.0	E980.4
ethacrynate	974.4	E858.5	E944.4	E950.4	E962.0	E980.4
fluoracetate (dust) (rodenticide)	989.4	E863.7	—	E950.6	E962.1	E980.7
fluoride — *see* Fluoride(s)						
free salt	974.5	E858.5	E944.5	E950.4	E962.0	E980.4
glucosulfone	961.8	E857	E931.8	E950.4	E962.0	E980.4
hydroxide	983.2	E864.2	—	E950.7	E962.1	E980.6
hypochlorite (bleach) NEC	983.9	E864.3	—	E950.7	E962.1	E980.6
disinfectant	983.9	E861.4	—	E950.7	E962.1	E980.6
medicinal (anti–infective) (external)	976.0	E858.7	E946.0	E950.4	E962.0	E980.4
vapor	987.8	E869.8	—	E952.8	E962.2	E982.8
hyposulfite	976.0	E858.7	E946.0	E950.4	E962.0	E980.4
indigotindisulfonate	977.8	E858.8	E947.8	E950.4	E962.0	E980.4
iodide	977.8	E858.8	E947.8	E950.4	E962.0	E980.4
iothalamate	977.8	E858.8	E947.8	E950.4	E962.0	E980.4
iron edetate	964.0	E858.2	E934.0	E950.4	E962.0	E980.4
lactate	963.3	E858.1	E933.3	E950.4	E962.0	E980.4
lauryl sulfate	976.2	E858.7	E946.2	E950.4	E962.0	E980.4
L–triiodothyronine	962.7	E858.0	E932.7	E950.4	E962.0	E980.4
metrizoate	977.8	E858.8	E947.8	E950.4	E962.0	E980.4
monofluoracetate (dust) (rodenticide)	989.4	E863.7	—	E950.6	E962.1	E980.7
morrhuate	972.7	E858.3	E942.7	E950.4	E962.0	E980.4
nafcillin	960.0	E856	E930.0	E950.4	E962.0	E980.4
nitrate (oxidizing agent)	983.9	E864.3	—	E950.7	E962.1	E980.6
nitrite (medicinal)	972.4	E858.3	E942.4	E950.4	E962.0	E980.4
nitroferricyanide	972.6	E858.3	E942.6	E950.4	E962.0	E980.4
nitroprusside	972.6	E858.3	E942.6	E950.4	E962.0	E980.4
para–aminohippurate	977.8	E858.8	E947.8	E950.4	E962.0	E980.4
perborate (non-medicinal) NEC	989.89	E866.8	—	E950.9	E962.1	E980.9
medicinal	976.6	E858.7	E946.6	E950.4	E962.0	E980.4
soap	989.6	E861.1	—	E950.9	E962.1	E980.9
percarbonate — *see* Sodium, perborate						
phosphate	973.3	E858.4	E943.3	E950.4	E962.0	E980.4
polystyrene sulfonate	974.5	E858.5	E944.5	E950.4	E962.0	E980.4
propionate	976.0	E858.7	E946.0	E950.4	E962.0	E980.4
psylliate	972.7	E858.3	E942.7	E950.4	E962.0	E980.4
removing resins	974.5	E858.5	E944.5	E950.4	E962.0	E980.4
salicylate	965.1	E850.3	E935.3	E950.0	E962.0	E980.0
sulfate	973.3	E858.4	E943.3	E950.4	E962.0	E980.4
sulfoxone	961.8	E857	E931.8	E950.4	E962.0	E980.4

Substance	Poisoning	External Cause (E-Code)				
		Accident	Therapeutic Use	Suicide Attempt	Assault	Undetermined
tetradecyl sulfate	972.7	E858.3	E942.7	E950.4	E962.0	E980.4
thiopental	968.3	E855.1	E938.3	E950.4	E962.0	E980.4
thiosalicylate	965.1	E850.3	E935.3	E950.0	E962.0	E980.0
thiosulfate	976.0	E858.7	E946.0	E950.4	E962.0	E980.4
tolbutamide	977.8	E858.8	E947.8	E950.4	E962.0	E980.4
tyropanoate	977.8	E858.8	E947.8	E950.4	E962.0	E980.4
valproate	966.3	E855.0	E936.3	E950.4	E962.0	E980.4
Solanine	977.8	E858.8	E947.8	E950.4	E962.0	E980.4
Solanum dulcamara	988.2	E865.4	—	E950.9	E962.1	E980.9
Solapsone	961.8	E857	E931.8	E950.4	E962.0	E980.4
Solasulfone	961.8	E857	E931.8	E950.4	E962.0	E980.4
Soldering fluid	983.1	E864.1	—	E950.7	E962.1	E980.6
Solid substance	989.9	E866.9	—	E950.9	E962.1	E980.9
specified NEC	989.9	E866.8	—	E950.9	E962.1	E980.9
Solvents, industrial	982.8	E862.9	—	E950.9	E962.1	E980.9
naphtha	981	E862.0	—	E950.9	E962.1	E980.9
petroleum	981	E862.0	—	E950.9	E962.1	E980.9
specified NEC	982.8	E862.4	—	E950.9	E962.1	E980.9
Soma	968.0	E855.1	E938.0	E950.4	E962.0	E980.4
Somatotropin	962.4	E858.0	E932.4	E950.4	E962.0	E980.4
Sominex	963.0	E858.1	E933.0	E950.4	E962.0	E980.4
Somnos	967.1	E852.0	E937.1	E950.2	E962.0	E980.2
Somonal	967.0	E851	E937.0	E950.1	E962.0	E980.1
Soneryl	967.0	E851	E937.0	E950.1	E962.0	E980.1
Soothing syrup	977.9	E858.9	E947.9	E950.5	E962.0	E980.5
Sopor	967.4	E852.3	E937.4	E950.2	E962.0	E980.2
Soporific drug	967.9	E852.9	E937.9	E950.2	E962.0	E980.2
specified type NEC	967.8	E852.8	E937.8	E950.2	E962.0	E980.2
Sorbitol NEC	977.4	E858.8	E947.4	E950.4	E962.0	E980.4
Sotradecol	972.7	E858.3	E942.7	E950.4	E962.0	E980.4
Spacoline	975.1	E858.6	E945.1	E950.4	E962.0	E980.4
Spanish fly	976.8	E858.7	E946.8	E950.4	E962.0	E980.4
Sparine	969.1	E853.0	E939.1	E950.3	E962.0	E980.3
Sparteine	975.0	E858.6	E945.0	E950.4	E962.0	E980.4
Spasmolytics	975.1	E858.6	E945.1	E950.4	E962.0	E980.4
anticholinergics	971.1	E855.4	E941.1	E950.4	E962.0	E980.4
Spectinomycin	960.8	E856	E930.8	E950.4	E962.0	E980.4
Speed	969.7	E854.2	E939.7	E950.3	E962.0	E980.3
Spermicides	976.8	E858.7	E946.8	E950.4	E962.0	E980.4
Spider (bite) (venom)	989.5	E905.1	—	E950.9	E962.1	E980.9
antivenin	979.9	E858.8	E949.9	E950.4	E962.0	E980.4
Spigelia (root)	961.6	E857	E931.6	E950.4	E962.0	E980.4
Spiperone	969.2	E853.1	E939.2	E950.3	E962.0	E980.3
Spiramycin	960.3	E856	E930.3	E950.4	E962.0	E980.4
Spirilene	969.5	E853.8	E939.5	E950.3	E962.0	E980.3
Spirit(s) (neutral) NEC	980.0	E860.1	—	E950.9	E962.1	E980.9
beverage	980.0	E860.0	—	E950.9	E962.1	E980.9
industrial	980.9	E860.9	—	E950.9	E962.1	E980.9
mineral	981	E862.0	—	E950.9	E962.1	E980.9
of salt — *see* Hydrochloric acid						
surgical	980.9	E860.9	—	E950.9	E962.1	E980.9
Spironolactone	974.4	E858.5	E944.4	E950.4	E962.0	E980.4
Sponge, absorbable (gelatin)	964.5	E858.2	E934.5	E950.4	E962.0	E980.4
Sporostacin	976.0	E858.7	E946.0	E950.4	E962.0	E980.4
Sprays (aerosol)	989.89	E866.8	—	E950.9	E962.1	E980.9
cosmetic	989.89	E866.7	—	E950.9	E962.1	E980.9
medicinal NEC	977.9	E858.9	E947.9	E950.5	E962.0	E980.5

Substance	Poisoning	External Cause (E-Code)				
		Accident	Therapeutic Use	Suicide Attempt	Assault	Undetermined
pesticides — *see* Pesticides						
specified content — *see* substance						
specified						
Spurge flax	988.2	E865.4	—	E950.9	E962.1	E980.9
Spurges	988.2	E865.4	—	E950.9	E962.1	E980.9
Squill (expectorant) NEC	975.5	E858.6	E945.5	E950.4	E962.0	E980.4
rat poison	989.4	E863.7	—	E950.6	E962.1	E980.7
Squirting cucumber (cathartic)	973.1	E858.4	E943.1	E950.4	E962.0	E980.4
Stains	989.89	E866.8	—	E950.9	E962.1	E980.9
Stannous — *see also* Tin						
fluoride	976.7	E858.7	E946.7	E950.4	E962.0	E980.4
Stanolone	962.1	E858.0	E932.1	E950.4	E962.0	E980.4
Stanozolol	962.1	E853.0	E932.1	E950.4	E962.0	E980.4
Staphisagria or stavesacre (pediculicide)	976.0	E858.7	E946.0	E950.4	E962.0	E980.4
Stelazine	969.1	E853.0	E939.1	E950.3	E962.0	E980.3
Stemetil	969.1	E853.0	E939.1	E950.3	E962.0	E980.3
Sterculia (cathartic) (gum)	973.3	E858.4	E943.3	E950.4	E962.0	E980.4
Sternutator gas	987.8	E869.8	—	E952.8	E962.2	E982.8
Steroids NEC	962.0	E858.0	E932.0	E950.4	E962.0	E980.4
ENT agent	976.6	E858.7	E946.6	E950.4	E962.0	E980.4
ophthalmic preparation	976.5	E858.7	E946.5	E950.4	E962.0	E980.4
topical NEC	976.0	E858.7	E946.0	E950.4	E962.0	E980.4
Stibine	985.8	E866.4	—	E950.9	E962.1	E980.9
Stibophen	961.2	E857	E931.2	E950.4	E962.0	E980.4
Stilbamide, stilbamidine	961.5	E857	E931.5	E950.4	E962.0	E980.4
Stilbestrol	962.2	E858.0	E932.2	E950.4	E962.0	E980.4
Stimulants (central nervous system)	970.9	E854.3	E940.9	E950.4	E962.0	E980.4
analeptics	970.0	E854.3	E940.0	E950.4	E962.0	E980.4
opiate antagonist	970.1	E854.3	E940.1	E950.4	E962.0	E980.4
psychotherapeutic NEC	969.0	E854.0	E939.0	E950.3	E962.0	E980.3
specified NEC	970.8	E854.3	E940.8	E950.4	E962.0	E980.4
Storage batteries (acid) (cells)	983.1	E864.1	—	E950.7	E962.1	E980.6
Stovaine	968.9	E855.2	E938.9	E950.4	E962.0	E980.4
infiltration (subcutaneous)	968.5	E855.2	E938.5	E950.4	E962.0	E980.4
nerve block (peripheral) (plexus)	968.6	E855.2	E938.6	E950.5	E962.0	E980.4
spinal	968.7	E855.2	E938.7	E950.4	E962.0	E980.4
topical (surface)	968.5	E855.2	E938.5	E950.4	E962.0	E980.4
Stovarsal	961.1	E857	E931.1	E950.4	E962.0	E980.4
Stove gas — *see* Gas, utility						
Stoxil	976.5	E858.7	E946.5	E950.4	E962.0	E980.4
STP	969.6	E854.1	E939.6	E950.3	E962.0	E980.3
Stramonium (medicinal) NEC	971.1	E855.4	E941.1	E950.4	E962.0	E980.4
natural state	988.2	E865.4	—	E950.9	E962.1	E980.9
Streptodornase	964.4	E858.2	E934.4	E950.4	E962.0	E980.4
Streptoduocin	960.6	E856	E930.6	E950.4	E962.0	E980.4
Streptokinase	964.4	E858.2	E934.4	E950.4	E962.0	E980.4
Streptomycin	960.6	E856	E930.6	E950.4	E962.0	E980.4
Streptozocin	960.7	E856	E930.7	E950.4	E962.0	E980.4
Stripper (paint) (solvent)	982.8	E862.9	—	E950.9	E962.1	E980.9
Strobane	989.2	E863.0	—	E950.6	E962.1	E980.7
Strophanthin	972.1	E858.3	E942.1	E950.4	E962.0	E980.4
Strophanthus hispidus or kombe	988.2	E865.4	—	E950.9	E962.1	E980.9
Strychnine (rodenticide) (salts)	989.1	E863.7	—	E950.6	E962.1	E980.7
medicinal NEC	970.8	E854.3	E940.8	E950.4	E962.0	E980.4
Strychnos (ignatii) — *see* Strychnine						
Styramate	968.0	E855.1	E938.0	E950.4	E962.0	E980.4
Styrene	983.0	E864.0	—	E950.7	E962.1	E980.6

Substance	Poisoning	Accident	Therapeutic Use	Suicide Attempt	Assault	Undetermined
			External Cause (E-Code)			
Succinimide (anticonvulsant)	966.2	E855.0	E936.2	E950.4	E962.0	E980.4
mercuric — *see* Mercury						
Succinylcholine	975.2	E858.6	E945.2	E950.4	E962.0	E980.4
Succinylsulfathiazole	961.0	E857	E931.0	E950.4	E962.0	E980.4
Sucrose	974.5	E858.5	E944.5	E950.4	E962.0	E980.4
Sulfacetamide	961.0	E857	E931.0	E950.4	E962.0	E980.4
ophthalmic preparation	976.5	E858.7	E946.5	E950.4	E962.0	E980.4
Sulfachlorpyridazine	961.0	E857	E931.0	E950.4	E962.0	E980.4
Sulfacytine	961.0	E857	E931.0	E950.4	E962.0	E980.4
Sulfadiazine	961.0	E857	E931.0	E950.4	E962.0	E980.4
silver (topical)	976.0	E858.7	E946.0	E950.4	E962.0	E980.4
Sulfadimethoxine	961.0	E857	E931.0	E950.4	E962.0	E980.4
Sulfadimidine	961.0	E857	E931.0	E950.4	E962.0	E980.4
Sulfaethidole	961.0	E857	E931.0	E950.4	E962.0	E980.4
Sulfafurazole	961.0	E857	E931.0	E950.4	E962.0	E980.4
Sulfaguanidine	961.0	E857	E931.0	E950.4	E962.0	E980.4
Sulfamerazine	961.0	E857	E931.0	E950.4	E962.0	E980.4
Sulfameter	961.0	E857	E931.0	E950.4	E962.0	E980.4
Sulfamethizole	961.0	E857	E931.0	E950.4	E962.0	E980.4
Sulfamethoxazole	961.0	E857	E931.0	E950.4	E962.0	E980.4
Sulfamethoxydiazine	961.0	E857	E931.0	E950.4	E962.0	E980.4
Sulfamethoxypyridazine	961.0	E857	E931.0	E950.4	E962.0	E980.4
Sulfamethylthiazole	961.0	E857	E931.0	E950.4	E962.0	E980.4
Sulfamylon	976.0	E858.7	E946.0	E950.4	E962.0	E980.4
Sulfan blue (diagnostic dye)	977.8	E858.8	E947.8	E950.4	E962.0	E980.4
Sulfanilamide	961.0	E857	E931.0	E950.4	E962.0	E980.4
Sulfanilylguanidine	961.0	E857	E931.0	E950.4	E962.0	E980.4
Sulfaphenazole	961.0	E857	E931.0	E950.4	E962.0	E980.4
Sulfaphenylthiazole	961.0	E857	E931.0	E950.4	E962.0	E980.4
Sulfaproxyline	961.0	E857	E931.0	E950.4	E962.0	E980.4
Sulfapyridine	961.0	E857	E931.0	E950.4	E962.0	E980.4
Sulfapyrimidine	961.0	E857	E931.0	E950.4	E962.0	E980.4
Sulfarsphenamine	961.1	E857	E931.1	E950.4	E962.0	E980.4
Sulfasalazine	961.0	E857	E931.0	E950.4	E962.0	E980.4
Sulfasomizole	961.0	E857	E931.0	E950.4	E962.0	E980.4
Sulfasuxidine	961.0	E857	E931.0	E950.4	E962.0	E980.4
Sulfinpyrazone	974.7	E858.5	E944.7	E950.4	E962.0	E980.4
Sulfisoxazole	961.0	E857	E931.0	E950.4	E962.0	E980.4
ophthalmic preparation	976.5	E858.7	E946.5	E950.4	E962.0	E980.4
Sulfomyxin	960.8	E856	E930.8	E950.4	E962.0	E980.4
Sulfonal	967.8	E852.8	E937.8	E950.2	E962.0	E980.2
Sulfonamides (mixtures)	961.0	E857	E931.0	E950.4	E962.0	E980.4
Sulfones	961.8	E857	E931.8	E950.4	E962.0	E980.4
Sulfonethylmethane	967.8	E852.8	E937.8	E950.2	E962.0	E980.2
Sulfonmethane	967.8	E852.8	E937.8	E950.2	E962.0	E980.2
Sulfonphthal, sulfonphthol	977.8	E858.8	E947.8	E950.4	E962.0	E980.4
Sulfonylurea derivatives, oral	962.3	E858.0	E932.3	E950.4	E962.0	E980.4
Sulfoxone	961.8	E857	E931.8	E950.4	E962.0	E980.4
Sulfur, sulfureted, sulfuric, sulfurous,						
sulfuryl (compounds) NEC	989.89	E866.8	—	E950.9	E962.1	E980.9
acid	983.1	E864.1	—	E950.7	E962.1	E980.6
dioxide	987.3	E869.1	—	E952.8	E962.2	E982.8
ether — *see* Ether(s)						
hydrogen	987.8	E869.8	—	E952.8	E962.2	E982.8
medicinal (keratolytic) (ointment) NEC	976.4	E858.7	E946.4	E950.4	E962.0	E980.4
pesticide (vapor)	989.4	E863.4	—	E950.6	E962.1	E980.7
vapor NEC	987.8	E869.8	—	E952.8	E962.2	E982.8

Substance	Poisoning	External Cause (E-Code)				
		Accident	Therapeutic Use	Suicide Attempt	Assault	Undetermined
Sulkowitch's reagent	977.8	E858.8	E947.8	E950.4	E962.0	E980.4
Sulph — *see also* Sulf–						
Sulphadione	961.8	E857	E931.8	E950.4	E962.0	E980.4
Sulthiame, sultiame	966.3	E855.0	E936.3	E950.4	E962.0	E980.4
Superinone	975.5	E858.6	E945.5	E950.4	E962.0	E980.4
Suramin	961.5	E857	E931.5	E950.4	E962.0	E980.4
Surfacaine	968.5	E855.2	E938.5	E950.4	E962.0	E980.4
Surital	968.3	E855.1	E938.3	E950.4	E962.0	E980.4
Sutilains	976.8	E858.7	E946.8	E950.4	E962.0	E980.4
Suxamethoniam (bromide) (chloride) (iodide)	975.2	E858.6	E945.2	E950.4	E962.0	E980.4
Suxethonium (bromide)	975.2	E858.6	E945.2	E950.4	E962.0	E980.4
Sweet oil (birch)	976.3	E858.7	E946.3	E950.4	E962.0	E980.4
Sym–dichloroethyl ether	982.3	E862.4	—	E950.9	E962.1	E980.9
Sympatholytics	971.3	E855.6	E941.3	E950.4	E962.0	E980.4
Sympathomimetics	971.2	E855.5	E941.2	E950.4	E962.0	E980.4
Synagis	979.6	E858.8	E949.6	E950.4	E962.0	E980.4
Synalar	976.0	E858.7	E946.0	E950.4	E962.0	E980.4
Synthroid	962.7	E858.0	E932.7	E950.4	E962.0	E980.4
Syntocinon	975.0	E858.6	E945.0	E950.4	E962.0	E950.4
Syrosingopine	972.6	E858.3	E942.6	E950.4	E962.0	E980.4
Systemic agents (primarily)	963.9	E858.1	E933.9	E950.4	E962.0	E980.4
specified NEC	963.8	E858.1	E933.8	E950.4	E962.0	E980.4
Tablets (see also specified substance)	977.9	E858.9	E947.9	E950.5	E962.0	E980.5
Tace	962.2	E858.0	E932.2	E950.4	E962.0	E980.4
Tacrine	971.0	E855.3	E941.0	E950.4	E962.0	E980.4
Talbutal	967.0	E851	E937.0	E950.1	E962.0	E980.1
Talc	976.3	E858.7	E946.3	E950.4	E962.0	E980.4
Talcum	976.3	E858.7	E946.3	E950.4	E962.0	E980.4
Tandearil, tanderil	965.5	E850.5	E935.5	E950.0	E962.0	E980.0
Tannic acid	983.1	E864.1	—	E950.7	E962.1	E980.6
medicinal (astringent)	976.2	E858.7	E946.2	E950.4	E962.0	E980.4
Tannin — *see* Tannic acid						
Tansy	988.2	E865.4	—	E950.9	E962.1	E980.9
TAO	960.3	E856	E930.3	E950.4	E962.0	E980.4
Tapazole	962.8	E858.0	E932.8	E950.4	E962.0	E980.4
Tar NEC	983.0	E864.0	—	E950.7	E962.1	E980.6
camphor — *see* Naphthalene						
fumes	987.8	E869.8	—	E952.8	E962.2	E982.8
Taractan	969.3	E853.8	E939.3	E950.3	E962.0	E980.3
Tarantula (venomous)	989.5	E905.1	—	E950.9	E962.1	E980.9
Tartar emetic (anti–infective)	961.2	E857	E931.2	E950.4	E962.0	E980.4
Tartaric acid	983.1	E864.1	—	E950.7	E962.1	E980.6
Tartrated antimony (anti–infective)	961.2	E857	E931.2	E950.4	E962.0	E980.4
TCA *see* Trichloroacetic acid						
TDI	983.0	E864.0	—	E950.7	E962.1	E980.6
vapor	987.8	E869.8	—	E952.8	E962.2	E982.8
Tear gas	987.5	E869.3	—	E952.8	E962.2	E982.8
Teclothiazide	974.3	E858.5	E944.3	E950.4	E962.0	E980.4
Tegretol	966.3	E855.0	E936.3	E950.4	E962.0	E980.4
Telepaque	977.8	E858.8	E947.8	E950.4	E962.0	E980.4
Tellurium	985.8	E866.4	—	E950.9	E962.1	E980.9
fumes	985.8	E866.4	—	E950.9	E962.1	E980.9
TEM	963.1	E858.1	E933.1	E950.4	E962.0	E980.4
Temazepan—*see* Benzodiazepines						
TEPA	963.1	E858.1	E933.1	E950.4	E962.0	E980.4
TEPP	989.3	E863.1	—	E950.6	E962.1	E980.7

Substance	Poisoning	Accident	Therapeutic Use	Suicide Attempt	Assault	Undetermined
			External Cause (E-Code)			
Terbutaline	971.2	E855.5	E941.2	E950.4	E962.0	E980.4
Teroxalene	961.6	E857	E931.6	E950.4	E962.0	E980.4
Terpin hydrate	975.5	E858.6	E945.5	E950.4	E962.0	E980.4
Terramycin	960.4	E856	E930.4	E950.4	E962.0	E980.4
Tessalon	975.4	E858.6	E945.4	E950.4	E962.0	E980.4
Testosterone	962.1	E858.0	E932.1	E950.4	E962.0	E980.4
Tetanus (vaccine)	978.4	E858.8	E948.4	E950.4	E962.0	E980.4
antitoxin	979.9	E858.8	E949.9	E950.4	E962.0	E980.4
immune globulin (human)	964.6	E858.2	E934.6	E950.4	E962.0	E980.4
toxoid	978.4	E858.8	E948.4	E950.4	E962.0	E980.4
with diphtheria toxoid	978.9	E858.8	E948.9	E950.4	E962.0	E980.4
with pertussis	978.6	E858.8	E948.6	E950.4	E962.0	E980.4
Tetrabenazine	969.5	E853.8	E939.5	E950.3	E962.0	E980.3
Tetracaine (infiltration) (topical)	968.5	E855.2	E938.5	E950.4	E962.0	E980.4
nerve block (peripheral) (plexus)	968.6	E855.2	E938.6	E950.4	E962.0	E980.4
spinal	968.7	E855.2	E938.7	E950.4	E962.0	E980.4
Tetrachlorethylene—*see* Tetrachloroethylene						
Tetrachlormethiazide	974.3	E858.5	E944.3	E950.4	E962.0	E980.4
Tetrachloroethane (liquid) (vapor)	982.3	E862.4	—	E950.9	E962.1	E980.9
paint or varnish	982.3	E861.6	—	E950.9	E962.1	E980.9
Tetrachloroethylene (liquid) (vapor)	982.3	E862.4	—	E950.9	E962.1	E980.9
medicinal	961.6	E857	E931.6	E950.4	E962.0	E980.4
Tetrachloromethane — *see* Carbon, tetrachloride						
Tetracycline	960.4	E856	E930.4	E950.4	E962.0	E980.4
ophthalmic preparation	976.5	E858.7	E946.5	E950.4	E962.0	E980.4
topical NEC	976.0	E858.7	E946.0	E950.4	E962.0	E980.4
Tetraethylammonium chloride	972.3	E858.3	E942.3	E950.4	E962.0	E980.4
Tetraethyl lead (antiknock compound)	984.1	E862.1	—	E950.9	E962.1	E980.9
Tetraethyl pyrophosphate	989.3	E863.1	—	E950.6	E962.1	E980.7
Tetraethylthiuram disulfide	977.3	E858.8	E947.3	E950.4	E962.0	E980.4
Tetrahydroaminoacridine	971.0	E855.3	E941.0	E950.4	E962.0	E980.4
Tetrahydrocannabinol	969.6	E854.1	E939.6	E950.3	E962.0	E980.3
Tetrahydronaphthalene	982.0	E862.4	—	E950.9	E962.1	E980.9
Tetrahydrozoline	971.2	E855.5	E941.2	E950.4	E962.0	E980.4
Tetralin	982.0	E862.4	—	E950.9	E962.1	E980.9
Tetramethylthiuram (disulfide) NEC	989.4	E863.6	—	E950.6	E962.1	E980.7
medicinal	976.2	E858.7	E946.2	E950.4	E962.0	E980.4
Tetronal	967.8	E852.8	E937.8	E950.2	E962.0	E980.2
Tetryl	983.0	E864.0	—	E950.7	E962.1	E980.6
Thalidomide	967.8	E852.8	E937.8	E950.2	E962.0	E980.2
Thallium (compounds) (dust) NEC	985.8	E866.4	—	E950.9	E962.1	E980.9
pesticide (rodenticide)	985.8	E863.7	—	E950.6	E962.1	E980.7
THC	969.6	E854.1	E939.6	E950.3	E962.0	E980.3
Thebacon	965.09	E850.2	E935.2	E950.0	E962.0	E980.0
Thebaine	965.09	E850.2	E935.2	E950.0	E962.0	E980.0
Theobromine (calcium salicylate)	974.1	E858.5	E944.1	E950.4	E962.0	E980.4
Theophylline (diuretic)	974.1	E858.5	E944.1	E950.4	E962.0	E980.4
ethylenediamine	975.7	E858.6	E945.7	E950.4	E962.0	E980.4
Thiabendazole	961.6	E857	E931.6	E950.4	E962.0	E980.4
Thialbarbital, thialbarbitone	968.3	E855.1	E938.3	E950.4	E962.0	E980.4
Thiamine	963.5	E858.1	E933.5	E950.4	E962.0	E980.4
Thiamylal (sodium)	968.3	E855.1	E938.3	E950.4	E962.0	E980.4
Thiazesim	969.0	E854.0	E939.0	E950.3	E962.0	E980.3
Thiazides (diuretics)	974.3	E858.5	E944.3	E950.4	E962.0	E980.4
Thiethylperazine	963.0	E858.1	E933.0	E950.4	E962.0	E980.4
Thimerosal (topical)	976.0	E858.7	E946.0	E950.4	E962.0	E980.4

Substance	Poisoning	External Cause (E-Code)				
		Accident	Therapeutic Use	Suicide Attempt	Assault	Undetermined
ophthalmic preparation	976.5	E858.7	E946.5	E950.4	E962.0	E980.4
Thioacetazone	961.8	E857	E931.8	E950.4	E962.0	E980.4
Thiobarbiturates	968.3	E855.1	E938.3	E950.4	E962.0	E980.4
Thiobismol	961.2	E857	E931.2	E950.4	E962.0	E980.4
Thiocarbamide	962.8	E858.0	E932.8	E950.4	E962.0	E980.4
Thiocarbarsone	961.1	E857	E931.1	E950.4	E962.0	E980.4
Thiocarlide	961.8	E857	E931.8	E950.4	E962.0	E980.4
Thioguanine	963.1	E858.1	E933.1	E950.4	E962.0	E980.4
Thiomercaptomerin	974.0	E858.5	E944.0	E950.4	E962.0	E980.4
Thiomerin	974.0	E858.5	E944.0	E950.4	E962.0	E980.4
Thiopental, thiopentone (sodium)	968.3	E855.1	E938.3	E950.4	E962.0	E980.4
Thiopropazate	969.1	E853.0	E939.1	E950.3	E962.0	E980.3
Thioproperazine	969.1	E853.0	E939.1	E950.3	E962.0	E980.3
Thioridazine	969.1	E853.0	E939.1	E950.3	E962.0	E980.3
Thio–TEPA, thiotepa	963.1	E858.1	E933.1	E950.4	E962.0	E980.4
Thiothixene	969.3	E853.8	E939.3	E950.3	E962.0	E980.3
Thiouracil	962.8	E858.0	E932.8	E950.4	E962.0	E980.4
Thiourea	962.8	E858.0	E932.8	E950.4	E962.0	E980.4
Thiphenamil	971.1	E855.4	E941.1	E950.4	E962.0	E980.4
Thiram NEC	989.4	E863.6	—	E950.6	E962.1	E980.7
medicinal	976.2	E858.7	E946.2	E950.4	E962.0	E980.4
Thonzylamine	963.0	E858.1	E933.0	E950.4	E962.0	E980.4
Thorazine	969.1	E853.0	E939.1	E950.3	E962.0	E980.3
Thornapple	988.2	E865.4	—	E950.9	E962.1	E980.9
Throat preparation (lozenges) NEC	976.6	E858.7	E946.6	E950.4	E962.0	E980.4
Thrombin	964.5	E858.2	E934.5	E950.4	E962.0	E980.4
Thrombolysin	964.4	E858.2	E934.4	E950.4	E962.0	E980.4
Thymol	983.0	E864.0	—	E950.7	E962.1	E980.6
Thymus extract	962.9	E858.0	E932.9	E950.4	E962.0	E980.4
Thyroglobulin	962.7	E858.0	E932.7	E950.4	E962.0	E980.4
Thyroid (derivatives) (extract)	962.7	E858.0	E932.7	E950.4	E962.0	E980.4
Thyrolar	962.7	E858.0	E932.7	E950.4	E962.0	E980.4
Thyrothrophin, thyrotropin	977.8	E858.8	E947.8	E950.4	E962.0	E980.4
Thyroxin(e)	962.7	E858.0	E932.7	E950.4	E962.0	E980.4
Tigan	963.0	E858.1	E933.0	E950.4	E962.0	E980.4
Tigloidine	968.0	E855.1	E938.0	E950.4	E962.0	E980.4
Tin (chloride) (dust) (oxide) NEC	985.8	E866.4	—	E950.9	E962.1	E980.9
anti–infectives	961.2	E857	E931.2	E950.4	E962.0	E980.4
Tinactin	976.0	E858.7	E946.0	E950.4	E962.0	E980.4
Tincture, iodine — *see* Iodine						
Tindal	969.1	E853.0	E939.1	E950.3	E962.0	E980.3
Titanium (compounds) (vapor)	985.8	E866.4	—	E950.9	E962.1	E980.9
ointment	976.3	E858.7	E946.3	E950.4	E962.0	E980.4
Titroid	962.7	E858.0	E932.7	E950.4	E962.0	E980.4
TMTD — *see* Tetramethylthiuram disulfide						
TNT	989.89	E866.8	—	E950.9	E962.1	E980.9
fumes	987.8	E869.8	—	E952.8	E962.2	E982.8
Toadstool	988.1	E865.5	—	E950.9	E962.1	E980.9
Tobacco NEC	989.84	E866.8	—	E950.9	E962.1	E980.9
Indian	988.2	E865.4	—	E950.9	E962.1	E980.9
smoke, second-hand	987.8	E869.4	—	—	—	—
Tocopherol	963.5	E858.1	E933.5	E950.4	E962.0	E980.4
Tocosamine	975.0	E858.6	E945.0	E950.4	E962.0	E980.4
Tofranil	969.0	E854.0	E939.0	E950.3	E962.0	E980.3
Toilet deodorizer	989.8	E866.8	—	E950.9	E962.1	E980.9
Tolazamide	962.3	E858.0	E932.3	E950.4	E962.0	E980.4
Tolazoline	971.3	E855.6	E941.3	E950.4	E962.0	E980.4

Substance	Poisoning	External Cause (E-Code)				
		Accident	Therapeutic Use	Suicide Attempt	Assault	Undetermined
Tolbutamide	962.3	E858.0	E932.3	E950.4	E962.0	E980.4
sodium	977.8	E858.8	E947.8	E950.4	E962.0	E980.4
Tolmetin	965.69	E850.6	E935.6	E950.0	E962.0	E980.0
Tolnaftate	976.0	E858.7	E946.0	E950.4	E962.0	E980.4
Tolpropamine	976.1	E858.7	E946.1	E950.4	E962.0	E980.4
Tolserol	968.0	E855.1	E938.0	E950.4	E962.0	E980.4
Toluene (liquid) (vapor)	982.0	E862.4	—	E950.9	E962.1	E980.9
diisocyanate	983.0	E864.0	—	E950.7	E962.1	E980.6
Toluidine	983.0	E864.0	—	E950.7	E962.1	E980.6
vapor	987.8	E869.8	—	E952.8	E962.2	E982.8
Toluol (liquid) (vapor)	982.0	E862.4	—	E950.9	E962.1	E980.9
Tolylene–2,4–diisocyanate	983.0	E864.0	—	E950.7	E962.1	E980.6
Tonics, cardiac	972.1	E858.3	E942.1	E950.4	E962.0	E980.4
Toxaphene (dust) (spray)	989.2	E863.0	—	E950.6	E962.1	E980.7
Toxoids NEC	978.8	E858.8	E948.8	E950.4	E962.0	E980.4
Tractor fuel NEC	981	E862.1	—	E950.9	E962.1	E980.9
Tragacanth	973.3	E858.4	E943.3	E950.4	E962.0	E980.4
Tramazoline	971.2	E855.5	E941.2	E950.4	E962.0	E980.4
Tranquilizers	969.5	E853.9	E939.5	E950.3	E962.0	E980.3
benzodiazepine–based	969.4	E853.2	E939.4	E950.3	E962.0	E980.3
butyrophenone–based	969.2	E853.1	E939.2	E950.3	E962.0	E980.3
major NEC	969.3	E853.8	E939.3	E950.3	E962.0	E980.3
phenothiazine–based	969.1	E853.0	E939.1	E950.3	E962.0	E980.3
specified NEC	969.5	E853.8	E939.5	E950.3	E962.0	E980.3
Trantoin	961.9	E857	E931.9	E950.4	E962.0	E980.4
Tranxene	969.4	E853.2	E939.4	E950.3	E962.0	E980.3
Tranylcypromine (sulfate)	969.0	E854.0	E939.0	E950.3	E962.0	E980.3
Trasentine	975.1	E858.6	E945.1	E950.4	E962.0	E980.4
Travert	974.5	E858.5	E944.5	E950.4	E962.0	E980.4
Trecator	961.8	E857	E931.8	E950.4	E962.0	E980.4
Tretinoin	976.8	E858.7	E946.8	E950.4	E962.0	E980.4
Triacetin	976.0	E858.7	E946.0	E950.4	E962.0	E980.4
Triacetyloleandomycin	960.3	E856	E930.3	E950.4	E962.0	E980.4
Triamcinolone	962.0	E858.0	E932.0	E950.4	E962.0	E980.4
ENT agent	976.6	E858.7	E946.6	E950.4	E962.0	E980.4
ophthalmic preparation	976.5	E858.7	E946.5	E950.4	E962.0	E980.4
topical NEC	976.0	E858.7	E946.0	E950.4	E962.0	E980.4
Triamterene	974.4	E858.5	E944.4	E950.4	E962.0	E980.4
Triaziquone	963.1	E858.1	E933.1	E950.4	E962.0	E980.4
Tribromacetaldehyde	967.3	E852.2	E937.3	E950.2	E962.0	E980.2
Tribromoethanol	968.2	E855.1	E938.2	E950.4	E962.0	E980.4
Tribromomethane	967.3	E852.2	E937.3	E950.2	E962.0	E980.2
Trichlorethane	982.3	E862.4	—	E950.9	E962.1	E980.9
Trichlormethiazide	974.3	E858.5	E944.3	E950.4	E962.0	E980.4
Trichloroacetic acid	983.1	E864.1	—	E950.7	E962.1	E980.6
medicinal (keratolytic)	976.4	E858.7	E946.4	E950.4	E962.0	E980.4
Trichloroethanol	967.1	E852.0	E937.1	E950.2	E962.0	E980.2
Trichloroethylene (liquid) (vapor)	982.3	E862.4	—	E950.9	E962.1	E980.9
anesthetic (gas)	968.2	E855.1	E938.2	E950.4	E962.0	E980.4
Trichloroethyl phosphate	967.1	E852.0	E937.1	E950.2	E962.0	E980.2
Trichlorofluoromethane NEC	987.4	E869.2	—	E952.8	E962.2	E982.8
Trichlorotriethylamine	963.1	E858.1	E933.1	E950.4	E962.0	E980.4
Trichomonacides NEC	961.5	E857	E931.5	E950.4	E962.0	E980.4
Trichomycin	960.1	E856	E930.1	E950.4	E962.0	E980.4
Triclofos	967.1	E852.0	E937.1	E950.2	E962.0	E980.2
Tricresyl phosphate	989.89	E866.8	—	E950.9	E962.1	E980.9
solvent	982.8	E862.4	—	E950.9	E962.1	E980.9

Substance	Poisoning	External Cause (E-Code)				
		Accident	Therapeutic Use	Suicide Attempt	Assault	Undetermined
Tricyclamol	966.4	E855.0	E936.4	E950.4	E962.0	E980.4
Tridesilon	976.0	E858.7	E946.0	E950.4	E962.0	E980.4
Tridihexethyl	971.1	E855.4	E941.1	E950.4	E962.0	E980.4
Tridione	966.0	E855.0	E936.0	E950.4	E962.0	E980.4
Triethanolamine NEC	983.2	E864.2	—	E950.7	E962.1	E980.6
detergent	983.2	E861.0	—	E950.7	E962.1	E980.6
trinitrate	972.4	E858.3	E942.4	E950.4	E962.0	E980.4
Triethanomelamine	963.1	E858.1	E933.1	E950.4	E962.0	E980.4
Triethylene melamine	963.1	E858.1	E933.1	E950.4	E962.0	E980.4
Triethylenephosphoramide	963.1	E858.1	E933.1	E950.4	E962.0	E980.4
Triethylenethiophosphoramide	963.1	E858.1	E933.1	E950.4	E962.0	E980.4
Trifluoperazine	969.1	E853.0	E939.1	E950.3	E962.0	E980.3
Trifluperidol	969.2	E853.1	E939.2	E950.3	E962.0	E980.3
Triflupromazine	969.1	E853.0	E939.1	E950.3	E962.0	E980.3
Trihexyphenidyl	971.1	E855.4	E941.1	E950.4	E962.0	E980.4
Triiodothyronine	962.7	E858.0	E932.7	E950.4	E962.0	E980.4
Trilene	968.2	E855.1	E938.2	E950.4	E962.0	E980.4
Trimeprazine	963.0	E858.1	E933.0	E950.4	E962.0	E980.4
Trimetazidine	972.4	E858.3	E942.4	E950.4	E962.0	E980.4
Trimethadione	966.0	E855.0	E936.0	E950.4	E962.0	E980.4
Trimethaphan	972.3	E858.3	E942.3	E950.4	E962.0	E980.4
Trimethidinium	972.3	E858.3	E942.3	E950.4	E962.0	E980.4
Trimethobenzamide	963.0	E858.1	E933.0	E950.4	E962.0	E980.4
Trimethylcarbinol	980.8	E860.8	—	E950.9	E962.1	E980.9
Trimethylpsoralen	976.3	E858.7	E946.3	E950.4	E962.0	E980.4
Trimeton	963.0	E858.1	E933.0	E950.4	E962.0	E980.4
Trimipramine	969.0	E854.0	E939.0	E950.3	E962.0	E980.3
Trimustine	963.1	E858.1	E933.1	E950.4	E962.0	E980.4
Trinitrin	972.4	E858.3	E942.4	E950.4	E962.0	E980.4
Trinitrophenol	983.0	E864.0	—	E950.7	E962.1	E980.6
Trinitrotoluene	989.89	E866.8	—	E950.9	E962.1	E980.9
fumes	987.8	E869.8	—	E952.8	E962.2	E982.8
Trional	967.8	E852.8	E937.8	E950.2	E962.0	E980.2
Trioxide of arsenic — *see* Arsenic						
Trioxsalen	976.3	E858.7	E946.3	E950.4	E962.0	E980.4
Tripelennamine	963.0	E858.1	E933.0	E950.4	E962.0	E980.4
Triperidol	969.2	E853.1	E939.2	E950.3	E962.0	E980.3
Triprolidine	963.0	E858.1	E933.0	E950.4	E962.0	E980.4
Trisoralen	976.3	E858.7	E946.3	E950.4	E962.0	E980.4
Troleandomycin	960.3	E856	E930.3	E950.4	E962.0	E980.4
Trolnitrate (phosphate)	972.4	E858.3	E942.4	E950.4	E962.0	E980.4
Trometamol	963.3	E858.1	E933.3	E950.4	E962.0	E980.4
Tromethamine	963.3	E858.1	E933.3	E950.4	E962.0	E980.4
Tronothane	968.5	E855.2	E938.5	E950.4	E962.0	E980.4
Tropicamide	971.1	E855.4	E941.1	E950.4	E962.0	E980.4
Troxidone	966.0	E855.0	E936.0	E950.4	E962.0	E980.4
Tryparsamide	961.1	E857	E931.1	E950.4	E962.0	E980.4
Trypsin	963.4	E858.1	E933.4	E950.4	E962.0	E980.4
Tryptizol	969.0	E854.0	E939.0	E950.3	E962.0	E980.3
Tuaminoheptane	971.2	E855.5	E941.2	E950.4	E962.0	E980.4
Tuberculin (old)	977.8	E858.8	E947.8	E950.4	E962.0	E980.4
Tubocurare	975.2	E858.6	E945.2	E950.4	E962.0	E980.4
Tubocurarine	975.2	E858.6	E945.2	E950.4	E962.0	E980.4
Turkish green	969.6	E854.1	E939.6	E950.3	E962.0	E980.3
Turpentine (spirits of) (liquid) (vapor)	982.8	E862.4	—	E950.9	E962.1	E980.9
Tybamate	969.5	E853.8	E939.5	E950.3	E962.0	E980.3
Tyloxapol	975.5	E858.6	E945.5	E950.4	E962.0	E980.4

Substance	Poisoning	External Cause (E-Code)				
		Accident	Therapeutic Use	Suicide Attempt	Assault	Undetermined
Tymazoline	971.2	E855.5	E941.2	E950.4	E962.0	E980.4
Typhoid vaccine	978.1	E858.8	E948.1	E950.4	E962.0	E980.4
Typhus vaccine	979.2	E858.8	E949.2	E950.4	E962.0	E980.4
Tyrothricin	976.0	E858.7	E946.0	E950.4	E962.0	E980.4
ENT agent	976.6	E858.7	E946.6	E950.4	E962.0	E980.4
ophthalmic preparation	976.5	E858.7	E946.5	E950.4	E962.0	E980.4
Undecenoic acid	976.0	E858.7	E946.0	E950.4	E962.0	E980.4
Undecylenic acid	976.0	E858.7	E946.0	E950.4	E962.0	E980.4
Unna's boot	976.3	E858.7	E946.3	E950.4	E962.0	E980.4
Uracil mustard	963.1	E858.1	E933.1	E950.4	E962.0	E980.4
Uramustine	963.1	E858.1	E933.1	E950.4	E962.0	E980.4
Urari	975.2	E858.6	E945.2	E950.4	E962.0	E980.4
Urea	974.4	E858.5	E944.4	E950.4	E962.0	E980.4
topical	976.8	E858.7	E946.8	E950.4	E962.0	E980.4
Urethan(e) (antineoplastic)	963.1	E858.1	E933.1	E950.4	E962.0	E980.4
Urginea (maritima) (scilla) — *see* Squill						
Uric acid metabolism agents NEC	974.7	E858.5	E944.7	E950.4	E962.0	E980.4
Urokinase	964.4	E858.2	E934.4	E950.4	E962.0	E980.4
Urokon	977.8	E858.8	E947.8	E950.4	E962.0	E980.4
Urotropin	961.9	E857	E931.9	E950.4	E962.0	E980.4
Urtica	988.2	E865.4	—	E950.9	E962.1	E980.9
Utility gas — *see* Gas, utility						
Vaccine NEC	979.9	E858.8	E949.9	E950.4	E962.0	E980.4
bacterial NEC	978.8	E858.8	E948.8	E950.4	E962.0	E980.4
with						
other bacterial component	978.9	E858.8	E948.9	E950.4	E962.0	E980.4
pertussis component	978.6	E858.8	E948.6	E950.4	E962.0	E980.4
viral–rickettsial component	979.7	E858.8	E949.7	E950.4	E962.0	E980.4
mixed NEC	978.9	E858.8	E948.9	E950.4	E962.0	E980.4
BCG	978.0	E858.8	E948.0	E950.4	E962.0	E980.4
cholera	978.2	E858.8	E948.2	E950.4	E962.0	E980.4
diphtheria	978.5	E858.8	E948.5	E950.4	E962.0	E980.4
influenza	979.6	E858.8	E949.6	E950.4	E962.0	E980.4
measles	979.4	E858.8	E949.4	E950.4	E962.0	E980.4
meningococcal	978.8	E858.8	E948.8	E950.4	E962.0	E980.4
mumps	979.6	E858.8	E949.6	E950.4	E962.0	E980.4
paratyphoid	978.1	E858.8	E948.1	E950.4	E962.0	E980.4
pertussis (with diphtheria toxoid) (with tetanus toxoid)	978.6	E858.8	E948.6	E950.4	E962.0	E980.4
plague	978.3	E858.8	E948.3	E950.4	E962.0	E980.4
poliomyelitis	979.5	E858.8	E949.5	E950.4	E962.0	E980.4
poliovirus	979.5	E858.8	E949.5	E950.4	E962.0	E980.4
rabies	979.1	E858.8	E949.1	E950.4	E962.0	E980.4
respiratory syncytial virus	979.6	E858.8	E949.6	E950.4	E962.0	E980.4
rickettsial NEC	979.6	E858.8	E949.6	E950.4	E962.0	E980.4
with						
bacterial component	979.7	E858.8	E949.7	E950.4	E962.0	E980.4
pertussis component	978.6	E858.8	E948.6	E950.4	E962.0	E980.4
viral component	979.7	E858.8	E949.7	E950.4	E962.0	E980.4
Rocky mountain spotted fever	979.6	E858.8	E949.6	E950.4	E962.0	E980.4
rotavirus	979.6	E858.8	E949.6	E950.4	E962.0	E980.4
rubella virus	979.4	E858.8	E949.4	E950.4	E962.0	E980.4
sabin oral	979.5	E858.8	E949.5	E950.4	E962.0	E980.4
smallpox	979.0	E858.8	E949.0	E950.4	E962.0	E980.4
tetanus	978.4	E858.8	E948.4	E950.4	E962.0	E980.4
typhoid	978.1	E858.8	E948.1	E950.4	E962.0	E980.4
typhus	979.2	E858.8	E949.2	E950.4	E962.0	E980.4

Substance	Poisoning	Accident	Therapeutic Use	Suicide Attempt	Assault	Undetermined
viral NEC	979.6	E858.8	E949.6	E950.4	E962.0	E980.4
with						
bacterial component	979.7	E858.8	E949.7	E950.4	E962.0	E980.4
pertussis component	978.6	E858.8	E948.6	E950.4	E962.0	E980.4
rickettsial component	979.7	E858.8	E949.7	E950.4	E962.0	E980.4
yellow fever	979.3	E858.8	E949.3	E950.4	E962.0	E980.4
Vaccinia immune globulin (human)	964.6	E858.2	E934.6	E950.4	E962.0	E980.4
Vaginal contraceptives	976.8	E858.7	E946.8	E950.4	E962.0	E980.4
Valethamate	971.1	E855.4	E941.1	E950.4	E962.0	E980.4
Valisone	976.0	E858.7	E946.0	E950.4	E962.0	E980.4
Valium	969.4	E853.2	E939.4	E950.3	E962.0	E980.3
Valmid	967.8	E852.8	E937.8	E950.2	E962.0	E980.2
Vanadium	985.8	E866.4	—	E950.9	E962.1	E980.9
Vancomycin	960.8	E856	E930.8	E950.4	E962.0	E980.4
Vapor (*see also* Gas)	987.9	E869.9	—	E952.9	E962.2	E982.9
kiln (carbon monoxide)	986	E868.8	—	E952.1	E962.2	E982.1
lead — *see* Lead						
specified source NEC (*see also* specific substance)	987.8	E869.8	—	E952.8	E962.2	E982.8
Varidase	964.4	E858.2	E934.4	E950.4	E962.0	E980.4
Varnish	989.89	E861.6	—	E950.9	E962.1	E980.9
cleaner	982.8	E862.9	—	E950.9	E962.1	E980.9
Vaseline	976.3	E858.7	E946.3	E950.4	E962.0	E980.4
Vasodilan	972.5	E858.3	E942.5	E950.4	E962.0	E980.4
Vasodilators NEC	972.5	E858.3	E942.5	E950.4	E962.0	E980.0
coronary	972.4	E858.3	E942.4	E950.4	E962.0	E980.4
Vasopressin	962.5	E858.0	E932.5	E950.4	E962.0	E980.4
Vasopressor drugs	962.5	E858.0	E932.5	E950.4	E962.0	E980.4
Venom, venomous (bite) (sting)	989.5	E905.9	—	E950.9	E962.1	E980.9
arthropod NEC	989.5	E905.5	—	E950.9	E962.1	E980.9
bee	989.5	E905.3	—	E950.9	E962.1	E980.9
centipede	989.5	E905.4	—	E950.9	E962.1	E980.9
hornet	989.5	E905.3	—	E950.9	E962.1	E980.9
lizard	989.5	E905.0	—	E950.9	E962.1	E980.9
marine animals or plants	989.5	E905.6	—	E950.9	E962.1	E980.9
millipede (topical)	989.5	E905.4	—	E950.9	E962.1	E980.9
plant NEC	989.5	E905.7	—	E950.9	E962.1	E980.9
marine	989.5	E905.6	—	E950.9	E962.1	E980.9
scorpion	989.5	E905.2	—	E950.9	E962.1	E980.9
snake	989.5	E905.0	—	E950.9	E962.1	E980.9
specified NEC	989.5	E905.8	—	E950.9	E962.1	E980.9
spider	989.5	E905.1	—	E950.9	E962.1	E980.9
wasp	989.5	E905.3	—	E950.9	E962.1	E980.9
Ventolin—*see* Salbutamol sulfate						
Veramon	967.0	E851	E937.0	E950.1	E962.0	E980.1
Veratrum						
album	988.2	E865.4	—	E950.9	E962.1	E980.9
alkaloids	972.6	E858.3	E942.6	E950.4	E962.0	E980.4
viride	988.2	E865.4	—	E950.9	E962.1	E980.9
Verdigris (*see also* Copper)	985.8	E866.4	—	E950.9	E962.1	E980.9
Veronal	967.0	E851	E937.0	E950.1	E962.0	E980.1
Veroxil	961.6	E857	E931.6	E950.4	E962.0	E980.4
Versidyne	965.7	E850.7	E935.7	E950.0	E962.0	E980.0
Viagra	972.5	E858.3	E942.5	E950.4	E962.0	E980.4
Vienna						
green	985.1	E866.3	—	E950.8	E962.1	E980.8
insecticide	985.1	E863.4	—	E950.6	E962.1	E980.7

Substance	Poisoning	External Cause (E-Code)				
		Accident	Therapeutic Use	Suicide Attempt	Assault	Undetermined
red	989.89	E866.8	—	E950.9	E962.1	E980.9
pharmaceutical dye	977.4	E858.8	E947.4	E950.4	E962.0	E980.4
Vinbarbital, vinbarbitone	967.0	E851	E937.0	E950.1	E962.0	E980.1
Vinblastine	963.1	E858.1	E933.1	E950.4	E962.0	E980.4
Vincristine	963.1	E858.1	E933.1	E950.4	E962.0	E980.4
Vinesthene, vinethene	968.2	E855.1	E938.2	E950.4	E962.0	E980.4
Vinyl						
bital	967.0	E851	E937.0	E950.1	E962.0	E980.1
ether	968.2	E855.1	E938.2	E950.4	E962.0	E980.4
Vioform	961.3	E857	E931.3	E950.4	E962.0	E980.4
topical	976.0	E858.7	E946.0	E950.4	E962.0	E980.4
Viomycin	960.6	E856	E930.6	E950.4	E962.0	E980.4
Viosterol	963.5	E858.1	E933.5	E950.4	E962.0	E980.4
Viper (venom)	989.5	E905.0	—	E950.9	E962.1	E980.9
Viprynium (embonate)	961.6	E857	E931.6	E950.4	E962.0	E980.4
Virugon	961.7	E857	E931.7	E950.4	E962.0	E980.4
Visine	976.5	E858.7	E946.5	E950.4	E962.0	E980.4
Vitamins NEC	963.5	E858.1	E933.5	E950.4	E962.0	E980.4
B_{12}	964.1	E858.2	E934.1	E950.4	E962.0	E980.4
hematopoietic	964.1	E858.2	E934.1	E950.4	E962.0	E980.4
K	964.3	E858.2	E934.3	E950.4	E962.0	E980.4
Vleminckx's solution	976.4	E858.7	E946.4	E950.4	E962.0	E980.4
Voltaren—*see* Diclofenac sodium						
Warfarin (potassium) (sodium)	964.2	E858.2	E934.2	E950.4	E962.0	E980.4
rodenticide	989.4	E863.7	—	E950.6	E962.1	E980.7
Wasp (sting)	989.5	E905.3	—	E950.9	E962.1	E980.9
Water						
balance agents NEC	974.5	E858.5	E944.5	E950.4	E962.0	E980.4
gas	987.1	E868.1	—	E951.8	E962.2	E981.8
incomplete combustion of — *see* Carbon, monoxide, fuel, utility						
hemlock	988.2	E865.4	—	E950.9	E962.1	E980.9
moccasin (venom)	989.5	E905.0	—	E950.9	E962.1	E980.9
Wax (paraffin) (petroleum)	981	E862.3	—	E950.9	E962.1	E980.9
automobile	989.89	E861.2	—	E950.9	E962.1	E980.9
floor	981	E862.0	—	E950.9	E962.1	E980.9
Weed killers NEC	989.4	E863.5	—	E950.6	E962.1	E980.7
Welldorm	967.1	E852.0	E937.1	E950.2	E962.0	E980.2
White						
arsenic — *see* Arsenic						
hellebore	988.2	E865.4	—	E950.9	E962.1	E980.9
lotion (keratolytic)	976.4	E858.7	E946.4	E950.4	E962.0	E980.4
spirit	981	E862.0	—	E950.9	E962.1	E980.9
Whitewashes	989.89	E861.6	—	E950.9	E962.1	E980.9
Whole blood	964.7	E858.2	E934.7	E950.4	E962.0	E980.4
Wild						
black cherry	988.2	E865.4	—	E950.9	E962.1	E980.9
poisonous plants NEC	988.2	E865.4	—	E950.9	E962.1	E980.9
Window cleaning fluid	989.89	E861.3	—	E950.9	E962.1	E980.9
Wintergreen (oil)	976.3	E858.7	E946.3	E950.4	E962.0	E980.4
Witch hazel	976.2	E858.7	E946.2	E950.4	E962.0	E980.4
Wood						
alcohol	980.1	E860.2	—	E950.9	E962.1	E980.9
spirit	980.1	E860.2	—	E950.9	E962.1	E980.9
Woorali	975.2	E858.6	E945.2	E950.4	E962.0	E980.4
Wormseed, American	961.6	E857	E931.6	E950.4	E962.0	E980.4
Xanthine diuretics	974.1	E858.5	E944.1	E950.4	E962.0	E980.4

Substance	Poisoning	External Cause (E-Code)				
		Accident	Therapeutic Use	Suicide Attempt	Assault	Undetermined
Xanthocillin	960.0	E856	E930.0	E950.4	E962.0	E980.4
Xanthotoxin	976.3	E858.7	E946.3	E950.4	E962.0	E980.4
Xylene (liquid) (vapor)	982.0	E862.4	—	E950.9	E962.1	E980.9
Xylocaine (infiltration) (topical)	968.5	E855.2	E938.5	E950.4	E962.0	E980.4
nerve block (peripheral) (plexus)	968.6	E855.2	E938.6	E950.4	E962.0	E980.4
spinal	968.7	E855.2	E938.7	E950.4	E962.0	E980.4
Xylol (liquid) (vapor)	982.0	E862.4	—	E950.9	E962.1	E980.9
Xylometazoline	971.2	E855.5	E941.2	E950.4	E962.0	E980.4
Yellow						
fever vaccine	979.3	E858.8	E949.3	E950.4	E962.0	E980.4
jasmine	988.2	E865.4	—	E950.9	E962.1	E980.9
Yew	988.2	E865.4	—	E950.9	E962.1	E980.9
Zactane	965.7	E850.7	E935.7	E950.0	E962.0	E980.0
Zaroxolyn	974.3	E858.5	E944.3	E950.4	E962.0	E980.4
Zephiran (topical)	976.0	E858.7	E946.0	E950.4	E962.0	E980.4
ophthalmic preparation	976.5	E858.7	E946.5	E950.4	E962.0	E980.4
Zerone	980.1	E860.2	—	E950.9	E962.1	E980.9
Zinc (compounds) (fumes) (salts)						
(vapor) NEC	985.8	E866.4	—	E950.9	E962.1	E980.9
anti–infectives	976.0	E858.7	E946.0	E950.4	E962.0	E980.4
antivaricose	972.7	E858.3	E942.7	E950.4	E962.0	E980.4
bacitracin	976.0	E858.7	E946.0	E950.4	E962.0	E980.4
chloride	976.2	E858.7	E946.2	E950.4	E962.0	E980.4
gelatin	976.3	E858.7	E946.3	E950.4	E962.0	E980.4
oxide	976.3	E858.7	E946.3	E950.4	E962.0	E980.4
peroxide	976.0	E858.7	E946.0	E950.4	E962.0	E980.4
pesticides	985.8	E863.4	—	E950.6	E962.1	E980.7
phosphide (rodenticide)	985.8	E863.7	—	E950.6	E962.1	E980.7
stearate	976.3	E858.7	E946.3	E950.4	E962.0	E980.4
sulfate (antivaricose)	972.7	E858.3	E942.7	E950.4	E962.0	E980.4
ENT agent	976.6	E858.7	E946.6	E950.4	E962.0	E980.4
ophthalmic solution	976.5	E858.7	E946.5	E950.4	E962.0	E980.4
topical NEC	976.0	E858.7	E946.0	E950.4	E962.0	E980.4
undecylenate	976.0	E858.7	E946.0	E950.4	E962.0	E980.4
Zoxazolamine	968.0	E855.1	E938.0	E950.4	E962.0	E980.4
Zygadenus (venenosus)	988.2	E865.4	—	E950.9	E962.1	E980.9

Substance	Poisoning	External Cause (E-Code)				
		Accident	Therapeutic Use	Suicide Attempt	Assault	Undetermined

SECTION 3

ALPHABETIC INDEX TO EXTERNAL CAUSES
OF INJURY AND POISONING (E CODE)

This section contains the index to the codes which classify environmental events, circumstances, and other conditions as the cause of injury and other adverse effects. Where a code from the section Supplementary Classification of External Causes of Injury and Poisoning (E800-E998) is applicable, it is intended that the E code shall be used in addition to a code form the main body of the classification, Chapters 1-17.

The alphabetic index to the E codes is organized by main terms which describe the *accident, circumstance, event,* or specific *agent* which caused the injury or other adverse effect.

> *Note—Transport accidents (E800-E848) include accidents involving:*
>   *aircraft and space craft (E840-E845)*
>   *watercraft (E830-E838)*
>   *motor vehicle (E810-E825)*
>   *railway (E800-E807)*
>   *other road vehicles (E826-E829)*
>
> *For definitions and examples related to transport accidents—see Volume 1, pages 571-585.*
>
> *The fourth-digit subdivisions for use with categories E800-E848 to identify the injured person are found on pages 1447-1451.*
>
> *For identifying the place in which an accident or poisoning occurred (circumstances classifiable to categories E850-E869 and E880-E928)—. see the listing in this section under "Accident, occurring."*

See the Table of Drugs and Chemicals (Section 2 of this volume) for identifying the specific agent involved in drug overdose or a wrong substance given or taken in error, and for intoxication or poisoning by a drug or other chemical substance.

The specific adverse effect, reaction, or localized toxic effect to a correct drug or substance properly administered in therapeutic or prophylactic dosage should be classified according to the nature of the adverse effect (e.g.: allergy, dermatitis, tachycardia) listed in Section 1 of this volume.

A

Assault—*continued*
  chemical from swallowing caustic,
    corrosive substance NEC E962.1
  hot liquid E968.3
  scalding E968.3
  vitriol E961
    swallowed E962.1
  caustic, corrosive substance E961
    swallowed E962.1
  cut, any part of body E966
  dagger E966
  drowning E964
  explosive(s) E965.9
    bomb (*see also* Assault, bomb) E965.8
    dynamite E965.8
  fight (hand) (fists) (foot) E960.0
    with weapon E968.9
      blunt or thrown E968.2
      cutting or piercing E966
      firearm—*see* Shooting, homicide
  fire E968.0
  firearm(s)—*see* Shooting, homicide
  garrotting E963
  gunshot (wound)—*see* Shooting, homicide
  hanging E963
  injury NEC E968.9
  knife E966
  late effect of E969
  ligature E963
  poisoning E962.9
    drugs or medicinals E962.0
    gas(es) or vapors, except drugs and
      medicinals E962.2
    solid or liquid substances, except drugs
      and medicinals E962.1
  puncture, any part of body E966
  pushing
    before moving object, train, vehicle
      E968.5
    from high place E968.1
  rape E960.1
  scalding E968.3
  shooting—*see* Shooting, homicide
  sodomy E960.1
  stab, any part of body E966
  strangulation E963
  submersion E964
  suffocation E963
  transport vehicle E968.5
  violence NEC E968.9
  vitriol E961
    swallowed E962.1
  weapon E968.9
    blunt or thrown E968.2
    cutting or piercing E966
    firearm—*see* Shooting, homicide
  wound E968.9
    cutting E966
    gunshot—*see* Shooting, homicide
    knife E966
    piercing E966
    puncture E966
    stab E966
Attack by animal NEC E906.9
Avalanche E909.2
  falling on or hitting
    motor vehicle (in motion) (on public
      highway) E909.2
    railway train E909.2
Aviators' disease E902.1

B

**Barotitis, barodontalgia, barosinusitis,
  barotrauma** (otitic) (sinus)—*see* Effects of,
  air pressure
Battered
  baby or child (syndrome)—*see* Abuse, child;
    category E967
  person other than baby or child—*see* Assault
Bayonet wound (*see also* Cut, by bayonet)
  E920.3
  in
    legal intervention E974
    terrorism E979.8
    war operations E995
Bean in nose E912
Bed set on fire NEC E898.0
Beheading (by guillotine)
  homicide E966
  legal execution E978
Bending, injury in E927
Bends E902.0
Bite
  animal (nonvenomous) NEC E906.5
    venomous NEC E905.9
  arthropod (nonvenomous) NEC E906.4
    venomous—*see* Sting
  black widow spider E905.1
  cat E906.3
  centipede E905.4
  cobra E905.0
  copperhead snake E905.0
  coral snake E905.0
  dog E906.0
  fer de lance E905.0
  gila monster E905.0
  human being
    accidental E928.3
    assault E968.7
  insect (nonvenomous) E906.4
    venomous—*see* Sting
  krait E905.0
  late effect of—*see* Late effect
  lizard E906.2
    venomous E905.0
  mamba E905.0
  marine animal
    nonvenomous E906.3
      snake E906.2
    venomous E905.6
      snake E905.0
  millipede E906.4
    venomous E905.4
  moray eel E906.3
  rat E906.1
  rattlesnake E905.0
  rodent, except rat E906.3
  serpent—*see* Bite, snake
  shark E906.3
  snake (venomous) E905.0
    nonvenomous E906.2
    sea E905.0
  spider E905.1
    nonvenomous E906.4
  tarantula (venomous) E905.1
  venomous NEC E905.9
    by specific animal—*see* category E905
  viper E905.0
  water moccasin E905.0

Burning, burns—*continued*
  internal, from swallowed caustic, corrosive liquid, substance—*see* Table of drugs and chemicals
  lamp (*see also* Fire, specified NEC) E898.1
  late effect of NEC E929.4
  lighter (cigar) (cigarette) (*see also* Fire, specified NEC) E898.1
  lightning E907
  liquid (boiling) (hot) (molten) E924.0
    caustic, corrosive (external) E924.1
      swallowed—*see* Table of drugs and chemicals
  local application of externally applied substance in medical or surgical care E873.5
  machinery—*see* Accident, machine
  matches (*see also* Fire, specified NEC) E898.1
  medicament, externally applied E873.5
  metal, molten E924.0
  object (hot) E924.8
    producing fire or flames—*see* Fire
  oven (electric) (gas) E924.8
  pipe (smoking) (*see also* Fire, specified NEC) E898.1
  radiation—*see* Radiation
  railway engine, locomotive, train (*see also* Explosion, railway engine) E803
  self-inflicted (unspecified whether accidental or intentional) E988.1
    caustic or corrosive substance NEC E988.7
    stated as intentional, purposeful E958.1
      caustic or corrosive substance NEC E958.7
  stated as undetermined whether accidental or intentional E988.1
    caustic or corrosive substance NEC E988.7
  steam E924.0
    pipe E924.8
  substance (hot) E924.9
    boiling or molten E924.0
    caustic, corrosive (external) E924.1
      swallowed—*see* Table of drugs and chemicals
  suicidal (attempt) NEC E958.1
    caustic substance E958.7
    late effect of E959
  tanning bed E926.2
  therapeutic misadventure
    overdose of radiation E873.2
  torch, welding (*see also* Fire, specified NEC) E898.1
  trash fire (*see also* Burning, bonfire) E897
  vapor E924.0
  vitriol E924.1
  x-rays E926.3
    in medical, surgical procedure—*see* Misadventure, failure, in dosage, radiation
Butted by animal E906.8

C

Cachexia, lead or saturnine E866.0
  from pesticide NEC (*see also* Table of drugs and chemicals) E863.4
Caisson disease E902.2
Capital punishment (any means) E978
Car sickness E903

Casualty (not due to war) NEC E928.9
  terrorism E979.8
  war (*see also* War operations) E995
Cat
  bite E906.3
  scratch E906.8
Cataclysmic (any injury)
  earth surface movement or eruption E909.9
    specified type NEC E909.8
  storm or flood resulting from storm E908.9
    specified type NEC E909.8
Catching fire —*see* Ignition
Caught
  between
    objects (moving) (stationary and moving) E918
    and machinery—*see* Accident, machine
  by cable car, not on rails E847
  in
    machinery (moving parts of)—*see* Accident, machine
    object E918
Cave-in (causing asphyxia, suffocation (by pressure)) (*see also* Suffocation, due to, cave-in) E913.3
  with injury other than asphyxia or suffocation E916
    with asphyxia or suffocation (*see also* Suffocation, due to, cave-in) E913.3
  struck or crushed by E916
    with asphyxia or suffocation (*see also* Suffocation, due to, cave-in) E913.3
Change(s) in air pressure—*see also* Effects of, air pressure
  sudden, in aircraft (ascent) (descent) (causing aeroneurosis or aviators' disease) E902.1
Chilblains E901.0
  due to manmade conditions E901.1
Choking (on) (any object except food or vomitus) E912
  apple E911
  bone E911
  food, any type (regurgitated) E911
  mucus or phlegm E912
  seed E911
Civil insurrection —*see* War operations
Cloudburst E908.8
Cold, exposure to (accidental) (excessive) (extreme) (place) E901.9
  causing chilblains or immersion foot E901.0
  due to
    manmade conditions E901.1
    specified cause NEC E901.8
    weather (conditions) E901.0
  late effect of NEC E929.5
  self-inflicted (undetermined whether accidental or intentional) E988.3
    suicidal E958.3
  suicide E958.3
Colic, lead, painters', or saturnine —*see* category E866
Collapse
  building E916 (movable)
    burning (uncontrolled fire) E891.8
      in terrorism E979.3
      private E890.8
  dam E909.3
  due to heat—*see* Heat
  machinery—*see* Accident, machine
  man-made structure E909.3
  postoperative NEC E878.9

Collapse—*continued*
  structure, burning NEC E891.8
    burning (uncontrolled fire)
      in terrorism E979.3
Collision (accidental)

> *Note—In the case of collisions between different types of vehicles, persons and objects, priority in classification is in the following order:*
>
> > *Aircraft*
> > *Watercraft*
> > *Motor vehicle*
> > *Railway vehicle*
> > *Pedal Cycle*
> > *Animal-drawn vehicle*
> > *Animal being ridden*
> > *Streetcar or other nonmotor road vehicle*
> > *Other vehicle*
> > *Pedestrian or person using pedestrian*
> >   *conveyance*
> > *Object (except where falling from or set in*
> >   *motion by vehicle etc. listed above)*
>
> *In the listing below, the combinations are listed only under the vehicle etc. having priority. For definitions, see Volume 1, page 477.*

  aircraft (with object or vehicle) (fixed)
    (movable) (moving) E841
    with
      person (while landing, taking off) (without
        accident to aircraft) E844
      powered (in transit) (with unpowered
        aircraft) E841
      while landing, taking off E840
      unpowered E842
      while landing, taking off E840
  animal being ridden (in sport or transport)
    E828
    and
      animal (being ridden) (herded)
        (unattended) E828
      nonmotor road vehicle, except pedal cycle
        or animal-drawn vehicle E828
      object (fallen) (fixed) (movable) (moving)
        not falling from or set in motion by
        vehicle of higher priority E828
      pedestrian (conveyance or vehicle) E828
  animal-drawn vehicle E827
    and
      animal (being ridden) (herded)
        (unattended) E827
      nonmotor road vehicle, except pedal cycle
        E827
      object (fallen) (fixed) (movable) (moving)
        not falling from or set in motion by
        vehicle of higher priority E827
      pedestrian (conveyance or vehicle) E827
      streetcar E827
  motor vehicle (on public highway) (traffic
    accident) E812
    after leaving, running off, public highway
      (without antecedent collision) (without
      re-entry) E816
    with antecedent collision on public
      highway—*see* categories E810-E815
    with re-entrance collision with another
      motor vehicle E811
    and
      abutment (bridge) (overpass) E815
      animal (herded) (unattended) E815

Collision—*continued*
    carrying person, property E813
  animal-drawn vehicle E813
  another motor vehicle (abandoned)
    (disabled) (parked) (stalled) (stopped)
    E812
    with, involving re-entrance (on same
      roadway) (across median strip) E811
  any object, person, or vehicle off the
    public highway resulting from a
    noncollision motor vehicle nontraffic
    accident E816
  avalanche, fallen or not moving E815
    falling E909
  boundary fence E815
  culvert E815
  fallen
    stone E815
    tree E815
  falling E909.2
  guard post or guard rail E815
  inter-highway divider E815
  landslide, fallen or not moving E815
    moving E909
  machinery (road) E815
  moving E909.2
  nonmotor road vehicle NEC E813
  object (any object, person, or vehicle off
    the public highway resulting from a
    noncollision motor vehicle nontraffic
    accident) E815
    off, normally not on, public highway
      resulting from a noncollision motor
      vehicle traffic accident E816
  pedal cycle E813
  pedestrian (conveyance) E814
  person (using pedestrian conveyance) E814
  post or pole (lamp) (light) (signal)
    (telephone) (utility) E815
  railway rolling stock, train, vehicle E810
  safety island E815
  street car E813
  traffic signal, sign, or marker (temporary)
    E815
  tree E815
  tricycle E813
  wall of cut made for road E815
  due to cataclysm—*see* categories E908,
    E909
  not on public highway, nontraffic accident
    E822
    and
      animal (carrying person, property)
        (herded) (unattended) E822
      animal-drawn vehicle E822
      another motor vehicle (moving), except
        off-road motor vehicle E822
        stationary E823
      avalanche, fallen, not moving E823
        moving E909
      landslide, fallen, not moving E823
        moving E909
      nonmotor vehicle (moving) E822
        stationary E823
      object (fallen) (normally) (fixed)
        (movable but not in motion)
        (stationary) E823
        moving, except when falling from, set
          in motion by, aircraft or cataclysm
          E822
      pedal cycle (moving) E822

Collision—*continued*

object (fallen) (fixed) (movable)
(moving) not falling from or set in
motion by aircraft, animal-drawn
vehicle, animal being ridden,
motor vehicle, nonmotor road
vehicle, pedal cycle, railway train,
or streetcar E848
road, except animal being ridden,
animal-drawn vehicle, or pedal cycle
E829
and
animal, herded, not being ridden,
unattended E829
another nonmotor road vehicle, except
animal being ridden, animal-drawn
vehicle, or pedal cycle E829
object (fallen) (fixed) (movable)
(moving) not falling from or set in
motion by, aircraft, animal-drawn
vehicle, animal being ridden,
motor vehicle, pedal cycle, or
railway train E829
pedestrian (conveyance) E829
person (using pedestrian conveyance)
E829
vehicle, nonmotor, nonroad E829
watercraft E838
and
person swimming or water skiing E838
causing
drowning, submersion E830
injury except drowning, submersion E831
Combustion, spontaneous —*see* Ignition
**Complication of medical or surgical
procedure or treatment**
as an abnormal reaction—*see* Reaction,
abnormal
delayed, without mention of
misadventure—*see* Reaction, abnormal
due to misadventure—*see* Misadventure
Compression
divers' squeeze E902.2
trachea by
food E911
foreign body, except food E912
Conflagration
building or structure, except private dwelling
(barn) (church) (convalescent or
residential home) (factory) (farm
outbuilding) (hospital) (hotel) (institution)
(educational) (dormitory) (residential)
(school) (shop) (store) (theatre) E891.9
with or causing (injury due to)
accident or injury NEC E891.9
specified circumstance NEC E891.8
burns, burning E891.3
carbon monoxide E891.2
fumes E891.2
polyvinylchloride (PVC) or similar
material E891.1
smoke E891.2
causing explosion E891.0
in terrorism E979.3
not in building or structure E892
private dwelling (apartment) (boarding house)
(camping place) (caravan) (farmhouse)
(home (private)) (house) (lodging house)
(private garage) (rooming house)
(tenement) E890.9

Conflagration—*continued*

with or causing (injury due to)
accident or injury NEC E890.9
specified circumstance NEC E890.8
burns, burning E890.3
carbon monoxide E890.2
fumes E890.2
polyvinylchloride (PVC) or similar
material E890.1
smoke E890.2
causing explosion E890.0
Contact with
dry ice E901.1
liquid air, hydrogen, nitrogen E901.1
Cramp(s)
Heat—*see* Heat
swimmers (*see also* category E910) E910.2
not in recreation or sport E910.3
Cranking (car) (truck) (bus) (engine), injury
by E917.9
Crash
aircraft (in transit) (powered) E841
at landing, take-off E840
in
terrorism E979.1
war operations E994
on runway NEC E840
stated as
homicidal E968.8
suicidal E958.6
undetermined whether accidental or
intentional E988.6
unpowered E842
glider E842
motor vehicle—*see also* Accident, motor
vehicle
homicidal E968.5
suicidal E958.5
undetermined whether accidental or
intentional E988.5
Crushed (accidentally) E928.9
between
boat(s), ship(s), watercraft (and dock or
pier) (without accident to watercraft)
E838
after accident to, or collision, watercraft
E831
objects (moving) (stationary and moving)
E918
by
avalanche NEC E909.2
boat, ship, watercraft after accident to,
collision, watercraft E831
cave-in E916
with asphyxiation or suffocation (*see also*
Suffocation, due to, cave-in) E913.3
crowd, human stampede E917.1
falling
aircraft (*see also* Accident, aircraft) E841
in
terrorism E979.1
war operations E994
earth, material E916
with asphyxiation or suffocation (*see
also* Suffocation, due to, cave-in)
E913.3
object E916
on ship, watercraft E838
while loading, unloading watercraft E838
landslide NEC E909.2
lifeboat after abandoning ship E831

Descent—*continued*
    due to accident to aircraft—*see* categories
      E840-E842
Desertion
  child, with intent to injure or kill E968.4
  helpless person, infant, newborn E904.0
    with intent to injure or kill E968.4
Destitution —*see* Privation
Disability, late effect or sequela of injury
    —*see* Late effect
Disease
  Andes E902.0
  aviators' E902.1
  caisson E902.2
  range E902.0
Divers' disease, palsy, paralysis, squeeze
    E902.0
Dog bite E906.0
Dragged by
  cable car (not on rails) E847
    on rails E829
  motor vehicle (on highway) E814
    not on highway, nontraffic accident E825
  street car E829
Drinking poison (accidental) —*see* Table of
  drugs and chemicals
Drowning —*see* Submersion
Dust in eye E914

E

Earth falling (on) (with asphyxia or
    suffocation (by pressure)) (*see also*
    Suffocation, due to, cave-in) E913.3
  as, or due to, a cataclysm (involving any
    transport vehicle)—*see* categories E908,
    E909
  not due to cataclysmic action E913.3
    motor vehicle (in motion) (on public
      highway) E818
      not on public highway E825
    nonmotor road vehicle NEC E829
    pedal cycle E826
    railway rolling stock, train, vehicle E806
    street car E829
    struck or crushed by E916
      with asphyxiation or suffocation E913.3
      with injury other than asphyxia,
        suffocation E916
Earthquake (any injury) E909.0
Effect(s) (adverse) of
  air pressure E902.9
    at high altitude E902.9
      in aircraft E902.1
      residence or prolonged visit (causing
        conditions classifiable to E902.0)
        E902.0
    due to
      diving E902.2
      specified cause NEC E902.8
    in aircraft E902.1
  cold, excessive (exposure to) (*see also* Cold,
    exposure to) E901.9
  heat (excessive) (*see also* Heat) E900.9
  hot
    place—*see* Heat
    weather E900.0
  insulation—*see* Heat
  late—*see* Late effect of
  motion E903

Effect(s) (adverse) of—*continued*
  nuclear explosion or weapon
    in
      terrorism E979.5
      war operations (blast) (fireball) (heat)
        (radiation) (direct) (secondary) E996
  radiation—*see* Radiation
  terrorism, secondary E979.9
  travel E903
Electric shock, electrocution (accidental)
    (from exposed wire, faulty appliance, high
    voltage cable, live rail, open socket) (by)
    (in) E925.9
  appliance or wiring
    domestic E925.0
    factory E925.2
    farm (building) E925.8
      house E925.0
    home E925.0
    industrial (conductor) (control apparatus)
      (transformer) E925.2
    outdoors E925.8
    public building E925.8
    residential institution E925.8
    school E925.8
    specified place NEC E925.8
  caused by other person
    stated as
      intentional, homicidal E968.8
      undetermined whether accidental or
        intentional E988.4
  electric power generating plant, distribution
    station E925.1
  homicidal (attempt) E968.8
  legal execution E978
  lightning E907
  machinery E925.9
    domestic E925.0
    factory E925.2
    farm E925.8
    home E925.0
  misadventure in medical or surgical procedure
    in electroshock therapy E873.4
  self-inflicted (undetermined whether
    accidental or intentional) E988.4
    stated as intentional E958.4
  stated as undetermined whether accidental or
    intentional E988.4
  suicidal (attempt) E958.4
  transmission line E925.1
Electrocution —*see* Electric shock
Embolism
  air (traumatic) NEC—*see* Air, embolism
Encephalitis
  lead or saturnine E866.0
    from pesticide NEC E863.4
Entanglement
  in
    bedclothes, causing suffocation E913.0
    wheel of pedal cycle E826
Entry of foreign body, material, any —*see*
  Foreign body
Execution, legal (any method) E978
Exhaustion
  cold—*see* Cold, exposure to
  due to excessive exertion E927
  heat—*see* Heat
Explosion (accidental) (in) (of) (on) E923.9
  acetylene E923.2
  aerosol can E921.8

Exposure (weather) (conditions) (rain) (wind)
E904.3
with homicidal intent E968.4
excessive E904.3
cold (*see also* Cold, exposure to) E901.9
self-inflicted—*see* Cold, exposure to,
self-inflicted
heat (*see also* Heat) E900.9
fire—*see* Fire
helpless person, infant, newborn due to
abandonment or neglect E904.0
noise E928.1
prolonged in deep-freeze unit or refrigerator
E901.1
radiation—*see* Radiation
resulting from transport accident—*see*
categories E800-E848
smoke from, due to
fire —*see* Fire
tobacco, second-hand E869.4
vibration E928.2

F

Fall, falling (accidental) E888.9
building E916
burning E891.8
private E890.8
down
escalator E880.0
ladder E881.0
in boat, ship, watercraft E833
staircase E880.9
stairs, steps—*see* Fall, from, stairs
earth (with asphyxia or suffocation (by
pressure)) (*see also* Earth, falling) E913.3
from, off
aircraft (at landing, take-off) (in-transit)
(while alighting, boarding) E843
resulting from accident to aircraft—*see*
categories E840-E842
animal (in sport or transport) E828
animal-drawn vehicle E827
balcony E882
bed E884.4
bicycle E826
boat, ship, watercraft (into water) E832
after accident to, collision, fire on E830
and subsequently struck by (part of)
boat E831
and subsequently struck by (part of) boat
E838
burning, crushed, sinking E830
and subsequently struck by (part of)
boat E831
bridge E882
building E882
burning (uncontrolled fire) E891.8
in terrorism E979.3
private E890.8
bunk in boat, ship, watercraft E834
due to accident to watercraft E831
cable car (not on rails) E847
on rails E829
car—*see* Fall from motor vehicle
chair E884.2
cliff E884.1
commode E884.6
curb (sidewalk) E880.1
elevation aboard ship E834

Fall, falling—*continued*
due to accident to ship E831
embankment E884.9
escalator E880.0
fire escape E882
flagpole E882
furniture NEC E884.5
gangplank (into water) (*see also* Fall,
from, boat) E832
to deck, dock E834
hammock on ship E834
due to accident to watercraft E831
haystack E884.9
high place NEC E884.9
stated as undetermined whether accidental
or intentional—*see* Jumping, from,
high place
horse (in sport or transport) E828
in-line skates E885.1
ladder E881.0
in boat, ship, watercraft E833
due to accident to watercraft E831
machinery—*see also* accident, machine
not in operation E884.9
motor vehicle (in motion) (on public
highway) E818
not on public highway E825
stationary, except while alighting,
boarding, entering, leaving E884.9
while alighting, boarding, entering,
leaving E824
stationary, except while alighting,
boarding, entering, leaving E884.9
while alighting, boarding, entering,
leaving, except off-road type motor
vehicle E817
off-road type—*see* Fall, from, off-road
type motor vehicle
nonmotor road vehicle (while alighting,
boarding) NEC E829
stationary, except while alighting,
boarding, entering, leaving E884.9
off road type motor vehicle (not on
public highway) NEC E821
on public highway E818
while alighting, boarding, entering,
leaving E817
snow vehicle—*see* Fall from snow
vehicle, motor-driven
one
deck to another on ship E834
due to accident to ship E831
level to another NEC E884.9
boat, ship, or watercraft E834
due to accident to watercraft E831
pedal cycle E826
playground equipment E884.0
railway rolling stock, train, vehicle (while
alighting, boarding) E804
with
collision (*see also* Collision, railway)
E800
derailment (*see also* Derailment,
railway) E802
explosion (*see also* Explosion, railway
engine) E803
rigging (aboard ship) E834
due to accident to watercraft E831
roller skates E885.1
scaffolding E881.1
scooter (nonmotorized) E885.0

Foreign body, object or material—*continued*
  nose (with asphyxia, obstruction,
     suffocation) E912
    causing injury without asphyxia,
      obstruction, suffocation E915
  alimentary canal (causing injury) (with
    obstruction) E915
  with asphyxia, obstruction respiratory
    passage, suffocation E912
    food E911
  mouth E915
    with asphyxia, obstruction, suffocation
     E912
     food E911
  pharynx E915
    with asphyxia, obstruction, suffocation
     E912
     food E911
  aspiration (with asphyxia, obstruction
    respiratory passage, suffocation) E912
    causing injury without asphyxia,
      obstruction respiratory passage,
      suffocation E915
    food (regurgitated) (vomited) E911
     causing injury without asphyxia,
       obstruction respiratory passage,
       suffocation E915
    mucus (not of newborn) E912
    phlegm E912
  bladder (causing injury or obstruction) E915
  bronchus, bronchi—*see* Foreign body, air
    passages
  conjunctival sac E914
  digestive system—*see* Foreign body,
    alimentary canal
  ear (causing injury or obstruction) E915
  esophagus (causing injury or obstruction) (*see
    also* Foreign body, alimentary canal) E915
  eye (any part) E914
  eyelid E914
  hairball (stomach) (with obstruction) E915
  ingestion—*see* Foreign body, alimentary canal
  inhalation—*see* Foreign body, aspiration
  intestine (causing injury or obstruction) E915
  iris E914
  lacrimal apparatus E914
  larynx—*see* Foreign body, air passage
  late effect of NEC E929.8
  lung—*see* Foreign body, air passage
  mouth—*see* Foreign body, alimentary canal,
    mouth
  nasal passage—*see* Foreign body, air passage,
    nose
  nose—*see* Foreign body, air passage, nose
  ocular muscle E914
  operation wound (left in)—*see* Misadventure,
    foreign object
  orbit E914
  pharynx—*see* Foreign body, alimentary canal,
    pharynx
  rectum (causing injury or obstruction) E915
  stomach (hairball) (causing injury or
    obstruction) E915
  tear ducts or glands E914
  trachea—*see* Foreign body, air passage
  urethra (causing injury or obstruction) E915
  vagina (causing injury or obstruction) E915
Found dead, injured
  from exposure (to)—*see* Exposure
  on
    public highway E819
    railway right of way E807

Fracture (circumstances unknown or
  unspecified) E887
  due to specified external means—*see* manner
    of accident
  late effect of NEC E929.3
  occurring in water transport NEC E835
Freezing —*see* Cold, exposure to
Frostbite E901.0
  due to manmade conditions E901.1
Frozen —*see* Cold, exposure to

G

Garrotting, homicidal (attempted) E963
Gored E906.8
Gunshot wound (*see also* Shooting) E922.9

H

Hailstones, injury by E904.3
Hairball (stomach) (with obstruction) E915
Hanged himself (*see also* Hanging,
  self-inflicted) E983.0
Hang gliding E842
Hanging (accidental) E913.8
  caused by other person
    in accidental circumstances E913.8
    stated as
      intentional, homicidal E963
      undetermined whether accidental or
        intentional E983.0
  homicide (attempt) E963
  in bed or cradle E913.0
  legal execution E978
  self-inflicted (unspecified whether accidental
    or intentional) E983.0
    in accidental circumstances E913.8
    stated as intentional, purposeful E953.0
  stated as undetermined whether accidental or
    intentional E983.0
  suicidal (attempt) E953.0
Heat (apoplexy) (collapse) (cramps) (effects of)
  (excessive) (exhaustion) (fever) (prostration)
  (stroke) E900.9
  due to
    manmade conditions (listed in E900.1,
      except boat, ship, watercraft) E900.1
    weather (conditions) E900.0
  from
    electric heating apparatus causing burning
      E924.8
    nuclear explosion
     in
      terrorism E979.5
      war operations E996
  generated in, boiler, engine, evaporator, fire
    room of boat, ship, watercraft E838
  inappropriate in local application or packing
    in medical or surgical procedure E873.5
  late effect of NEC E989
Hemorrhage
  delayed following medical or surgical
    treatment without mention of
     misadventure—*see* Reaction, abnormal
  during medical or surgical treatment as
    misadventure—*see* Misadventure, cut
High
  altitude, effects E902.9
  level of radioactivity, effects—*see* Radiation

I

Ictus
caloris—*see* Heat
solaris E900.0
Ignition (accidental)
anesthetic gas in operating theatre E923.2
bedclothes
with
conflagration—*see* Conflagration
ignition (of)
clothing—*see* Ignition, clothes
highly inflammable material (benzine)
(fat) (gasoline) (kerosene) (paraffin)
(petrol) E894
benzine E894
clothes, clothing (from controlled fire) (in
building) E893.9
with conflagration—*see* Conflagration
from
bonfire E893.2
highly inflammable material E894
sources or material as listed in E893.8
trash fire E893.2
uncontrolled fire—*see* Conflagration
in
private dwelling E893.0
specified building or structure, except
private dwelling E893.1
not in building or structure E893.2
explosive material—*see* Explosion
fat E894
gasoline E894
kerosene E894
material
explosive—*see* Explosion
highly inflammable E894
with conflagration—*see* Conflagration
with explosion E923.2
nightdress—*see* Ignition, clothes
paraffin E894
petrol E894
Immersion —*see* Submersion
Implantation of quills of porcupine E906.8
Inanition (from) E904.9
hunger—*see* Lack of, food
resulting from homicidal intent E968.4
thirst—*see* Lack of, water
Inattention after, at birth E904.0
homicidal, infanticidal intent E968.4
Infanticide (*see also* Assault)
Ingestion
foreign body (causing injury) (with
obstruction)—*see* Foreign body,
alimentary canal
poisonous substance NEC—*see* Table of
drugs and chemicals
Inhalation
excessively cold substance, manmade E901.1
foreign body—*see* Foreign body, aspiration
liquid air, hydrogen, nitrogen E901.1
mucus, not of newborn (with asphyxia,
obstruction respiratory passage,
suffocation) E912
phlegm (with asphyxia, obstruction respiratory
passage, suffocation) E912
poisonous gas—*see* Table of drugs and
chemicals
smoke from, due to
fire —*see* Fire

Inhalation—*continued*
tobacco, second-hand E869.4
vomitus (with asphyxia, obstruction
respiratory passage, suffocation) E911
Injury, injured (accidental(ly)) NEC E928.9
by, caused by, from
air rifle (B-B gun) E922.4
animal (not being ridden) NEC E906.9
being ridden (in sport or transport) E828
assault (*see also* Assault) E968.9
avalanche E909.2
bayonet (*see also* Bayonet wound) E920.3
being thrown against some part of, or
object in
motor vehicle (in motion) (on public
highway) E818
not on public highway E825
nonmotor road vehicle NEC E829
off-road motor vehicle NEC E821
railway train E806
snow vehicle, motor-driven E820
street car E829
bending E927
bite, human E928.3
broken glass E920.8
bullet—*see* Shooting
cave-in (*see also* Suffocation, due to,
cave-in) E913.3
without asphyxiation or suffocation E916
cloudburst E908.8
cutting or piercing instrument (*see also*
Cut) E920.9
cyclone E908.1
earth surface movement or eruption
E909.9
earthquake E909.0
electric current (*see also* Electric shock)
E925.9
explosion (*see also* Explosion) E923.9
fire—*see* Fire
flare, Very pistol E922.8
flood E908.2
foreign body—*see* Foreign body
hailstones E904.3
hurricane E908.0
landslide E909.2
law-enforcing agent, police, in course of
legal intervention—*see* Legal
intervention
lightning E907
live rail or live wire—*see* Electric shock
machinery—*see also* Accident, machine
aircraft, without accident to aircraft E844
boat, ship, watercraft (deck) (engine
room) (galley) (laundry) (loading) E836
missile
explosive E923.8
firearm—*see* Shooting
in
terrorism —*see* Terrorism, missile
war operations—*see* War operations,
missile
moving part of motor vehicle (in motion)
(on public highway) E818
not on public highway, nontraffic accident
E825
while alighting, boarding, entering,
leaving—*see* Fall, from, motor vehicle,
while alighting, boarding
nail E920.8

J

Late effect of—*continued*
  fire, accident caused by (accident classifiable to E890-E899) E929.4
  homicide, attempt (any means) E969
  injury
    due to terrorism E999.1
    undetermined whether accidentally or purposely inflicted (injury classifiable to E980-E988) E989
  legal intervention (injury classifiable to E970-E976) E977
  medical or surgical procedure, test or therapy as, or resulting in, or from
    abnormal or delayed reaction or complication—*see* Reaction, abnormal
    misadventure—*see* Misadventure
  motor vehicle accident (accident classifiable to E810-E825) E929.0
  natural or environmental factor, accident due to (accident classifiable to E900-E909) E929.5
  poisoning, accidental (accident classifiable to E850-E858, E860-E869) E929.2
  suicide, attempt (any means) E959
  transport accident NEC (accident classifiable to E800-E807, E826-E838, E840-E848) E929.1
  war operations, injury due to (injury classifiable to E990-E998) E999.0
Launching pad accident E845
Legal
  execution, any method E978
  intervention (by) (injury from) E976
    baton E973
    bayonet E974
    blow E975
    blunt object (baton) (nightstick) (stave) (truncheon) E973
    cutting or piercing instrument E974
    dynamite E971
    execution, any method E973
    explosive(s) (shell) E971
    firearms(s) E970
    gas (asphyxiation) (poisoning) (tear) E972
    grenade E971
    late effect of E977
    machine gun E970
    manhandling E975
    mortar bomb E971
    nightstick E973
    revolver E970
    rifle E970
    specified means NEC E975
    stabbing E974
    stave E973
    truncheon E973
Lifting, injury in E927
Lightning (shock) (stroke) (struck by) E907
Liquid (noncorrosive) in eye E914
  corrosive E924.1
Loss of control
  motor vehicle (on public highway) (without antecedent collision) E816
    with
      antecedent collision on public highway —see Collision, motor vehicle
      involving any object, person or vehicle not on public highway E816
      on public highway—*see* Collision, motor vehicle

Loss of control—*continued*
  not on public highway, nontraffic accident E825
    with antecedent collision—*see* Collision, motor vehicle, not on public highway
  off-road type motor vehicle (not on public highway) E821
    on public highway—*see* Loss of control, motor vehicle
  snow vehicle, motor-driven (not on public highway) E820
    on public highway—*see* Loss of control, motor vehicle
Lost at sea E832
  with accident to watercraft E830
  in war operations E995
Low
  pressure, effects—*see* Effects of, air pressure
  temperature, effects—*see* Cold, exposure to
Lying before train, vehicle or other moving object (unspecified whether accidental or intentional) E988.0
  stated as intentional, purposeful, suicidal (attempt) E958.0
Lynching (*see also* Assault) E968.9

M

Malfunction, atomic power plant in water transport E838
Mangled (accidentally) NEC E928.9
Manhandling (in brawl, fight) E960.0
  legal intervention E975
Manslaughter (nonaccidental)—*see* Assault
Marble in nose E912
Mauled by animal E906.8
Medical procedure, complication of
  delayed or as an abnormal reaction without mention of misadventure—*see* Reaction, abnormal
  due to or as a result of misadventure—*see* Misadventure
Melting of fittings and furniture in burning in terrorism E979.3
Minamata disease E865.2
Misadventure(s) to patient(s) during surgical or medical care E876.9
  contaminated blood, fluid, drug or biological substance (presence of agents and toxins as listed in E875) E875.9
    administered (by) NEC E875.9
      infusion E875.0
      injection E875.1
      specified means NEC E875.2
      transfusion E875.0
      vaccination E875.1
  cut, cutting, puncture, perforation or hemorrhage (accidental) (inadvertent) (inappropriate) (during) E870.9
    aspiration of fluid or tissue (by puncture or catheterization, except heart) E870.5
    biopsy E870.8
      needle (aspirating) E870.5
    blood sampling E870.5
    catheterization E870.5
      heart E870.6
    dialysis (kidney) E870.2
    endoscopic examination E870.4
    enema E870.7
    infusion E870.1

Reduction in—*continued*
    deep water diving causing caisson or
        divers' disease, palsy or paralysis
        E902.2
    underground E902.8
Residual (effect)—*see* Late effect
Rock falling on or hitting (accidentally)
    motor vehicle (in motion) (on public
        highway) E818
        not on public highway E825
    nonmotor road vehicle NEC E829
    pedal cycle E826
    person E916
    railway rolling stock, train, vehicle E806
Running off, away
    animal (being ridden) (in sport or transport)
        E828
        not being ridden E906.8
    animal-drawn vehicle E827
    rails, railway (*see also* Derailment) E802
    roadway
        motor vehicle (without antecedent
            collision) E816
            nontraffic accident E825
            with antecedent collision—*see* Collision,
                motor vehicle, not on public highway
        with
            antecedent collision—*see* Collision motor
                vehicle
            subsequent collision
                involving any object, person or vehicle
                    not on public highway E816
                    on public highway E811
        nonmotor road vehicle NEC E829
        pedal cycle E826
Run over (accidentally) (by)
    animal (not being ridden) E906.8
        being ridden (in sport or transport) E828
    animal-drawn vehicle E827
    machinery—*see* Accident, machine
    motor vehicle (on public highway)—*see* Hit
        by, motor vehicle
    nonmotor road vehicle NEC E829
    railway train E805
    street car E829
    vehicle NEC E848

S

Saturnism E866.0
    from insecticide NEC E863.4
Scald, scalding (accidental) (by) (from) (in)
        E924.0
    acid—*see* Scald, caustic
    boiling tap water E924.2
    caustic or corrosive liquid, substance E924.1
        swallowed—*see* Table of drugs and
            chemicals
    homicide (attempt)—*see* Assault, burning
    inflicted by other person
        stated as
            intentional or homicidal E968.3
            undetermined whether accidental or
                intentional E988.2
    late effect of NEC E929.8
    liquid (boiling) (hot) E924.0
    local application of externally applied
        substance in medical or surgical care
        E873.5
    molten metal E924.0

Scald, scalding—*continued*
    self-inflicted (unspecified whether accidental
        or intentional) E988.2
    stated as intentional, purposeful E958.2
    stated as undetermined whether accidental or
        intentional E988.2
    steam E924.0
    tap water (boiling) E924.2
    transport accident—*see* categories E800-E848
    vapor E924.0
Scratch, cat E906.8
Sea
    sickness E903
Self-mutilation —*see* Suicide
Sequelae (of)
    in
        terrorism E999.1
        war operations E999.0
Shock
    anaphylactic (*see also* Table of drugs and
        chemicals) E947.9
        due to
            bite (venomous)—*see* Bite, venomous NEC
            sting—*see* Sting
    electric (*see also* Electric shock) E925.9
    from electric appliance or current (*see also*
        Electric shock) E925.9
Shooting, shot (accidental(ly)) E922.9
    air gun E922.4
    BB gun E922.4
    hand gun (pistol) (revolver) E922.0
    himself (*see also* Shooting, self-inflicted)
        E985.4
        hand gun (pistol) (revolver) E985.0
        military firearm, except hand gun E985.3
            hand gun (pistol) (revolver) E985.0
        rifle (hunting) E985.2
            military E985.3
        shotgun (automatic) E985.1
        specified firearm NEC E985.4
        Verey pistol E985.4
    homicide (attempt) E965.4
        air gun E968.6
        BB gun E968.6
        hand gun (pistol) (revolver) E965.0
        military firearm, except hand gun E965.3
            hand gun (pistol) (revolver) E965.0
        paintball gun E965.4
        rifle (hunting) E965.2
            military E965.3
        shotgun (automatic) E965.1
        specified firearm NEC E965.4
        Verey pistol E965.4
    inflicted by other person
        in accidental circumstances E922.9
            hand gun (pistol) (revolver) E922.0
            military firearm, except hand gun E922.3
                hand gun (pistol) (revolver) E922.0
            rifle (hunting) E922.2
                military E922.3
            shotgun (automatic) E922.1
            specified firearm NEC E922.8
            Verey pistol E922.8
        stated as
            intentional, homicidal E965.4
                hand gun (pistol) (revolver) E965.0
                military firearm, except hand gun E965.3
                    hand gun (pistol) (revolver) E965.0
                paintball gun E965.4
                rifle (hunting) E965.2
                    military E965.3

War operations—*continued*
  bayonet E995
  biological warfare agents E997.1
  blast (air) (effects) E993
    from nuclear explosion E996
    underwater E992
  bomb (mortar) (explosion) E993
    after cessation of hostilities E998
    fragments, injury by E991.9
      antipersonnel E991.3
  bullet(s) (from carbine, machine gun, pistol,
    rifle, shotgun) E991.2
    rubber E991.0
  burn from
    chemical E997.2
    fire, conflagration (caused by
      fire-producing device or conventional
      weapon) E990.9
      from nuclear explosion E996
      petrol bomb E990.0
    gas E997.2
  burning aircraft E994
  chemical E997.2
  chlorine E997.2
  conventional warfare, specified form NEC
    E995
  crushing by falling aircraft E994
  depth charge E992
  destruction of aircraft E994
  disability as sequela one year or more after
    injury E999.0
  drowning E995
  effect (direct) (secondary) nuclear weapon
    E996
  explosion (artillery shell) (breech block)
    (cannon shell) E993
    after cessation of hostilities of bomb,
      mine placed in war E998
    aircraft E994
    bomb (mortar) E993
      atom E996
      hydrogen E996
      injury by fragments from E991.9
        antipersonnel E991.3
      nuclear E996
    depth charge E992
    injury by fragments from E991.9
      antipersonnel E991.3
    marine weapon E992
    mine
      at sea or in harbor E992
      land E993
        injury by fragments from E991.9
      marine E992
    munitions (accidental) (being used in
      war) (dump) (factory) E993
    nuclear (weapon) E996
    own weapons (accidental) E993
      injury by fragments from E991.9
        antipersonnel E991.3
    sea-based artillery shell E992
    torpedo E992
  exposure to ionizing radiation from nuclear
    explosion E996
  falling aircraft E994
  fire or fire-producing device E990.9
    petrol bomb E990.0
  fireball effects from nuclear explosion E996
  fragments from
    antipersonnel bomb E991.3

War operations—*continued*
  artillery shell, bomb NEC, grenade,
    guided missile, land mine, rocket,
    shell, shrapnel E991.9
  fumes E997.2
  gas E997.2
  grenade (explosion) E993
    fragments, injury by E991.9
  guided missile (explosion) E993
    fragments, injury by E991.9
    nuclear E996
  heat from nuclear explosion E996
  injury due to, but occurring after cessation of
    hostilities E998
  lacrimator (gas) (chemical) E997.2
  land mine (explosion) E993
    after cessation of hostilities E998
    fragments, injury by E991.9
  laser(s) E997.0
  late effect of E999.0
  lewisite E997.2
  lung irritant (chemical) (fumes) (gas) E997.2
  marine mine E992
  mine
    after cessation of hostilities E998
    at sea E992
    in harbor E992
    land (explosion) E993
      fragments, injury by E991.9
    marine E992
  missile (guided) (explosion) E993
    fragments, injury by E991.9
    marine E992
    nuclear E996
  mortar bomb (explosion) E993
    fragments, injury by E991.9
  mustard gas E997.2
  nerve gas E997.2
  phosgene E997.2
  poisoning (chemical) (fumes) (gas) E997.2
  radiation, ionizing from nuclear explosion
    E996
  rocket (explosion) E993
    fragments, injury by E991.9
  saber, sabre E995
  screening smoke E997.8
  shell (aircraft) (artillery) (cannon) (land
    based) (explosion) E993
    fragments, injury by E991.9
    sea-based E992
  shooting E991.2
    after cessation of hostilities E998
    bullet(s) E991.2
      rubber E991.0
    pellet(s) (rifle) E991.1
  shrapnel E991.9
  submersion E995
  torpedo E992
  unconventional warfare, except by nuclear
    weapon E997.9
    biological (warfare) E997.1
    gas, fumes, chemicals E997.2
    laser(s) E997.0
    specified type NEC E997.8
  underwater blast E992
  vesicant (chemical) (fumes) (gas) E997.2
  weapon burst E993
Washed
  away by flood—*see* Flood
  away by tidal wave—*see* Tidal wave
  off road by storm (transport vehicle) E908.9
  overboard E832

Weather exposure —*see also* Exposure
  cold E901.0
  hot E900.0
Weightlessness (causing injury) (effects of) (in
    spacecraft, real or simulated) E928.0
Wound (accidental) NEC (*see also* Injury)
    E928.9
  battle (*see also* War operation) E995
  bayonet E920.3
    in
      legal intervention E974
      war operations E995
  gunshot—*see* Shooting
  incised—*see* Cut
  saber, sabre E920.3
    in war operations E995

RAILWAY ACCIDENTS (E800–E807)

The following fourth–digit subdivisions are for use with categories E800–E807 to identify the injured person.

.0 Railway employee

Any person who by virtue of his employment in connection with a railway, whether by the railway company or not, is at increased risk of involvement in a railway accident, such as:

catering staff on train	postal staff on train
driver	railway fireman
guard	shunter
porter	sleeping car attendant

.1 Passenger on railway

Any authorized person traveling on a train, except a railway employee

Excludes: intending passenger waiting at station (.8)
            unauthorized rider on railway vehicle (.8)

.2 Pedestrian

See definition (r), Vol. 1, page 479

.3 Pedal cyclist

See definition (p), Vol. 1, page 479

.8 Other specified person

Intending passenger waiting at station

Unauthorized rider on railway vehicle

.9 Unspecified person

MOTOR VEHICLE TRAFFIC AND NONTRAFFIC ACCIDENTS
(E810–825)

The following fourth–digit subdivisions are for use with categories E810–E819 and E820–E825 to identify the injured person:

.0 Driver of motor vehicle other than motorcycle

    See definition (l), Vol. 1, page 479

.1 Passenger in motor vehicle other than motorcycle

    See definition (l), Vol. 1, page 479

.2 Motorcyclist

    See definition (l), Vol. 1, page 479

.3 Passenger on motorcycle

    See definition (l), Vol. 1, page 479

.4 Occupant of streetcar

.5 Rider of animal; occupant of animal–drawn vehicle

.6 Pedal cyclist

    See definition (p), Vol. 1, page 479

.7 Pedestrian

    See definition (r), Vol. 1, page 479

.8 Other specified person

    Occupant of vehicle other than above

    Person in railway train involved in accident

    Unauthorized rider of motor vehicle

.9 Unspecified person

OTHER ROAD VEHICLE ACCIDENTS (E826–E829)

(animal–drawn vehicle, streetcar, pedal cycle, and other nonmotor road vehicle accidents)

The following fourth–digit subdivisions are for use with categories E826–E829 to identify the injured person:

.0 Pedestrian

 See definition (r), Vol. 1, page 479

.1 Pedal cyclist (does not apply to codes E827, E828, E829)

 See definition (p), Vol. 1, page 479

.2 Rider of animal (does not apply to code E829)

.3 Occupant of animal–drawn vehicle (does not apply to codes E828, E829)

.4 Occupant of streetcar

.8 Other specified person

.9 Unspecified person

WATER TRANSPORT ACCIDENTS (E830–E838)

The following fourth–digit subdivisions are for use with categories E830–E838 to identify the injured person:

.0 Occupant of small boat, unpowered

.1 Occupant of small boat, powered

    See definition (t), Vol. 1, page 479

    Excludes: water skier (.4)

.2 Occupant of other watercraft — crew

    Persons:

        engaged in operation of watercraft

        providing passenger services [cabin attendants, ship's physician, catering personnel]

        working on ship during voyage in other capacity [musician in band, operators of shops and beauty parlors]

.3 Occupant of other watercraft — other than crew

    Passenger

    Occupant of lifeboat, other than crew, after abandoning ship

.4 Water skier

.5 Swimmer

.6 Dockers, stevedores

    Longshoreman employed on the dock in loading and unloading ships

.8 Other specified person

    Immigration and custom officials on board ship

    Person:

        accompanying passenger or member of crew

        visiting boat

    Pilot (guiding ship into port)

.9 Unspecified person

AIR AND SPACE TRANSPORT ACCIDENTS (E840–E845)

The following fourth–digit subdivisions are for use with categories E840–E845 to identify the injured person:

.0 Occupant of spacecraft

.1 Occupant of military aircraft, any

> Crew
> Passenger (civilian) (military)   in military aircraft [air force] [army]
> Troops   [national guard] [navy]

> *Excludes:* occupants of aircraft operated under jurisdiction of police departments (.5)
> parachutist (.7).

.2 Crew of commercial aircraft (powered) in surface to surface transport

.3 Other occupant of commercial aircraft (powered) in surface to surface transport

> Flight personnel:

> > not part of crew
> > on familiarization flight

> Passenger on aircraft (powered) NOS

.4 Occupant of commercial aircraft (powered) in surface to air transport

> Occupant [crew] [passenger] of aircraft (powered) engaged in activities, such as:

> > aerial spraying (crops) (fire retardants)
> > air drops of emergency supplies
> > air drops of parachutists, except from military craft
> > crop dusting
> > lowering of construction material [bridge or telephone pole]
> > sky writing

.5 Occupant of other powered aircraft

> Occupant [crew] [passenger] of aircraft (powered) engaged in activities, such as:

> > aerobatic flying
> > aircraft racing
> > rescue operation
> > storm surveillance
> > traffic surveillance

> Occupant of private plane NOS

.6 Occupant of unpowered aircraft, except parachutist

> Occupant of aircraft classifiable to E842

.7 Parachutist (military) (other)

> Person making voluntary descent

> *Excludes:* person making descent after accident to aircraft (.1–.6)

.8 Ground crew, airline employee

> Persons employed at airfields (civil) (military) or launching pads, not occupants of aircraft

.9 Other person

SUMMARY OF ADDITIONS, DELETIONS, AND REVISIONS TO VOLUME 1 IN 2003

038   **Septicemia**
Exclusion added

040.82   **Toxic shock syndrome**
New code

062.8   **Other specified mosquito-borne viral encephalitis**
Exclusion added

066.3   **Other mosquito-borne fever**
Description revised

066.4   **West Nile fever**
New code

256.2   **Postablative ovarian failure**
Description added, exclusion term revised

256.3   **Other ovarian failure**
Description revised

277.00   **Without mention of meconium ileus**
Description added

277.02   **With pulmonary manifestations**
New code

277.03   **With gastrointestinal manifestations**
New code

277.09   **With other manifestations**
New code

277.7   **Dysmetabolic syndrom X**
Description revised

337.3   **Autonomic dysreflexia**
Description revised

357.8   **Other**
Description deleted

357.81   **Chronic inflammatory demyelinating polyneuritis**
New code

357.82   **Critical illness polyneuropathy**
New code

357.89   **Other inflammatory and toxic neuropathy**
New code

359.81   **Critical illness myopathy**
New code

359.89   **Other myopathies**
New code

365.83   **Aqueous misdirection**
New code

368.6   **Night blindness**
Description deleted

402   **Hypertensive heart disease**
Description added

402.00   **Without heart failure**
Revised code

402.01   **With heart failure**
Revised code

402.10   **Without heart failure**
Revised code

402.11   **With heart failure**
Revised code

402.90   **Without heart failure**
Revised code

402.91   **With heart failure**
Revised code

404   **Hypertensive heart and renal disease**
Description added, revised

411.81   **Acute coronary occlusion without myocardial infarction**
Exclusion term revised

414.06   **Of coronary artery of transplanted heart**
New code

414.1   **Aneurysm and dissection of heart**
Revised code

414.10   **Aneurysm of heart (wall)**
Revised code

414.11   **Aneurysm of coronary vessels**
Revised code

414.12   **Dissection of coronary artery**
New code

414.19   **Other aneurysm of heart**
Revised code

427.89   **Other**
Exclusion added

428   **Heart failure**
Exclusion deleted, description added

428.0   **Congestive heart failure, unspecified**
Revised code

428.2   **Systolic heart failure**
New subcategory

428.20   **Unspecified**
New code

428.21   **Acute**
New code

428.22   **Chronic**
New code

428.23   **Acute on chronic**
New code

428.3   **Diastolic heart failure**
New subcategory

428.30   **Unspecified**
New code

428.31   **Acute**
New code

428.32   **Chronic**
New code

428.33   **Acute on chronic**
New code

428.4   **Combined systolic and diastolic heart failure**
New subcategory

428.40   **Unspecified**
New code

428.41   **Acute**
New code

428.42   **Chronic**
New code

428.43   **Acute on chronic**
New code

430-438   **CEREBROVASCULAR DISEASE**
Exclusion added

436   **Acute, but ill-defined, cerebrovascular disease**
Exclusion added

438.6   **Alterations of sensations**
New code

438.7   **Disturbances of vision**
New code

438.83   **Facial weakness**
New code

438.84   **Ataxia**
New code

438.85   **Vertigo**
New code

440   **Atherosclerosis**
Exclusion added

440.8   **Of other specified arteries**
Exclusion term revised

441.0   **Dissection of aorta**
Description deleted

443.2   **Other arterial dissection**
New subcategory

443.21   **Dissection of carotid artery**
New code

43.22   **Dissection of iliac artery**
New code

443.23   **Dissection of renal artery**
New code

443.24   **Dissection of vertebral artery**
New code

443.29   **Dissection of other artery**
New code

444   **Arterial embolism and thrombosis**
Exclusion added

445   **Atheroembolism**
New category

445.0   **Of extremities**
New subcategory

445.01   **Upper extremity**
New code

445.02   **Lower extremity**
New code

445.8   **Of other sites**
New subcategory

445.81   **Kidney**
New code

445.89   **Other site**
New code

447.6   **Arteritis, unspecified**
Exclusion term revised

454.8   **With other complications**
New code

454.9   **Asymptomatic varicose veins**
Revised code

459.1   **Postphlebetic syndrome**
Description added, exclusion added

459.10   **Postphlebetic syndrome without complications**
New code

459.11   **Postphlebetic syndrome with ulcer**
New code

459.12   **Postphlebetic syndrome with inflammation**
New code

459.13   **Postphlebetic syndrome with ulcer and inflammation**
New code

459.19   **Postphlebetic syndrome with other complication**
New code

459.3   **Chronic venous hypertension (idiopathic)**
New subcategory

459.30   **Chronic venous hypertension without complications**
New code

459.31   **Chronic venous hypertension with ulcer**
New code

459.32   **Chronic venous hypertension with inflammation**
New code

459.33   **Chronic venous hypertension with ulcer and inflammation**
New code

459.39   **Chronic venous hypertension with other complication**
New code

491.2   **Obstructive chronic bronchitis**
Description deleted

491.20   **Without mention of acute exacerbation**
Description deleted

491.21   **With acute exacerbation**
Description deleted

493.2   **Chronic obstructive asthma**
Description added, exclusion added

518.81   **Acute respiratory failure**
Exclusion term revised

518.82   **Other pulmonary insufficiency, not elsewhere classified**
Exclusion term revised

521.0   **Dental caries**
Description deleted

537.84   **Dieulafoy lesion (hemorrhagic) of stomach and duodenum**
New code

569.86   **Dieulafoy lesion (hemorrhagic) of intestine**
New code

577.8   **Other specified diseases of pancreas**
Exclusion term revised

590.0   **Chronic pyelonephritis**
Description added, deleted

593.7   **Vesicoureteral reflux**
Description deleted

599.0   **Urinary tract infection, site not specified**
Exclusion added

602.3   **Dysplasia of prostate**
Description revised, exclusion term revised

622.1   **Dysplasia of cervix (uteri)**
Description added

627.2   **Symptomatic menopausal or female climacteric states**
Revised code